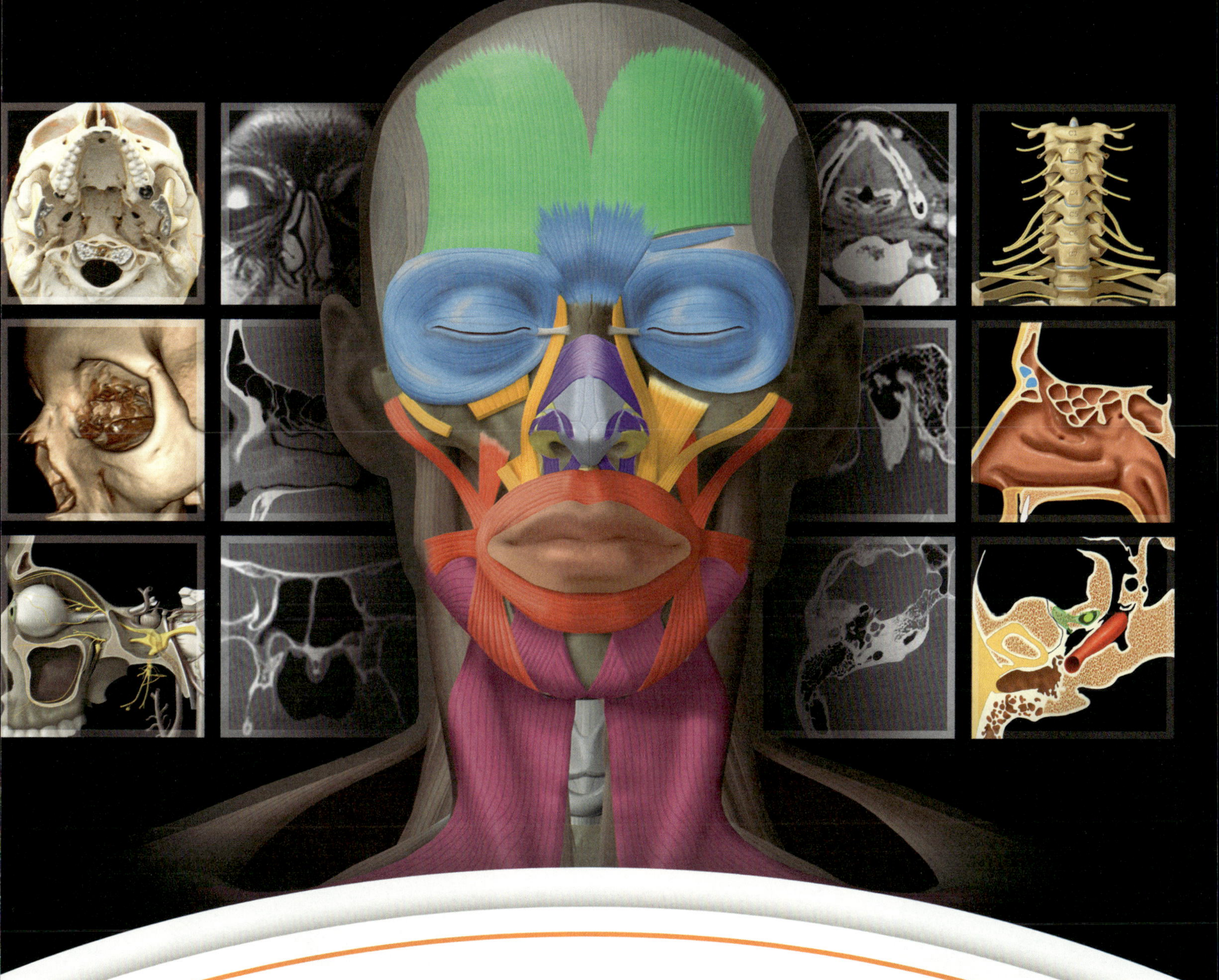

SECOND EDITION

IMAGING ANATOMY

Head and Neck

Vattoth

Chapman | Harnsberger

Gaddikeri | Jhaveri | Meltzer | Muttikkal | Singhal

ELSEVIER

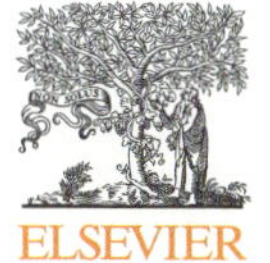

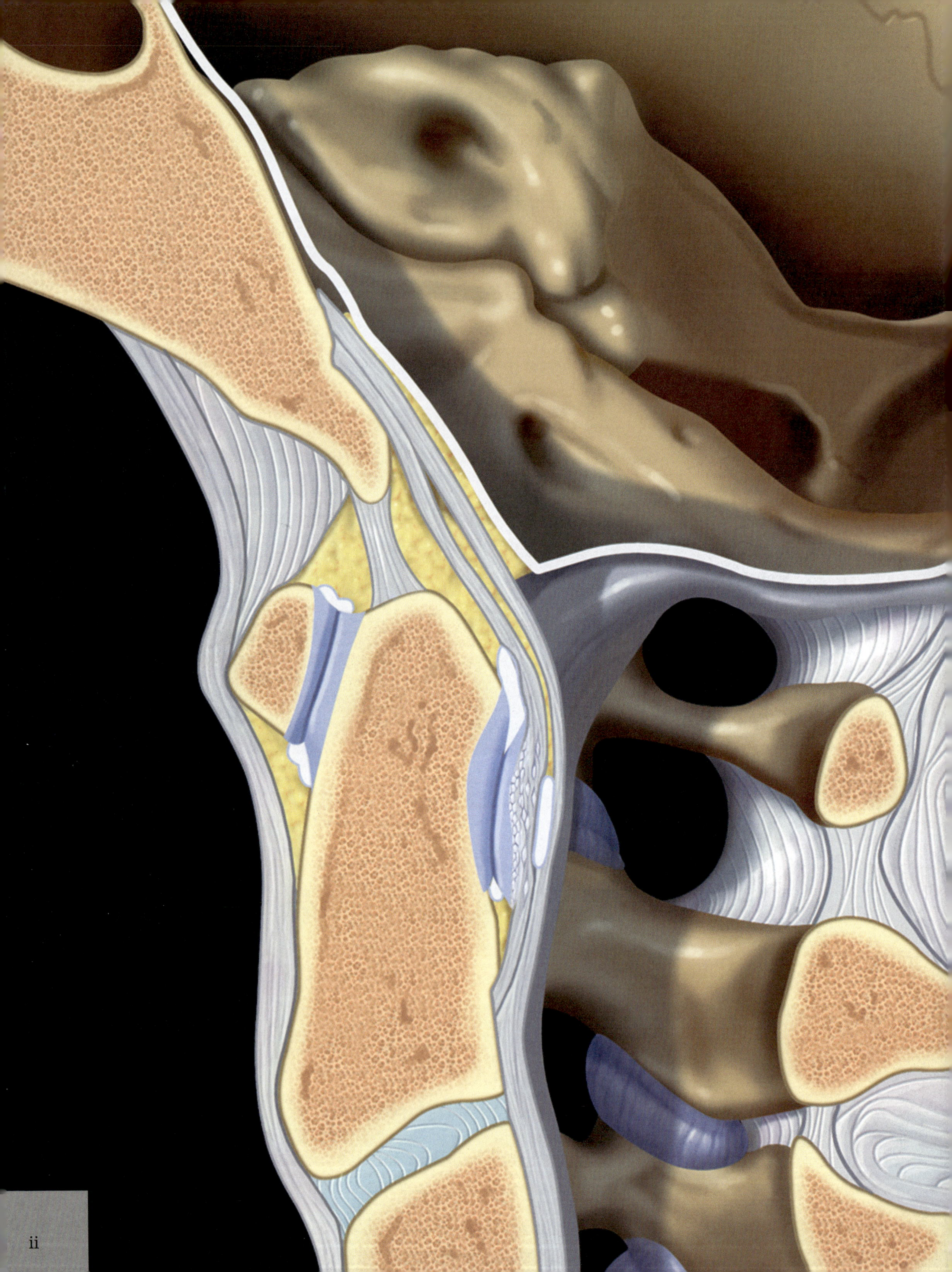

IMAGING ANATOMY

Head and Neck

SECOND EDITION

Surjith Vattoth, MD, FRCR
Professor of Radiology
Department of Diagnostic Radiology and Nuclear Medicine
Division of Neuroradiology
Rush University Medical Center
Chicago, Illinois

Philip R. Chapman, MD
Professor of Radiology
Director of Head and Neck Radiology
Duke University
Durham, North Carolina

H. Ric Harnsberger, MD
Professor Emeritus, Radiology and Otolaryngology
Department of Radiology and Imaging Sciences
University of Utah School of Medicine
Salt Lake City, Utah

Elsevier
1600 John F. Kennedy Blvd.
Ste 1800
Philadelphia, PA 19103-2899

IMAGING ANATOMY: HEAD AND NECK, SECOND EDITION

ISBN: 978-0-443-24964-8

Previous edition copyrighted 2019.

Library of Congress Control Number: 2024930463

Printed in Canada by Friesens, Altona, Manitoba, Canada

Last digit is the print number: 9 8 7 6 5 4 3 2 1

Dedication

Dedicated to Fiju (Dr. Fathima Fijula P. Manzil), my wife and soulmate since childhood; son, Lazim, and daughters, Lamis and Liya, who happily sacrificed their precious countless hours of evening and weekend family time with me while I was deeply indulged in the work of this book and other projects as a passionate educator.

I am also indebted to my parents and sisters on the other side of the world, who let me fly high and far away from them to fulfill my career dreams and disperse my knowledge in radiology for the betterment of patient care.

And last but not least, to all my current/former residents, fellows, medical students, and social media followers around the world, who keep me motivated and passionate as an educator.

SV

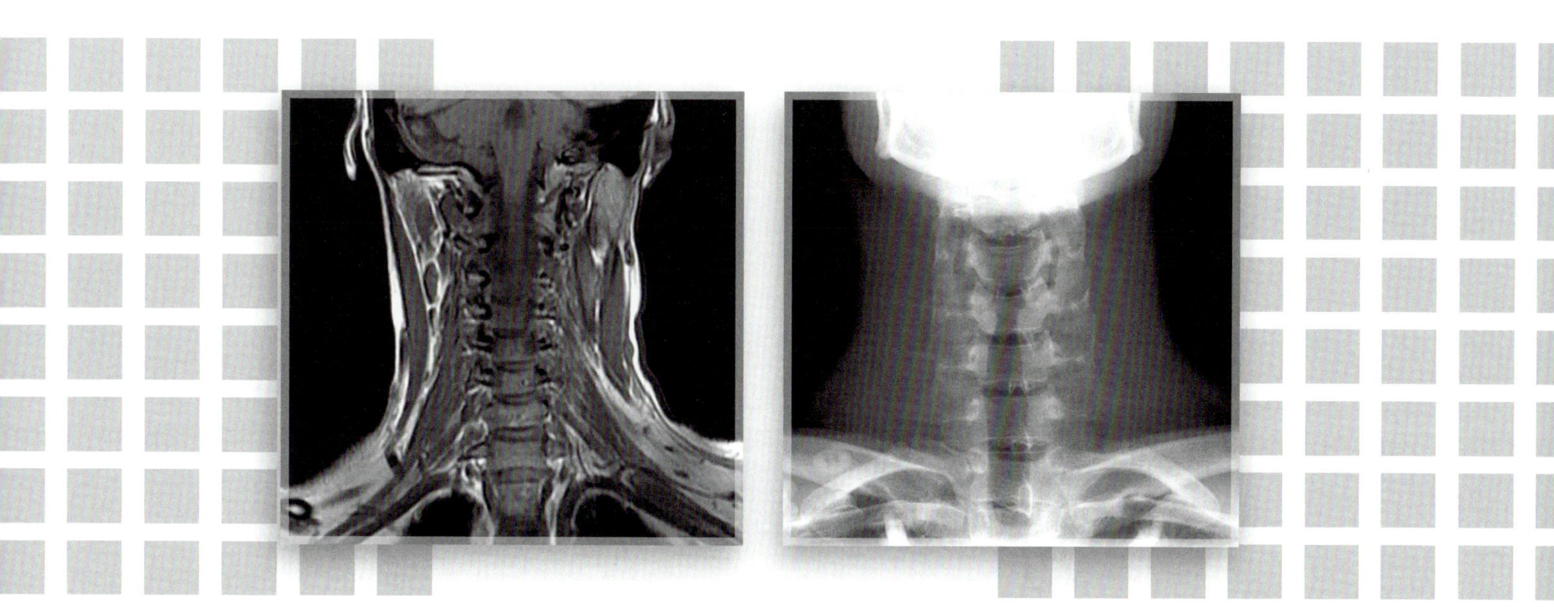

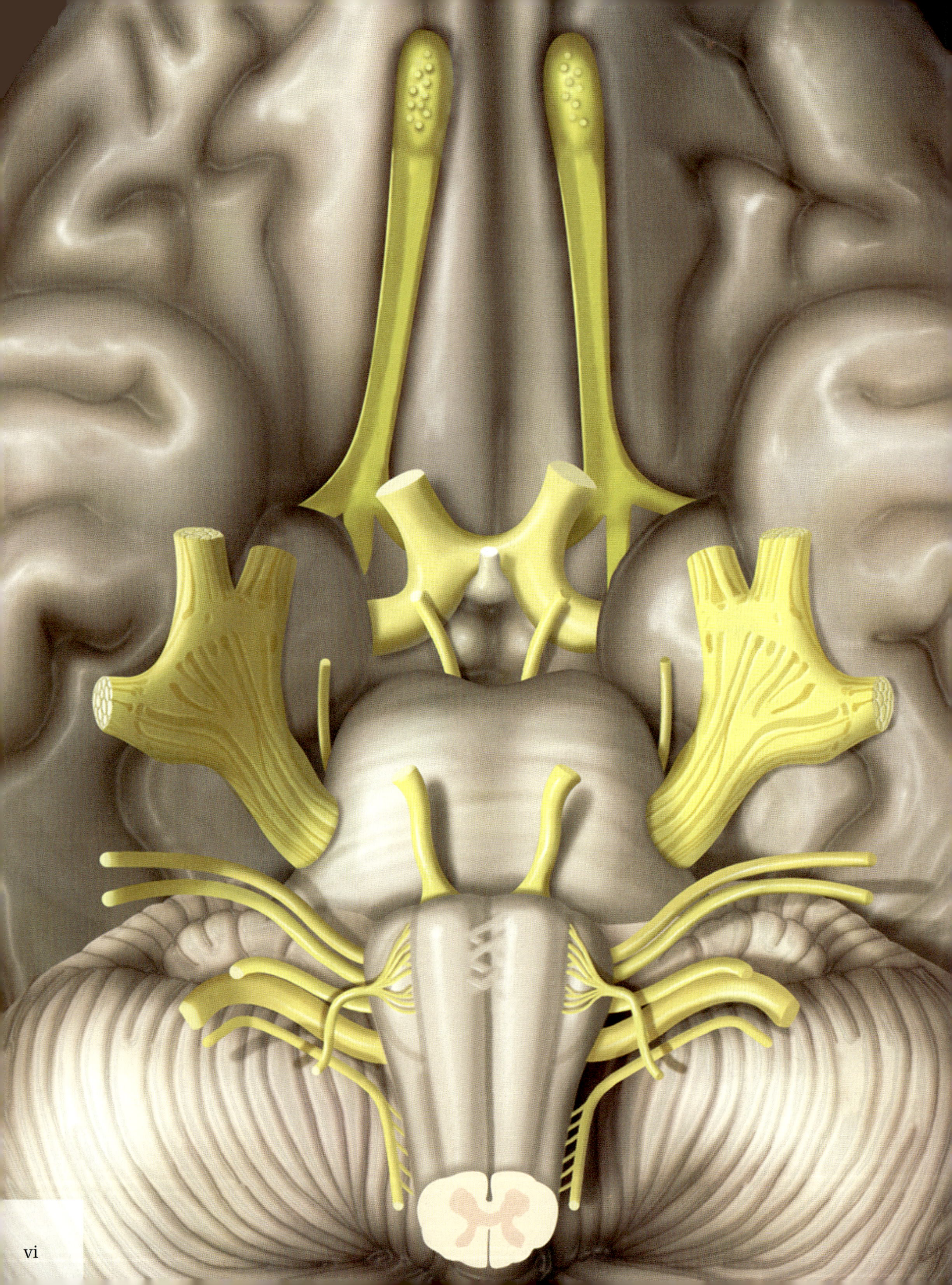

Contributing Authors

Santhosh Gaddikeri, MD
Associate Professor
Department of Diagnostic Radiology and Nuclear Medicine
Rush University Medical Center
Chicago, Illinois

Miral D. Jhaveri, MD, MBA
Professor
Division Head, Neuroradiology
Interim Chair, Department of Diagnostic Radiology and Nuclear Medicine
Rush University Medical Center
Chicago, Illinois

Daniel E. Meltzer, MD
Associate Professor of Radiology
Division of Neuroradiology
Department of Radiology
Icahn School of Medicine at Mount Sinai
New York, New York

Thomas Jose Eluvathingal Muttikkal, MD
Associate Professor
Neuroradiology Division
Department of Radiology and Medical Imaging
University of Virginia Health System
Charlottesville, Virginia

Aparna Singhal, MD
Associate Professor
Neuroradiology Section
Department of Radiology
University of Alabama at Birmingham
Birmingham, Alabama

Additional Contributors

H. Christian Davidson, MD
Siddhartha Gaddamanugu, MD
Anthony B. Morlandt, MD, DDS
Jeffrey S. Ross, MD

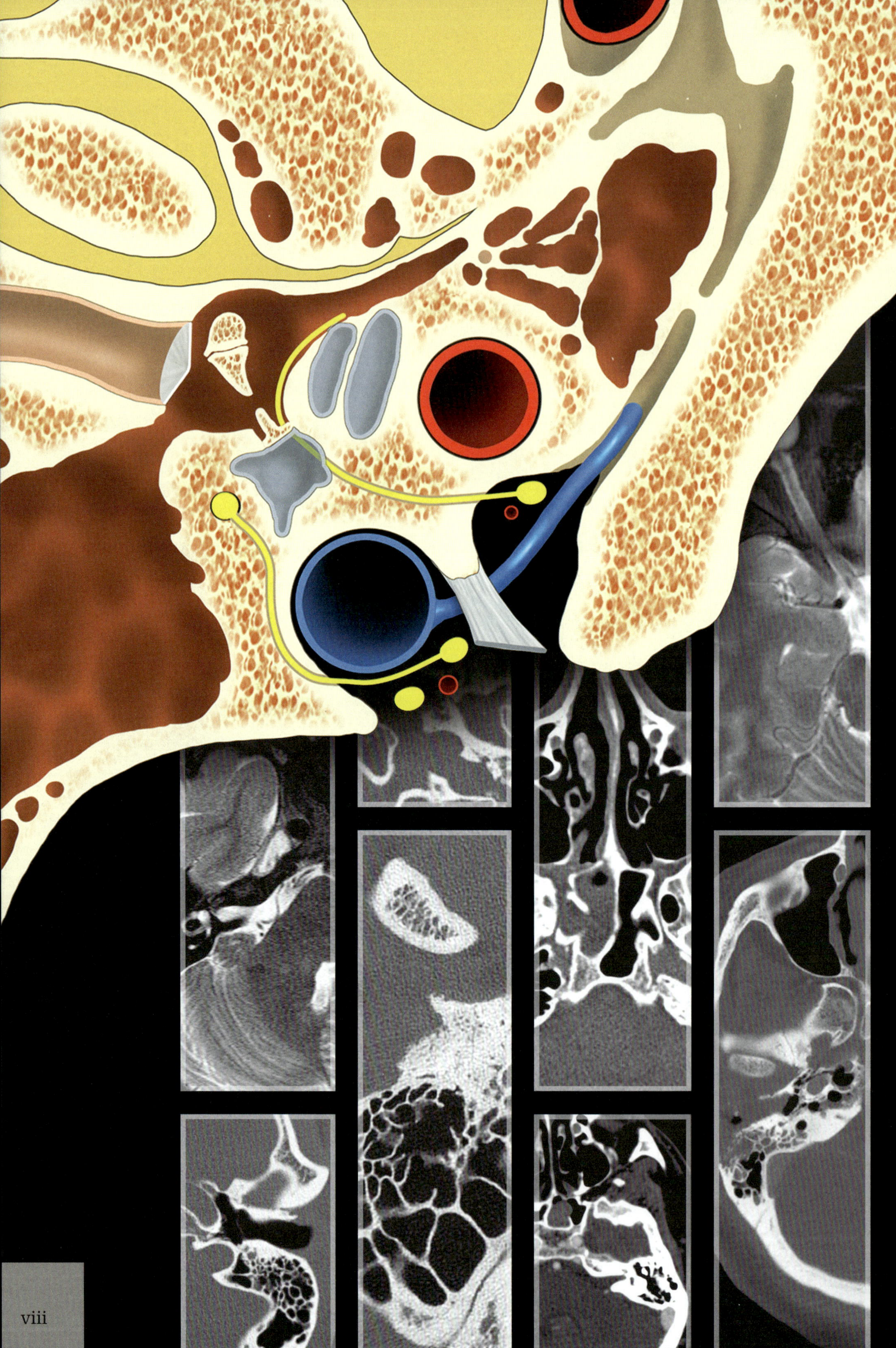

Preface

I am honored and proud to welcome you to the 2nd edition of *Imaging Anatomy: Head and Neck* as its lead author. The 1st edition, led by Phil Chapman, MD, took its origin from the landmark publication, *Diagnostic and Surgical Imaging Anatomy: Brain, Head and Neck, Spine*, published in 2006 under the leadership of Ric Harnsberger, MD. In this new edition, we approach head and neck anatomy as a critically important standalone subject for radiologists and other professionals who rely on head and neck imaging for patient evaluation and treatment. Anatomy is the key in head and neck imaging. Knowledge of the subdivision of head and neck spaces and the anatomic structures living in those individual spaces forms the solid foundation to evaluate for pathology involving and spreading out of these spaces, and this is what brings us to a meaningful diagnosis for patient care.

This book not only targets the radiologist and radiology resident/fellow, but also head and neck surgeons, neurosurgeons, medical and radiation oncologists, anatomists, and medical or technological sciences students in these fields. The text is offered in a formatted design with concise, bulleted content and state-of-the-art images that identify the clinical entities in each anatomic area. It is easy to use and understand, with each series of successive imaging slices in standard planes of imaging (coronal, sagittal, and axial) as is seen during evaluation of CT or MR scans in clinical practice. The book allows for rapid reference and comprehensive review of clinically relevant head and neck anatomy. In each section, the critical foundation of normal anatomy is provided along with imaging recommendations and imaging correlations. Radiologic-pathologic correlation is provided when appropriate to emphasize anatomic relationships.

The text is accompanied by hundreds of full-color graphic illustrations created by our expert medical illustrators as well as hundreds of high-resolution multiplanar CT, MR, and ultrasound images, which include new images and graphics and preexisting images that have undergone further scrutiny and editing. Each illustration and image is labeled and comes with its own legend to expedite the learning experience. The result is an organized and readily accessible anatomic atlas of head and neck anatomy.

The purchase of this book comes with an electronic version that provides the ultimate in accessibility, whether the reader is at home, in the reading room, or in the clinic. The content is also available in Elsevier STATdx.

When I was approached by Elsevier to lead this project just 5 years after the 1st edition, there was concern that there would not be enough new advancements and literature in anatomy to bring out a new edition of this high-end reference book. However, the team was pleasantly surprised that we had to edit and add a substantial amount of text material, images, graphics, and pages in most of the chapters, as well as add many new chapters. This edition contains new chapters on external nose anatomy, facial nerve in temporal bone, minor fissures and sutures around the temporal bone, and temporal bone anatomy on photon-counting detector (PCD) CT.

The authors and Elsevier publishing team are extremely pleased to present the 2nd edition of our book, and we hope that the readers will find it as or even more pleasing and enjoyable than we did delivering it to you.

Surjith Vattoth, MD, FRCR
Professor of Radiology
Department of Diagnostic Radiology and Nuclear Medicine
Division of Neuroradiology

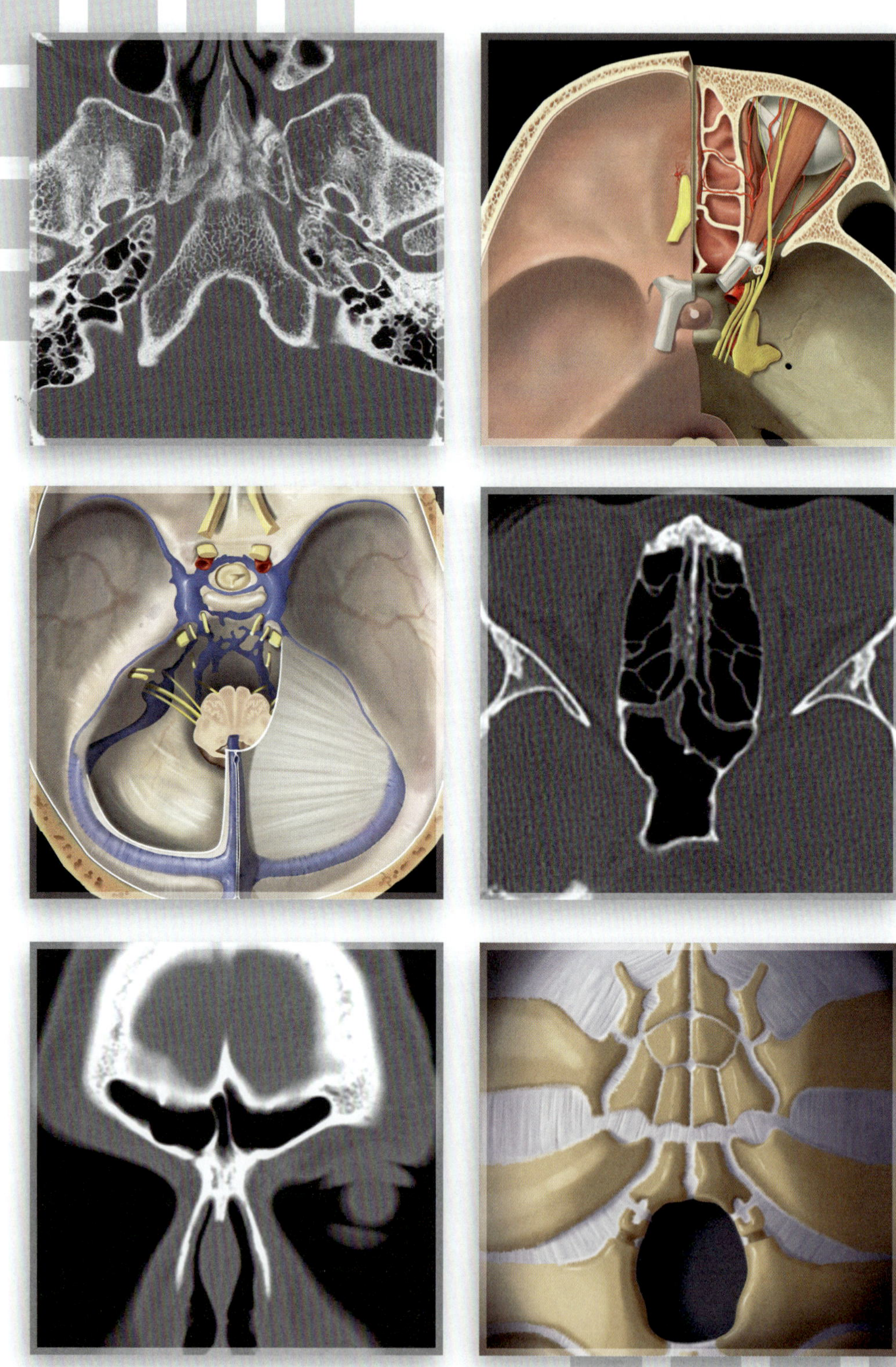

Acknowledgments

LEAD EDITOR
Nina Themann, BA

LEAD ILLUSTRATOR
Richard Coombs, MS

TEXT EDITORS
Arthur G. Gelsinger, MA
Rebecca L. Bluth, BA
Terry W. Ferrell, MS
Megg Morin, BA
Kathryn Watkins, BA
Shannon Kelly, MA

ILLUSTRATIONS
Lane R. Bennion, MS
Laura C. Wissler, MA

IMAGE EDITORS
Jeffrey J. Marmorstone, BS
Lisa A. M. Steadman, BS

ART DIRECTION AND DESIGN
Cindy Lin, BFA

PRODUCTION EDITORS
Emily C. Fassett, BA
John Pecorelli, BS

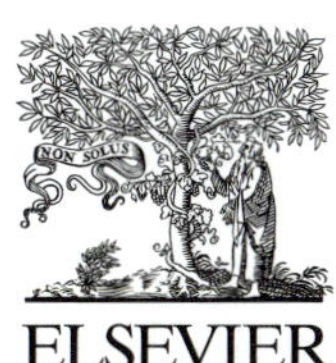

ELSEVIER

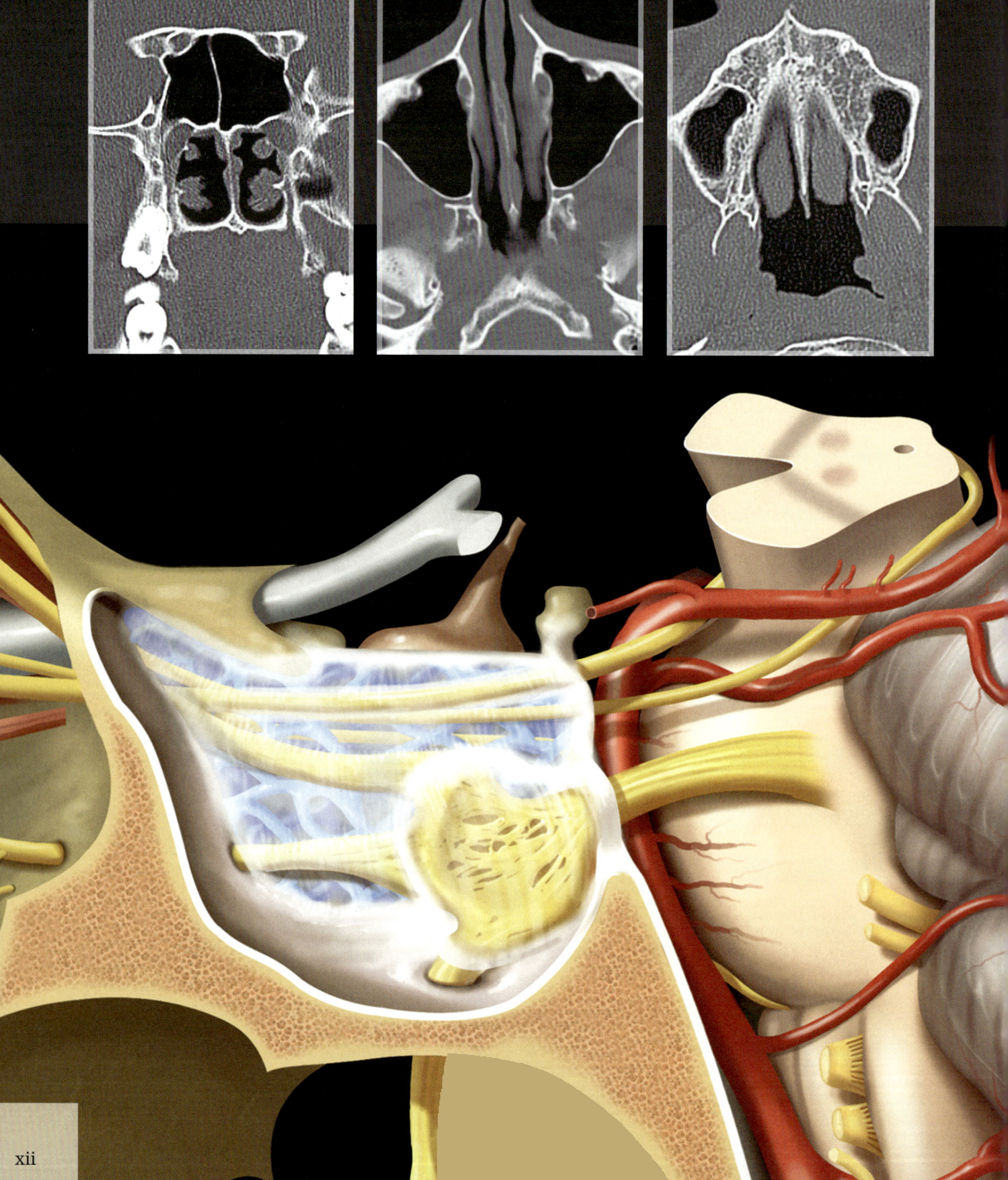

Sections

TABLE OF CONTENTS

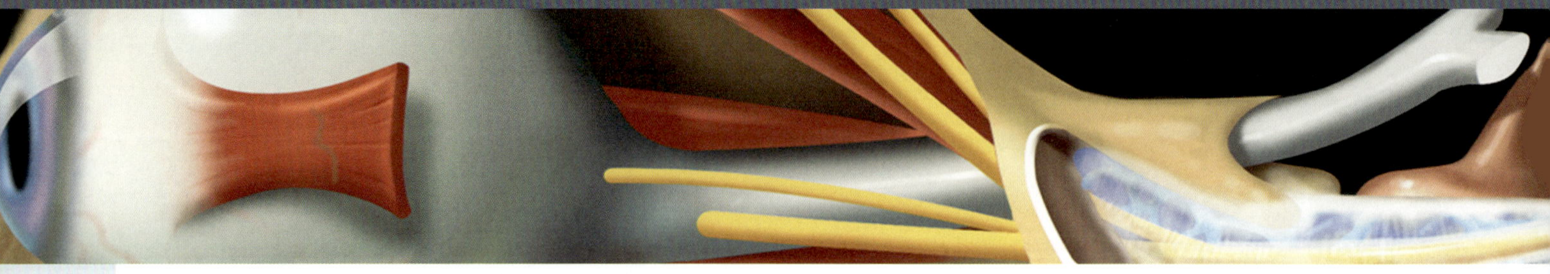

TABLE OF CONTENTS

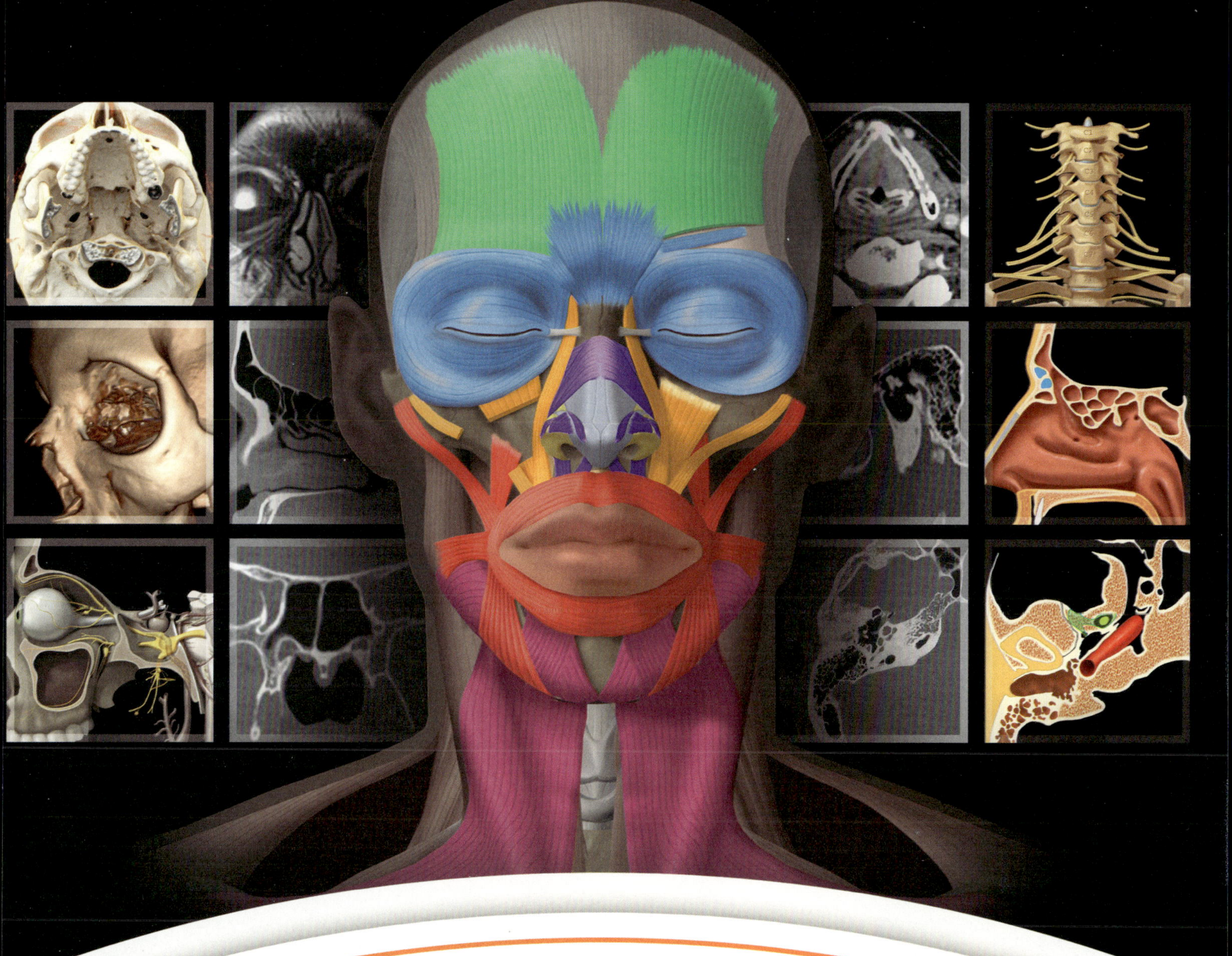

SECOND EDITION

IMAGING ANATOMY

Head and Neck

Vattoth

Chapman | Harnsberger

Gaddikeri | Jhaveri | Meltzer | Muttikkal | Singhal

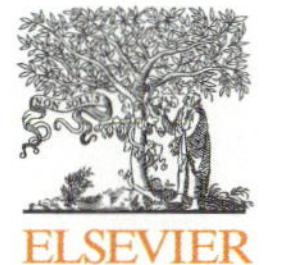

ELSEVIER

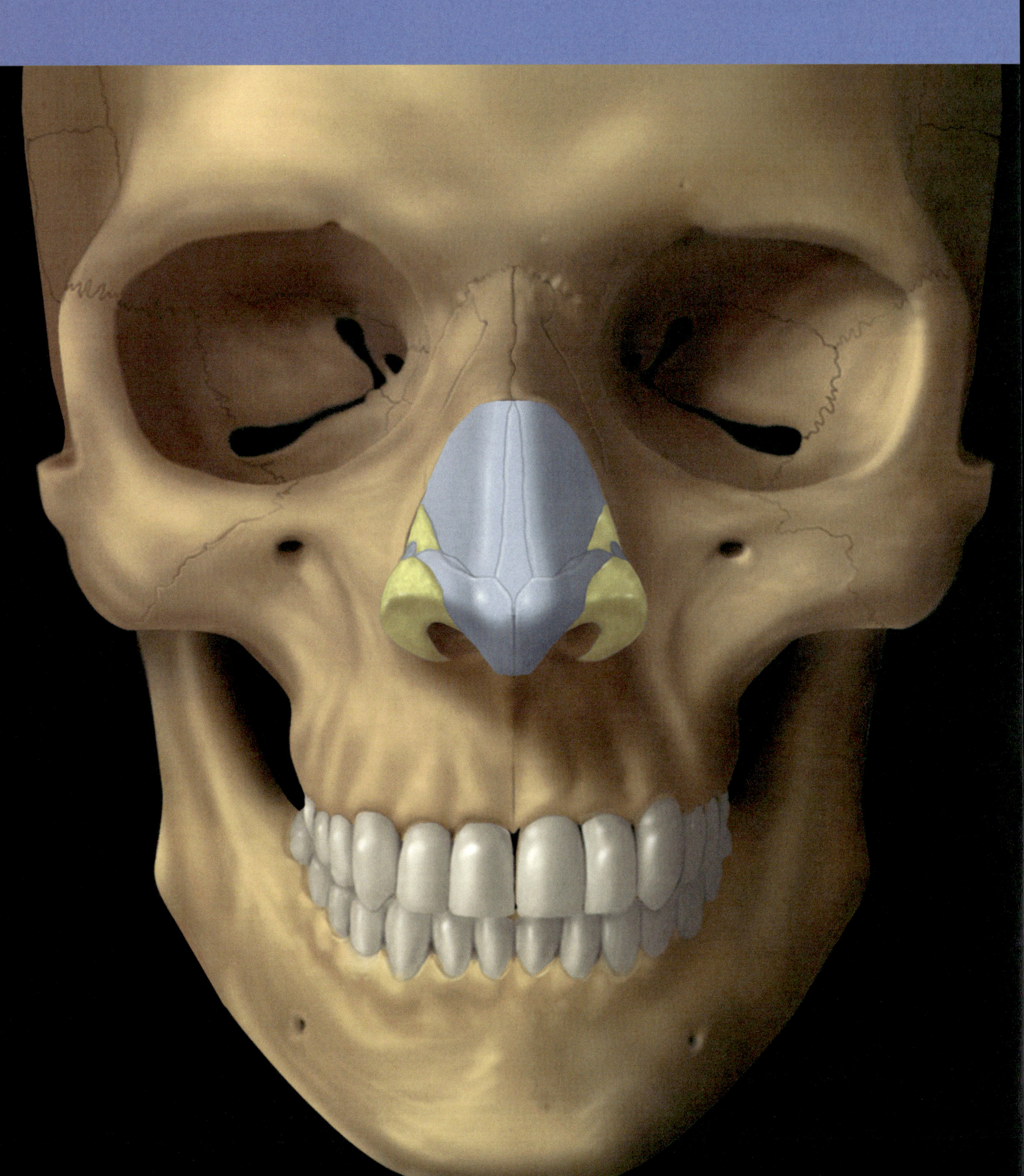

SECTION 1

Face

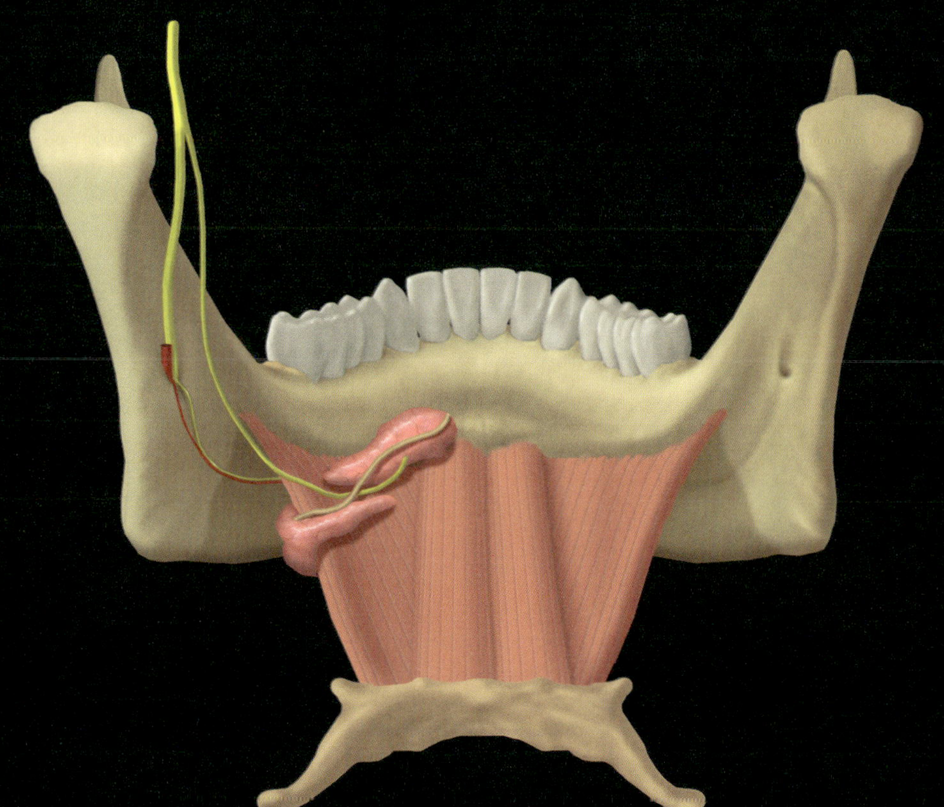

TERMINOLOGY

Abbreviations

- Superficial musculoaponeurotic system (SMAS)

Definitions

- Mimetic muscles/mimic muscles/muscles of facial mimicry: Primary function is facial expression
  - Muscles insert directly into dermis via SMAS facilitating facial expression (in rest of body, investing layer of fascia separates muscle from subcutaneous tissue)
- SMAS: Continuous organized fibrous network connecting facial muscles to dermis
- Modiolus: Dense fibromuscular structure formed at corner of mouth lateral border by attached muscles convergence

IMAGING ANATOMY

Overview

- Muscles of facial mimicry have their origin on bone but insert directly into dermis (through SMAS)
- Exceptions are inconsistently found in risorius & malaris muscles with both origin & insertion in soft tissue
- Other exceptions are tiny nasal muscles, namely, compressor narium minor, dilator naris anterior (DNA) (both have origin from nasal cartilages & insert into skin)
- Mimetic muscles act as sphincters & dilators of facial orifices & elevators & depressors of facial structures
- Adjacent muscles closely intertwined due to their common origin from mesoderm of 2nd branchial arch; large muscular sheets later differentiate into individual muscles
- Groups of facial muscles share common insertion sites; therefore, identification is often easiest by tracing them back from their insertion to less crowded origins
- 6 groups for purpose of easy identification, namely, muscles inserting at: (1) Scalp, (2) orbit, (3) nose, (4) upper lip, (5) modiolus/angle of mouth, & (6) lower lip

Anatomy Relationships

- Layers of face, from superficial to deep
  - **(1) Skin**
  - **(2) Subcutaneous fat**
    - Extensive in cheek region (**malar fat pad**); less in eyelid, lips, & nose
    - Malar fat pad slides downward & inward over SMAS with aging, deepening nasolabial crease
    - Malar fat pad firmly fixed to dermis & also to thicker superior part of SMAS but loosely attached to thinner inferior SMAS
    - Zygomatic ligament: Osteocutaneous ligament on zygoma lateral to zygomaticus minor (ZMi) muscle origin, anchors malar fat to deeper tissue layers
    - Fat pad beneath orbicularis oculi (OOc) muscle called **suborbicularis oculi fat pad**
  - **(3) SMAS (superficial fascia)**
    - Connects facial muscles to skin dermis
    - SMAS continuous above with **temporoparietal fascia** (TpF) as it passes over zygomatic arch
    - **TpF** a.k.a. superficial **temporal fascia** or **epicranial aponeurosis**
    - TpF, in turn, continuous with galea aponeurotica in scalp superiorly, frontalis muscle anteriorly, & occipitalis muscle posteriorly
    - TpF usually fibrous, sometimes contains vestigial muscles, namely, **temporoparietal muscle** & **superior auricular muscle**
    - SMAS extremely thin beyond anterior border of masseter as it enters cheek area, barely traceable by position of split peripheral part of platysma
    - SMAS blends with platysma inferiorly & begins fading medially as it reaches lateral nasal margin
    - Lower 1/2 of SMAS is extremely thin & somewhat discontinuous with no mechanical bearing capacity
    - SMAS invests in & extends into external aspects of facial muscles, mainly frontalis, OOc, ZMi, zygomaticus major (Zmj), risorius, orbicularis oris (OOr), & platysma
    - SMAS composed of 3D scaffold of collagen & elastic fibers with interspersed fat cells
    - 2 distinct histologic subtypes of SMAS described
      - **Type 1**: SMAS lateral to nasolabial fold (NLF)
      - Meshwork of fibrous septa that envelop large lobules of fat cells & allow for connections with both facial muscles as well as periosteum
      - More susceptible to aging process than type 2
      - **Type 2**: SMAS medial to NLF, mainly in lips
      - Meshwork of intermingled collagen, elastic & muscle fibers reaching up into dermis
      - Much firmer connection to skin than type 1, fat cells lie dispersed unlike distinct fat lobules in type 1
      - Transition between types 1 & 2 SMAS at NLF: Challenge for facial rejuvenation surgeries
      - CT: Hyperdense line between superficial & deep fibroadipose tissue; MR: T1-/T2-hypointense line
  - **(4) Superficial facial muscles ("mimic muscles")**: 6 groups
  - **(5) Parotideomasseteric fascia (deep fascia)**: Investing fascia enveloping parotid gland, duct, & masseter muscle
    - Also envelop facial nerve branches in parotid gland & part of buccal fat pad
      - Note: **Buccal fat pad** lies just outside corners of mouth; deeper layer than **malar fat pad** lying in front part of cheek
    - Continues to superficial layer of deep cervical fascia inferiorly & superiorly to temporalis fascia (a.k.a. deep temporal fascia)
      - Temporalis fascia, in turn, covers temporalis muscle, splits inferiorly attaching around zygomatic arch, & attaches superiorly to pericranium at and above superior temporal line on skull
  - **(6) Retaining ligaments**: Connects overlying structures to underlying periosteum of facial bones
  - **Facial nerve branches in parotid gland** lie **deep** underneath parotideomasseteric fascia (deep fascia in cheek deep to SMAS), making **sub-SMAS dissection safe during facelift surgery** at this level
    - Facial nerve branches eventually traverse deep fascia in their anteromedial superficial course to innervate muscles of SMAS, most of which receive innervation from their deep surfaces
    - Facial nerve fibers become more superficial medially beyond facial artery & vein; important anatomy note to avoid injury during face lift surgery

- **Facial nerve (CNVII) branches course in face**
  - **Zygomatic arch level**: In loose areolar tissue plane between TpF & zygomatic arch periosteum
  - **1 cm above zygomatic arch**: In loose areolar plane between superficial TpF & deep temporalis fascia
  - **2 cm above zygomatic arch**: Penetrates TpF to run along anterior branch of superficial temporal artery
- **Facial artery** curves upward over body of mandible at anteroinferior angle of masseter muscle → pass anterosuperiorly across cheek to ~ 8-23 mm lateral to labial commissure → ascends along side of nose to end at medial commissure of eye as **angular artery**
  - Accompanied by **facial & angular veins**
- **Internal maxillary artery**, including its **infraorbital artery** branch lying in between levator labii superioris (LLS) & levator anguli oris (LAO) muscles, & **superficial temporal artery** also supplies face

Internal Contents

- 6 groups of facial muscles based on insertion site

I: Muscles Inserting at Scalp

- **Frontal belly of occipitofrontalis (frontalis muscle):** Origin from epicranial aponeurosis near coronal suture & insertion at skin of frontal region & galea aponeurotica
  - Partially intertwined with muscle fibers of adjacent corrugator supercilii (CS), procerus, & OOc
  - Furrows forehead, raises eyebrows, & widens eyes
  - Can cause **horizontal hyperfunctional facial lines on forehead**; treatment with botulinum toxin injection

II: Muscles Inserting at Orbit

- **OOc**: Origins: **Palpebral** part from medial palpebral ligament, a.k.a. medial canthal tendon, **orbital** part from medial orbital rim, & **lacrimal** part from lacrimal bone
  - Palpebral part inserts on lateral palpebral raphe, orbital part inserts laterally to palpebral portion, & lacrimal part inserts at upper & lower eyelids
  - Medially, muscle is deep to medial canthal tendon
  - Palpebral part helps in light closure of eyelids
  - Orbital part used for more forceful closure along with medial displacement of eyelids
    - Compress eye globe & lacrimal sac to initiate flow of tears into nasolacrimal duct
  - Hyperactivity of lateral OOc can produce radial lines stemming from lateral canthus ("**crow's feet**")
  - **Malaris** muscle: Inconsistent lateral muscular band of OOc originating from TpF & terminates at either zygomatic arch or cheek region or angle of mouth
    - Plays role in facial animation
  - Inconsistent medial muscular bands may be present
    - Preventing drooping of OOc
  - Many muscular connections between OOc & ZMi
    - May play role in facial expression
- CS: Origin on frontal bone at medial supraorbital margin & inserts into frontalis; deep to frontalis; 2 bellies
  - Deep transverse belly & superficial oblique belly
  - Deep to frontalis
  - Depresses brow, pulls it medially, & **creates vertical skin creases as in frowning**
- **Depressor supercilii (DS)**: Origin in region of medial orbital rim on frontal process of maxilla (FPM) 2-5 mm below frontomaxillary suture; some fibers from lacrimal sac
  - Inserts into dermis 14-15 mm superior to medial canthal tendon (medial palpebral ligament)
  - DS interdigitates with adjacent OOc & CS
  - Depresses medial aspect of brow during frowning
- **Procerus**: Origin on lower end of nasal bone & upper part of upper lateral nasal cartilage
  - Inserts on forehead skin medial to eye & interdigitates with frontalis muscle
  - Displaces medial angle of eyebrow inferiorly, which also causes **horizontal facial skin creases, frowning**
  - Elevator of nose

III: Muscles Inserting at Nose

- Nasal **elevators**: Anomalous nasi & 2 extrinsic muscles, namely, procerus (inserting at orbit) & LLS alaeque nasi (LLSAN) (inserting at upper lip with medial slip inserting into greater alar cartilage)
- Nasal **depressors**: Alar nasalis & depressor septi nasi
- Nasal **compressors**: Transverse nasalis & compressor narium minor
- Nasal **dilators**: DNA, dilator naris vestibularis (DNV), & contribution from alar nasalis & LLSAN
- **Anomalous nasi**: Origin on FPM & inserts into nasal bone, upper lateral nasal cartilage, procerus, & transverse nasalis; is nasal elevator
- **Transverse nasalis**: Nasalis muscle has 2 parts, namely, transverse nasalis & alar nasalis
  - Origin of transverse nasalis on canine eminence of maxilla superolateral to incisive fossa
  - Inserts, expanding into thin aponeurosis continuous on bridge of nose with that of opposite side transverse nasalis & with aponeurosis of procerus
  - Main nasal compressor; hyperactivity can cause radial lines along dorsum of nose as far down to lower border of greater alar cartilage called "**bunny lines**"
- **Alar nasalis**: Origin on maxilla just medial to transverse nasalis above lateral incisor tooth, located anterior to transverse nasalis
  - Ascends anterolaterally to insert on alar-facial crease & adjacent deep surface of external skin of alar lobule
  - Is nasal depressor; also helps to dilate nares (hence, sometimes called **dilator naris posterior**)
- **Depressor septi nasi**: Origin in incisive fossa of maxilla located further medial to origin of alar nasalis
  - Inserts on base & lateral surface of medial crus of greater alar cartilage; is nasal depressor
  - Medially, attach to dermocartilagenous ligament, which gets sandwiched by medial crus of greater alar cartilage
- **DNA**: Origin on frontal surface of lateral 1/2 of lateral crus of greater alar cartilage & adjacent lesser alar cartilage
  - Inserts on skin of nose superior to alar groove (supraalar crease); is nasal dilator
- **DNV**: Origin on external skin of alar lobule, radiates along dome of nasal vestibule
  - Inserts on vestibular skin of alar lobule; dilator of nasal vestibule (nasal vestibule: Most anterior nasal cavity)
- **Compressor narium minor**: Origin on anterior part of greater alar cartilage

- Inserts into skin near margin of nostril; is nasal compressor

IV: Muscles Inserting at Upper Lip

- **LLS**: Origin on inferior margin of orbit just above infraorbital foramen deep to OOc & inserts on upper lip; raises upper lip
- **LLSAN**: Origin on FPM & inserts in 2 places
  - Insertion at greater alar cartilage & skin of nose: Elevates nose & dilates nares
  - Insertion at muscles of upper lip: Displaces upper lip superomedially
  - LLSAN & LLS can be injected with botulinum toxin to decrease **gingival show** or "**gummy smile**" whereby they are prevented from contracting, which, in turn, decreases superior displacement of upper lip
- **ZMi**: Origin on anterior aspect of zygomatic bone posterior to zygomaticomaxillary suture & inserts on upper lip
  - Inserts to both upper lip & ala of nose in ~ 1/4 of cases
  - Displaces upper lip superiorly, resulting in deepening of nasolabial furrow during expression of contempt
  - LLS, LLSAN, & ZMi pass through OOr at upper lip insertion contributing to **NLF**

V: Muscles Inserting at Modiolus/Angle of Mouth

- Tendinous tissue nodule in modiolus seen in 20%; facial artery passes 1 mm lateral to lateral border of modiolus
- **ZMj**: Origin on zygoma (behind ZMi origin) anterior to zygomaticotemporal suture & inserts at modiolus
  - At modiolar insertion, deep to LAO
  - If ZMj is bifid, then LAO passes between its 2 heads
  - Main insertion of deep muscle band of ZMj **at anterior margin of buccinator** muscle & its fascia
    - Key relationship in facial animation (even though buccinator not classified as muscle of facial mimicry)
  - Raises angle of mouth superiorly & posteriorly & helps to smile or laugh
  - **Bifid ZMj** can cause **cheek "dimple"** due to fascial strands inserting into dermis & causing dermal tethering effect
- **OOr**: Origin from other facial muscles converging to mouth; bony origin of upper portion on alveolar border of maxilla & lower portion on mandible lateral to mentalis; insert at angle of mouth
  - Sphincter of mouth, which brings lips close to teeth & alveoli, brings lips together & protrudes lips forward
  - Hyperactivity can result in radial lines around mouth, a.k.a. "**lipstick lines**" or "**smoker's lines**"; treated with botulinum toxin in combination with lip fillers
- **LAO**: Origin in canine fossa of maxilla well below infraorbital foramen & inserts at modiolus just superficial to ZMj insertion
  - Displaces lip angle superiorly & results in deepening of nasolabial furrow
  - In its superior aspect, LAO lies deep to LLS; **infraorbital vessels & nervous plexus** lie between them
- **Depressor anguli oris (DAO)**: Origin on oblique line of mandible lateral & inferior to depressor labii inferioris (DLI)
  - Also interdigitates with platysma & inserts at corner of mouth as narrow fasciculus
  - Depresses angle of mouth during grief & displaces angle medially on simultaneous contraction with LAO
  - Some fibers may continue below mental tubercle joining contralateral DAO & creating **transversus menti** muscle
- **Risorius**: Inconsistent muscle, most fibers originating from SMAS (superficial fascia), some fibers from parotidomasseteric fascia (deep fascia); in some cases receives platysma fibers
  - Inserts at modiolus in 3 distinct superficial, flush, & deep layers in relation to DAO
  - Displaces skin of cheek posteriorly, stretches lower lip & displaces corner of mouth inferolaterally during grinning

VI: Muscles Inserting at Lower Lip

- **DLI**: Origin on oblique line of mandible between mental foramen & symphysis (superomedial to DAO origin), also interdigitates with platysma
  - Inserts on skin of lower lip & OOr
  - Displaces lower lip inferiorly & slightly laterally
- **Mentalis**: Origin in incisive fossa of mandible & inserts on skin of chin; only elevator of lower lip
  - Elevates & protrudes lower lip & can wrinkle chin; if deep, is treated with botulinum toxin
- **Platysma**: Origin on superficial pectoral & deltoid fascia & inserts on inferior body of mandible, skin, & hypodermis
  - Depresses lower mandible & lower lip

ANATOMY IMAGING ISSUES

Imaging Recommendations

- Most "mimic muscles" identified in thin-section CT & 3-mm T1 & T2 MR with accurate knowledge of anatomy

CLINICAL IMPLICATIONS

Clinical Importance

- Important landmarks for surgical procedures: Facial rejuvenation, rhytidectomy (face lift), cleft lip/palate repair
- Facial wrinkles occur perpendicular to muscle action there; important for injection treatment, such as botulinum toxin
- Atrophy of facial fat pads plays significant role in aging
- "**Marionette lines**" or "**melomental folds**": Long vertical lines laterally circumscribing chin, extending downward from oral commissures; appear with aging
  - When ligaments, skin, & fat around mouth & chin sag
  - Treated with injectable fillers & surgeries, such as face lift
- Imaging identification of denervation changes in facial muscles: Numerous etiologies, including neoplasms
- Involved in tumors, including lesions along SMAS & facial muscles & perineural spread along CNV & CNVII in relation to SMAS: Lymphoma, squamous cell carcinoma

Major Contributor Muscles to Common Facial Expressions

- **Surprise**: Frontalis
- **Frowning**: CS, DS, & procerus
- **Anger**: DNA, DNV, depressor septi nasi
- **Contempt**: ZMi
- **Smiling & laughing**: ZMj
- **Grinning:** Risorius
- **Sadness**: LLS, LAO; grief: DAO
- **Doubt**: Mentalis
- **Whistling**: Buccinator, OOr
- **Horror, terror, & fright**: Platysma

FACIAL MUSCLES: GRAPHIC & 3D BONE CT REFORMAT OF SKULL

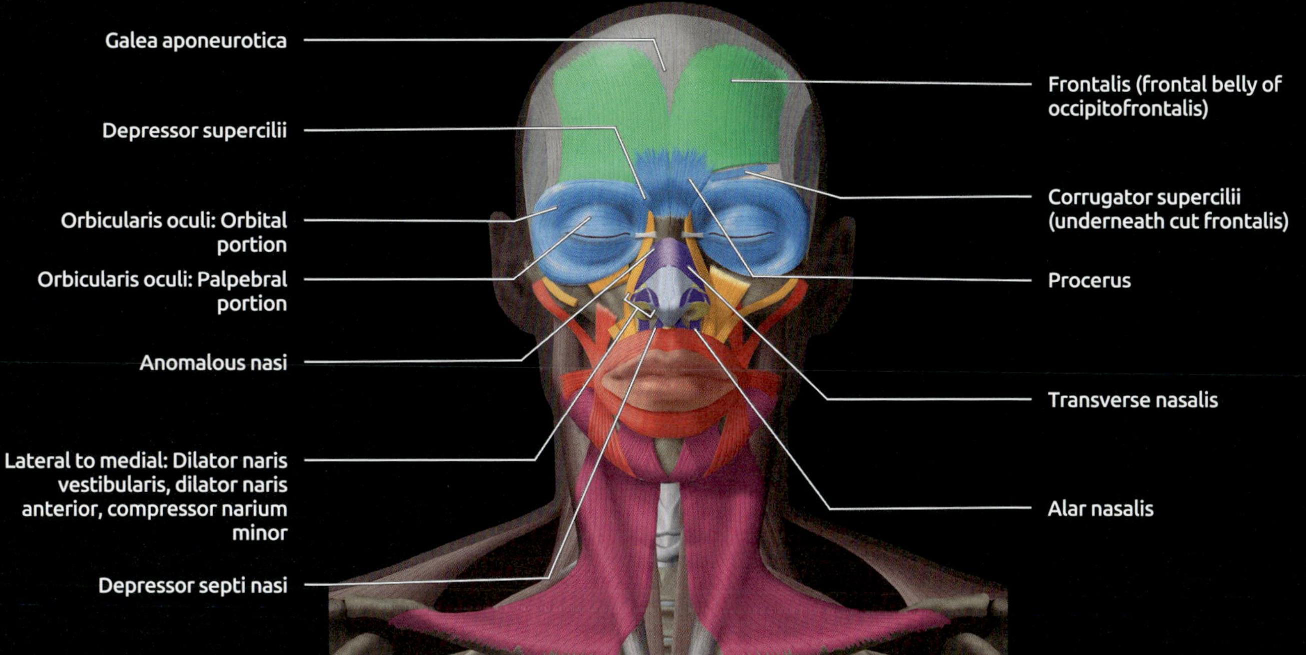

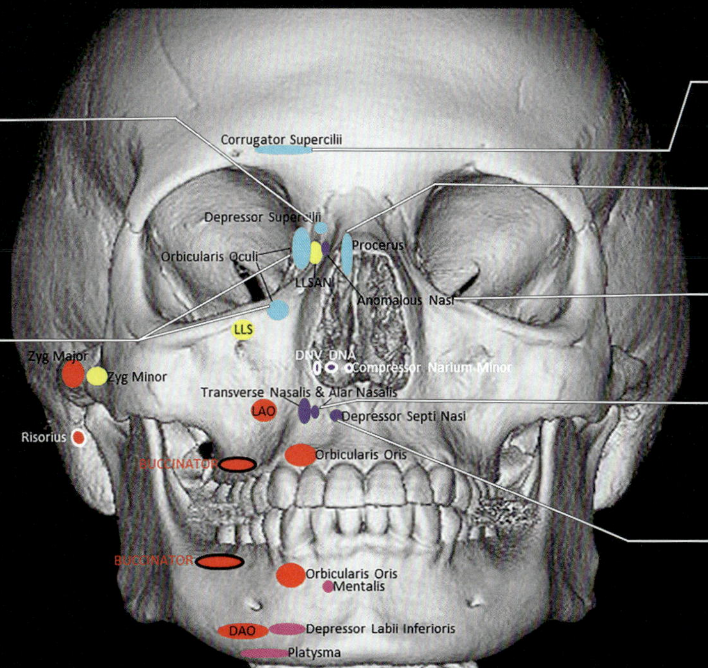

(Top) *Frontal graphic shows facial mimic muscles color-coded into 6 groups according to common insertion sites: The scalp is green, orbit is blue, nose is purple, upper lip is yellow, modiolus/angle of mouth is red, & lower lip is magenta. Muscles inserting around the scalp, orbit, & nose only are marked with line captions in this image.* **(Bottom)** *The origin of facial muscles is painted on this 3D skull CT. Muscle groups follow color coding seen on the previous graphic according to their insertion sites. Muscles of facial mimicry have their origin on bone & insert into the dermis through the superficial musculoaponeurotic system (SMAS). Exceptions are inconsistently found in the risorius & malaris muscles, having both origin and insertion in soft tissue, & also the tiny nasal muscles, namely, the compressor narium minor, dilator naris anterior (DNA) (both have origin from nasal cartilages and insert into skin), & dilator naris vestibularis (DNV) (origin and insertion in skin). In this image, these muscle origins are painted with white outlines outside their respective internal color coding. The origin of muscles inserting around the orbit (blue) & nose (purple) only are explained with line captions.*

FACIAL MUSCLES: GRAPHIC & 3D BONE CT REFORMAT OF SKULL

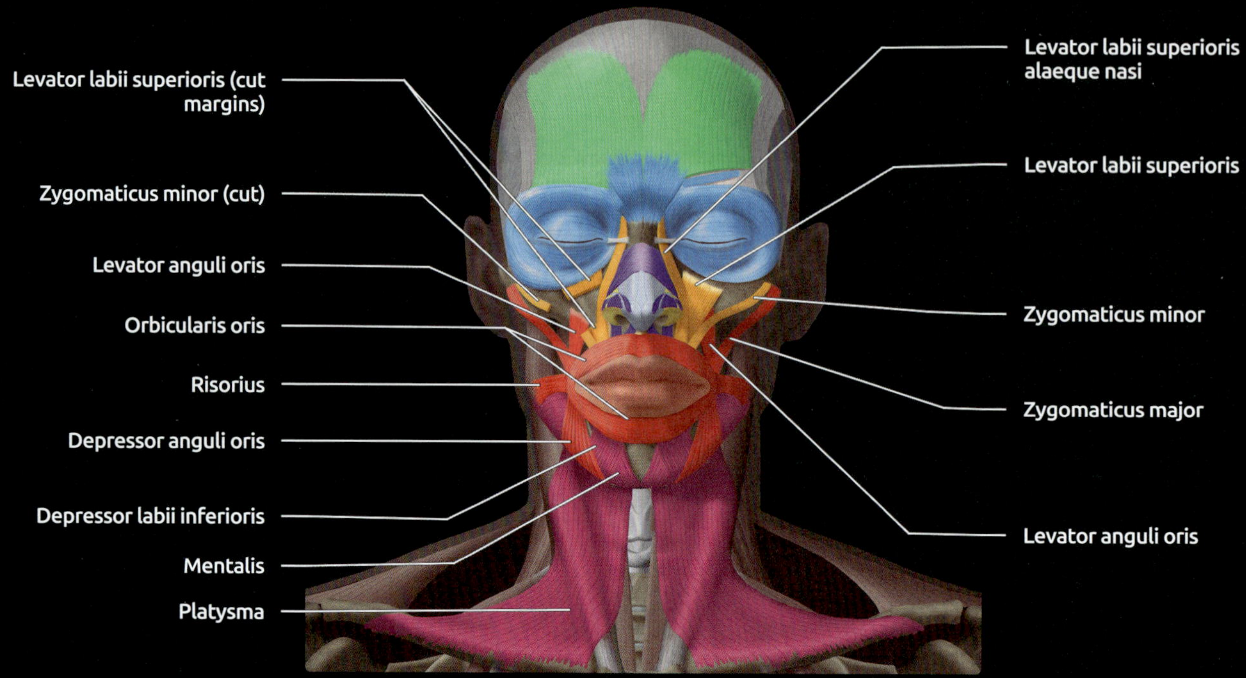

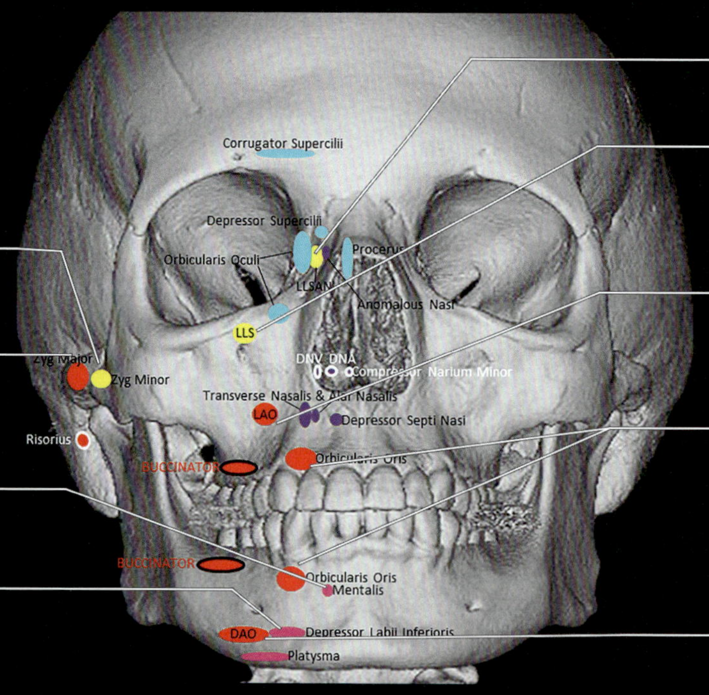

(Top) *Color-coded frontal graphic shows muscles inserting around the upper lip (yellow), modiolus/angle of mouth (red), & lower lip (magenta) marked with line captions. A tiny part of the lower aspect of the orbicularis oculi muscle is removed on the left to show the infraorbital origin of the levator labii superioris (LLS) underneath the orbicularis oculi. Zygomaticus minor (ZMi) is cut on right to show the underlying levator anguli oris (LAO) (also partially cut on right), originating from the canine fossa of the maxilla, seen underneath the cut midportion of LLS. Infraorbital neurovascular bundle courses in between LAO & LLS & is a potential route for perineural tumor spread from the face to the pterygopalatine fossa along the infraorbital canal.* **(Bottom)** *Origin of facial muscles painted on a 3D skull CT shows the muscles inserting around the upper lip (yellow), modiolus/angle of mouth (red), & lower lip (magenta) marked with line captions. Buccinator muscle makes up the bulk of the cheek & forms the lateral wall of the oral cavity; it is not classified as a muscle of facial mimicry. It originates on the alveolar processes of mandible & maxilla near the molar teeth & from the pterygomandibular raphe.*

AXIAL T1 MR

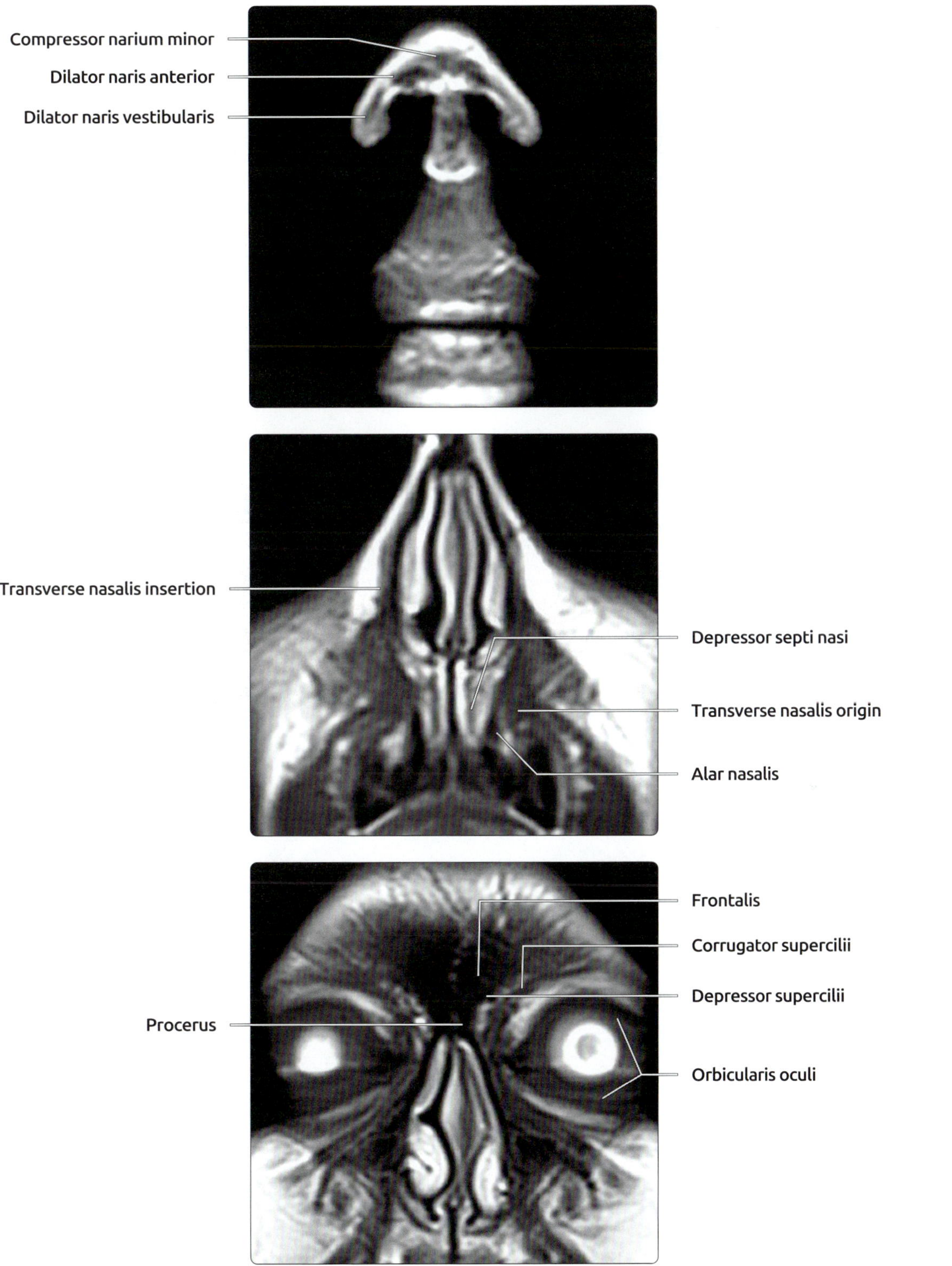

(Top) *The 1st of 3 coronal 3-mm T2 MR images from anterior to posterior shows the tiny compressor narium minor, DNA, and DNV, which do not have bony origins.* **(Middle)** *Coronal T2 MR though the soft tissues of the nose shows the depressor septi nasi originating in the maxillary incisive fossa; just laterally is the alar nasalis originating above the maxillary lateral incisor, & further laterally is the transverse nasalis originating from the maxillary canine eminence. As their name implies, the depressor septi nasi inserts near the nasal septum into the medial crus of the greater alar cartilage, the alar nasalis lies anterior to the transverse nasalis & inserts into the nasal alar lobule skin & alar-facial crease, & the transverse nasalis continues superiorly across the bridge of the nose.* **(Bottom)** *Coronal T2 MR though the anterior orbital level shows the frontalis inserting at the scalp, along with the corrugator supercilii, depressor supercilii, procerus, & orbicularis oculi, which are muscles inserting around the eye region. Intrinsic nasal muscles are functionally grouped as elevators, depressors, compressors, & dilators. The procerus & LLS alaeque nasi (LLSAN) are extrinsic nasal elevators.*

AXIAL T1 MR

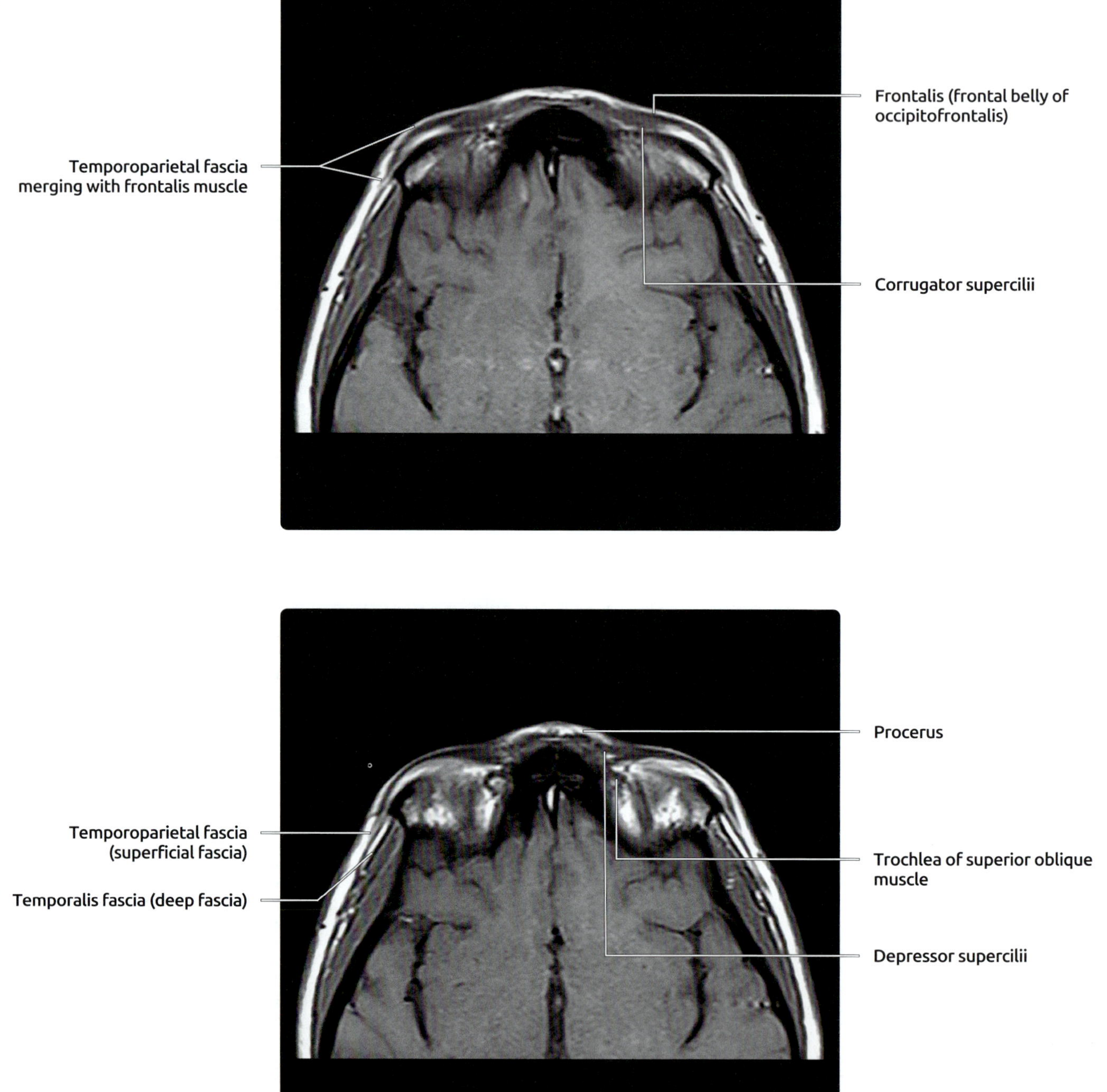

(Top) *Axial 3-mm T1 MR series from superior to inferior is shown. MR at the forehead shows the corrugator supercilii originating from the frontal bone at the medial supraorbital rim & lying deep to the frontalis to which it attaches. Note the temporoparietal fascia (TpF) (superficial fascia) merging with the frontalis muscle. The TpF is continuous with the galea aponeurotica in the scalp superiorly, frontalis muscle anteriorly, occipitalis muscle posteriorly, & SMAS inferiorly. The SMAS (superficial fascia) is a continuous fibrous network connecting facial muscles to dermis, helping facial expressions, & is continuous above with TpF as it passes over the zygomatic arch. The SMAS blends with the platysma muscle inferiorly & begins fading medially as it reaches the lateral nasal margin. The SMAS is extremely thin beyond the anterior border of the masseter as it enters the cheek area & is also so at its lower 1/2.* **(Bottom)** *Axial T1 MR at the topmost orbital level shows insertion of the procerus muscle into the skin & frontalis muscle & that of depressor supercilii muscle into the dermis. Also note the trochlea of the superior oblique muscle near its attachment on the superior nasal aspect of frontal bone.*

AXIAL T1 MR

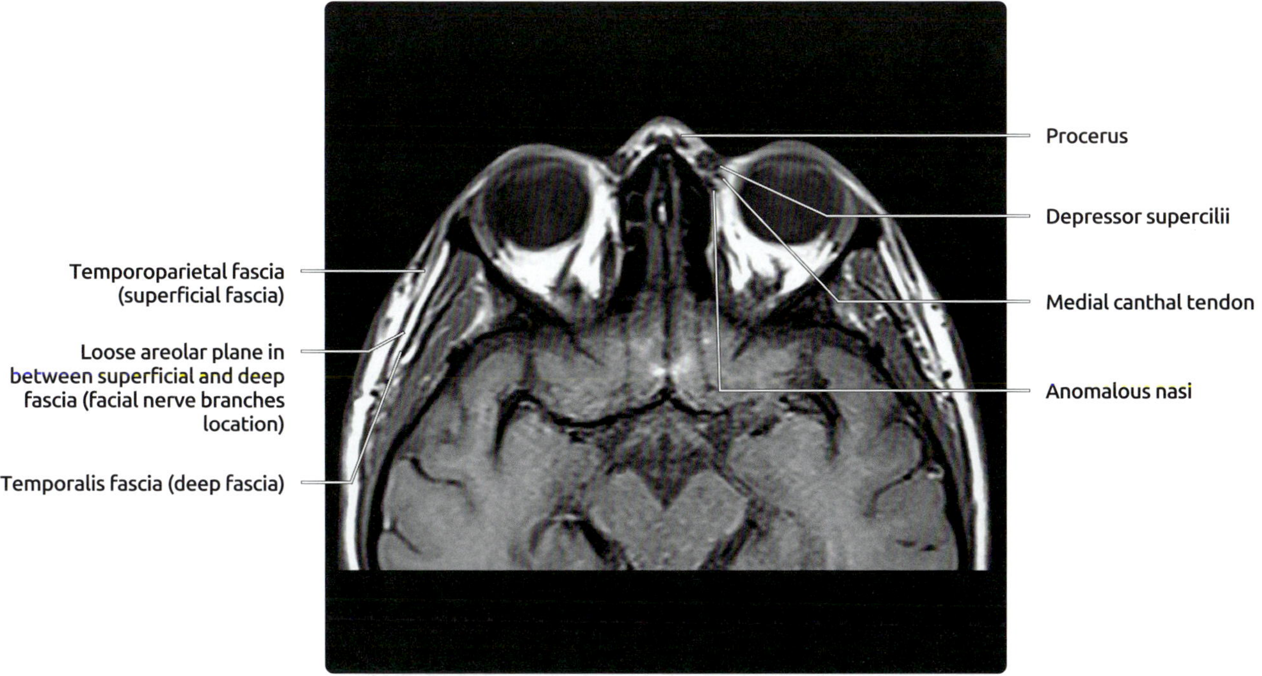

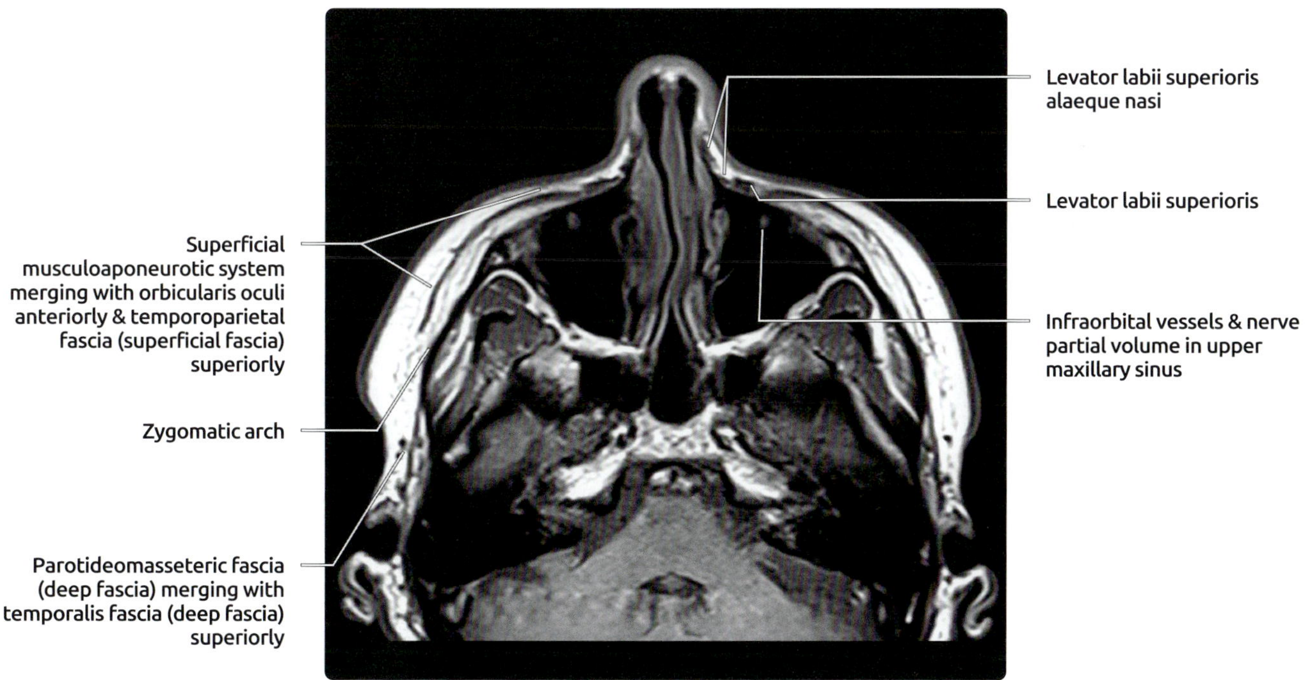

(Top) *Axial T1 MR at the level of the eye lens shows the origin of the procerus muscle on the nasal bone (inserts around the orbit but also acts as a nasal elevator) & depressor supercilii (inserts around the orbit) & anomalous nasi (inserts at the nose) on the frontal process of the maxilla (FPM). Note the delineation of the superficial TpF, deep temporalis fascia, & the loose areolar plane in between them; facial nerve branches at the temple lie in the fat of the loose areolar plane until 2 cm above the zygomatic arch and then pierce the TpF.* **(Bottom)** *Axial T1 MR just below the inferior orbital margin at the upper maxillary sinus level shows 2 main muscles inserting at the upper lip: The LLSAN, a nasal elevator also, to the nose anteriorly and upper lip posteriorly, & the LLS. The LLSAN can be easily tracked down from its origin on FPM, a readily identifiable bony landmark. The LLS is shown just below its origin on the infraorbital margin above the infraorbital foramen; therefore, the infraorbital vessels and nerve run down deep to it over the maxilla. Superficial (SMAS, TpF) & deep (parotidomasseteric fascia, temporalis fascia) fascial derivatives merging is shown.*

AXIAL T1 MR

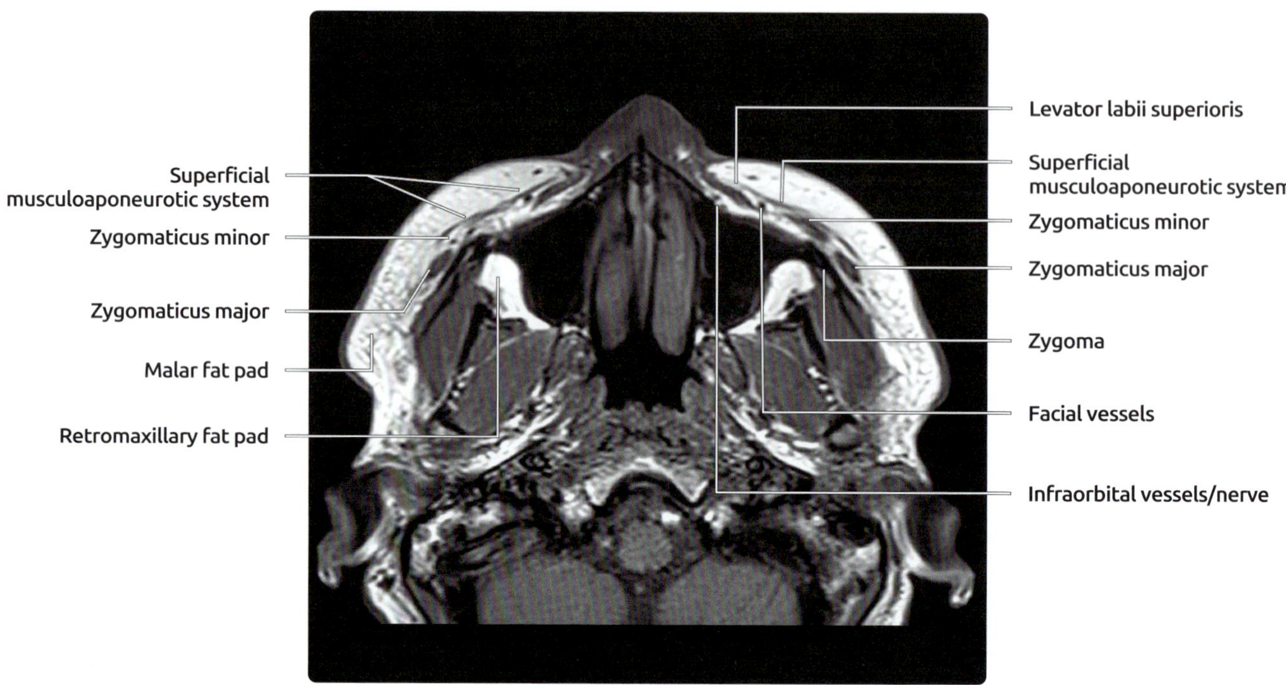

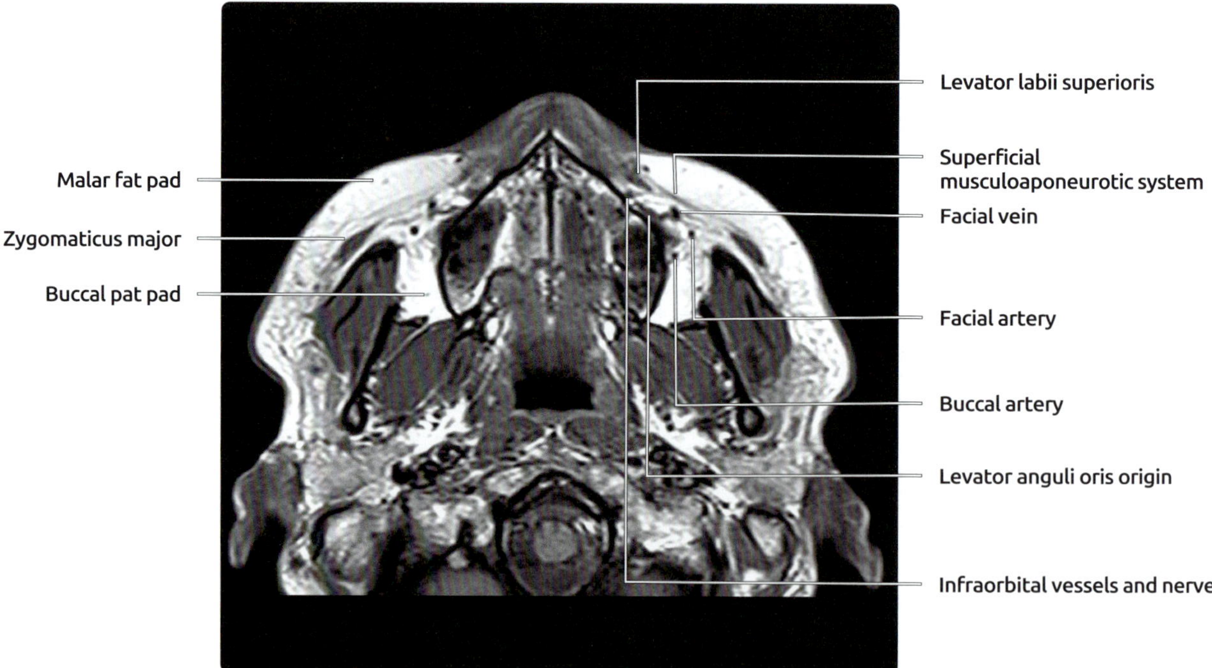

(Top) *Axial T1 MR at the lower zygomatic arch level shows the 3rd upper lip muscle, ZMi. ZMi is seen originating on the zygoma anterior to the origin of the zygomaticus major (ZMj), which attaches at the modiolus/angle of mouth. ZMi can be extremely thin unilaterally or bilaterally & is thin on the right in this patient. Note retromaxillary fat pad, a part of buccal space.* **(Bottom)** *Axial T1 MR just above the maxillary alveolus shows LAO muscle origin from the canine fossa of the maxilla. LAO is the deepest muscle seen anterior to the maxilla, & this deep location can be used as a key identifier to separate this muscle (inserting into the modiolus/angle of mouth region) from the more superficial LLS & LLSAN muscles (which can be traced toward their insertion in the upper lip). Infraorbital vessels & nerves running down deep to the LLS now lie in between the LLS & LAO, whereas the facial vessels run more laterally. The facial vein is larger & has a more predictable course than the smaller but tortuous facial artery. A tiny buccal artery is seen. Note that the malar fat pad is subcutaneous in front of the cheek, whereas the buccal fat pad is deeper just outside the corners of the mouth.*

AXIAL T1 MR

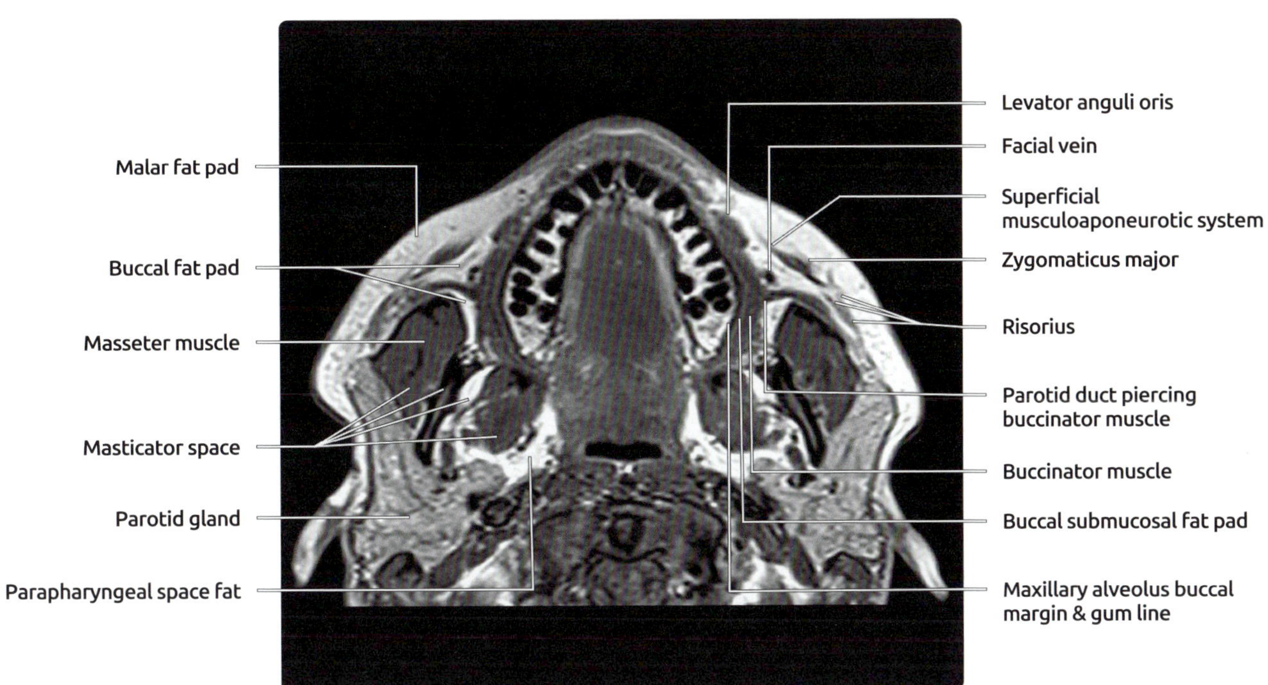

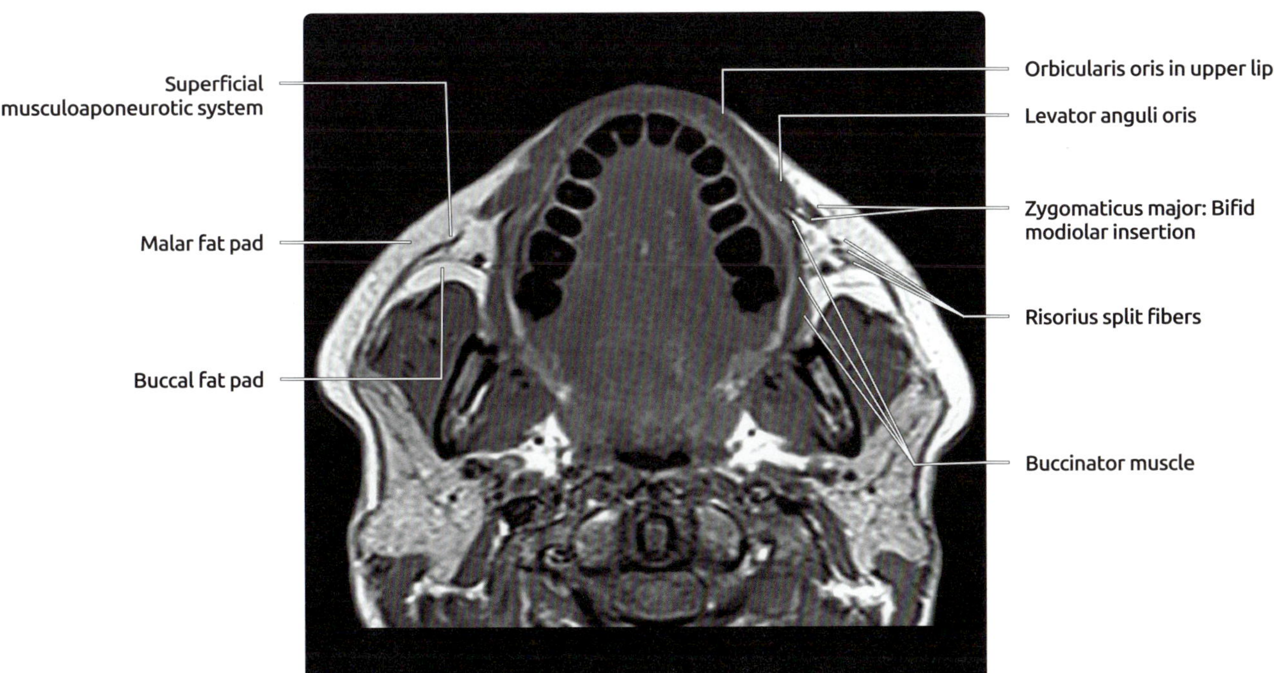

(Top) *Axial T1 MR at the maxillary alveolus level shows the parotid duct (PD) dividing the fat-filled buccal space into 2 compartments. The ZMj is seen anterior to the PD, or the risorius muscle originating from the SMAS anteriorly & parotidomasseteric fascia posteriorly (prongs of forked line) could be confused for the PD. The PD pierces the buccinator muscle opposite the maxillary 2nd molar tooth. The buccal submucosal fat pad is seen as a thin, bright line lateral to the potential space of the oral cavity, whereas the maxillary alveolus buccal margin & gum are seen as dark & soft tissue lines medial to the oral cavity. The masseter muscle is part of the masticator space, & buccinator muscle is part of the buccal space.* **(Bottom)** *Axial T1 MR through the upper lip shows the orbicularis oris muscle making up the bulk of the lip. ZMj insertion is bifid, & the LAO passes between its 2 heads at modiolar insertion (if not bifid, ZMj insertion is deep to LAO). The main insertion of deep muscle band of the ZMj is at the anterior margin of buccinator muscle/fascia (buccopharyngeal fascia); key for facial animation. Note risorius split fibers going toward modiolar insertion around depressor anguli oris (not shown) inferiorly.*

AXIAL T1 MR

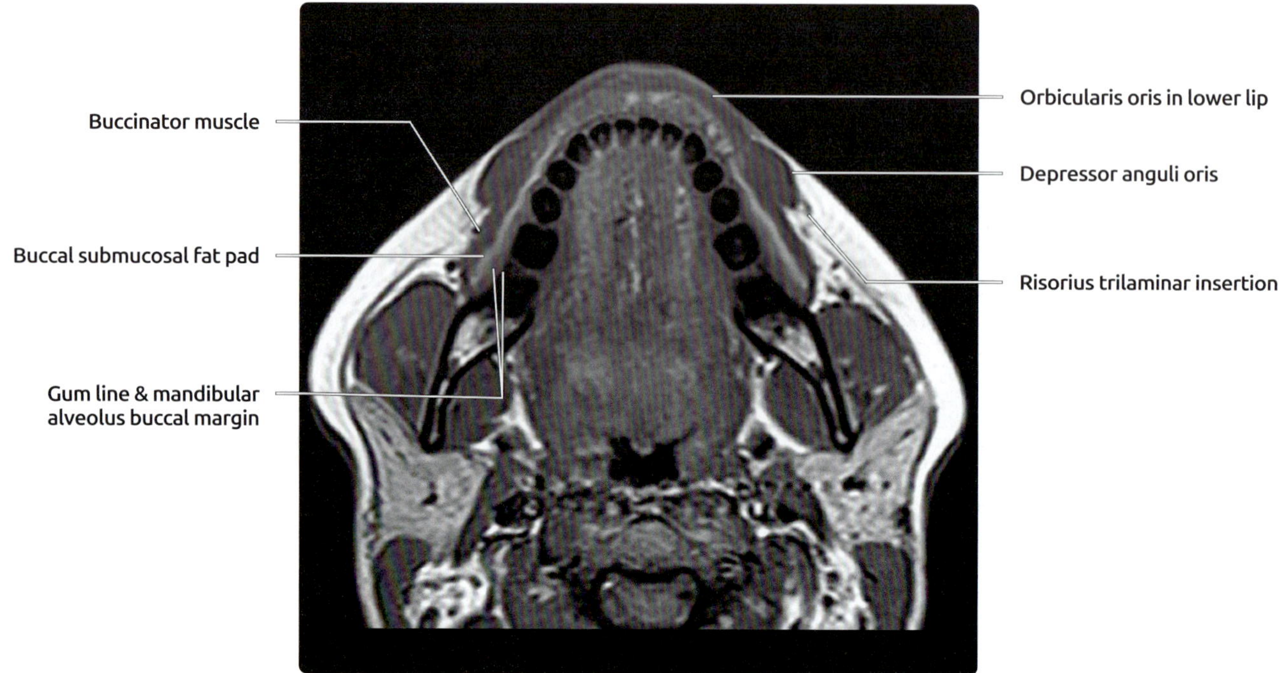

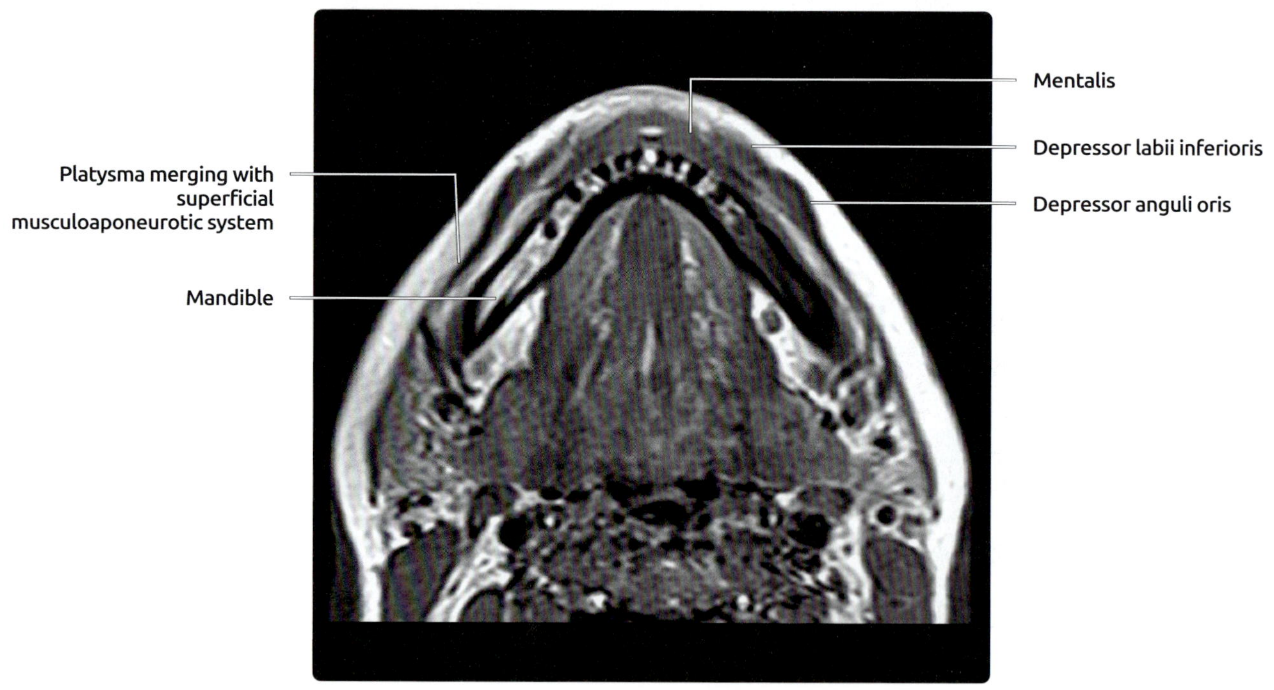

(Top) *Axial T1 MR through the lower lip shows the orbicularis oris muscle making up the bulk of the lip. The depressor anguli oris & split trilaminar insertion of risorius around the DAO are seen. Risorius, an inconsistent muscle with most fibers originating from SMAS, some fibers from parotidomasseteric fascia, and, in some cases, receiving platysma muscle fibers, inserts at the modiolus in 3 distinct superficial, flush, & deep layers in relation to DAO. Even though DAO prominently stands out at lower lip & mandibular levels, it is not a muscle inserting at the lower lip. DAO can be traced superiorly to its modiolar insertion. The mandibular alveolus buccal margin & gum line are seen as a dark line & soft tissue intensity, respectively, medial to the potential space of the oral cavity.* **(Bottom)** *Axial T1 MR at lower mandible level shows muscles inserting at the lower lip, namely, depressor labii inferioris, mentalis, & platysma. Platysma originates from the superficial pectoral & deltoid fascia, inserts on inferior body of mandible, skin, & hypodermis, & is continuous with SMAS in face. Some fibers of DAO may continue below mental tubercle, joining contralateral DAO & creating transversus menti muscle.*

CORONAL T1 MR

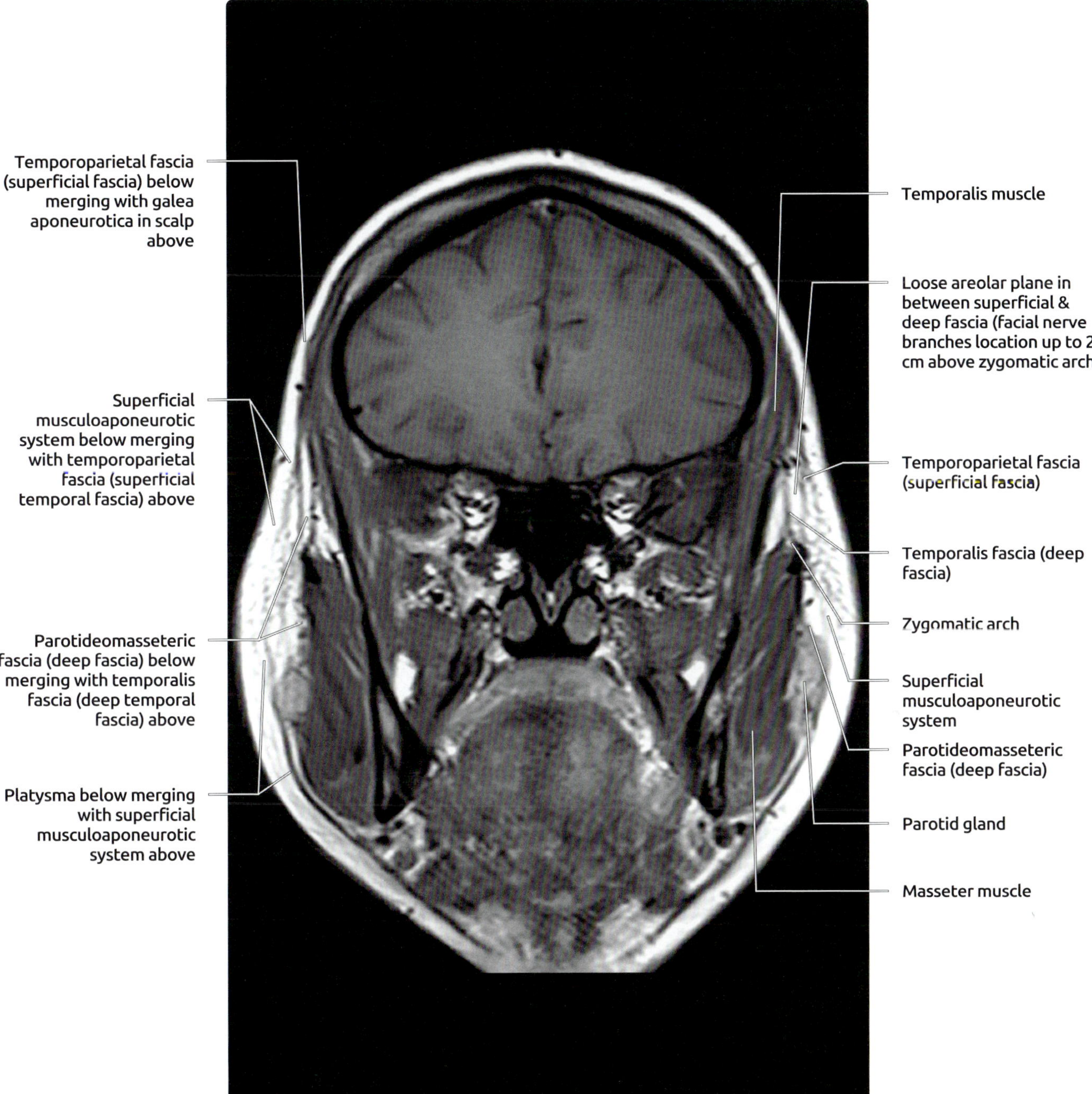

Coronal T1 MR shows fascial reflections. In the face, muscles insert directly into the dermis via the SMAS, facilitating facial expression (in the rest of the body, an investing layer of fascia separates muscle from subcutaneous tissue). The SMAS is continuous above with the TpF (a.k.a. superficial temporal fascia) as it passes over the zygomatic arch, which, in turn, is continuous with galea aponeurotica in the scalp superiorly, frontalis muscle anteriorly, & occipitalis muscle posteriorly. Parotidomasseteric fascia (deep fascia in the cheek deep to the SMAS) is continuous above with temporalis fascia (a.k.a. deep temporal fascia), which, in turn, covers the temporalis muscle, splits over the zygomatic arch superficial & deep surfaces inferiorly, & attaches to the pericranium at & above the superior temporal line on the skull superiorly. The facial nerve branches in the parotid gland lie deep underneath parotideomasseteric fascia, then in the loose areolar tissue plane between the TpF & zygomatic arch, in the loose areolar plane between the superficial TpF & deep temporalis fascia ~ 1 cm above the zygomatic arch, & penetrates TpF ~ 2 cm above the zygomatic arch to run along the superficial temporal artery.

TERMINOLOGY

Definitions

- Angle of mandible: Obtuse angle of mandible where inferior segment of ramus meets posterior mandible body

IMAGING ANATOMY

Internal Contents

- Mandible anatomy: Bony
  - 2 vertical rami attached to horizontal horseshoe-shaped body
  - Each ramus has 2 upwardly directed processes
    - **Condylar process**: Condylar head & neck contains articular surface of TMJ
    - **Coronoid process**: Temporalis muscle inserts here
    - Mandibular notch separates these 2 processes
    - Mandibular ramus divides masticator space into lateral & medial compartments
  - **Mandibular foramen**
    - Location: Center medial surface of mandible ramus
    - Nerve transmitted: Inferior alveolar nerve
    - Lingula: Small osseous lip extending from anterior aspect of mandibular foramen
  - Mandibular body
    - U-shaped, horizontal body composed of 2 halves; fuses in anterior midline at **symphysis menti**
    - Alveolar process consists of external buccal & internal lingual plates, covered by periosteum
    - **Mental foramen**: Paired external openings of mandibular canal that transmits mental nerve
    - **Mylohyoid ridge**: Bony ridge on lingual mandible body; site of attachment of mylohyoid muscle
  - Mandibular canal
    - Lies within distal ramus & proximal body of mandible
    - Extends from mandibular to mental foramen
    - Contains inferior alveolar nerve & vessels
- Mandible anatomy: Nerves
  - **Inferior alveolar nerve**
    - Extends from mandibular foramen, through mandibular canal to mental foramen
    - Innervates ipsilateral premolars & molars
    - Divides into mental & incisive branches
  - **Mental nerve**
    - Exits mental foramen
    - Provides sensory innervation to skin & mucosa of lower lip & labial gingiva
  - **Incisive nerve**
    - Innervates ipsilateral canine & incisors
- Maxillary alveolar & palatine processes: Bony
  - Represents inferior aspect of maxillary bone
  - Maxillary alveolar ridge (arch)
    - Adult version contains 16 teeth
  - **Premaxilla**: Anterior hard palate & alveolar ridge
    - Contains **incisive foramen** (nasopalatine nerve)
    - Nasopalatine canals converge as incisive foramen
  - Palatine process of maxillary bone
    - Forms anterior 2/3 of hard palate
  - Posterior 1/3 of hard palate formed by horizontal plate of palatine bone
- Maxillary alveolar & palatine processes: Nerves
  - **Nasopalatine nerve** (V2 sensory branch) travels through incisive foramen
    - Supplies sensory fibers to anterior hard palate
  - **Greater palatine nerve** comes down greater palatine canal in palatine bone
    - Supplies sensation to posterior 2/3 of hard palate
    - Exits greater palatine foramen anteriorly to hard palate mucosa
  - **Lesser palatine nerve** comes down lesser palatine canal in palatine bone
    - Exits lesser palatine foramen posterior to greater palatine foramen
    - Supplies sensory fibers to palatine tonsil
- Dental anatomy, mandible, & maxilla
  - 32 total permanent teeth in mandible (16) & maxilla (16)
    - Each tooth has crown, root, & pulp
  - 16 adult teeth in each "dental arch"
    - Each arch consists of 2 quadrants
    - Each quadrant contains 3 molars, 2 premolars, 1 canine, 1 lateral incisor, & 1 central incisor
  - **Universal Numbering System for teeth (ADA approved, most common in USA)**
    - Maxillary alveolar ridge: Begin with right 3rd molar, 1-16 across to left 3rd molar
    - Mandibular alveolar ridge: Begin with left 3rd molar, 17-32 across to right 3rd molar
  - Each crown: Outer enamel surrounding dentin; pulp in center
    - **Enamel**: Densest material in body
    - **Dentin**: Encases pulp
    - **Pulp**: Nourishes dentin
  - Tooth root covered by cementum
    - Cementum acts as medium for attaching fibers of periodontal ligament to tooth
    - Periodontal ligament located in periodontal space
    - Periodontal space is radiolucency surrounding root

ANATOMY IMAGING ISSUES

Questions

- Is **V2** perineural malignant tumor?
  - If malignancy affects skin of upper lip, **hard palate**, soft palate, check for V2 perineural tumor (PNT)
  - Major locations to identify V2 PNT extend from incisive canal-greater palatine foramen to root entry zone of V in lateral pons
  - If imaging for V2 PNT, check incisive canal, greater & lesser palatine foramen, pterygopalatine canal & fossa, foramen rotundum, Meckel cave, preganglionic segment of CNV, & root entry zone
- Is **V3** perineural malignant tumor?
  - If malignant tumor of skin of chin, mandibular alveolar ridge, or masticator space, check for V3 PNT
  - If imaging for V3 PNT, check entire length of V3 to root entry zone
    - Pay special attention to inferior alveolar canal, mandibular foramen, masticator space

GRAPHICS

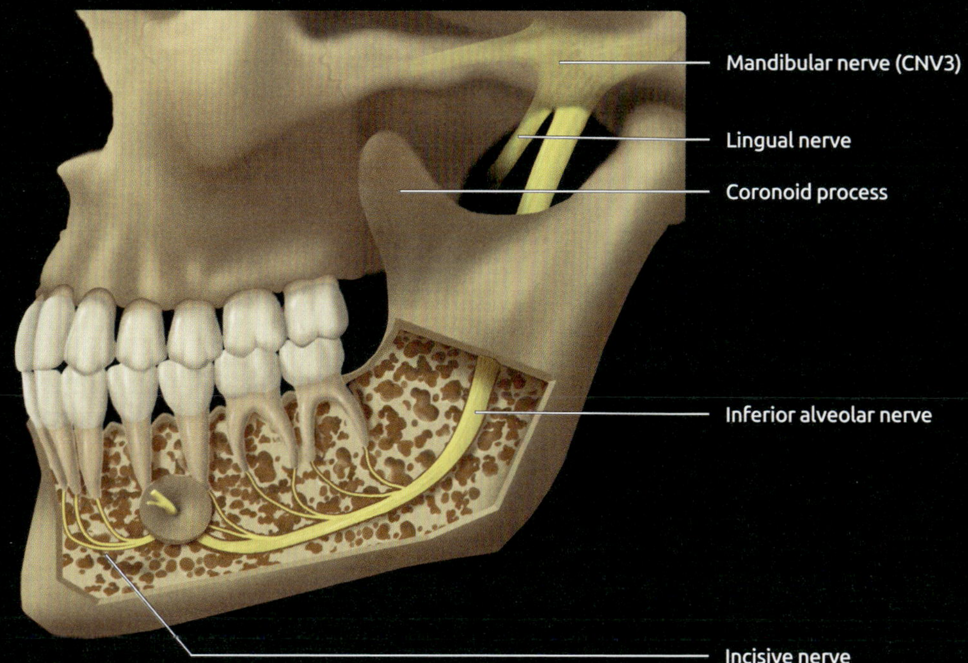

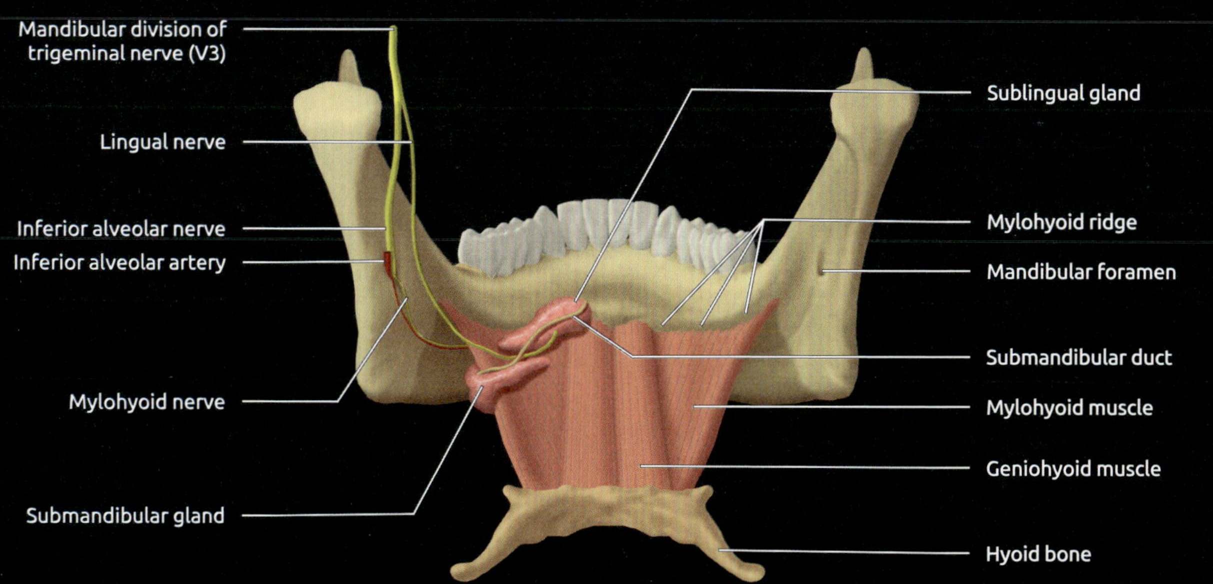

(Top) *Lateral graphic of the mandible with its lateral cortex removed reveals the mandibular nerve divides into the lingual and inferior alveolar nerves. The inferior alveolar nerve divides distally into the mental and incisive branches. The mental nerve branch reaches the superficial chin through the mental foramen.* **(Bottom)** *Graphic of the posterior view of the floor of mouth and mandible shows the S-shaped mylohyoid ridge where the mylohyoid muscle attaches to the mandible. Also note the mandibular division of the trigeminal nerve bifurcates into the lingual nerve and the inferior alveolar nerve. Just prior to entering the mandibular foramen, the inferior alveolar nerve gives off the mylohyoid motor branch that innervates the mylohyoid and anterior belly of the digastric muscles.*

GRAPHICS

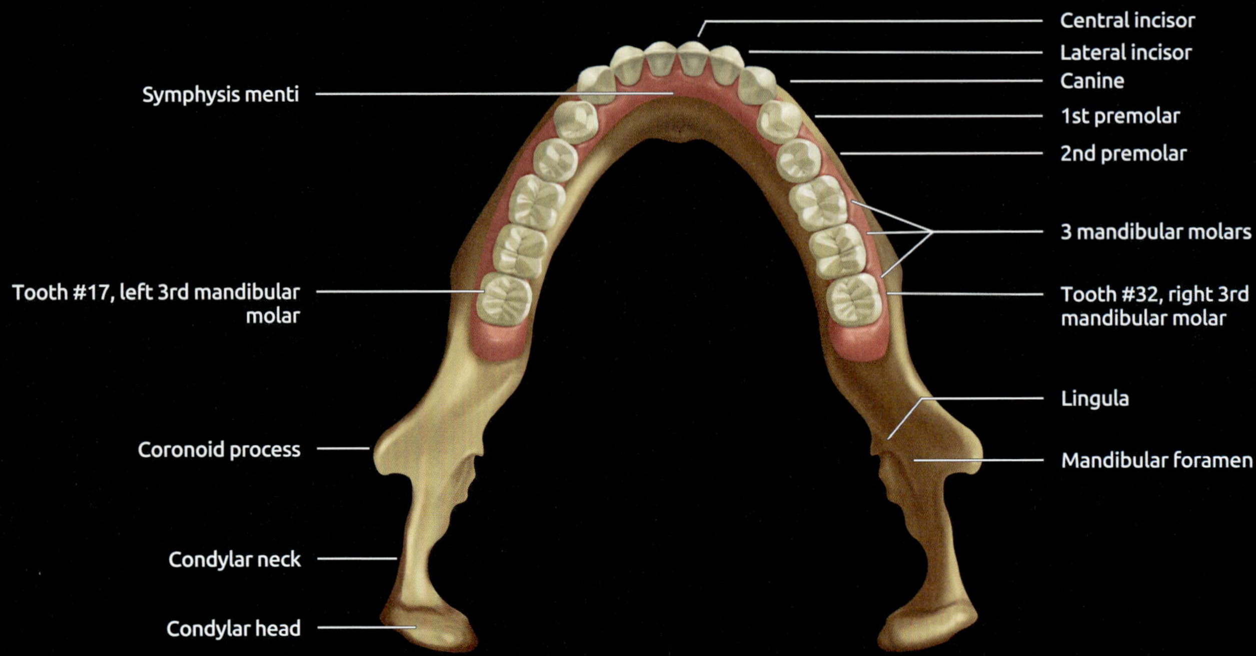

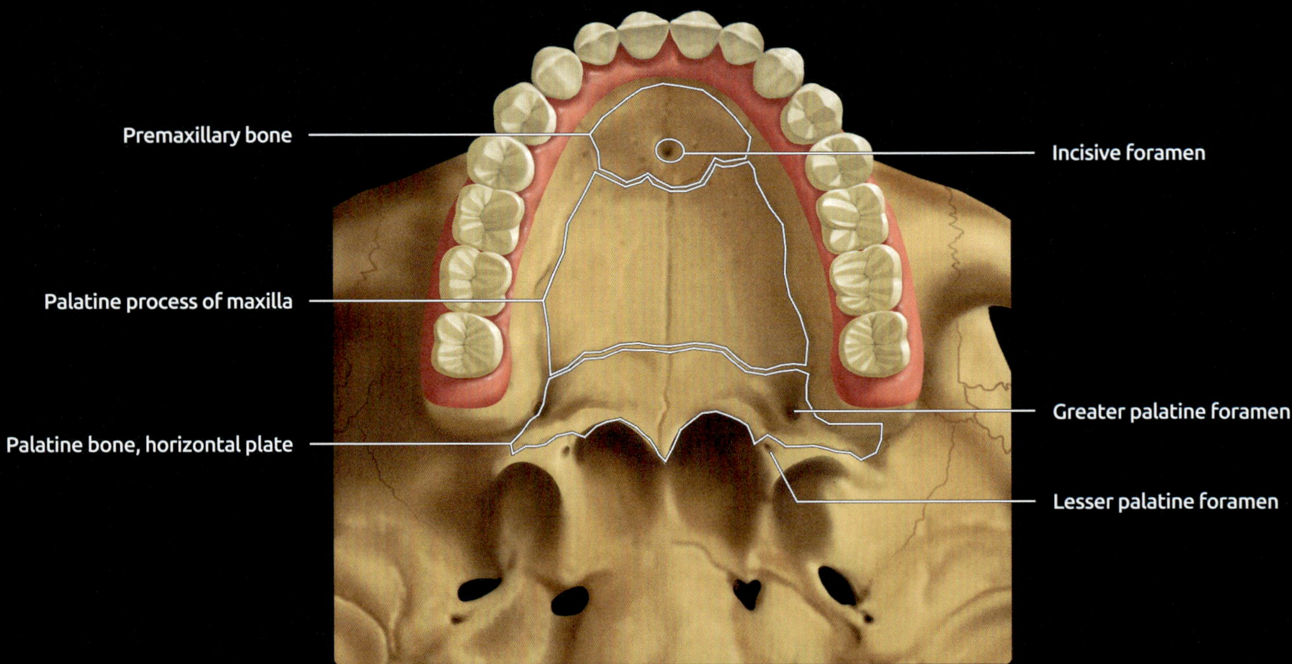

(Top) *Axial graphic of the mandible seen from above demonstrates the cephalad condylar head and neck leading to the more inferior ramus. The mandibular foramen is seen on the inner surface of the mandibular ramus. The cephalad projecting coronoid processes attach to the temporalis muscle tendons. The U-shaped mandibular bodies fuse in the midline at the symphysis menti. Notice there are 16 adult teeth, numbered 17-32, from the left 3rd molar to the right 3rd molar.* **(Bottom)** *Axial graphic of the hard palate and maxillary alveolar ridge viewed from below shows the anterior premaxillary bone and the larger, more posterior palatine process of the maxillary bone. The horizontal plate of the palatine bone completes the hard palate picture. Notice the anterior midline incisive canal and the posterolateral greater and lesser palatine foramina.*

GRAPHIC & BONE CT

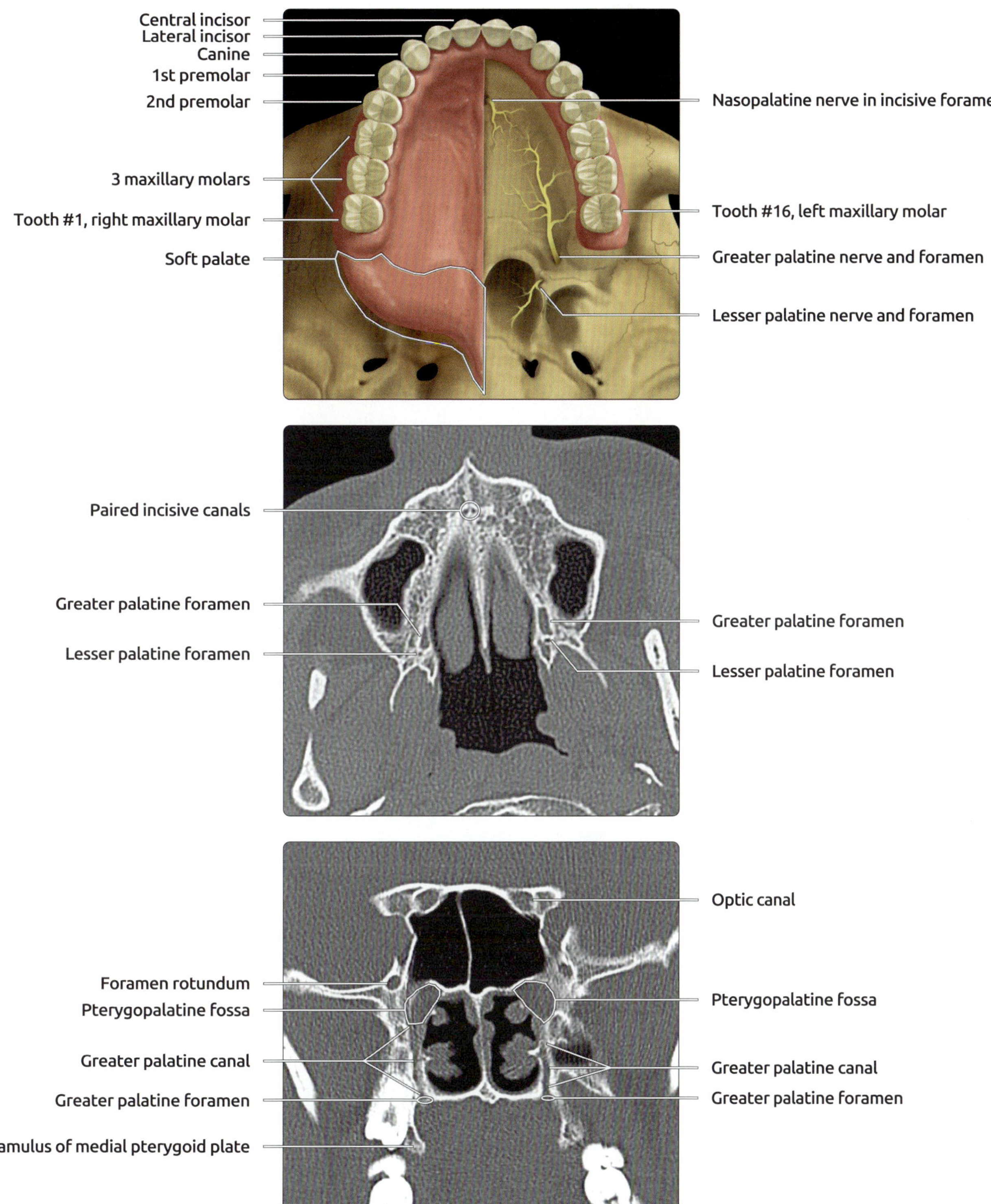

(Top) *Axial graphic of the hard palate viewed from below with mucosa removed on the right side is shown. Hard palate sensory innervation is shown on the right with the anterior 1/3 of the hard palate supplied by the nasopalatine nerve and the posterior 2/3 of the hard palate supplied by the greater palatine nerve. Notice there are 16 adult teeth, numbered beginning at the right 3rd molar from 1-16.* **(Middle)** *Axial bone CT depicts foramina carrying nerves to the hard palate. Anterior paired incisive canals lead to more inferior incisive foramen (not shown). Greater and lesser palatine foramina transmit greater and lesser palatine nerves, respectively.* **(Bottom)** *Coronal bone CT through the vertical aspect of the greater palatine canal shows this canal connecting the pterygopalatine fossa above with the greater palatine foramen below. The greater palatine nerve uses the greater palatine canal to access the palate.*

AXIAL BONE CT

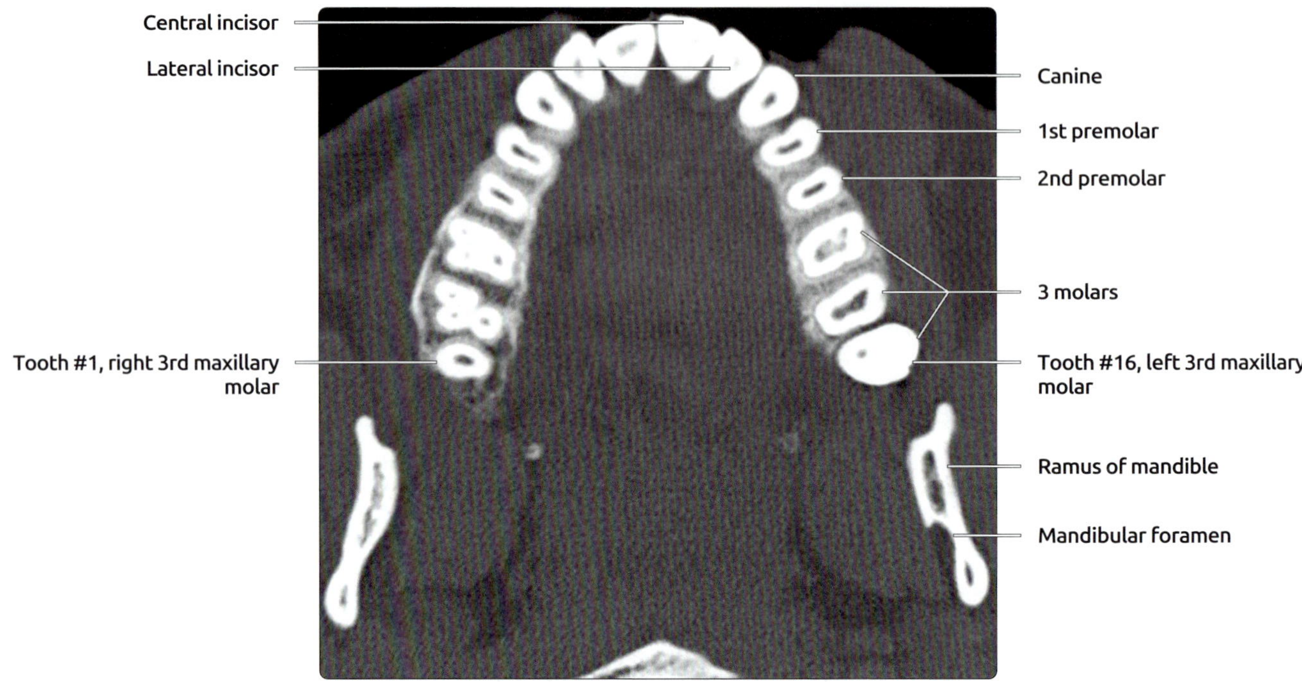

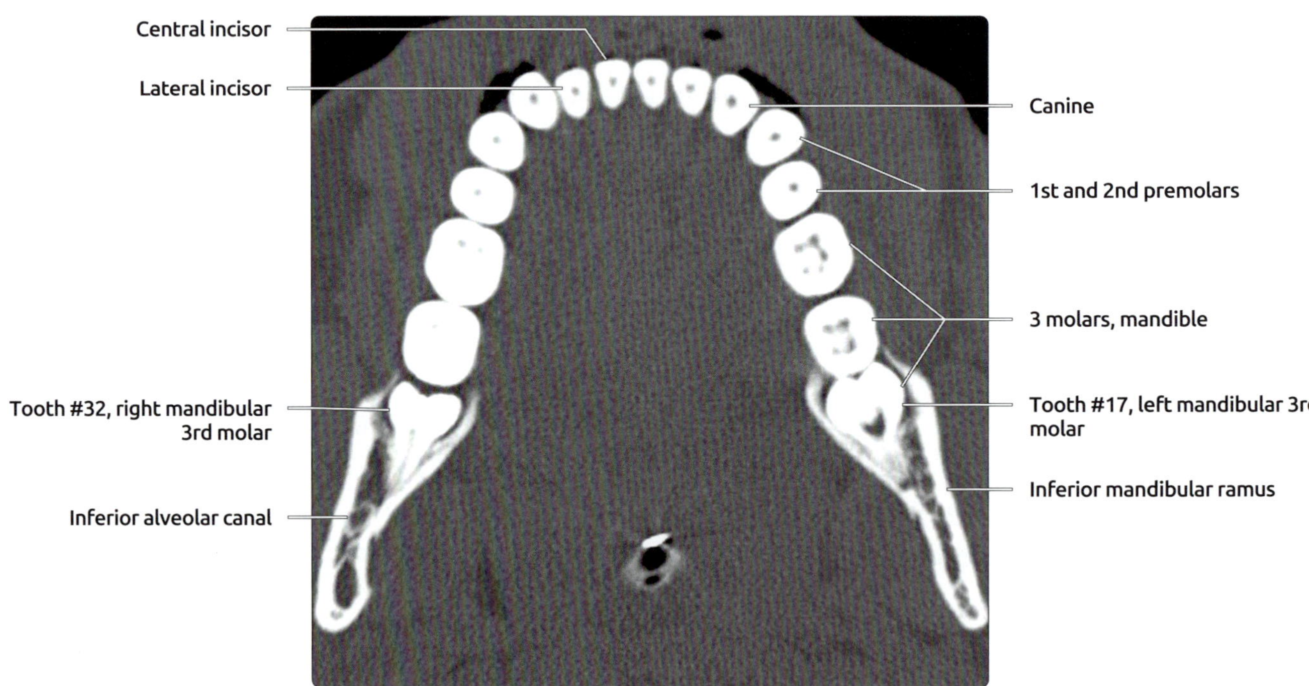

(Top) *Axial bone CT at the level of the maxillary ridge delineates the 16 upper teeth. Numbering convention begins with tooth #1 (upper posterior right molar tooth), extending from there across to the opposite left posterior maxillary molar, which is designated as tooth #16. Note that there are 2 each of medial and lateral incisors, canine, 1st and 2nd premolars, and 3 molar teeth.* **(Bottom)** *Axial bone CT of the 16 mandibular teeth is shown. Continuing the numbering convention for the mandibular teeth, the left 3rd molar is considered tooth #17 with numbering moving across to the opposite right 3rd mandibular molar designated as tooth #32. Note again that there are paired central and lateral incisors, canines, 1st and 2nd premolars, and 3 molar teeth in the mandible.*

3D CT OF MANDIBLE

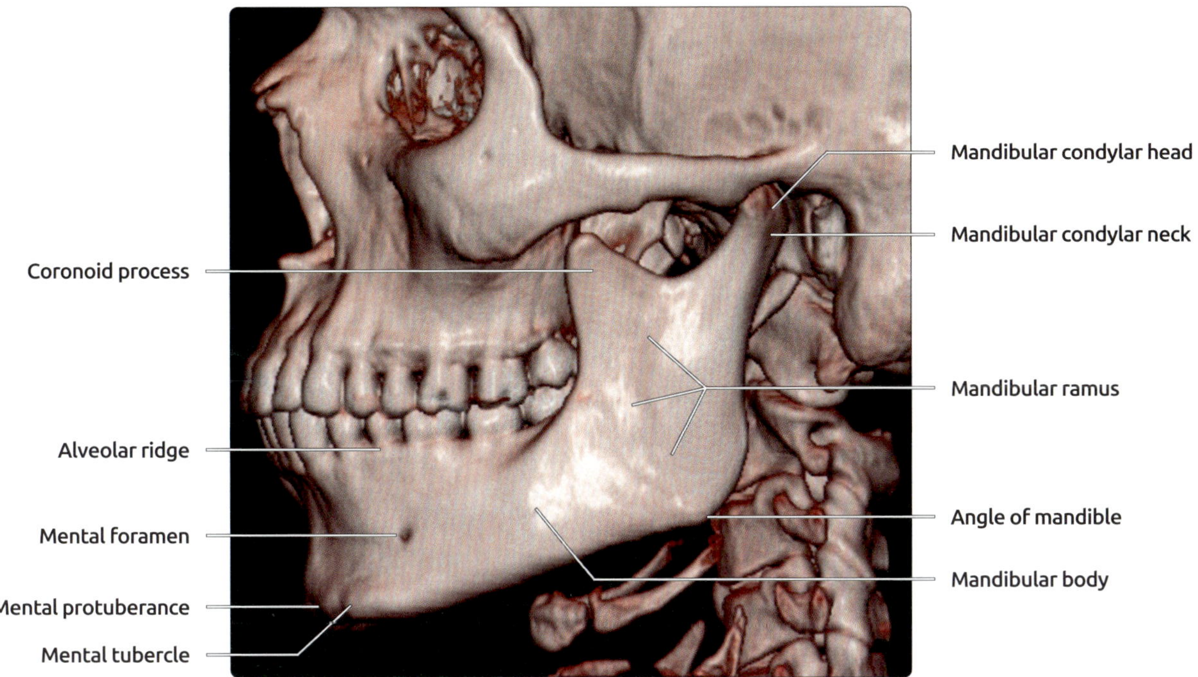

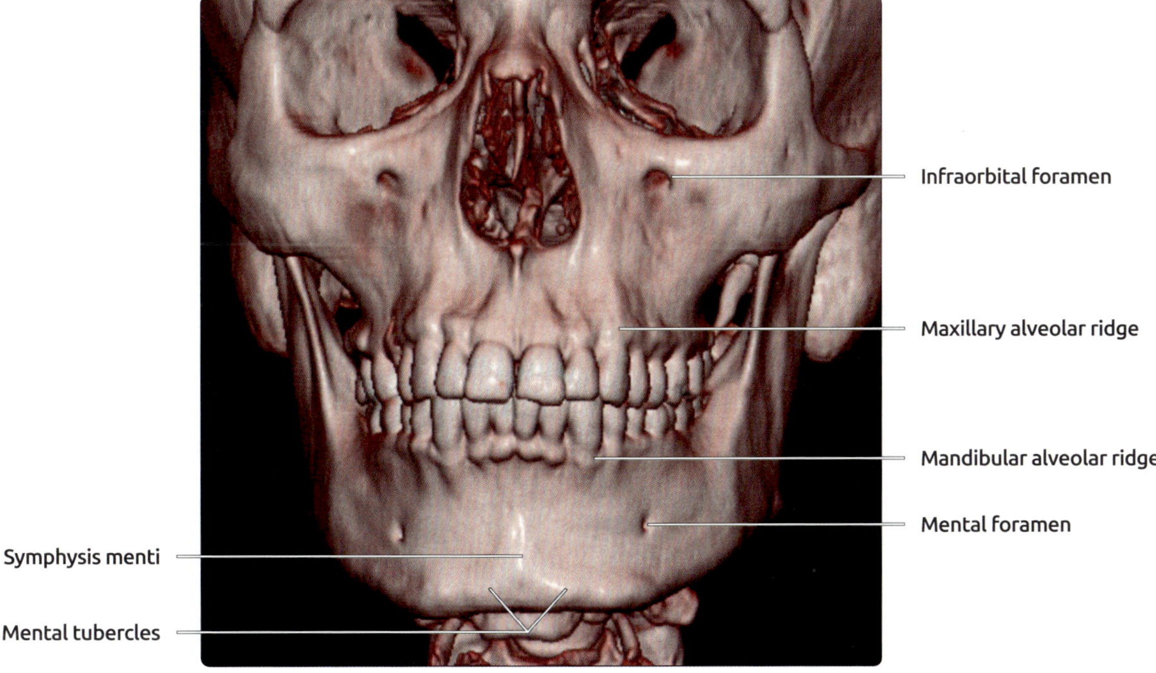

(Top) *Lateral view of a 3D reconstruction of the facial bones is shown. The mandible can be divided into the condyle, neck, ramus, coronoid process, body, and alveolar ridge. The mental foramen is seen in the anterior body and transmits the mental nerve, a sensory nerve to the chin.* **(Bottom)** *Frontal view of a 3D reconstruction of the facial bones is shown. The mandible anterior body is best delineated with the paired mental foramina evident. The infraorbital nerves are transmitted via the paired infraorbital foramina.*

TERMINOLOGY

Definitions

- Articulation between mandible & T-bone

IMAGING ANATOMY

Overview

- Complex diarthrodial synovial joint between mandibular fossa & mandibular condyle, which allows mobility of mandible for speech & mastication
- Located on each side at skull base anterior to external auditory canal

Internal Contents

- **Articular surfaces of TMJ**
  - Undersurface of squamous T-bone contains mandibular fossa & articular eminence
    - **Mandibular fossa** (glenoid/articular fossa)
      - Concave-shaped articular surface, petrosquamous & petrotympanic fissures together form posterior articular ridge
      - Posterior articular ridge lateral pole called **postglenoid process** & medial pole called **entoglenoid process**
    - **Articular eminence** (articular tubercle)
      - Transverse bony bar at root of zygoma with convex surface located anterior to mandibular fossa
  - **Mandibular condyle**: Condylar H&N: Posterior protrusion from ramus of mandible
- **Articular cartilage**: 2- to 5-mm thick **fibrous cartilage** covers articular surface (as opposed to hyaline cartilage in other synovial joints)
- **Articular disc**: Most important anatomic structure providing cushion & absorbing stress in TMJ
  - Biconcave, oval, dumbbell-shaped fibrocartilaginous structure, which enables compatibility of articular surfaces
  - **Intermediate zone** (avascular): 1-mm thick zone between anterior & posterior bands
  - **Anterior band**: 2-mm thick band attaches to anterior joint capsule & is partially integrated into superior belly of lateral pterygoid muscle
  - **Posterior band**: 3-mm thick bilaminar band
  - **Bilaminar zone**: Connects articular disc to retrodiscal tissue
    - **Superior lamina** composed of **loose** elastin; attached to postglenoid process & prevents slipping of disc during excessive mouth opening
    - **Inferior lamina** composed of **taut** collagen material; attached to posterior margin of mandibular condyle & prevents excessive rotation of disc over condyle
  - Medially & laterally, disc attaches to joint capsule & medial & lateral condyle through collateral ligaments
- **TMJ compartments**: Disc creates superior & inferior compartments
  - **Superior joint compartment**: Between disc & mandibular fossa of T-bone
    - Volume: 1-2 mL normally but can increase up to 6 mL with pathology
  - **Inferior joint compartment**: Between disc & condyle; 2 distinct recesses
    - Volume: < 1 mL normally but can increase up to 2 mL with pathology
- **TMJ capsule & ligaments**
  - **Joint capsule**: Funnel-shaped; extends T-bone to condylar neck
  - **TMJ ligaments**: Holds joint together & restricts its movement
    - **Temporomandibular ligament**: Lateral ligament attached to zygomatic arch articular eminence above & lateral surface of mandibular neck below
    - **Sphenomandibular ligament**: Medial ligament attaches above on spine of sphenoid & below to lingula of mandibular foramen
    - **Stylomandibular ligament**: Thickened band-shaped deep cervical fascia; extends from styloid process to posterior edge of mandibular ramus & angle

MR Appearances of TMJ

- **Articular disc**: Low signal on T1 & T2
- **Articular disc movement**
  - Intermediate zone, always interposed between mandibular condyle & fossa during open- & closed-mouth positions
  - Initially upon mouth opening, inferior (discomandibular) joint rotates
  - When mouth fully opens, mandibular condyle slides forward & downward onto articular eminence
  - Articular disc slides in same direction until its posterior fibroelastic attachments are stretched to their limits
- **Closed-mouth sagittal MR**: Sigmoid-shaped disc in anterior 1/2 of joint space
  - Junction between low-signal posterior band & intermediate-signal bilaminar zone at 12-o'clock position relative to mandibular condyle
- **Open-mouth sagittal MR**: Bow tie-shaped disc anteroinferior to articular eminence & above mandibular condyle
  - Posterior band, posterior to condyle's posterior margin

ANATOMY IMAGING ISSUES

Imaging Recommendations

- Most TMJ imaging requested for internal derangement (abnormal disc position) or TMJ degenerative disorders
- MR best imaging modality; coronal closed-mouth T1, sagittal T1 & T2 with closed- & open-mouth positions; T2 FS best for evaluation of joint effusion
- Bone CT: NECT with ≤ 1-mm axial images; sagittal & coronal reformations helpful to assess osseous structures

Imaging Sweet Spots

- If posterior band anterior to 12-o'clock position of condyle, consider anterior displacement
- Review coronal images to evaluate lateral displacement of articular disc
- Assess disc T2 signal, especially at posterior attachment in patients with TMJ pain

GRAPHICS

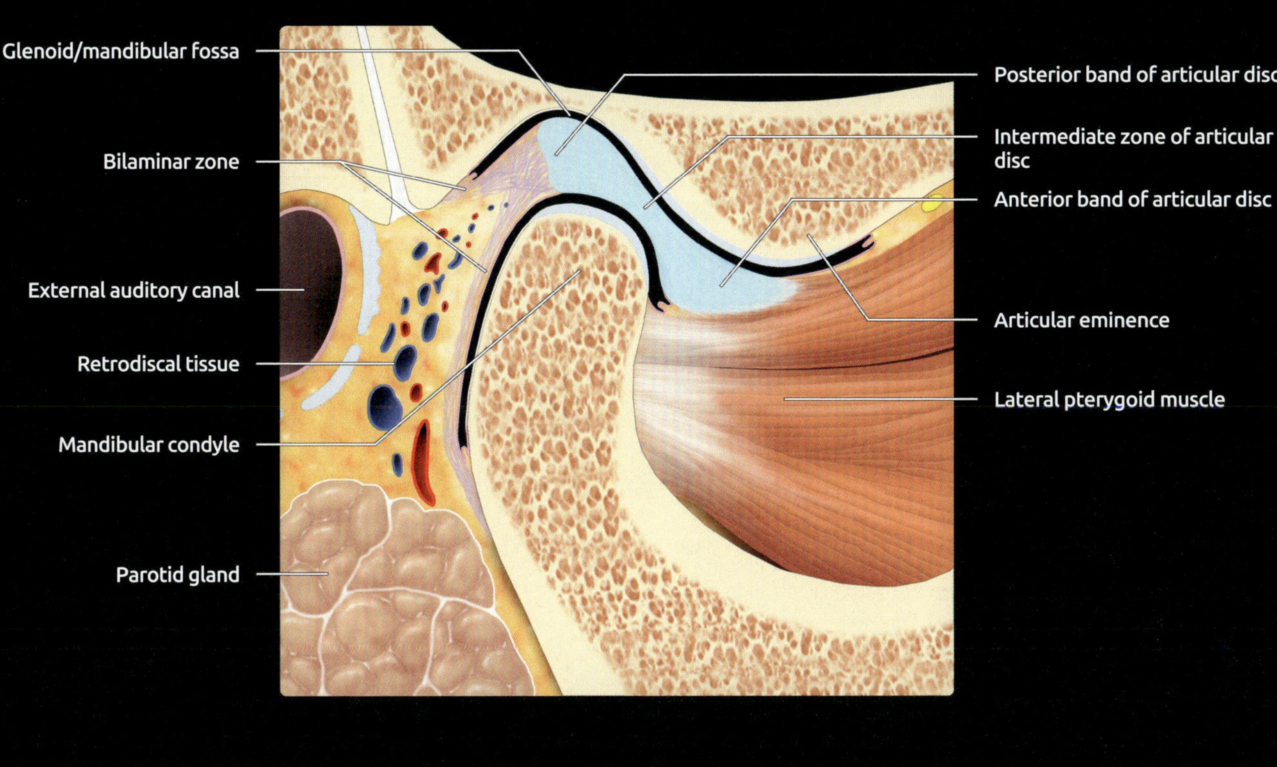

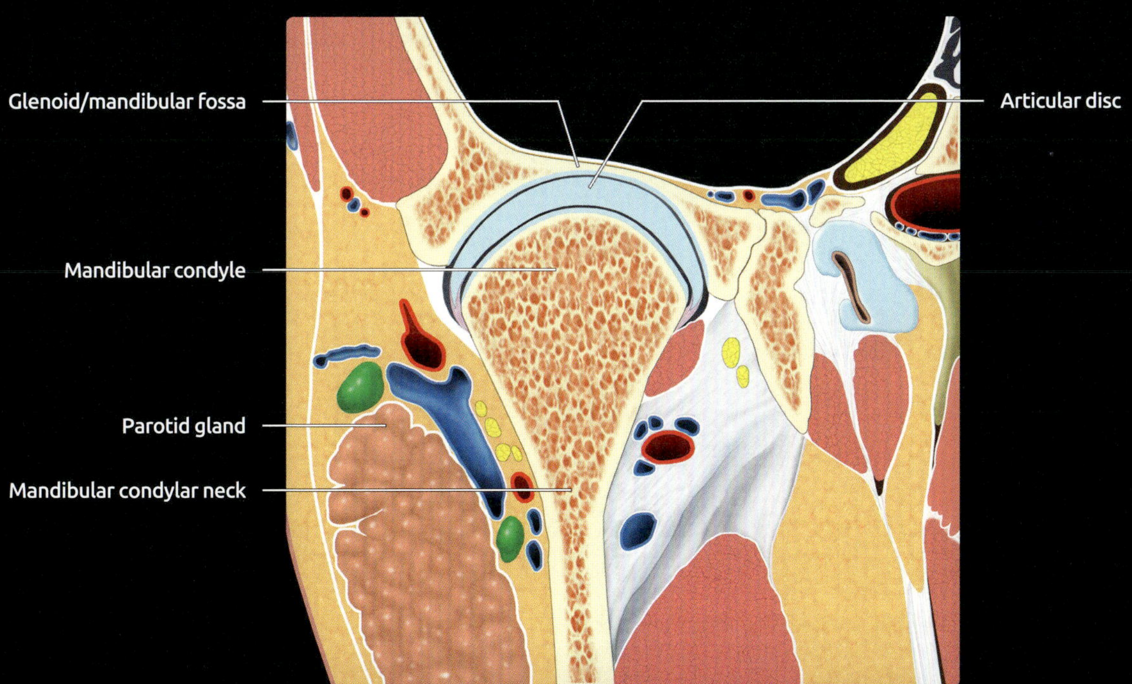

(Top) *Lateral graphic of the TMJ demonstrates the mandibular condyle articulating in the glenoid fossa in the closed-mouth position. Anterior to the glenoid fossa is the articular eminence to which the mandibular condyle slides in the open-mouth position (not shown). Note the biconcave articular disc with anterior & posterior bands & an intermediate zone. The lateral pterygoid muscle is attached to the mandibular condyle & articular disc.* **(Bottom)** *Frontal graphic of the TMJ demonstrates the mediolateral relation of the articular disc with the mandibular condyle. (Courtesy D. Tamimi, BDS, DMSc.)*

BONE CT

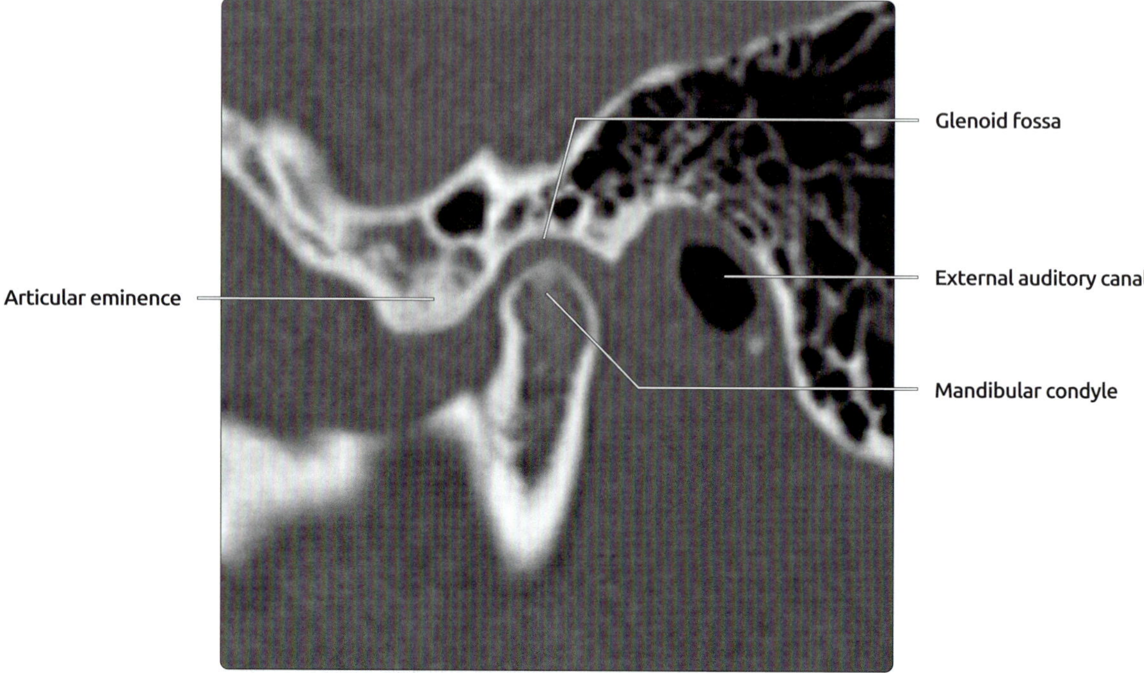

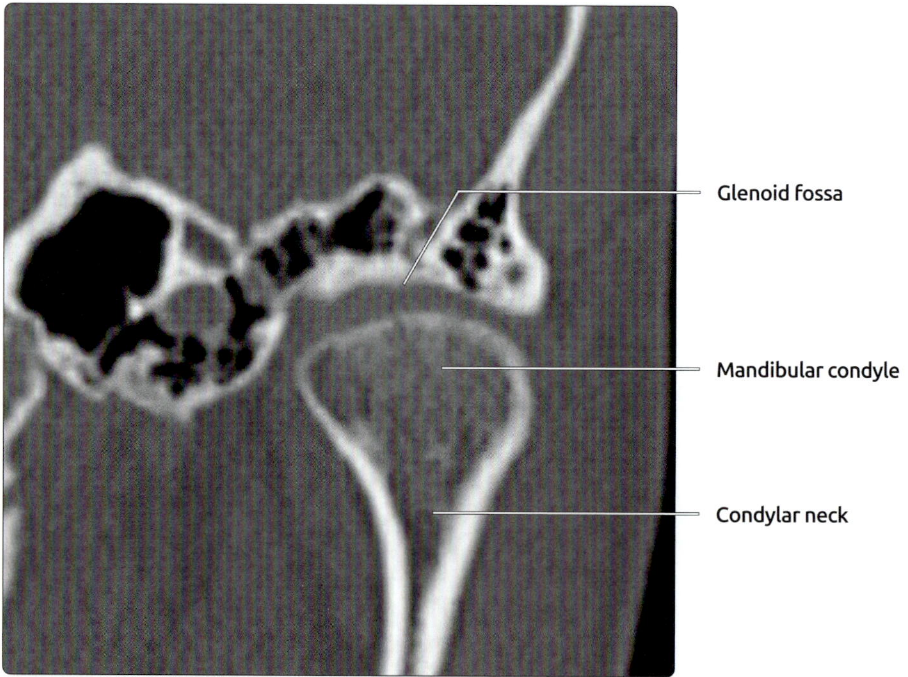

(Top) *Sagittal reformat of a thin-section bone algorithm NECT of the TMJ in the closed-mouth position demonstrates the mandibular condyle articulating with the glenoid fossa. The articular eminence is located immediately anterior to the glenoid fossa & the external auditory canal posterior to it.* **(Bottom)** *Coronal reformat of a thin-section bone algorithm NECT of the TMJ in the closed-mouth position demonstrates the mediolateral dimension of the mandibular condyle (15-20 mm) wider than its anteroposterior dimension (8-10 mm). The long axis of the mandibular condyle is directed posteromedially.*

3D VRT BONE CT & CORONAL T1 MR

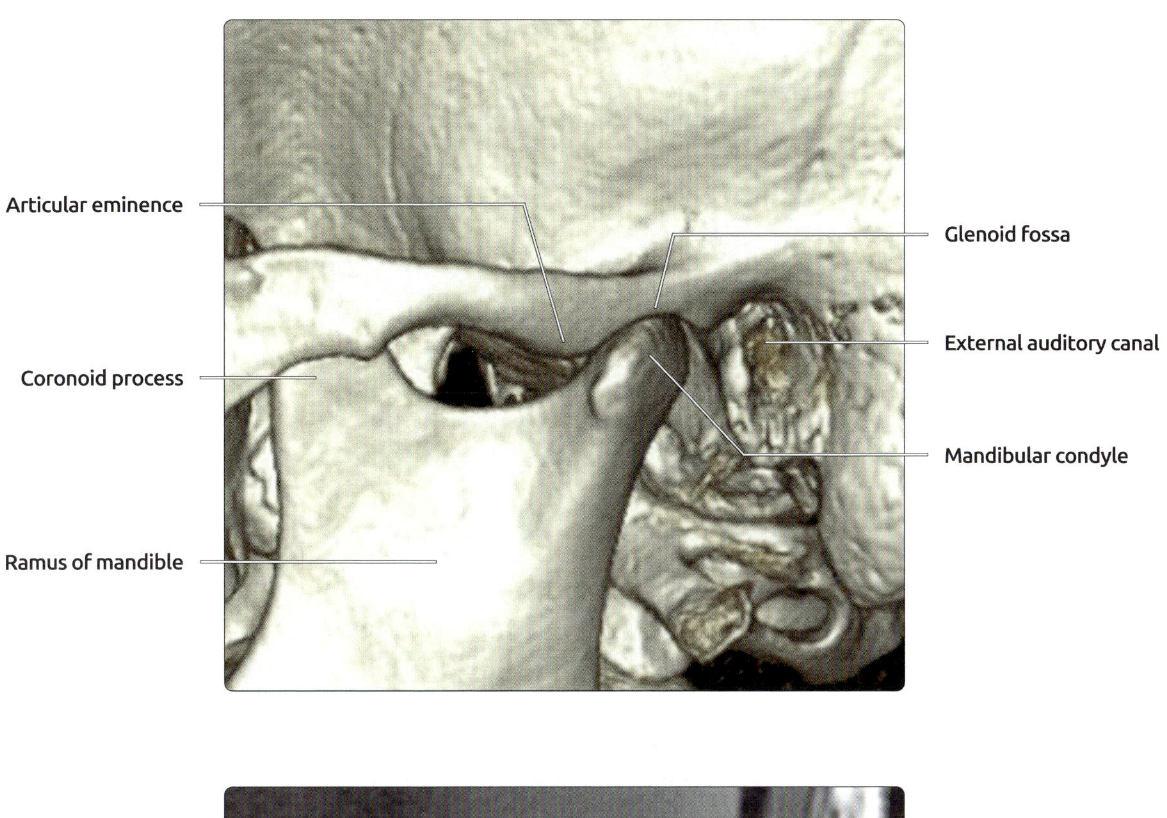

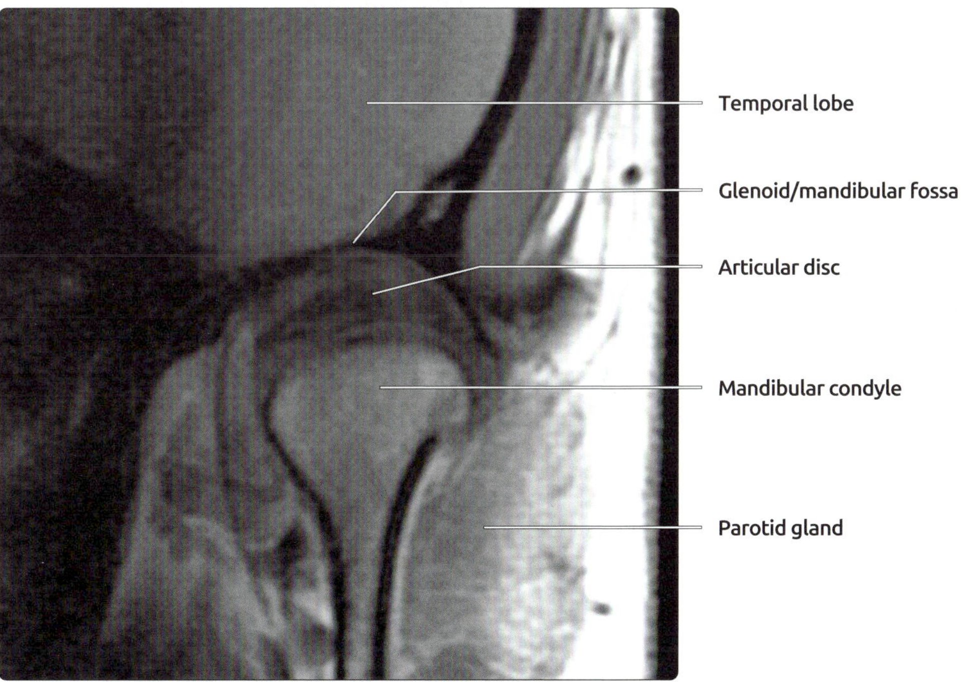

(Top) *3D volume-rendered reconstruction of a thin-section bone algorithm NECT demonstrates a normal TMJ in the closed-mouth position. Note the mandibular condyle articulating with the glenoid fossa with the articular eminence anterior & external auditory canal posterior to the TMJ.* **(Bottom)** *Coronal noncontrast PD MR of the TMJ in the closed-mouth position demonstrates mediolaterally bipolar mandibular condyle articulating with the glenoid fossa. Hypointense concavoconvex articular disc is seen in the joint space, which is an important structure of the TMJ, providing cushion & absorbing stress in the joint. (Courtesy D. Singhal, MD.)*

SAGITTAL T1 MR: CLOSED-MOUTH POSITION

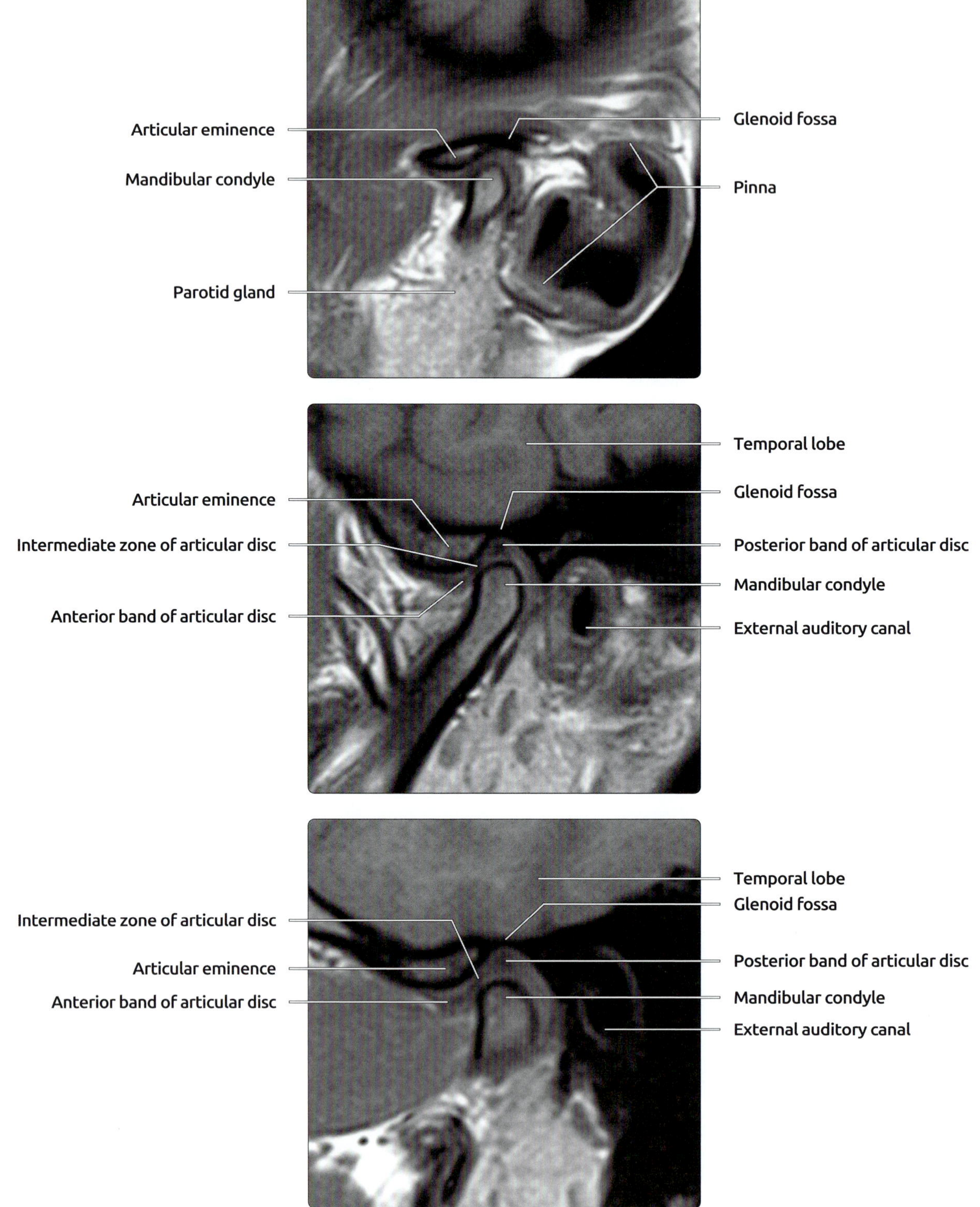

(Top) *First in a series of 3 noncontrast sagittal T1 MR images of the left TMJ from lateral to medial in the closed-mouth position demonstrates condylar head seated in the glenoid fossa.* **(Middle)** *The low- to intermediate-signal articular disc has a sigmoid shape & is seen in the anterior 1/2 of the joint space.* **(Bottom)** *The junction between the low-signal posterior band of the disc & the intermediate-signal bilaminar zone is normally found at the 12-o'clock position relative to the condylar head in the closed-mouth position. (Courtesy K. Sargar, MD.)*

SAGITTAL T1 MR: OPEN-MOUTH POSITION

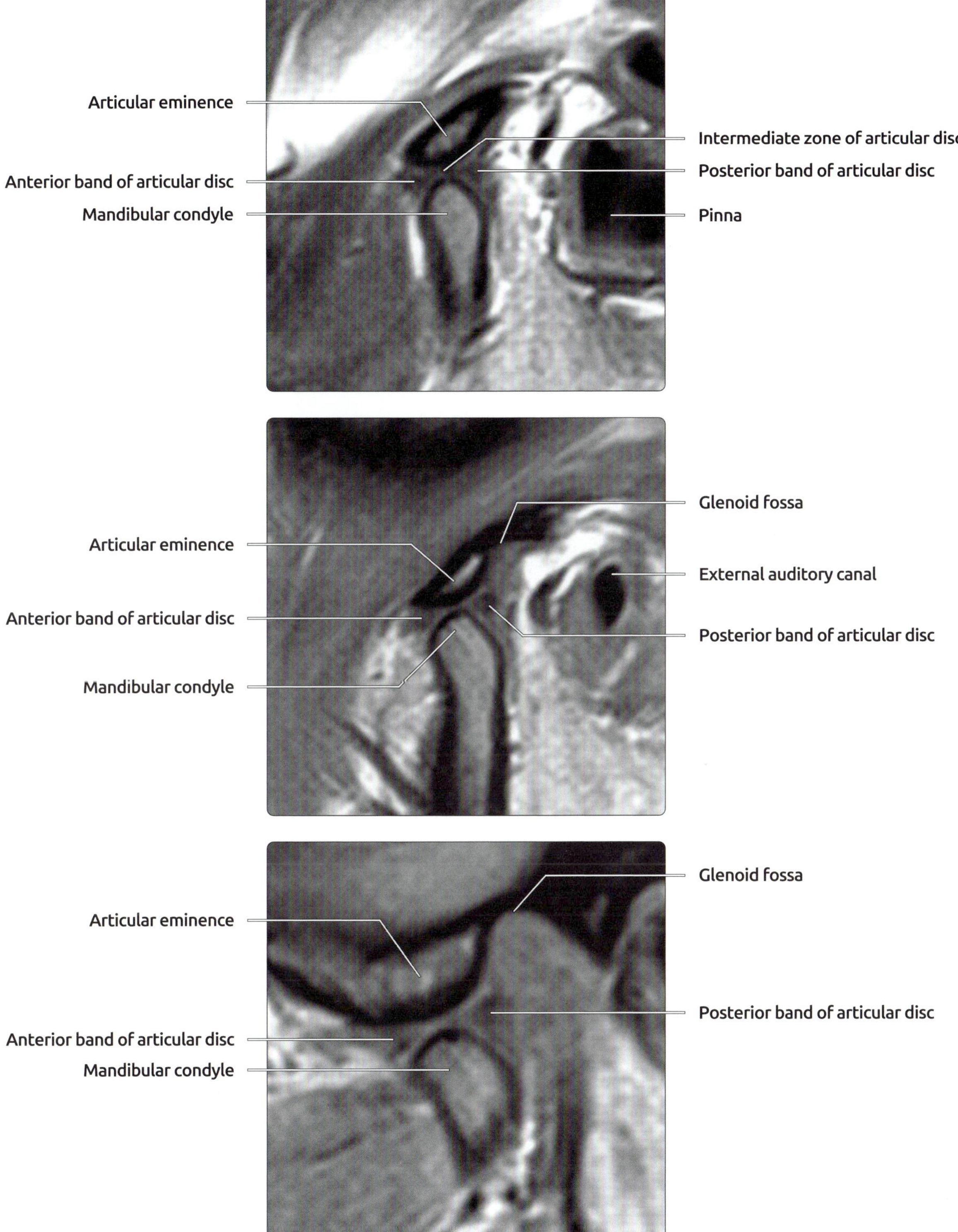

(Top) *First in a series of 3 noncontrast sagittal T1 MR images of the left TMJ from lateral to medial in the open-mouth position demonstrates that the condylar head has translated anteroinferiorly onto the articular eminence.* **(Middle)** *The articular disc has moved to a position between the articular eminence & mandibular condyle, taking on a bow tie appearance.* **(Bottom)** *Both disc & mandibular condyle must complete this anterior movement for the TMJ to function normally. When the disc fails to complete this movement, internal derangement of the TMJ results. (Courtesy K. Sargar, MD.)*

SAGITTAL T2 MR: CLOSED-MOUTH POSITION

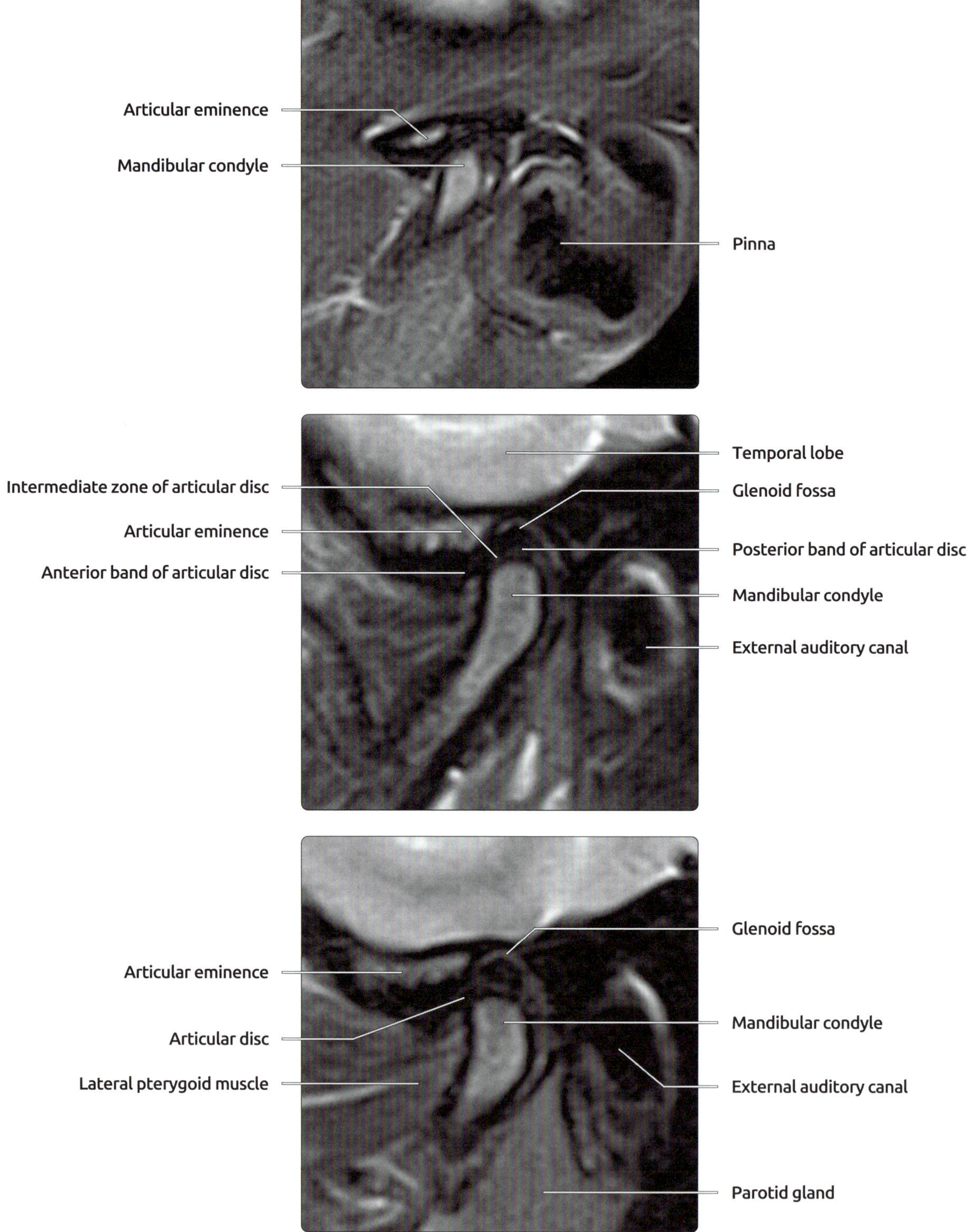

(Top) *First in a series of 3 noncontrast sagittal T2 fat-suppressed MR images of the left TMJ from lateral to medial in the closed-mouth position demonstrates condylar head seated in the glenoid fossa.* **(Middle)** *The low-signal articular disc has a sigmoid shape & is seen in the anterior 1/2 of the joint space. Fat-suppressed T2 images are useful in assessing signal abnormality in articular disc, bone marrow edema, & joint effusion.* **(Bottom)** *The posterior band of the disc & bilaminar zone junction is normally found at 12 o'clock relative to the condylar head in the closed-mouth position. (Courtesy K. Sargar, MD.)*

SAGITTAL T2 MR: OPEN-MOUTH POSITION

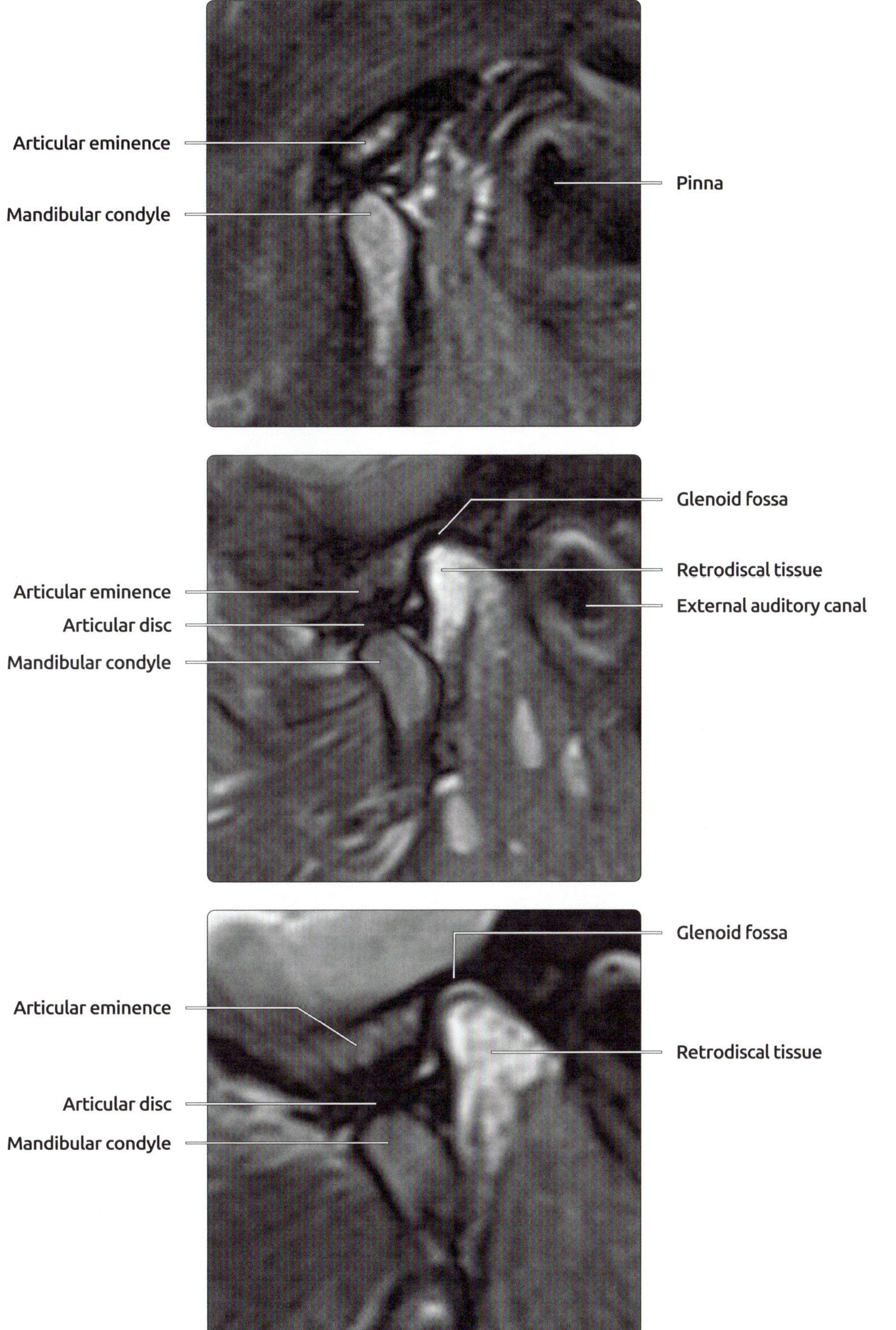

(Top) *First in a series of 3 noncontrast sagittal T2 fat-suppressed MR images of the left TMJ from lateral to medial in the open-mouth position demonstrates that the condylar head has translated anteroinferiorly onto the articular eminence.* **(Middle)** *The articular disc has moved to a position between the articular eminence & mandibular condyle, taking on a bow tie appearance. Hyperintense retrodiscal tissue can be seen in the glenoid fossa posterior to the mandibular condyle.* **(Bottom)** *Both disc & mandibular condyle must complete this anterior movement for the TMJ to function normally. If the posterior band is anterior to the 12-o'clock position of the condyle, consider anterior displacement. Disc T2 signal should be assessed, especially at the posterior attachment in patients with TMJ pain. (Courtesy K. Sargar, MD.)*

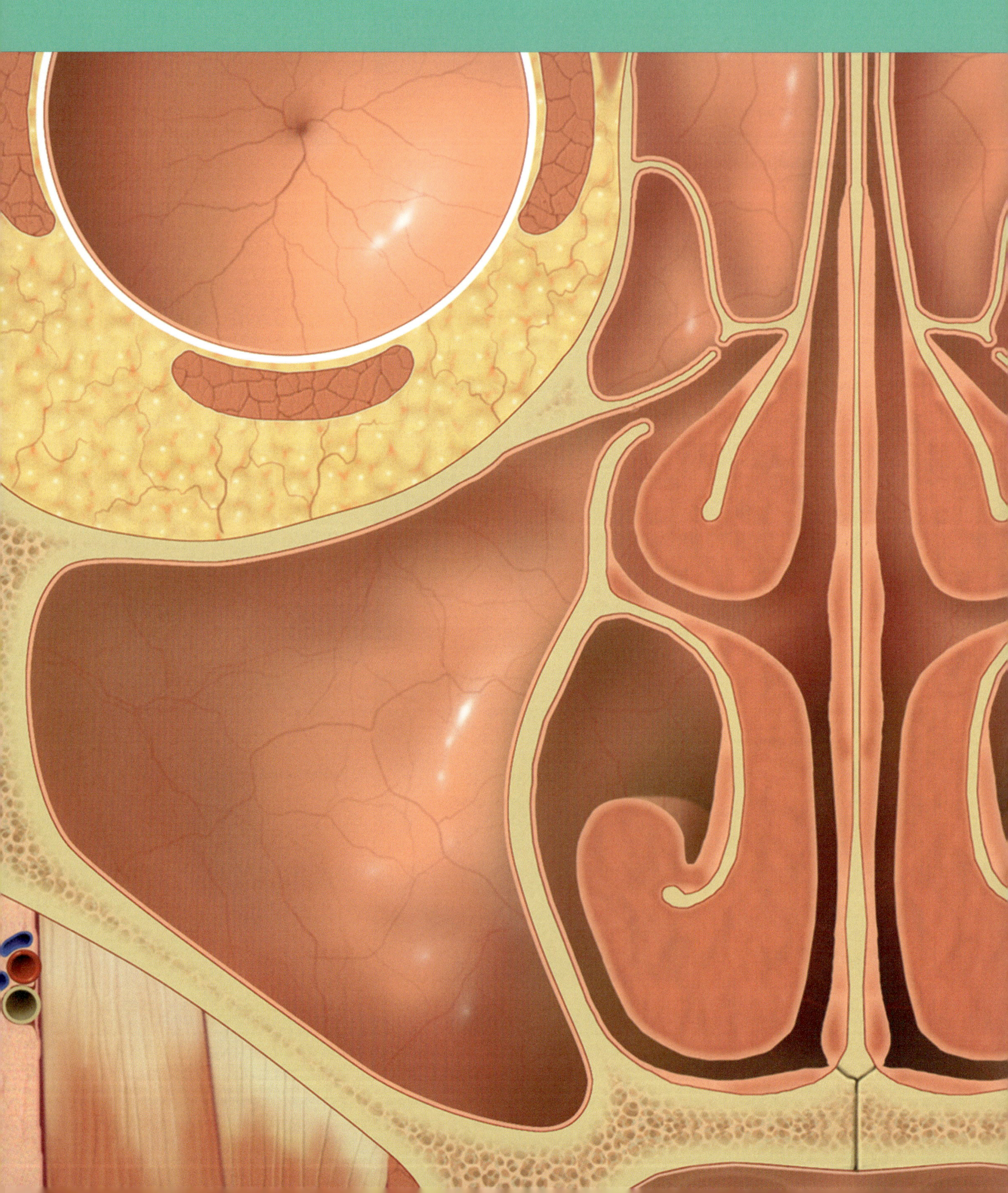

SECTION 2

Nose and Sinuses

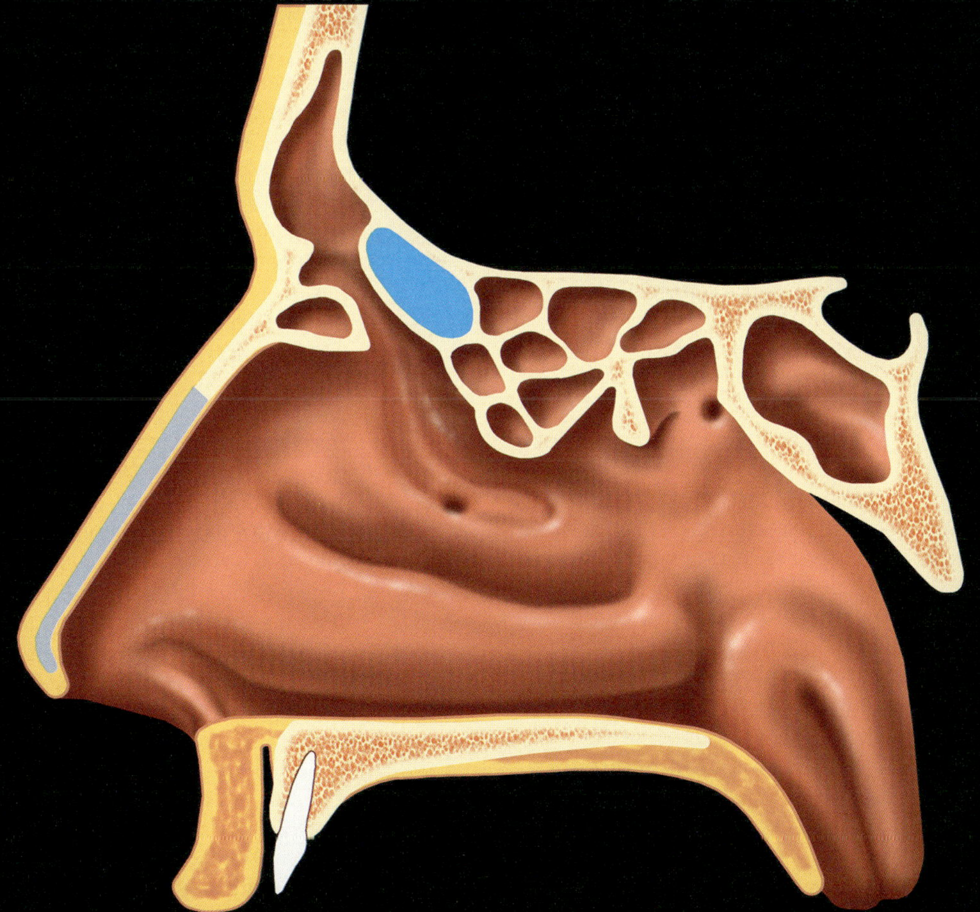

TERMINOLOGY

Abbreviations

- Frontal process of maxilla (FPM)
- Anterior lacrimal crest (ALC)
- Posterior lacrimal crest (PLC)
- Internal nasal valve (INV)
- Nasal vestibular body (NVB)
- External nasal valve (ENV)

Definitions

- **Glabella**: Smooth area between eyebrows, above nose
- **Nasion**: Most anterior aspect of frontonasal suture, situated just below glabella
    - Midpoint of frontonasal suture intersection with upper end of median internasal suture (joining nasal bones)
- **Sellion**: Soft tissue equivalent of nasion
    - Deepest point of nasofrontal angle at intersection of forehead slope & upper aspect of bridge of nose
- **Radix (root of nose)**: Origin of nose from glabella, extends equal distance superiorly & inferiorly centered at nasion
    - Extends inferiorly from nasion to level of horizontal line drawn through lateral canthi
    - Height of radix at nasion ideally between 9-14 mm as measured from anterior corneal plane
- **Rhinion**: Point at lower end of median internasal suture where nasal bones join with nasal septal cartilage

IMAGING ANATOMY

Overview

- **Dorsum of nose (nasal ridge)**: Outer surface between root & tip of nose
- **Ala (wing) of nose**: Lower lateral surface of external nose, kept in shape by alar cartilage & dense connective tissue; flare out around nostril
- **Nasal cavity**: Divided into 2 cavities by nasal septum, opens outside through external **nostril**
- **Nasal vestibule**: Most anterior aspect of nasal cavity lined with skin, hair follicles, & sebaceous glands, & surrounded by cartilages
    - **Limen nasi (mucocutaneous junction)**: Mucous ridge separating skin-lined vestibule from respiratory epithelium-lined larger nasal cavity proper; contains dense microvasculature
- **Pyriform aperture of nose**: Pear-shaped anterior aperture at limen nasi level; anterior bony margin of nasal skeleton
    - Superior margin: Nasal bone lower margin
    - Inferolateral margin: Maxillary bone thin, sharp margins separating anterior from nasal surfaces of maxilla
        - Curve medially joining premaxilla to form **anterior nasal spine of maxilla**
- **INV**: Narrowest portion of nasal cavity located ~ 1.3 cm from nares
    - Area bordered inferiorly by head of inferior turbinate, medially by dorsal nasal septum, & laterally by caudal portion of upper lateral cartilage
    - Static INV obstruction: Structural, lesion-like, enlarged turbinate or high nasal septal deviation
    - Dynamic INV obstruction: Collapse of upper lateral cartilage/lateral nasal wall on inspiration due to weakness in their integrity
- **NVB**: Small mound of dynamic soft tissue in lateral aspect of INV, situated anteroinferior to head of inferior turbinate
    - May contribute to nasal obstruction in some patients
- **ENV**: Area in nasal vestibule bordered by alar rim & columella, including medial crus, nasal spine, & soft tissues covering nostril sill
    - Static ENV obstruction: Vestibular stenosis
    - Dynamic ENV obstruction: Collapse of floppy, weak alar rim on inspiration

Internal Contents

- **Nasal cartilages**: Septal, lateral, major (greater) alar, minor (lesser) alar, & vomeronasal
    - **Septal** cartilage: In midline, from nasal bones anteroinferior meeting point (rhinion) anteriorly to bony nasal septum posteriorly; pass along nasal cavity floor
        - Attached by loose ligaments laterally to bony margin of nasal pyriform aperture
    - **Lateral** cartilage: Anterior margin thicker, attaches with & continues laterally from septal cartilage
        - a.k.a. **upper lateral** cartilage
        - Superior margin attaches to nasal bone & FPM; inferior margin to greater alar cartilage by fibrous tissue
    - **Major (greater) alar** cartilage: Thin, U-shaped cartilage plate attached to lateral cartilage superiorly & also anteroinferior aspect of septal cartilage
        - a.k.a. **lower lateral** cartilage
        - Bends along walls of vestibule: Medial & lateral crura
        - Bilateral medial crura attaches to septal cartilage: Forms fleshy medial crural footpads in front of nostrils
        - Medial crura meet in midline below end of septum to form columella & lobule
            - **Columella**: Bridge of tissue at undersurface of nasal septum separating nostrils
            - **Lobule**: **Tip of nose** & **nostrils** at its base
            - **Alar domes**: Tip-defining points of nose at peaks of medial crural folds separated by notch
            - Tip rhinoplasty or tip plasty: Shaping tip of nose by mainly reshaping greater alar cartilage
        - Cartilage bends superolaterally around nostrils, forming lateral crura
        - **Nasal scroll**: Formed by lateral & major cartilage edge interlocking by one scrolling upward & other inward
            - Prevents internal nasal lumen collapse from airflow pressure during breathing
    - **Minor (lesser or accessory) alar** cartilage: 3 or 4 cartilages within connective tissue membrane attaching lateral & major (greater) alar cartilages to FPM
    - **Vomeronasal** (Jacobson) cartilage: Narrow cartilage strip in inferior nasal septum between septal cartilage & vomer of bony septum
        - Lies below rudimentary vomeronasal (Jacobson) organ (VNO), which is accessory olfactory organ with blind sac & duct opening anteriorly
        - VNO contains esthesiocytes (specialized olfactory sensory cells)
        - VNO esthesiocytes may have role in afferent neurons of pheromone reception & in sexual gonadotropin-releasing hormone production
        - VNO may be ectopic esthesioneuroblastoma origin site (usually originate in upper nasal cavity)

- **Areas with no cartilage support**: Small areas around septum, lateral cartilage, top of nostril, & in nasal ala
- Irregular notches on lower ends of nasal bones on either side of rhinion due to developmental variations at osteocartilaginous junction may mimic fractures

- **Bones: Nasal bone**, **FPM, lacrimal bone, & nasal septum**
  - Common mistake: Misnaming FPM as nasal bone
- **Nasal septum**: Anterior septal cartilage & posterior bone
  - Bony septum: **Perpendicular plate of ethmoid** posterosuperiorly, **vomer** posteroinferiorly, & **maxillary crest** at undersurface
  - Maxillary crest: Narrow bone strip projecting superiorly from maxilla anteriorly & palatine bone posteriorly along anteroposterior length of septum
    - Articulates above with septal cartilage anteriorly & vomer posteriorly
  - Columella: Forms external undersurface of nasal septum, composed of cartilage & soft tissue
  - **Philtrum**: Vertical groove in midline of upper lip, just below columella
  - Nasal septum divides triangular nasal cavity in 2
- **Sutures**
  - **Internasal** suture: Between nasal bones of both sides
    - Top point meets nasion & bottom point forms rhinion
  - **Nasomaxillary** suture: Between nasal bone & FPM
  - **Frontonasal** suture: Between nasal bones of both sides & frontal bone superiorly
    - Nasion forms its most anterior aspect where it meets internasal suture
  - **Frontomaxillary** suture: Between FPM & nasal process of frontal bone superiorly
    - Continuous medially with frontonasal suture
- **Lacrimal fossa**: Formed by thick **ALC** of FPM & thin **PLC** of lacrimal bone
- **Lacrimal sac**: Lies within lacrimal fossa, invested by superficial & deep parts of orbicularis oculi muscle
  - Lacrimal sac below **medial canthal tendon (MCT)** not covered by muscle, potential site of weakness for intraorbital spread of infection
- **Medial orbital septum** & check ligament of medial rectus muscle attach just posterior to PLC of lacrimal bone
  - Therefore, **lacrimal fossa & lacrimal sac** considered **preseptal** structures
    - Preseptal location important in treatment plan of lacrimal sac infection, mainly antibiotics
  - Orbital septum attaches to orbital margin at "arcus marginale," thickening where periorbita joins periosteum
- **MCT injury &** status of central fragment of fractured bone extremely important in **nasoorbitoethmoid (NOE) fracture** management
- MCT injury can lead to medial telecanthal deformities, such as shortened palpebra, obtuse angled medial canthi with infraplacement, increased intercanthal distance, & absent nasoorbital valley
- MCT: 3 limbs attached to bones (fractures of these bones important to assess in every trauma CT scan)
  - Anterior (strongest limb) attaches to ALC of FPM & continues into periosteum of nasal bone
  - Posterior limb attaches to PLC of lacrimal bone (difficult to fix injury as PLC & lacrimal bone are delicate)
  - Superior limb attaches to medial orbital rim few mm above anterior limb

Muscles Inserting at Nose

- Nasal **elevators**: Anomalous nasi & 2 extrinsic muscles, namely, procerus (inserting at orbit) & levator labii superioris alaeque nasi (LLSAN), (inserting at upper lip with medial slip inserting into greater alar cartilage)
- Nasal **depressors**: Alar nasalis & depressor septi nasi
- Nasal **compressors**: Transverse nasalis & compressor narium minor
- Nasal **dilators**: Dilator naris anterior (DNA), dilator naris vestibularis (DNV), & contribution from alar nasalis & LLSAN
- **Procerus**: Origin on lower end of nasal bone & upper part of lateral nasal cartilage
  - Inserts on forehead skin medial to eye & interdigitates with frontalis muscle
  - Displace medial angle of eyebrow down & elevates nose
- **LLSAN**: Origin on FPM & inserts in 2 places: One at greater alar cartilage & skin of nose, other at muscles of upper lip
  - Elevates nose & dilates nares, displaces upper lip superomedially
- **Anomalous nasi**: Origin on FPM & inserts into nasal bone, lateral nasal cartilage, & procerus & transverse nasalis; is nasal elevator
- **Transverse nasalis**: Nasalis muscle has 2 parts, namely, transverse nasalis & alar nasalis
  - Origin of transverse nasalis on canine eminence of maxilla superolateral to incisive fossa
  - Inserts, expanding into thin aponeurosis continuous on bridge of nose with that of opposite side transverse nasalis & with aponeurosis of procerus
  - Main nasal compressor; hyperactivity can cause radial lines along dorsum of nose as far down to lower border of greater alar cartilage, called "bunny lines"
- **Alar nasalis**: Origin on maxilla just medial to transverse nasalis above lateral incisor tooth, located anterior to transverse nasalis
  - Ascends anterolaterally to insert on alar-facial crease & adjacent deep surface of external skin of alar lobule
  - Is nasal depressor & also helps to dilate nares (hence, sometimes called dilator naris posterior)
- **Depressor septi nasi**: Origin in incisive fossa of maxilla located further medial to origin of alar nasalis
  - Inserts on base & lateral surface of medial crus of greater alar cartilage; is nasal depressor
  - Medially, attaches to dermocartilagenous ligament, which is sandwiched by medial crus of greater alar cartilage
- **DNA**: Origin on frontal surface of lateral 1/2 of lateral crus of greater alar cartilage & adjacent lesser alar cartilage
  - Inserts on skin of nose superior to alar groove (supraalar crease); is nasal dilator
- **DNV**: Origin on external skin of alar lobule, radiates along dome of nasal vestibule
  - Inserts on vestibular skin of alar lobule; is dilator of nasal vestibule
- **Compressor narium minor**: Origin on anterior part of greater alar cartilage
  - Inserts into skin near margin of nostril; is nasal compressor

3D RECONSTRUCTIONS OF EXTERNAL NOSE

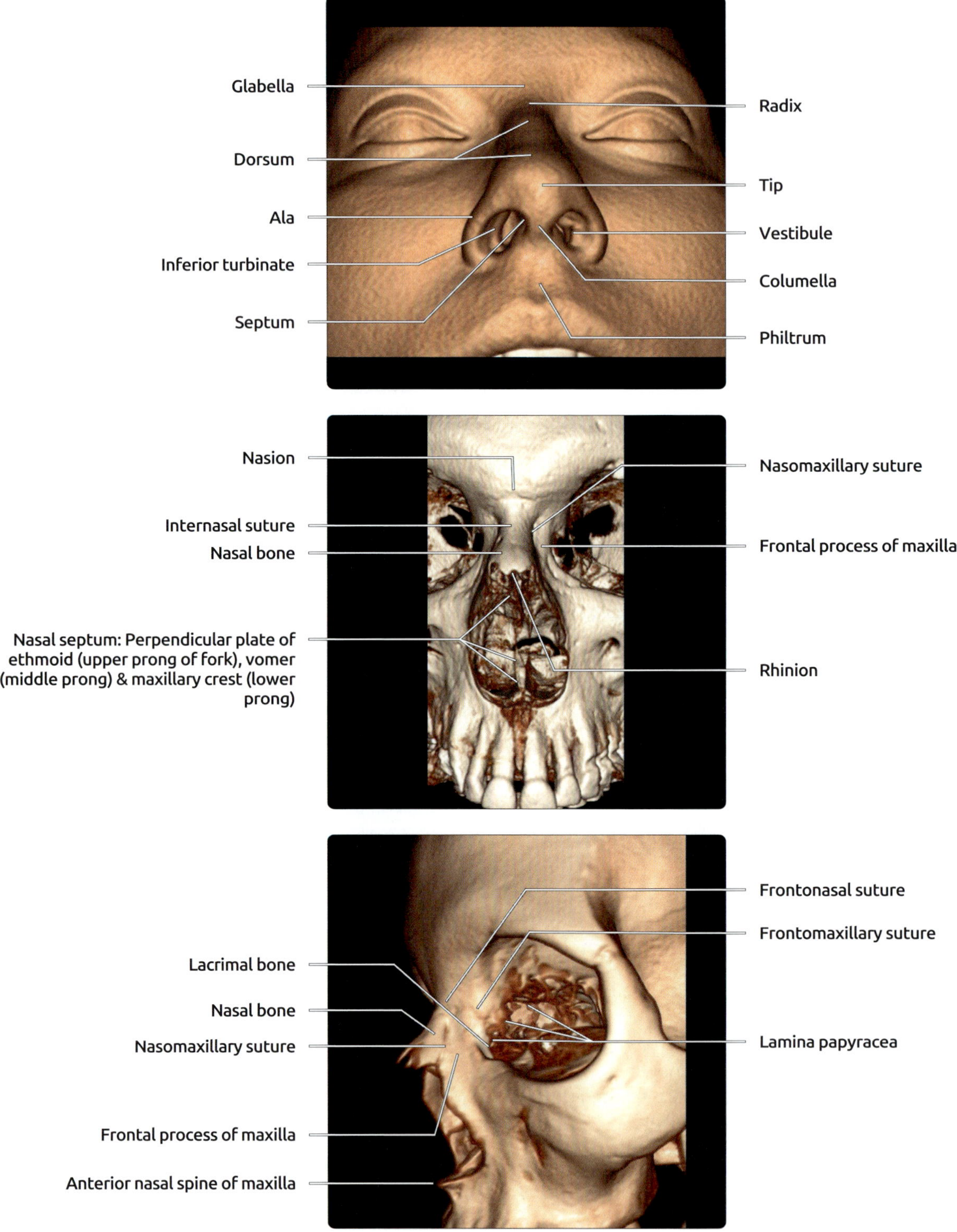

(Top) *3D soft tissue CT shows the important surface markings of the external nose.* **(Middle)** *Anterior 3D bone CT of external nose skeleton shows the paired nasal bones with an internasal suture between them, & the frontal process of maxilla (FPM) lateral to it separated by a nasomaxillary suture. The nasion is the most anterior aspect of frontonasal suture, & the rhinion is the point at the lower end of the median internasal suture where nasal bones join with nasal septal cartilage. Bony nasal septum consists of the perpendicular plate of ethmoid posterosuperiorly, vomer posteroinferiorly, & narrow bony strip, known as maxillary crest, at its undersurface.* **(Bottom)** *Anterior oblique 3D bone CT of external nose skeleton shows the nasal bone & FPM of the left side separated by a nasomaxillary suture. The more posteriorly situated lacrimal bone, which forms posterior lacrimal crest (PLC) of lacrimal fossa in the medial orbit, is also shown. Note anterior nasal spine of maxilla situated inferiorly. Lamina papyracea forms medial wall of orbit/lateral wall of ethmoid air cells & is seen posterior to lacrimal bone. Frontonasal suture is continuous laterally with frontomaxillary suture.*

AXIAL CT SCAN OF BONES OF EXTERNAL NOSE

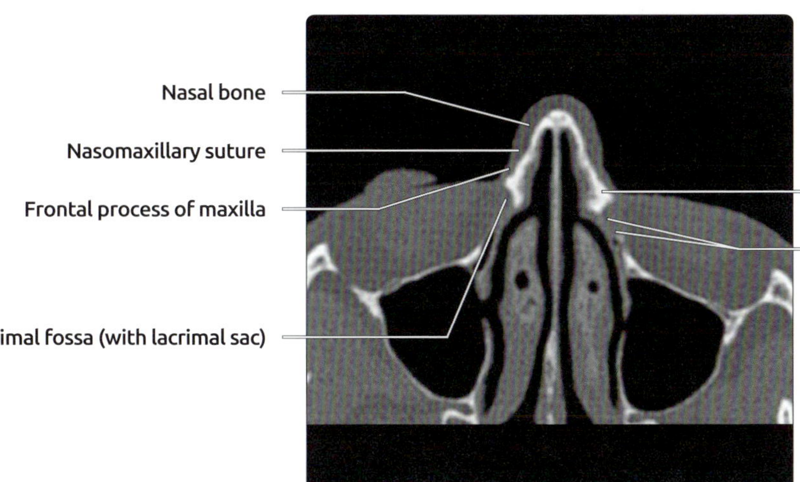

Anterior lacrimal crest (from frontal process of maxilla)

Posterior lacrimal crest (from lacrimal bone)

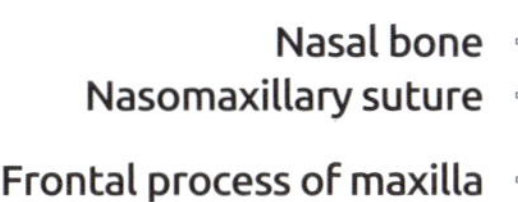

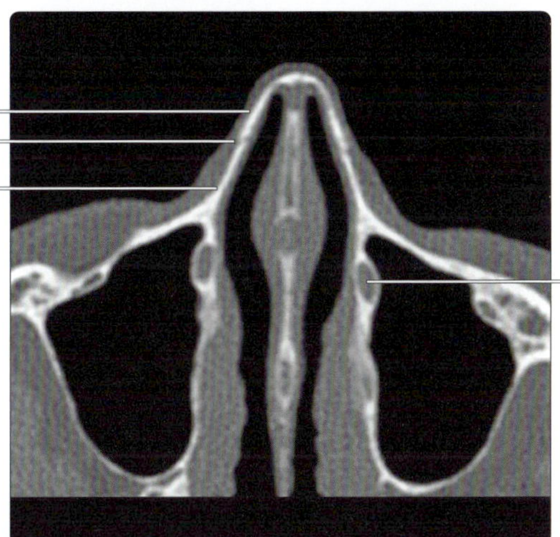

Nasolacrimal duct

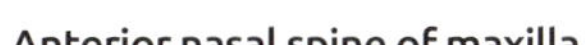

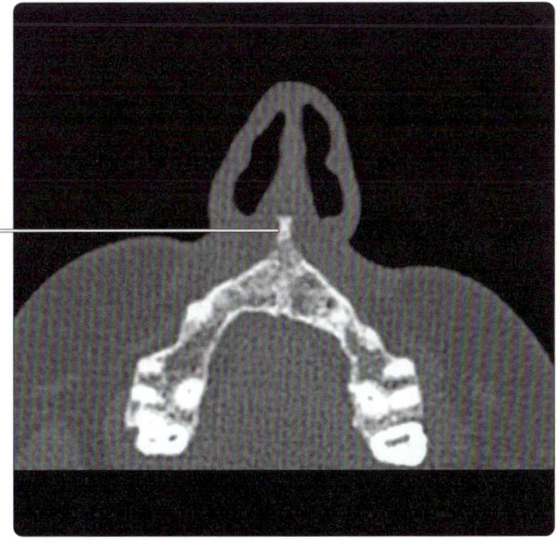

(Top) *Axial bone CT of the external nose at the orbital level shows the 3 bones forming its skeleton, namely, the nasal bone, FPM, & lacrimal bone. It is a common mistake in radiology reports to call an FPM fracture a nasal bone fracture. The lacrimal fossa is formed by the thick anterior lacrimal crest of the FPM & thin PLC of the lacrimal bone. The lacrimal sac lies within the lacrimal fossa & is invested by superficial & deep parts of the orbicularis oculi muscle. Lacrimal sac below the medial canthal tendon (MCT) is not covered by muscle & is a potential weakness site for intraorbital infection spread. Look for MCT/bony attachment injury in nasoorbitoethmoid fractures. Medial orbital septum & check ligament of medial rectus muscle attach just posterior to PLC of lacrimal bone, hence, the lacrimal fossa & lacrimal sac are preseptal structures.* **(Middle)** *Axial bone CT further inferiorly shows nasomaxillary suture separating the nasal bone from the FPM. Note the nasolacrimal duct, which continues inferiorly from the lacrimal sac, & opens in the inferior meatus of the nose (not shown).* **(Bottom)** *Axial bone CT through the lower aspect of the nose shows the anterior nasal spine of maxilla.*

CARTILAGES & BONES OF EXTERNAL NOSE

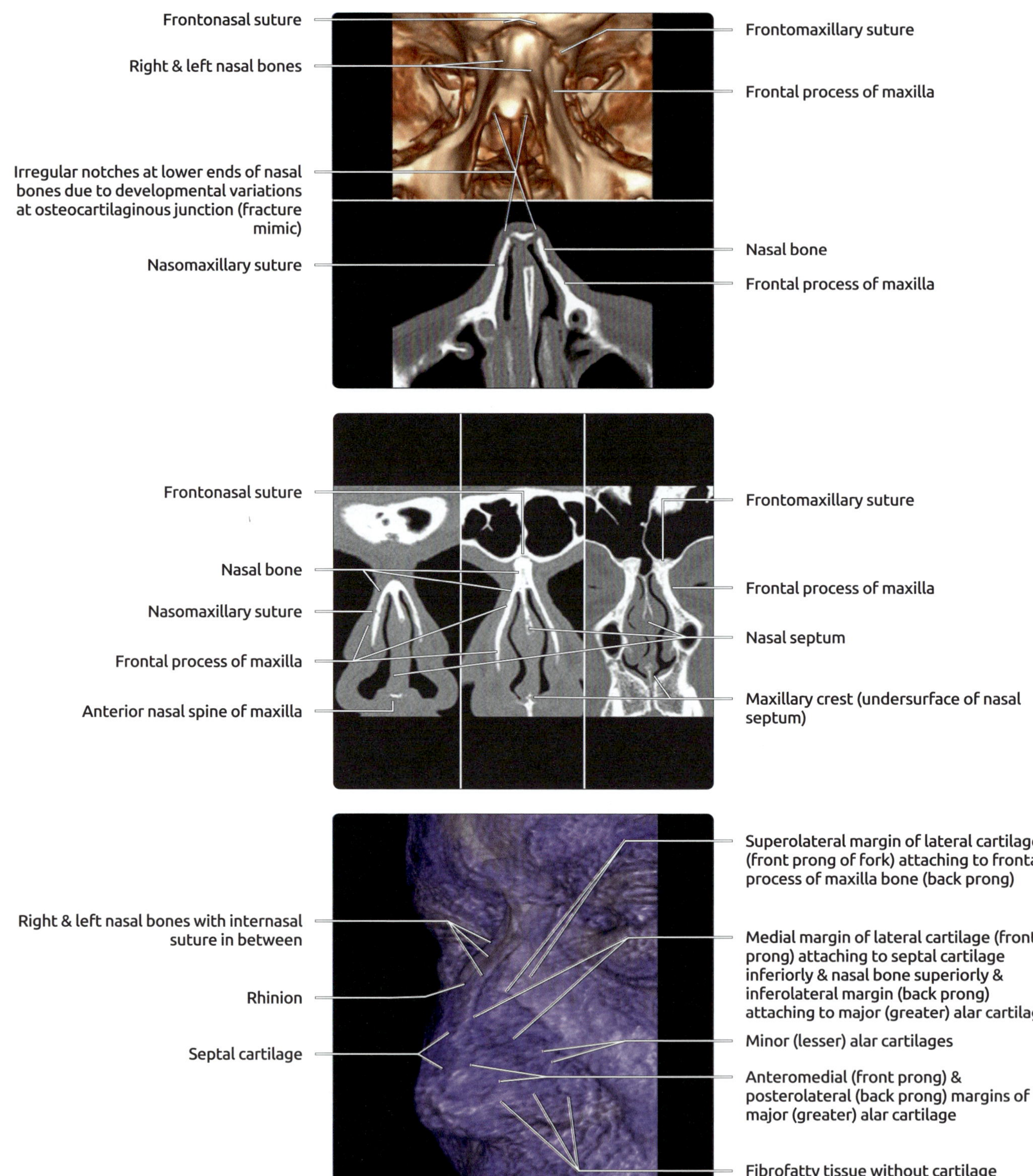

(Top) *Anterior 3D bone CT (above) and axial bone CT (below) show irregular notches at the lower ends of the nasal bones due to developmental variations at the osteocartilaginous junction, which should not be mistaken for fractures.* **(Middle)** *Coronal bone CT images from anterior to posterior show the anteriorly located nasal bone & anteroinferior aspect of the FPM separated by the nasomaxillary suture in the most anterior image. Also note the anterior nasal spine of the maxilla projecting anteriorly. The slightly posterior CT through the frontonasal suture level shows less portions of nasal bones & more of FPM. Further posterior CT behind the level of nasal bones shows the FPM & frontomaxillary suture. Note the nasal septum in midline in all the images, which is predominantly cartilaginous anteriorly & bony posteriorly.* **(Bottom)** *3D CT scan windowed to show cartilage and bone: Septal cartilage extends from rhinion (lower end of median internasal suture) anteriorly to bony nasal septum posteriorly. Three or 4 minor (lesser/accessory) alar cartilages lie within the connective tissue membrane attaching upper lateral and major/greater alar (lower lateral) cartilages to FPM.*

MUSCLES ATTACHING AROUND EXTERNAL NOSE

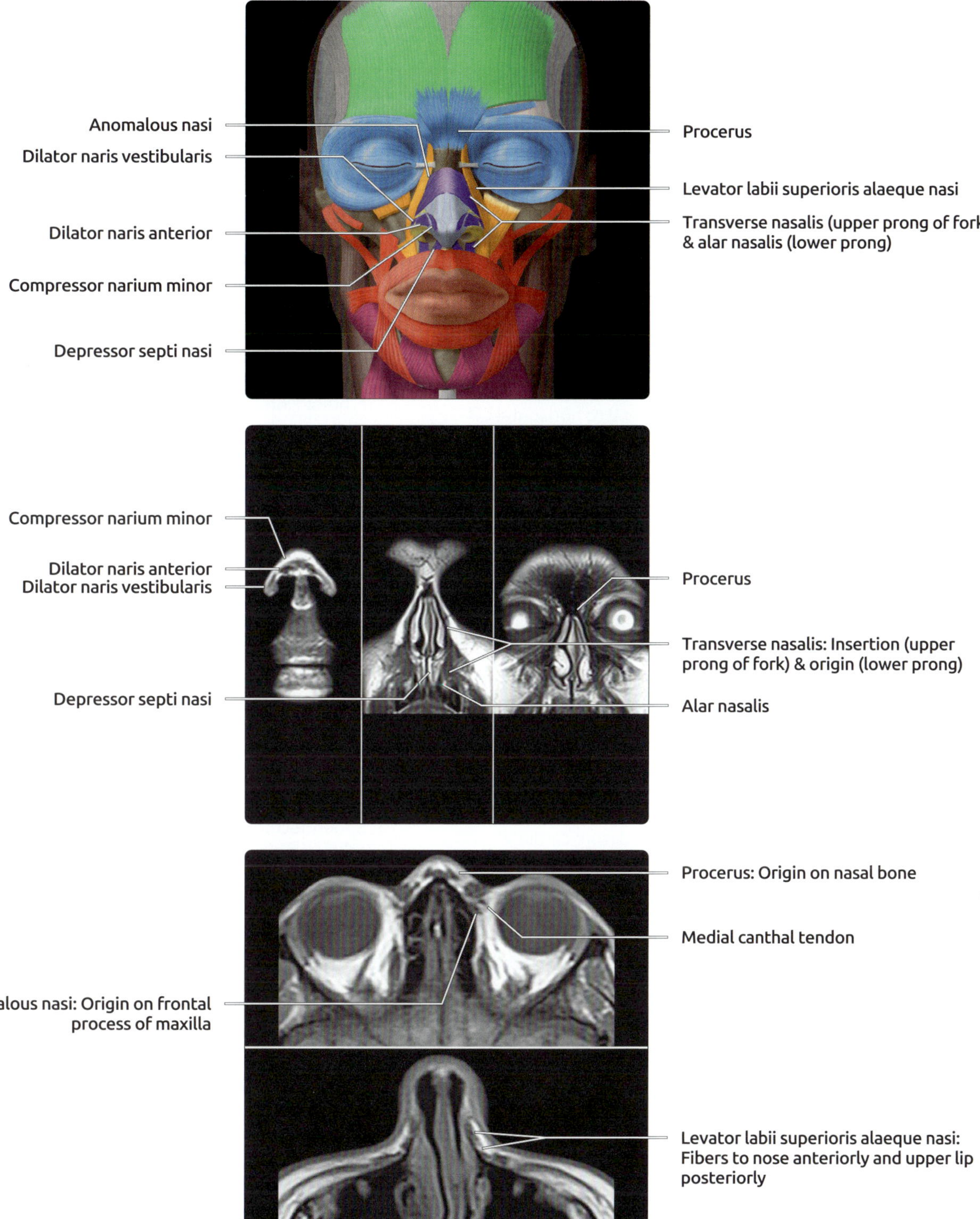

(Top) *Frontal graphic shows facial muscles attaching into external nose (purple). Note that 2 extrinsic muscles, namely, procerus (blue, attaching around eye) & levator labii superioris alaeque nasi [(LLSAN), yellow, attaching at upper lip] are also nasal elevators.* **(Middle)** *Coronal 3-mm T2 MRs from anterior to posterior are shown. First MR shows tiny nasal muscles, which do not have bony origins. Second MR shows depressor septi nasi originating in maxillary incisive fossa; just lateral to this lies alar nasalis originating above maxillary lateral incisor, & further laterally is transverse nasalis (TN) originating from maxillary canine eminence. As their name implies, depressor septi nasi inserts near nasal septum into medial crus of greater alar cartilage, alar nasalis lies anterior to TN & inserts into nasal alar lobule skin & alar-facial crease, & TN continues superiorly across bridge of nose. Third image shows procerus inserting around eye.* **(Bottom)** *Axial T1 MR at level of eye lens (top) shows origin of procerus muscle on the nasal bone & anomalous nasi on FPM. Axial T1 MR just below inferior orbital margin at upper maxillary sinus level (bottom) shows levator labii superioris alaeque nasi origin on FPM.*

IMAGING ANATOMY

Overview

- All paranasal sinuses lined by respiratory pseudostratified epithelium attached directly to bone (mucoperiosteum)
- **Nasal cavity**: Triangle divided in midline by septum
  - Roof formed by horizontal **cribriform plate (CP) of ethmoid**, floor by hard & soft palate, lateral aspect by lateral nasal wall with attached turbinates
  - Nasal mucosa & sensory nerves traverse CP into anterior cranial fossa & synapse intracranially with secondary neurons in olfactory bulb & tract
  - Anteriorly, **nasal pyriform aperture**; posteriorly, **posterior choana** connecting to nasopharynx
  - Polyps obstructing inferomedial nasal airway removed first at endoscopic surgery for good visualization of choana & blood drainage route into nasopharynx
- Ethmoid roof formed by horizontal **fovea ethmoidalis** of orbital plate of frontal bone superolaterally & vertical **lateral lamella** of CP medially (just lateral to horizontal CP of nasal roof)
  - Lateral lamella 10x thinner than fovea ethmoidalis
- **Keros classification** of ethmoid roof/olfactory fossa into 3 types according to increasing vertical height of lateral lamella & resultant depth of olfactory fossa
  - 1-3 mm type I, 4-7 mm type II, & 8-16 mm type III
  - Type III: Maximum risk of iatrogenic injury to lateral lamella & CSF leak at endoscopic surgery
- **Pyriform aperture** of nose: Pear-shaped anterior aperture at mucocutaneous junction (limen nasi) level; anterior bony margin of nose
  - Superior margin: Nasal bone lower margin
  - Inferolateral margin: Maxillary bone, thin sharp margins separating anterior from nasal surfaces of maxilla
    - Curve medially, joining premaxilla to form **anterior nasal spine of maxilla**
- **Nasal septum**: Anterior septum formed from cartilage
  - Bony septum: **Perpendicular plate of ethmoid** posterosuperiorly, **vomer** posteroinferiorly, & **maxillary crest** at undersurface
- **Nasal turbinates (conchae)**: Occasional supreme turbinate
  - Bony superior, middle (part of ethmoidal complex), & inferior (separate bone) turbinates
  - Project medially into nasal cavity; define region below & lateral as superior, middle, & inferior meati, respectively
  - Tail of superior turbinate points medially toward natural ostium of sphenoid sinus in sphenoethmoid recess; very important surgical landmark here
  - Vertical portion of basal lamella of middle turbinate attaches to CP (coronal CT), middle & posterior portions laterally to lamina papyracea (sagittal CT)
  - Concha bullosa: Pneumatized (usually middle) turbinate
- **Nasal meati**
  - **Superior meatus**: Receives drainage from posterior ethmoid & sphenoid sinus at sphenoethmoidal recess (known as posterior ostiomeatal complex)
    - Sphenopalatine foramen (site of origin of juvenile nasopharyngeal angiofibroma) connects superior meatus with pterygopalatine fossa lateral to it
  - **Middle meatus: Ethmoid bulla**: Large ethmoid air cell at superior aspect of ostiomeatal complex
    - **Hiatus semilunaris (HS)**: Semilunar region between uncinate process & ethmoid bulla, receives drainage from anterior ethmoid air cells & maxillary sinus via ethmoid (maxillary) infundibulum
  - **Inferior meatus**: Receives drainage from nasolacrimal duct anteriorly, covered by mucosal (Hasner) valve

Anatomy Relationships

- **Maxillary sinus**: Paired air cells within maxillary bone
  - Drain via **maxillary ostium** at its superomedial aspect, into **infundibulum**, then into **HS** at middle meatus
- **Ethmoid sinus**: Paired groups of 3-18 air cells within ethmoid labyrinths
  - **Anterior & posterior cells separated** by basal lamella of middle turbinate lateral attachment to lamina papyracea
  - Ethmoid bulla: Dominant anterior ethmoid air cell that protrudes inferomedially into infundibulum or HS
  - Anterior ethmoid air cells drainage: Anterior recess of HS & middle meatus around ethmoid bulla & some into ethmoid infundibulum
  - Posterior ethmoid air cells drainage: Superior meatus & sphenoethmoidal recess
- **Frontal sinus**: Paired air cells in frontal bone; drain along funnel-shaped frontal recess (FR) into middle meatus
- **Sphenoid sinus**: Paired air cells within sphenoid bone; drainage into sphenoethmoidal recess
- **Extramural paranasal air cells**
  - **Infraorbital ethmoid cells (Haller)**: Ethmoid cells that extend into inferomedial orbital floor
  - **Agger nasi cell**: Most anterior air cell that involves lacrimal bone or frontal process of maxilla
  - **FR Kuhn cells (4 types)**: FR bordered **anteriorly** by agger nasi inferiorly, & Kuhn cells superiorly
  - **Bulla ethmoidalis & frontal bullar, suprabullar (intramural), & supraorbital ethmoid (extramural) cells**: FR bordered **posteriorly** by these cells
  - **Sphenoethmoidal cells (Onodi)**: Posterior ethmoid air cells with prominent superolateral pneumatization
    - Close relationship to optic nerve
    - Look for horizontal septum in upper sphenoid sinus on coronal CT & trace its continuity with posterior ethmoid air cell in sagittal or axial images

ANATOMY IMAGING ISSUES

Imaging Recommendations

- CT scan ideally delayed in URIs & done after 4-6 weeks of starting sinusitis medications, as mucosal thickening can be nonspecific & changes due to simple sinusitis may be seen
- Unenhanced, thin 0.625-mm volumetric images with sagittal & coronal reconstructions at 1- to 2-mm intervals
- Both high-resolution bone & soft tissue algorithm reconstructions in all 3 planes
- No gantry tilt; include ears, maxilla, tip of nose, chin, & frontal sinuses to be compatible with functional endoscopic sinus surgery image navigation guidance systems
- Sinusitis complications can be imaged with CECT; CE MR better for adjacent orbits, dura, brain, & cavernous sinuses
- MR best to differentiate solid internal enhancement of tumor from peripheral mucosal enhancement of polyp, retention cyst, or retained secretions filling sinus
- Fat suppression on at least 1 postcontrast sequence

GRAPHICS

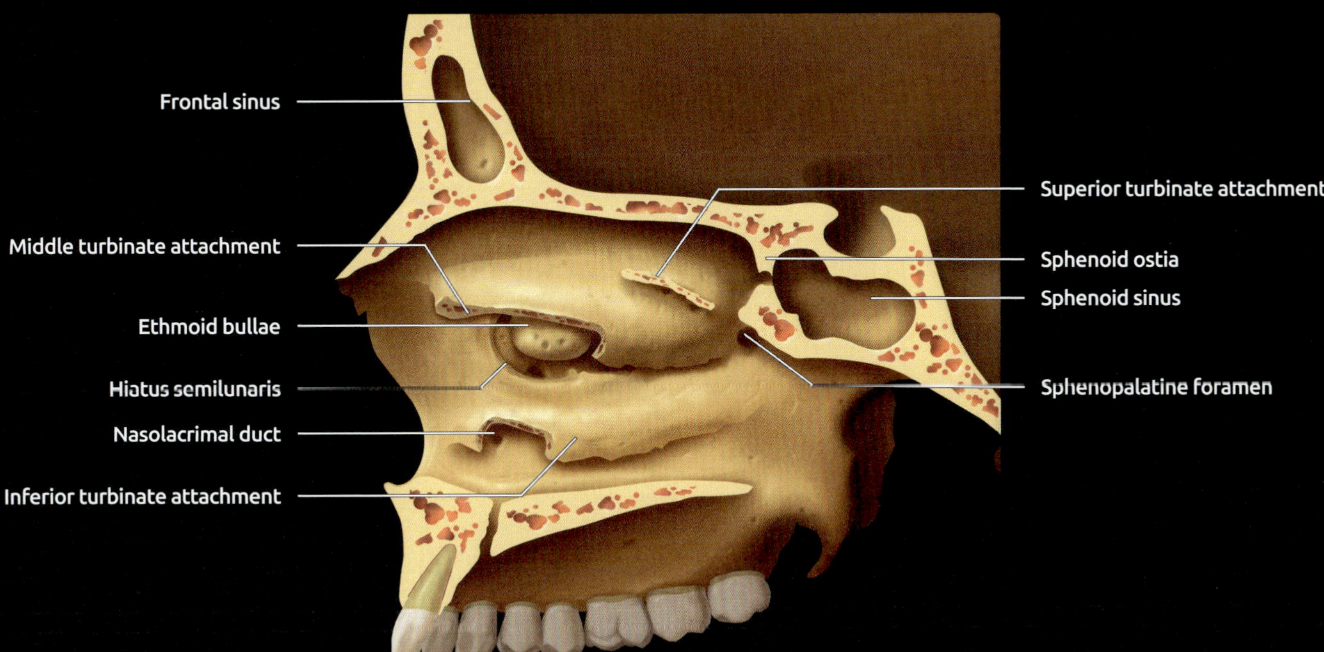

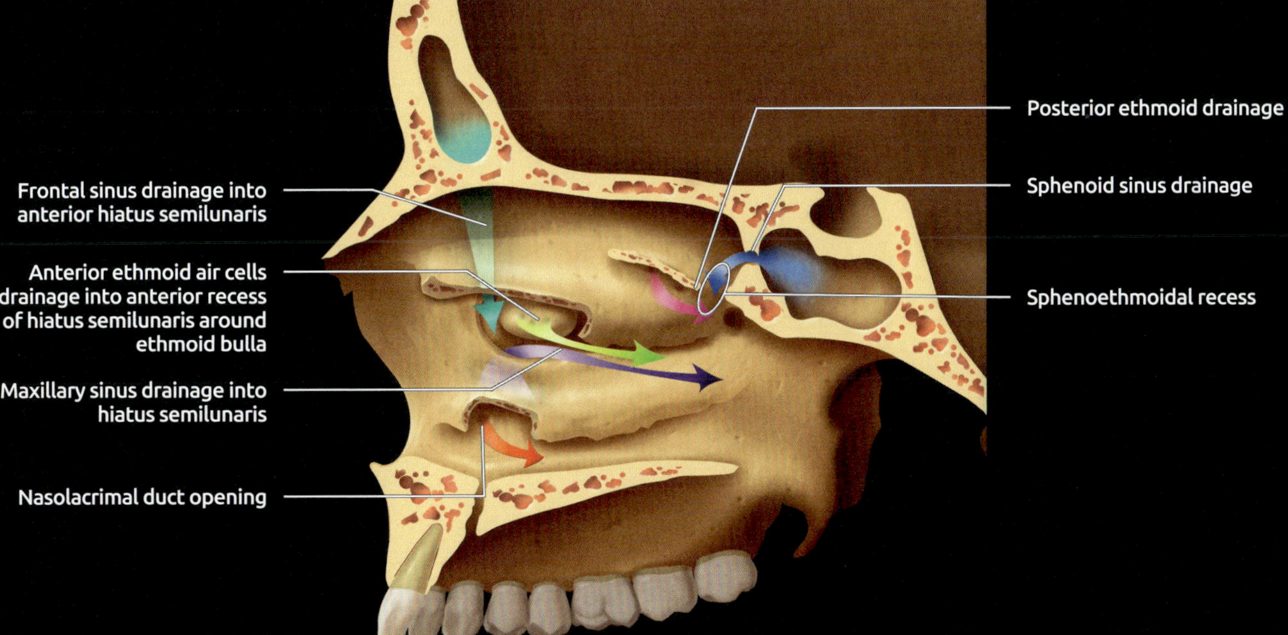

(Top) *Sagittal graphic shows osseous anatomy of the lateral wall of the nose. The superior & middle turbinates have been resected. The ethmoid bullae & hiatus semilunaris are below the middle turbinate attachment. The nasolacrimal duct empties into the anterior aspect of the inferior meatus.* **(Bottom)** *Sagittal graphic shows drainage pathways of the sinuses, ultimately directed towards nasopharynx. Sphenoid & posterior ethmoid sinuses drain into the sphenoethmoidal recess in the posterior nasal cavity; maxillary sinus drains via the ethmoid infundibulum, while the anterior ethmoids mostly drain into the anterior recess of hiatus semilunaris in middle meatus around ethmoid bulla (some into ethmoid infundibulum). Frontal sinus drains into the anterior middle meatus through the frontal recess. Well-pneumatized sphenoid sinus (sellar-type pneumatization) is seen. "Conchal" (rudimentary or absent sphenoid sinus where area below sella is a solid block of bone; extremely rare) & "presellar" (sphenoid pneumatized to level of anterior plane of sella & not beyond, where posterior sphenoid sinus wall is separated from sella by thick bone; seen in 1%) are other types of sphenoid sinus pneumatization.*

AXIAL BONE CT

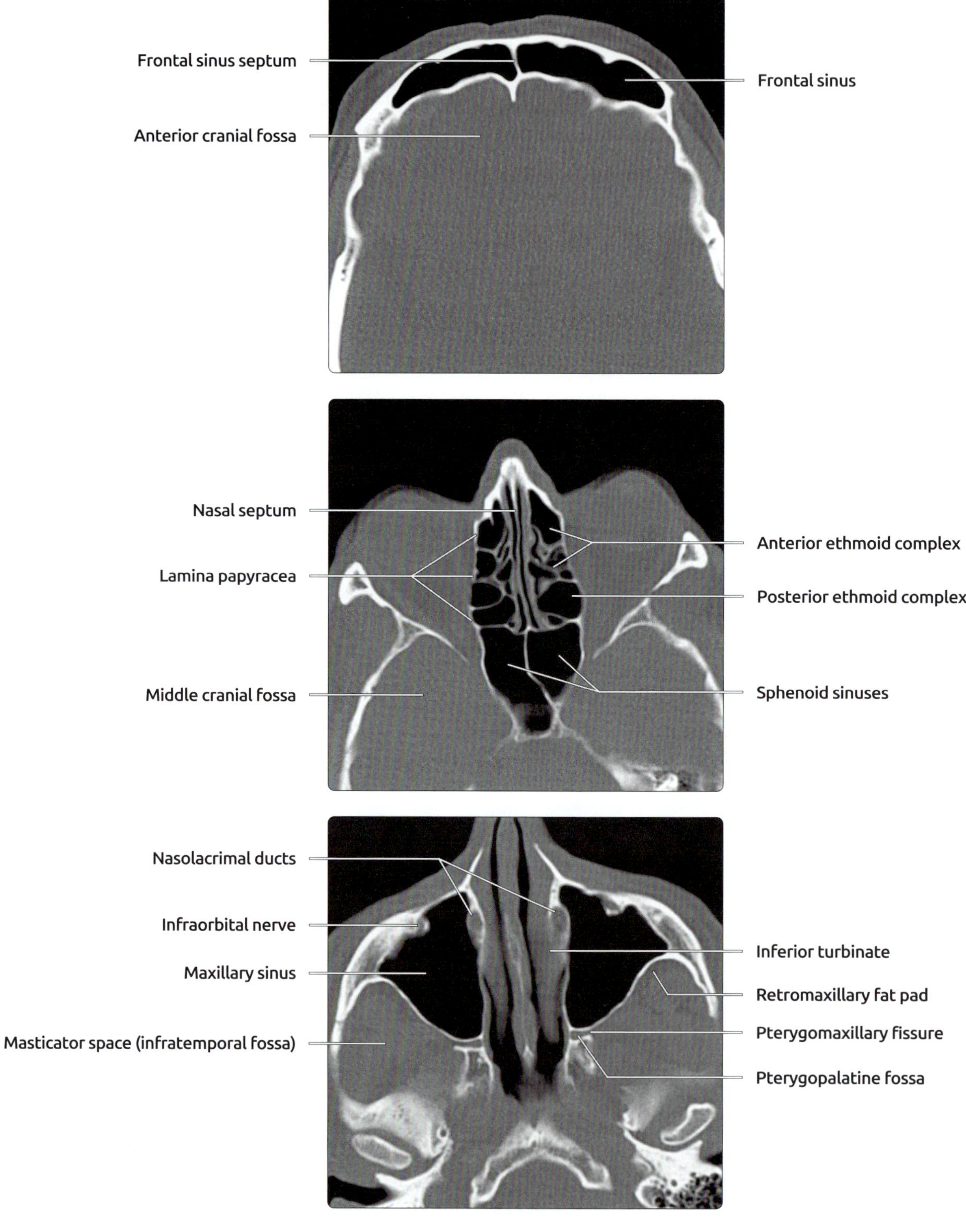

(Top) *First of 3 axial bone CT images of the sinuses presented from superior to inferior is shown. This image shows the frontal sinuses with their midline septum & thin posterior wall separating the sinuses from the anterior cranial fossa. Frontal sinus disease can extend posteriorly into the cranial vault.* **(Middle)** *This image shows the ethmoid air cells & sphenoid sinuses. The thin lamina papyracea is the lateral wall of the ethmoid sinuses. Ethmoid air cell disease can extend through the lamina papyracea to create a postseptal subperiosteal orbital abscess.* **(Bottom)** *This image through the maxillary sinuses shows their intimate relationship to the nasolacrimal ducts, pterygopalatine fossa (PPF), & retromaxillary fat pad. Notice the infraorbital nerve anteriorly just before it exits through the infraorbital foramen.*

CORONAL BONE CT

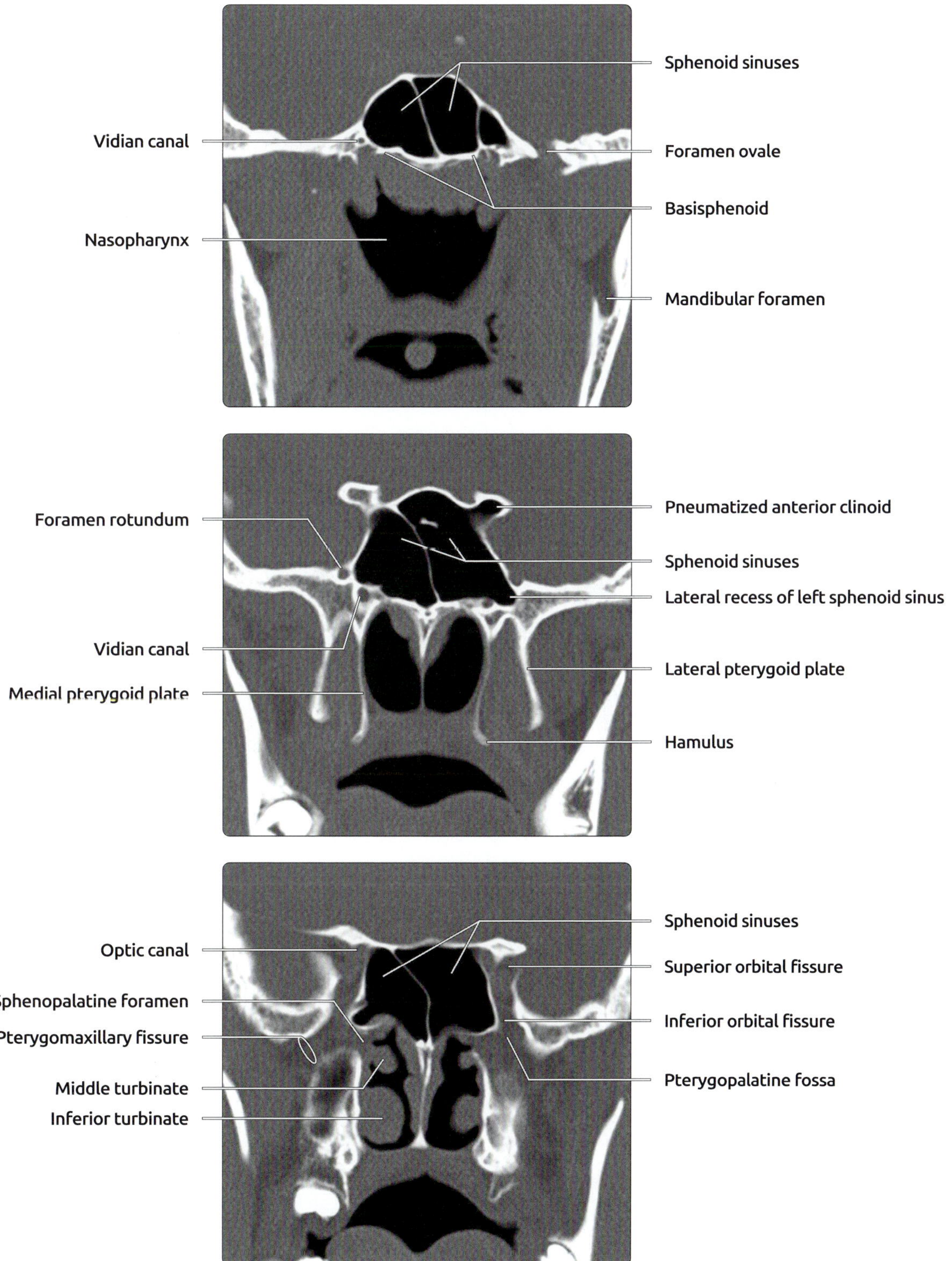

(Top) *First of 9 coronal bone NECTs through the paranasal sinuses presented from posterior to anterior shows sphenoid sinuses superior to the nasopharynx.* **(Middle)** *Image shows pterygoid plates posterior to maxillary sinuses. Inferolateral to the sphenoid sinus, note the foramen rotundum & vidian canal. Note lateral (pterygoid) recess of the sphenoid sinus on the left side separating vidian canal in the body of sphenoid bone inferomedially from foramen rotundum superolaterally. Best practical method to identify skull base foramina on coronal images is by identifying them in relation to lateral recess of sphenoid sinus. Lateral recess may hinder endoscopic repair of sphenoid sinus CSF leak, as pterygoid process acts like a pillar, blocking access to recess, & will need a transpterygoid approach with partial pterygoid process excision to facilitate sinus obliteration by complete removal of sinus mucosa.* **(Bottom)** *Image shows complex anatomic landscape surrounding PPF. Lateral exit of the PPF is pterygomaxillary fissure through which it exits into masticator space. Superiorly, PPF exits into inferior orbital fissure. Medial exit from PPF is through sphenopalatine foramen into posterolateral nose.*

CORONAL BONE CT

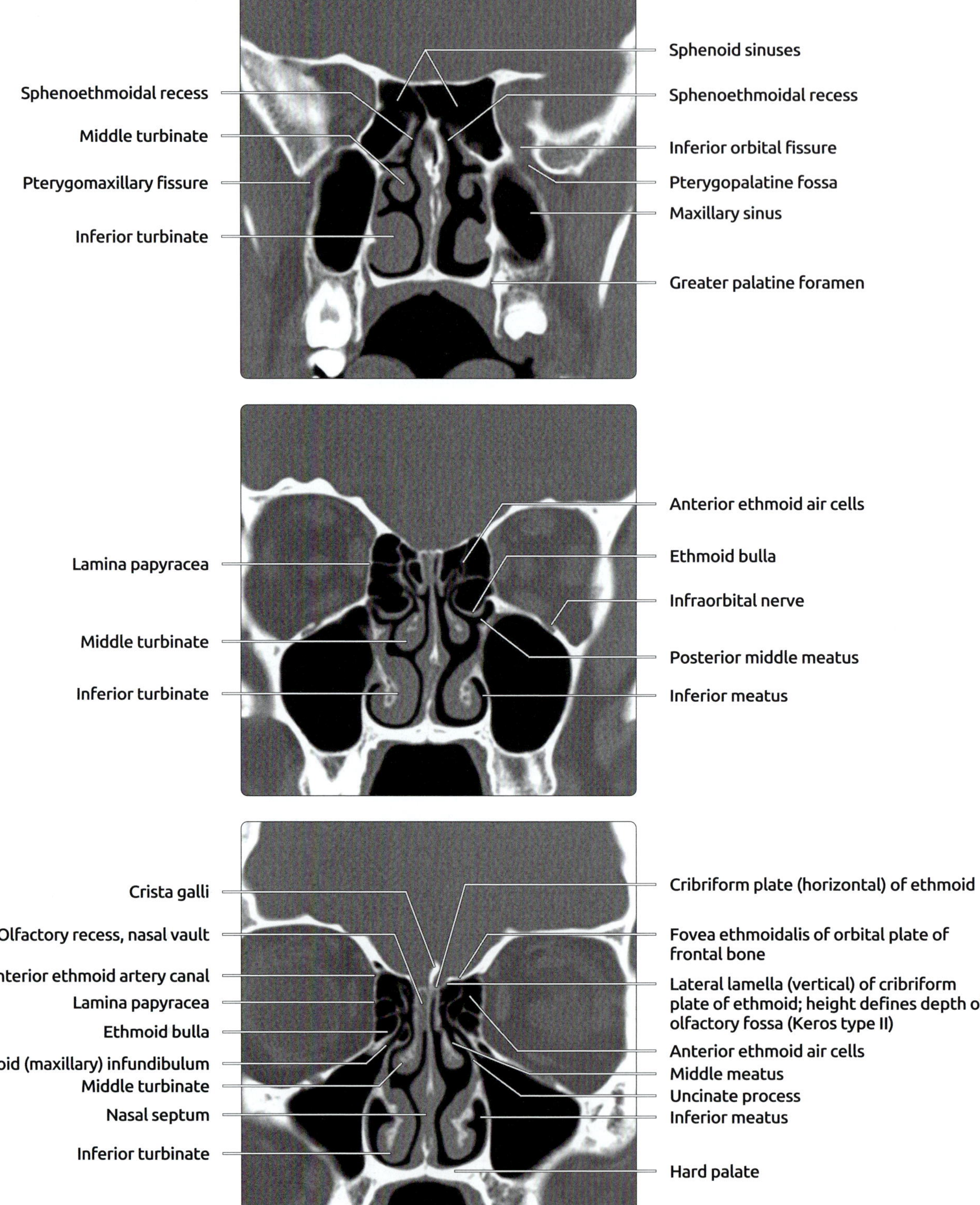

(Top) *In this image, sphenoethmoidal recess is seen as vertical air-filled slits in the posterosuperior nose into which both the posterior ethmoid & sphenoid sinuses empty. Note the greater palatine canal exiting the lateral hard-soft palate junction. Perineural malignancy may travel from the palate to the pterygopalatine fossa via this.* **(Middle)** *In this image through anterior ethmoid air cells, ethmoid bulla is seen projecting inferiorly into the middle meatus. The shared wall between the anterior ethmoid air cells and the orbit is paper thin, hence the term lamina papyracea.* **(Bottom)** *Image through ostiomeatal complex (OMC) shows maxillary infundibulum draining the maxillary sinuses into middle meatus. Uncinate process, middle meatus, maxillary infundibulum, & ethmoid bulla are the components of OMC. The olfactory fossa depth corresponds to Keros type II (4-7 mm), which is the most common. Note that there is a lateral to medial slope of the anterior skull base, which is extremely important during transethmoidal surgical approach to anterior skull base lesions. The same axial plane of dissection that was safe along the more lateral ethmoid roof could injure the skull base if extended medially.*

CORONAL BONE CT

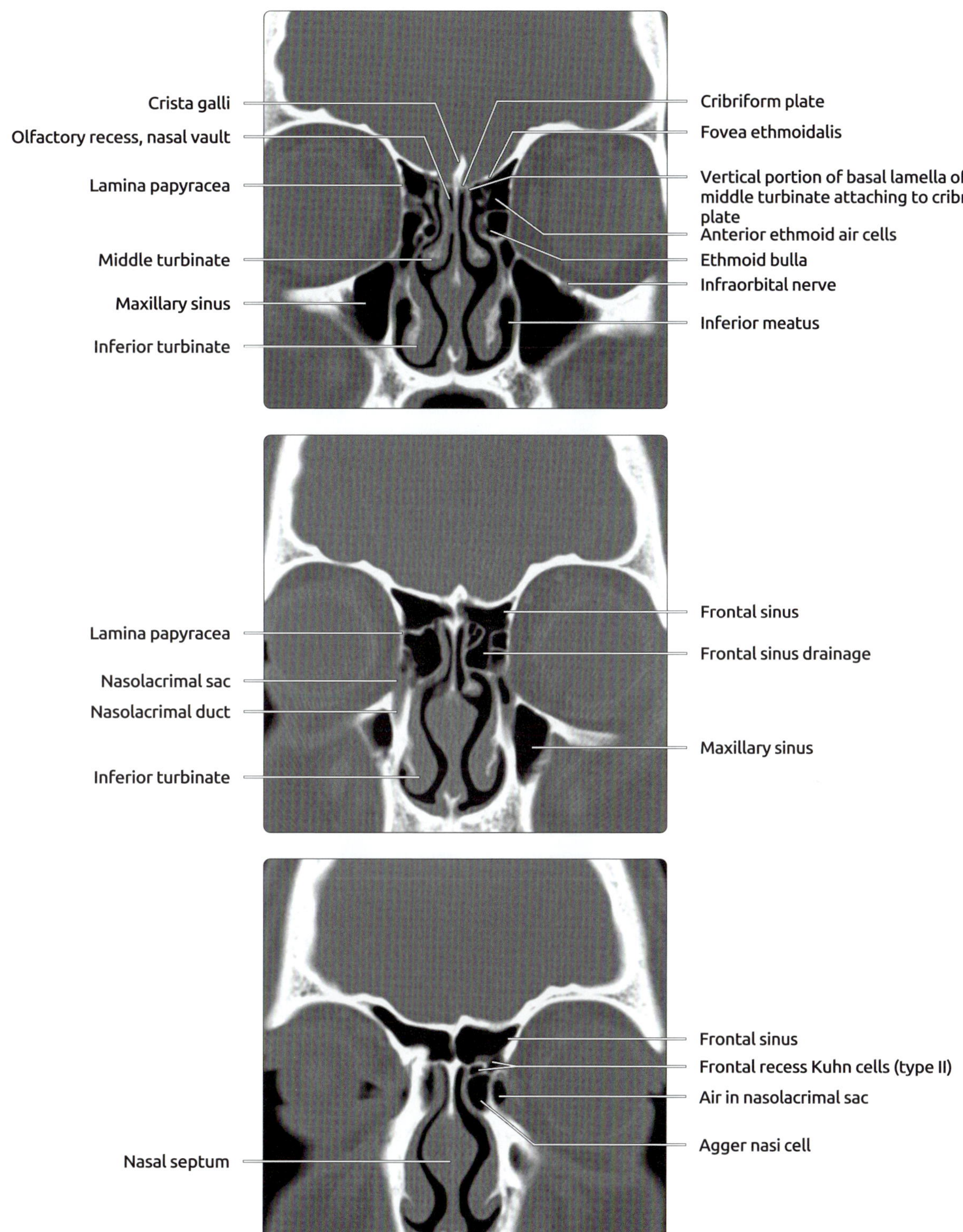

(Top) *Image through anterior aspect of anterior ethmoid complex, fovea ethmoidalis (ethmoid roof), cribriform plate, & crista galli along roof of sinuses & nose from lateral to medial is shown. Olfactory recess of nasal vault contains nasal mucosa from which esthesioneuroblastoma arise. Foveal plane is horizontal plane passing through junction of fovea ethmoidalis with medial orbital wall. Foveal angle is between fovea & lamina papyracea. A low-sloping fovea predisposes anterior skull base injury & intracranial penetration during functional endoscopic sinus surgery (FESS). Safest anatomy is when horizontal line from ethmoid roof crosses upper 1/3 of orbit. Precautions to avoid skull base injury should be taken when horizontal plane of ethmoid roof crosses below vertical midpoint of orbit.* **(Middle)** *Image shows close relationship of nasolacrimal duct (NLD) to maxillary sinuses. NLD drains into inferior meatus.* **(Bottom)** *Frontal sinuses & anteroinferior extramural ethmoid air cell (agger nasi) are shown. Kuhn cells are frontal recess air cells seen above agger nasi (type I single, type II multiple in recess, & type III single, reaching sinus). Type IV is a single isolated cell within frontal sinus.*

SAGITTAL BONE CT

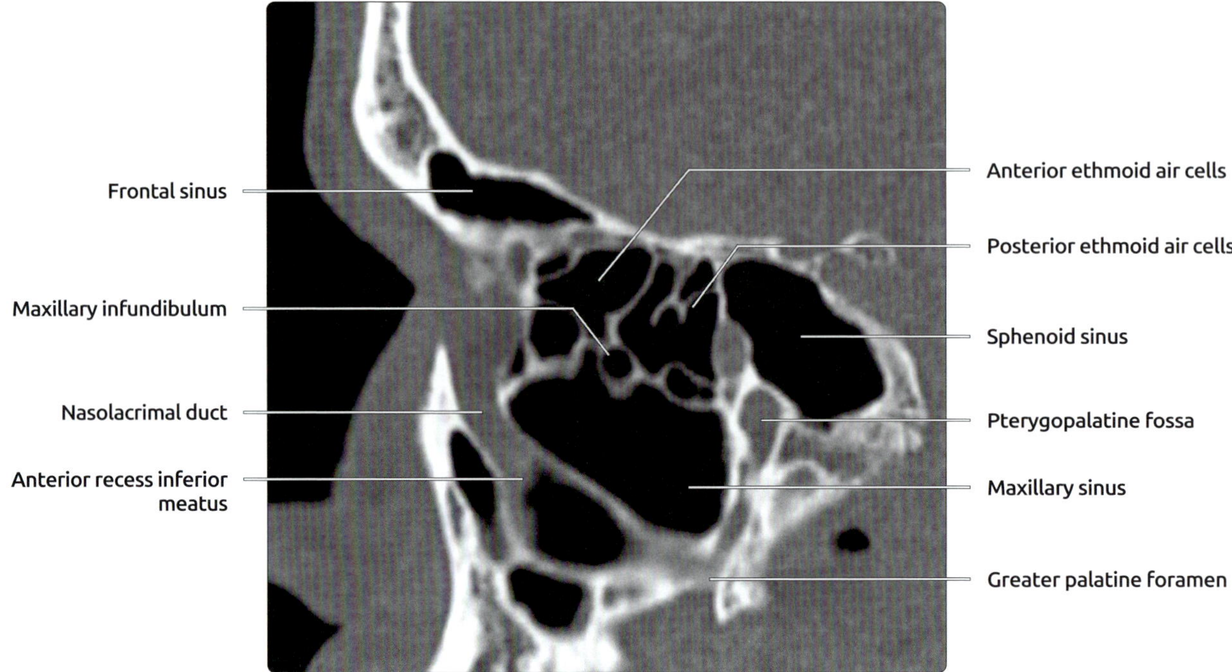

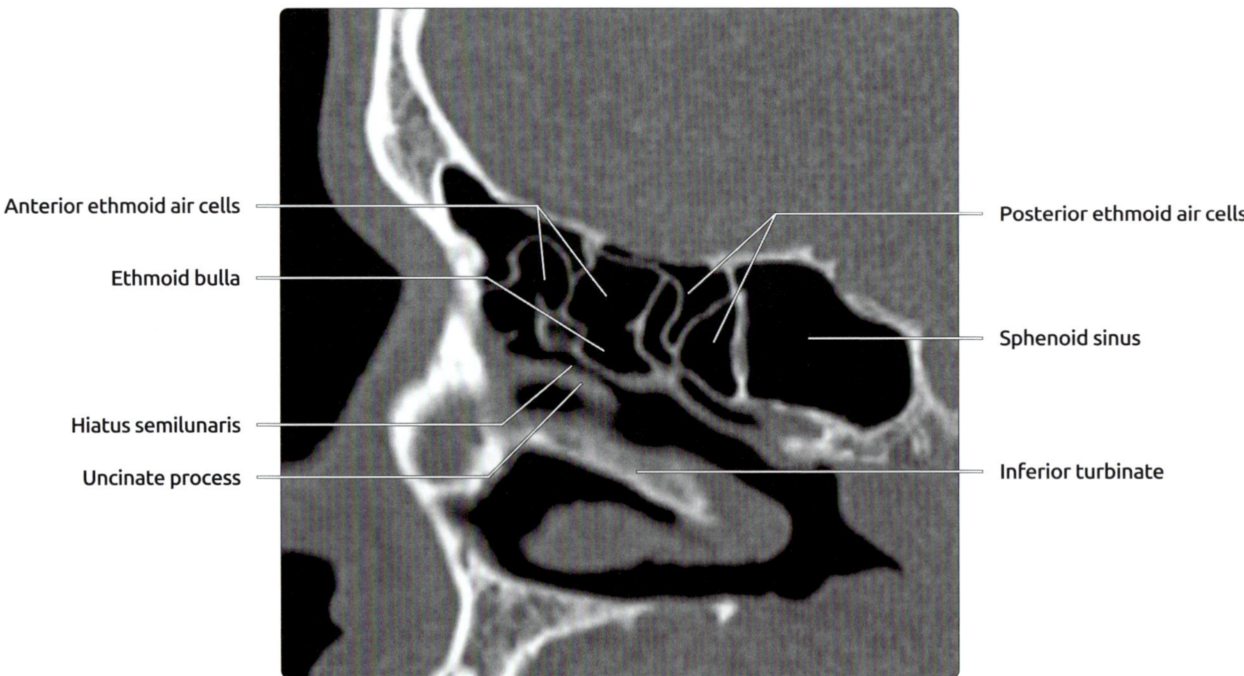

(Top) *First of 4 sagittal bone NECT images through the paranasal sinuses presented from lateral to medial shows the nasolacrimal duct draining into the inferior meatus. Also note the PPF posterior to the maxillary sinus.* **(Bottom)** *In this image, the uncinate process can be seen just inferior to the ethmoid bulla. The gap between these 2 structures is the hiatus semilunaris. Note that there is a concept of a series of 5 obliquely oriented parallel lamellae (derived from the ridges in the lateral nasal wall of the fetus called ethmoturbinals), which are easy to recognize at surgery. The 1st lamella is the uncinate process, the 2nd is ethmoid bulla, the 3rd is ground or basal lamella of the middle turbinate, the 4th is basal lamella of the superior turbinate, and the 5th lamella is the basal lamella of the supreme turbinate. Most important is the 3rd lamella (ground or basal lamella of the middle turbinate), which is a bony septation that separates the anterior and posterior ethmoid air cells with separate drainage pathways.*

SAGITTAL BONE CT

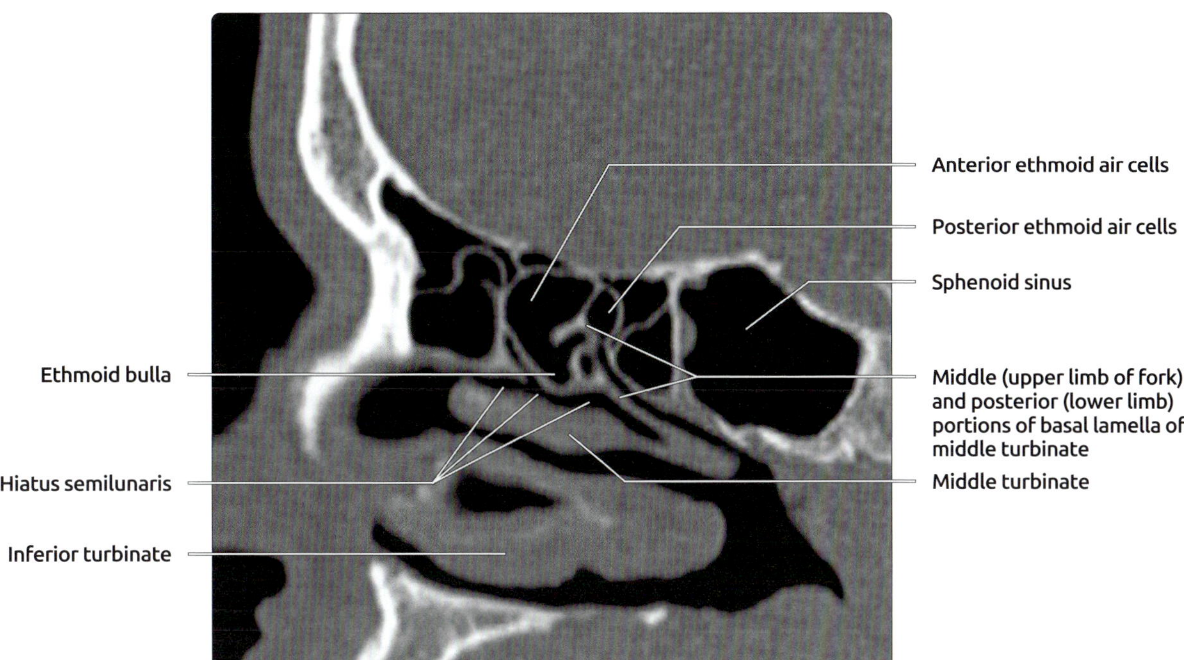

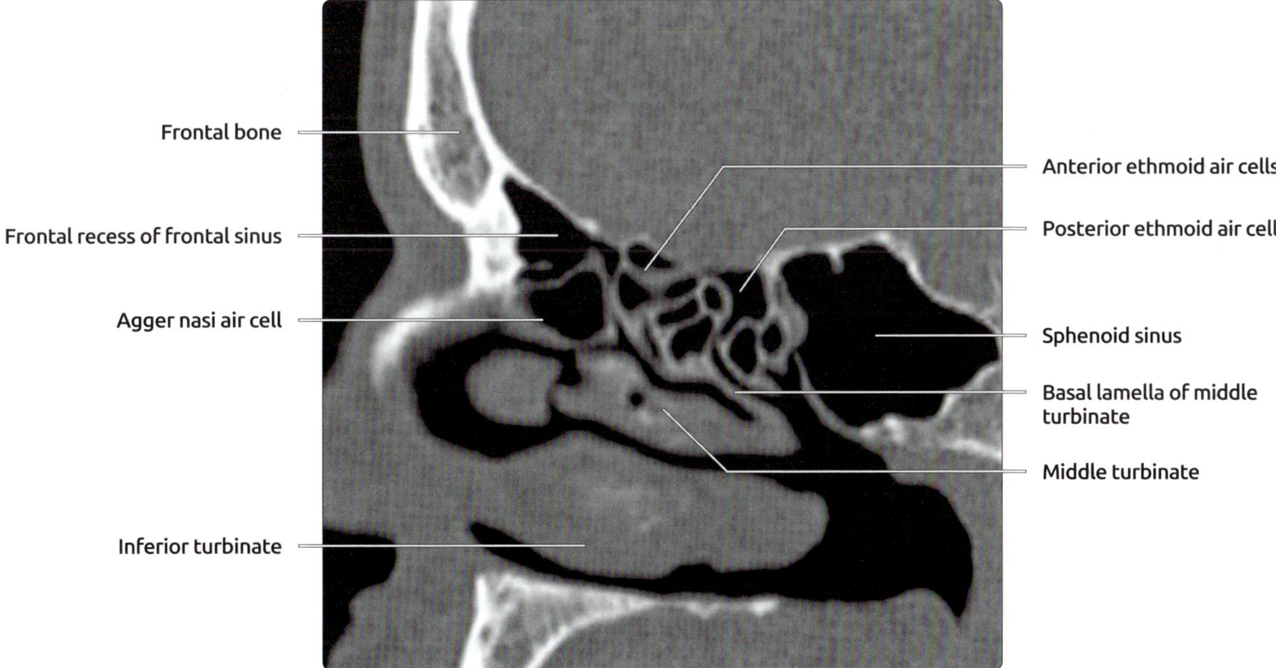

(Top) *Image shows middle & inferior turbinates & basal lamella of middle turbinate. Vertical portion of basal lamella attaches to cribriform plate & is best seen in coronal CTs; is very delicate, & detachment at surgery in this region could damage dura with resultant CSF leak. Middle & posterior portions of basal lamella extend laterally to join lamina papyracea & divide anterior from posterior ethmoid air cells. Posterior margin of basal lamella attaches to perpendicular plate of palatine bone.* **(Bottom)** *Image shows anteroinferior ethmoid air cell (agger nasi cell) extending anteroinferiorly to frontal recess of frontal sinus. If this cell is infected, frontal sinus recess & frontal sinus will also become infected secondarily. Sphenoid sinus is well pneumatized, which is most common pattern (sellar type where pneumatization extends into body of sphenoid with posterior sphenoid sinus wall adjacent to sellar floor or beyond & may even reach clivus; incomplete sellar in 22% & complete sellar in 76%). Sphenoid sinus can be classified into 3 types based on extent of pneumatization: Conchal, presellar, & sellar.*

AXIAL T1 MR

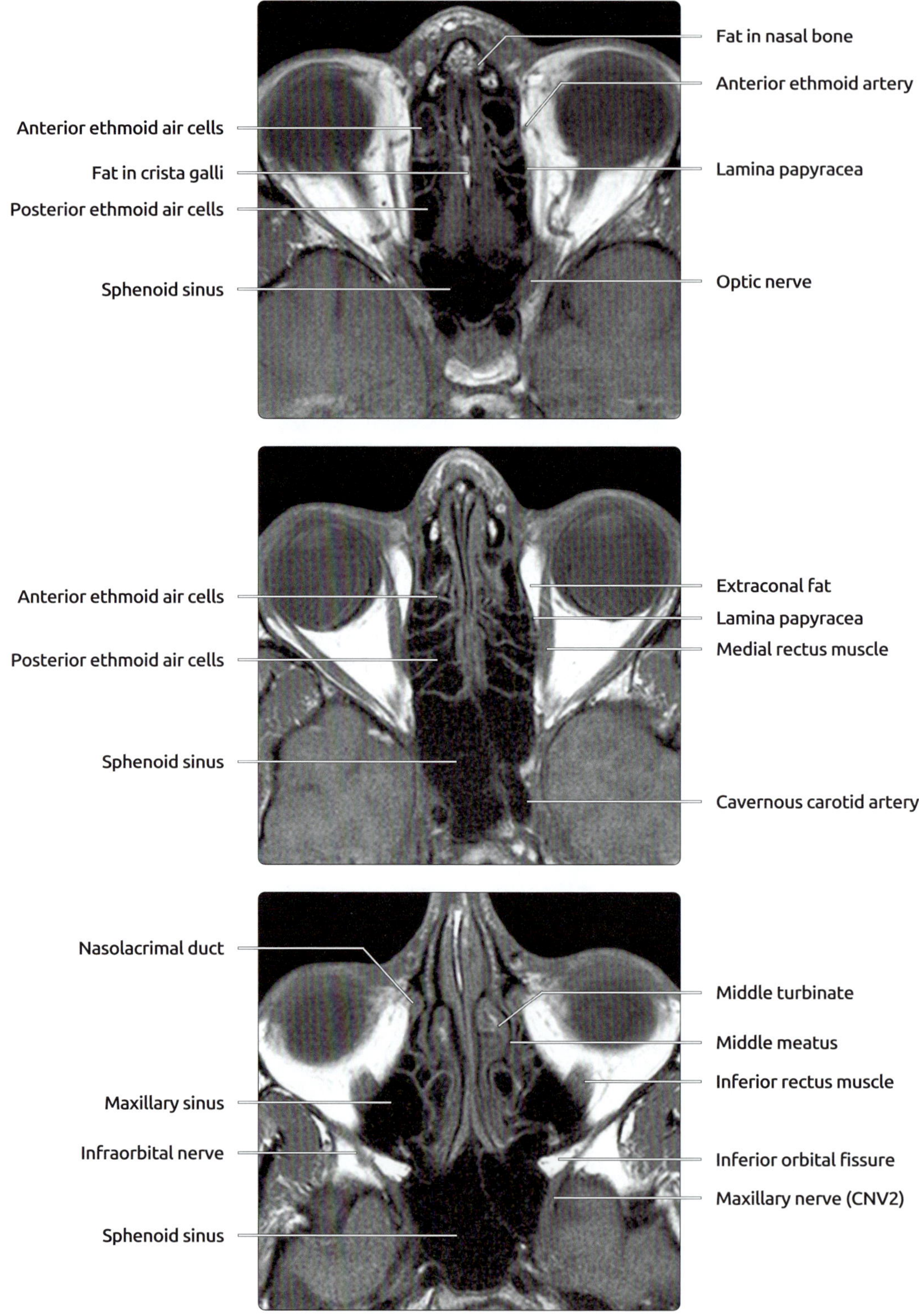

(Top) *First of 6 axial precontrast T1 MR images through the paranasal sinuses from superior to inferior shows the anterior ethmoidal artery (AEA) is visible piercing the lamina papyracea into the anterior ethmoid air cells. The AEA (along with the vein & nerve) travels from the orbit through a canal piercing the lamina papyracea into the anterior ethmoid sinus 6-15 mm posterior to the frontal recess, crosses the sinus, & enters the anterior cranial fossa.* **(Middle)** *In this image through the midglobes, the close relationship of the ethmoid air cells to extraconal fat & medial rectus muscle is seen. The thin lateral wall of the ethmoid sinus (lamina papyracea) is all that separates the orbit from the sinus. If the ethmoid sinuses become infected, inadequate treatment can lead to orbital infection.* **(Bottom)** *In this image through the superior portion of the maxillary sinus, the middle meatus & middle turbinate are seen in the axial plane. Note the fluid-filled normal NLD in the anterior aspect of the lateral nasal wall.*

AXIAL T1 MR

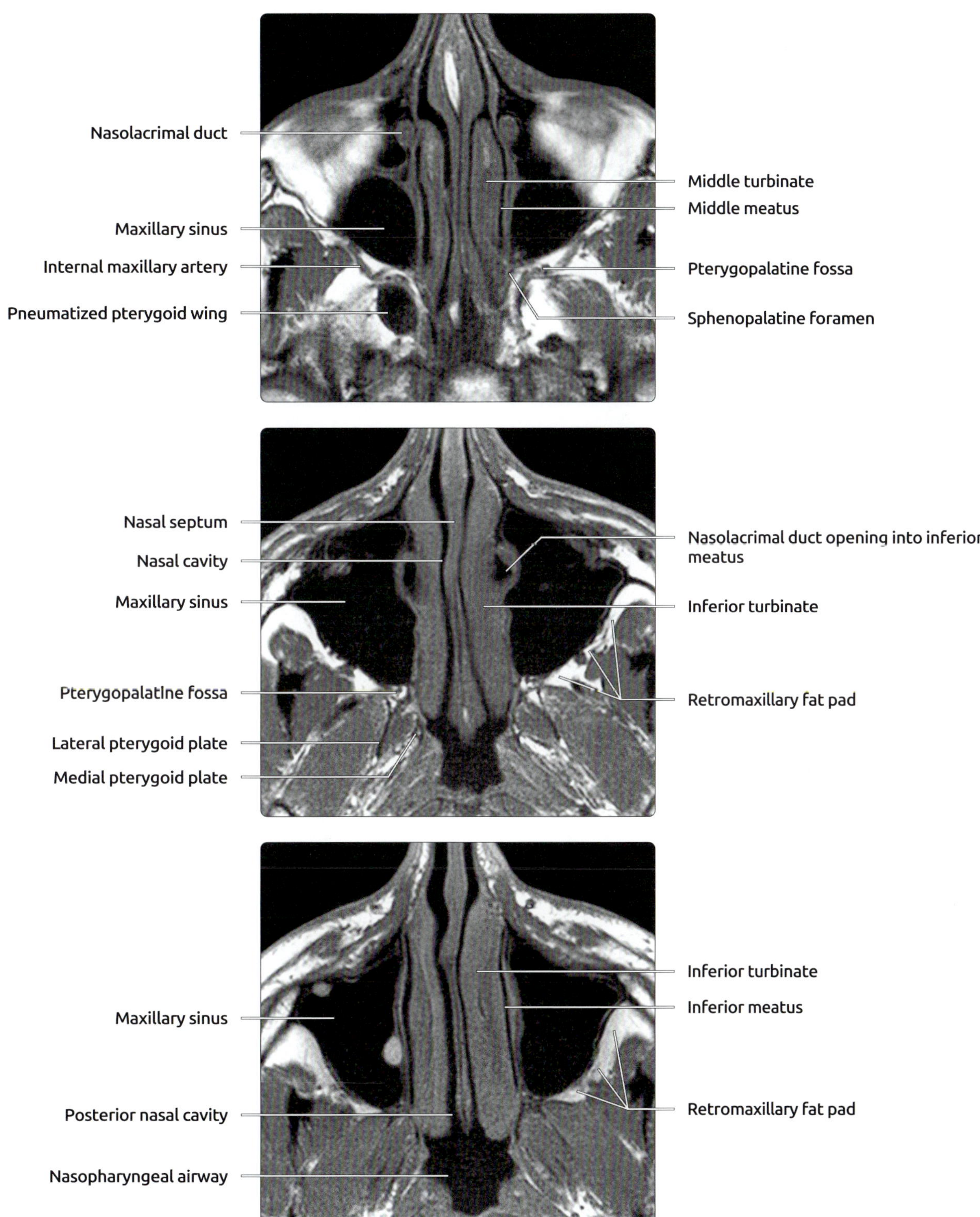

(Top) *At the level of the PPF, the internal maxillary artery can be seen as its principal occupant. The medial exit from the PPF is the sphenopalatine foramen. Juvenile angiofibroma originates along the nasal margin of the sphenopalatine foramen. Often the 1st route of spread for this tumor is through this foramen into the PPF.* **(Middle)** *In this image, the nasolacrimal duct is visible emptying inferiorly into the anterior recess of the inferior meatus. The inferior turbinate is the largest of the turbinates & can be mistaken for a mass when large and asymmetric.* **(Bottom)** *At the level of the midmaxillary sinus, the posterior nasal cavity can be seen in direct continuity with the nasopharyngeal airway. The retromaxillary fat pad sits behind the maxillary sinus & is an extension of the buccal space fat.*

SAGITTAL & CORONAL BONE CT

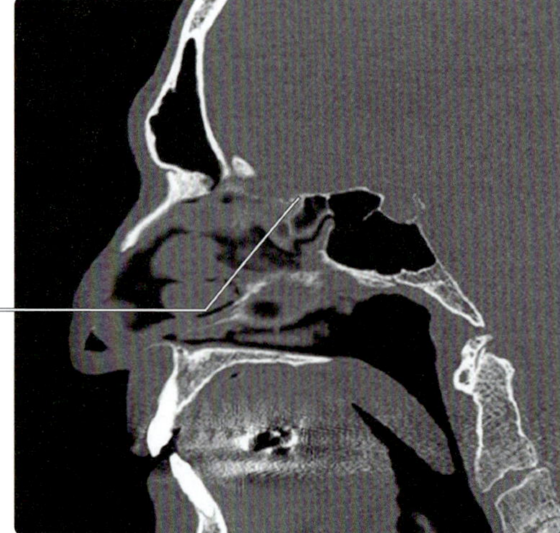

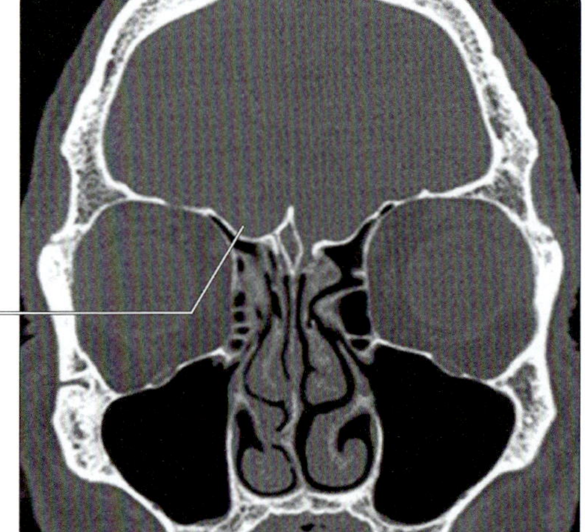

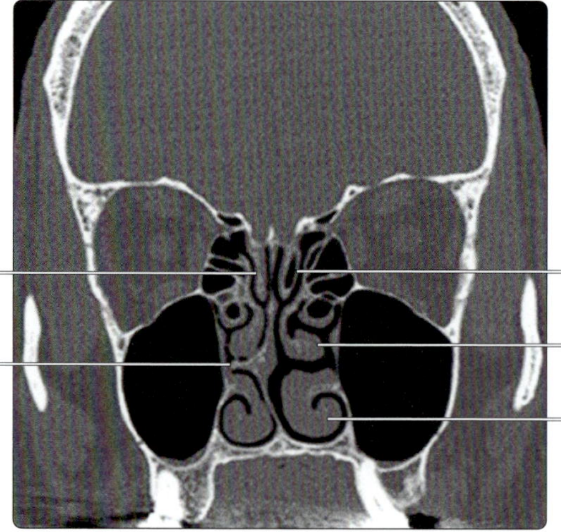

(Top) *Sagittal bone NECT shows the "anterior to posterior sloping down" of the skull base from the frontal recess to the planum sphenoidale along the ethmoid roof. This slope is variable among different people. During FESS, skull base injury can be avoided by assessment of the skull base slope in preoperative CT & surgery using the "back-to-front technique," whereby first the lower-lying posterior skull base is located & operated at the sphenoid sinus roof after identifying the superior meatus & sphenoid sinus ostium.* **(Middle)** *Coronal bone NECT shows the "lateral to medial slope" of the anterior skull base during transethmoidal surgery. The same safe axial dissection plane along lateral ethmoid roof could injure the skull base if extended medially to the cribriform plate region.* **(Bottom)** *Coronal bone NECT shows pneumatized left superior turbinate. Posteriorly, the tail of the superior turbinate points medially toward natural ostium of sphenoid sinus in the sphenoethmoid recess, an important surgical landmark. Sphenoid sinus ostium is located medial to the posteroinferior attachment of the supreme turbinate (Santorini concha, present in 50-60%) behind its vertical part.*

CORONAL MR & CT & SAGITTAL CT

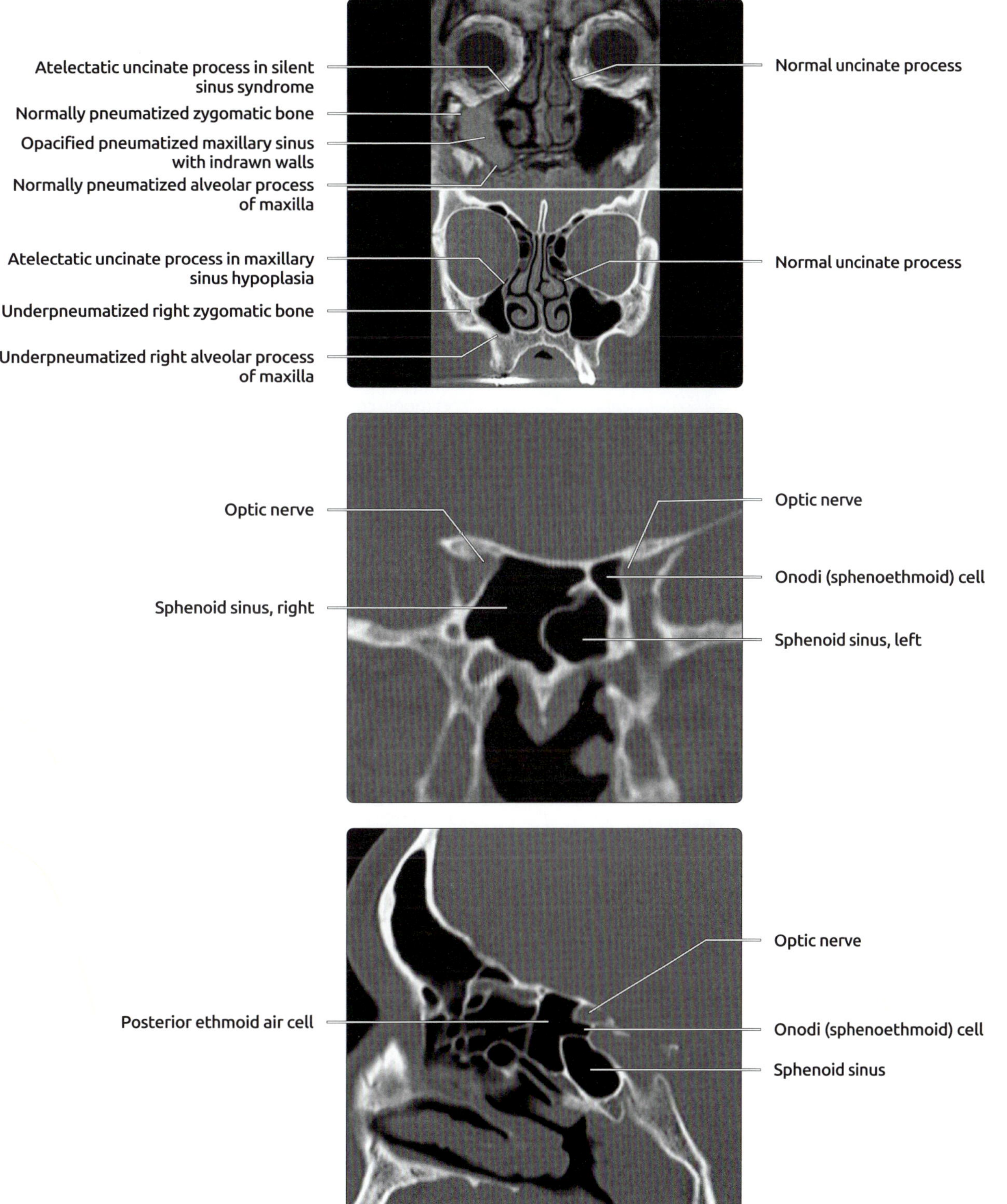

(Top) *Coronal T1WI MR in a patient with right silent sinus syndrome & coronal bone NECT in another patient with right maxillary sinus hypoplasia shows an atelectatic uncinate process, which is located more superolateral than expected, apposed to the inferomedial orbital wall. Note the normal location of uncinate process on the left side. Normal pneumatization of zygomatic bone & alveolar process of maxilla in silent sinus syndrome helps in its differentiation from maxillary sinus hypoplasia where there is reduced pneumatization.* **(Middle)** *Coronal bone NECT shows an air cell above a septation in the superior aspect of left sphenoid sinus, which could be due to an Onodi (sphenoethmoid) cell or just a septated sphenoid sinus. Evaluation of sagittal or axial images will help to differentiate between them. Onodi cell surgical manipulation during FESS may lead to optic nerve injury.* **(Bottom)** *Sagittal bone NECT in the same patient shows that the air cell above the septation is continuous with a posterior ethmoid air cell, confirming that it is an Onodi cell. Note the optic nerve/canal along the posterosuperior aspect of the Onodi cell.*

TERMINOLOGY

Abbreviations

- Ostiomeatal unit (OMU); ostiomeatal complex (OMC); uncinate process (UP); hiatus semilunaris (HS)

IMAGING ANATOMY

Overview

- OMU includes superomedial maxillary sinus, maxillary ostium, maxillary (ethmoid) infundibulum (EI), UP, ethmoid bulla (bulla ethmoidalis) & HS/middle meatus

Anatomy Relationships

- **Middle meatus** receives anterior ethmoid, maxillary, & frontal sinus drainage into crescent-shaped groove called **HS** between tip of UP & ethmoid bulla
  - **HS** best seen from endoscopic vantage point; difficult to see on coronal sinus CT, but sagittal CT reconstruction somewhat demonstrates it
  - **Anterior ethmoid air cells** drain mostly into middle meatus around ethmoid bulla & some into EI
  - **Maxillary sinus** drains through maxillary ostium into EI & then into middle meatus
  - **Frontal sinus** drains through frontal recess (FR) into anterior middle meatus
    - If **UP inserts on middle turbinate or skull base**, FR drains into EI & then middle meatus
      - Obstruction in EI may cause combined frontal, anterior ethmoid, & maxillary sinusitis
    - If **UP inserts on lamina papyracea**, FR drains into middle meatus directly, & EI closed superiorly by blind-ending pouch called **recessus terminalis**
      - Obstruction in EI results in anterior ethmoid & maxillary sinusitis (without frontal sinusitis)
    - Paradoxically, presence of recessus terminalis increases incidence of frontal sinusitis
      - Presumably due to lack of anatomic barrier between FR & middle meatus against ascent of predisposing factors like allergens, irritants, & infections from nasal cavity
    - Disease in recessus terminalis can displace UP medially against middle turbinate obstructing FR drainage
    - **FR**: Frontal sinus drainage funnel
      - Bordered anteriorly by agger nasi & FR Kuhn cells
      - Bordered posteriorly by bulla ethmoidalis & frontal bullar, suprabullar, & supraorbital ethmoid cells

Internal Contents

- **UP**: Upper medial maxillary sinus wall, projects anterosuperiorly from palate & inferior turbinate
  - Defines medial wall of EI & endoscopically hides HS
  - UP removal (uncinectomy) is 1st step of most functional endoscopic sinus surgeries (FESS)
  - UP anterior insertion to lamina papyracea should be kept in mind to avoid medial orbital wall injury
  - Atelectatic UP: Located more superolateral than expected, apposed to inferomedial orbital wall
    - In silent sinus syndrome & maxillary sinus hypoplasia
  - Nasal mass (inverted papilloma) displaces UP laterally toward orbit, while maxillary sinus mass (antrochoanal polyp) displaces it medially toward nasal cavity
- **Ethmoid bulla**: Dominant anterior ethmoid air cell protruding inferomedially into EI & upper middle meatus, defining EI lateral wall
  - When nonpneumatized, rarely results in bony projection from lamina papyracea called **torus lateralis**
- **Middle meatus**: Space between middle turbinate & medial wall of maxillary sinus
- **EI**: Drainage channel of maxillary sinus
  - Defined laterally by bulla ethmoidalis/orbit & UP medially
  - Drains into middle meatus via natural **maxillary ostium**
  - Superior border of maxillary sinus ostium identifies orbital floor level after uncinectomy
  - **Accessory ostium** of maxillary sinus lies behind HS & under ethmoid bulla between tails of middle & inferior turbinates in area called **posterior fontanelle**
    - Can be mistaken for natural ostium during FESS if uncinectomy incomplete
- **Potentially obstructing aeration & variants near OMU**
  - **Concha bullosa**: Aeration of nasal turbinate, most commonly **conchal cells** by ethmoid air cells invading anterior aspect of **middle turbinate**
    - When inflamed, may compress UP & obstruct OMU
    - **Complete** obstructive **OMU pattern** with frontal, maxillary, & anterior ethmoid opacification
    - **Interlamellar cells** arise from superior meatus, pneumatizing vertical lamella of middle turbinate
      - Called lamellar concha bullosa
  - **Paradoxical middle turbinate**: Middle turbinate oriented convex toward lateral nasal wall (instead of usual concave orientation)
    - May compress UP & obstruct OMU
  - **Turbinate sinus**: Exaggerated normal lateral concave curve of middle turbinate may envelope middle meatus
    - Space under its concavity frequently filled by large ethmoid bulla, called turbinate sinus
  - **Haller cell** (infraorbital ethmoid air cell): Air cell located inferomedial to orbit & lateral to EI
    - When inflamed, may obstruct posteroinferior EI → **infundibular pattern** of **isolated maxillary** sinusitis
  - **Agger nasi** air cell: Most anterior of ethmoid air cells
    - Found medial to lamina papyracea, adjacent to FR
    - When inflamed, agger nasi air cell may obstruct FR → **isolated frontal** sinusitis
  - **Deviated nasal septum with spurring**: May displace middle turbinate laterally, narrowing middle meatus
  - **Mucosal contact point headache (MCPH)**: Sinonasal headache most commonly from contact between MT & nasal septum &/or between MT & lateral nasal wall, called **middle turbinate (MT) squeeze syndrome**
  - Diagnostic criteria of MCPH: Endoscopic & imaging evidences of MCP; local anesthetic significantly reduce/abolish headache in 5 minutes compared to placebo, or headaches disappear in 7 days after surgery
  - Nasal septum deviation (41%), MT concha bullosa (32%), superior turbinate pneumatization (21%), abnormal curve of MT (20%), nasal septal pneumatization (16%), inferior turbinate hypertrophy (9%), Haller cell (5%), UP pneumatization (4%) or multiple anatomic abnormalities
  - Theories: Negative pressure, anterior or posterior ethmoidal nerve compression, & neuropeptide release (substance P, calcitonin gene-related peptide, & NK-1R)

GRAPHICS

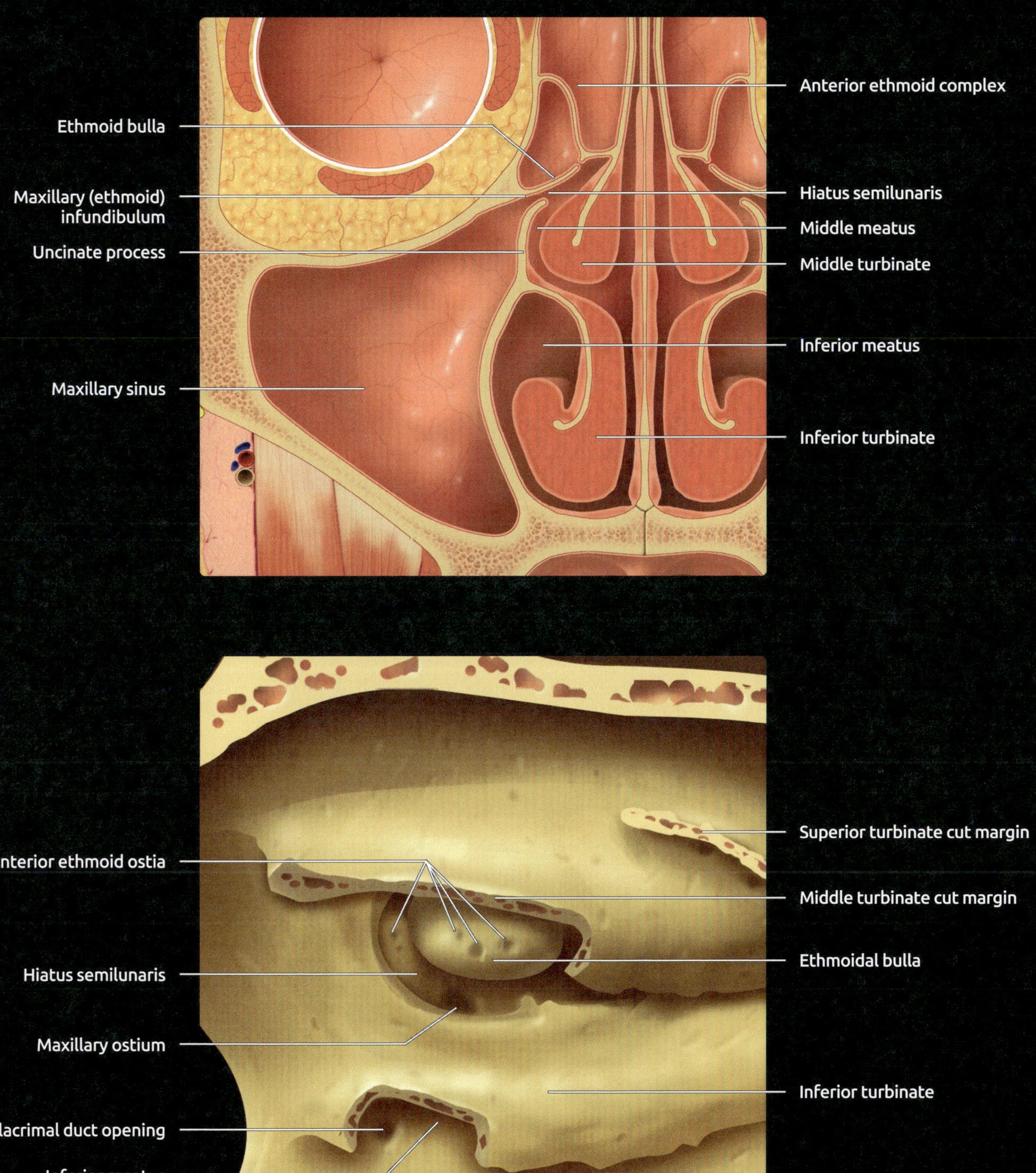

(Top) *Coronal graphic of magnified right sinonasal area illustrates the important structures of the ostiomeatal unit (OMU). Note that the maxillary (ethmoid) infundibulum provides drainage for the maxillary sinus, while the ethmoid bulla (dominant ethmoid air cell of the anterior ethmoid complex) protrudes inferomedially into the upper middle meatus. The middle meatus is the key area of drainage of normal secretions of the anterior ethmoid sinuses and the maxillary sinus.* **(Bottom)** *Graphic of the lateral wall of the nose focused on the region of the middle meatus with the superior turbinate removed as well as part of the middle turbinate is shown. Note anterior ethmoid ostia drain into the middle meatus, as does the maxillary sinus via maxillary infundibulum. The nasolacrimal duct drains into the inferior meatus.*

CORONAL BONE CT

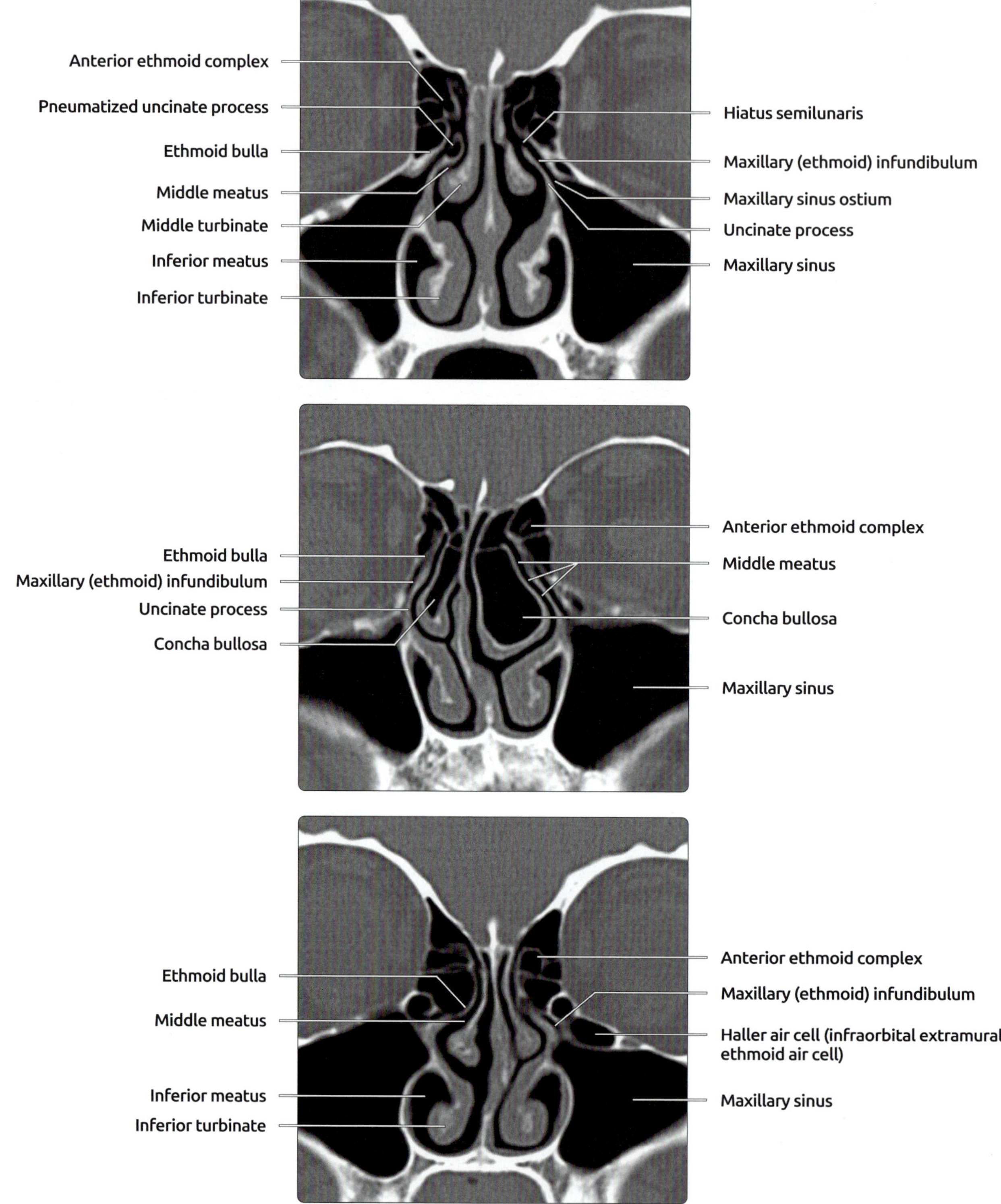

(Top) *First of 3 coronal bone CT images through the OMU is shown. This image shows the typical appearance of the maxillary (ethmoid) infundibulum & ethmoid bulla. Note that the superior tip of the right uncinate process is pneumatized, which, if large or inflamed, may compress the OMU, producing complete OMU pattern sinusitis.* **(Middle)** *In this image, bilateral, aerated, uncomplicated concha bullosa are visible. Notice the attenuated maxillary (ethmoid) infundibulum. If the concha bullosa becomes infected (complicated), early obstruction of the middle meatus causes opacification of the ipsilateral maxillary, anterior ethmoid, and frontal sinuses (complete OMU pattern).* **(Bottom)** *Image through a normal OMU with Haller air cell (infraorbital air cell) seen protruding into maxillary infundibulum is shown. If the Haller cell becomes infected, it can cause an infundibular pattern of sinus disease where there is isolated maxillary sinus opacification without ethmoid or frontal sinus involvement. This occurs when only the posteroinferior aspect of the ethmoid infundibulum is occluded by Haller cell, as anterior ethmoid and frontal sinuses drain via ethmoid infundibulum more anterosuperiorly.*

SAGITTAL BONE CT

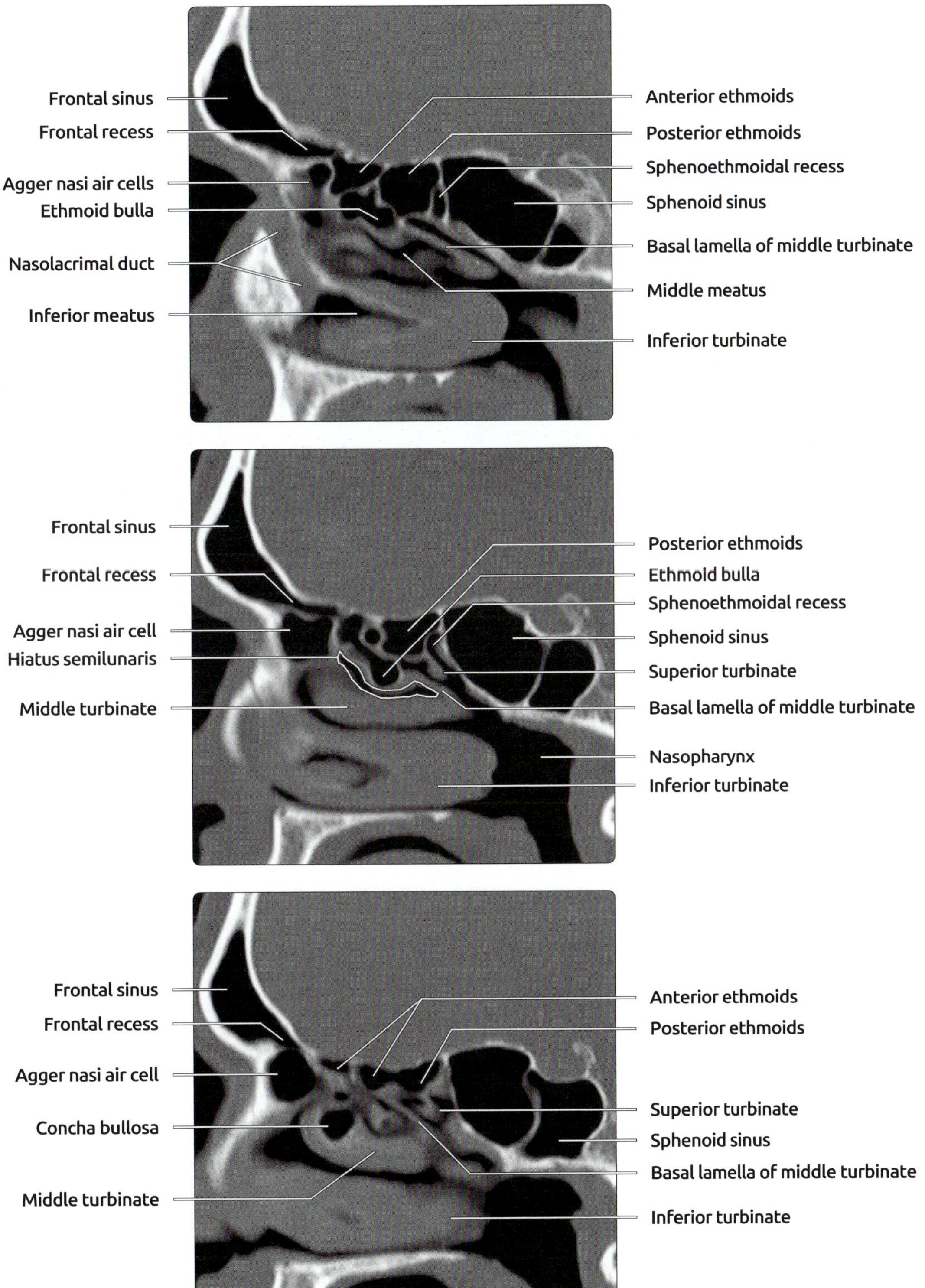

(Top) *First of 3 sagittal bone CT reformations of the sinonasal region presented from lateral to medial demonstrating the structures of the OMU and its vicinity is shown. In this image, the middle meatus can be seen just inferior to the ethmoid bulla. The nasolacrimal duct is visible emptying inferiorly into the anterior aspect of the inferior meatus.* **(Middle)** *In this image, middle and inferior turbinates as well as the basal lamella of the middle turbinate are seen. Also note the curvilinear hiatus semilunaris. The frontal recess is visible extending around the agger nasi air cell. The sphenoethmoidal recess receives the secretions of the posterior ethmoid and sphenoid sinuses.* **(Bottom)** *Notice the air cell in the anterior middle turbinate (concha bullosa) in this image. The basal lamella of the middle turbinate is also visible.*

CORONAL BONE CT

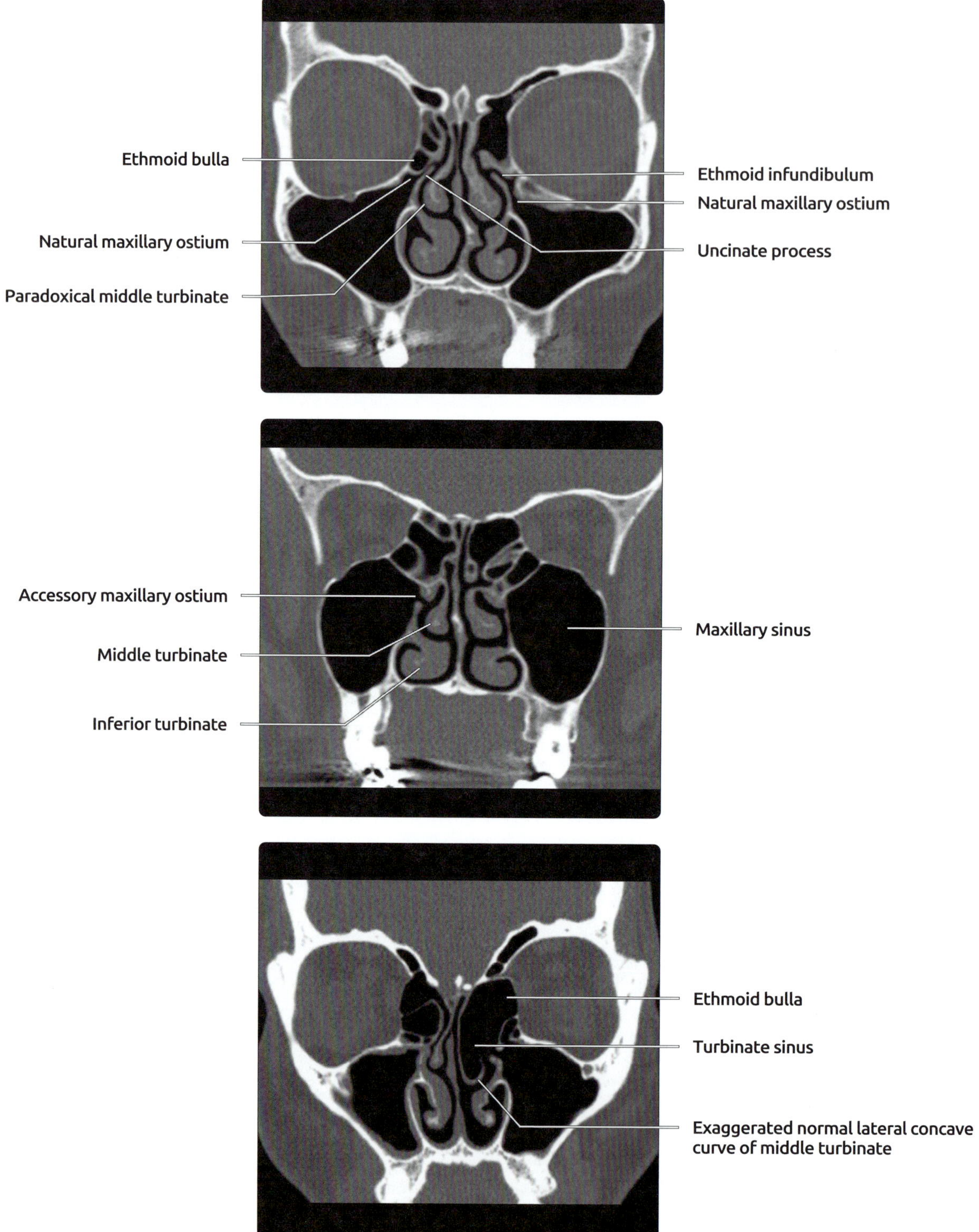

(Top) *Coronal bone NECT through the OMU shows natural maxillary sinus ostium around the orbital floor axial level, leading into the ethmoid infundibulum (which is bordered laterally by uncinate process and medially by ethmoid bulla). The superior border of maxillary sinus ostium identifies the orbital floor level after uncinectomy. Note the paradoxical middle turbinate oriented convex towards the lateral nasal wall instead of usual concave orientation. Paradoxical middle turbinate may compress the uncinate process and obstruct OMU, producing a complete OMU pattern of frontal, maxillary, and ethmoid sinusitis. Other anatomic variants that may produce a complete OMU pattern of sinusitis include concha bullosa and pneumatized uncinate process.* **(Middle)** *Coronal bone CT slightly posteriorly in the same patient shows an accessory ostium of the right maxillary sinus, which can be mistaken for natural ostium during FESS if uncinectomy is incomplete.* **(Bottom)** *Coronal bone CT shows exaggerated normal lateral concave curve of the left middle turbinate enveloping the middle meatus; "turbinate sinus" is the space under its concavity frequently filled by large ethmoid bulla.*

CORONAL BONE CT

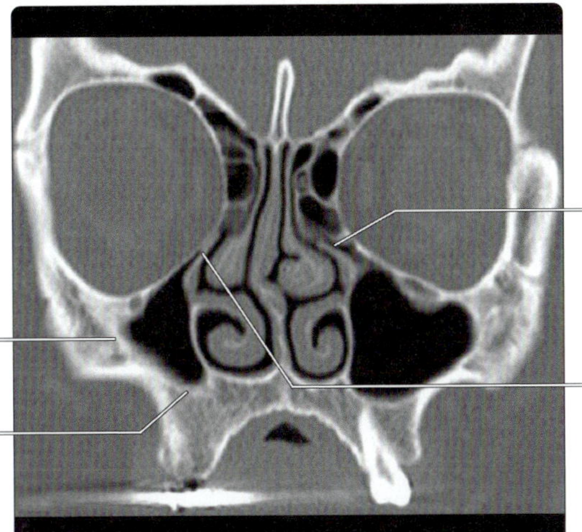

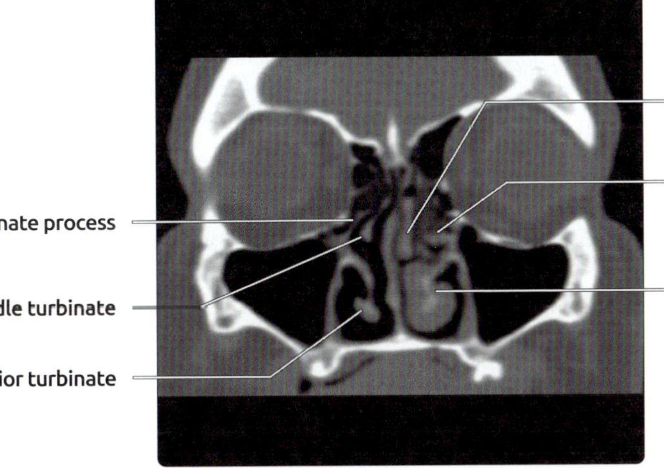

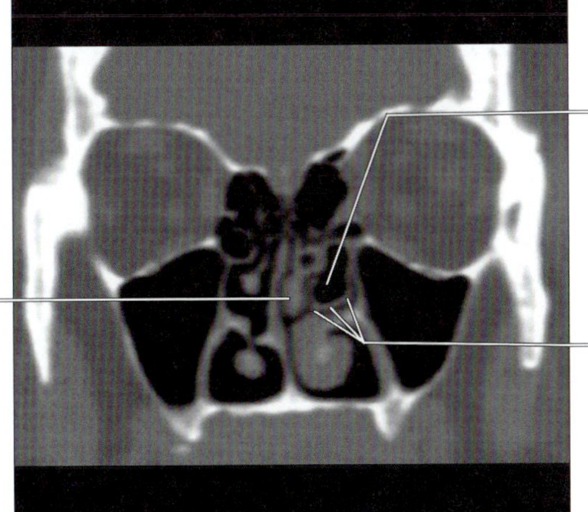

(Top) *Coronal bone NECT in a patient with right maxillary sinus hypoplasia shows an atelectatic uncinate process, which is located more superolateral than expected, apposed to the inferomedial orbital wall. Note the normal location of the uncinate process on the left side. Underpneumatization of zygomatic bone and alveolar process of the maxilla in maxillary sinus hypoplasia help to differentiate it from silent sinus syndrome, which is another condition having atelectatic uncinate process, but will show normal pneumatization of the above-described areas in it.* **(Middle)** *Coronal bone NECT shows a medially bent left uncinate process, which is known as an accessory middle turbinate. This may resemble bifid inferior or middle turbinate.* **(Bottom)** *Coronal bone NECT slightly posteriorly in the same patient shows a bony projection covered by soft tissue that originates from the lateral wall of the middle meatus, which is known as a secondary middle turbinate. Interestingly, this secondary middle turbinate is pneumatized and expanded, making it a concha bullosa of the secondary middle turbinate. Note the usual normal left middle turbinate being pushed slightly medially.*

Pterygopalatine Fossa

TERMINOLOGY

Abbreviations

- Pterygopalatine fossa (PPF)

Definitions

- Major crossroads deep within face between nose, mouth, orbit, masticator space, skull base, nasopharynx, & middle cranial fossa
- Name derived from bones at its posterior wall (pterygoid) & medial wall (perpendicular plate of palatine bone)

IMAGING ANATOMY

Overview

- Narrow space (fossa) roughly shaped like inverted pyramid
- Predominantly fat-filled but contains pterygopalatine ganglion (PPG) as well as several small nerves & vessels that communicate between nose, mouth, orbit, masticator space, skull base, nasopharynx, & middle cranial fossa
- Within PPF, **arteries** are usually located in **anterior plane** separate from more **posteriorly located nerves**
  - **Except** occasional **pterygovaginal artery** posterior to neural plane in PPF to enter palatovaginal canal (PVC)

Extent

- Anterior wall: Posterior wall of maxillary sinus
- Posterior wall: Base of pterygoid process superiorly & ventral aspect of pterygoid process inferiorly (fused medial & lateral pterygoid plates)
- Roof: Inferior orbital fissure (IOF)
- Floor: Narrowing to pterygopalatine (greater palatine) canal
- Lateral wall: Pterygomaxillary fissure
- Medial wall: Perpendicular plate of palatine bone with sphenopalatine foramen

Internal Contents

- **Fat**
  - Look for CT-hypodense & T1 MR-hyperintense small, fat-filled fossa behind maxillary sinus on axial images
- **PPG**
  - Small parasympathetic ganglion in upper PPF hung down by 2 sensory roots from maxillary nerve (CNV2) in front of vidian canal & lateral to sphenopalatine foramen
  - PPG receives synapsing preganglionic parasympathetic & nonsynapsing postganglionic sympathetic fibers from **vidian nerve** & tiny sensory nerves from CNV2
- **Vidian nerve**
  - Mixed nerve entering posteroinferomedial aspect of PPF from **vidian canal**
  - Formed in vidian canal by confluence of parasympathetic fibers from **greater superficial petrosal nerve (GSPN)** & sympathetic fibers from **deep petrosal nerve (DPN)**
  - **Parasympathetic fibers** from **pontine superior salivatory/lacrimatory nuclei** pass through nervus intermedius, **facial nerve**, geniculate ganglion, **GSPN**, & **vidian** nerve to reach **PPG**
    - Postganglionic fibers supply secretomotor nerves to lacrimal gland & to mucous glands of nose, paranasal sinuses, palate, & nasopharynx
  - **Sympathetic postganglionic fibers** from **superior cervical sympathetic ganglion** pass through **internal carotid plexus**, **DPN**, & **vidian nerve** to reach **PPG**
    - Supply vasomotor nerves to mucous membrane of nose, paranasal sinuses, palate, & nasopharynx
- **Maxillary nerve (CNV2)**
  - Largest nerve in PPF, enters posterosuperolateral aspect of PPF from cavernous sinus lateral wall in middle cranial fossa through **foramen rotundum**
  - Provides sensory innervation to cheek, maxillary sinus, nasal cavity, maxillary alveolar ridge, palate, & posterior wall of nasopharynx
  - CNV2 passes anteriorly & laterally through **upper aspect of PPF**, giving off its branches namely zygomatic nerve & posterior superior alveolar nerves
  - Continues anteriorly along roof of PPF into **IOF**, gives off anterior & middle superior alveolar nerve branches
  - Then enters infraorbital canal to become **infraorbital nerve**, which is terminal branch of CNV2
  - CNV2 in PPF inferior branches passing through PPG
    - Nasopalatine (long sphenopalatine) nerve & posterior superior nasal nerve: Exit PPF medially through sphenopalatine foramen
    - Greater palatine nerve & lesser palatine nerves: Exit PPF inferiorly through pterygopalatine (greater palatine) canal
    - Pharyngeal nerve: Exits PPF posteroinferomedially through PVC
- **Vessels**
  - Vessels can be seen normally on CT & MR as variable linear & curvilinear structures in fat-filled PPF
  - **Veins**: Enhancement in PPF seen on postcontrast fat-suppressed T1 MR
  - **Distal internal maxillary artery (IMAX)** from masticator space enters lateral PPF via **pterygomaxillary fissure**
    - **Sphenopalatine artery (epistaxis)**, which is IMAX branch, enters nose from PPF via sphenopalatine foramen
  - Arteries lie anterior to nerves in PPF except occasional pterygovaginal artery
  - **Pterygovaginal artery** may arise early from IMAX lateral to pterygomaxillary fissure & course posterior to neural plane in PPF, hiding it from view during surgery
    - Pterygovaginal artery then enters PVC to reach nasopharynx & anastomoses with ascending pharyngeal & ascending palatine arteries
    - May carry blood retrogradely, increasing epistaxis ligation failure
    - Lateral selective IMAX DSA: **Descending posterior course from PPF** along PVC

Communications of Pterygopalatine Fossa

- **Superior/anterior**: IOF, orbit, & infraorbital canal
  - **IOF**: Roof/anterosuperior opening of PPF into orbit
  - Transmits infraorbital nerve (CNV2 terminal branch) & artery, zygomatic branch of CNV2, & ascending branches of PPG
  - Infraorbital nerve continues anteriorly in infraorbital canal of orbital floor then enters face
    - In face, infraorbital neurovascular bundle courses between levator labii superioris & levator anguli oris facial muscles
- **Posterior**: Postero**superolaterally** foramen rotundum & postero**inferomedially** vidian canal; inconsistent palatovaginal & vomerovaginal canals

- On coronal CT/MR, utilize **lateral (pterygoid) recess of sphenoid sinus** (or even imaginary recess) to separate superolateral foramen rotundum from inferomedial vidian, palatovaginal, & vomerovaginal canals
- **Foramen rotundum**: Posterosuperolateral canal along which intracranial maxillary nerve (CNV2) pass into PPF
  - Look for canal connecting PPF to middle cranial fossa (cavernous sinus lateral wall)
- **Vidian (pterygoid) canal**: Posteroinferomedial thinner canal below foramen rotundum, connecting PPF to foramen lacerum
  - Vidian canal lies in sphenoid bone body/medial pterygoid junction
  - Foramen lacerum: Cartilaginous floor anteroinferomedial to horizontal petrous internal carotid artery canal between sphenoid & temporal bones; transmits vidian artery, nerve, & vein
- **Palatovaginal (palatinovaginal) canal** (inconsistent): Posteroinferior communication of PPF, further medial to vidian canal
  - Short, very thin bony canal formed by articulation of sphenoidal process of **palatine** bone anteriorly to **vaginal** process of sphenoid bone posteriorly
    - Vaginal process is medial extension from upper end of medial pterygoid plate inferior to body of sphenoid to articulate with ala of vomer of posteroinferior nasal septum
  - Opens into roof of nasopharynx & transmits pterygovaginal artery & pharyngeal nerve
  - On axial CT, posteroinferior aspect of PPF splits into anteroposteriorly oriented vidian canal & medially oblique PVC
    - Further inferiorly, PVC posterior groove orients anteroposteriorly & ends in roof of nasopharynx
- **Vomerovaginal canal** (inconsistent): Posteroinferior communication of PPF medial to PVC connected to it or, rarely, to vidian canal
  - Located between ala of vomer of nasal septum & vaginal process of sphenoid
  - Opens into roof of nasopharynx & transmits branch of sphenopalatine artery
  - On axial CT, vomerovaginal canal seen as extremely thin medially oblique canal where PVC posterior groove is anteroposteriorly oriented

- **Lateral**
  - **Pterygomaxillary fissure**: Lateral opening of PPF into masticator space located between lateral aspect of pterygoid posteriorly & posterolateral maxillary sinus wall anteriorly; fat in PPF gets continuous with fat in masticator space & retromaxillary fat pad also here
- **Medial**
  - **Sphenopalatine foramen**: Medial opening of PPF into superior meatus of nose; within perpendicular plate of palatine bone
    - Transmits nasopalatine nerve & posterior superior nasal nerve (CNV2 branches) & sphenopalatine artery (artery of epistaxis)
    - Covered with mucosa; juvenile nasopharyngeal angiofibroma (JNA) may arise here; other reported potential sites of JNA origin are PPF, vidian canal, choana, nasopharynx, & pterygoid wedge (anterior junction of lateral & medial pterygoid plates)
- **Inferior**: Greater palatine (pterygopalatine) canal, greater palatine foramen, & lesser palatine canals/foramina
  - **Pterygopalatine (greater palatine) canal**: Inferior canal from PPF leading through **greater palatine foramen** to open into hard palate
    - Formed by vertical groove on posterior part of maxillary surface of palatine bone & converted into canal by articulation with maxilla
    - Transmits descending palatine artery, vein, & greater & lesser palatine nerves
  - Accessory canals branch off from this canal known as **lesser palatine canals**, opening in hard palate in variable number of (usually 2) **lesser palatine foramina** located posterior to greater palatine foramen

ANATOMY IMAGING ISSUES

Imaging Recommendations

- **CT**
  - Thin-slice bone CT with coronal & sagittal reformations best for demonstrating bony erosion or destruction involving adjacent regions of hard palate, pterygoid process, sinuses, or sphenoid bone
  - CECT shows replacement of normal fat in PPF & presence of enhancing inflammatory/neoplastic process
- **MR**
  - T1 precontrast images in axial & coronal planes best for demonstrating normal PPF fat
  - Fat-suppressed T1-weighted images with contrast best demonstrates abnormal enhancing pathology in PPF
  - Complete evaluation for perineural tumor spread (PNTS) requires imaging from distal nerve back to brainstem

Imaging Pitfalls

- Beware of fat-saturation artifact on MR; blooming at air-tissue interface may obscure PPF (or result in incomplete fat saturation) as result of maxillary sinus air
- Dental amalgam artifact may obscure subtle lesions of PPF
- Normal asymmetric neurovascular structures in PPF

CLINICAL IMPLICATIONS

Clinical Importance

- Primary tumors of PPF are rare (like schwannoma)
- Neoplasms involve PPF by direct invasion or by PNTS
- Tumors involving PPF are more difficult to treat surgically & carry worse prognosis
- Tumors in PPF can access central skull base & cavernous sinus by PNTS (foramen rotundum) or direct invasion
- **PNTS most commonly involves CNV2**
  - **Infraorbital nerve**: Cheek skin, maxillary sinus, orbit
  - **Palatine nerves**: Hard/soft palate
  - **Pharyngeal nerve**: Nasopharynx
  - **Vidian nerve**: If nasopharyngeal/skull base tumor erodes into vidian canal, PNTS may extremely rarely reach **facial nerve (CNVII)** via **GSPN** from vidian nerve
- Intractable **epistaxis** usually from sphenopalatine artery
- Other branches of IMAX PPF, such as posteriorly lying enlarged **pterygovaginal artery**, can cause epistaxis
  - May cause arterial ligation failure, as its posterior to neural plane location in PPF (arteries usually anterior to nerves in PPF) could hide it from view during surgery

GRAPHICS

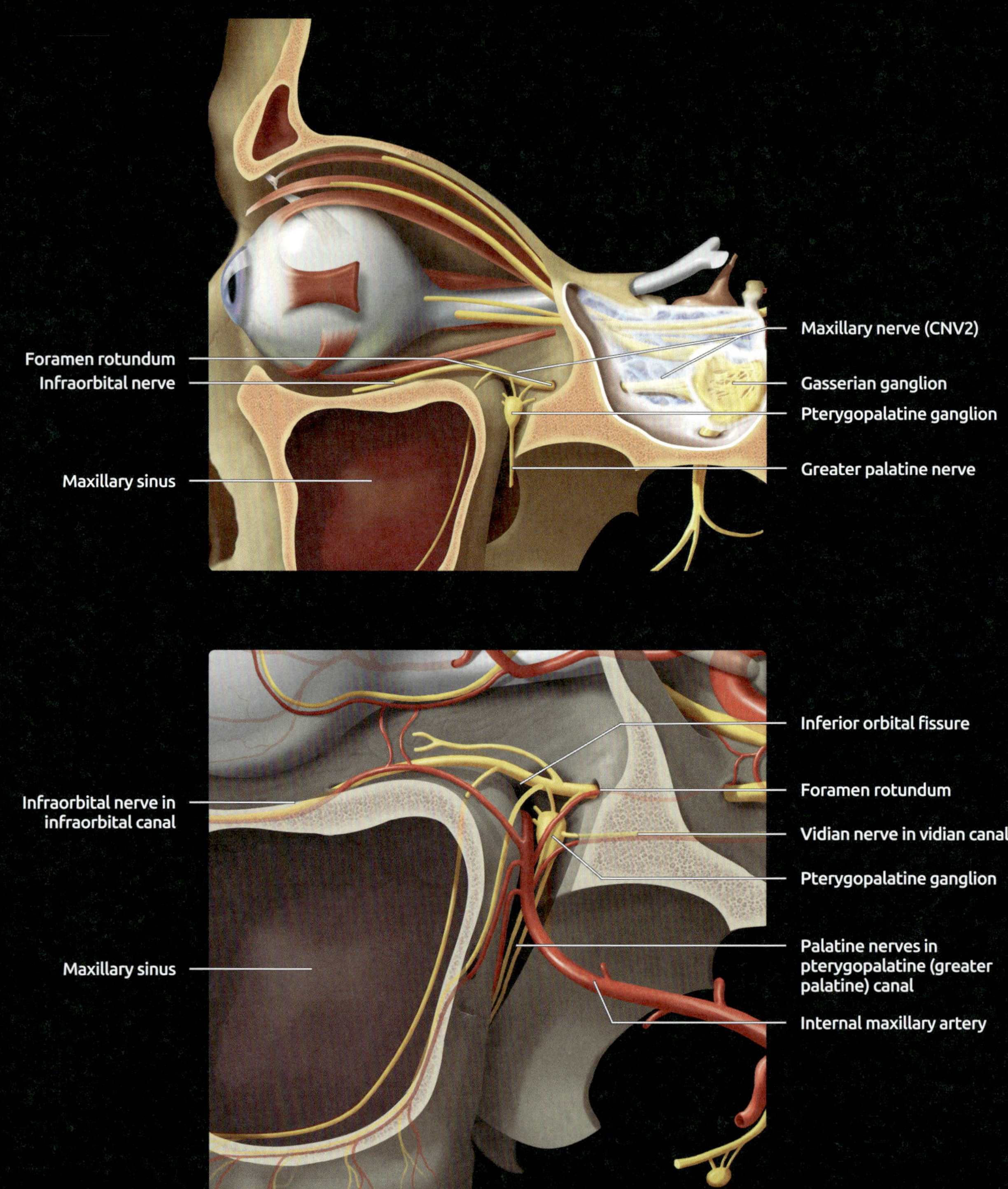

(Top) *Sagittal graphic demonstrates the anatomic landscape surrounding the pterygopalatine fossa (PPF). Pterygopalatine ganglion is hung down by 2 sensory roots from maxillary nerve (CNV2).* **(Bottom)** *Magnified sagittal graphic shows contents of the PPF. The inferior orbital fissure (IOF) forms its roof & connects the PPF anterosuperiorly with the orbit & infraorbital canal. Foramen rotundum connects the PPF with cavernous sinus lateral wall posterosuperolaterally. Vidian canal connects PPF to foramen lacerum posteroinferomedially. Inconsistent posteroinferomedial canals, namely palatovaginal & vomerovaginal canals, leading to the nasopharynx are not shown. The pterygopalatine (greater palatine) canal leads inferiorly through the greater palatine foramen & lesser palatine canals/foramina to the oral cavity. The pterygomaxillary fissure leading to the masticator space laterally & sphenopalatine foramen to superior meatus of nose medially are not shown. Note that the major arteries are located anterior to the neural plane in PPF. An enlarged pterygovaginal artery can be an exception to this rule, coursing posterior to the neural plane in the PPF, hiding it from view during epistaxis ligation surgery.*

AXIAL BONE CT

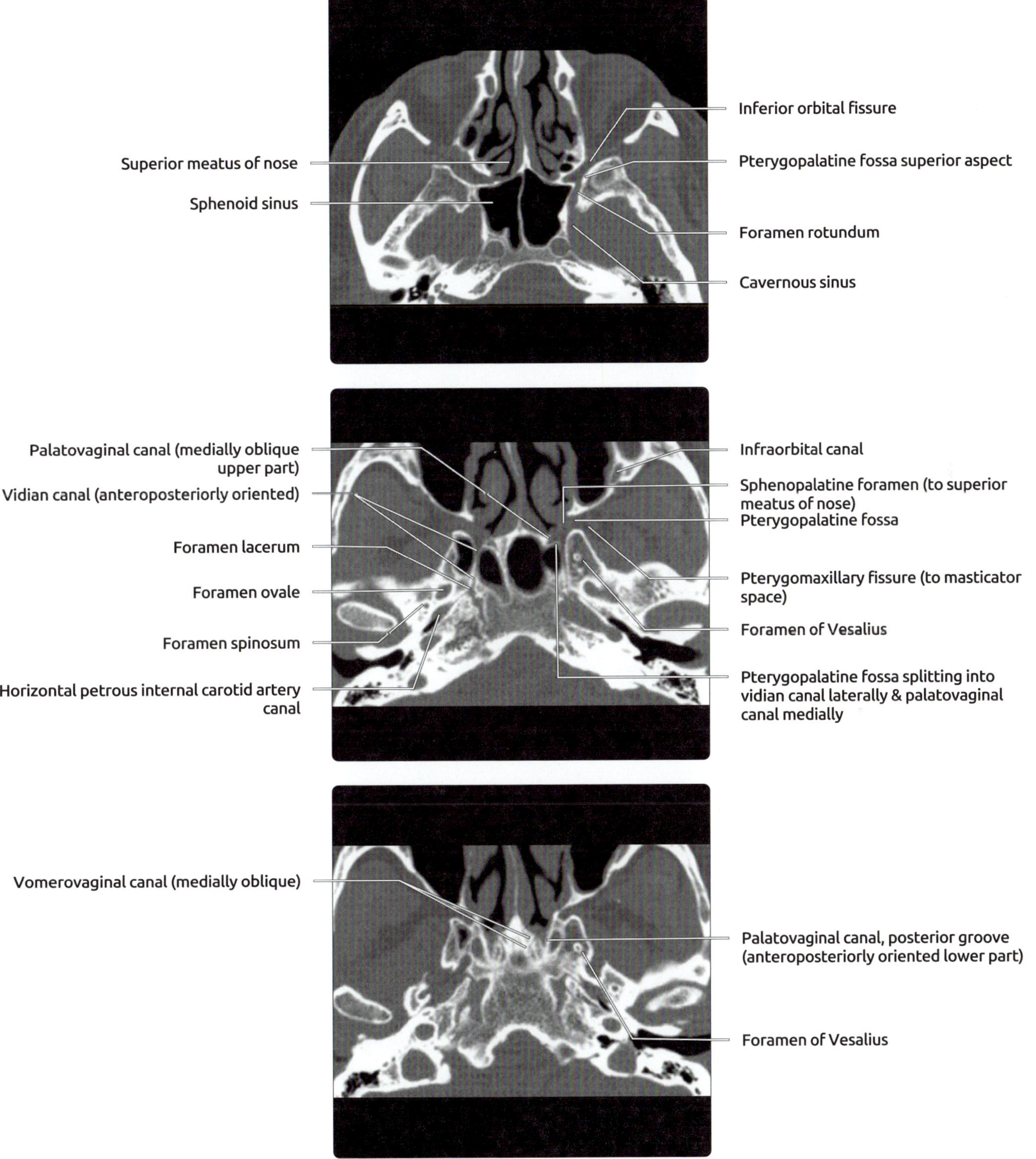

(Top) *Axial bone CT at the superior aspect of the PPF shows the IOF (roof & anterosuperior communication of the PPF connecting to the orbit; contains infraorbital nerve) & foramen rotundum posteriorly [connecting the PPF posterosuperolaterally to the lateral wall of cavernous sinus in middle cranial fossa; contains maxillary (CNV2) nerve].* **(Middle)** *Axial bone CT through the PPF shows the vidian canal passing through the body of the sphenoid bone body/medial pterygoid junction, connecting the PPF to the foramen lacerum. The foramen lacerum is the anteroinferomedial cartilaginous floor of the horizontal petrous internal carotid artery (ICA) canal between sphenoid & temporal bones. Note that the posteroinferomedial aspect of the PPF splits into the anteroposteriorly oriented vidian canal & medially oblique upper aspect of thin palatovaginal canal (PVC). Foramen of Vesalius is lateral to vidian canal & anterior to foramen ovale.* **(Bottom)** *Image shows the lower aspect of the PVC (posterior groove), which is anteroposteriorly oriented. Note extremely thin medially oblique vomerovaginal canal connected to PVC. Both these inconsistently seen canals open into the roof of the nasopharynx.*

CORONAL BONE CT

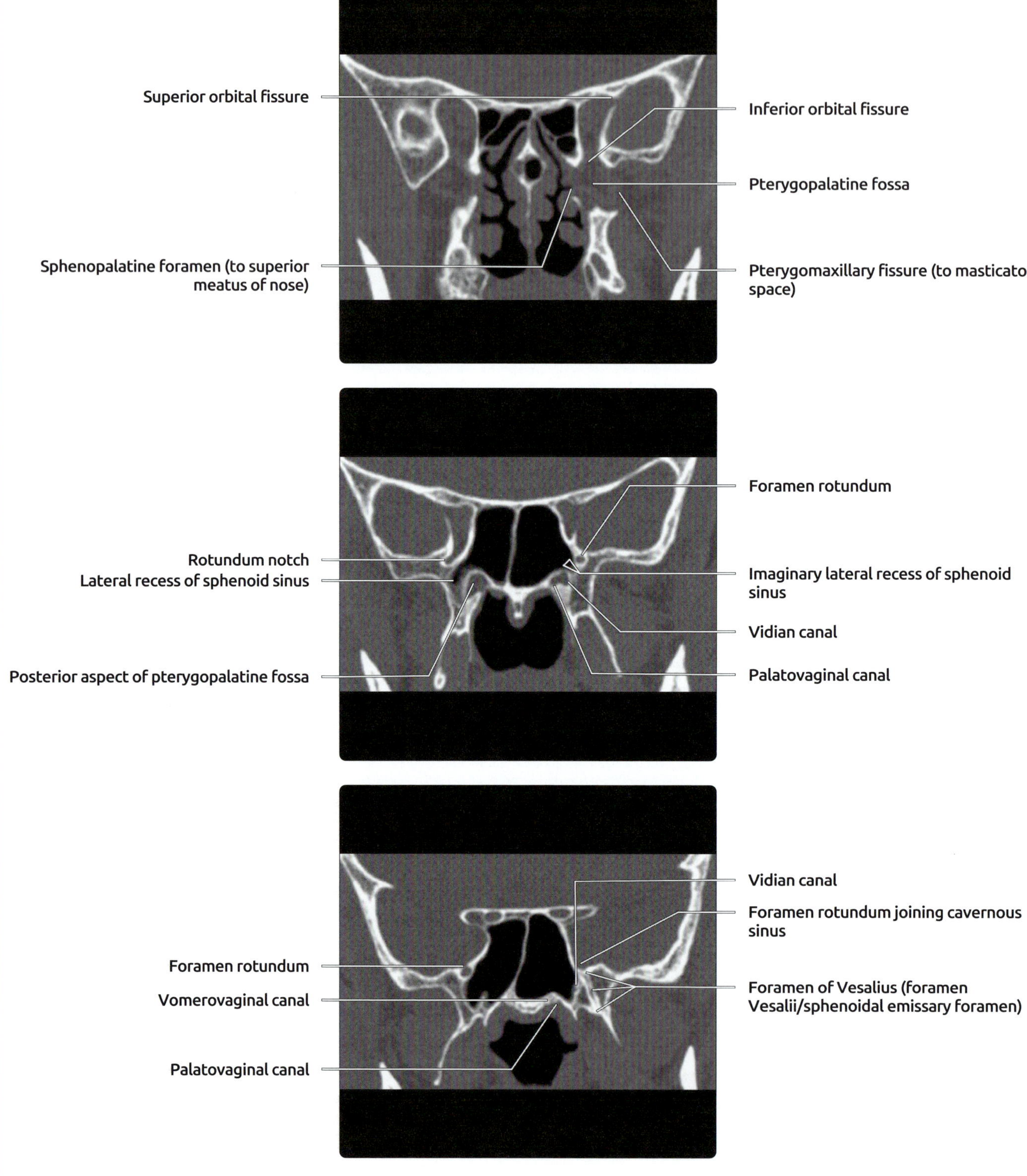

(Top) *Anterior coronal CT at PPF level shows the IOF forming its roof, the pterygomaxillary fissure leading to the masticator space laterally, & the sphenopalatine foramen opening to the superior meatus of the nose medially.* **(Middle)** *Slightly posterior coronal CT shows the foramen rotundum at the base of the greater wing of sphenoid, superolateral to the vidian canal in the body of the sphenoid. Practically identify these foramina on coronal images by their relation to sphenoid sinus lateral (pterygoid) recess. If no lateral recess, draw an imaginary recess at the inferolateral aspect of the sinus. Posteriorly, inferior PPF divides into vidian canal & tiny PVC.* **(Bottom)** *Further posterior coronal CT shows the posterior aspect of the vidian canal on its way toward the foramen lacerum. Note PVC & vomerovaginal canal opening into roof of nasopharynx. Foramen Vesalii is an inconsistent channel in greater wing of sphenoid, lateral to vidian canal & anterior to foramen ovale, containing an emissary vein connecting cavernous sinus superiorly near the foramen rotundum to masticator space pterygoid venous plexus inferiorly; infection may spread from upper face/orbit/sinus to cavernous sinus.*

SAGITTAL BONE CT

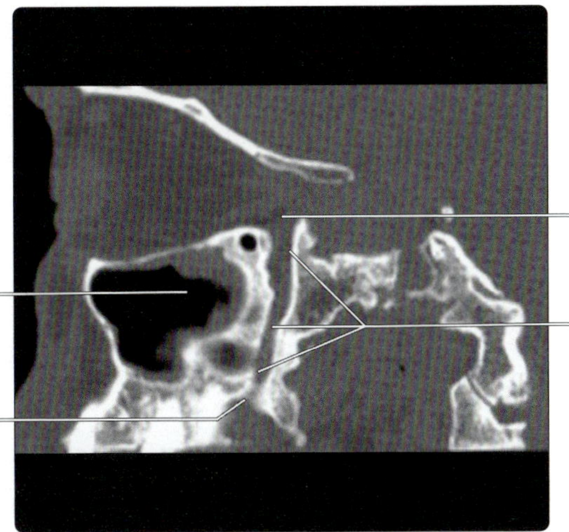

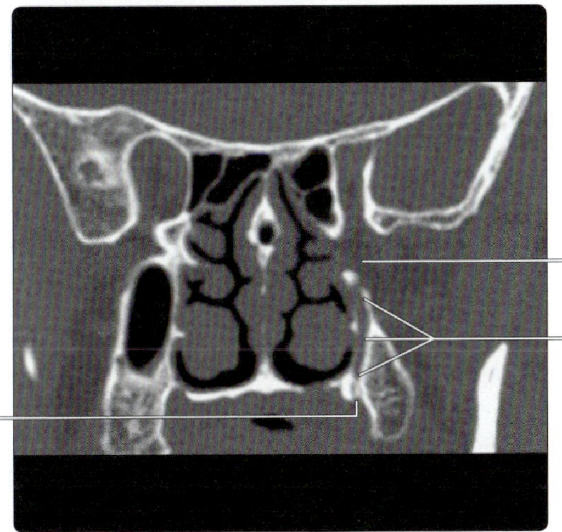

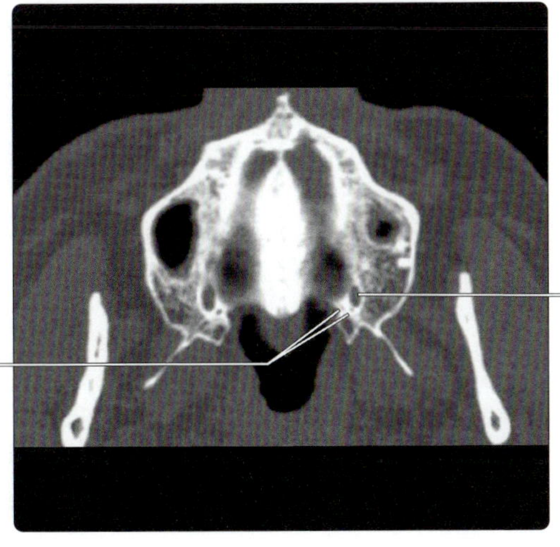

(Top) *Left parasagittal CT reconstruction of the pterygopalatine (greater palatine) canal connecting PPF inferiorly through greater palatine foramen to hard palate/oral cavity is shown. Accessory canals branch off from this canal (known as lesser palatine canals), opening in the hard palate into a variable number of (usually 2) lesser palatine foramina located posterior to greater palatine foramen. Pterygopalatine (greater palatine) canal is formed by a vertical groove on the posterior part of maxillary surface of palatine bone & converted into a canal by articulation with maxilla. It transmits the descending palatine artery, vein, & greater & lesser palatine nerves.* **(Middle)** *Coronal oblique reconstruction demonstrates the course of the pterygopalatine (greater palatine) canal.* **(Bottom)** *Axial bone CT at hard palate level shows the lower end of pterygopalatine (greater palatine) canal in the greater palatine foramen. Also note the accessory canals from this canal ending in lesser palatine foramina posteriorly. Oral cavity tumors in the palate can reach PPF through these foramina & canals. Oropharyngeal carcinoma may also rarely invade the palate & spread into PPF through these channels.*

AXIAL T1 MR

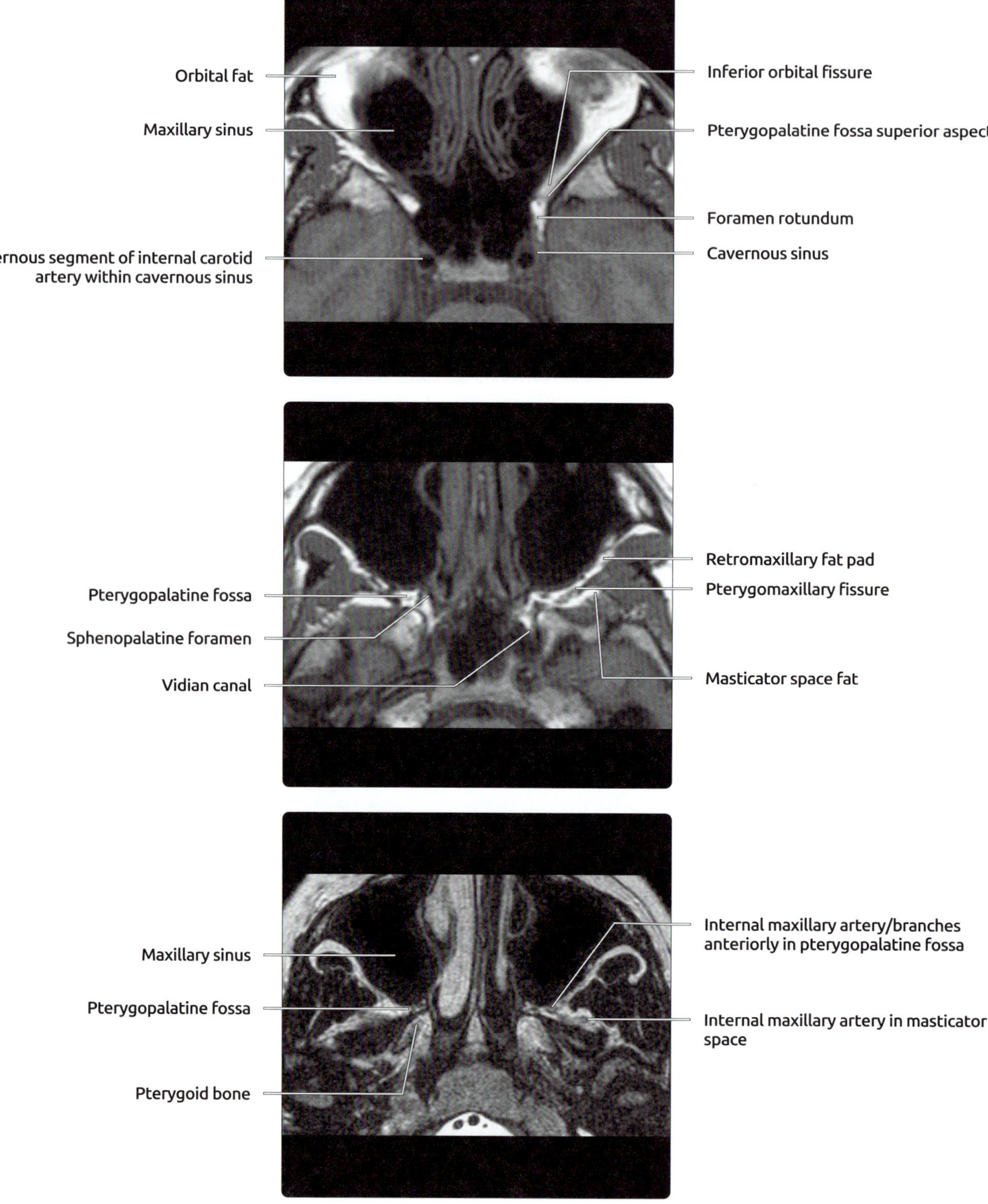

(Top) *Axial T1WI MR at the superior aspect of the PPF shows the T1-hyperintense fat in the IOF (roof & anterosuperior communication of PPF connecting to orbit; contains infraorbital nerve) & foramen rotundum posteriorly [connecting PPF posterosuperolaterally to the lateral wall of cavernous sinus in middle cranial fossa; contains maxillary (CNV2) nerve].* **(Middle)** *Axial T1WI MR at a slightly lower level through the PPF shows the pterygomaxillary fissure leading to masticator space laterally, sphenopalatine foramen opening to superior meatus of nose medially, & the vidian canal posteriorly passing through body of sphenoid bone body/medial pterygoid junction toward the foramen lacerum. Note that the hyperintense fat in the PPF gets continuous with masticator space fat & also the retromaxillary fat pad along the pterygomaxillary fissure. In turn, retromaxillary fat becomes continuous with the buccal space fat.* **(Bottom)** *Axial high-resolution 3D T2WI MR shows vascular flow voids of the internal maxillary artery in the masticator space extending into PPF; its major branch in PPF is the sphenopalatine artery. Within PPF, arteries are usually located in an anterior plane with posteriorly located nerves.*

ANATOMIC-RADIOLOGIC CORRELATION

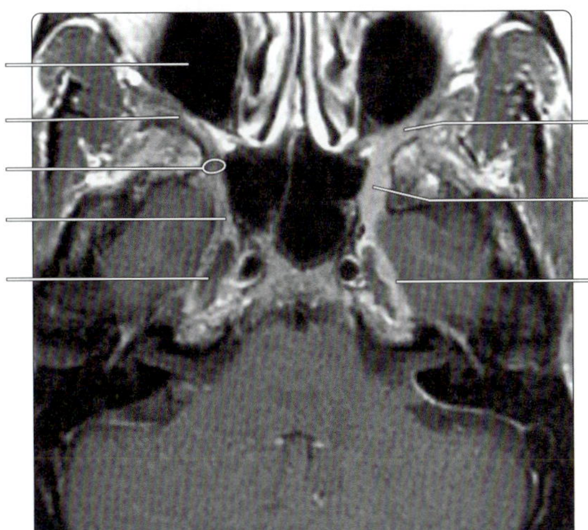

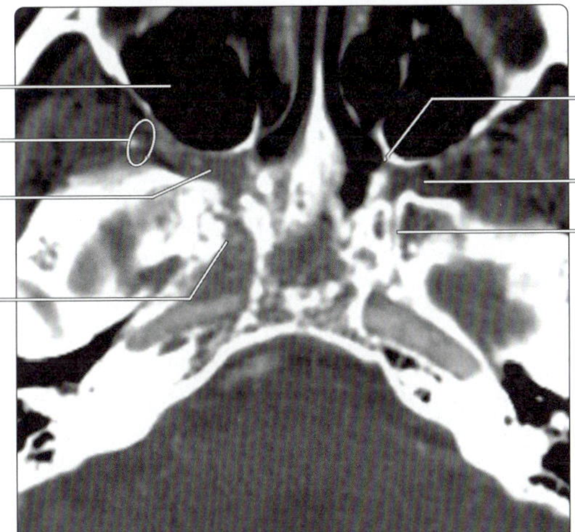

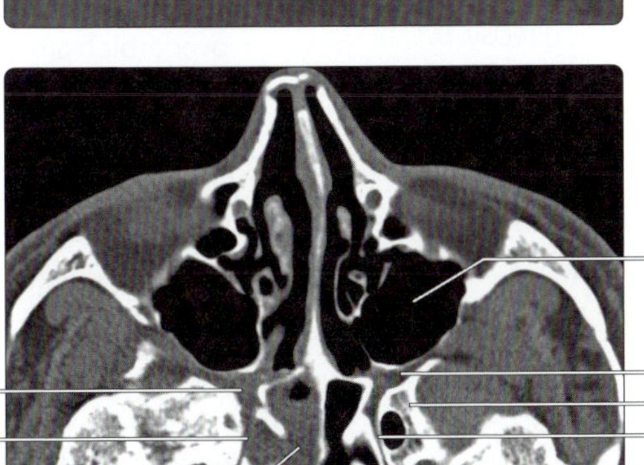

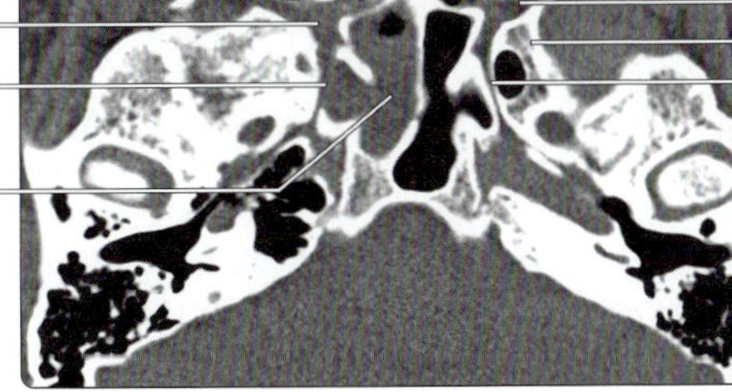

(Top) *Schwannoma of CNV2 is shown. Axial T1 C+ MR through the upper PPF demonstrates an enhancing lesion along the left CNV2. Abnormal enhancement extends from the Meckel cave posterior, through the expanded foramen rotundum, & into the proximal IOF.* **(Middle)** *Axial CECT through the central skull base in a patient with known nasopharyngeal carcinoma & new right-sided facial pain demonstrates enhancing soft tissue within the right PPF, extending posteriorly along the vidian nerve to the foramen lacerum. CT demonstrates replacement of normal fat density in the PPF & bony erosion & widening of the right vidian canal.* **(Bottom)** *Invasive fungal sinusitis in a chemotherapy patient is shown. Axial CT through the level of the mid-PPF demonstrates opacification of the sphenoid sinus, indicative of sinusitis. The medial wall of the vidian canal is eroded & there is abnormal soft tissue density infiltrating the PPF, consistent with invasion by fungal sinusitis.*

TERMINOLOGY

Abbreviations

- Frontal recess (FR); agger nasi cell (AN); ethmoid bulla (EB); suprabullar cell (SBC); frontal bullar cell (FBC); supraorbital ethmoid cell (SOEC); anterior ethmoidal artery (AEA)

Definitions

- **FR**: Frontal sinus drainage pathway (FSDP) (inverted funnel shape) bordered anteriorly by AN & FR Kuhn cells, posteriorly by bulla ethmoidalis, FBCs, & SBCs, & posterolaterally by SOECs

IMAGING ANATOMY

Overview

- **Frontal sinus** lies within frontal bone (right & left sinuses develop independently) with thick anterior table & thinner posterior table; medial wall intersinus septum; thin floor corresponds to anterior aspect of orbital roof
  - Thin posterior wall & floor can be eroded by mucocele
- Funnel-shaped posteroinferomedial aspect of frontal sinus (often called **frontal infundibulum**) superiorly & inverted funnel-shaped FR inferiorly likened to hourglass with its waist in between at frontal sinus ostium
- **Frontal beak (nasofrontal process)** forms floor of inferior frontal sinus & is identifier for anterior landmark of **frontal sinus ostium**
- FR formed by opposition of adjacent air cells at anteroinferior aspect of frontal bone superiorly & anterosuperior aspect of ethmoid bone inferiorly
- Upper border of FR by frontal sinus ostium; inferior drainage from FR can be either to **middle meatus** directly or via **ethmoid infundibulum**

Extent

- If uncinate process turns laterally to insert on **lamina papyracea**, FR drains into middle meatus directly, & ethmoid infundibulum is closed superiorly by blind-ending pouch called **recessus terminalis**
- If uncinate process turns medially to insert on **middle turbinate** or runs superiorly to insert on **skull base**, FR drains into ethmoid infundibulum & then middle meatus

Anatomy Relationships

- Anteriorly: AN below & Kuhn cells above
- Laterally: Lamina papyracea (or intervening AN & Kuhn cells when present)
- Posterolaterally: SOECs when present
- Medially: Middle turbinate vertical portion
- Posteriorly: EB, SBCs, & FBCs when present

Internal Contents

- **Middle & posterior portions of basal lamella of middle turbinate**: Extend laterally to join lamina papyracea & divide anterior from posterior ethmoid air cells
  - Vertical portion of basal lamella attaches to cribriform plate of ethmoid & is best seen in coronal CT; very delicate, & its detachment at surgery in this region could damage dura with resultant CSF leak
  - EB, SBCs, & FBCs are intramural anterior ethmoid air cells anterior to basal lamella of middle turbinate & form posterior boundary of FR
  - Posterior margin of basal lamella attaches to perpendicular plate of palatine bone
- **EB (bulla ethmoidalis)**: Dominant anterior ethmoid air cell formed by pneumatization of bulla lamella (seen anterior to basal lamella of middle turbinate)
  - Forms lateral margin of ethmoid infundibulum & posterior margin of FR
- **SBCs**: Anterior ethmoid cells seen above EB; extends behind FR but lies entirely below level of frontal sinus ostium (no extension into frontal sinus)
  - SBC superior wall: **Skull base**
  - CT correlate of suprabullar recess; seen as cleft above EB when viewed endoscopically
- **Suprabullar & retrobullar recesses**: Previously less correctly called **sinus lateralis** or **lateral sinus of Grunwald**
  - Located between ethmoid roof superiorly, EB anteriorly & inferiorly, lamina papyracea laterally, & basal lamella of middle turbinate posteriorly
  - Recesses typically separated by bony crest or mucosal projection from basal lamella of middle turbinate to EB
  - Recesses communicate medially with middle meatus through hiatus semilunaris superior
  - Suprabullar recess separated from FR by bulla lamella/EB reaching & attaching to skull base; 2 recesses do not typically communicate with FR
  - FR may rarely drain directly into suprabullar recess when bulla lamella/EB does not extend to skull base
  - **AEA** at roof of suprabullar recess in majority (85%)
- **FBCs**: Anterior ethmoid cells above EB; extends behind FR & **also into frontal sinus** above frontal sinus ostium
  - FBC posterosuperior wall: **Skull base**
- Both SBCs & FBCs may be mistaken for skull base during endoscopic surgery → incomplete surgical dissection
  - SBC/FBC presence should be determined before surgery by assessing preoperative scans
- **SOECs**: Anterior ethmoid air cells extending superolaterally over orbit from FR & seen posterolateral to FR
  - Posterior wall: **Skull base**
  - Pneumatization of orbital plate of frontal bone posterior to frontal sinus & posterolateral to FR
  - SOEC ostium can be mistaken for frontal sinus ostium during functional endoscopic sinus surgery (FESS)
  - Transillumination of **SOECs** with telescope during FESS shows transmitted **light in inner canthal area**, while that of frontal sinus shows light in supraorbital area
  - Drain into lateral aspect of FR; SOEC ostium seen just anterior to AEA canal on sequential coronal CT images
  - **SOECs** can be mistaken for **septated frontal sinus** on coronal images
  - **SOECs** can be differentiated by their location posterior to frontal sinus separated by **horizontally oriented septum** on **axial** images
  - **AEA** runs in **anterior ethmoidal notch (foramen)** along medial orbital wall (lamina papyracea); crosses anterior ethmoid air cells in bony **anterior ethmoidal canal**
  - AEA enters anterior cranial fossa at point in lateral lamella of cribriform plate called **ethmoidal sulcus**
  - AEA found endoscopically by tracing anterior wall of EB towards ethmoid roof; 11 mm (range 6-15 mm) behind posterior wall of FR (in suprabullar recess in 85%)

- AEA usually in contact with skull base, can be 1-3 mm below skull base within bony mesentery
- **Anterior ethmoidal canal** ~ 8 mm in length; 40% show partial or total bony dehiscence, especially inferiorly
- **AEA** runs obliquely in skull base behind anterior wall of EB where skull base turns from vertical (posterior frontal sinus wall) to horizontal (cribriform plate of ethmoid)
- **Intact bulla technique** for FR surgery can protect AEA
- If anterior wall of EB does not reach skull base with presence of suprabullar recess, then AEA may be damaged even with intact bulla technique
- **SOECs** immediately above anterior ethmoidal notch/canal/sulcus predisposes **AEA at risk during FESS**
  - AEA travels freely in ethmoid sinus/suprabullar recess
- If no SOECs, anterior ethmoidal notch/canal/sulcus abuts fovea ethmoidalis/lateral lamella of cribriform plate
  - AEA considered relatively protected during FESS
- AEA injury → rapidly enlarging retroorbital hematoma due to retraction of transected artery into orbit
- Cut AEA should be prophylactically cauterized to avoid enlarging orbital hematoma
- **Posterior ethmoidal artery** ~ 10 mm behind AEA

- **Interfrontal sinus septal cell**: Pneumatized interfrontal sinus septum; can extend into crista galli when extensive
  - Drains into medial aspect of FR
  - Can obstruct frontal sinus ostium
- **AN**: Latin for nasal mound
  - Most anterior ethmoid air cell that involves **lacrimal bone** or **frontal process of maxilla**
  - Forms anterior & lateral **boundary of FR inferiorly**
  - Key to surgical access to FR
  - Open AN & palpate with probe to identify posterior wall of frontal sinus away from & in front of AEA for good, safe visualization of frontal sinus
- **FR Kuhn cells**: Anterior & lateral **boundary of FR superiorly**
  - **Types 1-3** Kuhn cells: FR air cells seen **above AN** (type 1 single & type 2 multiple in FR, & type 3 single reaching sinus), but **type 4** single isolated cell within frontal sinus **not abutting AN**
  - Type 1: Single cell above AN
    - Posterior wall: Free partition in FR
  - Type 2: Tier of 2 or more cells above AN
    - Posterior wall: Free partition in FR
  - Type 3: Single large cell above AN; extends superiorly into frontal infundibulum/sinus proper
    - Posterior wall: Free partition in FR **& frontal sinus**
  - FBCs also extend from FR into frontal sinus & cannot be differentiated in coronal CT from type 3 Kuhn cell
  - **FBCs (posterior to FR)** sagittal CT: **Skull base** forms **posterosuperior wall**
  - **Type 3 Kuhn cells (anterior to FR)** sagittal CT: **Free partition in frontal sinus & FR** forms posterosuperior wall with air gap of frontal sinus/recess between type 3 Kuhn cells & skull base
  - Type 4: Rare, isolated cell in frontal sinus; **anterior table or floor of frontal sinus** forms anterior/inferior margin
    - Free partition in frontal sinus forms posterior wall
  - Called "cell within cell"; sometimes isolated aerated type 4 cell may be seen with opacification of surrounding diseased frontal sinus
  - **Modified Kuhn classification** defines type 3 cell as extending up from FR above frontal beak but < 50% of vertical height of frontal sinus, whereas type 4 cell extends from FR into frontal sinus > 50% of its height
- **International frontal sinus anatomy classification (IFAC)**
  - **Anterior cells**: Push FSDP medially, posteriorly, or posteromedially
    - AN, supraagger cell (corresponds to types 1 & 2 Kuhn cells) & supraagger frontal cell (corresponds to types 3 & 4 Kuhn cells))
  - **Posterior cells**: Push FSDP anteriorly
    - SBC, suprabulla frontal cell (corresponds to FBC), & SOEC
  - **Medial cells**: Push FSDP laterally
    - Frontal septal cell (corresponds to interfrontal sinus septal cell)

CLINICAL IMPLICATIONS

Clinical Importance

- Primary surgery of FR usually avoided initially; anterior ethmoid/ostiomeatal unit (OMU) primary surgery done 1st
  - To reduce risk of injury to critical structures adjacent to FR, such as orbit, AEA, & anterior skull base, & due to susceptibility of FR region to postsurgical scar formation
- Frontal sinus surgeries mostly revision procedures after failed OMU surgeries, such as uncinectomy, anterior ethmoidectomy, middle meatal antrostomy, & septoplasty
- Anterior ethmoid/OMU surgeries usually enough to clear FR & frontal sinus disease
- Small **size of FR** limits enlargement of FSDP during frontal sinus FESS & more extensive frontal sinusotomy will have to be done
- Size of FR should be evaluated on preoperative scans
- Frontal beak (nasofrontal process) anterior to frontal sinus ostium has no important structures; drilling anterior to frontal ostium with angled burr relatively safe
- Posterior margin of frontal sinus ostium should be never breached due to its close relationship with cribriform plate & anterior cranial fossa
- **Inadequate removal** of air cells in relation to FR is most common cause of failed frontal FESS: AN or other anterior (Kuhn), medial (intersinus cell), posterior (EB, SBC, FBC), or posterolateral (SOEC)
  - Residual air cells obstruct FR & also serve as scaffold for scar tissue formation
- Disease in recessus terminalis in cases where inferior FR drains into middle meatus directly (when uncinate process turns laterally to insert on lamina papyracea) can displace uncinate process medially towards FR
  - **Retained medialized uncinate process** predisposes to FR restenosis after FESS
- **Lateralized middle turbinate** amputated anterior stump may obstruct FR after FESS
- **Bolgerization**: Process of medialization of middle turbinate by surgically creating small abrasions on its medial aspect & adjacent nasal septum to correct floppy lateralized middle turbinate rather than resecting it
  - Medialized middle turbinate normal expected postsurgical finding in this scenario

CORONAL AND SAGITTAL GRAPHICS OF TYPES 1 & 2 KUHN CELLS

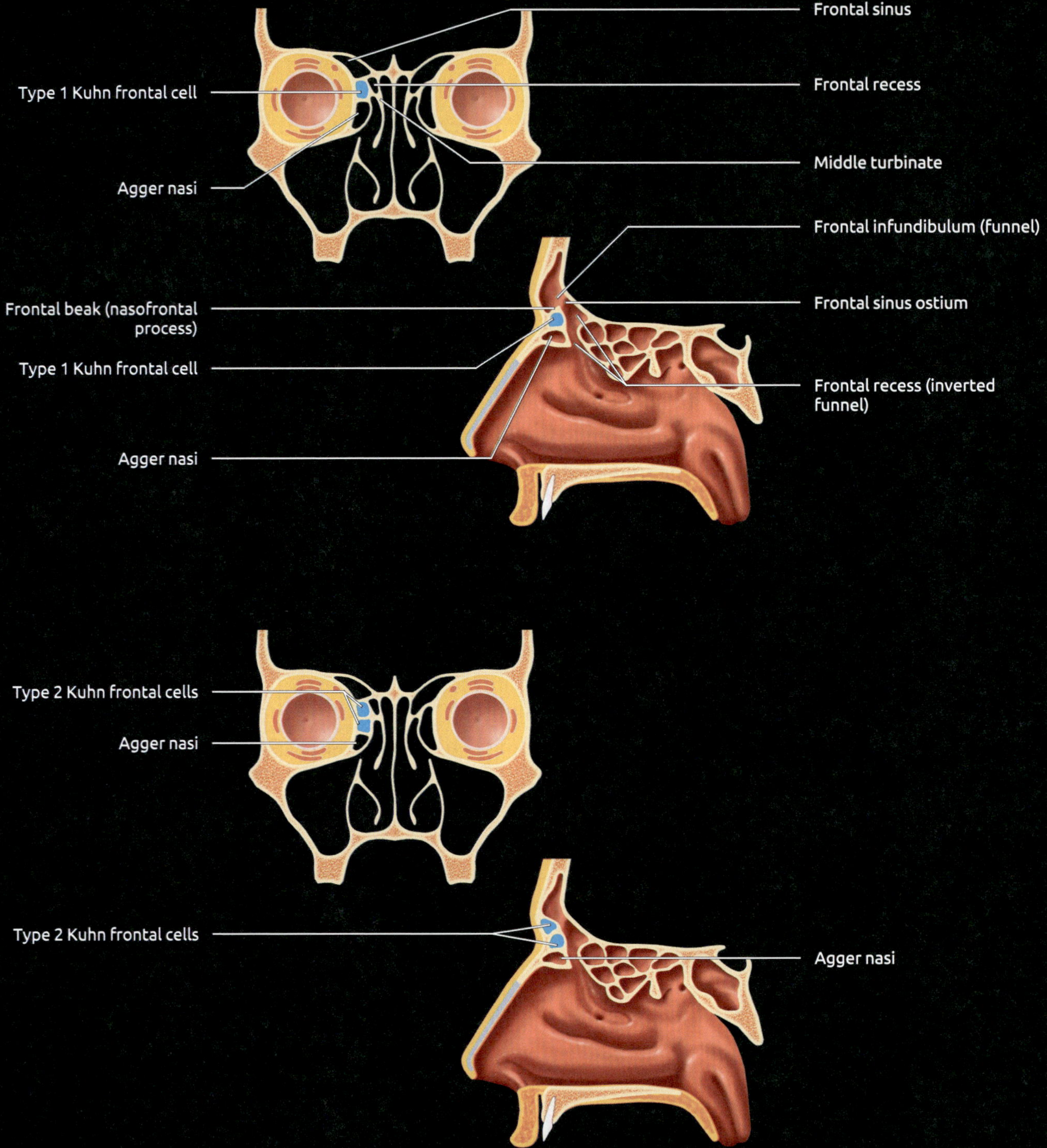

Frontal sinus
Type 1 Kuhn frontal cell
Frontal recess
Middle turbinate
Agger nasi
Frontal infundibulum (funnel)
Frontal beak (nasofrontal process)
Frontal sinus ostium
Type 1 Kuhn frontal cell
Frontal recess (inverted funnel)
Agger nasi

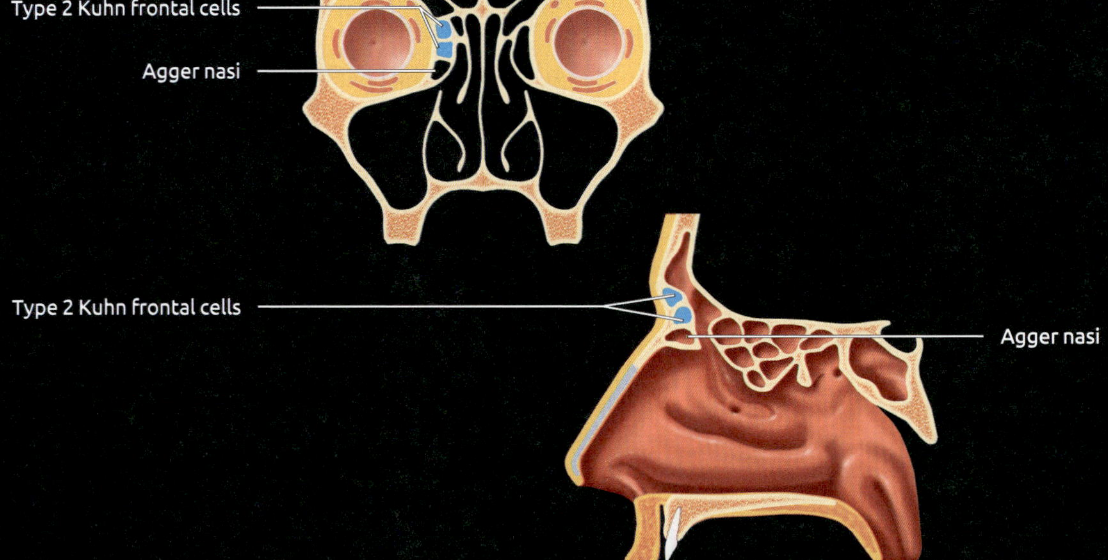

(Top) *Graphics show frontal sinus drainage pathway anatomy & a right type 1 Kuhn frontal cell (supraagger cell [SAC] as per International Frontal Sinus Anatomy Classification [IFAC]). Frontal sinus drainage is through a funnel-shaped posteroinferomedial frontal sinus (frontal infundibulum) superiorly & an inverted funnel-shaped frontal recess (FR) inferiorly; together they resemble an hourglass with a waist in between at the frontal sinus ostium. Frontal beak (nasofrontal process) forms the inferior frontal sinus floor & serves as the anterior landmark of the frontal sinus ostium. FR is bordered anterolaterally by agger nasi & FR Kuhn cells, posteriorly by bulla ethmoidalis, frontal bullar, & suprabullar cells, & posterolaterally by supraorbital ethmoid cells (SOEC). The upper border of the FR is the frontal sinus ostium, & its inferior drainage can be either directly to the middle meatus or via ethmoid infundibulum according to attachment pattern of uncinate process. Type 1 Kuhn cell is a single cell above agger nasi.* **(Bottom)** *Graphics show type 2 Kuhn cells (SAC as per IFAC), a tier of 2 or more cells above agger nasi. Posterior walls of both types 1 & 2 Kuhn cells are free partitions in the FR.*

CORONAL AND SAGITTAL GRAPHICS OF TYPES 3 & 4 KUHN CELLS

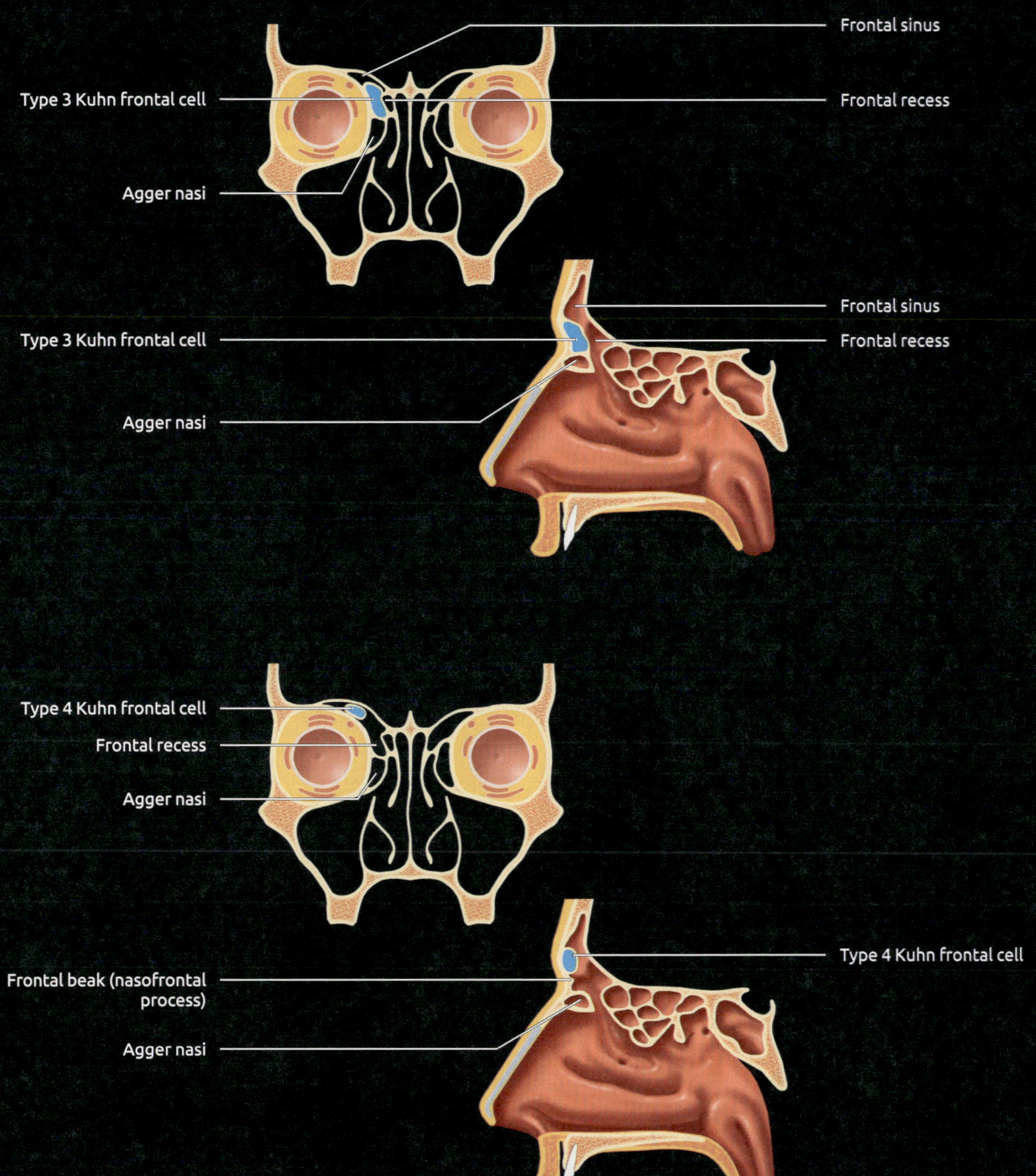

(Top) *Graphics show a type 3 Kuhn frontal cell (SAC frontal cell [SAFC] as per IFAC), a single large cell above agger nasi. It extends superiorly beyond the FR into the frontal infundibulum/sinus proper. Posterior wall of a type 3 cell is a free partition in the FR & frontal sinus.* **(Bottom)** *Graphics show a type 4 Kuhn frontal cell (SAFC as per IFAC), a rare, isolated cell in the frontal sinus. Its anterior or inferior margin is formed by the anterior table or floor of the frontal sinus, & the posterior wall is a free partition in the frontal sinus. Note that types 1-3 Kuhn cells are FR air cells seen above agger nasi (type 1 single & type 2 multiple in FR, & type 3 single reaching sinus) & form the anterior and lateral boundary of the FR superiorly, whereas type 4 is a single isolated cell within the frontal sinus not abutting agger nasi air cell.*

CORONAL AND SAGITTAL GRAPHICS OF SUPRABULLAR CELLS & BULLAR CELLS

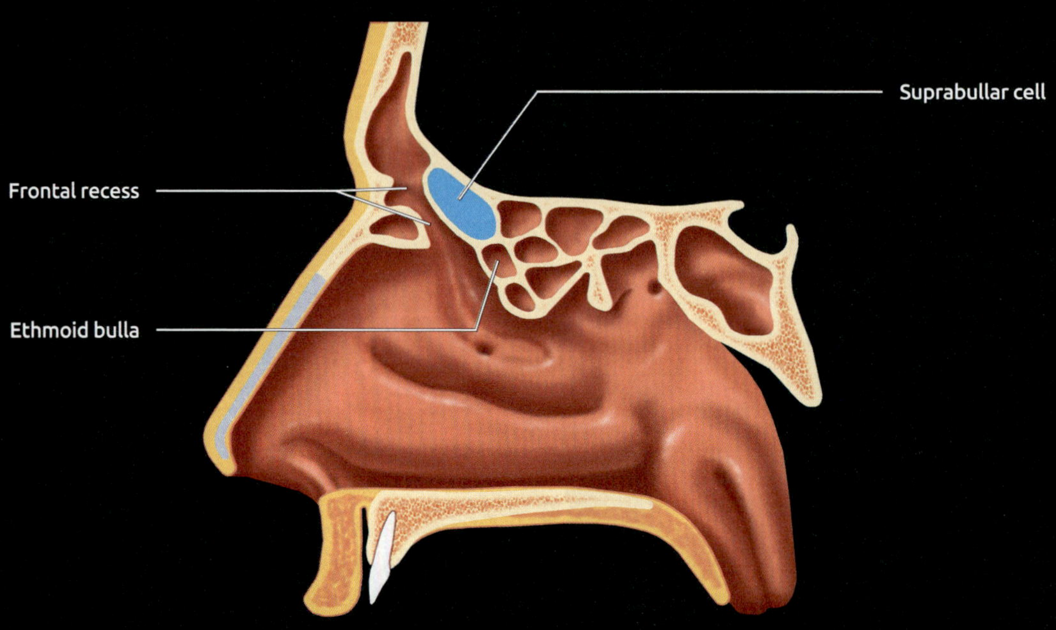

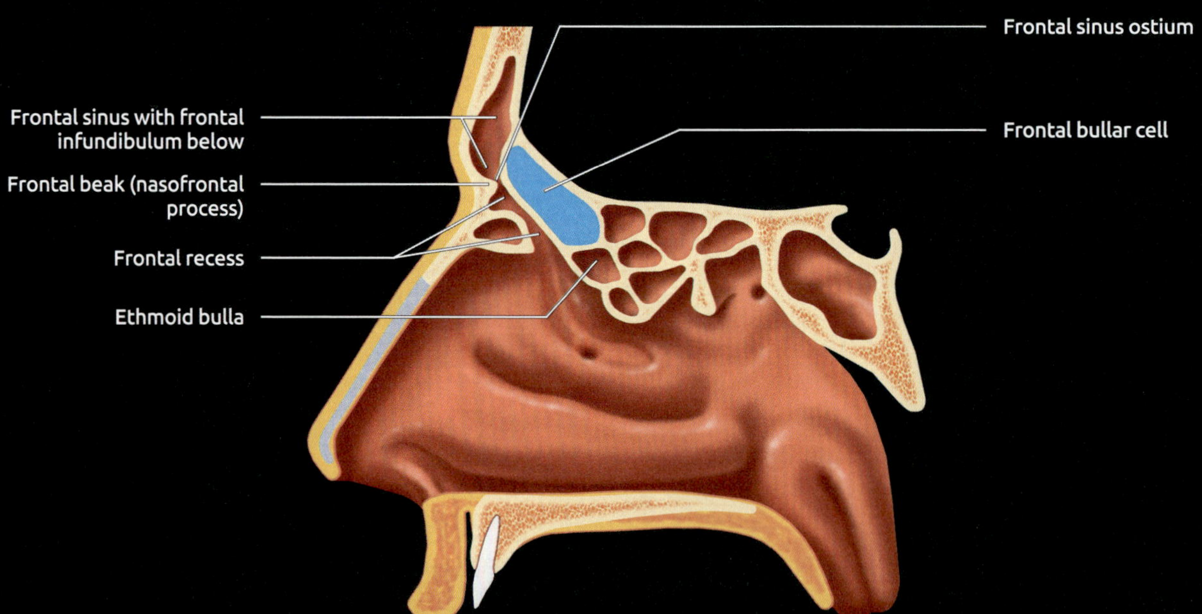

(Top) *Sagittal graphic shows a suprabullar cell ([SBC] as per IFAC), which are anterior ethmoid air cells seen above the bulla ethmoidalis extending behind the FR & lying entirely below the level of frontal sinus ostium (with no extension into the frontal sinus); its superior wall is the skull base. An SBC is the CT scan correlate of a suprabullar recess, which is seen as a cleft above the ethmoid bulla when viewed endoscopically. Suprabullar & retrobullar recesses were previously known as sinus lateralis or the lateral sinus of Grunwald. The anterior ethmoidal artery is located at the roof of the suprabullar recess in the majority (85%).* **(Bottom)** *Sagittal graphic shows a frontal bullar cell (FBC). FBCs (suprabulla frontal cell [SBFC] as per IFAC) are also anterior ethmoid air cells above the bulla ethmoidalis extending behind the FR, but unlike SBCs, extend into the frontal sinus above frontal sinus ostium; its posterosuperior wall is also the skull base. Both SBCs and SBFCs may be mistaken for the skull base during endoscopic surgery, resulting in incomplete surgical dissection. Their presence should be determined before surgery by assessing preoperative scans.*

CORONAL GRAPHICS

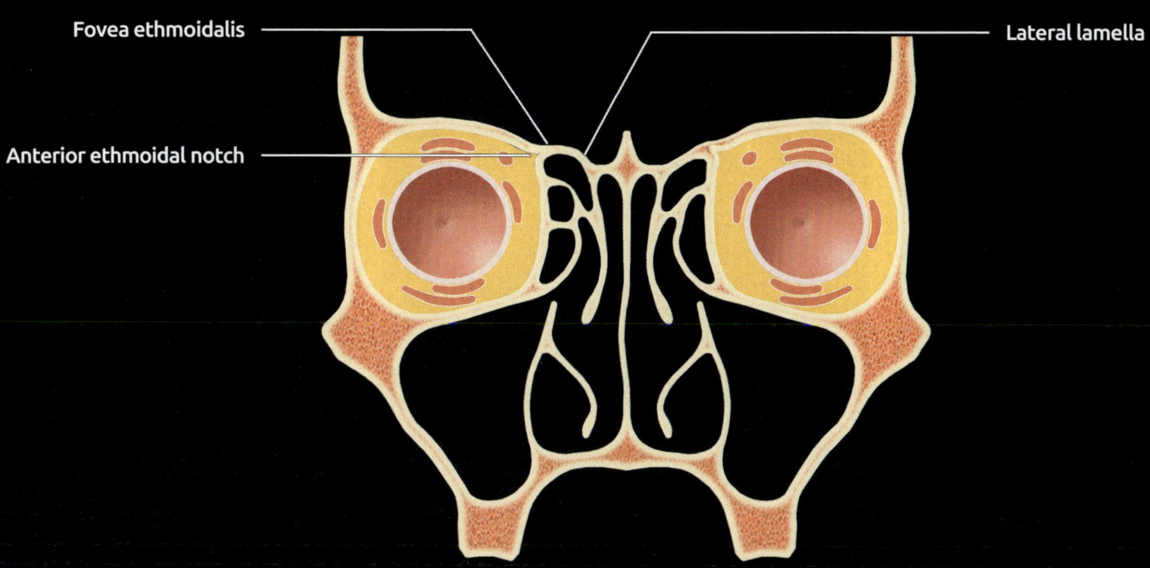

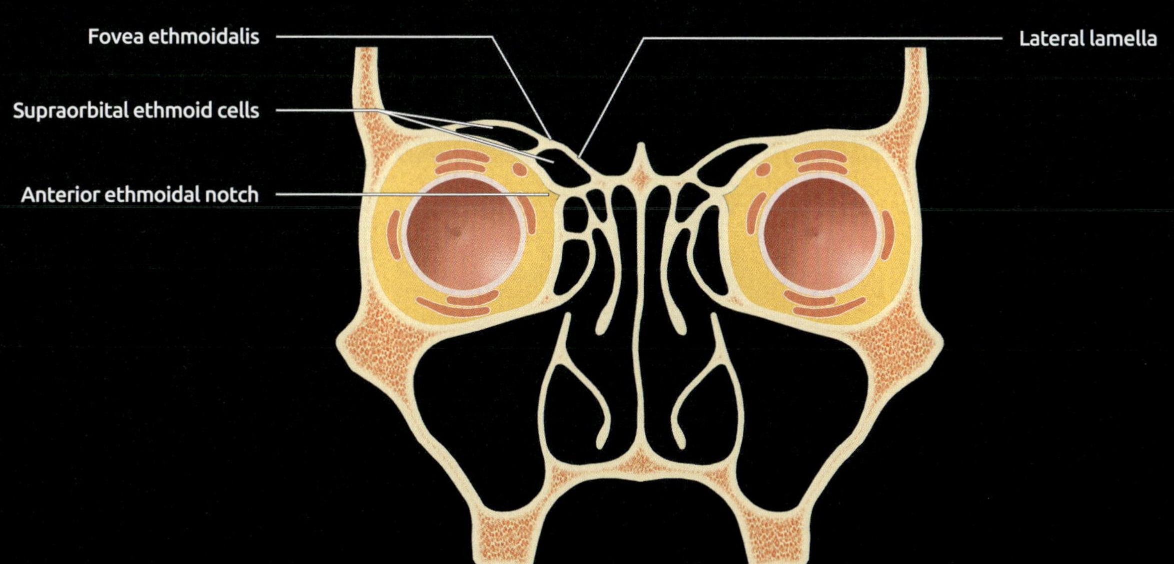

(Top) *Coronal graphic shows the anterior ethmoidal notch/canal/sulcus (containing the anterior ethmoid artery) abutting the fovea ethmoidalis/lateral lamella of the cribriform plate. The anterior ethmoid artery is considered relatively protected during functional endoscopic sinus surgery (FESS) with this anatomy.* **(Bottom)** *Coronal graphic shows supraorbital ethmoid cells [(SOECs) as per IFAC] immediately above the anterior ethmoidal notch/canal/sulcus. This anatomy predisposes anterior ethmoid artery injury risk during FESS, since the artery travels freely within the air cells, ethmoid sinus/suprabullar recess. SOECs are anterior ethmoid air cells that extend superolaterally over the orbit from the FR & are seen posterolateral to the FR. They are formed by pneumatization of the orbital plate of the frontal bone posterior to the frontal sinus & posterolateral to FR. SOECs drain into the lateral aspect of the FR; SOEC ostium is seen just anterior to the anterior ethmoidal artery canal in sequential coronal CT images. The ostium can be mistaken for the frontal sinus ostium during FESS.*

SAGITTAL AND CORONAL BONE CT

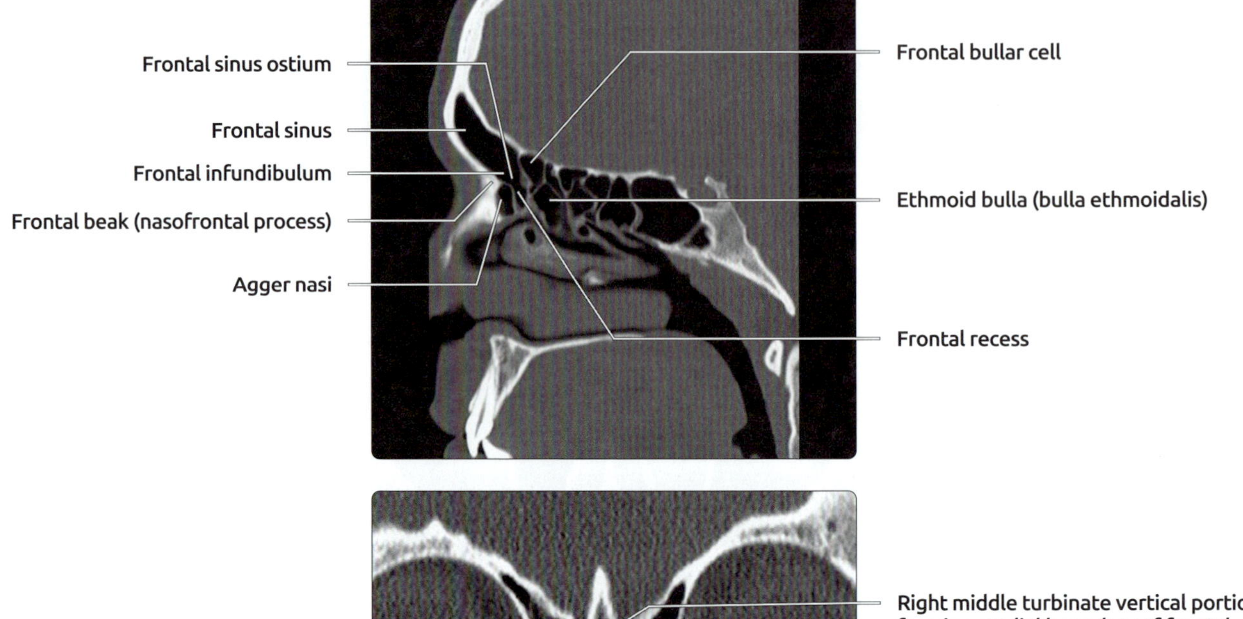

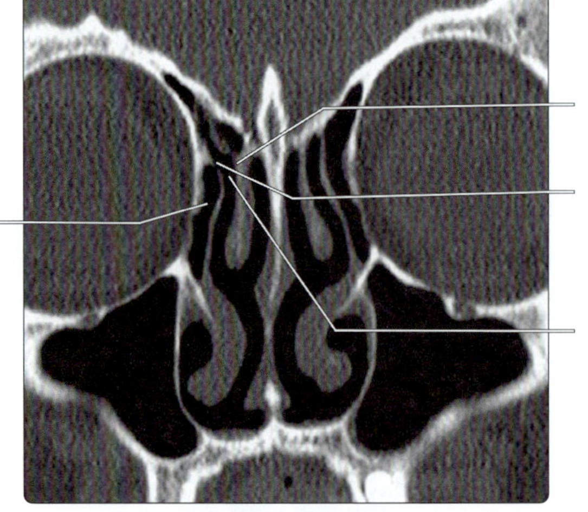

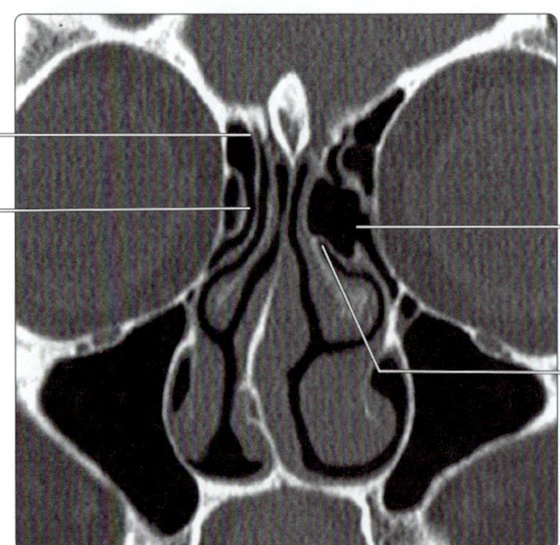

(Top) *Sagittal CT shows the frontal sinus drainage pathway, which is likened to an hourglass with the superior part formed by the funnel-shaped posteroinferomedial frontal sinus & inferior part by the inverted funnel-shaped FR; the waist of the hourglass is at frontal sinus ostium level. The frontal beak (the nasofrontal process) is the anterior landmark of the frontal sinus ostium. The FR is bordered anterolaterally by agger nasi & Kuhn cells (no Kuhn cells are present here).* **(Middle)** *Coronal bone NECT shows inferior drainage of the FR. If the uncinate process (UP) turns laterally to insert on the lamina papyracea, the FR drains into the middle meatus directly, & the ethmoid infundibulum is closed superiorly by a blind-ending pouch called "recessus terminalis," as seen on the right side of this patient.* **(Bottom)** *Coronal bone NECT shows inferior drainage of the FR. If the UP runs superiorly to insert on the skull base (labeled on the right side of this patient) or turns medially to insert on middle turbinate (labeled on left side of this patient), the FR drains into the ethmoid infundibulum & then the middle meatus.*

SAGITTAL BONE CT

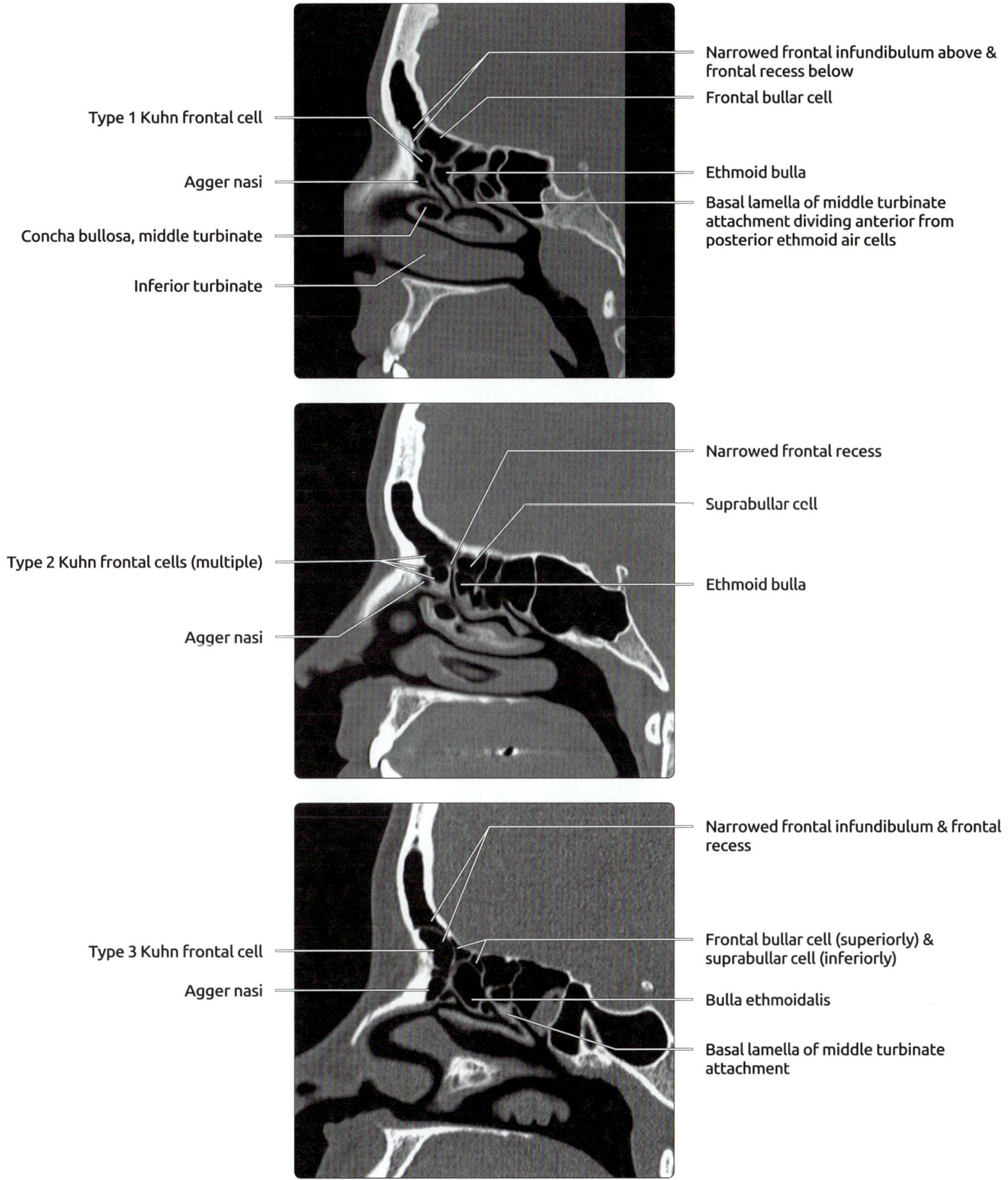

(Top) *Sagittal CT shows a type 1 Kuhn cell, a single cell above agger nasi.* **(Middle)** *Sagittal CT shows type 2 Kuhn frontal cells. Kuhn cells form the anterior & lateral boundary of the superior aspect of FR. Types 1-3 Kuhn cells are FR air cells just above agger nasi, but type 4 is a single, isolated cell within the frontal sinus not abutting agger nasi. Type 1 is single & type 2 are multiple cells in the FR, whereas a type 3 cell is a single air cell in FR extending superiorly into the frontal infundibulum/frontal sinus proper.* **(Bottom)** *Sagittal CT shows a type 3 Kuhn frontal cell. Its posterior wall is a free partition in FR & frontal infundibulum/frontal sinus & can narrow these structures from the anterior aspect. In contrast, the frontal bullar cell narrows the FR & frontal infundibulum/frontal sinus from its posterior aspect; a suprabullar cell narrows only the FR from the posterior aspect.*

SAGITTAL & CORONAL BONE CT

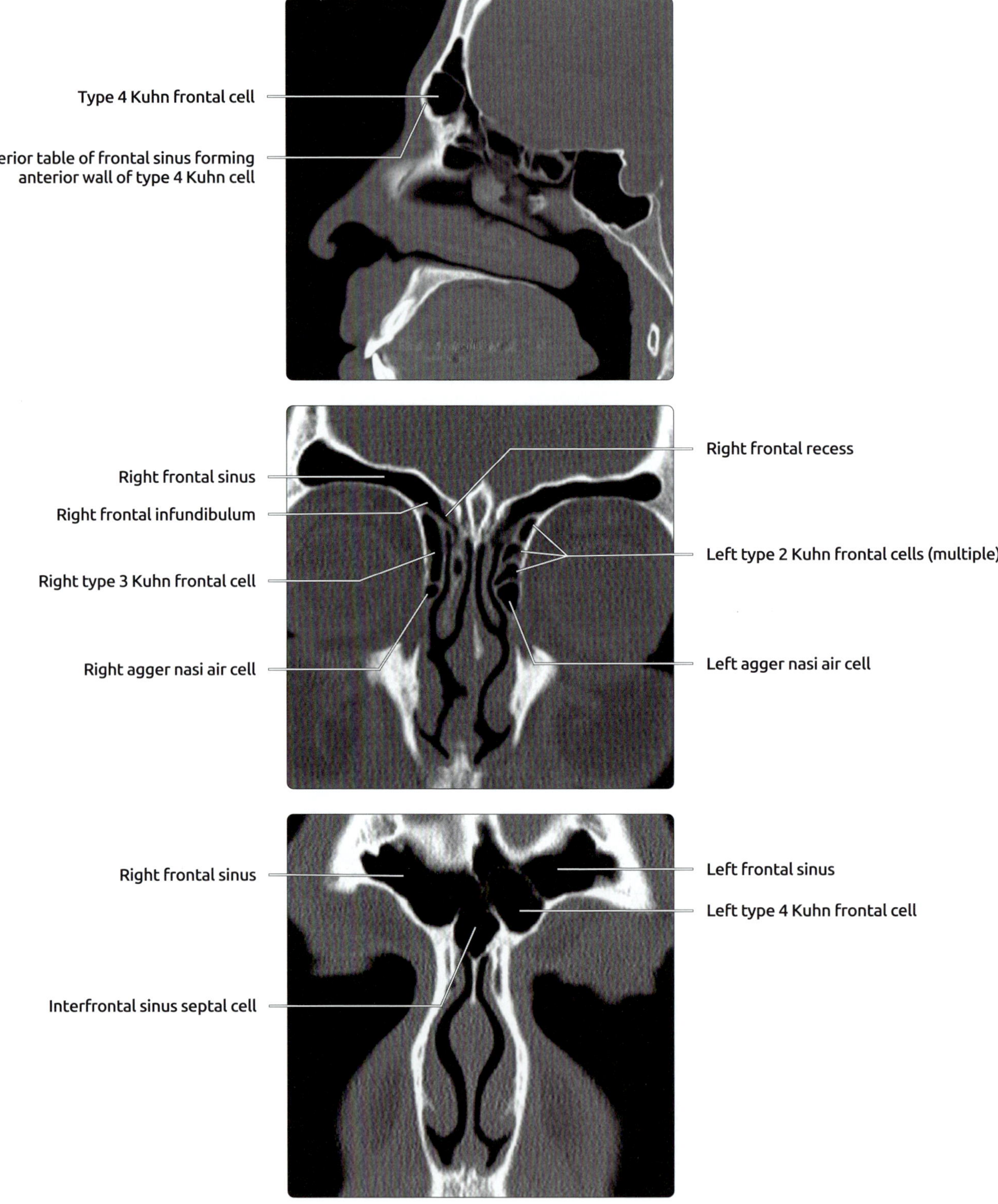

(Top) *Sagittal CT shows a type 4 Kuhn cell, a rare, isolated cell in the frontal sinus. Its anterior/inferior margin is the anterior table/floor of the frontal sinus; the posterior wall is a free partition in that sinus. Note that the Modified Kuhn classification defines a type 3 cell as extending up from the FR above the frontal beak but < 50% of vertical height of the frontal sinus, whereas a type 4 cell extends from the FR into the frontal sinus > 50% of its height.* **(Middle)** *Coronal bone NECT shows a right type 3 FR Kuhn cell extends superiorly beyond the FR into the frontal infundibulum/sinus proper, & multiple left type 2 FR Kuhn cells lie below the frontal sinus ostium. Types 1-3 Kuhn cells lie lateral to the FR, just above agger nasi.* **(Bottom)** *Coronal bone NECT shows an interfrontal sinus septal cell (frontal septal cell [FSC] as per IFAC); it can extend into crista galli when extensive, drains into the medial aspect of the FR, & can obstruct the frontal sinus ostium. Also shown is a left type 4 Kuhn cell.*

SAGITTAL & CORONAL BONE CT OF FRONTAL BULLAR CELL TYPE 3 KUHN CELL

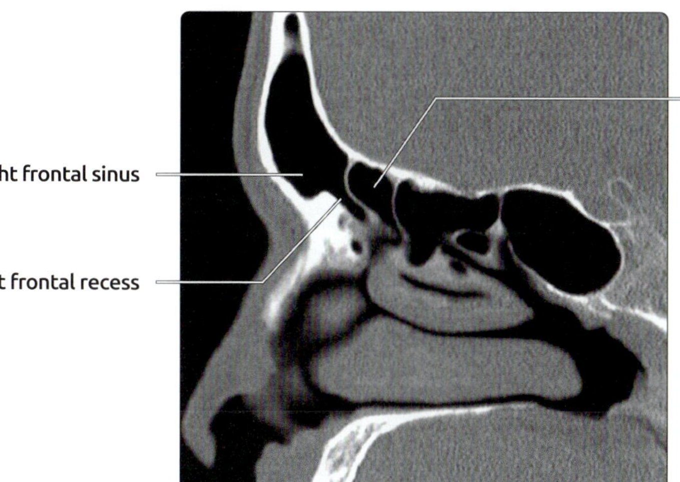

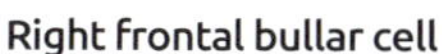

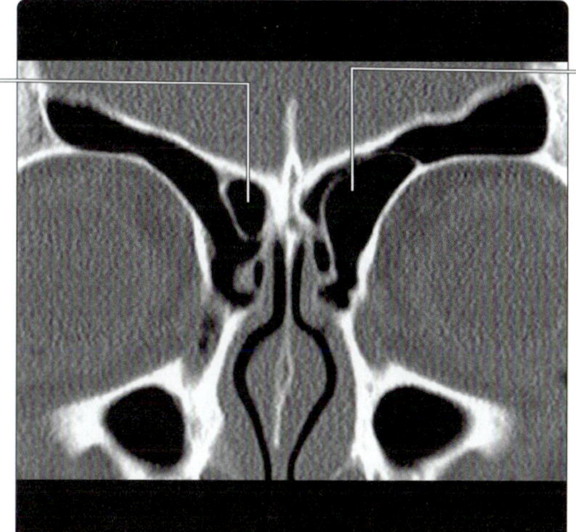

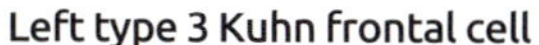

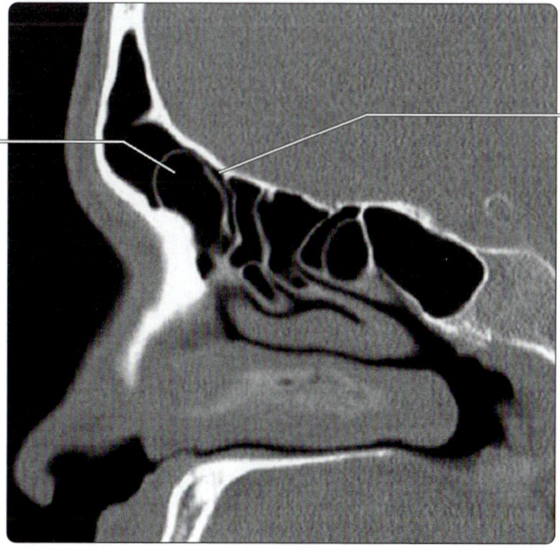

(Top) *Right parasagittal bone NECT shows a right FBC. On sagittal images, the posterosuperior wall of an FBC (posterior to frontal sinus/recess) is formed by the skull base.* **(Middle)** *Coronal NECT in the same patient shows a right FBC (confirmed by right parasagittal CT images) & a larger left type 3 Kuhn cell (confirmed by evaluating left parasagittal CT images). Both extend from the FR into the frontal sinus & cannot be differentiated on coronal CT.* **(Bottom)** *Left parasagittal bone NECT in the same patient shows a left type 3 Kuhn cell. On sagittal images, the posterosuperior wall of a type 3 Kuhn cell (anterior to the frontal sinus/recess) is a free partition in the FR & frontal sinus with an air gap of the frontal sinus/recess between it & the skull base.*

CORONAL BONE CT

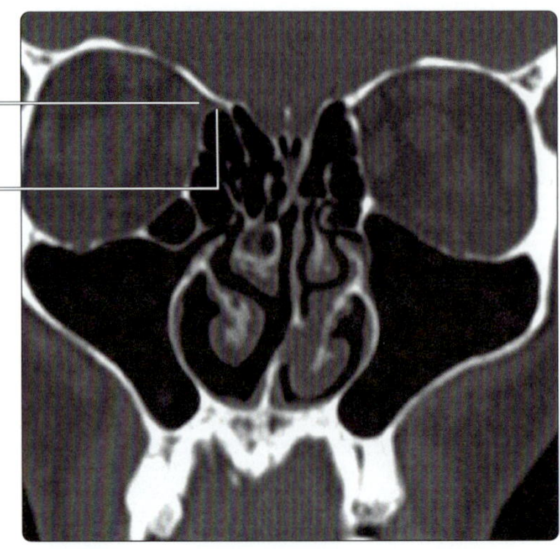

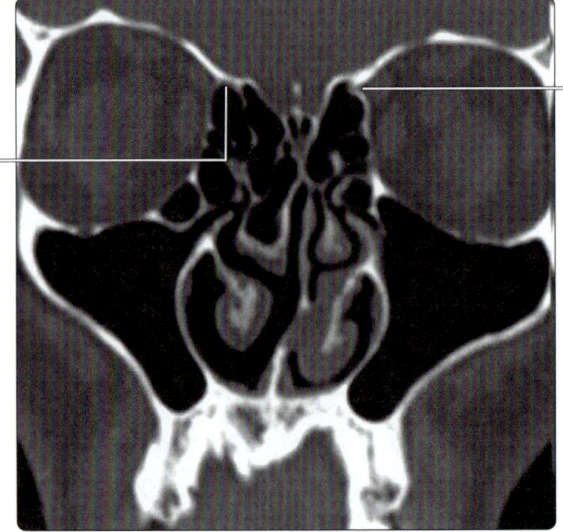

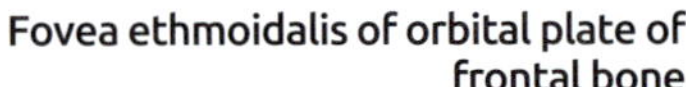
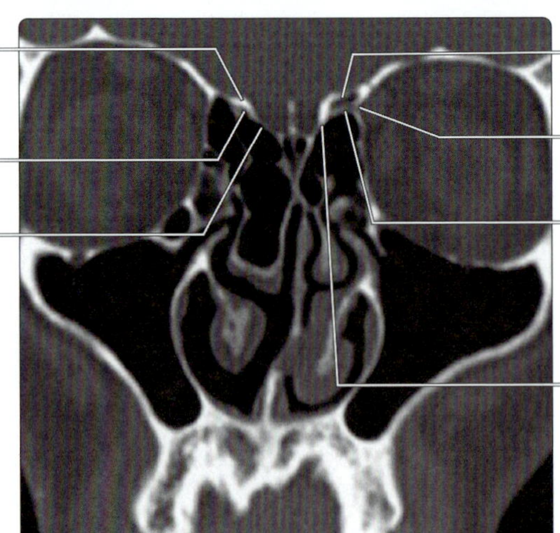

(Top) *The 1st of 3 coronal CT images presented from posterior to anterior shows the course of the anterior ethmoidal arteries that run in the "anterior ethmoidal notch" along the medial orbital wall, crossing anterior ethmoid cells in the anteromedial oblique bony canal called the "anterior ethmoidal canal," & then entering the anterior cranial fossa at a point in the lateral lamella of the cribriform plate (near its junction with fovea ethmoidalis) called the "ethmoidal sulcus." The anterior ethmoidal canal is ~ 8 mm long with 40% showing some bony dehiscence & lies ~ 11 mm (range: 6-15 mm) behind the posterior wall of the FR (in the suprabullar recess in 85%). It is usually in contact with the skull base (right side in this patient), but is sometimes 1-3 mm below the skull base within a bony mesentery (left side). The anterior ethmoidal artery usually lies well posterior to the anterior wall of the ethmoid bulla, so the "intact bulla" technique for FR surgery can protect it to some extent.* **(Middle)** *The 2nd coronal CT shows the course of the anterior ethmoidal arteries.* **(Bottom)** *The 3rd coronal CT shows the course of the anterior ethmoidal arteries.*

AXIAL, SAGITTAL, & CORONAL BONE CT

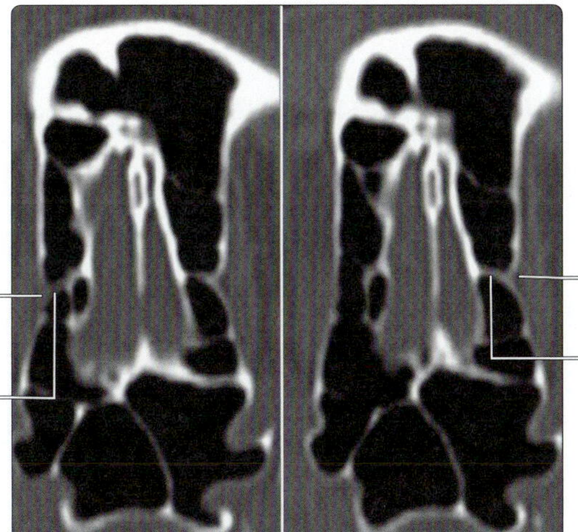

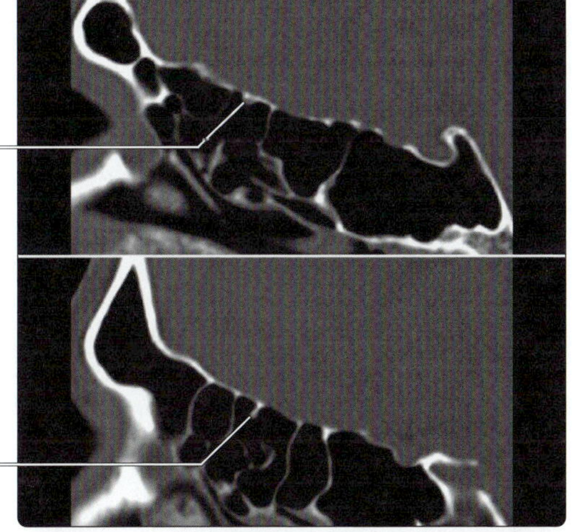

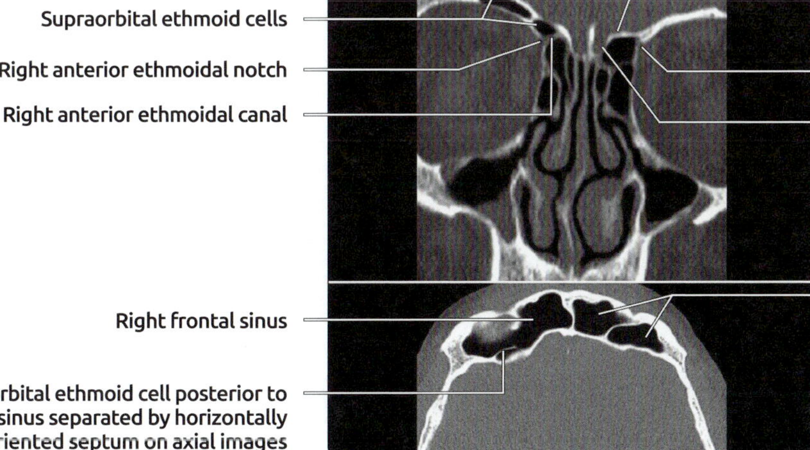

(Top) *Axial CT images in the same patient show bilateral anterior ethmoidal notches & canals containing anterior ethmoidal arteries.* **(Middle)** *Sagittal CT images in the same patient show the right anterior ethmoidal canal in contact with the skull base, & the left canal hanging down a few millimeters below the skull base within a bony mesentery. The posterior ethmoidal artery lies ~ 10 mm posterior to the anterior ethmoidal artery.* **(Bottom)** *Coronal bone NECT shows SOECs immediately above the anterior ethmoidal notch/canal/sulcus on the right; this predisposes anterior ethmoid artery injury at FESS. The anterior ethmoid artery is relatively safer in this patient on the left side without SOECs where the anterior ethmoidal notch/canal/sulcus abuts the fovea ethmoidalis/lateral lamella. SOECs can mimic a septated frontal sinus on coronal CT, but axial CT shows its location posterior to the frontal sinus, separated by a horizontally oriented septum. Note that the left frontal sinus septation is anteroposteriorly/obliquely oriented.*

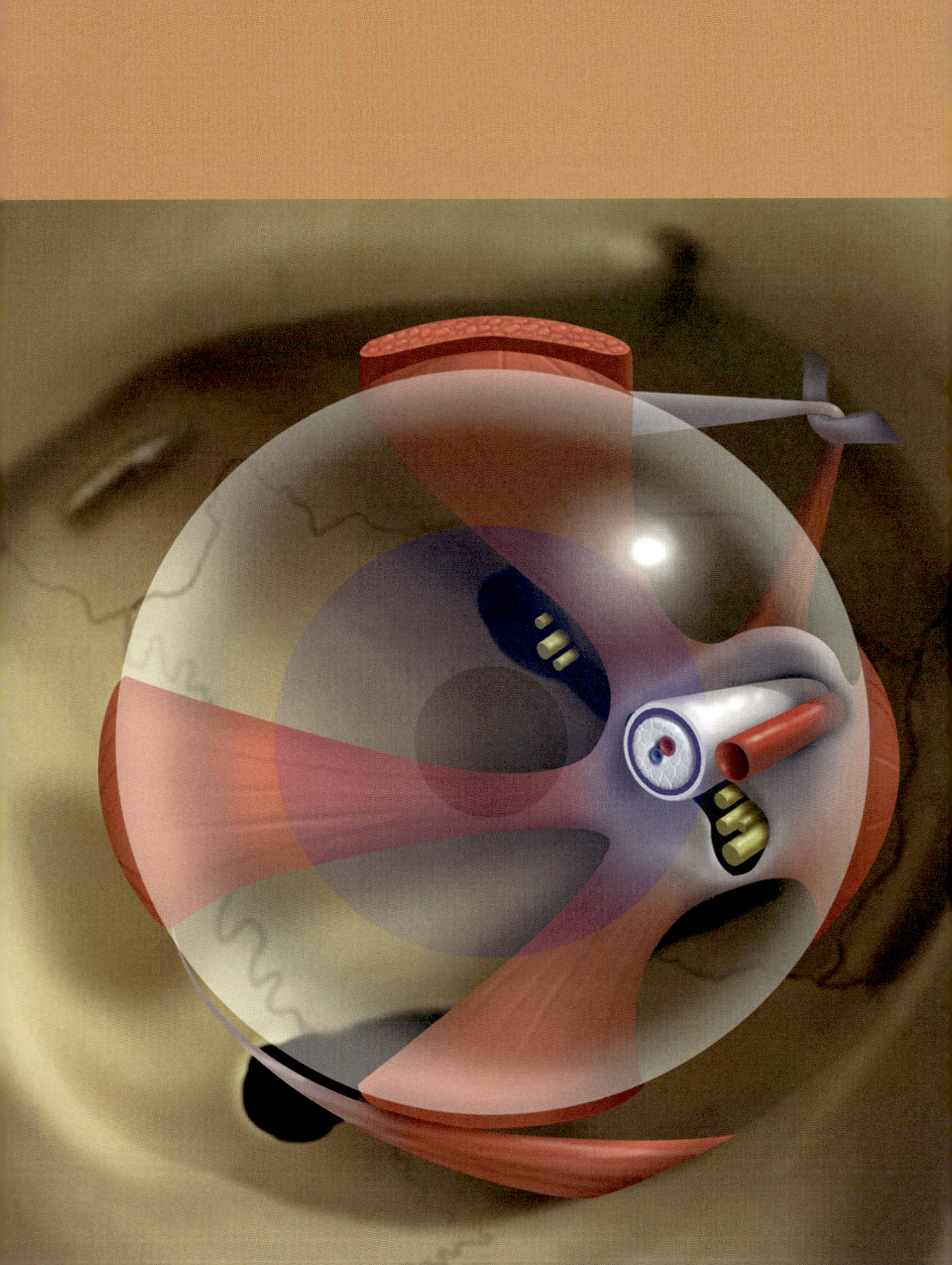

SECTION 3
Orbit

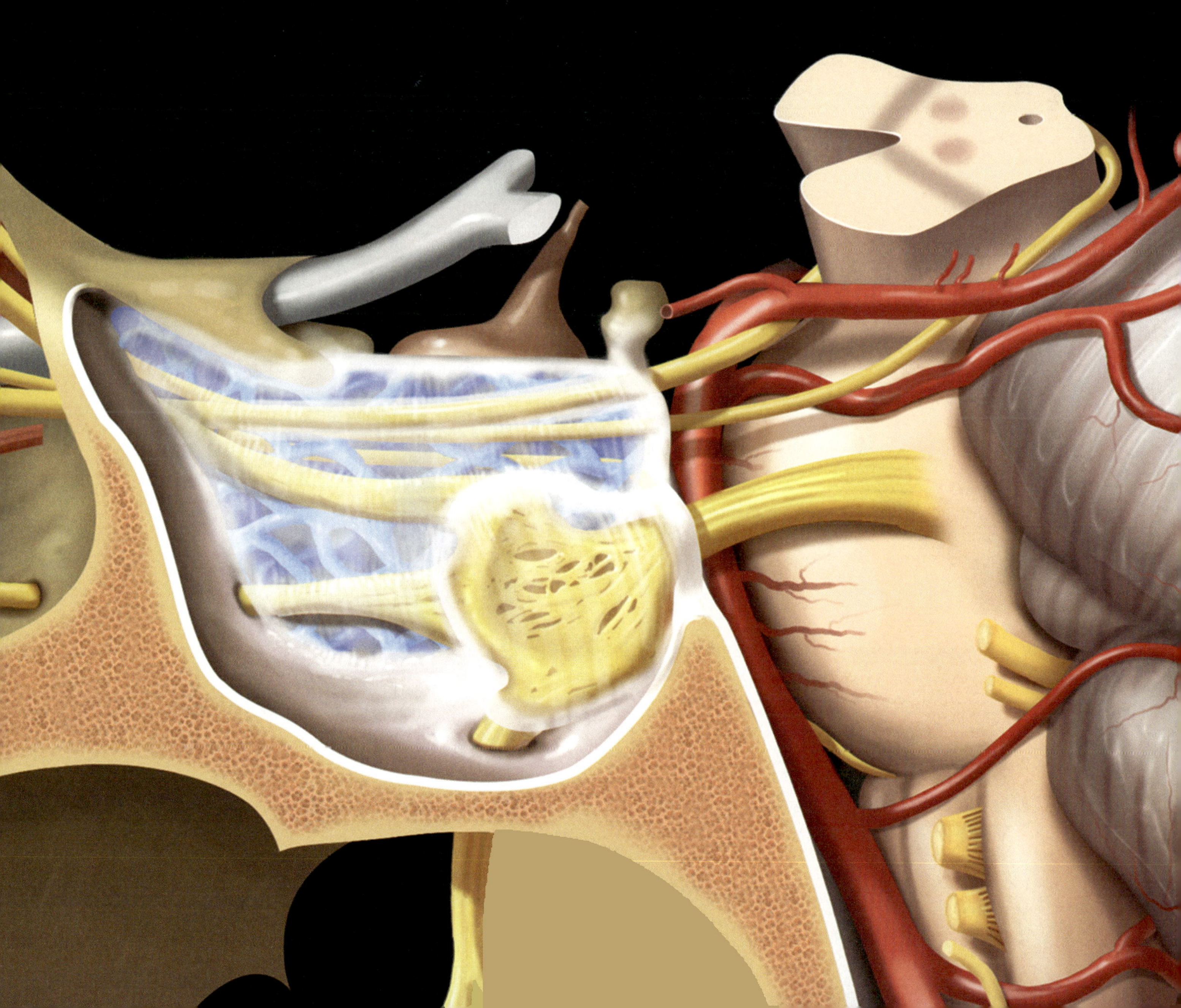

TERMINOLOGY

Abbreviations

- Cranial nerves
  - Optic nerve (CNII)
  - Oculomotor nerve (CNIII)
  - Trochlear nerve (CNIV)
  - Trigeminal nerve (CNV)
    - Branches (V1, V2, and V3)
  - Abducens nerve (CNVI)
- Orbital structures
  - Superior ophthalmic veins (SOV), inferior ophthalmic veins (IOV)
  - Superior orbital fissures (SOF), inferior orbital fissures (IOF)
  - Extraocular muscles (EOM)
  - Ophthalmic artery (OphA)

IMAGING ANATOMY

Overview

- Each orbit consists of conical-shaped bony cavity or socket (bony orbit) and its internal contents that extend from eyelids anteriorly to orbital apex posteriorly
- Orbit contains globe and intraorbital optic nerve
- Also contains lacrimal gland, EOM, various nerves (motor, autonomic, and sensory), fat, arteries, and veins

Extent

- Margins of orbit largely determined by bony orbital walls arranged in cone or pyramid shape
- Ventral aspect of orbit (or base) formed by orbital rim peripherally and soft tissues centrally; anterior soft tissue margin defined by orbital septum
- 7 different bones that contribute to bony orbit
  - Roof of orbit: Sphenoid and frontal bones
  - Medial wall: Formed from lesser wing of sphenoid bone, ethmoid bone, lacrimal bone, and frontal process of maxilla (FPM)
  - Orbital floor: Formed from sphenoid bone, orbital process of palatine bone, and orbital process of maxillary bone
  - Lateral wall: Greater wing of sphenoid bone near apex and frontal and zygomatic bones anteriorly toward face
- Size and extent of orbit influenced by age, race, and sex of individual
  - Height of orbit measured anteriorly at rim: ~ 3.5 cm
  - Width of orbit: ~ 4 cm
  - Medial orbital wall measures ~ 4.5 cm from rim to apex
  - Lateral wall shorter than medial wall, measuring ~ 3.5 cm
  - Volume of each orbit variable but ranges 16-30 cm^3

Anatomy Relationships

- Orbit superior to maxillary sinus and lateral to ethmoid sinus
- Roof of orbit forms floor of anterior cranial fossa
- Apex of orbit is at transition zone between anterior skull base and central skull base

Internal Contents

- **Globe**
  - Occupies 1/3 of volume of orbit
  - Spherical organ of vision; functions in refraction of light so that photons focused on retina
  - Retina specialized layer of globe that contains neurons sensitive to light
  - Uveal tract consists of choroid (posterior) and ciliary body and iris (anterior)
  - Globe is mobile and maneuvered by EOMs
- **CNII (optic nerve)**
  - Transmits nerve impulses from retina to visual center of brain
  - Arises from posterior margin of globe at optic disc
  - Contains nerve fibers from nerve cells in retina
  - Covered by pia, arachnoid, and dura
- **EOMs**
  - Responsible for movement of eye
    - Lateral and medial rectus are pure abductor and pure adductor, respectively
    - Other EOMs have component of torsion that must be coordinated with other EOM
  - Most EOMs arise from annulus of Zinn and insert upon globe
  - Inferior rectus originates from anterior floor of orbit, not annulus
  - Levator palpebrae superioris originates from annulus but inserts on upper eyelid, not globe
  - Have similar density on CT and similar signal on MR as other skeletal muscle
  - Demonstrate prominent gadolinium enhancement on MR
  - **Superior rectus**
    - Located at upper aspect of orbit, inferior to levator palpebrae muscle
    - Originates from superior rim of annulus
    - Primary function upward gaze, rotation of superior margin globe posteriorly
    - Innervated by CNIII (oculomotor)
  - **Medial rectus**
    - Located along medial orbital wall, just lateral to lamina papyracea
    - Originates along medial aspect of annulus and attaches to medial margin of globe
    - Medial rectus rotates medial margin of globe posteriorly allowing for medial gaze
    - Innervated by CNIII (oculomotor)
  - **Lateral rectus**
    - Located along lateral orbital wall
    - Originates along lateral margin of of annulus and attaches to lateral margin of globe
    - Contraction results in posterior rotation of lateral margin of globe for lateral gaze
    - Innervated by abducens CNVI (abducens)
  - **Inferior rectus**
    - Located along floor of orbit
    - Originates along inferior margin of annulus and attaches to inferior margin of globe
    - Rotates inferior margin of globe posteriorly for downward gaze
    - Innervated by CNIII (oculomotor)
  - **Superior oblique**
    - Origin at medial margin of annulus of Zinn

- Passes through trochlea at superomedial rim of bony orbit
- Inserts posterolaterally on sclera superiorly
- Rotates globe inferiorly
- Innervated by CNIV (trochlear nerve)
- **Inferior oblique**
  - Origin at anteroinferior orbital rim
  - Insertion posterolaterally on sclera inferiorly
  - Rotates eye superiorly
  - Innervated by CNIII (oculomotor)
- **Levator palpebrae superioris**
  - Unlike other EOMs, does not attach to or move globe
  - Origin at annulus of Zinn
  - Courses above superior rectus, divides in 2
  - Superior aponeurosis insertion at upper eyelid
  - Inferior Müller insertion at tarsal plate
  - Elevates upper eye lid
  - Innervated by CNIII (oculomotor)

- **Orbital fat**
  - Occupies ~ 50% of orbital volume
  - Functions to stabilize globe, cushion globe, and facilitates movement of intraorbital structures
  - Fat can be divided into intraconal (behind globe and within conical boundaries of rectus muscles) and extraconal components
  - Normal orbital fat density on CT and fat signal on MR allow for delineation of most important intraorbital structures
- **Intraorbital nerves**
  - CNII: Optic nerve represents collection of axons derived from retinal ganglion cells that transmit visual information from retina to brain
  - CNIII: Motor to medial, superior and inferior recti, and levator palpebrae; parasympathetic motor to iris
  - CNIV: Motor to superior oblique
  - CNVI: Motor to lateral rectus
  - CNV: Sensory from orbit and eyelids (V1)
- **OphA**
  - Major arterial supply of orbit
  - 1st intradural branch of internal carotid artery (ICA); measures 0.7- to 1.5-mm diameter at origin
  - Typical origin just above distal dural ring
  - **Variant origin**: 1-2% originate from middle meningeal artery; < 1% originate from cavernous ICA
  - OphA courses along inferolateral optic canal, piercing proximal dural sleeve of CNII laterally
  - Intraorbital course
    - At apex (1st segment), passes along inferolateral aspect on CNII
      - Then passes medially (becoming 2nd segment), most often **over** CNII
      - Finally extends forward (3rd segment) in medial aspect of orbit, medial to CNII
  - OphA branches can be classified into ocular, orbital, extraorbital, and dural branches
  - **Ocular** branches include **central retinal artery**, lateral posterior ciliary artery, and medial posterior ciliary artery
    - These arteries arise near junction of 1st and 2nd segments of intraorbital OphA
  - **Orbital** branches include muscular and lacrimal
  - **Extraorbital**: Supraorbital, anterior and posterior ethmoidal, palpebral, dorsal nasal, and supratrochlear branches
  - **Dural**: Recurrent branches of OphA, one superficial and other deep, course back through SOF and supply dura of cavernous sinus
- **Ophthalmic veins**
  - **SOV**
    - Formed by confluence of angular vein and supraorbital vein at medial margin of supraorbital rim
    - Passes by trochlea and medial to superior oblique muscle, crosses anterior portion of CNII, and passes posteriorly along superolateral border of CNII
    - Extends through SOF before draining into cavernous sinus
  - **IOV**
    - Smaller and more variable than SOV
    - Located just superior to inferior rectus
    - Usually anastomoses with SOV but may drain into cavernous sinus directly or drain through IOF into pterygoid venous plexus
- **Connective tissue and supporting structures**
  - **Periorbita**
    - a.k.a. orbital periosteum or orbital fascia
    - Dense connective tissue membrane that covers inner margins of bones of orbit, serves as attachment for muscles, tendons, and ligaments
    - Continuous anteriorly with periosteal covering of facial bones
    - Continuous posteriorly through orbital foramina and fissures with periosteal layer of dura mater
    - Posteriorly, periorbita thickens to form fibrous ring that encircles optic nerve canal and portions of SOF, annulus of Zinn
    - Attached loosely to underlying bone except at orbital margins, along sutures, and at edges of fissures and foramina
  - **Annulus of Zinn**
    - Tendinous ring formed by thickened periorbita at apex of orbit
    - Ring passes over optic nerve canal and partially encircles medial aspect of SOF
    - 4 rectus and superior oblique muscles and levator palpebrae superioris arise from annulus
    - CNIII (upper and lower divisions of oculomotor), CNVI (abducens), and nasociliary branch of ophthalmic division of CNV (trigeminal) all enter apex of orbit through annulus of Zinn
    - CNII (optic nerve) also passes through annulus as nerve passes through optic canal
  - **Tenon capsule**
    - Dense elastic and vascular fibrous connective tissue that surrounds globe and separates globe from retrobulbar fat
    - Extends from insertion site of optic nerve to margins of cornea
    - Capsule separated from episclera by loose potential space providing smooth inner surface; allows for ocular motility
    - EOMs must penetrate capsule before inserting on globe

- **Orbital septum**
  - Thin anterior band of connective tissue arising from orbital periosteum of orbital rim
  - Orbital septum attaches to orbital margin at "arcus marginale," thickening where periorbita joins periosteum
  - Inserts into levator palpebrae aponeurosis, superior tarsal plate (upper lid), and inferior tarsal plate (lower lid)
  - Essentially separates orbital contents from lid structures
  - Location inferred on routine CT and MR scans
  - High-resolution MR scans can occasionally demonstrate septum
- **Tarsal plates**
  - Dense connective tissue that adds rigidity to upper and lower eyelids
  - Contain large sebaceous glands (meibomian glands)
- **Lateral canthal ligament**
  - Anchors tarsal plates of both lids to zygomatic bone laterally at Whitnall tubercle
- **Medial canthal ligament (medial canthal tendon)**
  - Medial tendinous attachment of orbicularis oculi and upper and lower tarsal plates
  - Anchor primarily at anterior lacrimal crest (ALC), located on FPM
- **Whitnall ligament (superior transverse ligament)**
  - Primary suspensory support for upper lid found at intersection of muscular and aponeurotic portions of levator palpebrae
  - Extends from trochlea medially to lateral orbit wall
  - Attaches to levator aponeurosis and superior rectus muscle as well as conjunctiva and Tenon capsule
  - May function as fulcrum for levator palpebrae superioris
  - Passes between orbital and palpebral lobes of lacrimal gland
- **Intermuscular transverse ligament (ITL)**
  - Also originates from trochlea and inserts into lateral orbital wall on deeper part of Whitnall ligament
  - ITL passes only behind palpebral lobe
- **Lockwood ligament**
  - Thickened lower part of Tenon capsule
  - Serves as suspensory ligament for globe
  - Blends with lateral canthus and lateral check ligament laterally and attaches to lacrimal crest medially

- **Müller muscle**
  - Sympathetically innervated smooth muscle that functions as upper eyelid retractor
  - Extends from inferior aspect of levator palpebra muscle to superior edge of tarsal plate, posterior to levator aponeurosis
- **Nasolacrimal apparatus**
  - **Lacrimal gland**
    - Orbital lobe: Larger, lies in bony fossa at anterior aspect of superotemporal orbit
    - Palpebral lobe: Smaller, lies inferiorly, separated by levator aponeurosis
  - Drainage via puncta at medial lower lids → canaliculi → lacrimal sac → nasolacrimal duct
  - **Lacrimal fossa and lacrimal sac**
    - Lacrimal fossa formed by thick ALC of FPM and thin posterior lacrimal crest (PLC) of lacrimal bone
    - Lacrimal sac lies within lacrimal fossa, invested by superficial and deep parts of orbicularis oculi muscle
    - Lacrimal sac below medial canthal tendon not covered by muscle, potential site of weakness for intraorbital spread of infection
    - Medial orbital septum and check ligament of medial rectus muscle attach posterior to PLC of lacrimal bone
      - Hence, lacrimal fossa and lacrimal sac preseptal structures

ANATOMY IMAGING ISSUES

Questions

- Approach to orbital lesions
  - Localize to region and involved structures
    - Globe: Intraocular vs. transscleral
    - Optic nerve vs. nerve-sheath complex
    - Intraconal vs. conal vs. extraconal orbit
    - Lacrimal gland: Unilateral vs. bilateral (systemic)
    - Isolated vs. multifocal vs. transspatial process
    - Intracranial: Direct extension vs. secondary
  - Assess CT, MR, &/or ultrasound characteristics
    - Solid or cystic; heterogeneity
    - Fluid, fat, blood, or soft tissue
    - Bony remodeling vs. destruction
    - Well defined vs. infiltrative
    - Degree and homogeneity of enhancement

Imaging Recommendations

- CT
  - Axial + coronal planes; thin sections (≤ 2 mm)
  - Multislice isovoxel acquisition with MPR
  - Soft tissue algorithm; bone in at least 1 plane
  - Excellent evaluation of orbit aided by natural contrast between fat, bone, air, and soft tissues
  - Easily detects calcifications
  - Noncontrast CT alone for thyroid orbitopathy
  - Bone windows for evaluation of fracture, hyperostosis, or permeative changes
- MR
  - Optimal soft tissue contrast for globe, optic nerve, orbital structures, and intracranial findings
  - Stronger gradients, faster sequences, surface coils, fat suppression + gadolinium improve image quality
  - Axial: Above orbital roof to orbital floor
  - Coronal: Back of pons through globe
  - Thin section (3-4 mm); small FOV (12-16 cm)
  - T1 precontrast (axial + coronal)
  - STIR or T2 FSE fat saturation (axial + coronal)
  - T1 C+ fat saturation (axial + coronal)
  - Routine postcontrast brain MR protocol usually inadequate to evaluate ON and sheath; need thinner sections and fat saturation
- Ultrasound
  - 1st-line modality for intraocular lesions
  - Noninvasive, readily available

BONY ORBIT

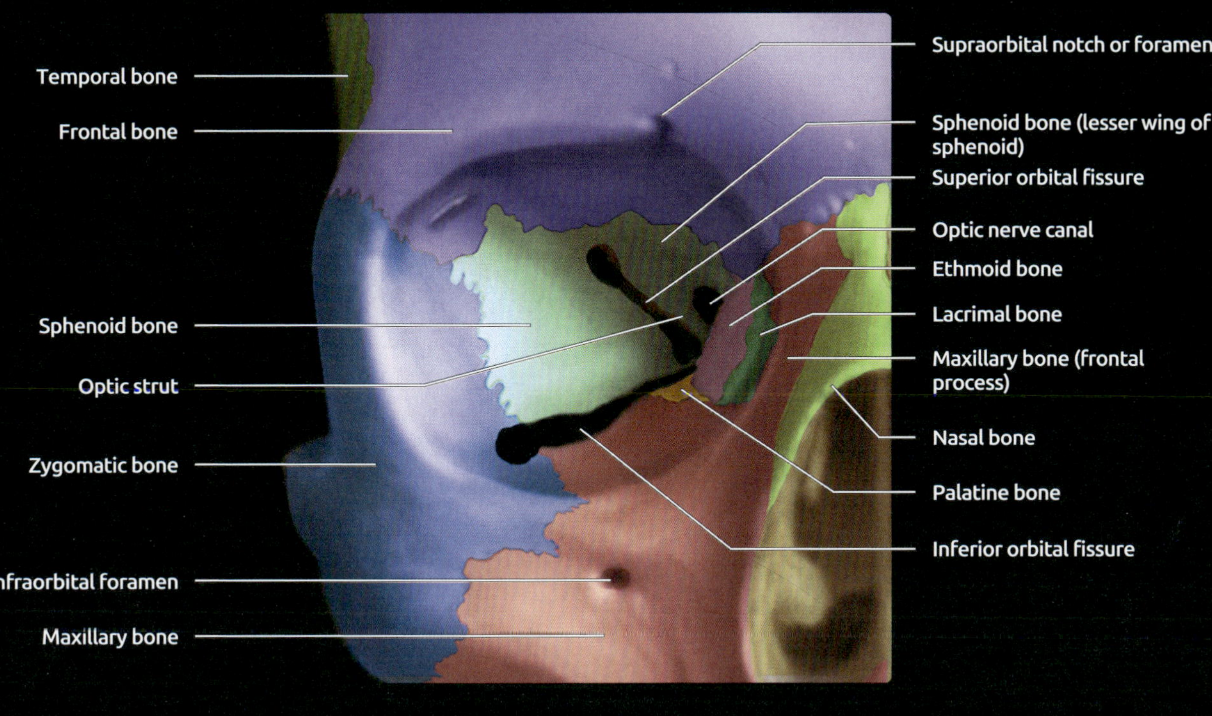

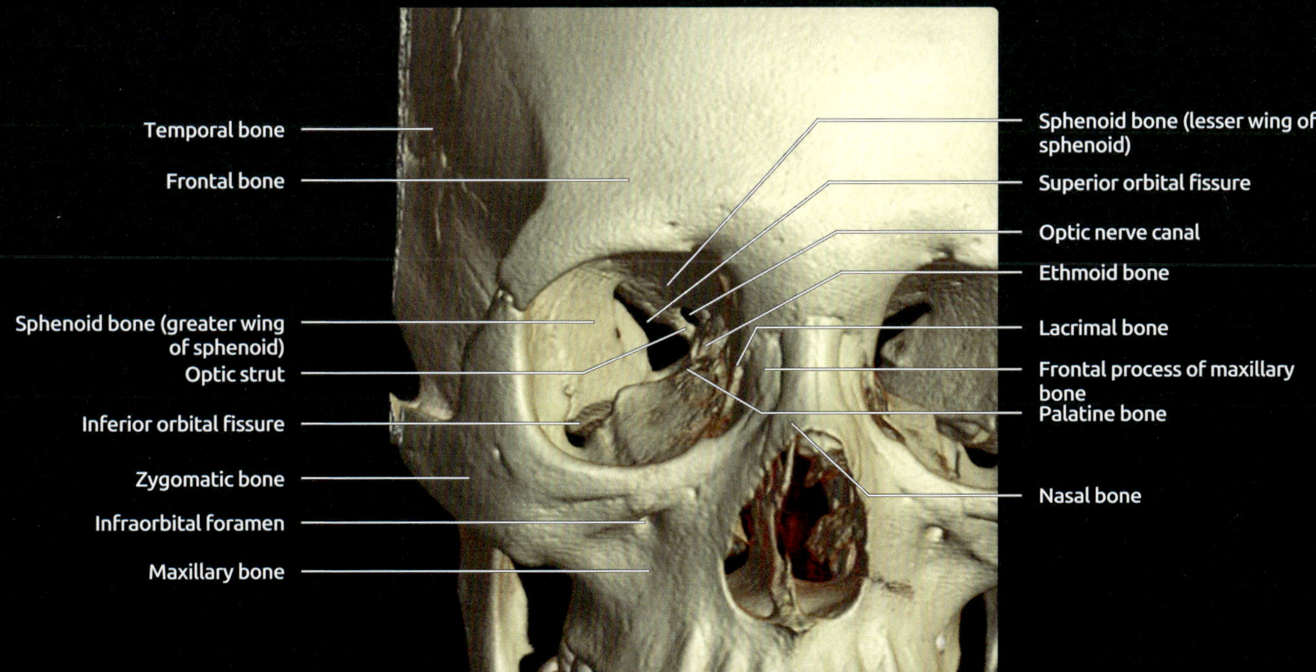

(Top) *Frontal graphic shows the bones of the right orbit. A total of 7 embryologically distinct bones contribute to the bony orbit (lacrimal, ethmoid, palatine, maxillary, zygomatic, sphenoid, and frontal bones). The sphenoid bone has greater and lesser sphenoid wings. The complex orbital fissures and optic canal at the apex are formed largely by the wings of the sphenoid bone and associated relationships. Notice that the optic canal has the lesser wing of sphenoid and ethmoid bone components.* **(Bottom)** *Oblique frontal projection through the right orbit demonstrates the 3D characteristics of the cone-shaped bony confines of the orbit and illustrates several of the important foramina and fissures. Notice that the optic canal is separated from the superior orbital fissure by the optic strut.*

GRAPHIC AND AXIAL STIR MR

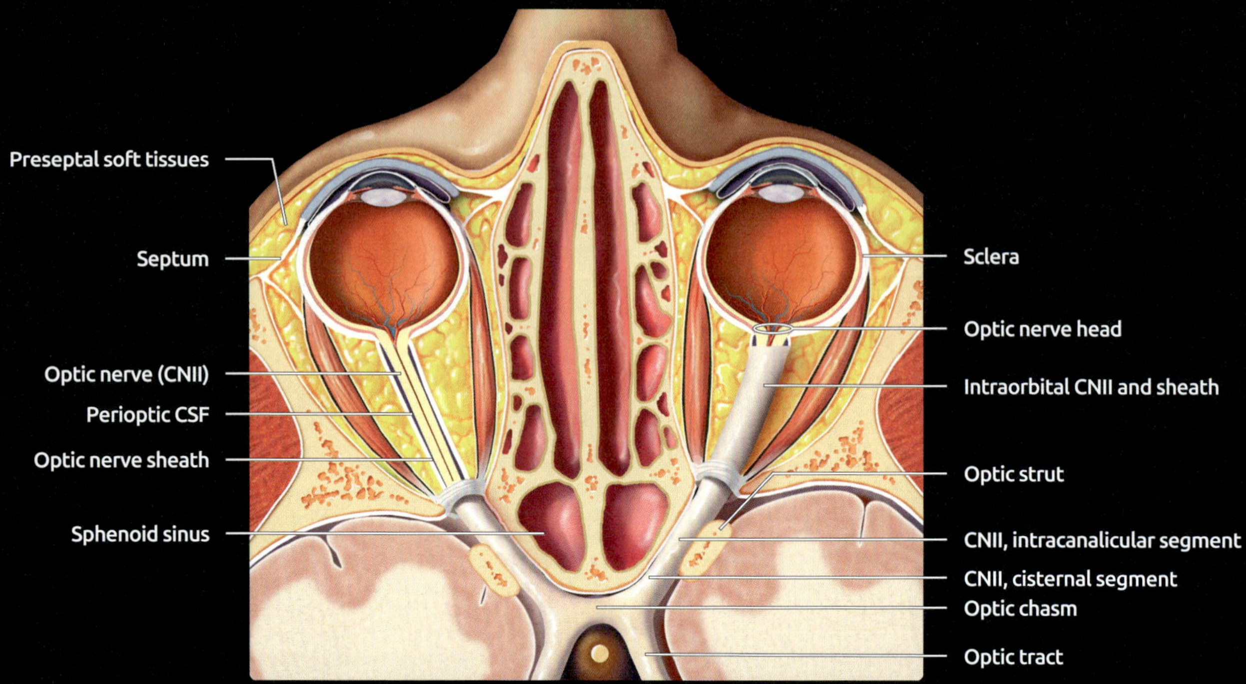

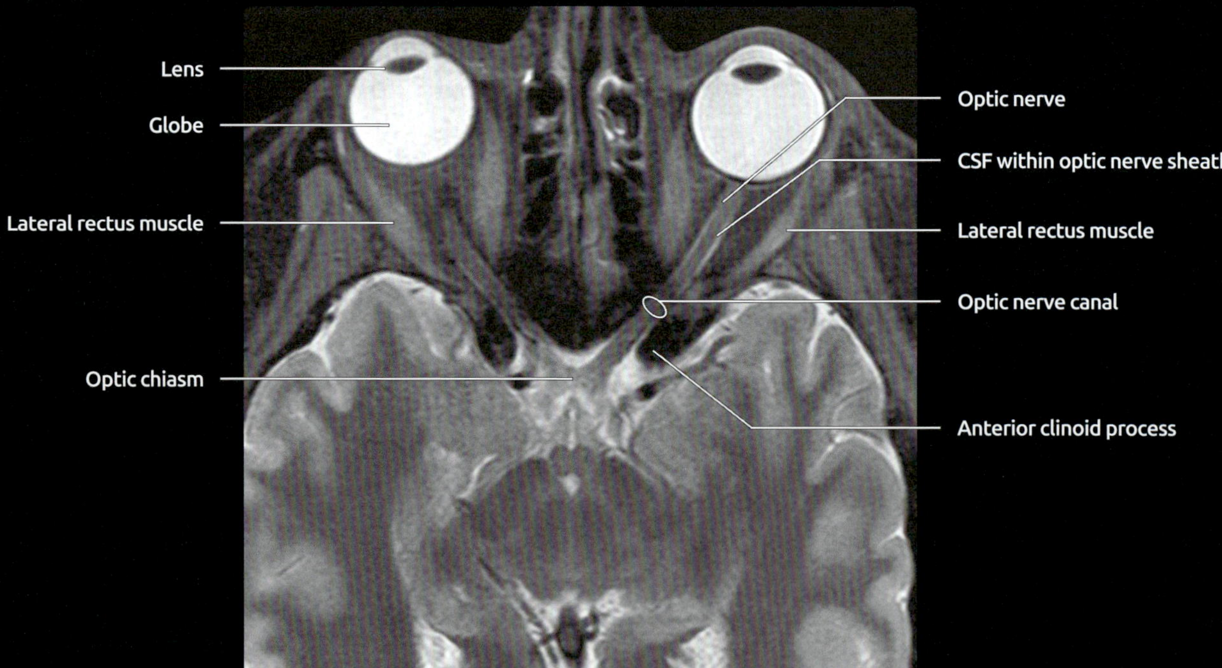

(Top) *Axial graphic shows the intraorbital and intracranial segments of CNII. The extraaxial optic pathways can be segmented (posterior to anterior) into the optic tract, optic chiasm, cisternal nerve, intracanalicular nerve, and intraorbital nerve. The optic sheath is a dural reflection that is contiguous with intracranial dura mater. Optic glioma, optic melanoma, and retinoblastoma may all follow the orbital segment of the optic nerve to reach intracranial structures.* **(Bottom)** *Axial STIR MR through the level of the optic nerves is shown. In this sequence, the fat is suppressed so that all fat is hypointense. Fluid signal is hyperintense. Muscle is intermediate in signal.*

GRAPHICS AND OBLIQUE SAGITTAL T1 MR

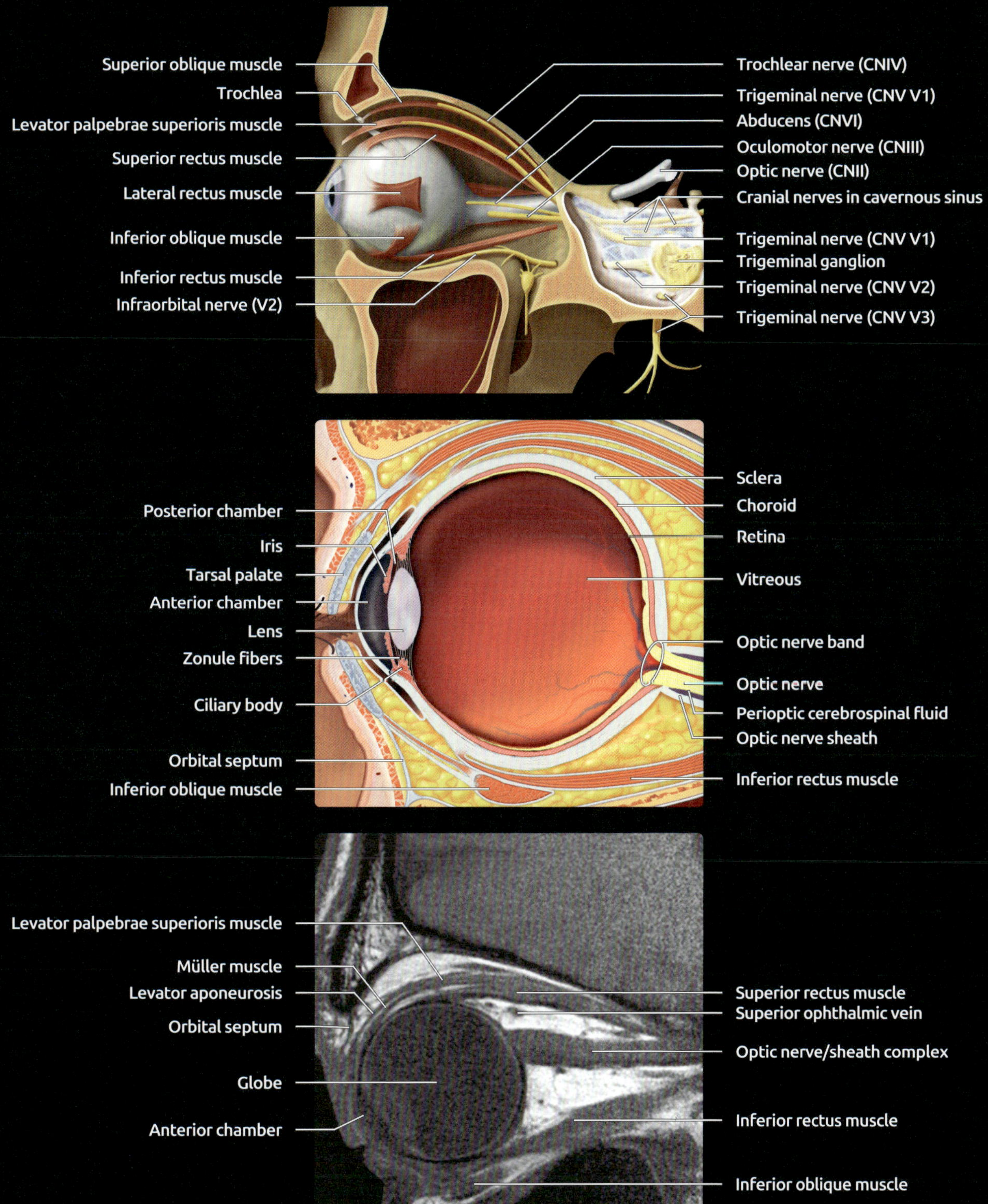

(Top) *Lateral graphic of the left orbit is shown. Intricate mechanics and innervation of the extraocular muscles provide for complementary and complex control of eye motion. CNII-VI enter the orbit via the complex foramina.* **(Middle)** *Sagittal graphic reveals an anterior segment composed of anterior and posterior chambers, which are contiguous through the pupil. The choroid, ciliary body, and iris comprise the uveal tract. The posterior segment is filled by the vitreous chamber. The retina and sclera are contiguous with the optic nerve and sheath, respectively, at the nerve head.* **(Bottom)** *Oblique sagittal T1 MR at the midorbit shows the intimate relationship between the superior oblique and levator palpebrae superioris muscles. The distinct division of the Müller muscle and levator aponeurosis anteriorly is evident. Inferiorly, the inferior oblique muscle is seen in oblique cross section, distinct from the inferior rectus muscle.*

EXTRAOCULAR MUSCLES

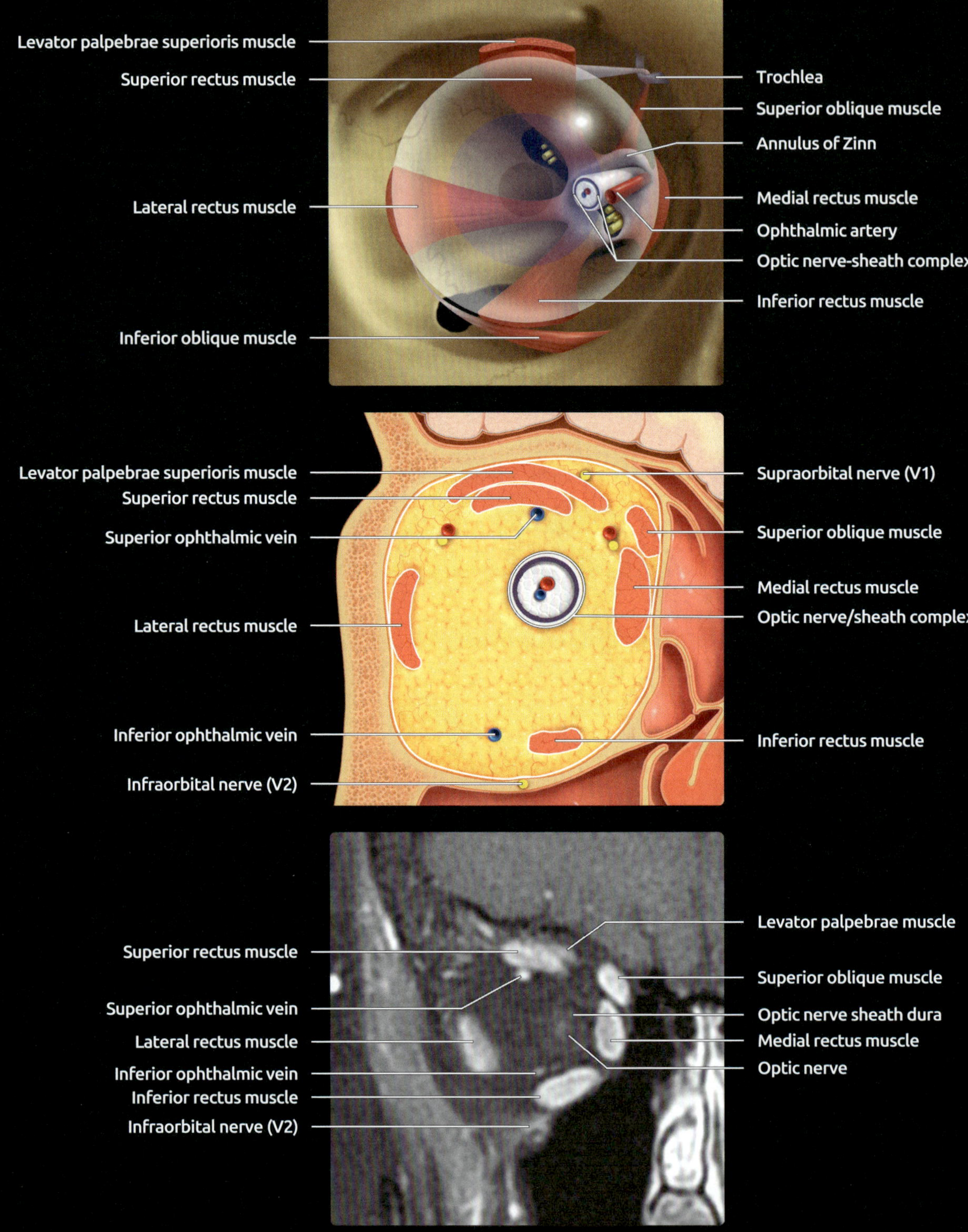

(Top) *Frontal graphic of the right orbit is shown. The rectus muscles originate at the annulus of Zinn at the orbital apex and insert at the corneoscleral junction of the eye, forming a muscle cone. The superior oblique muscle courses through the trochlea, providing for the angled pulley motion of this muscle. The inferior oblique inserts at the inferolateral aspect of the eye.* **(Middle)** *Coronal graphic of the right orbit is shown. The optic nerve-sheath complex courses in the intraconal space behind the eye. Branches of CNIII-VI, branches of the ophthalmic artery, and ophthalmic veins are located in the intraconal and extraconal spaces.* **(Bottom)** *Coronal T1 C+ FS MR demonstrates normal enhancement of the extraocular muscles. The optic nerve should not enhance. Normally, the optic nerve sheath dura can have subtle enhancement.*

CORONAL T1 MR

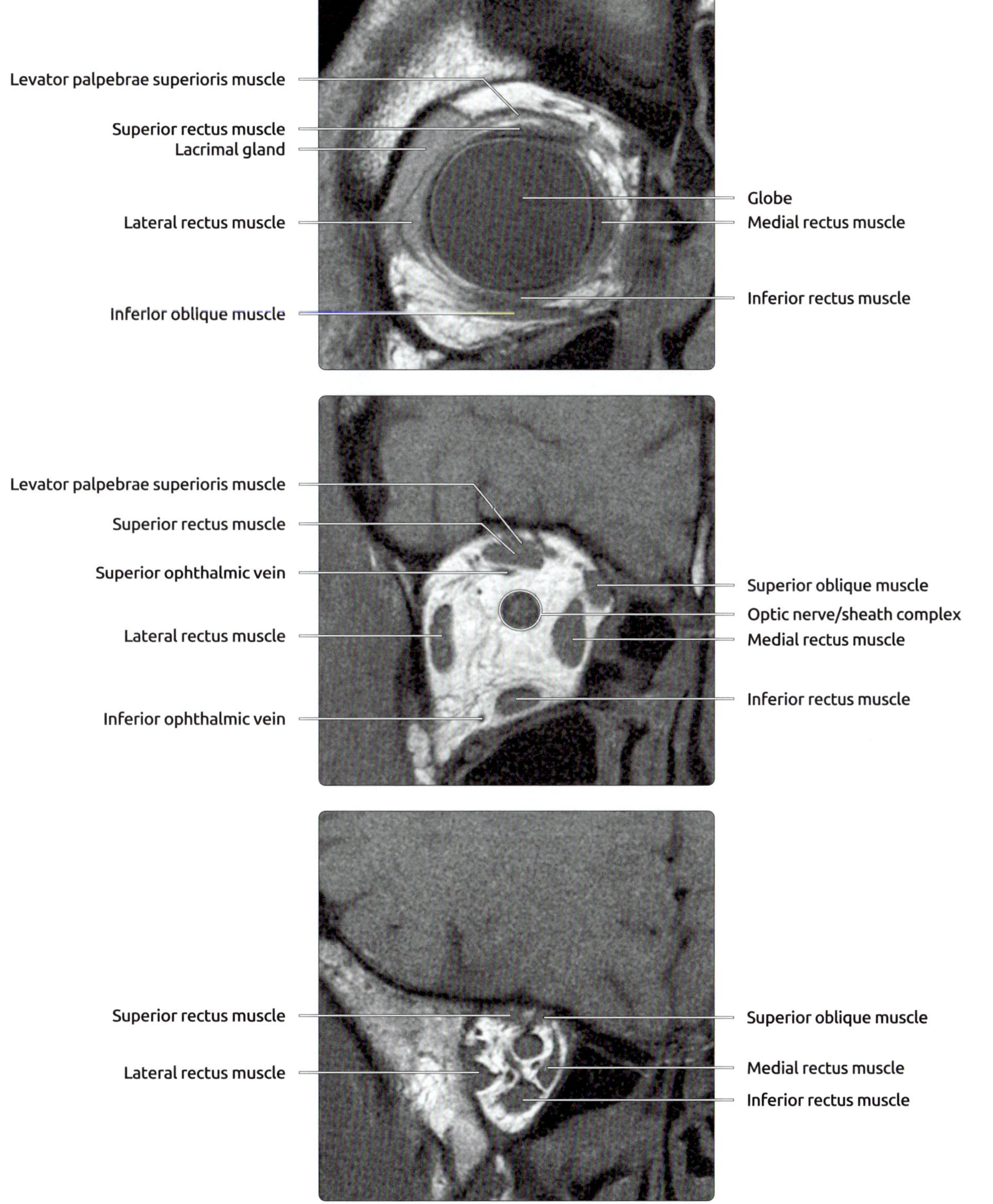

(Top) *Coronal T1 MR at the level of the globe shows the flattened and thinned tendinous contours of the extraocular muscles near their insertions. The inferior oblique muscle is evident at this level. The lacrimal gland has signal similar to muscle and is located in the anterior aspect of the superotemporal extraconal space.* **(Middle)** *Coronal T1 MR in the midorbit shows the muscle cone formed by the extraocular muscles with the nerve-sheath complex centrally in the intraconal space. Complex and variable branches of the ophthalmic artery are seen as small flow voids within the intraconal and extraconal fat.* **(Bottom)** *Coronal T1 MR at the orbital apex shows the close proximity of the extraocular muscles, nerve-sheath complex, and ophthalmic vessels.*

AXIAL ANATOMY CECT

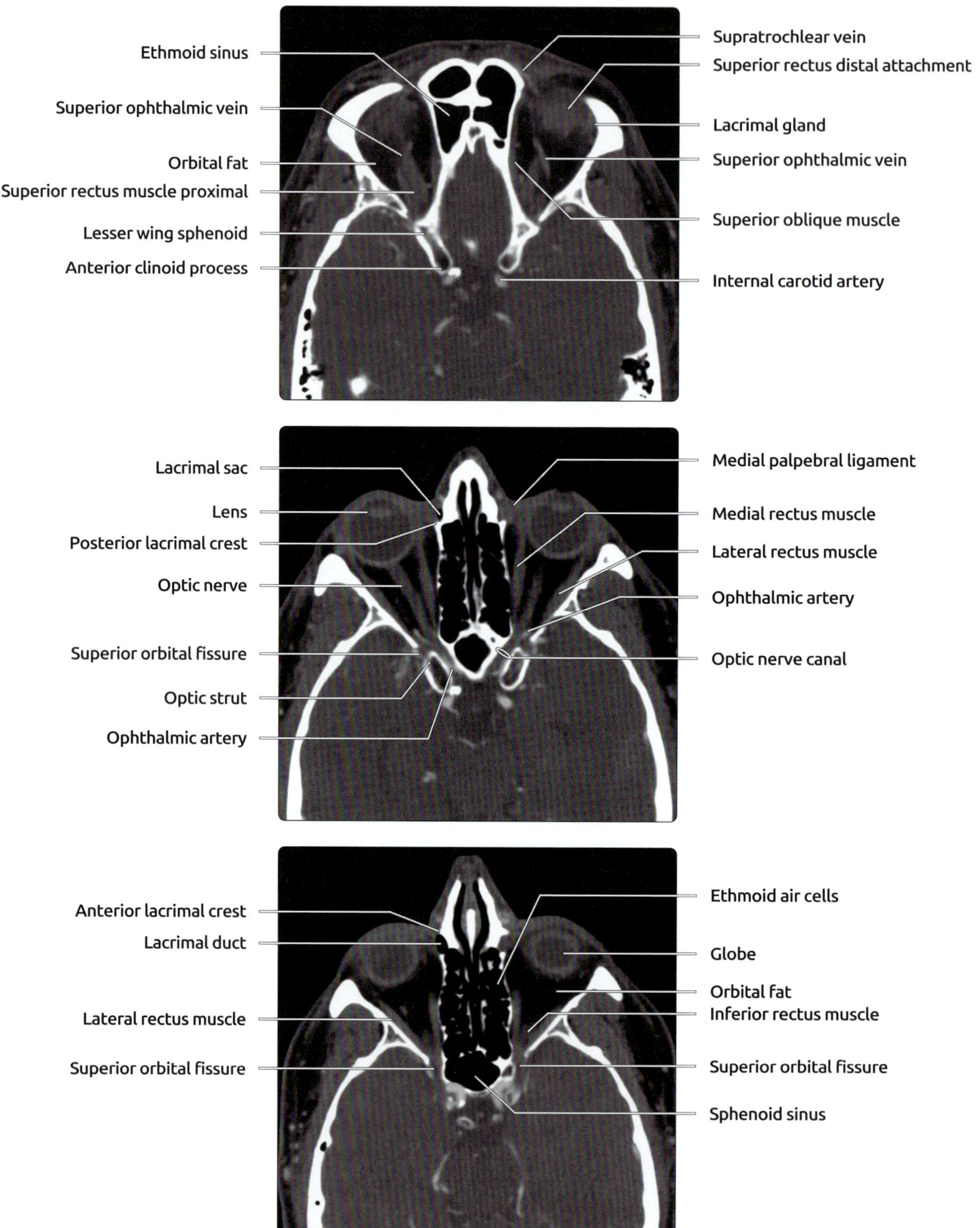

(Top) *Axial CECT through the superior aspect of the orbit demonstrates partial inclusion of the superior rectus muscle (and levator palpebrae muscle) in the plane as well as the superior ophthalmic vein that is quite variable in size and can be asymmetric normally. Anterior tributaries to the superior ophthalmic vein include the supraorbital and supratrochlear veins. The superior oblique muscle is seen medially within the superior orbit, en route to the trochlea. Notice the extensive orbital fat.* **(Middle)** *Axial CECT through the midorbit includes most of the intraorbital optic nerve on the left side of the image. The proximal ophthalmic arteries are seen within the optic nerve canals bilaterally, traveling just below the optic nerves. The optic strut is part of the lesser wing of the sphenoid that separates the optic nerve canal from the superior orbital fissure.* **(Bottom)** *Axial CECT through the inferior aspect of the orbit is shown. The proximal inferior rectus muscles are seen partially. The inferior ophthalmic veins are less consistent and often consist of groups of small veins. The superior orbital fissure is more conspicuous at this level.*

ANATOMIC-PATHOLOGIC CORRELATION

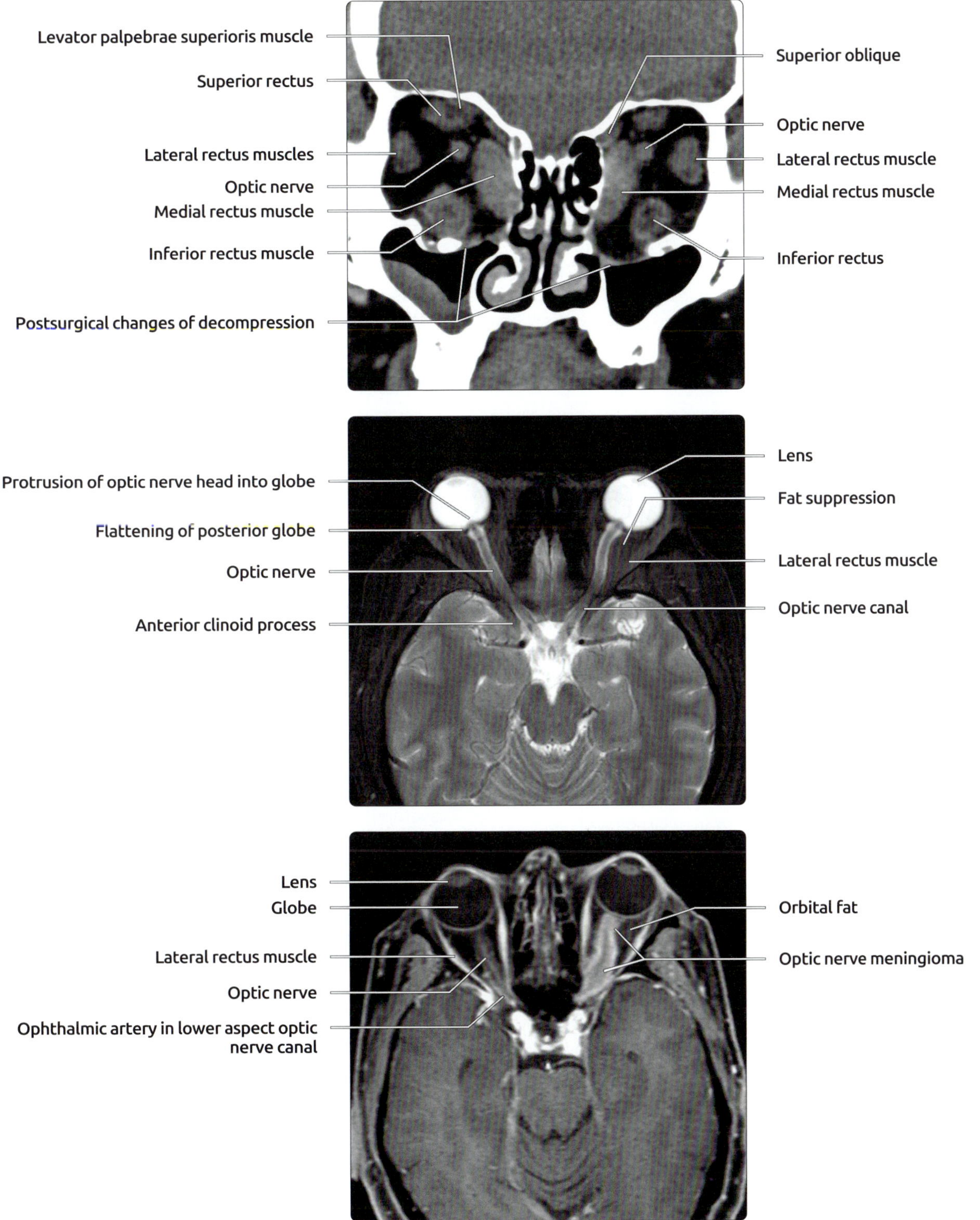

(Top) *Coronal CT through the orbits in a patient with thyroid-associated orbitopathy associated with Graves disease is shown. In this disease, autoimmune response leads to inflammation and enlargement of the extraocular muscles. The muscles are involved bilaterally but asymmetrically. The mass effect from extraocular muscle enlargement can create considerable proptosis and lead to optic nerve compression. This patient has undergone decompression surgery that essentially expands the bony volume of the orbits inferomedially.* **(Middle)** *Axial STIR MR of papilledema in the setting of idiopathic intracranial hypertension shows excellent fat suppression and nice delineation of the optic nerves. There is mild prominence of the optic nerve sheaths bilaterally and prominent swelling of the optic nerve head, which protrudes into the posterior globe.* **(Bottom)** *Axial T1 C+ FS MR through the orbit demonstrates a typical optic nerve meningioma of the left optic nerve. The meningioma arises from the dura along the optic nerve. In this case, the enhancing meningioma extends the entire length of the intraorbital optic nerve.*

Bony Orbit and Foramina

TERMINOLOGY

Abbreviations

- **Bones, foramina, and fissures**
  - Greater wing of sphenoid (GWS)
  - Lesser wing of sphenoid (LWS)
  - Optic canal (OpC)
  - Superior orbital fissure (SOF)
  - Inferior orbital fissure (IOF)
  - Foramen rotundum (FR)
  - Foramen ovale (FO)
  - Vidian canal (VC)
  - Pterygopalatine fossa (PPF)
- **Cranial nerves**
  - Optic nerve (CNII)
  - Oculomotor nerve (CNIII)
  - Trochlear nerve (CNIV)
  - Trigeminal nerve (CNV)
    - Ophthalmic branch (V1)
    - Maxillary branch (V2)
    - Mandibular branch (V3)
  - Abducens nerve (CNVI)
- **Vessels**
  - Ophthalmic artery (OA)
  - Superior ophthalmic vein (SOV)
  - Inferior ophthalmic vein (IOV)

Definitions

- MPR: 2D multiplanar reformations

GROSS ANATOMY

Bones of Orbit

- **Frontal bone**
  - Forms superior rim and anterior roof (orbital process)
- **Zygomatic bone**
  - Forms inferolateral rim, anterior portion of lateral wall (orbital process), anterolateral floor (maxillary process)
- **Maxillary bone**
  - Forms inferomedial rim (frontal process) and anterior portion of inferomedial wall (orbital surface)
- **Nasal bone**
  - Forms bridge of nose
  - Anteromedial to frontal process of maxillary bone
- **Ethmoid bone**
  - Forms midportion of medial wall: Lamina papyracea (in Latin means paper-like sheet)
  - Contributes to medial walls of several apical fissures
- **Lacrimal bone**
  - Forms anterior portion of medial wall, just posterior to frontal process of maxillary bone
  - Fossa for lacrimal sac
- **Sphenoid bone**
  - Forms posterior portion of lateral wall (GWS) and posterior portion of medial roof (LWS)
  - Contours between GWS and LWS create apical fissures
- **Palatine bone**
  - Forms small portion of inferomedial wall posteriorly
  - Located between orbital portions of ethmoid and maxillary bones

IMAGING ANATOMY

Anatomy Relationships

- **Major foramina**
  - **OpC**
    - Formed predominantly by LWS with medial contribution from ethmoid bone
    - Separated from SOF by optic strut, which arises from LWS
  - **SOF**
    - Formed by LWS and ethmoid bone medially, GWS laterally
    - Main pathway from orbit to intracranial compartment
  - **IOF**
    - Formed by GWS and zygomatic bone laterally, maxillary and ethmoid bones medially
    - Mostly contiguous with SOF, separated only at posterior aspect by short bony roof of FR
    - Anterior continuation of FR

Internal Contents

- **Contents of foramina**
  - **OpC**: CNII and OA
  - **SOF**: CNIII, IV, V (V1), and VI, SOV
  - **IOF**: CNV (V2), IOV
  - **FR**: CNV (V2)-proximal segment
  - **FO**: CNV (V3)
  - **Supraorbital foramen**: Supraorbital nerve (V1)
  - **Infraorbital foramen and canal**: Infraorbital nerve (V2)

ANATOMY IMAGING ISSUES

Questions

- **Pathways of orbit-sinus disease spread**
  - Orbit → intracranial
    - SOF and IOF: Common pathway; extends into cavernous sinus and Meckel cave, involves CNIII-VI
    - OpC: Involves CNII, dura
  - Orbit → deep face
    - SOF and IOF: Communicate with PPF
    - Infraorbital canal to PPF
    - Supraorbital canal to SOF (rare)
  - Sinus → orbit
    - Ethmoid: Common pathway through lamina papyracea
    - Frontal: Especially postobstructive process

Imaging Recommendations

- CT
  - Preferred for assessing bony structures and foramina
- MR
  - Preferred for evaluation of tumor and inflammation

Imaging Pitfalls

- Assessing foramina
  - OpC oriented obliquely
    - MPR orthogonal to long axis may be required to demonstrate intact canal
  - FR and VC often mistaken
    - FR superolateral to VC on coronals, shorter than VC

GRAPHICS

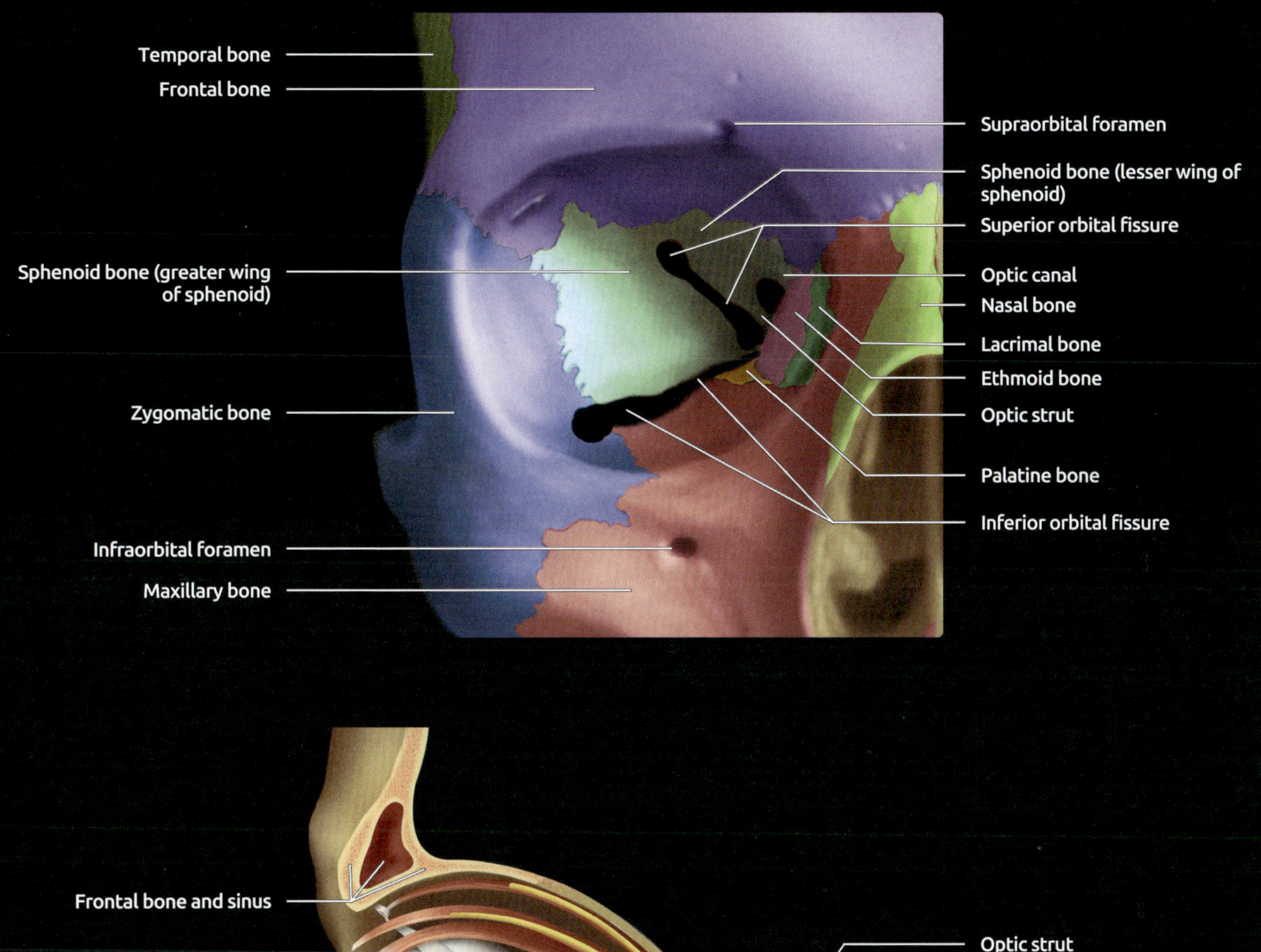

(Top) *Frontal graphic of the bones of the right orbit is shown. A total of 7 embryologically distinct bones contribute to the bony orbit (lacrimal, ethmoid, palatine, maxillary, zygomatic, sphenoid, and frontal bones). The sphenoid bone has greater and lesser sphenoid wings. The complex orbital fissures and optic canal at the apex are formed largely by the wings of the sphenoid bone and associated relationships. Notice that the optic canal has lesser wing of sphenoid and ethmoid bone components.* **(Bottom)** *Lateral graphic of the left orbit is shown. The optic nerve (CNII) is relatively isolated in the optic canal, whereas the superior orbital fissure transmits CNIII, IV, V1, and VI as they course forward from the cavernous sinus and Meckel cave. The other branches of CNV also contribute to the complexity of the central skull base as they pass through their respective foramina.*

AXIAL BONE CT

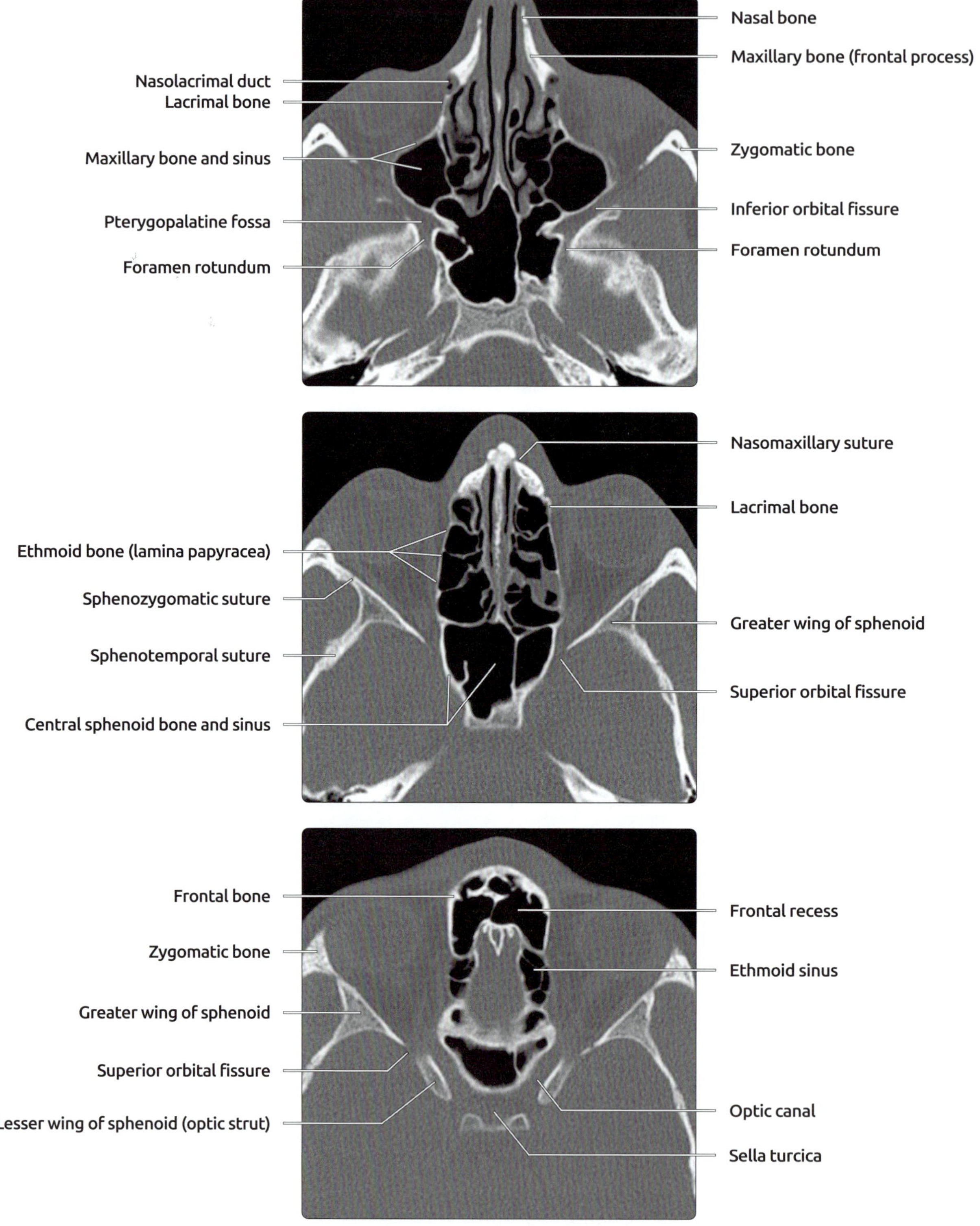

(Top) *First of 3 axial bone CT images presented from inferior to superior is shown. The short, horizontally oriented foramen rotundum is seen at the posterior margin of the pterygopalatine fossa with the inferior orbital fissure extending anterolaterally in roughly the same plane. Anteriorly, relationships between the medial bony orbit and nasolacrimal structures are evident.* **(Middle)** *Image at the level of the midorbit is shown. The superior orbital fissure is seen as a gap at the orbital apex. The thin ethmoid bone forms the bulk of the medial orbital wall.* **(Bottom)** *Image at the level of the upper orbit is shown. The optic canals show characteristic angles as the nerves approach the chiasm, which is located above the sella. The superior orbital fissure is inferior and lateral to the optic canal, from which it is separated by the bony optic strut of the lesser wing of sphenoid. Sinus air space within the paramedian portions of the frontal bones is seen anteriorly.*

CORONAL BONE CT

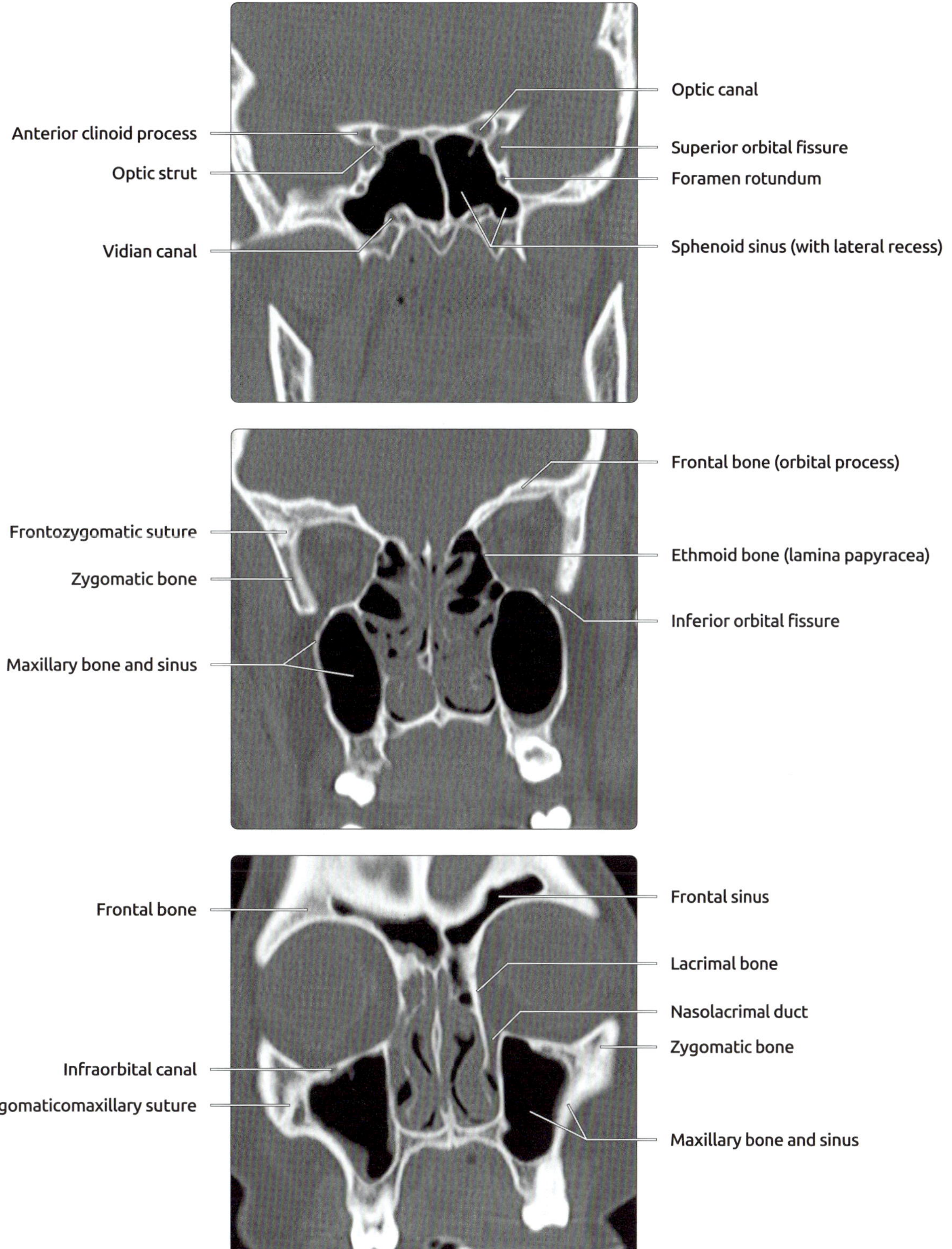

(Top) *First of 3 coronal bone CT images presented from posterior to anterior is shown. The obliquely oriented optic canals show the characteristic ovoid shape. The superior orbital fissure is located inferolaterally relative to the optic canal with the optic strut and attached clinoid process of the lesser wing of sphenoid separating the 2. Further inferolaterally is the foramen rotundum. The vidian canal is inferior and medial to rotundum, noting a prominent lateral recess of the sphenoid sinus separating the 2 foramina.* **(Middle)** *Image at the level of the midorbit is shown. Contours of the bony orbit, including integrity of the thin lamina papyracea of the medial wall, are best seen in this plane.* **(Bottom)** *Image at the level of the anterior orbit is shown. Contours of the bony orbital rim are best evaluated in the coronal plane. The nasolacrimal structures as well as anterior sinonasal spaces are well demonstrated.*

Optic Nerve/Sheath Complex

TERMINOLOGY

Abbreviations

- Optic nerve/sheath complex (ONSC)
- Ophthalmic artery (OA)

Synonyms

- Optic nerve (CNII)

Definitions

- Optic nerve, chiasm, and tract: Afferent visual CNS pathways from retina to visual nuclei of midbrain
- Optic sheath: Dural encasement of intraorbital CNII

GROSS ANATOMY

Optic Nerve

- Each optic nerve contains ~ 1 million axons that originate in ganglion cell layer of retina
- Nonmyelinated axons converge at optic nerve head, organize into fascicles, and then cross lamina cribrosa
- Axons then enter intraorbital segment and become myelinated from oligodendrocytes, **not** Schwann cells
- Anatomically CNS tract; differs from other cranial nerves

Optic Sheath

- All 3 membrane layers of meninges present, including pia, arachnoid, and dura mater
- Layers separated by subarachnoid and subdural spaces
- Layers and spaces contiguous with intracranial counterparts
  - Subarachnoid space contiguous with suprasellar cistern, transmits intracranial pressure

IMAGING ANATOMY

Extent

- **Optic nerve**
  - From optic nerve head to chiasm
  - Optic nerve segments
    - **Intraocular**: Within nerve head (1 mm)
    - **Orbital**: Nerve head to optic canal (30 mm)
    - **Canalicular**: Within optic canal (10 mm)
    - **Cisternal**: Optic canal to optic chiasm (10 mm)
- **Optic chiasm**
  - Within suprasellar cistern just anterior to pituitary stalk
  - Decussation of 1/2 of axons
    - Represents nasal portion of retina
    - Each 1/2 of visual field from each eye afferent to contralateral visual cortex
- **Optic tract**
  - From optic chiasm to visual nuclei of midbrain

Anatomy Relationships

- Optic canal
  - Transmits ONSC and OA
  - Separated from superior orbital fissure by optic strut

Internal Contents

- **Vascular supply**
  - **OA**
    - 1st intradural branch of internal carotid artery
    - Major arterial supply to orbit
    - Passes through optic canal in dural sheath
    - Exits sheath laterally at orbital apex
  - **Central retinal artery**
    - Major branch of OA, supplies retina
    - Enters CNII ~ 1 cm posterior to nerve head
  - **Central retinal vein**
    - Accompanies central retinal artery
    - Drains directly into cavernous sinus

ANATOMY IMAGING ISSUES

Questions

- **Orientation of optic nerve**
  - **Intraorbital segment**
    - Posteromedial oblique sagittal long axis
    - Roughly horizontal plane
    - Position varies with eye movement
    - Nerve longer than distance from apex to globe, tends to form S-shaped contour
  - **Canalicular segment**
    - Oblique axis results in nonorthogonal "ovoid" cross-sectional appearance on coronal images
  - **Cisternal segment**
    - Angle changes relative to intraorbital segment as it courses posteriorly
    - Oblique sagittal long axis ~ 30° medially and superiorly

Imaging Recommendations

- Routine orbital approach appropriate for most nerve/sheath lesions
- Special circumstances
  - **Sheath mass** (possible meningioma)
    - May benefit from noncontrast CT to detect calcification
    - Additional brain imaging may be necessary to define extent of intraaxial tumor
  - **Inflammatory nerve work-up** (optic neuritis)
    - Requires concomitant brain imaging
    - High incidence of demyelinating disease

Imaging Approaches

- Dedicated optic nerve MR imaging
  - Axial sequences
    - 3.0 mm, anterior fossa floor through floor of orbit
  - Coronal sequences
    - 3.5-4.0 mm, back of pons through globe
  - T1WI, STIR, and T1 C+ with fat suppression
    - Both axial and coronal
    - May substitute axial T2WI FSE + fat suppression for STIR
  - Routine brain protocols not adequate to evaluate ONSC

Imaging Pitfalls

- Motion artifacts on MR
  - Common due to irrepressible eye motion
- Surface coils
  - Generally not adequate to visualize entire ONSC

CLINICAL IMPLICATIONS

Nerve vs. Sheath Lesions

- Important distinction, different DDx and prognoses
- Best with coronal STIR and T1 C+ with fat suppression

GRAPHICS

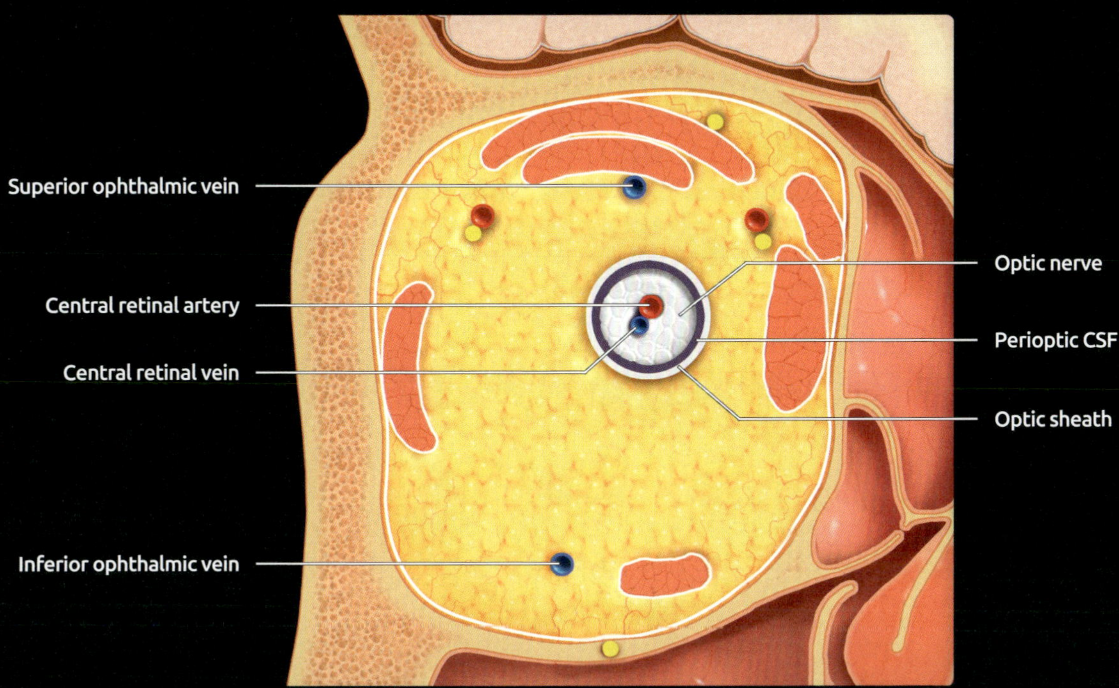

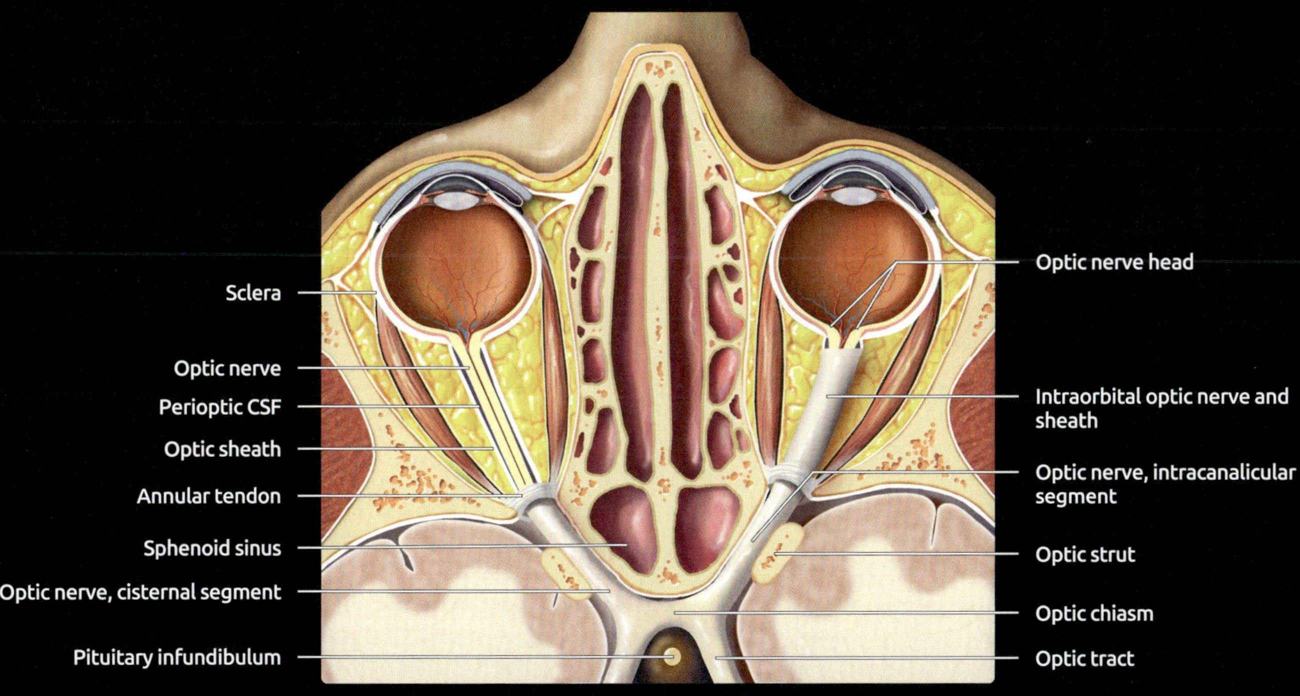

(Top) *Coronal graphic of the midorbit depicts the optic nerve/sheath complex. The nerve is bathed by a thin layer of CSF, which is contained by the dural optic sheath. The central retinal vessels are external to the optic sheath posteriorly in the orbit and pierce the dura in the midportion of the nerve to travel within the substance of the nerve anteriorly.* **(Bottom)** *Axial graphic of the intraorbital and intracranial segments of CNII is shown. The extraaxial optic pathways can be segmented (posterior to anterior) into the optic tract, optic chiasm, cisternal nerve, intracanalicular nerve, and intraorbital nerve. The optic sheath is a dural reflection that is contiguous with intracranial dura mater. Note the relationship of the pituitary infundibulum to the optic chiasm.*

CORONAL AND AXIAL T1 MR

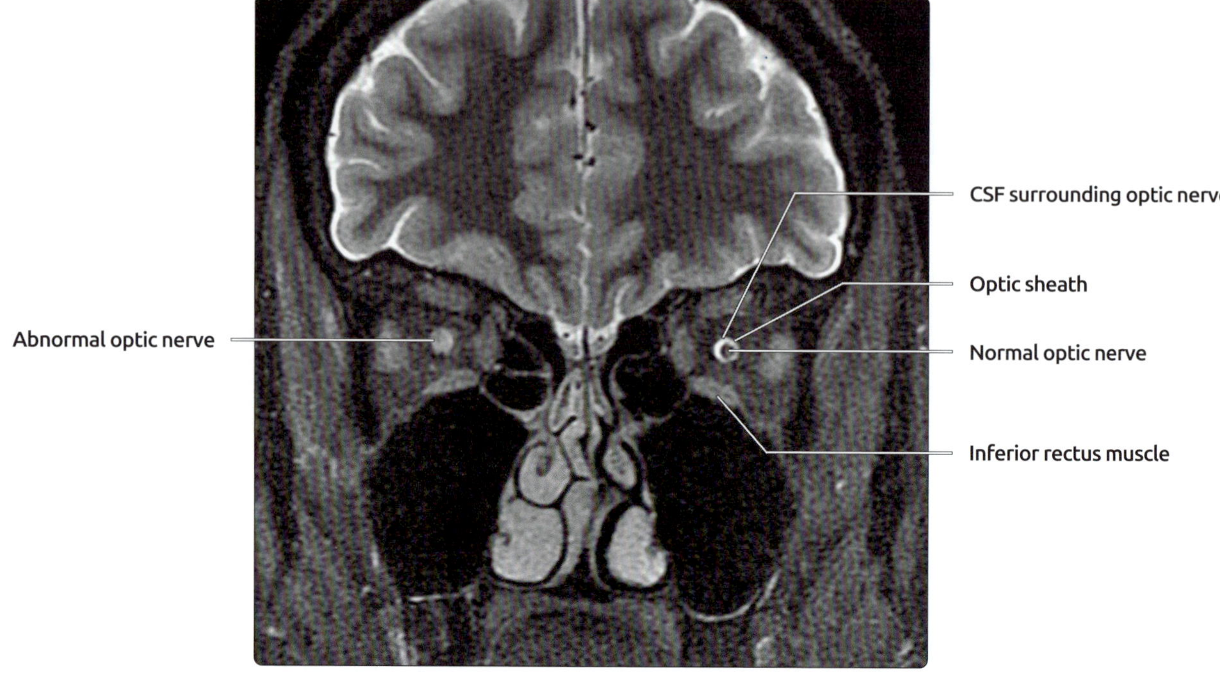

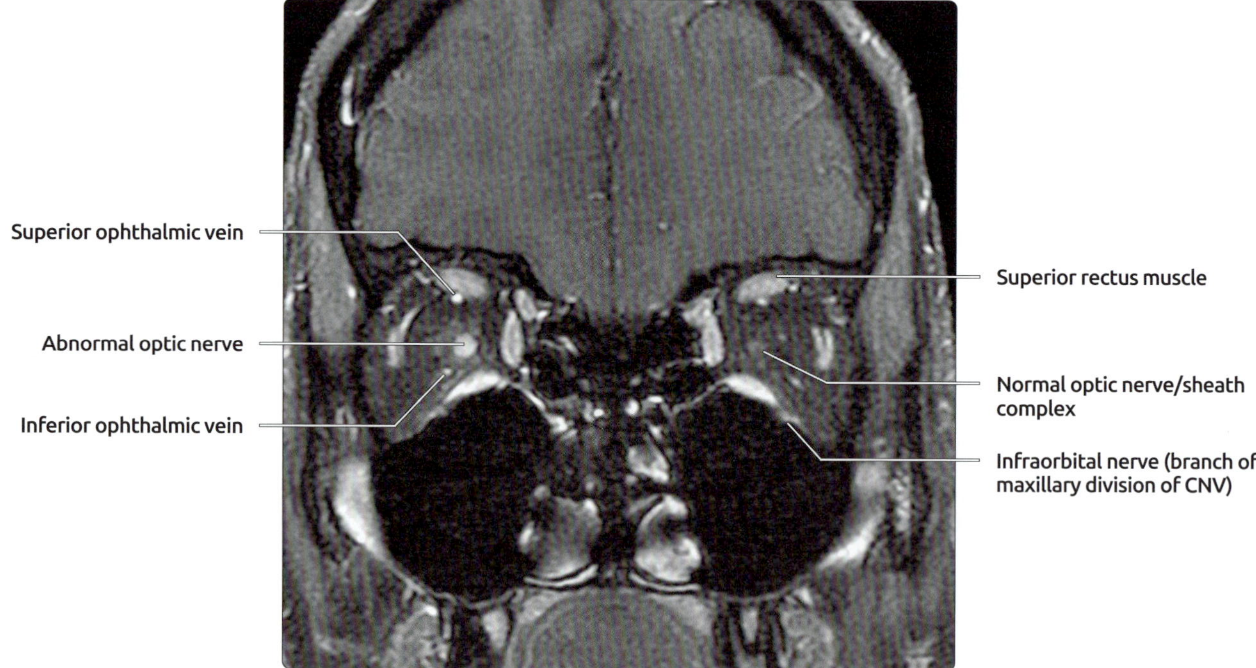

(Top) *A 36-year-old woman with acute onset of right eye pain and blurry vision underwent MR imaging. The right optic nerve is abnormally hyperintense on this STIR MR. Given the acute onset of symptoms, these findings are consistent with optic neuritis. Note the normal left optic nerve/sheath complex.* **(Bottom)** *Coronal postcontrast T1 C+ FS MR in the same patient is shown. Corresponding to the abnormal signal in the right optic nerve on the previous STIR MR, there is abnormal enhancement in the right optic nerve, consistent with optic neuritis.*

CORONAL AND AXIAL STIR MR

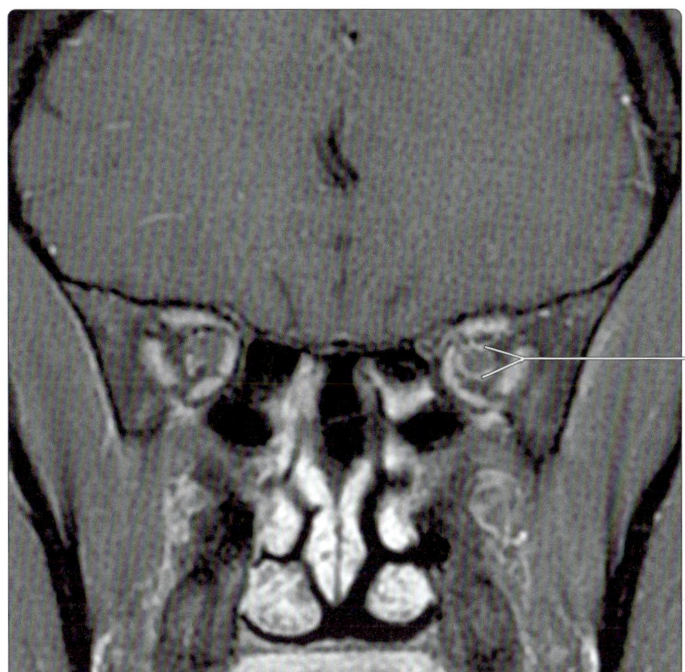

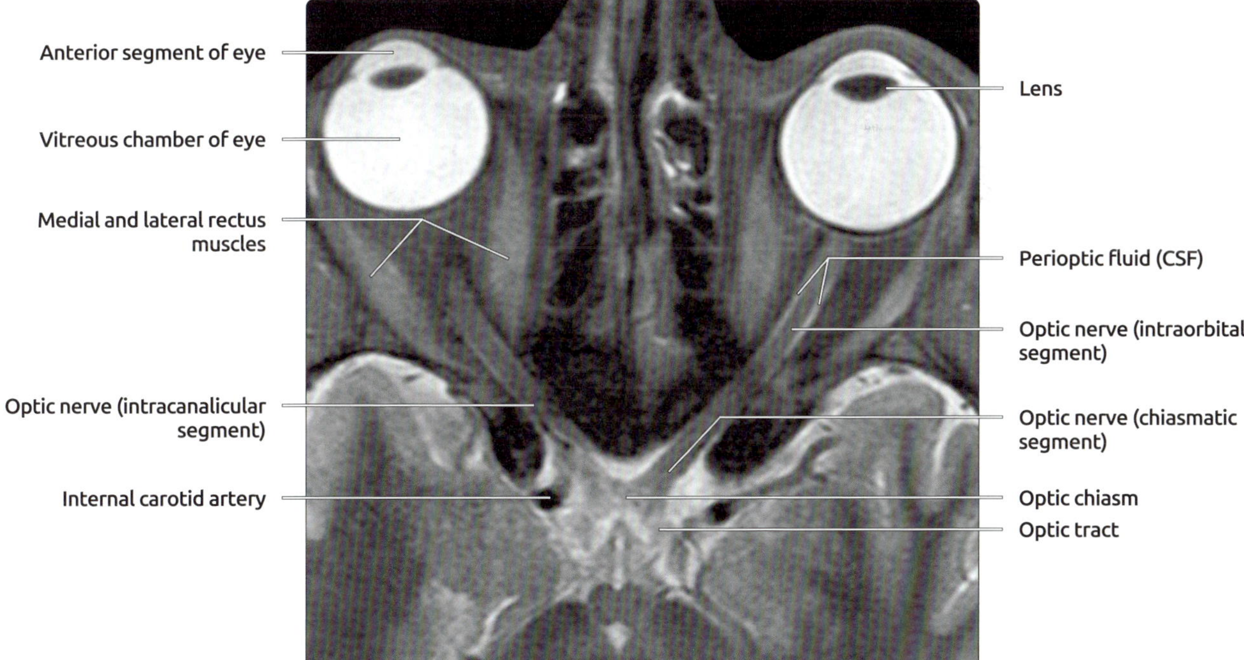

(Top) *Coronal T1 C+ FS MR in a 44-year-old man who presented with acute-onset left-sided orbital pain and blurry vision is shown. This patient's coronal STIR sequence (not shown) demonstrated abnormal T2 signal in the left optic nerve at this level, consistent with edema. While the symptoms and presence of edema in the nerve are similar to optic neuritis, the peripheral enhancement is more consistent with perineuritis, and raises diagnostic and prognostic considerations that differ from optic neuritis.* **(Bottom)** *Axial T2 STIR MR of the orbits is shown. A slightly oblique plane allows for demonstration of both intraorbital and cisternal segments of CNII. Because of the normal angulation of the nerves proximally, the chiasm and tracts are usually demonstrated on images superior to those depicting the intraorbital nerves. The anterior segment of the eye includes both the anterior and posterior chambers in front of the lens.*

GROSS ANATOMY

Segments

- **Anterior segment of globe**
  - Portion of eye in front of anterior margin of vitreous (hyaloid face)
    - Ciliary body, suspensory ligaments, and lens
    - Anterior and posterior chambers
    - Iris
    - Cornea
- **Posterior segment of globe**
  - Vitreoretinal portion of eye and its layers
    - Vitreous chamber
    - Retina
    - Choroid
    - Sclera

Chambers

- **Anterior chamber**
  - Major chamber of anterior segment
  - Between cornea and iris
  - Filled with aqueous humor, which provides nutrition and structure
- **Posterior chamber**
  - Small potential space posterior to iris and anterior to lens/ligament complex
  - Contiguous with anterior chamber through pupil
- **Vitreous chamber**
  - Large chamber that fills posterior segment
  - Filled with viscoelastic transparent gel

Tunicae

- **Tunica interna (retina)**
  - Multilayered sensorineural organ
    - Photoreceptor cells (rods and cones) overlie pigment epithelium at outermost layer
    - Bipolar and ganglion cells form inner layer (next to vitreous) and assemble and convey sensory signals
  - Regions and extent
    - **Macula**: Central portion, daylight and color vision
    - **Fovea**: Macular center, highest spatial resolution
    - **Peripheral**: Outer portion, night vision and motion
    - **Ora serrata**: Anterior margin of retina
- **Tunica vasculosa (uvea)**
  - Pigmented, vascular loose connective tissue
  - **Choroid**
    - Layer between retina and sclera
    - Vascular supply to photoreceptor layer
  - **Ciliary body**
    - Uveal structure anterior to ora serrata
    - Attached to lens via zonule fibers
    - Contractile function provides for lens accommodation
    - Source of aqueous production
  - **Iris**
    - Thin elastic tissue overlying lens
    - Sphincter muscle provides pupillary response
- **Tunica fibrosa (sclera)**
  - Outer fibrous layer
  - Attachment site for extraocular muscles
  - Contiguous with dura of optic sheath as well as fibrous diaphragm (lamina cribrosa) at nerve head
  - Contiguous with cornea anteriorly

IMAGING ANATOMY

Overview

- Primary imaging approaches
  - Direct funduscopy is 1st-line technique
  - Sonography readily available at most eye clinics
- Cross-sectional modalities (MR and CT)
  - Particularly useful in eyes with opaque media (i.e., obscured by vitreous or aqueous opacity)
  - Routine imaging as part of orbital evaluation
    - Extraocular extension of ocular disease
    - Ocular involvement of orbital process

Internal Contents

- **Anterior segment**
  - Aqueous chambers exhibit fluid signal
  - Lens moderately hyperdense on CT, isointense on T1WI, hypointense relative to fluid on T2WI
  - Ciliary body and iris variably distinguishable but not diagnostic detail
- **Posterior segment**
  - Vitreous chamber exhibits fluid signal

ANATOMY IMAGING ISSUES

Imaging Recommendations

- CT
  - Evaluation of calcification (e.g., retinoblastoma)
  - Evaluation in child without sedation
- MR
  - Preferred for evaluation of extraocular extent of disease
  - T2WI useful for evaluating vitreous and aqueous chambers; otherwise limited utility in eye
  - T1WI pre- and postcontrast better for assessing uveoretinal structures
  - Surface coils improve signal and resolution in globe but may be limited in assessment of posterior orbit

Imaging Pitfalls

- MR
  - Irrepressible globe movement results in ubiquitous motion artifact

EMBRYOLOGY

Embryologic Events

- **Optic fissure**
  - Extends along inferonasal aspect of optic disc and stalk
  - Fissure fusion (~ 5th week) required for normal globe and nerve formation
  - Failure of fusion results in coloboma
- **Primary vitreous**
  - Embryonic fibrovascular hyaloid with hyaloid artery in Cloquet canal
  - Normally regresses ~ 7 months gestation
    - Visible in premature infant
  - Failure of regression results in persistent hyperplastic primary vitreous

GRAPHIC AND SAGITTAL T1 MR

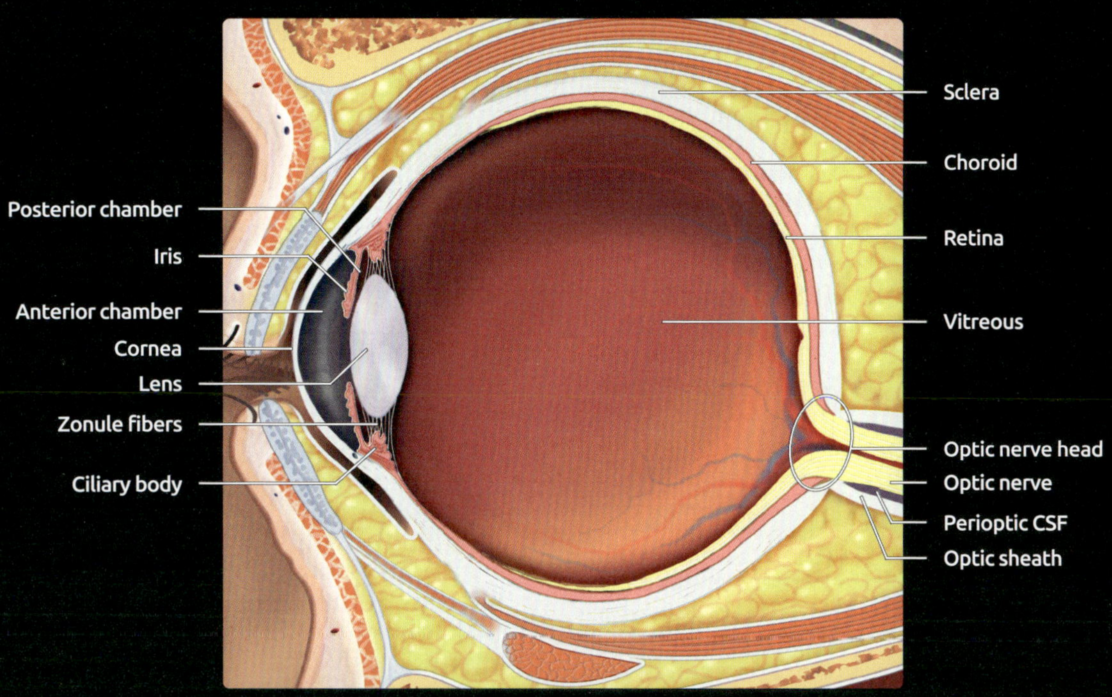

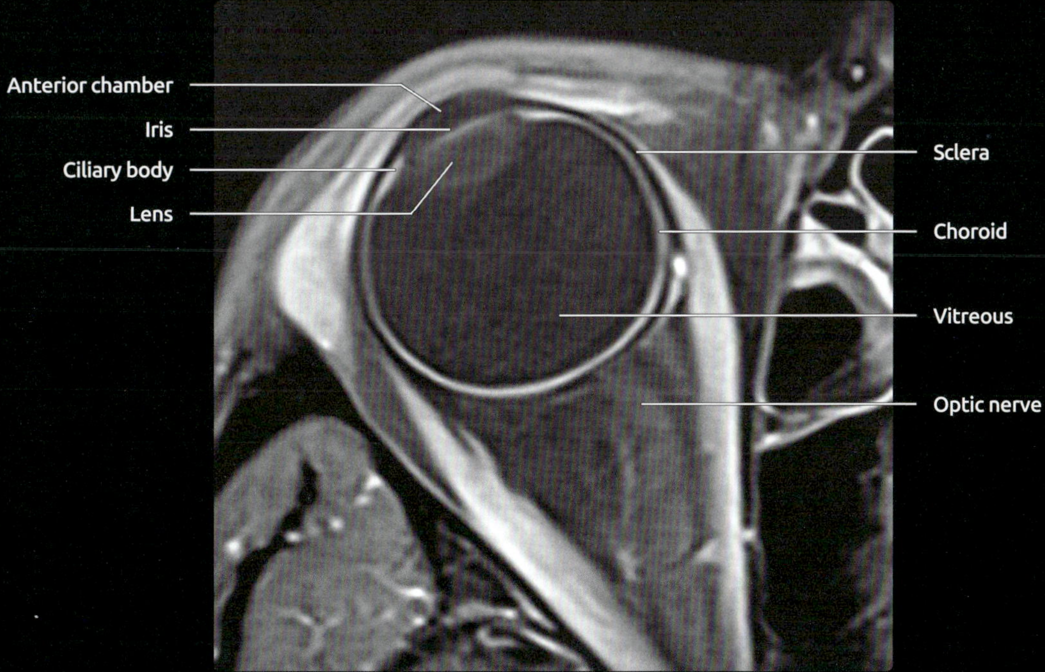

(Top) *Sagittal graphic shows that the anterior and posterior chambers of the anterior segment are contiguous through the pupil. The choroid and iris are anterior extensions of the uveal tract. The posterior segment is filled by the vitreous chamber. The retina and sclera are contiguous with the optic nerve and sheath, respectively, at the nerve head.* **(Bottom)** *Axial T1 C+ FS MR shows that the aqueous-filled anterior chamber and vitreous-filled posterior chamber exhibit essentially pure fluid signal. The lens is visible; the iris and ciliary body are identifiable but not reliably diagnostic on routine MR imaging. There is normal enhancement of the choroid, ciliary body, and iris (the components of the uveal tract). In its normal state, the retina is not clearly distinguishable from the choroid on routine MR imaging.*

TERMINOLOGY

Abbreviations

- Cavernous sinus (CS)

Definitions

- Paired venous lakes with multiple septa within located lateral to sella turcica, pituitary & sphenoid sinus, & medial to mesial temporal lobe
- CSs drain multiple veins from orbit, sylvian fissure, middle & anterior fossa; ultimately provide venous drainage posteriorly & inferiorly via inferior petrosal, superior petrosal, & basilar venous sinuses
- Described as anatomic jewel box due to its complex contents, including several cranial nerves & internal carotid artery (ICA)
- Term cavernous sinus 1st used by Winslow in 1734

IMAGING ANATOMY

Overview

- Valveless, septated dural venous sinuses of central skull base, present on either side of sella
- Extradural in location communicating with extradural space of spine & orbits, in contrast to other venous sinuses, which are located between 2 layers of dura
- Important given location, relationship to sella, pituitary gland, & internal contents, including multiple cranial nerves & cavernous ICA

Anatomy Relationships

- **Boundaries**
  - Boat-shaped structure, narrowest anteriorly & widest posteriorly, bounded by dura with 5 walls, including anterior, posterior, medial, lateral, & superior/roof
  - **Superior**: Extends from base of anterior clinoid process to posterior clinoid process
  - **Lateral**: Bordered by 2 layers of dura
  - **Medial**: Bordered by lateral margin of sella & lateral wall of sphenoid sinus with carotid sulcus
  - **Anterior**: Extends to anterior clinoid process & superior orbital fissure (SOF) below it
  - **Posterior**: Extends to posterior clinoid process, lateral margin of upper clivus, & petroclival junction, extending laterally to point just medial to trigeminal impression
- **Superior wall/roof**
  - Extends from optic strut & SOF anteriorly to petrous apex (PA) & tentorial incisura posteriorly
  - Medial margin of roof contiguous with diaphragma sellae
  - **Oculomotor triangle**, triangular-shaped portion of CS roof created by 3 dural folds
    - Lateral margin of roof separated from lateral wall of CS by cord-like thickening of dura called **anterior petroclinoid fold** that extends from tentorial edge at PA to anterior clinoid process
    - Separate fold extends from tentorial edge at PA to posterior clinoid process, **posterior petroclinoid fold**
    - Thin band of dura, **interclinoid fold**, extends from anterior clinoid process to posterior clinoid process
    - CNIII, along with its sleeve of arachnoid (oculomotor cistern), pierces roof at oculomotor triangle
    - CNIV enters posterolateral aspect of oculomotor triangle just posterior to CNIII
  - Small portion of roof passes inferomedial to anterior clinoid process where dural roof merges with dura, forming proximal & distal dural rings
- **Lateral wall**
  - Sail-shaped dural sheet that extends from SOF & anterior clinoid process anteriorly to PA posteriorly; faces medial temporal lobe
  - Consists of thick dural membrane that typically can be dissected into 2 distinct layers
    - Thin outer (meningeal) layer
    - Thicker inner (endosteal)
  - Inner layer envelops oculomotor nerve (CNIII), trochlear nerve (CNIV), ophthalmic (V1) & maxillary (V2) segments of trigeminal nerve
  - Lateral & medial walls of CS merge inferiorly along lateral margin of sphenoid, just above maxillary nerve (V2)
  - While V3 invested by contiguous dura, not considered component of CS wall
  - V2 similar to V3 in regards to CS lateral wall; lies at inferior margin of CS or just outside CS envelope rather than being true component of wall
  - Lateral wall merges inferiorly & posteriorly with dura covering Meckel cave
- **Medial wall**
  - Consists of upper sellar component & lower sphenoid component
  - Upper sellar component of medial wall formed by thin dural membrane, typically single cell layer in thickness that separates venous compartment from lateral margin of pituitary gland
  - Inherent weakness of upper sellar component makes it susceptible to invasion from pituitary tumors
  - Thicker lower medial wall adherent to carotid sulcus of sphenoid bone
- **Anterior wall**
  - Rectangular in shape extending from optic strut, beneath anterior clinoid process laterally to include SOF
  - Inferior margin formed by foramen rotundum
  - Anterior CS merges with venous plexus in SOF
- **Posterior wall**
  - Extends from lateral margin of dorsum sellae to medial aspect of trigeminal impression of PA & superomedial aspect of Meckel cave
  - Limited inferiorly by junction of PA & body of sphenoid bone at superomedial aspect of petroclival fissure
  - **Dorello canal & CNVI**
    - Small gap that separates PA from clivus near medial & superior tip of PA
    - Small petrosphenoid ligament of Gruber, crosses from PA tip to base of posterior clinoid process
    - Contains venous tissue at confluence of posterior CS & petrosal sinuses
    - CNVI passes from prepontine cistern through Dorello canal to enter CS
  - **Petrolingual ligament (PLL)**
    - Extends from PA to lingula of sphenoid bone
    - Invariably surrounds dorsal & lateral walls of lacerum segment of ICA

- Important surgical landmark that marks point at which ICA lacerum segment transitions to cavernous segment
- Also marks inferior & posterior margin of CS

- **Venous communications**
  - Venous tributaries
    - Superior, inferior ophthalmic veins
    - Sphenoparietal sinus
  - Communicate with each other via intercavernous plexus (anterior, posterior, & inferior across sella) & basilar venous plexus (across clivus)
  - Communicates posteriorly with inferior petrosal sinus, superior petrosal sinus, & basilar venous sinus
  - Additional communications with veins of pterygoid venous plexus & skull base foramina (foramen ovale, rotundum, & spinosum, carotid canal, & sphenoidal emissary foramen)
- **Meckel cave**
  - Dural outpouching that begins in posterior fossa (porus trigeminus) & extends over petrosphenoid junction into medial & posterior aspect of middle cranial fossa
  - Contains part of trigeminal nerve, including trigeminal ganglion
  - Superior, anterior, & medial portions of Meckel cave are immediately adjacent to posterior & lateral aspects of CS
  - Medial & inferior aspect of Meckel cave is just lateral to ICA as it arises from medial opening of carotid canal & begins to turn vertically & anteriorly into CS
  - Trigeminal ganglion positioned in anterior & inferior aspect of Meckel cave, divides into 3 divisions: Ophthalmic (V1), maxillary (V2), & mandibular (V3)
  - Ophthalmic division (V1) extends medially & anteriorly & enters lateral wall of CS
  - Maxillary division (V2) extends anteriorly, along inferior margin of CS to enter foramen rotundum
  - Mandibular division (V3) extends inferiorly & laterally through foramen ovale

Internal Contents

- **CNIII**
  - Pierces roof of CS in oculomotor cistern & gets embedded in lateral wall
  - Surrounded by thin sleeve of arachnoid & CSF (oculomotor cistern) that travels with nerve for several millimeters to anterior clinoid process
- **CNIV**
  - Also pierces roof of CS, & nerve positioned in lateral wall below CNIII
- **V1** (ophthalmic division of CNV) in lateral wall below CNIV
- **V2** (maxillary division of CNV), most inferior cranial nerve in lateral CS wall
- **V3** (mandibular division of CNV) does **not** enter CS proper (passes from Meckel cave inferiorly into foramen ovale)
- **CNVI** lies within CS proper, next to ICA
- Sympathetic fibers travel along ICA within CS
- **Cavernous ICA**
  - Bouthillier et al described 7-segment classification system for ICA
    - Cervical
    - Petrous
    - Lacerum
    - Cavernous
    - Clinoid
    - Ophthalmic
    - Communicating segments
  - Cavernous segment begins as lacerum segment of ICA passes beneath PLL
  - Initially ascends & then turns (posterior genu) anteriorly to assume horizontal course through CS
  - Posterior genu, usual site of origin for **meningohypophyseal trunk**
  - Horizontal portion of cavernous ICA lies within carotid sulcus along lateral margin of sphenoid bone
  - Carotid sulcus occasionally dehiscent, allowing ICA to protrude into sphenoid sinus
  - Horizontal segment gives rise to **inferolateral trunk,** which supplies tiny branches to intracavernous cranial nerves & tentorium
  - Near anterior margin of CS, ICA turns cephalad (anterior genu) & continues medial to anterior clinoid process
  - Along this anterior vertical course, ICA passes through 2 anatomically distinct dural rings: Proximal dural ring, which forms true roof of CS anteriorly, & distal dural ring
  - Short vertical clinoid segment medial to anterior clinoid process & corresponds to interdural segment of artery between proximal & distal dural rings

ANATOMY IMAGING ISSUES

Imaging Recommendations

- Due to high soft tissue contrast resolution & multiplanar capabilities, MR ± contrast remain imaging modality of choice
  - Coronal thin-section high-resolution T2 & T1 weighted sequences
  - Axial & coronal T1 fat-saturated thin-section high-resolution sequence after intravenous gadolinium contrast injection
- CT angiogram best for identifying pathology of cavernous ICA & for carotid cavernous fistula
- CT venogram can produce adequate venous-phase contrast enhancement to evaluate for CS thrombosis or thrombophlebitis
- High-resolution bone CT imaging, complementary in evaluation of erosive or destructive pathologies of central skull base
- Conventional angiogram often necessary for diagnosis & treatment of direct & indirect carotid cavernous fistulas as well as cavernous carotid aneurysms

Imaging Pitfalls

- Enhancement of CS can be asymmetric, especially in arterial phase or early venous phase, & should not be mistaken for pathology
- Given presence of multiple potentially enhancing structures in & around CS (CS, pituitary, & ICA), small enhancing lesion, such as perineural tumor spread, may be difficult to discriminate
- Fat can be normally seen anterior in CS near SOF & posterior ICA
- Air foci in CS can be seen on CT from venous emboli resulting from peripheral IV catheter placement

GRAPHICS

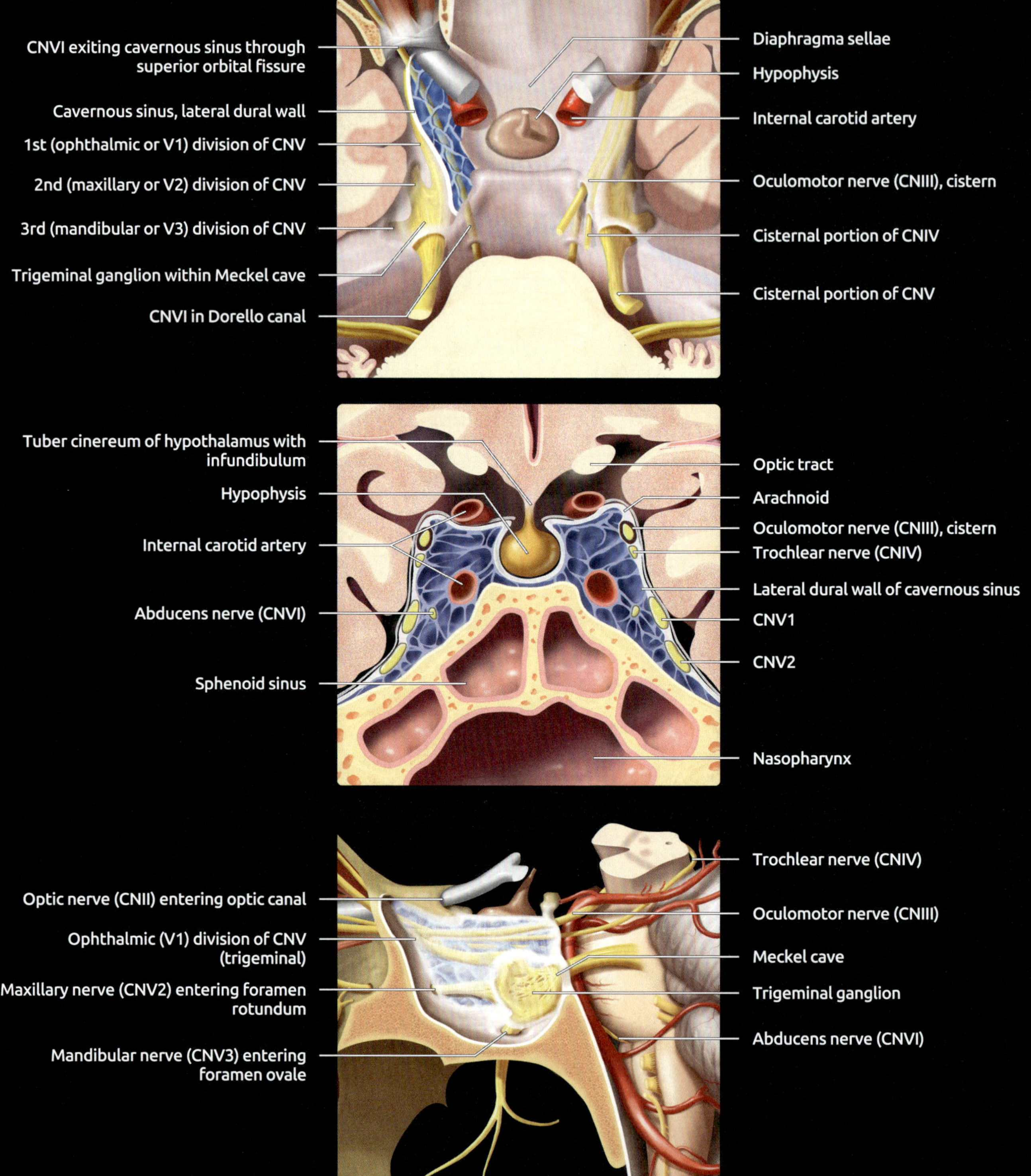

(Top) *Axial graphic of sella turcica, as viewed from above, depicts normal sellar and parasellar anatomy. Dura covering right cavernous sinus (CS) is removed to show CNV and CNVI. All cranial nerves are shown in left CS. Mandibular division of CNV does not run through CS but exits from Meckel cave inferiorly to enter foramen ovale. Note CS is not a single venous channel but is extensively septated.* **(Middle)** *Coronal graphic depicts contents of CSs. The following cranial nerves traverse CS within lateral wall of CS, from superior to inferior: Oculomotor (CNIII), trochlear (CNIV), 1st (ophthalmic or V1) and 2nd (maxillary or V2) divisions of trigeminal (CNV) nerves. The only cranial nerve actually within venous sinusoids of CS is abducens nerve (CNVI).* **(Bottom)** *Lateral graphic demonstrates cranial nerve detail in sellar region. CNIII, CNIV, CNV1, and CNV2 are in lateral dural wall of CS. CNVI courses within venous sinusoids of CS, adjacent to internal carotid artery (not shown). Meckel cave is CSF-filled, dural and arachnoid-lined invagination that communicates freely with prepontine cistern. It contains fascicles of trigeminal nerve (CNV) and trigeminal (gasserian) ganglion.*

AXIAL T1 C+ MR

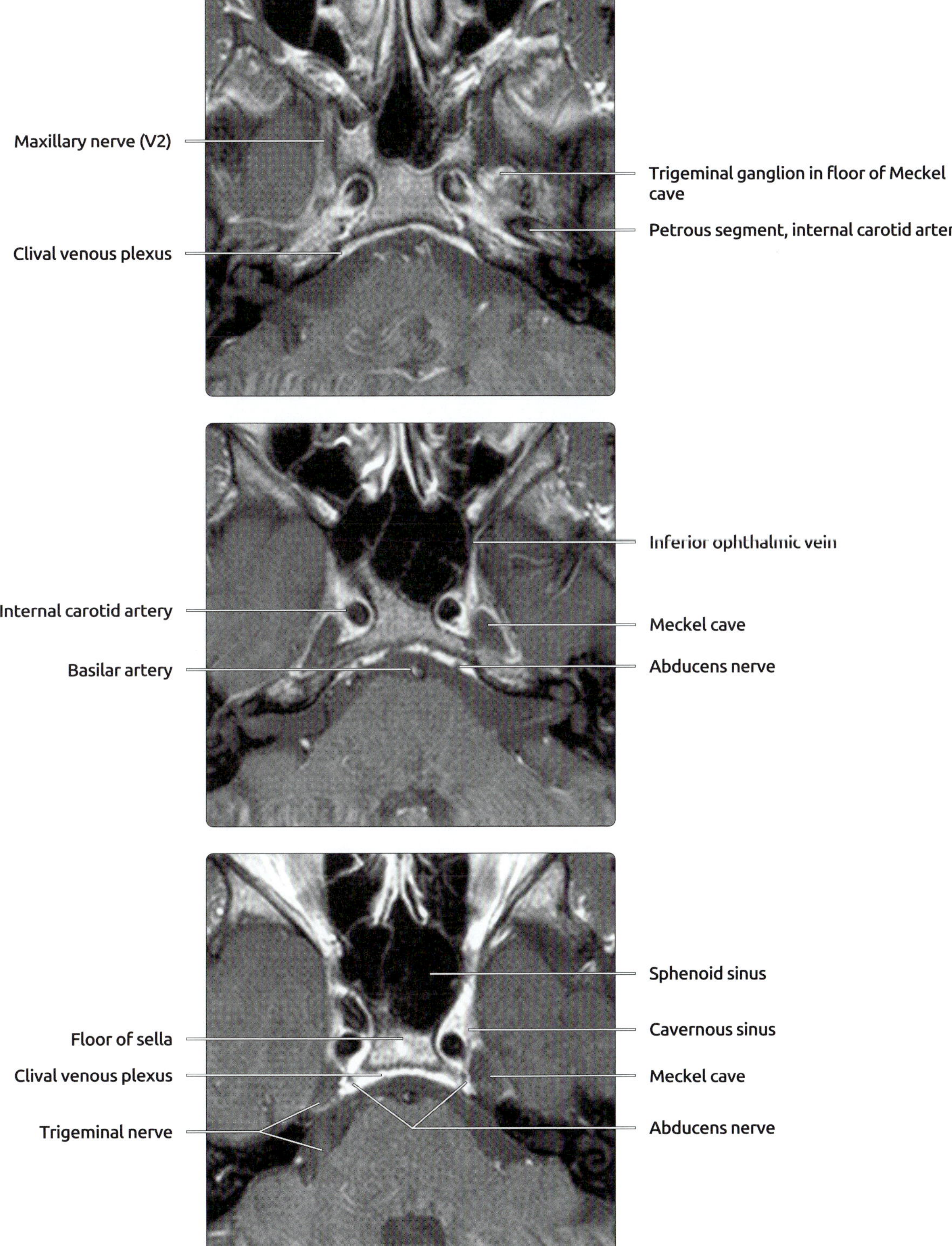

(Top) *Series of 6 axial contrast-enhanced T1 MR images, presented from inferior to superior through the skull base and CS, demonstrates the right maxillary nerve (V2) passing anteriorly into the foramen rotundum and the left trigeminal ganglion. The mandibular nerve (V3) will exit inferiorly through the foramen ovale (not shown).* **(Middle)** *The Meckel cave is located posterior, inferior, and lateral relative to the CS. Dura forming the posterior part of the lateral wall of the CS also forms the upper medial 1/3 of the Meckel cave, separating the 2 structures. Note the abducens nerve (CNVI) seen here as a filling defect within the clival venous plexus, just before entering the Dorello canal.* **(Bottom)** *Both abducens nerves are seen coursing through the Dorello canal to enter the posterior CS. The right trigeminal nerve is seen entering the Meckel cave.*

AXIAL T1 C+ MR

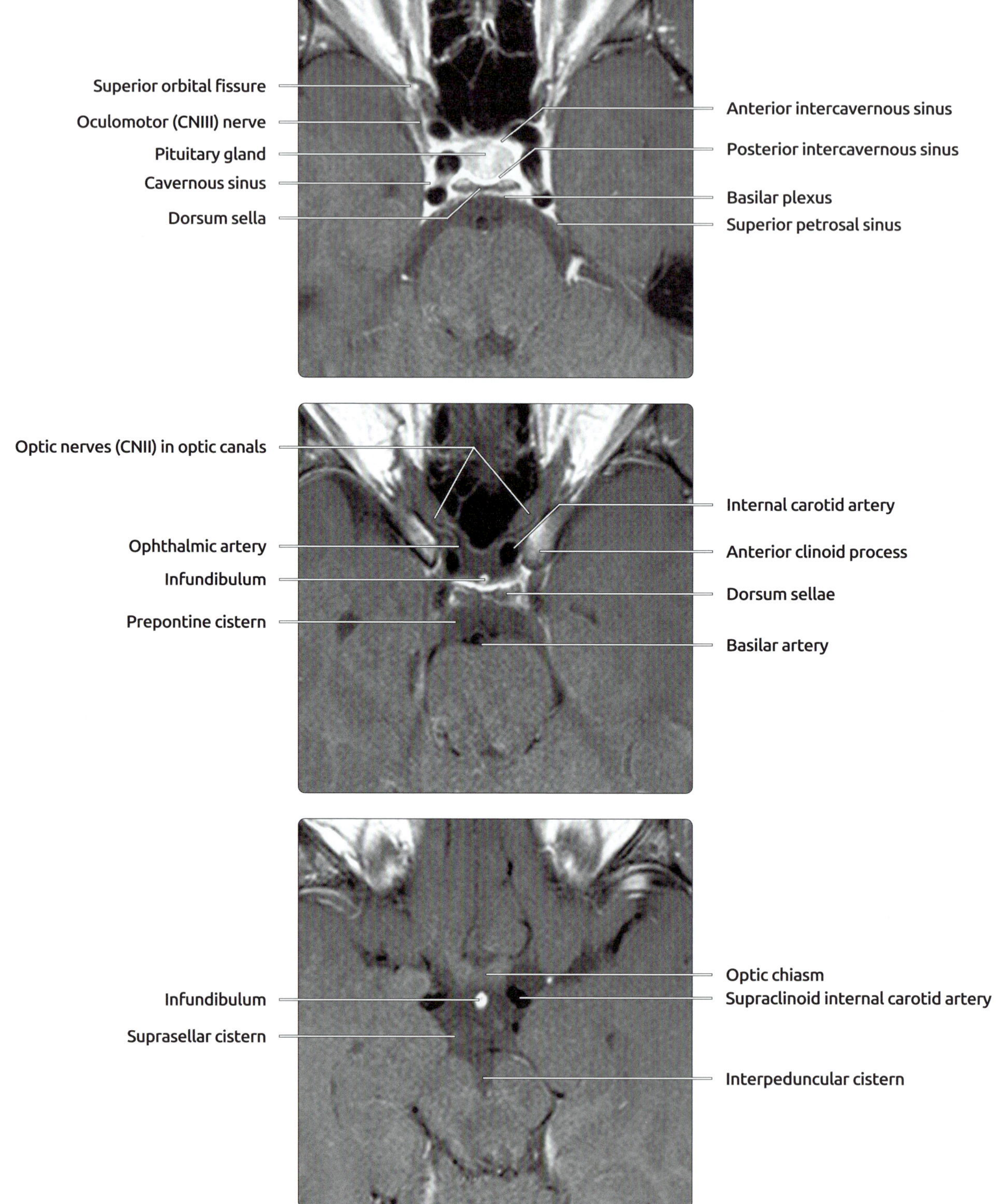

(Top) *Cranial nerves exiting the CS through the superior orbital fissure (SOF) are CNIII, CNIV, CNVI, and the 1st (ophthalmic or V1) division of CNV.* **(Middle)** *The optic nerve in the optic canal is located anteromedial to the anterior clinoid and superomedial to the SOF. It is separated from the SOF by a thin, bony strut, the "optic strut." The cavernous carotid is posteromedial to the anterior clinoid. Note the origin of the ophthalmic artery from the internal carotid artery, just above the transition from the intracavernous carotid (below) to the intradural carotid (above) segments.* **(Bottom)** *Pituitary infundibulum is seen within the suprasellar cistern posterior to the optic chiasm; avid enhancement seen here is typical. The supraclinoid internal carotid artery (or terminal segment) is seen laterally.*

CORONAL T2 MR

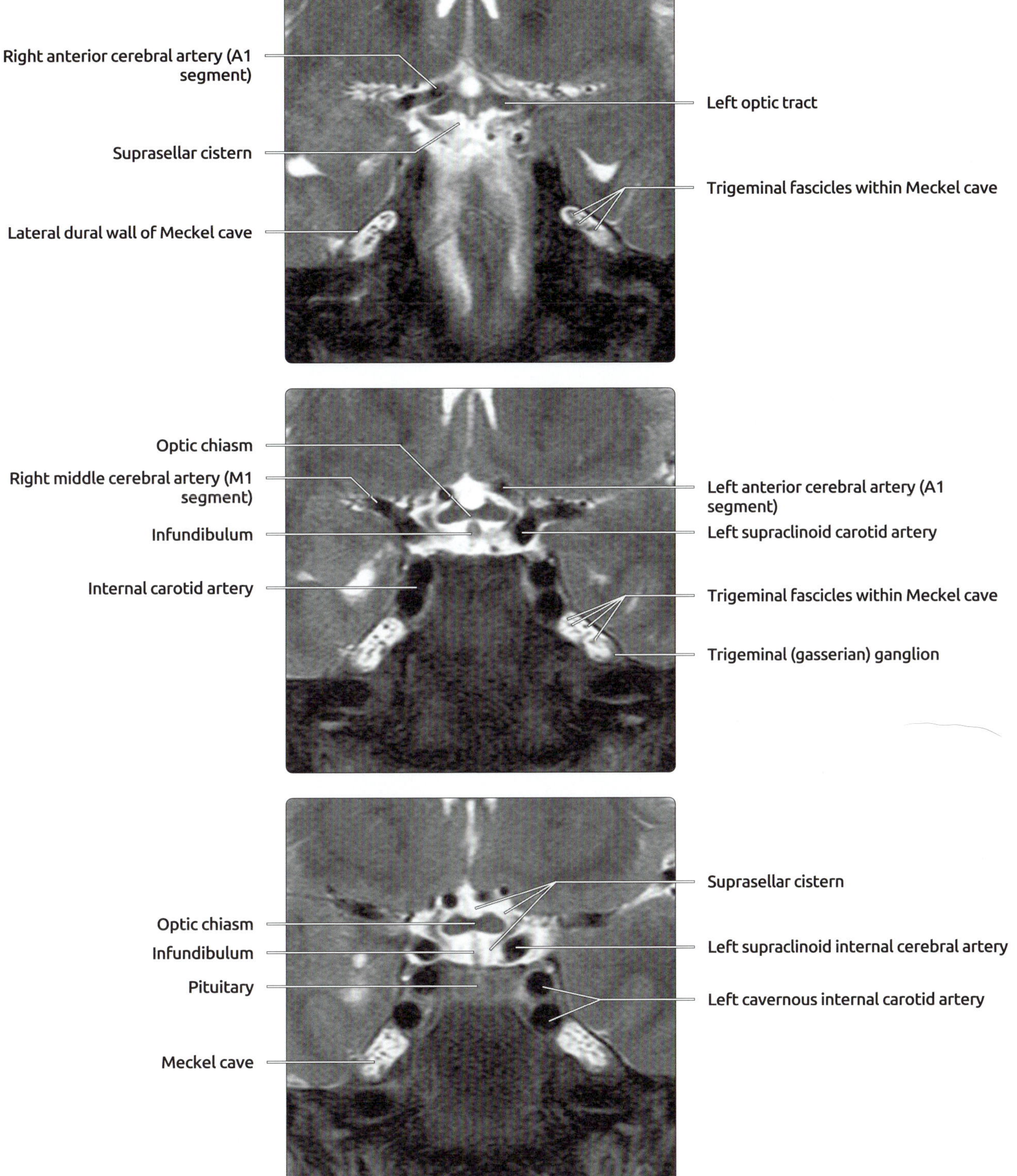

(Top) *First of 6 sequential coronal T2 MR images, presented from posterior to anterior, demonstrates the optic tracts within the posterior aspect of the suprasellar cistern and the anterior cerebral and supraclinoid internal carotid arteries.* **(Middle)** *The posterior optic chiasm and part of the pituitary infundibulum are seen here. Note the internal carotid, middle cerebral, and anterior cerebral arteries. Individual trigeminal nerve rootlets are well demonstrated within the Meckel cave on thin-section imaging.* **(Bottom)** *Image at the level of the optic chiasm within the suprasellar cistern demonstrates normal pituitary gland and regional vascular anatomy. Note the normal location and appearance of the Meckel cave, seen inferior and lateral. The pituitary gland and venous blood within the CS are nearly isointense with each other on T2.*

CORONAL T2 MR

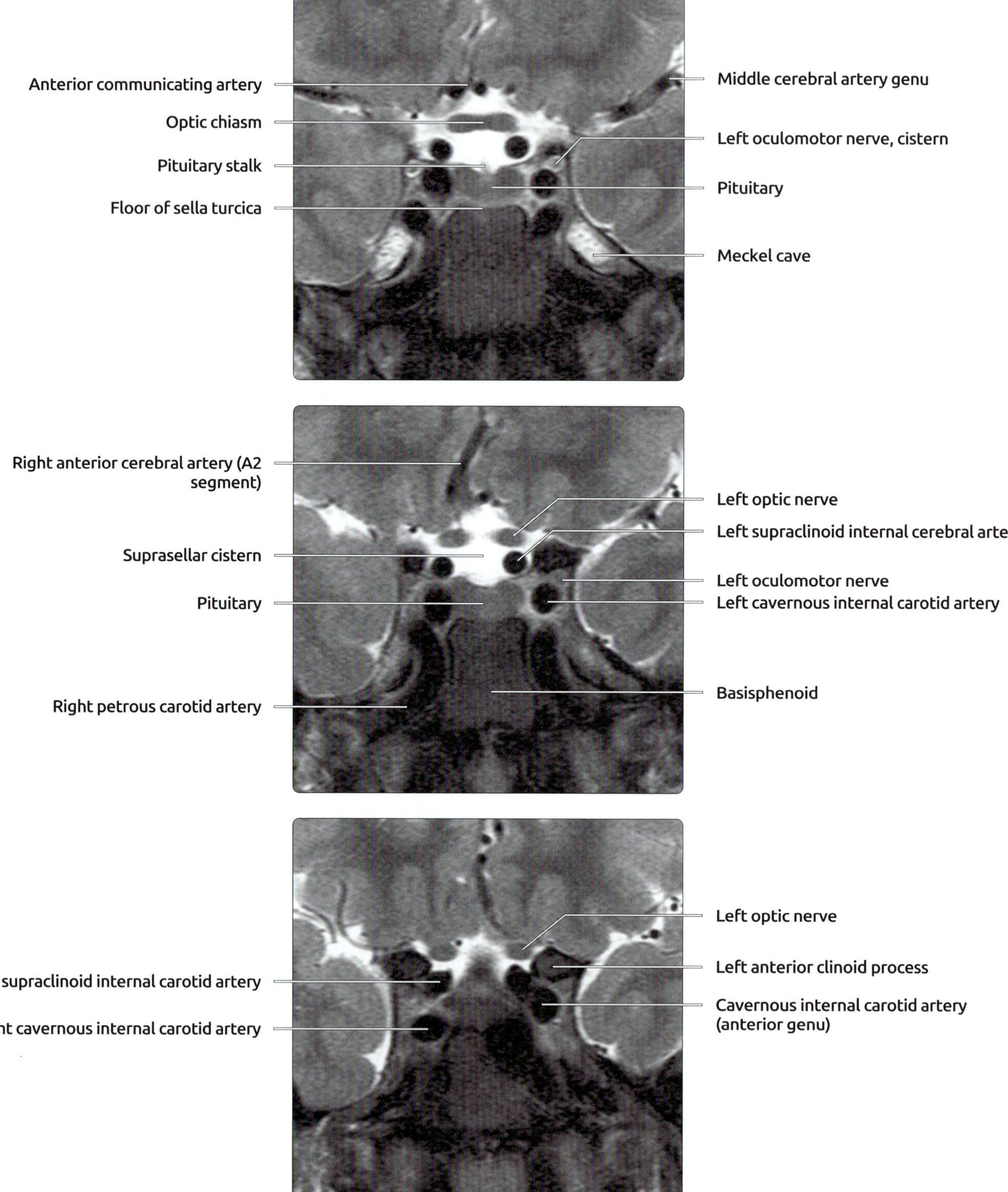

(Top) *Normal appearances of the anterior pituitary gland, CS, Meckel cave, and suprasellar cistern are shown. The oculomotor nerves (CNIII) and optic nerves (CNII) are well seen. The anterior communicating artery, which connects the 2 anterior cerebral arteries and the left middle cerebral artery genu, are visible.* **(Middle)** *The most anterior aspect of the suprasellar cistern demonstrates normal optic nerves (CNII), oculomotor nerves (CNIII), cavernous internal carotid arteries, and the anterior cerebral artery within the anterior interhemispheric fissure.* **(Bottom)** *The anterior clinoid processes seen here form the anterolateral boundaries of the sella turcica. Note the normal optic nerves, located medial to the anterior clinoids, and the anterior genu of the cavernous internal carotid artery on the left.*

CORONAL T1 C+ MR

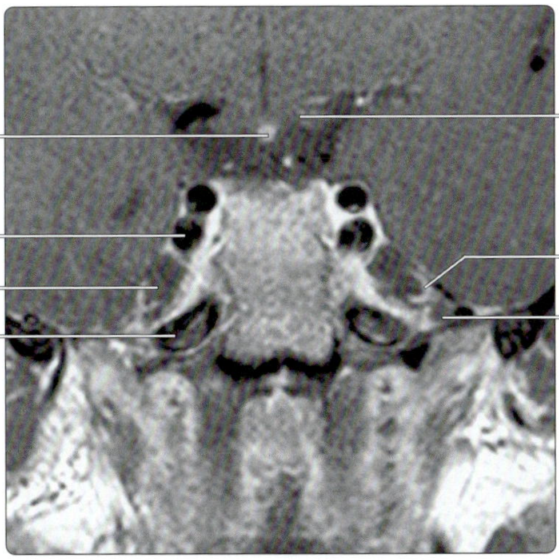

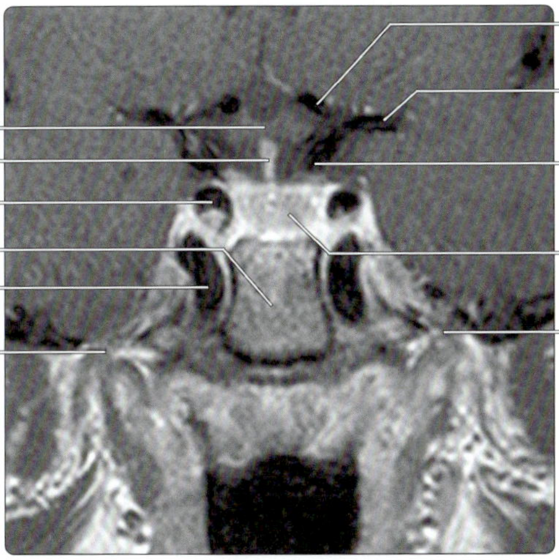

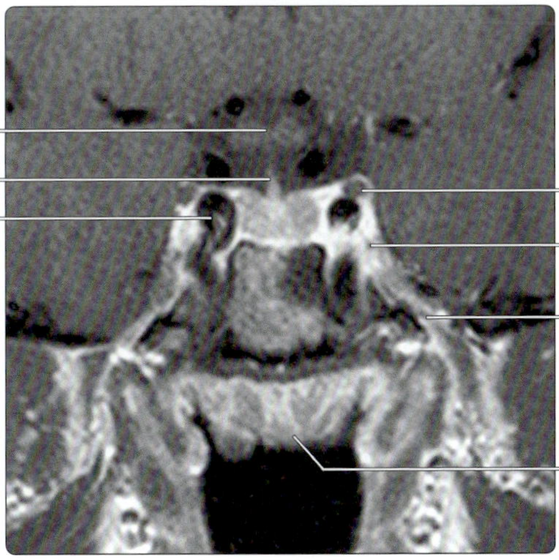

Infundibulum (pituitary stalk) upper aspect
Optic chiasm
Posterior cavernous internal carotid artery
Gasserian ganglion
Meckel cave
Mandibular nerve (V3)
Petrous internal carotid artery

Left anterior cerebral artery (A1 segment)
Left middle cerebral artery (M1 segment)
Optic chiasm
Infundibulum (pituitary stalk)
Supraclinoid left internal carotid artery
Cavernous internal carotid artery
Pituitary gland
Basisphenoid
Petrous internal carotid artery
Left foramen ovale
Mandibular nerve (V3) exiting foramen ovale

Optic chiasm
Infundibulum (pituitary stalk)
Oculomotor nerve (CNIII)
Cavernous internal carotid artery
Abducens nerve within cavernous sinus sinusoids
Mandibular nerve (V3)
Nasopharyngeal/adenoidal tissue

(Top) *First of 6 sequential contrast-enhanced T1 MR images through the sella, presented from posterior to anterior, demonstrates details of the Meckel cave. The mandibular (V3) division of the trigeminal nerve is seen inferior to the normally enhancing gasserian ganglion.* **(Middle)** *The pituitary infundibulum insertion into the gland is well seen. Note the mandibular nerve (3rd division of trigeminal nerve or V3), best seen on the right as it exits through foramen ovale, entering the high masticator space. It is easy to see how extracranial tumors may gain access to the intracranial compartment without destroying the skull base, either through direct extension or via perineural spread.* **(Bottom)** *The left foramen ovale is well seen. Note the 3rd and 6th cranial nerves within the CS. All of the cranial nerves are not well seen on this image.*

CORONAL T1 C+ MR

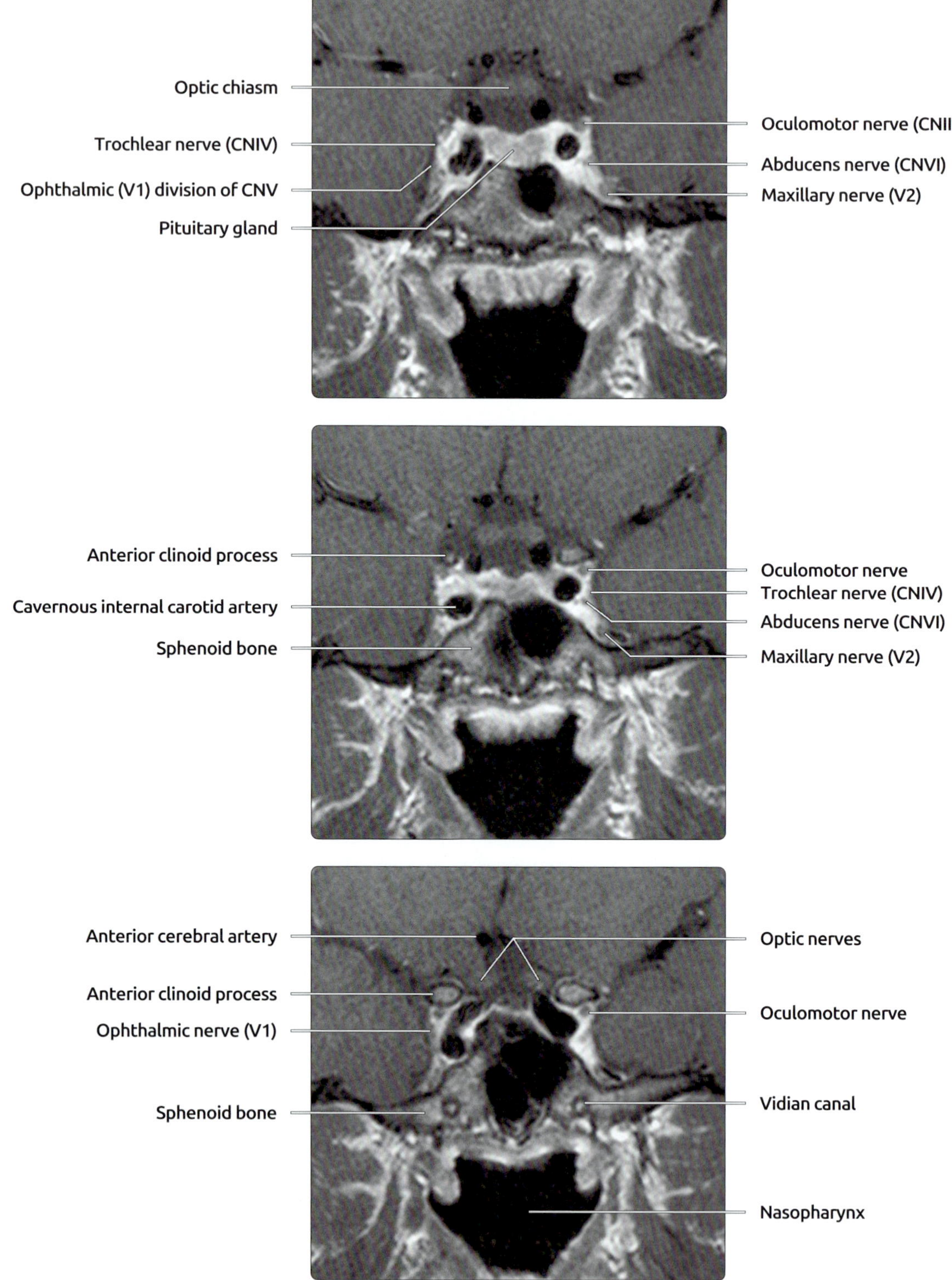

(Top) *This image demonstrates the oculomotor, abducens, and maxillary nerves. The pituitary gland enhances less strongly than venous blood in the CS.* **(Middle)** *Normal cranial nerves traversing the CS from superior to inferior include the oculomotor nerve, trochlear nerve, abducens nerve, ophthalmic nerve (V1), and maxillary nerve (V2). The 4th cranial nerve (trochlear) is small and difficult to visualize but is normally located in the lateral CS between the oculomotor and trigeminal nerves, lateral to the abducens.* **(Bottom)** *The oculomotor nerve is again well seen in the anterior CS before it traverses the SOF. The vidian canal, which contains the vidian artery and nerve, is seen in the sphenoid bone. Note the optic nerves medial to the anterior clinoids before entering the optic canals.*

ANATOMIC-PATHOLOGIC CORRELATION

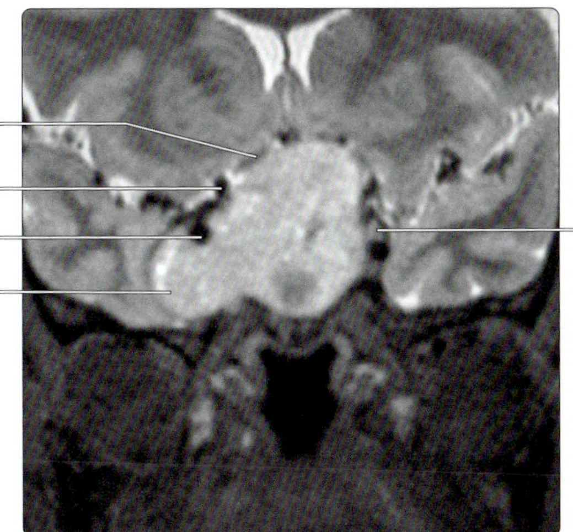

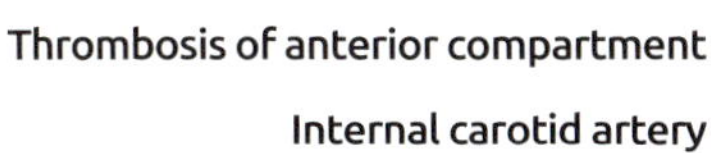

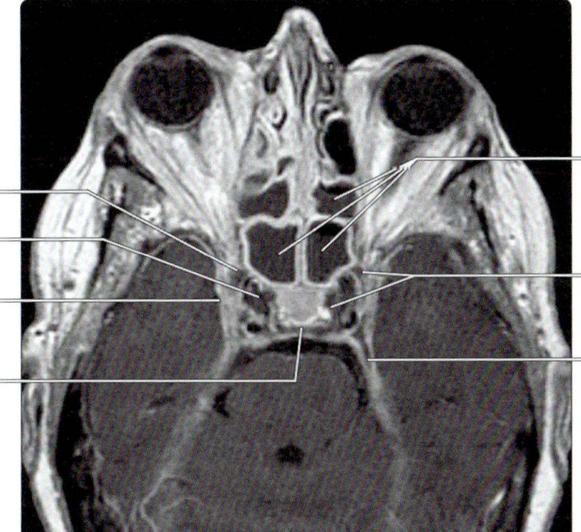

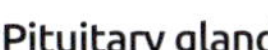

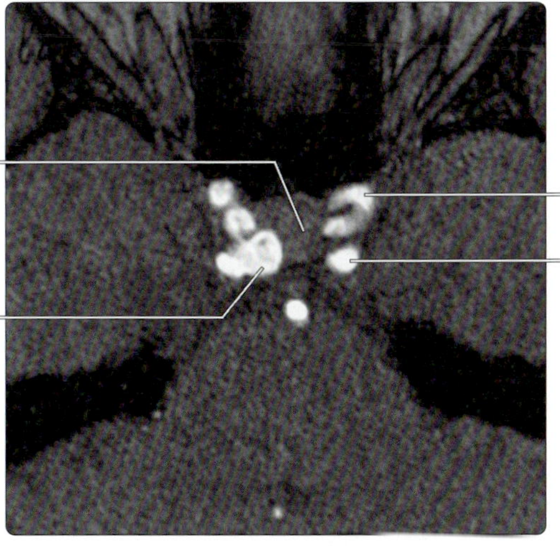

(Top) *Coronal T2 MR at the level of the CS demonstrates pituitary macroadenoma in the sella with suprasellar extension invading into the right CS. There is encasement of the right cavernous carotid with preserved flow void. There is significant mass effect on the optic apparatus. Note the normal left CS.* **(Middle)** *Axial MR performed in the same patient with bacterial sinusitis and bilateral CS thrombosis is shown. The flow voids in the internal carotid arteries are less distinct but present. The CS walls enhance normally, but the internal venous compartments of the CSs fail to enhance bilaterally due to venous sinus thrombosis.* **(Bottom)** *Axial 3D time-of-flight MRA demonstrates a saccular aneurysm arising from posterior genu of right cavernous carotid projecting medially with mild mass effect on the pituitary gland. Note normal left cavernous carotid flow-related signal.*

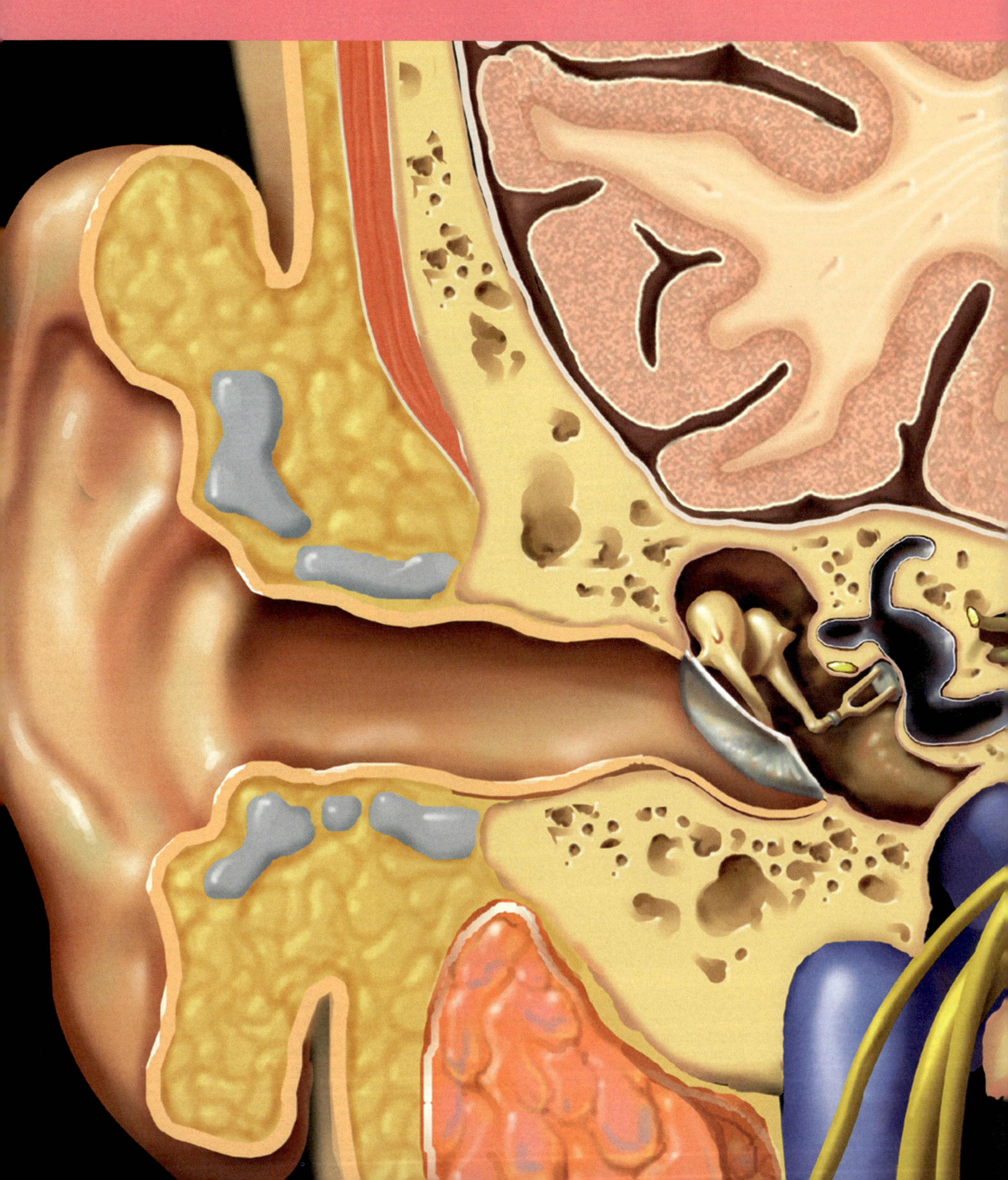

SECTION 4

Temporal Bone

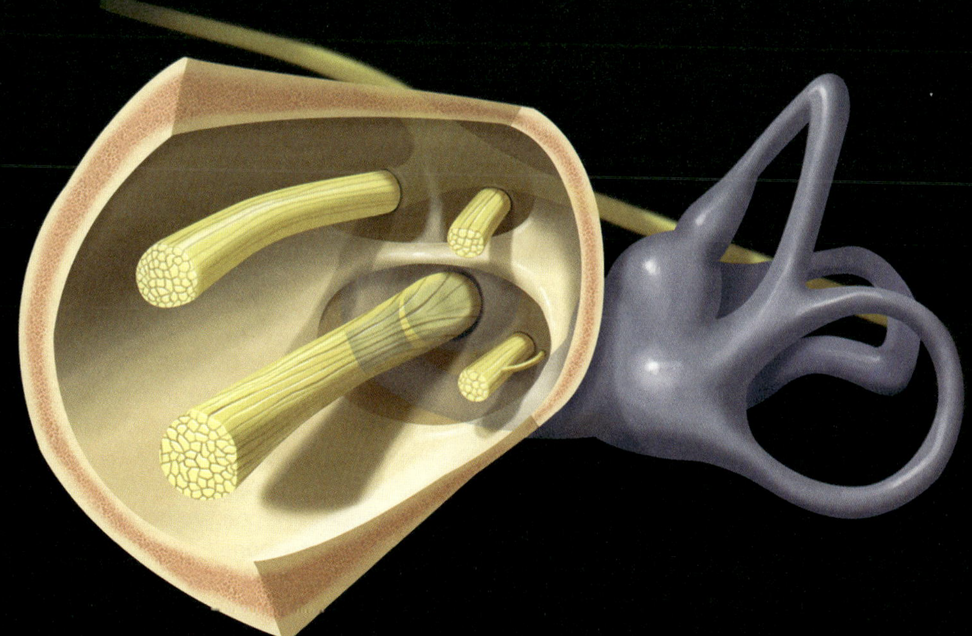

TERMINOLOGY

Abbreviations

- Temporal bone (T-bone)

IMAGING ANATOMY

Overview

- 5 bony parts to T-bone
  - **Squamous**: Forms lateral wall of middle cranial fossa
  - **Mastoid**: Aerated posterolateral T-bone
  - **Petrous**: Pyramidal-shaped medial T-bone with inner ear (IE), internal auditory canal (IAC), petrous apex (PA)
  - **Tympanic**: U-shaped bone forming bony external auditory canal (EAC)
  - **Styloid**: Forms styloid process after birth

Internal Contents

- **EAC**
  - Tympanic bone medially, fibrocartilage laterally
  - Medial border tympanic membrane
  - Nodal drainage to parotid chain
- **Middle ear (ME)-mastoid**
  - **Epitympanum** (attic): ME above line from superior EAC margin/scutal tip to tympanic CNVII on coronal CT/MR
    - **Tegmen tympani**: Roof of ME cavity
    - **Prussak space**: Lower lateral epitympanic recess below lateral malleal ligament
  - **Mesotympanum**: ME proper
    - Between epitympanum & hypotympanum
    - Medial wall: Lateral semicircular canal (SCC), tympanic segment CNVII, oval & round window craniocaudally
    - Posterior wall [retrotympanum (RT)]: Classic anatomy: Divided by **pyramidal eminence** into **facial recess** laterally & **sinus tympani** medially
      - Endoscopic anatomy much more complex
  - **RT endoscopic anatomy**: Divided by **pyramidal eminence** into lateral RT & medial RT
    - **Lateral RT**: Divided by **chordal eminence** into **facial recess** medially & **lateral tympanic sinus** laterally
      - **Styloid eminence** separates lateral RT superiorly from hypotympanum inferiorly
    - **Medial RT**: Divided by **subiculum** into **superior RT** & **inferior RT**
      - **Superior RT**: Divided by **ponticulus** into **posterior tympanic sinus** above & **sinus tympani** below
      - One or both of these sinuses may communicate with inconsistent **subpyramidal space** extending posteromedial to pyramidal eminence
      - **Inferior RT**: **Sinus subtympanicus** between lower otic capsule medially & styloid eminence laterally
      - **Finiculus** separates medial RT (sinus subtympanicus) posterosuperiorly from hypotympanum anteroinferiorly
  - **Hypotympanum**: Shallow trough in ME floor below line from inferomedial margin of EAC (tympanic annulus) to base of cochlear promontory on coronal CT/MR
  - **Protympanum**: ME compartment that lies anterior to frontal plane drawn through anterior margin of EAC/tympanic anulus on axial images
    - Opens posteriorly into mesotympanum
    - Leads anteriorly into eustachian tube & semicanal for tensor tympani muscle
  - **ME ossicles**: Malleus, incus, & stapes
    - Ice cream & cone appearance in epitympanum on axial CT: Malleus head & incus body/short process
  - **Mastoid** sinus: 4 key structures
    - **Aditus ad antrum**: Connects epitympanum to mastoid antrum
    - **Mastoid antrum**: Large, central mastoid air cell
    - **Körner septum**: Part of petrosquamosal suture running posterolaterally through mastoid air cells
    - **Tegmen mastoideum**: Roof of mastoid air cells
- **IE components**
  - **Bony labyrinth**: Bone lodging cochlea, vestibule, & SCCs
  - **Perilymphatic spaces**
    - **Perilymph** = fluid within bony labyrinth that surrounds & "bathes" endolymph-containing membranous labyrinth (ML) structures
    - In cochlea **within** scala tympani & scala vestibuli
    - In vestibule **surrounding** utricle & saccule
    - In SCCs **surrounding** semicircular ducts
    - Within perilymphatic duct inside cochlear aqueduct
  - **ML/endolymphatic spaces**
    - **Endolymph** = fluid within structures of ML
    - In cochlea **within** scala media (cochlear duct)
    - In vestibule **within** utricle & saccule
    - In SCCs **within** semicircular ducts
    - In vestibular aqueduct **within** endolymphatic duct/sac
  - **Cochlea**: ~ 2.5 turns; modiolus; 3 spiral chambers (scala tympani, scala vestibuli, & scala media)
  - SCCs: Superior, lateral, & posterior
    - Superior SCC (SSCC): Bony ridge over SSCC in roof of petrous pyramid called **arcuate eminence**
    - Lateral SCC: In medial ME just above tympanic CNVII
    - Posterior SCC: Along posterior petrous bone
- **PA**
  - Anteromedial to IE
  - Pneumatized or nonpneumatized (marrow)
- **Intratemporal facial nerve**
  - CNVII segments: IAC, labyrinthine, tympanic, mastoid
  - **Geniculate ganglion** = anterior genu
  - Posterior genu: Tympanic segment bends inferiorly to become mastoid segment
  - **Stylomastoid foramen**: CNVII exits skull base here
- **Petrous internal carotid artery (ICA): C2 segment**
  - ICA: Vertical & horizontal T-bone segments
  - Vertical segment: Rises to genu beneath cochlea
  - Horizontal segment: Projects anteromedially to turn cephalad as precavernous & cavernous ICA
- **Muscles of T-bone**
  - **Tensor tympani muscle**
    - Dampens sound; hyperacusis if injured
    - Innervation: V3 branch
    - Location: Anteromedial wall, mesotympanum
    - Attachment: Tendon inserts on malleus handle
  - **Stapedius muscle**
    - Dampens sound; hyperacusis if injured
    - Innervation: CNVII
    - Location: Muscle belly in pyramidal eminence
    - Attachment: Tendon attaches on neck of stapes

GRAPHICS: EXTERNAL EAR AND MIDDLE EAR

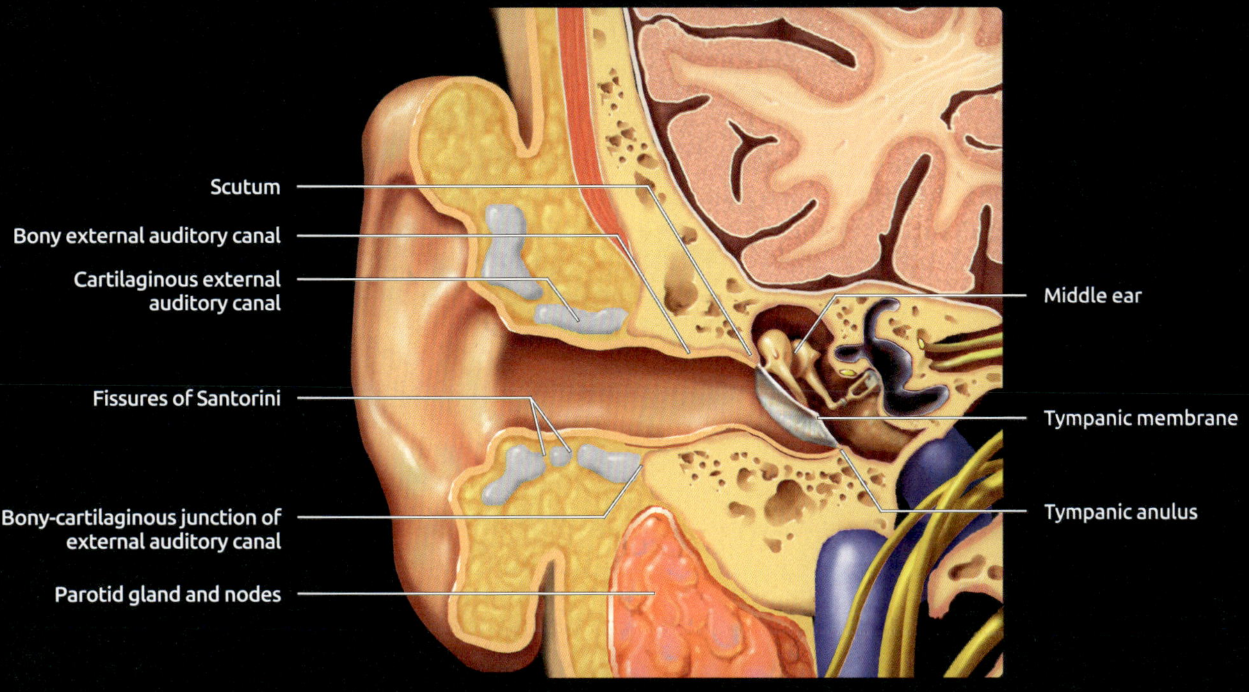

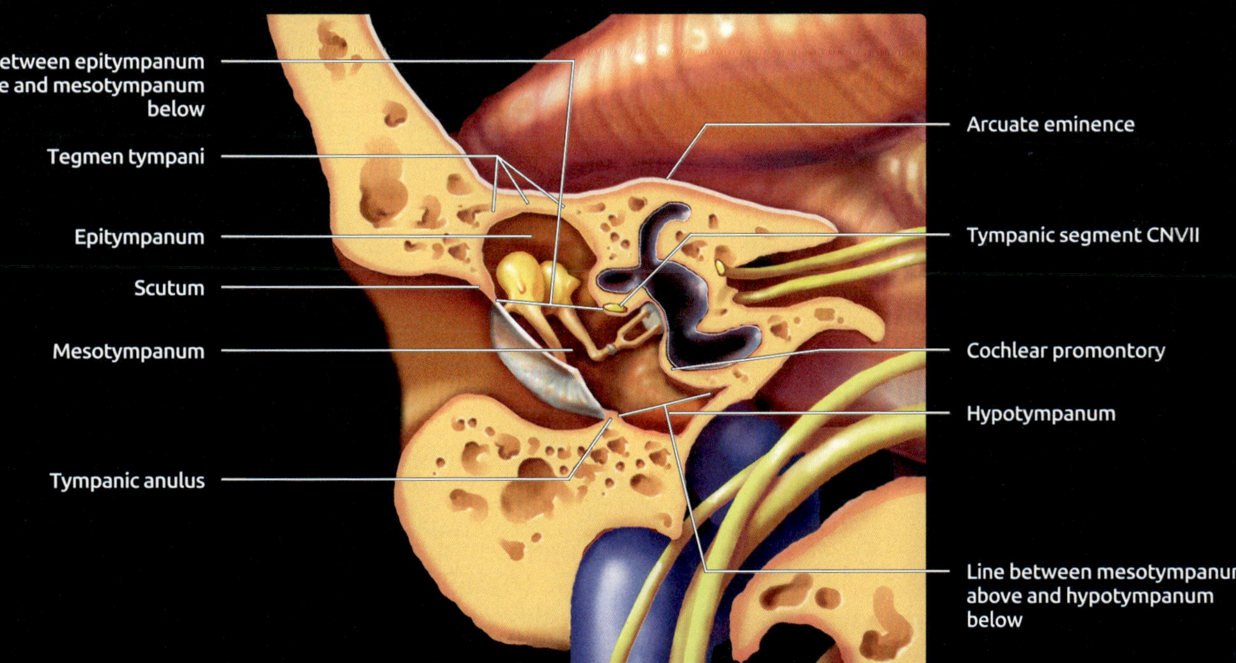

(Top) *Coronal graphic shows the external and middle ear. The external auditory canal (EAC) is made up of lateral cartilaginous and medial bony components. Infection of the EAC can penetrate inferomedially to the skull base and associated spaces via the fissures of Santorini (gaps in the EAC cartilage). External ear and EAC lymphatic drainage is to the parotid nodal chain. The medial margin of the EAC is the tympanic membrane, which attaches to the scutum and tympanic anulus.* **(Bottom)** *Coronal graphic shows the middle ear, which is divided into 3 components: Epitympanum, mesotympanum, and hypotympanum. Epitympanum is the middle ear cavity above a line drawn from the medial roof of EAC/scutal tip and tympanic segment of CNVII. Its roof is called the tegmen tympani. The mesotympanum extends from this line inferiorly to a line connecting the medial inferior margin of EAC/tympanic anulus to the base of the cochlear promontory. Hypotympanum lies inferior to this line. Protympanum lies anterior to a frontal plane drawn through anterior margin of EAC/tympanic anulus on axial images and leads anteriorly into eustachian tube and semicanal for tensor tympani muscle.*

GRAPHICS: FACIAL NERVE AND CRANIAL NERVE

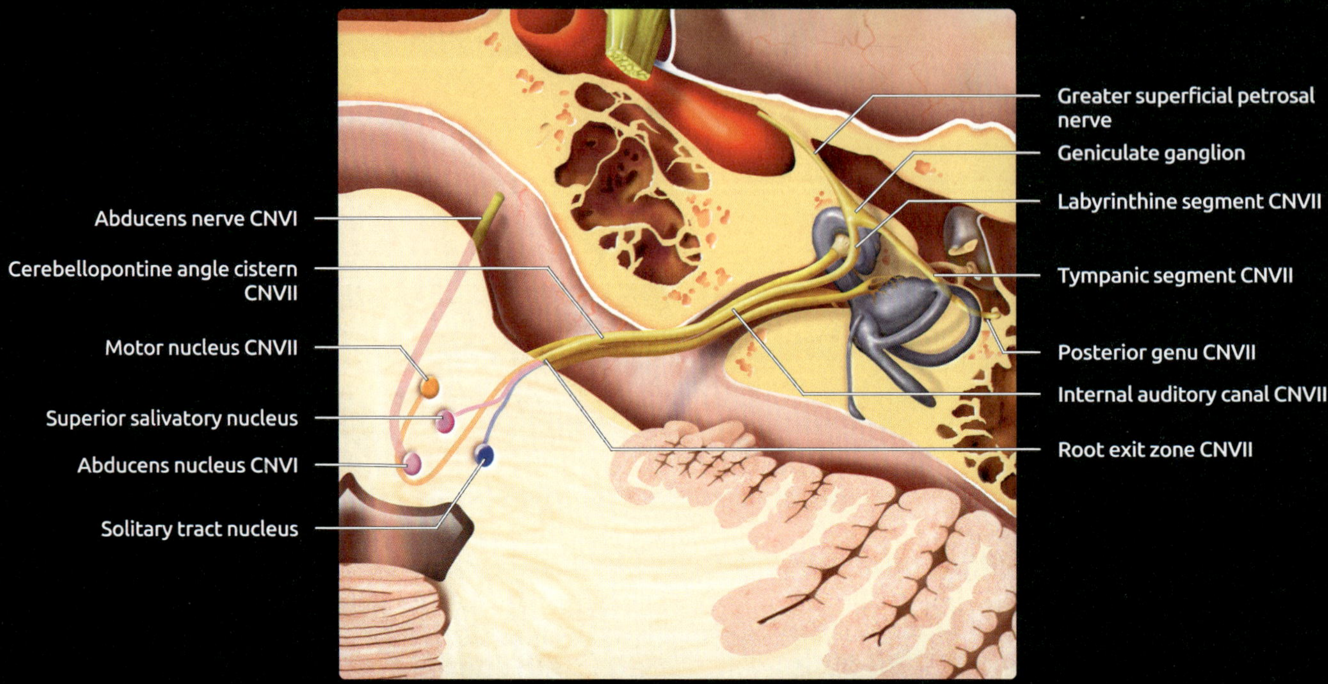

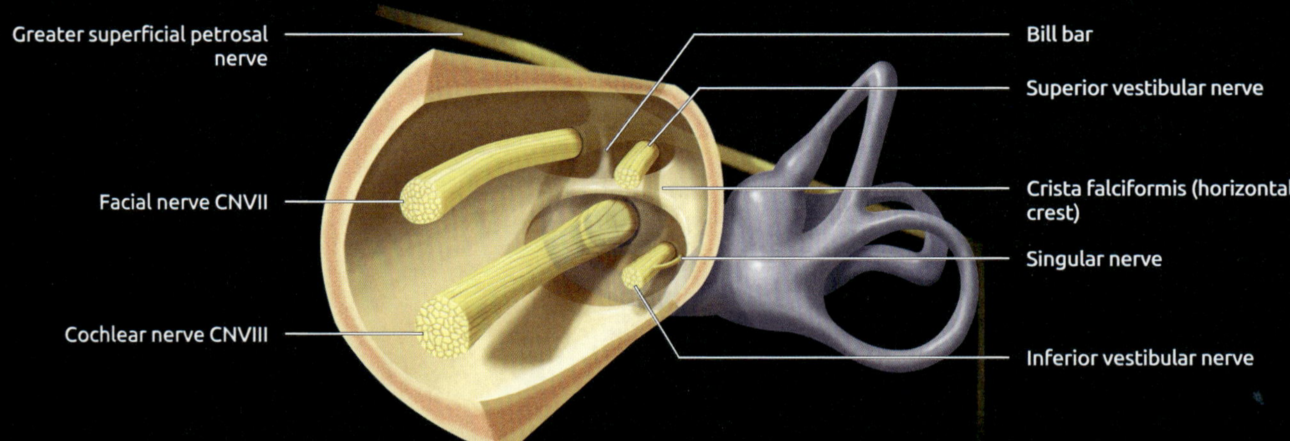

(Top) *Axial graphic shows the facial nerve from the brainstem nuclei to the posterior genu of the temporal bone. Motor nucleus sends out its fibers to circle CNVI nucleus (facial colliculus) before reaching root exit zone at pontomedullary junction. Superior salivatory nucleus sends parasympathetic secretomotor fibers to lacrimal and nasal glands [through nervus intermedius of Wrisberg (NIW) → facial nerve → greater superficial petrosal nerve (GSPN) → vidian nerve → pterygopalatine ganglion], and submandibular, sublingual (through NIW → facial nerve → chorda tympani nerve → lingual nerve → submandibular ganglion) salivary glands. Solitary tract nucleus receives anterior 2/3 of tongue taste information through chorda tympani and from palate through GSPN.* **(Bottom)** *Graphic shows nerves at internal auditory canal fundus. Note that horizontal crista falciformis separates facial nerve and superior vestibular nerve (SVN) above from cochlear nerve and inferior vestibular nerve (IVN) below, while the vertical crest (Bill bar) separates the facial nerve from the SVN. Anteriorly: "7up (CNVII)/coke (cochlear) down." Posteriorly: Vestibular nerves; SVN up, IVN down.*

GRAPHICS: MEMBRANOUS LABYRINTH AND PETROUS INTERNAL CAROTID ARTERY

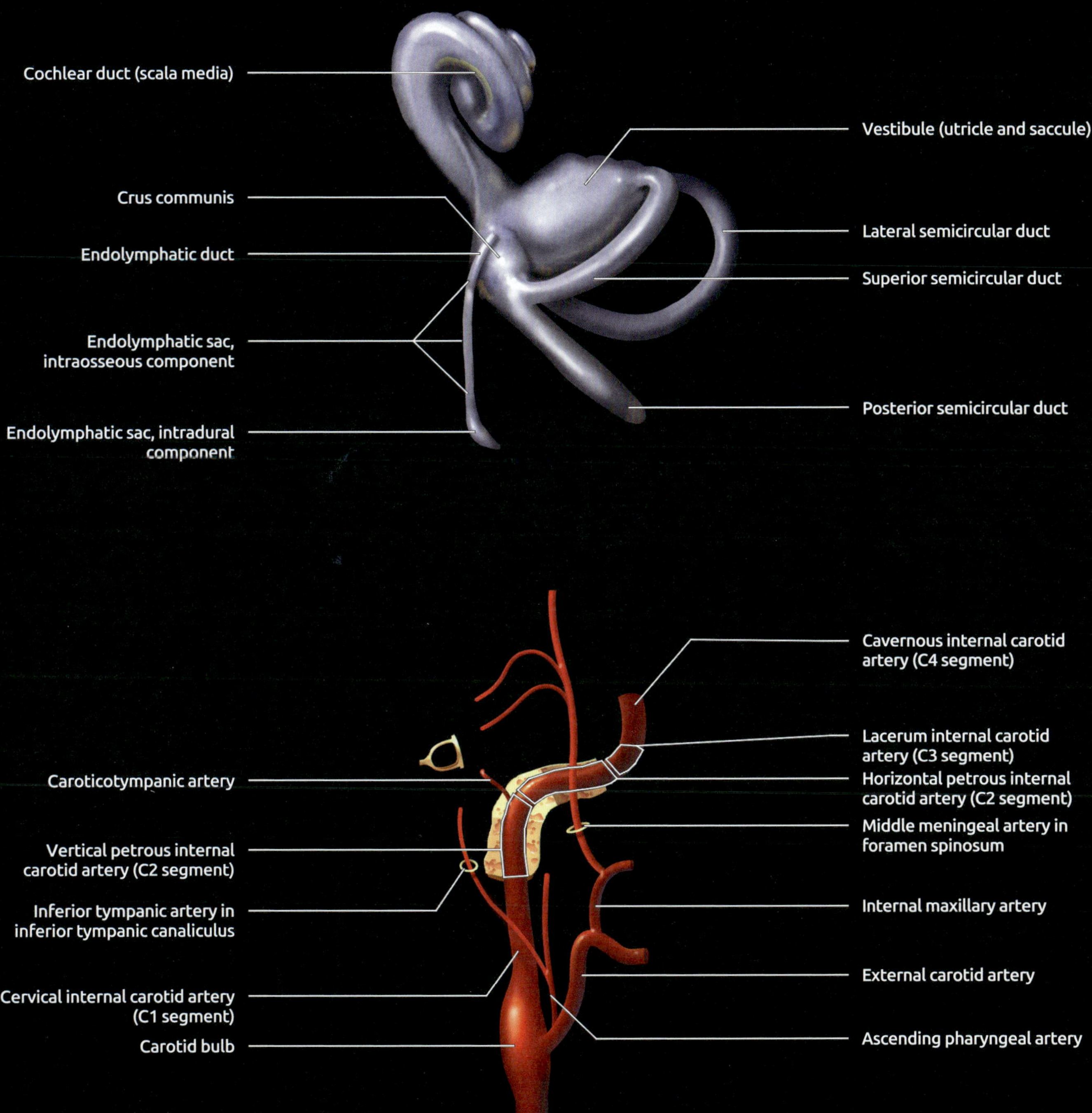

(Top) *Graphic of membranous labyrinth from above is shown. Key elements of membranous labyrinth to consider include ~ 2.5 turns of cochlea, the meeting point of the superior and posterior semicircular ducts (crus communis), and endolymphatic duct and sac. Note that endolymphatic duct has intraosseous and intradural components. Vestibule has sac-like components named utricle posterosuperiorly and saccule anteroinferiorly. Ductus reuniens connects the base of scala media of cochlea to the adjacent anteroinferiorly situated saccule of vestibule.* **(Bottom)** *Graphic emphasizes the petrous internal carotid artery (ICA). The cervical ICA enters the carotid canal of the skull base to become the vertical petrous ICA (C2 subsegment ICA). It then turns anteromedially to become the horizontal petrous ICA. The segment of the intracranial ICA just above the foramen lacerum is called the lacerum segment (C3 ICA segment). Note the inferior tympanic artery arising from the ascending pharyngeal artery and passing through the inferior tympanic canaliculus, and the middle meningeal artery arising from the internal maxillary artery and passing through the foramen spinosum.*

AXIAL BONE CT

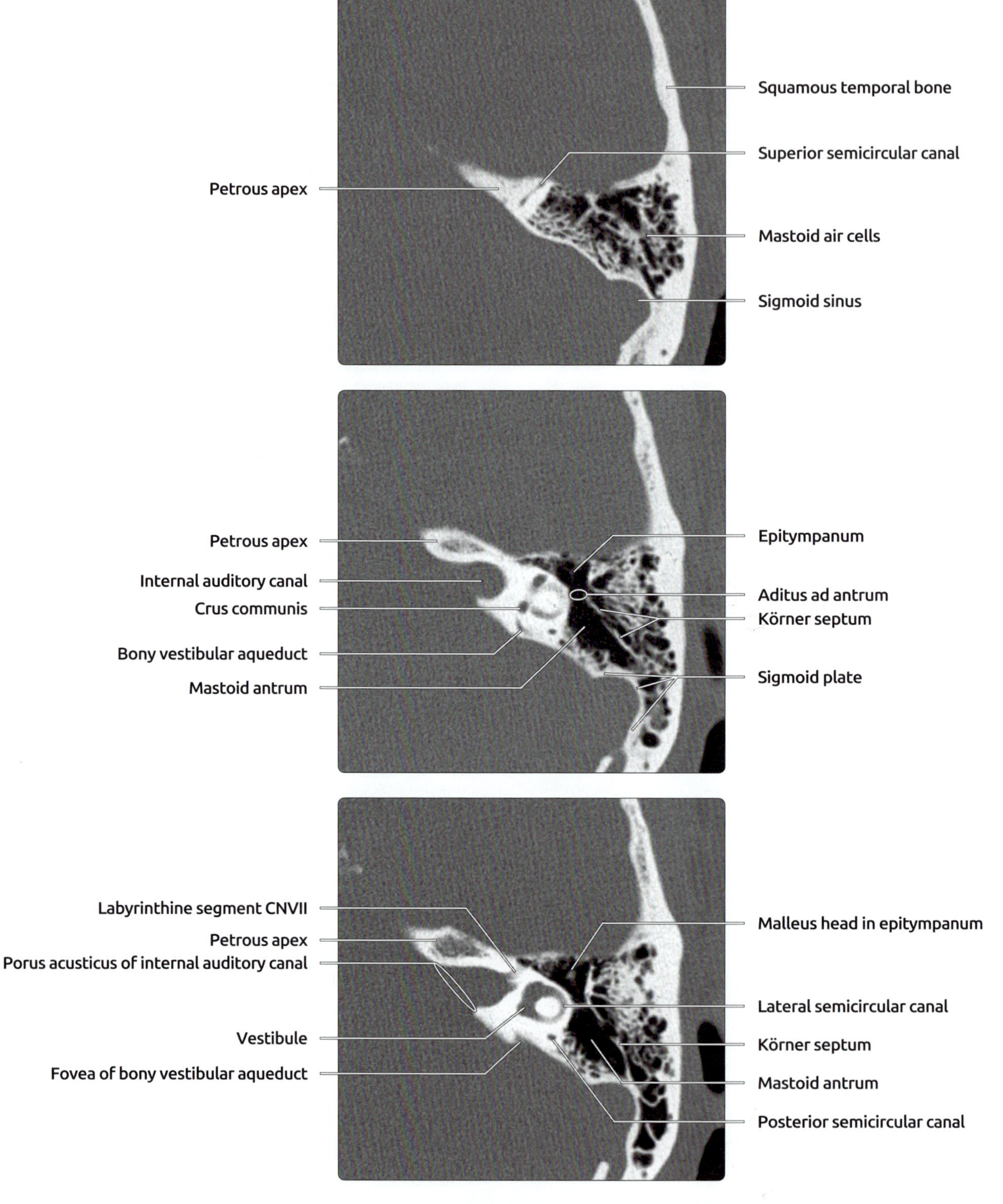

(Top) *First of 12 axial bone CT images of the left temporal bone from superior to inferior is shown. The superior semicircular canal projects cephalad from the inner ear. The bony cover over the top of the semicircular canal is called the arcuate eminence.* **(Middle)** *At the level of the upper internal auditory canal, the aditus ad antrum (Latin: "Entrance to the cave") is seen connecting the epitympanum to the mastoid antrum (Latin: "Cave"). Notice the Körner septum separating the mastoid antrum from the squamous portion of the mastoid air cells. Sigmoid plate is the thin bony plate separating the sigmoid sinus from adjacent structures like the mastoid air cells. Some authors describe the sigmoid plate more specifically as the thin bone between the jugular bulb and middle ear cavity (jugular floor/wall/plate or paries jugularis).* **(Bottom)** *At the level of the lateral semicircular canal, the opening to the internal auditory canal, the porus acusticus, is particularly well seen. The fovea of the bony vestibular aqueduct along the posterior wall of the temporal bone houses the intradural endolymphatic sac.*

AXIAL BONE CT

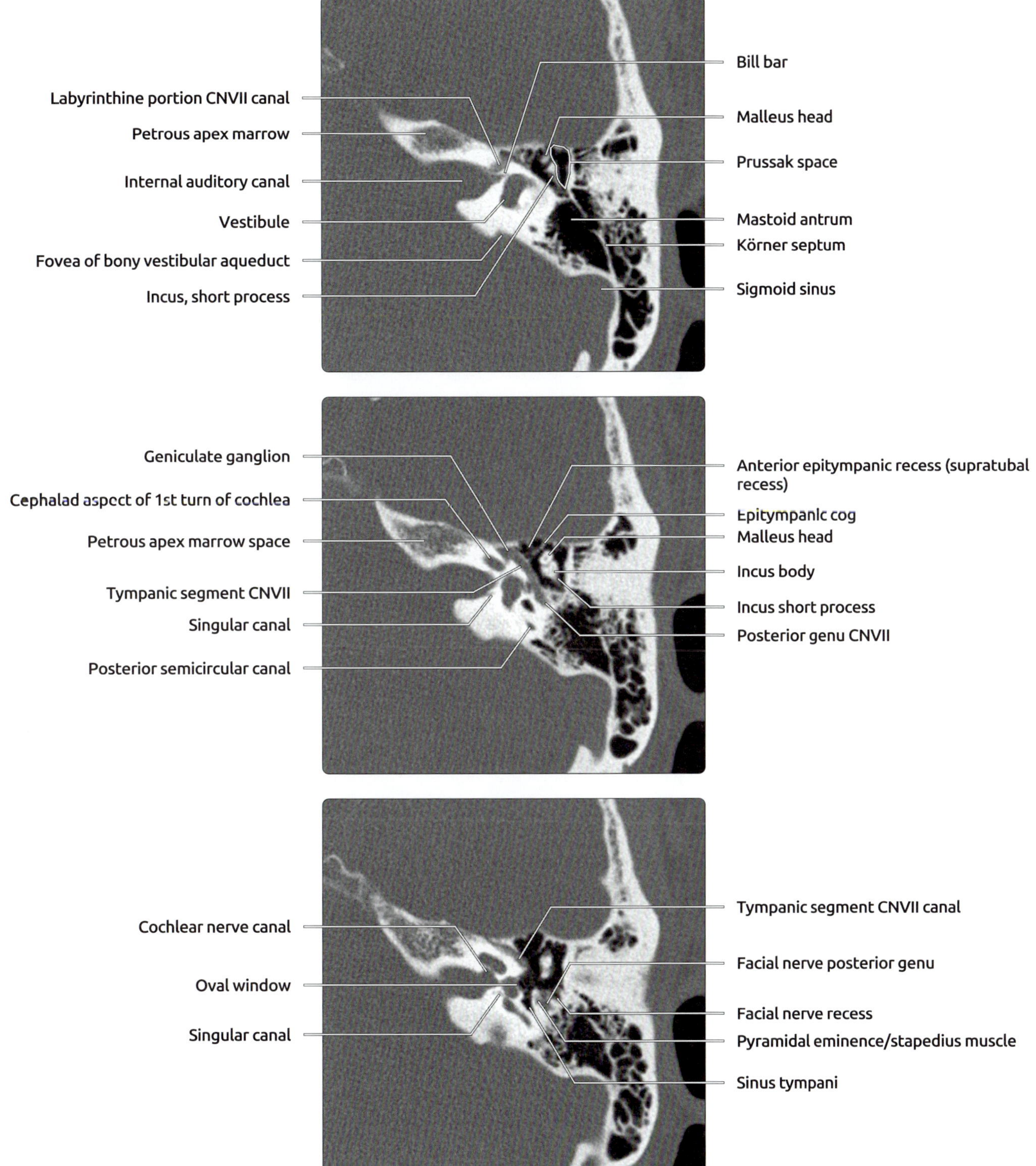

(Top) *Image through the labyrinthine segment of the facial nerve shows this structure just cephalad to the cochlea. The Prussak space is now visible, which is the lower lateral epitympanic recess below lateral malleal ligament. This is the 1st area that the typical pars flaccida cholesteatoma involves in the middle ear.* **(Middle)** *Tympanic segment of the facial nerve is seen from anteromedial geniculate ganglion to the posterior genu, where it changes to become the mastoid segment. Note the epitympanic cog (anterior attic bony plate), which is a coronally oriented bony septum, suspended from the anterior tegmen tympani. Cog partitions the anterior epitympanic recess (supratubal recess) from epitympanum proper.* **(Bottom)** *Three key structures on the posterior wall of the middle ear cavity are well seen. From medial to lateral, they are the sinus tympani, pyramidal eminence, and facial nerve recess. Endoscopic anatomy of the retrotympanum is more complex and includes other air spaces, namely, lateral tympanic sinus, posterior tympanic sinus, subpyramidal space and sinus subtympanicus, and bony bars, such as, chordiculus, ponticulus, subiculum, finiculus, and styloid eminence.*

AXIAL BONE CT

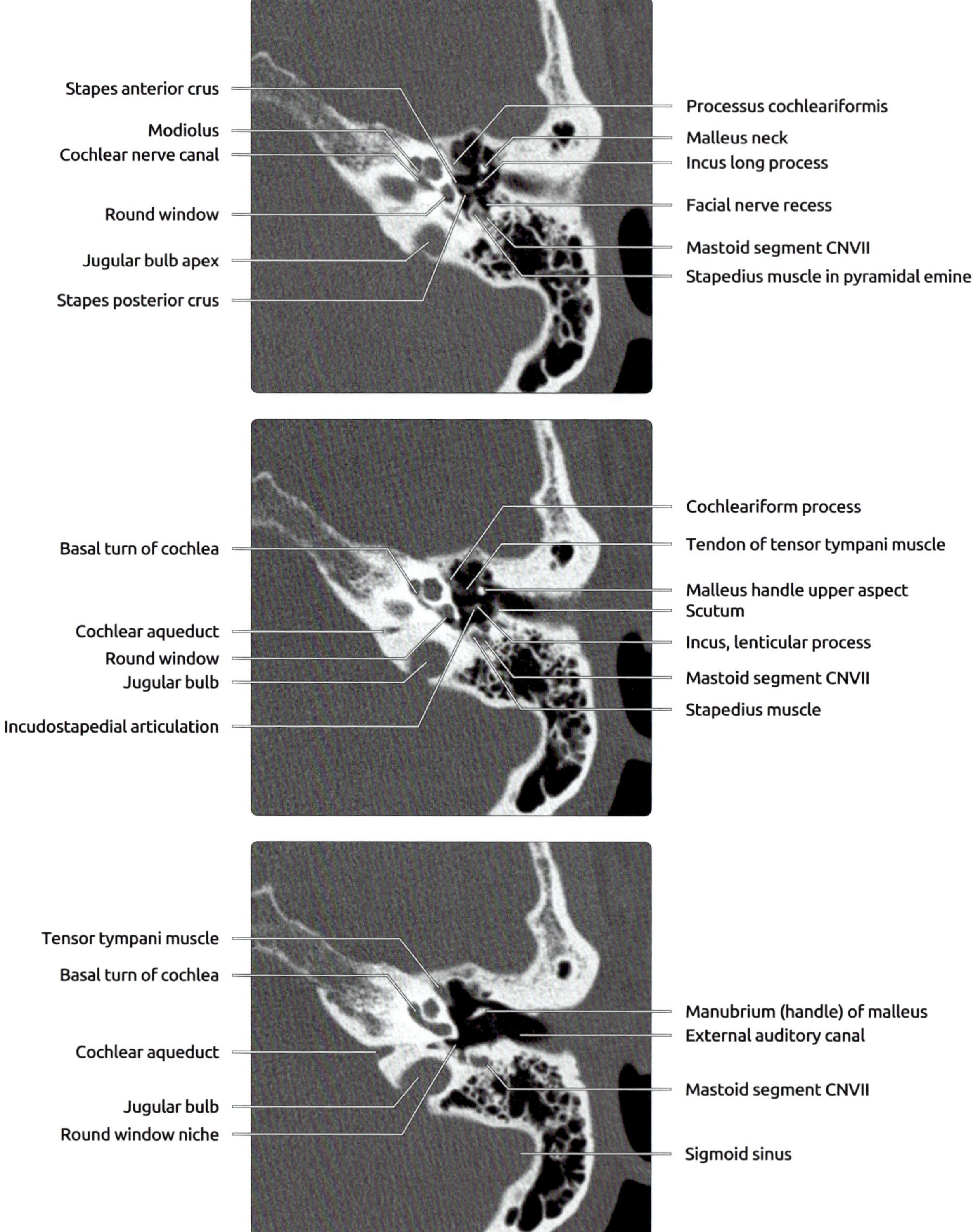

(Top) *This image at the level of the cochlear nerve canal shows the cochleariform process high on the cochlear promontory. The cochleariform process (processus cochleariformis) is the anulus through which the tendon of the tensor tympani muscle turns toward the more lateral malleus handle (manubrium). Stapes crura are visible. The stapedius muscle in the pyramidal eminence is now distinguishable from the mastoid segment of the facial nerve.* **(Middle)** *Midcochlear image shows both the cochleariform process and the tendon of the tensor tympani muscle extending over to the upper proximal aspect of the handle of malleus. The incudostapedial articulation is visible between the lenticular process of the incus and the stapes head. Also note the round window at the base of the basal turn of the cochlea. Cochlear aqueduct arises superolaterally from the scala tympani at the basal turn of cochlea and runs through the otic capsule and petrous apex; difficult to see on CT.* **(Bottom)** *At the level of the low mesotympanum, note the cochlear aqueduct on the medial wall parallel and inferior to the internal auditory canal. The manubrium (handle) of the malleus is also visible.*

AXIAL BONE CT

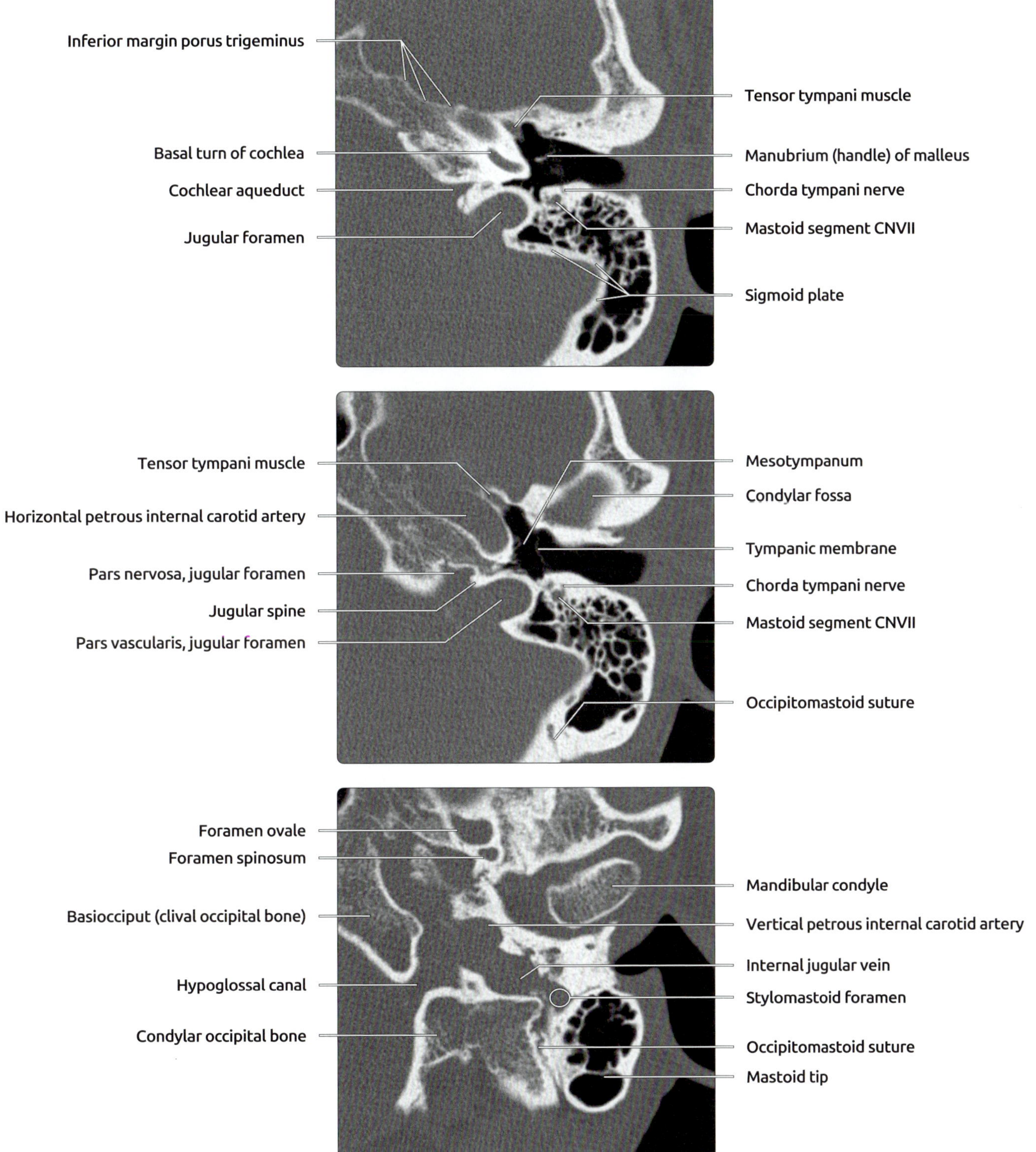

(Top) *In this image, the normal cortex of the sigmoid plate is well seen. The sigmoid plate separates the mastoid air cells from the sigmoid sinus. Notice the cochlear aqueduct on the medial temporal bone wall. The funnel-shaped inferomedial end of cochlear aqueduct opens at a part of the roof of pars nervosa of jugular foramen called pyramidal fossa.* **(Middle)** *At the level of the mesotympanum, the normal tympanic membrane is just barely visible. The horizontal petrous ICA canal is seen running anteromedial towards the cavernous sinus. Notice the pars nervosa (just below cochlear aqueduct) and pars vascularis of the jugular foramen partially separated by the jugular spine.* **(Bottom)** *The mastoid tip is seen in this inferior image. Just anteromedial to the mastoid tip is the stylomastoid foramen where the facial nerve exits the skull base. Notice the entrance to the vertical segment of the petrous ICA canal just medial to the condylar fossa. The occipitomastoid suture should not be mistaken for a fracture line.*

CORONAL BONE CT

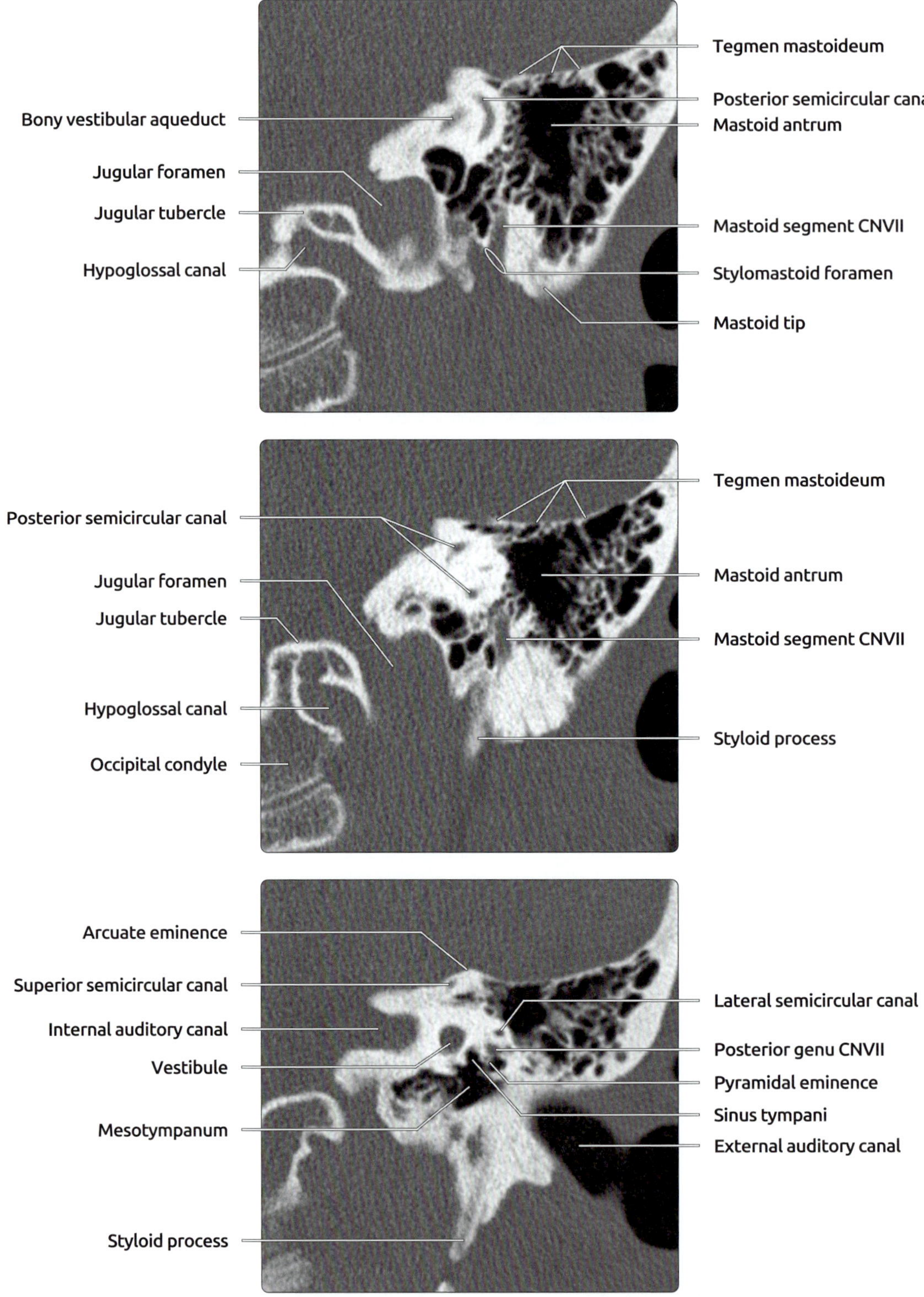

(Top) *First of 12 coronal bone CT images from posterior to anterior is shown. In this most posterior image, the stylomastoid foramen and distal mastoid segment of the facial nerve can be seen to be protected by the mastoid tip. The mastoid sinus grows into this protective position in the 1st decade of life.* **(Middle)** *In this image, the midmastoid segment of the facial nerve is seen. The jugular foramen and the hypoglossal canal are separated by the "eagle's beak," a portion of the jugular tubercle. Jugular foramen lies superolateral to the "beak," and hypoglossal canal lies underneath the "beak."* **(Bottom)** *In this image of the posterior mesotympanum, the 3 critical posterior wall structures are seen. From medial to lateral, these structures are the sinus tympani, the pyramidal eminence, and the facial nerve recess with the posterior genu of CNVII in its depth. Note that it is possible to see the stapedius muscle as a small, round soft tissue density within pyramidal eminence.*

CORONAL BONE CT

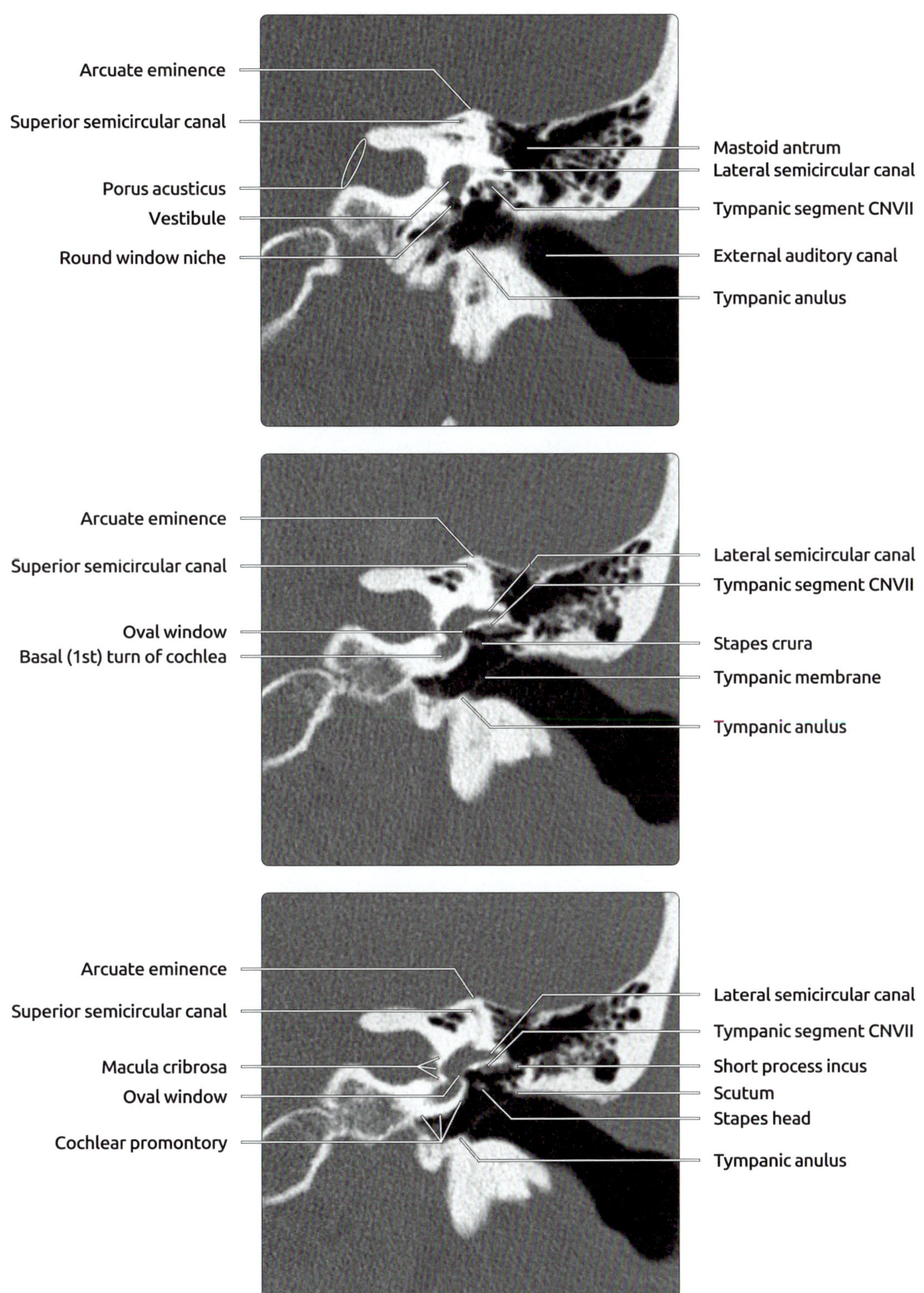

(Top) *In this image, the posterior tympanic segment of the facial nerve is visible under the lateral semicircular canal. The round window niche is a small bony pouch defined by thin overhanging bone that extends from the cochlear promontory. The small, air-filled area off the medial mesotympanum here leads to the round window membrane.* **(Middle)** *At the level of the oval window niche, the basal turn of the cochlea becomes visible. Notice the tympanic membrane is barely seen when it is normal. Its inferior attachment, the tympanic anulus, is a useful landmark separating the middle ear from the medial external ear.* **(Bottom)** *In this image, the short process of the incus is seen projecting posteriorly towards the aditus ad antrum. Both the tympanic membrane attachments can be seen: The superior scutum and the inferior tympanic anulus. Notice that the cochlear promontory projects out into the mesotympanum. Glomus tympanicum paragangliomas occur here.*

CORONAL BONE CT

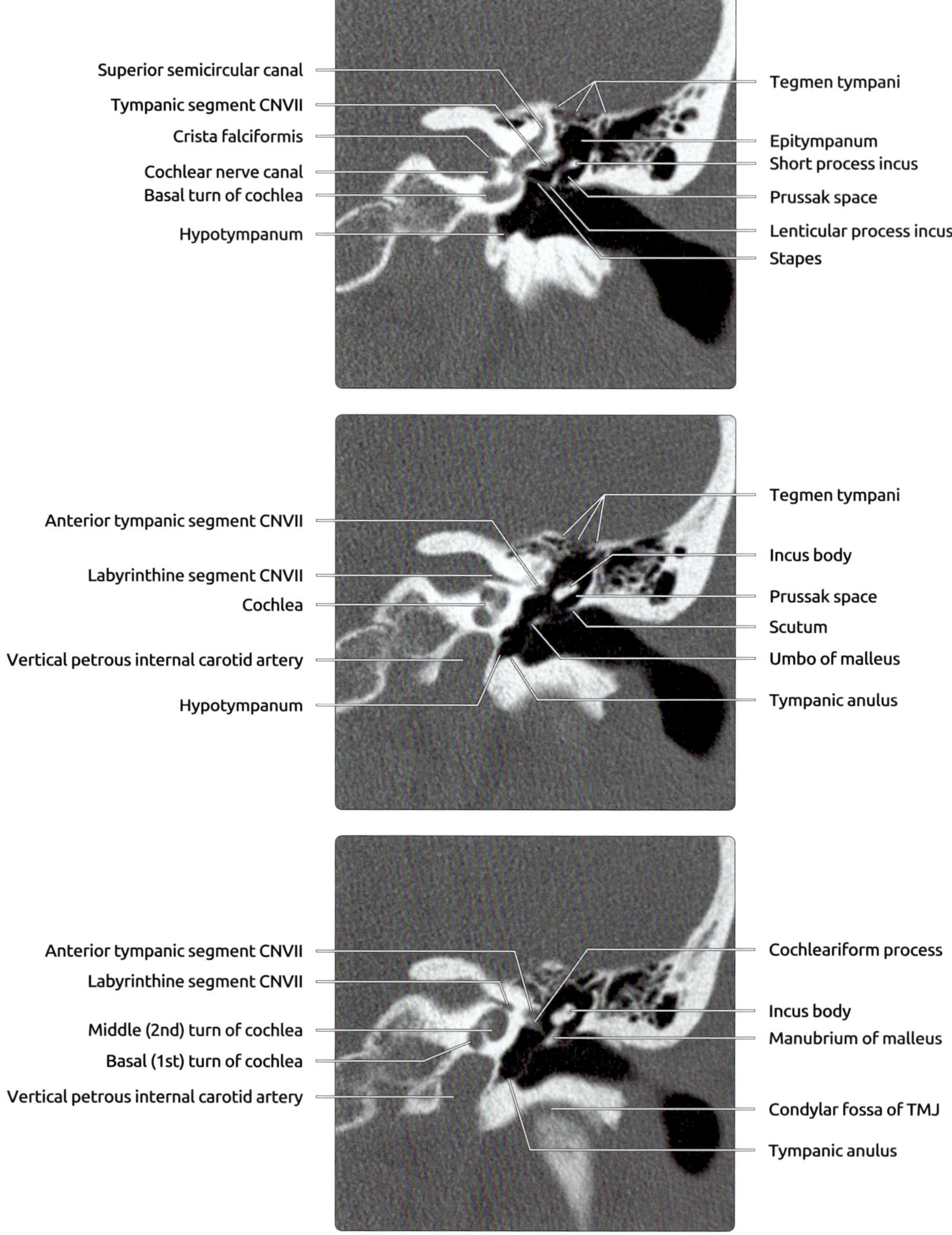

(Top) *Image through the midmesotympanum shows the more superior epitympanum with the long and short processes of the incus forming the medial margin and the lower lateral epitympanic wall forming the lateral margin of Prussak space. Pars flaccida cholesteatoma involves the middle ear cavity, initially in Prussak space.* **(Middle)** *In this image, the tegmen tympani (Latin: "Roof of the cave") can be seen as the superior wall of the epitympanum. Note its normal variable thickness. Just above the cochlea, the facial nerve canal is seen emerging from the fundus of the internal auditory canal to become the labyrinthine segment CNVII.* **(Bottom)** *Three key structures are seen together in this image: The labyrinthine segment CNVII, anterior tympanic CNVII, and the cochleariform process. Note the tendon of the tensor tympani muscles projecting from the cochleariform process to attach to the upper aspect of manubrium (handle) of malleus.*

CORONAL BONE CT

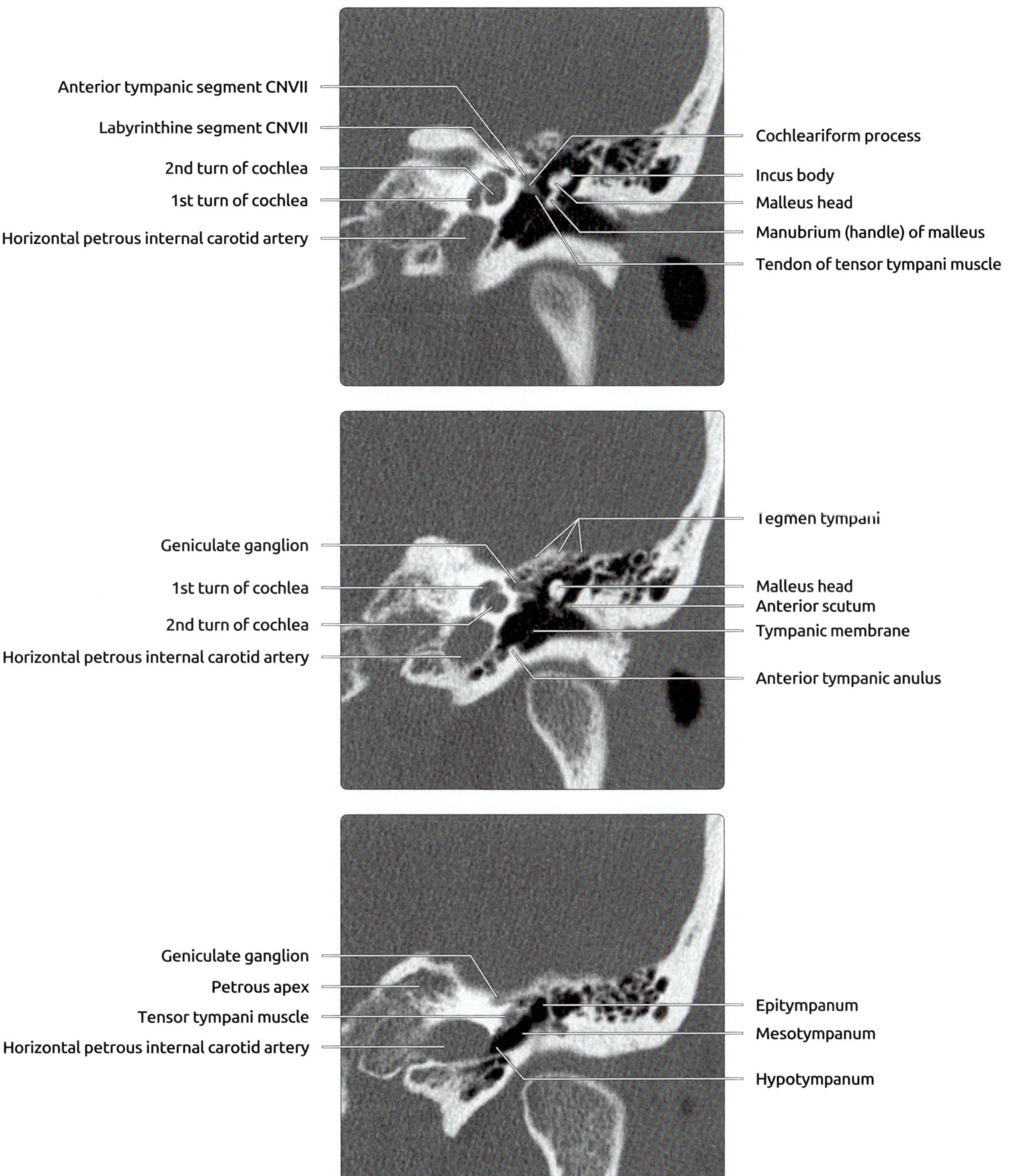

(Top) *The labyrinthine segment of CNVII is seen here merging together with the anterior tympanic CNVII above the cochlea. The cochleariform process and tendon of the tensor tympani muscle are both visible. The petrous ICA horizontal segment can be seen below the cochlea.* **(Middle)** *In this image, the tegmen tympani is thick and well defined. The geniculate ganglion in the geniculate fossa is seen on the superolateral cochlea with the horizontal petrous ICA below the cochlea. Both the scutum and tympanic anulus are visible between the gossamer thin tympanic membrane.* **(Bottom)** *In the most anterior middle ear cavity, the ossicles are not seen. The geniculate ganglion in the geniculate fossa, along with the tensor tympani muscle, are visible. The horizontal petrous ICA is now projecting anteromedially.*

SAGITTAL T2 MR

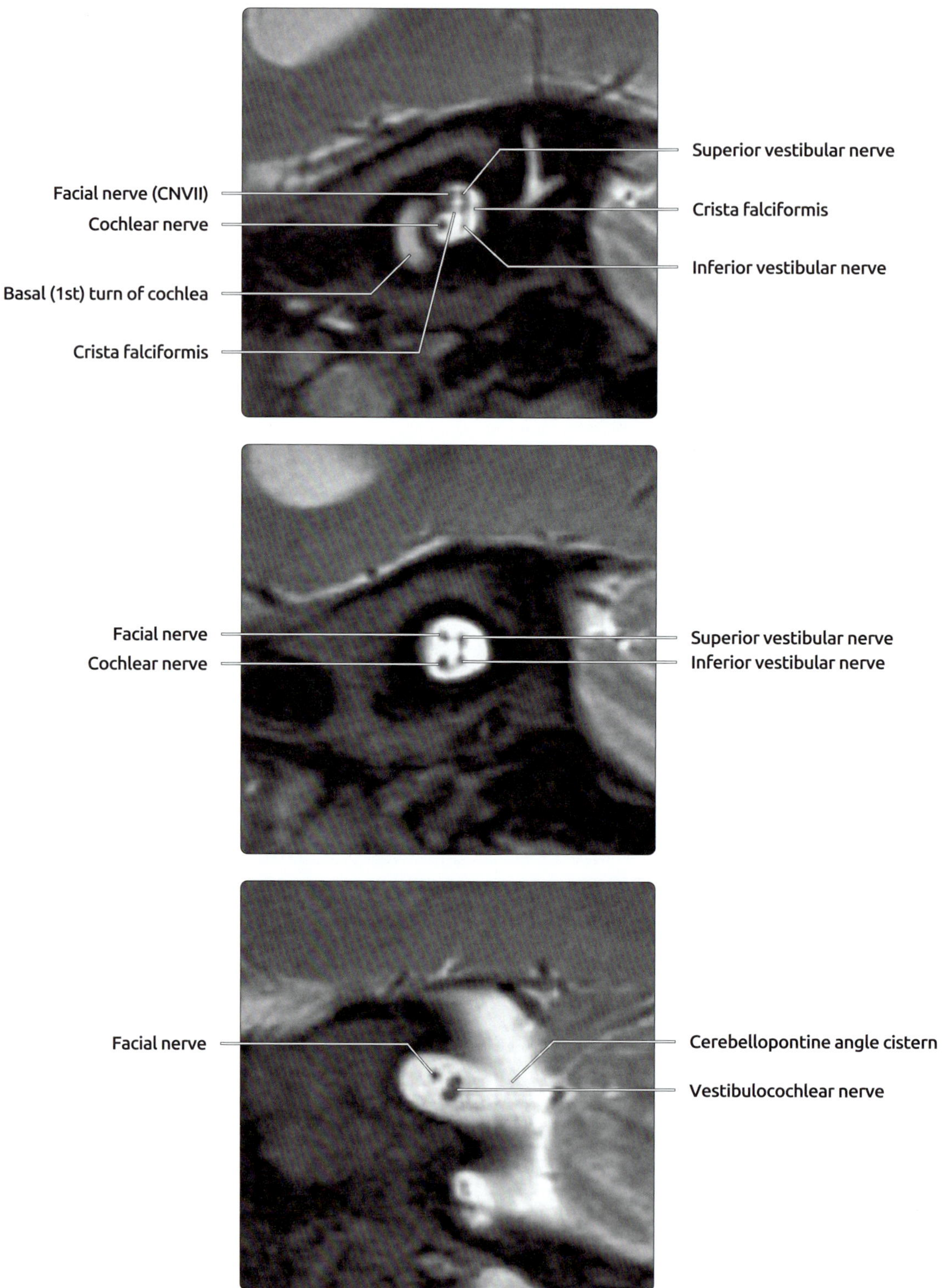

(Top) *First of 3 high-resolution oblique sagittal T2 MR images of the internal auditory canal, presented from lateral to medial, shows the facial nerve to be anterosuperior and the cochlear nerve to be anteroinferior. This fundal view reveals the crista falciformis, seen as a vague, low-signal line dividing CNVII and the SVN above from the cochlear and IVN below.* **(Middle)** *In the midinternal auditory canal, 4 discrete nerves are visible. Anteriorly: "7up (CNVII)/coke (cochlear) down." Posteriorly: Vestibular nerves; SVN up, IVN down. Notice that the anterosuperior facial nerve is normally slightly smaller than the anteroinferior cochlear nerve. The SVN and IVN are often joined by connecting fibers, as in this example.* **(Bottom)** *At the level of the porus acusticus, the vestibulocochlear nerve has the appearance of a "catcher's mitt" with the facial nerve looking like the "ball in the mitt."*

AXIAL T2 MR

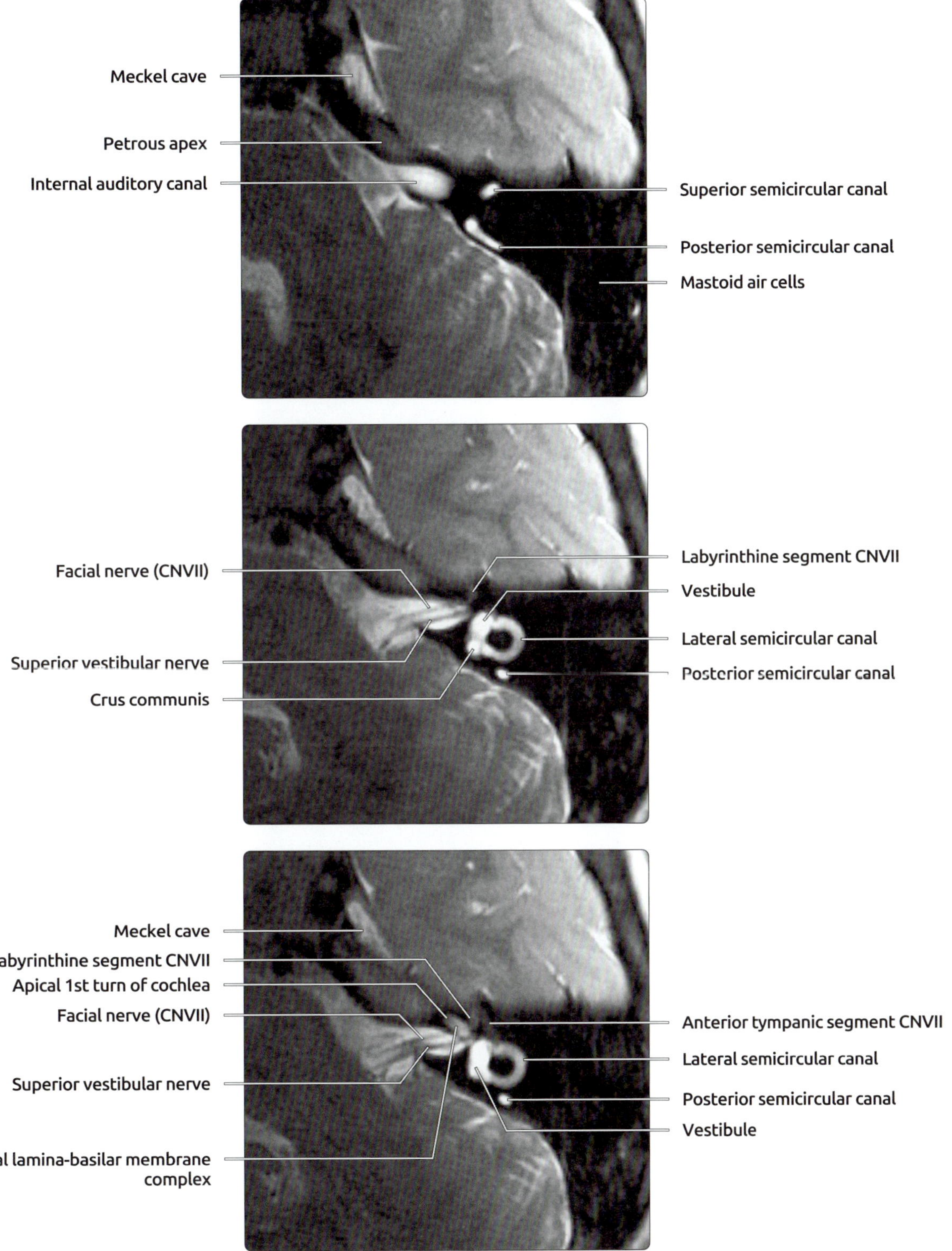

(Top) *First of 6 high-resolution axial thin-section T2 MR images, presented from superior to inferior through the left temporal bone, shows the superior internal auditory canal and semicircular canals.* **(Middle)** *In this image, the facial nerve is visible anterior and parallel to the SVN in the superior aspect of the internal auditory canal. The fluid spaces of the membranous labyrinth are high signal within the dark signal of the bony labyrinth.* **(Bottom)** *In this image, the labyrinthine and anterior tympanic segments of the facial nerve are visible. As they are not surrounded by CSF, as is CNVII in the internal auditory canal, they are more difficult to see.*

AXIAL T2 MR

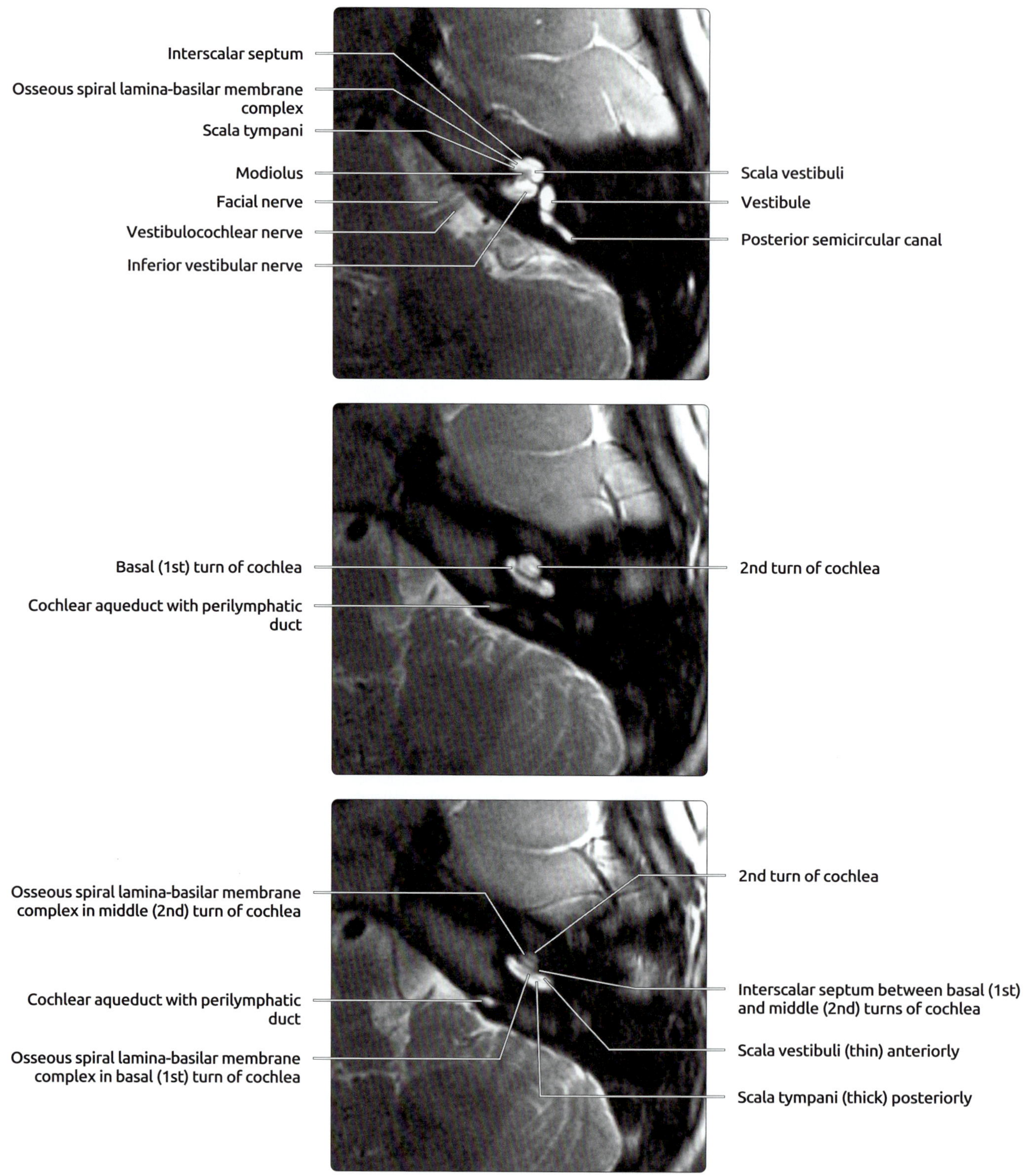

(Top) *In this image through the cochlear nerve canal, the modiolus of the cochlea is seen as an intermediate-signal structure at the hub of the cochlea. The 2 larger cochlear chambers are visible. The anterior thin chamber is the scala vestibuli, and the posterior thicker chamber is the scala tympani. Scala media is not routinely resolvable. Osseous spiral lamina-basilar membrane complex is seen within each cochlear turn in between the scala, and the interscalar septum (ISS) is seen separating different cochlear turns. Note that unlike what its name sounds like, ISS is not between the scala of cochlea.* **(Middle)** *In this image, both the 1st and 2nd turns of the cochlea are visible.* **(Bottom)** *The cochlear aqueduct is a tubular-shaped structure on the medial wall of the temporal bone inferior to the internal auditory canal. No definite function can be assigned to this structure. Cochlear aqueduct is a small canal in bony labyrinth harboring the perilymphatic (periotic) duct and draining perilymph into posterior cranial fossa subarachnoid space CSF.*

CORONAL T2 MR

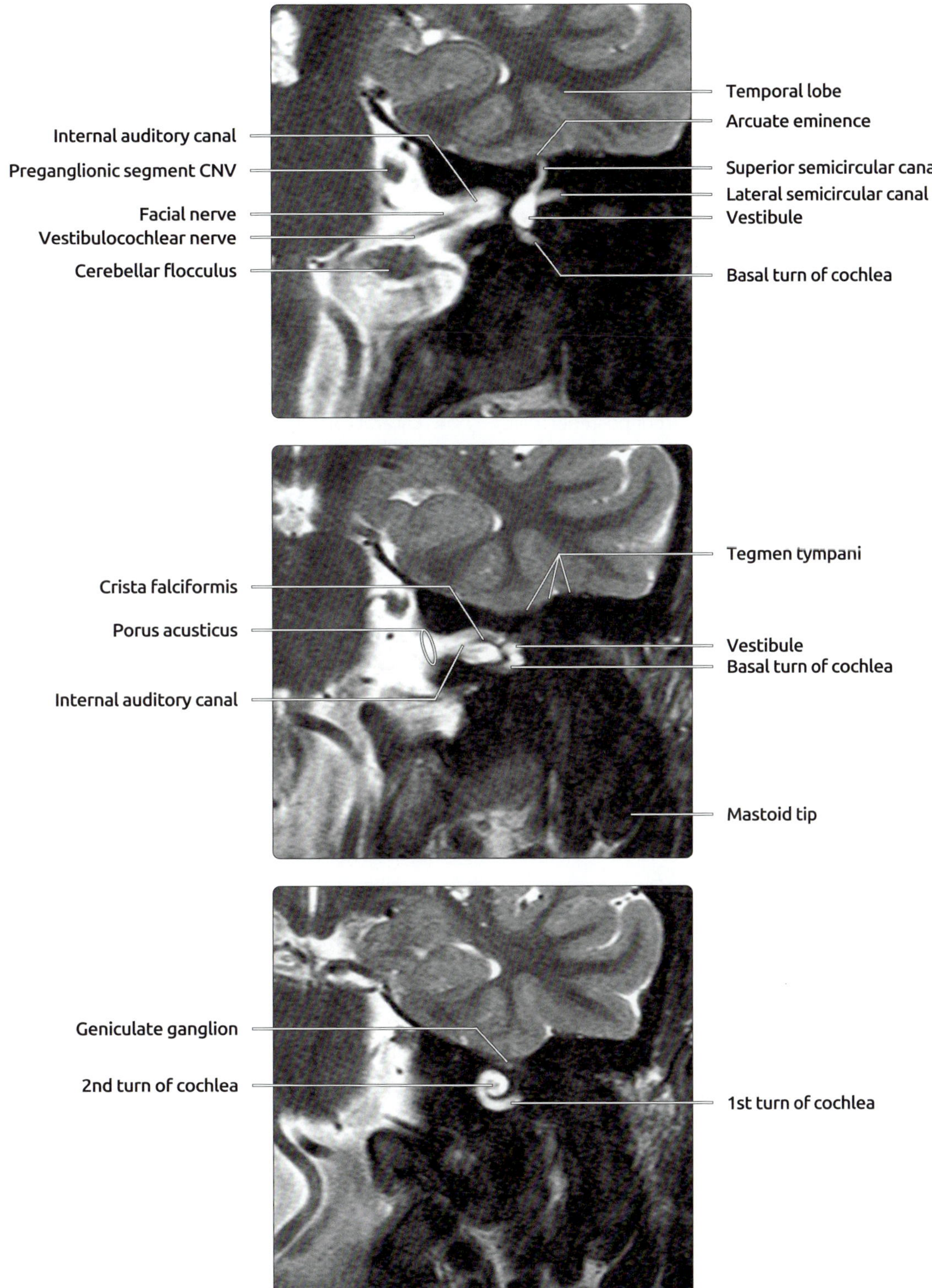

(Top) *First of 3 coronal T2 MR images of the left ear from posterior to anterior is shown. The membranous labyrinth of the inner ear is visible as high-signal fluid. Notice the superior and lateral semicircular canals adjacent to the vestibule.* **(Middle)** *In this image through the internal auditory canal, an unusually long crista falciformis is seen in the fundus. The area of the tegmen tympani is marked, but no landmarks in the middle ear are visible because both air and bone are low signal on MR imaging.* **(Bottom)** *At the level of the cochlea, the snail shape is particularly obvious, displaying both the 1st and 2nd turns. The geniculate ganglion is barely visible above and lateral to the cochlea. Again, note the lack of middle ear definable structures.*

TERMINOLOGY

Abbreviations

- External auditory canal (EAC); external acoustic meatus (EAM)

Definitions

- External ear: Pinna (auricle) and cartilaginous and bony EAC

IMAGING ANATOMY

Overview

- External ear
  - Pinna (auricle): Visible external ear
    - Major components: Helix, antihelix, tragus, antitragus, concha, lobule, and external meatus of EAC
  - EAC: Cartilaginous and bony parts
    - Lateral 1/3 of EAC formed by fibrocartilage
    - Medial 2/3 of EAC formed by cortical bone
      - Anterior, inferior, and lower part of posterior wall formed by tympanic component of temporal bone
      - Posterior wall and roof formed by squamous portion
    - Both cartilaginous and bony EAC **lined by skin**
      - Lateral cartilaginous EAC covered with thicker hair bearing skin
      - Medial bony EAC lined with very thin stratified squamous epithelium layer without dermal elements
      - Skin in EAC susceptible to common skin pathologies, including infection and neoplasm (squamous cell carcinoma, basal cell neoplasm)

Extent

- EAC extends from meatus of pinna laterally to tympanic membrane (TM)
- Measures 2-3 cm in length, 7-10 mm in diameter
- 2 normal sites of relative narrowing of EAC
  - Isthmus (junction of cartilaginous and bony portions)
  - Medial end of EAC, adjacent to TM
- Medial border of bony EAC
  - **TM** forms medial wall of EAC and separates EAC from middle ear proper
    - Semitransparent membrane with 2 general regions
    - **Pars flaccida**: Small upper region attaching to scutum
      - Forms lateral border of Prussak space (PS)
    - **Pars tensa**: Forms most of TM, relatively tight
    - Central portion (**umbo**) tented inward where tip of malleus attaches
    - 3 layers of TM from lateral to medial
      - Stratified squamous epithelium
      - Fibrous layer of lamina propria with radial and circumferential collagen bundles
      - Mucosal layer continuous with middle ear epithelium
  - **Scutum**: Relatively sharp bony spur continuation of medial roof of EAC and forms at junction of roof of EAC and lateral wall of middle ear cavity
    - Pars flaccida of TM attaches to scutum superiorly
    - Scutum commonly eroded in cases of acquired cholesteatoma initiated from pars flaccida
  - **PS**: Lowermost aspect of lateral epitympanic recess
    - PS lateral margin: Scutum, pars flaccida of TM, and manubrium (handle) of malleus bone leading to umbo
    - PS upper margin: Lateral malleal ligament
  - **Tympanic annulus**: Fibrocartilaginous ring that attaches to tympanic sulcus (narrow bony rise along floor of EAC) along medial margin of EAC; serves as anchor for TM
    - Ring incomplete anteriorly and superiorly

Anatomy Relationships

- EAC relationships
  - Anterior: Tympanosquamous suture and TMJ
    - Anterior wall of bony EAC also serves as posterior wall of TMJ fossa
  - Posterior: Tympanomastoid suture and mastoid air cells
  - Superior: Superolateral mastoid air cells
  - Inferior: Parotid space
  - Medial: Middle ear cavity

Internal Contents

- **Lateral cartilaginous component of EAC**
  - Circumferential fibrocartilage extension of cartilage of concha; supports and maintains patency of EAC
  - Skin thicker and contains sebaceous glands, ceruminous glands, and hair follicles
  - **Fissures of Santorini** (incisurae cartilaginis meatus acustici)
    - Multiple small vertical gaps in anterior cartilaginous wall of EAC; provide increased flexibility to canal
    - Fissures not identified on routine CT or MR imaging
    - Fissures may represent gateway for infection from EAC into parotid space and other proximal deep spaces of neck
    - Malignant otitis externa thought to utilize this pathway in some cases to spread to adjacent infratemporal regions and to skull base
- **Medial bony component of EAC**
  - U-shaped tympanic bone forms bony EAC
  - Skin relatively thin, devoid of significant subcutaneous tissue, and tightly adherent to underlying bone
  - Skin in medial canal continuous with outer layer of TM
  - Medial margin defined by TM, which attaches superiorly to scutum and inferiorly to tympanic annulus
  - Anterior wall shared with TMJ fossa
  - **Tympanosquamous suture**: Anterior to bony EAC
    - Continues medially into petrotympanic and petrosquamous sutures
  - Posterior bony EAC wall shared with mastoid complex
  - **Tympanomastoid suture**: Posterior to bony EAC
    - Auricular branch of vagus (CNX) nerve (Arnold nerve) passes through mastoid canaliculus and emerges through tympanomastoid fissure
    - Arnold nerve supplies part of TM and EAC: Cause Arnold nerve cough reflex when mechanically stimulating ear
  - **Persistent foramen of Huschke (foramen tympanicum)**
    - Dehiscence in anteroinferior bony EAC wall posteromedial to TMJ
    - Anatomic variant normally closing by 5 years age; sometimes persist into adulthood

- Seen in 50% of ears with necrotizing external otitis (malignant otitis externa), but only in 11.5% controls
- Rarely associated with salivary discharge into EAC during mastication/salivary fistula
- Rarely TMJ soft tissue herniates into foramen/EAC, or scope enters during TMJ arthroscopy

- **Sensory innervation to external ear**
  - 4 cranial nerves and 2 upper cervical nerves contribute to sensory innervation
    - Considerable overlap and ambiguity in sensory distribution of these nerves
  - CNV3 supplies tragus, helical crus, anterosuperior wall of EAC, adjacent TM, and TMJ
  - CNVII: Supplies posteroinferior portion of EAC and adjacent TM
  - CNIX: Supplies inner ear and inner surface of TM
  - CNX: Supplies inner ear, inner surface of TM, and concha (hollow next to ear canal)
  - C2 and C3: Innervate skin in front of and behind ear
    - Also skin of medial and lateral pinna and lobule
- **Arterial supply to external ear**
  - Posterior auricular artery gives off auricular branch
    - Auricular artery ascends behind ear to supply cartilage of pinna
  - Superficial temporal artery gives off anterior auricular artery branch
    - Anterior auricular artery supplies anterior portion of pinna, lobule, and part of EAC
  - Occipital artery gives off auricular branch
    - Auricular artery branch supplies back of concha
- **External ear nodal drainage**
  - Pre- and postauricular nodal groups
  - Parotid nodal group

ANATOMY IMAGING ISSUES

Questions

- What 2 bony structures help radiologists identify medial border of EAC?
  - 2 bony structures that mark medial wall of EAC are scutum and tympanic annulus
    - On coronal CT imaging of temporal bone, normal TM barely visible
    - Bony attachments of TMs always visible
    - Superior point of TM attachment: Scutum
    - Inferior point of TM attachment: Tympanic annulus
- What characteristic of cartilaginous EAC permits EAC infection to spread into subjacent deep facial space?
  - Fissures of Santorini (multiple cartilaginous gaps in lateral EAC) permit EAC infection to readily spread into adjacent deep facial spaces
- If skin malignancy (squamous cell carcinoma, melanoma) affects external ear or adjacent scalp, where do nodal metastases 1st appear?
  - Pre- and postauricular nodes (clinically apparent) along with intraparotid nodes (may be subclinical)
  - Bone CT of EAC may not show parotid lymph nodes
    - Acquire soft tissue algorithm image sequences for review of parotid and adjacent soft tissues
- What are most common causes of primary otalgia (origin of pain arises from ear itself)?
  - Otomastoiditis, cholesteatoma, and foreign bodies lodged within ear canal
- Define term referred otalgia (ear pain)
  - In referred otalgia, source of ear pain does not reside within ear but originates from sources distant from ear
    - 50% of otalgia cases are referred
    - In referred otalgia (convergence of common sensory pathways between complex sensory innervation supplying both ear and cranial nerves innervating head and neck), CNS unable to correctly pinpoint location of pathology
- What are most common causes of referred otalgia?
  - Any pathology residing within sensory net of CNV, CNVII, CNIX, CNX, and upper cervical nerves C2 and C3 potentially cause pain (referred otalgia)
  - Major areas include nose and sinus, pharynx, and oral cavity, including mandible and maxilla

Imaging Recommendations

- Axial high-resolution bone CT with coronal and sagittal reformations best study to evaluate bony integrity of temporal bone, including medial bony component of EAC
- High-resolution multiplanar MR to include T1 without fat saturation, T1 + gadolinium with fat saturation, and STIR images most comprehensive approach for evaluation of temporal bone/skull base pathology
  - Images should include TMJ, parotid gland, nasopharyngeal carotid space, clivus, and preclival region

Imaging Approaches

- High-resolution CT with reformations provides preoperative mapping in cases of congenital external ear malformation (auricle/EAC atresia)
- For presumed mass in EAC or lateral temporal bone
  - CT and MR complimentary for evaluation of invasive neoplasm (skin or parotid) of temporal bone and surrounding structures
  - T1 MR + gadolinium with fat saturation best to demonstrate entire extent of tumor
    - Mastoid invasion
    - TMJ involvement
    - Marrow space invasion
    - Perineural tumor spread of CNVII
  - CT soft tissue neck completes evaluation for local adenopathy
- Malignant otitis externa and skull base osteomyelitis
  - Infection may spread well beyond EAC in soft tissues of suprahyoid neck, extending to preclival soft tissues
  - MR required to evaluate marrow of petrous apex and clivus
- Referred otalgia
  - CECT best for evaluation of mucosal lesion of pharynx
  - Scan needs to extend from skull base through hypopharynx

Imaging Pitfalls

- Clinical and imaging findings of neoplasm and invasive infection of EAC can overlap
- On CT, fibrocartilage and soft tissues near EAC (including parotid tissue) are difficult to differentiate from adjacent invasive neoplasm, and tumor extent may be overestimated

AURICLE AND EXTERNAL AUDITORY CANAL: NORMAL ANATOMY

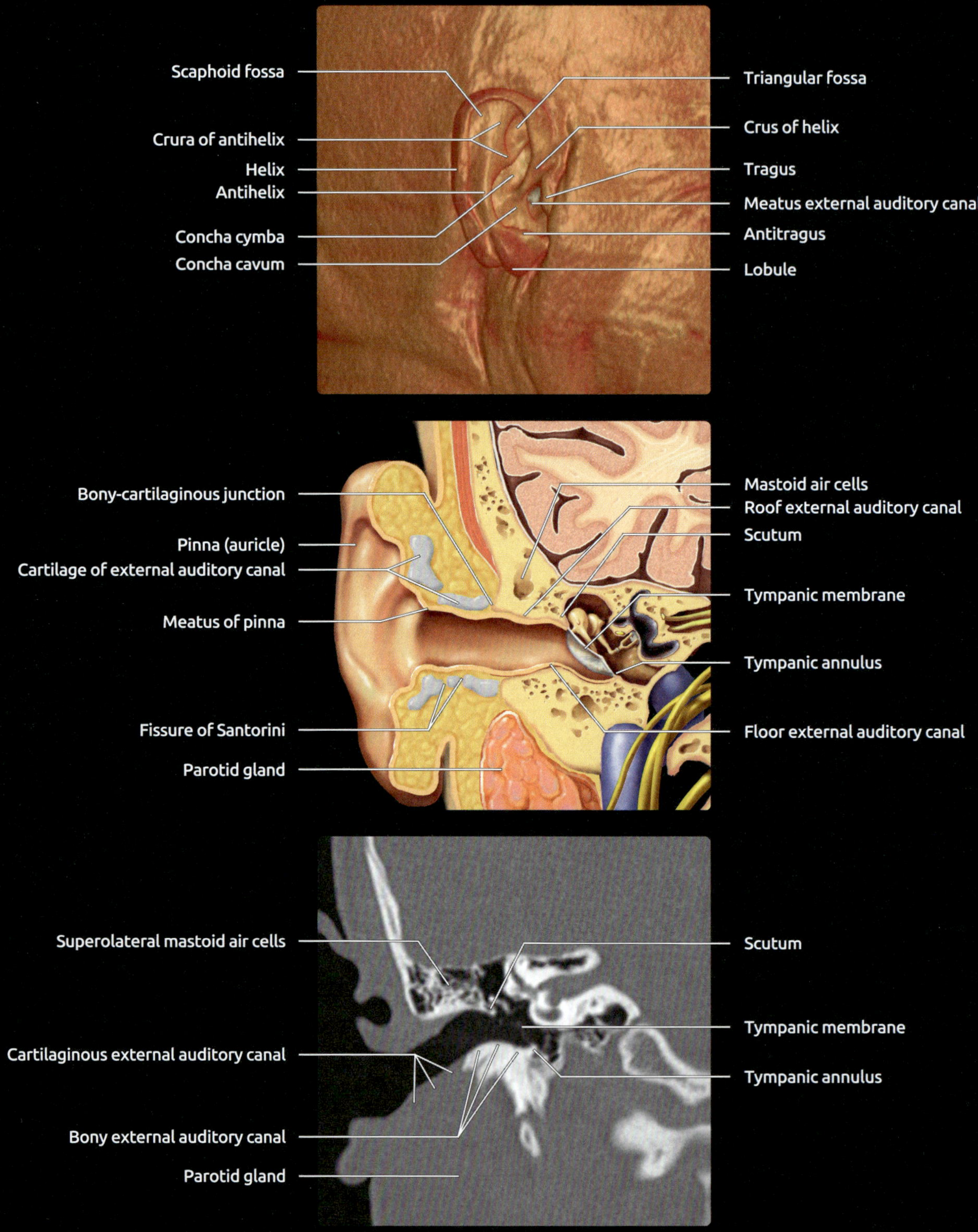

(Top) *3D surface rendering of the right auricle in a patient demonstrates normal surface anatomy of the external ear. The peripheral fold is called the helix, and the inner smaller fold is called the antihelix. Named depressions include triangular fossa, scaphoid fossa, and the concha composed of the cymba and the cavum.* **(Middle)** *Coronal graphic shows the external and middle ear. The external auditory canal (EAC) is made up of lateral cartilaginous and medial bony components. Infection of the EAC can penetrate inferomedially to the skull base and associated spaces via the fissures of Santorini (gaps in the EAC cartilage). External ear and EAC lymphatic drainage is generally to the parotid nodal chain. The medial margin of the EAC is the tympanic membrane, which attaches to the scutum and tympanic annulus.* **(Bottom)** *Coronal bone CT shows the medial wall of the EAC with its barely visible tympanic membrane attached to the scutum superiorly and to the tympanic annulus inferiorly. Notice that the inferior cartilaginous EAC abuts the parotid space. The superior bony EAC abuts the superolateral mastoid air cells.*

EXTERNAL AUDITORY CANAL: AXIAL CT

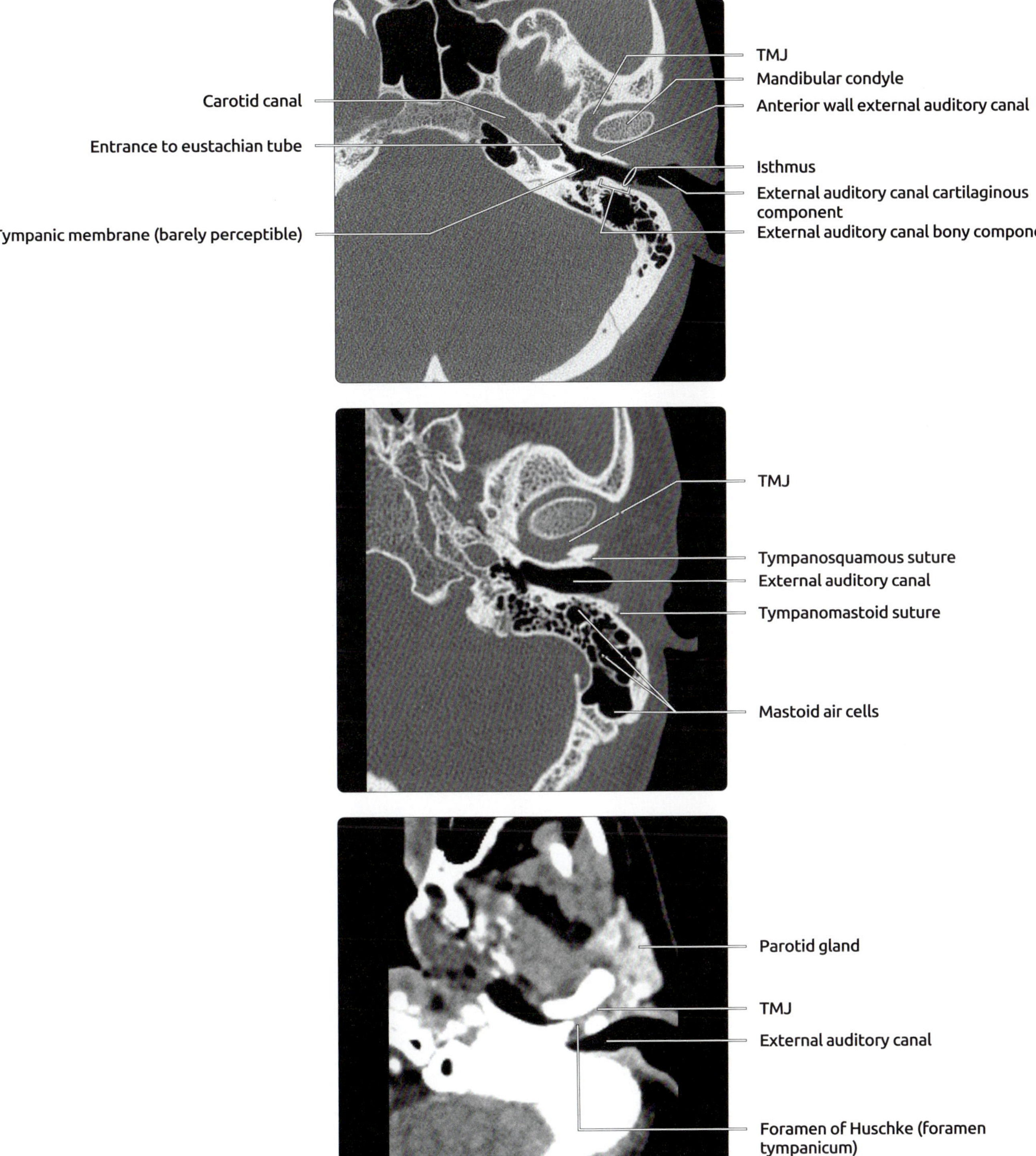

(Top) *Axial bone CT through the EAC shows cartilaginous EAC representing the lateral 1/3 of the canal and bony EAC representing the medial 2/3. There is mild narrowing of the canal at the bony-cartilaginous junction called the isthmus. The tympanic membrane (normally barely perceptible) separates the EAC from the middle ear. The anterior wall of the EAC is relatively thin cortical bone and forms the posterior wall of the mandibular fossa.* **(Middle)** *Axial bone CT shows the tympanosquamous (TS) and tympanomastoid (TM) sutures. TS suture lies anterior to bony EAC and continues medially into petrotympanic and petrosquamous sutures (not shown). TM suture lies posterior to bony EAC and is inconsistently seen. Auricular branch of vagus (CNX) nerve (Arnold nerve) passes through mastoid canaliculus and emerges through TM fissure. Arnold nerve supplies part of TM and EAC and causes Arnold nerve cough reflex when mechanically stimulating the external ear.* **(Bottom)** *Axial bone CT shows persistent foramen of Huschke (foramen tympanicum), which is a dehiscence in the anteroinferior EAC wall located posteromedial to TMJ.*

EXTERNAL AUDITORY CANAL: SAGITTAL CT

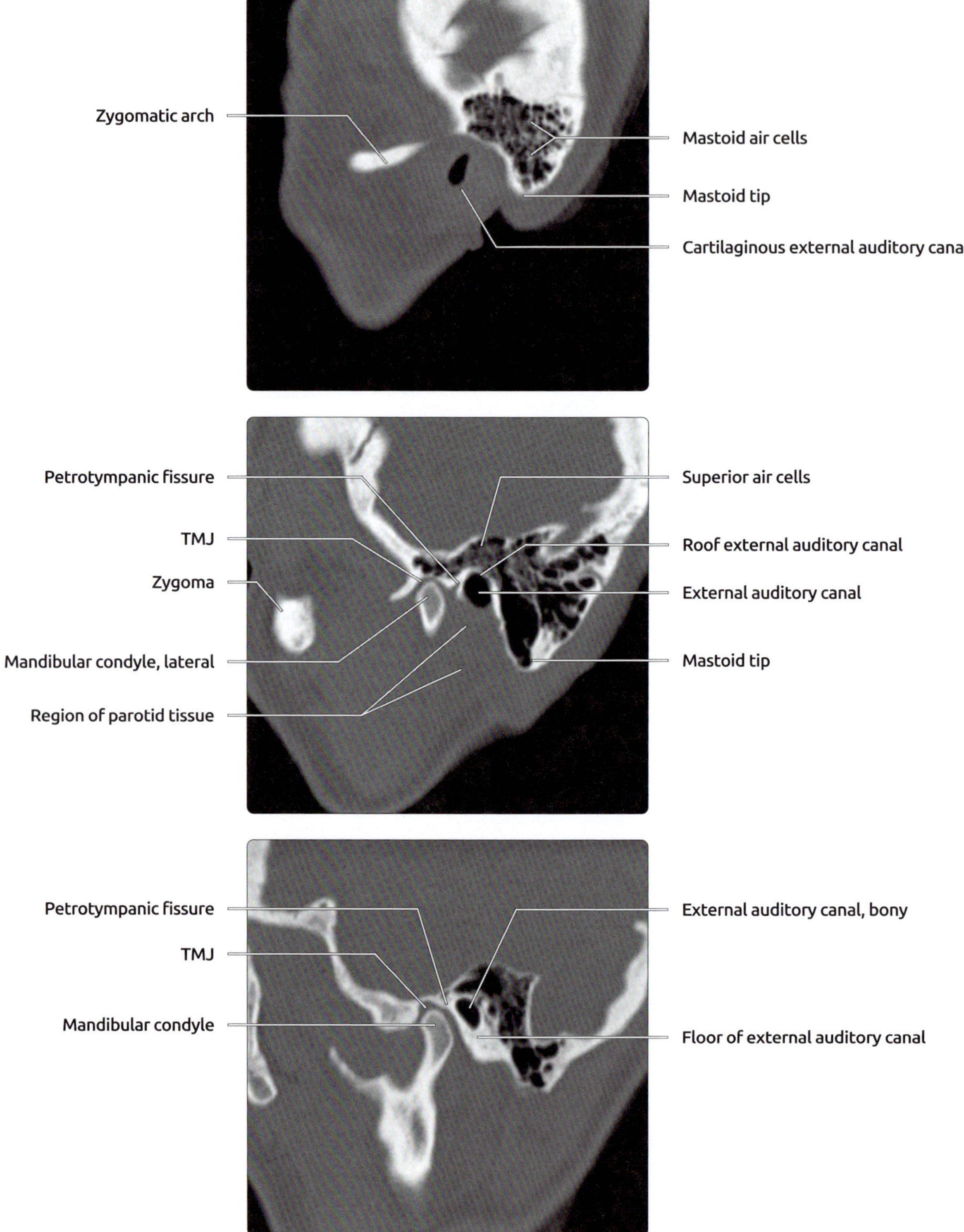

(Top) *Sagittal CT through the lateral aspect of the EAC is shown. Notice the cartilaginous component angles anteriorly as it moves laterally. With bone windows, it is difficult to appreciate the relationship of the parotid gland to the inferior margin of the cartilaginous EAC.* **(Middle)** *Sagittal bone CT through the EAC and TMJ is obtained near the junction of the cartilaginous and bony components of the EAC.* **(Bottom)** *Sagittal bone CT through the EAC and TMJ demonstrates the U-shaped tympanic bone bordered posteriorly by the TM suture/mastoid air cells and anteriorly by the petrotympanic fissure and TMJ. A blow to the mandible may readily fracture the bony EAC.*

EXTERNAL AUDITORY CANAL: SAGITTAL MR

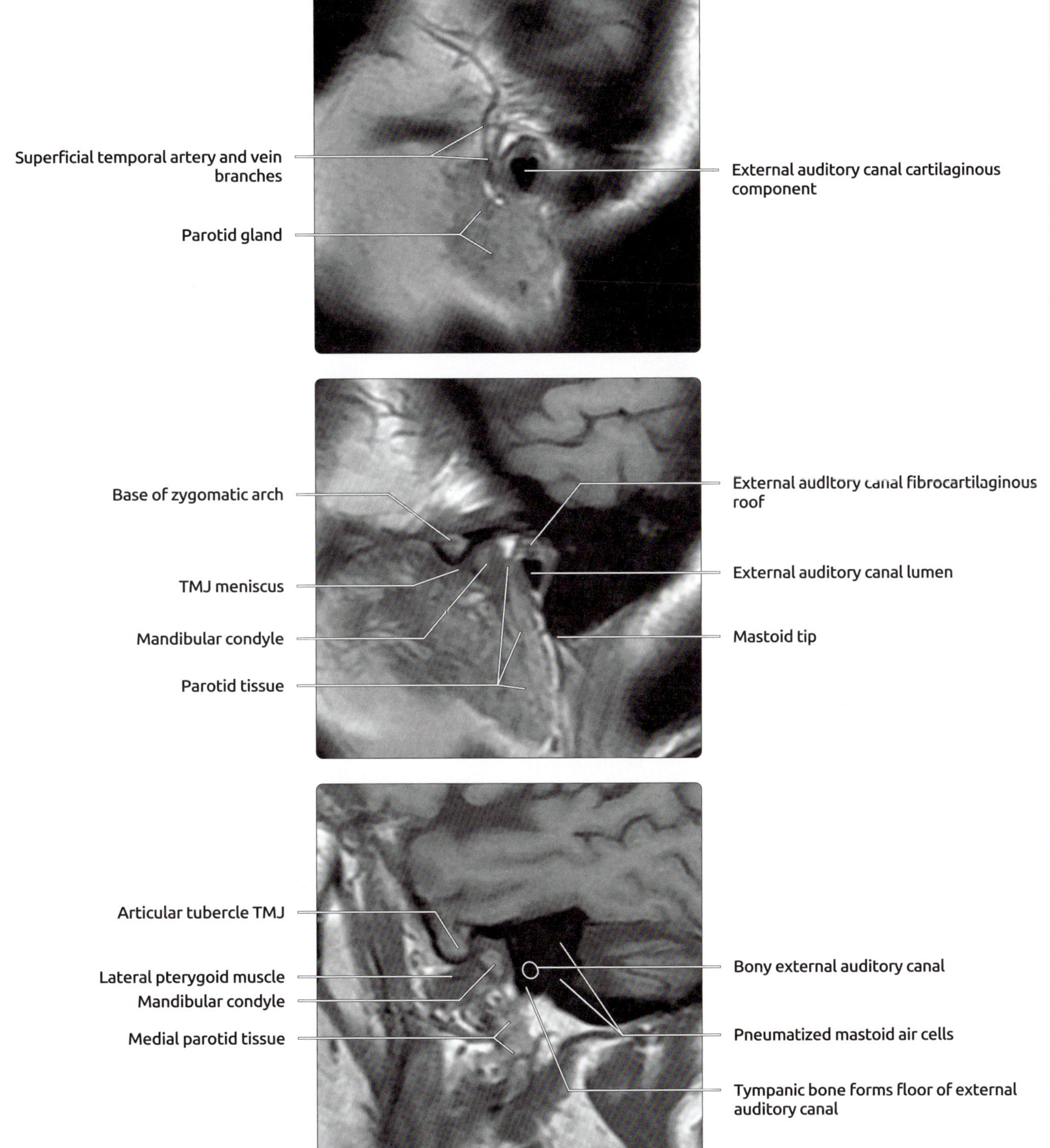

(Top) *Sagittal T1 MR though the lateral aspect of the EAC shows the ring of fibrocartilaginous tissue surrounding the EAC that is patent and contains air. Notice the proximity of the EAC with the superior margin of the parotid gland. It may be difficult to differentiate an invasive skin malignancy of the EAC from invasive parotid malignancy.* **(Middle)** *Sagittal T1 MR through the TMJ near the junction of the cartilaginous and bony EAC shows the intimate relationship of the EAC to the TMJ, the mastoid air cells, and the superior medial parotid tissue.* **(Bottom)** *Sagittal T1 MR obtained through the TMJ is shown. The EAC is difficult to separate from the surrounding hypointensity created by pneumatized air cells and surrounding cortical bone of the tympanic bone. Some minimal parotid tissue can still be observed along the bony floor of the EAC.*

TERMINOLOGY

Abbreviations

- Middle ear (ME); tympanic membrane (TM); external auditory canal (EAC); semicircular canal (SCC)

IMAGING ANATOMY

Anatomy Relationships

- **ME (tympanic cavity)**: Located in petrous temporal bone between external & inner ears
- **Mastoid cavity**: Mastoid antrum superiorly & extensive air cells located in mastoid temporal bone
  - Variably pneumatizes into petrous temporal bone
- ME subdivisions: Epitympanum, mesotympanum with protympanum & retrotympanum (RT), & hypotympanum
- **Tegmen (roof)**: Anterior ME bony roof: **Tegmen tympani**
  - Posterior roof above mastoid: **Tegmen mastoideum**
- Line drawn from superior EAC margin/scutal tip to tympanic CNVII on coronal CT/MR separates
  - **Epitympanum** above & **mesotympanum** below
- Line drawn from medial inferior margin of EAC (tympanic annulus) to base of cochlear promontory on coronal CT/MR
  - **Mesotympanum** above & **hypotympanum** below
- **Protympanum**: **Anterior** aspect of **meso**tympanum that lies anterior to frontal plane drawn through anterior margin of EAC/tympanic annulus on axial images
- **RT**: **Posterior** aspect of **meso**tympanum

Internal Contents

- **Epitympanum** (attic): Above mesotympanum
  - **Prussak space (PS)**: Lower **lateral epitympanic recess below lateral malleal ligament**
    - Extending from level of scutum to umbo
    - **Scutum**: Sharp, bony spur separating superior aspect of EAC from ME
    - **Umbo**: Deepest point of concavity of TM where tip of manubrium of malleus attaches
    - Lateral margin of PS: **Pars flaccida** (upper part) of TM
    - Medial margin of PS: **Manubrium (handle) of malleus** leading to umbo
    - Common site of acquired cholesteatoma formation
  - **Tegmen tympani** ("roof of cavity"): Thin, bony roof between epitympanum & middle cranial fossa dura
  - **Körner septum** (KS) (**petrosquamous lamina**): Bony lamina dividing mastoid cavity at level of mastoid antrum
    - Into superficial mastoid air cells pneumatizing squamosal portion & deeper petrosal portion
    - Due to developmental interruption resulting in persistence of lamina between squamous & petrous parts of temporal bone; seen in 6-45%
    - Continuation of persistent **petrosquamous suture**
    - **Petrosquamous fissure**: Small defect in tegmen tympani continuous with KS
    - KS can be eroded by cholesteatoma
  - **Epitympanic cog** (anterior attic bony plate): Coronal bony septum, suspended from anterior tegmen tympani
    - Complete thin, bony plate (type I), small, incomplete (type II), or nonvisualized on CT (type III)
    - Middle portion of **petrosquamous lamina**
    - Cog partitions **anterior epitympanic recess (AER)** from epitympanum proper
  - **AER (supratubal recess)**: Small aerated epitympanic recess anterior to head of malleus; partitioned from epitympanum proper by cog
    - AER could have single cell or multiple air cells
    - Bordered medially by facial nerve geniculate fossa & facial nerve anterior tympanic canal
    - Diseases affecting AER & surgical removal of bony cog could result in facial nerve paralysis
    - **Cholesteatoma may hide in AER**
  - **Aditus ad antrum** ("entrance to cave"): Connects epitympanum of ME to mastoid antrum
- **Mesotympanum**: (ME proper): Between epitympanum & hypotympanum
  - **ME medial wall**: Includes tympanic segment of CNVII, oval & round windows, & cochlear promontory
  - **Processus cochleariformis (Pc)**: Tiny angulated bony process above cochlear promontory
    - Pc forms pulley over which tendon of tensor tympani muscle swings into mesotympanum from posterior end of semicanal for tensor tympani
    - Pc lies anterosuperior to oval window (OW), inferolateral to proximal tympanic segment of facial nerve canal, & forms floor of AER
  - **Protympanum**: **Anterior** aspect of **mesotympanum**
    - Opens posteriorly into mesotympanum proper
    - Leads anteriorly into eustachian tube (ET) below & semicanal for tensor tympani muscle just above ET
    - ET separated from semicanal for tensor tympani by thin, bony plate called **septum canalis musculotubarii**
  - **RT**: **Posterior** aspect of **mesotympanum**, including posterior wall
    - **Classic teaching**: Medial RT **sinus tympani (ST)** separated by **pyramidal eminence (PE)** from lateral RT **CNVII (facial) recess**
    - Endoscopic anatomy depicted on photon-counting detector (PCD) CT much more complex
  - **Medial RT**: Divided by **subiculum** into superior & inferior
    - **Subiculum**: Bony crest from posterior round window niche to styloid eminence
    - **Superior medial RT**: Divided by **ponticulus** into **posterior tympanic sinus** above & **ST** below
      - One or both of these sinuses may communicate with inconsistent **subpyramidal space** extending posteromedial to PE
      - **Ponticulus**: Bony bar extending from cochlear promontory to PE
    - **Inferior medial RT**: **Sinus subtympanicus** between otic capsule medially & styloid eminence laterally
      - Finiculus separates medial RT (sinus subtympanicus) posterosuperiorly from hypotympanum anteroinferiorly
      - **Finiculus**: Bony crest connecting anterior pillar of round window superiorly & jugular foramen roof (hypotympanum floor) inferiorly
  - **Lateral RT**: Divided by **chordal eminence** into **facial recess** medially & **lateral tympanic sinus** laterally
    - **Chordal eminence**: Bony prominence on posterior wall of tympanic cavity formed by chorda tympani nerve (CTN) posterior canaliculus

- **Chordiculus**: Bony crest between chordal eminence inferolaterally & PE superomedially
- **Styloid eminence** separates lateral RT superiorly from hypotympanum inferiorly

- **Hypotympanum**: Shallow trough in floor of ME below mesotympanum
- **ME muscles**
  - **Tensor tympani muscle**
    - Originates from cartilaginous margin of ET, passes through its own bony semicanal in wall of protympanum just above & parallel to bony ET
    - On coronal CT, found anteroinferior to anterior tympanic segment of CNVII
    - Tendon curves around **Pc** (cochleariform process), turns laterally across ME, & attaches to upper part of **malleus handle (manubrium)**
  - **Stapedius muscle**
    - Originates from fasciculi of **posterior belly of digastric** muscle, which inserts in mastoid groove, then fasciculi pass through **stylomastoid foramen** towards **PE base**
    - Muscle belly found just medial to upper mastoid segment CNVII in base of **PE**
    - Tendon emerges from apex of PE & attaches to **neck of stapes**
- **Ossicles of ME**
  - **Malleus** (hammer)
    - Location: Anterior epitympanum & mesotympanum
      - **"Ice cream cone" in epitympanum**: Malleus head forms "**Ice cream**" anteriorly
    - Components: Head, neck, lateral process, anterior process & handle (manubrium) with tip
    - Ligaments & tendons: **Superior, anterior, & lateral mallear ligaments**; tendon of tensor tympani muscle
  - **Incus** (anvil)
    - Location: Posterior epitympanum & mesotympanum
      - "Ice cream cone" in epitympanum: Incus body forms wider part & short process tip of **cone** posteriorly
    - Components: Body; short, long, & lenticular processes
    - Ligament: **Posterior incudal ligament**
  - **Stapes** (stirrup)
    - Location: Medial mesotympanum
    - Components: Head (capitulum), neck (hub), anterior & posterior crura, & footplate (base)
    - Tendon: Stapedius muscle tendon
    - **Stapes superstructure**: 2nd branchial arch-derived portions: Head, crura, tympanic portion of footplate
    - Vestibular portion of footplate of stapes & annular ligament: Otic capsule derived
- **TM**: Separates external ear from ME
  - Upper 1/3 = **pars flaccida**; lower 2/3 = **pars tensa**
  - Malleus tip (at umbo) & lateral process (at apex of pars flaccida) embedded in TM
  - Superior attachment: **Scutum** (Latin for shield)
  - Inferior attachment: **Tympanic annulus**
    - Separates hypotympanum medially & EAC laterally
- **ME medial wall relationships from top to bottom**
  - **Lateral SCC (LSCC)**
    - Projects horizontally & laterally from vestibule, creating bony ridge along epitympanic medial wall
  - **CNVII nerve canal (tympanic segment)**
    - Tympanic segment of facial nerve canal: Tubular bony covering of tympanic segment of nerve itself
    - Begins at geniculate ganglion & runs posteriorly, passing above Pc
    - Runs parallel to & below LSCC, above OW
    - Posterior part of nerve canal lies superolateral to PE of RT wall & passes into 2nd genu
    - Focal dehiscence of undersurface of tympanic canal considered normal variant, occurring in as much as 20-25% of adults; most common just above OW
  - **OW (fenestra vestibuli)**
    - OW: Opening between ME & vestibule; covered by OW membrane
    - **Stapes footplate** occupies OW; circumferentially attached by **annular ligament**
    - Stapes moves in & out against OW, causing vibrations of vestibular perilymph, then sound waves transmit into scala vestibuli of cochlea perilymph
    - Tympanic facial canal forms roof of OW niche
    - Includes tiny space surrounding footplate and stapes
  - **Cochlear promontory**
    - Rounded, shallow protrusion arising from central aspect of medial wall projecting into mesotympanum
    - Lateral bony covering of **basal turn of cochlea**
    - Located anterior & inferior to OW; anterior to round window (RW) niche
  - **RW (fenestra cochleae)**
    - RW covered by RW membrane (a.k.a. secondary TM), separating ME from scala tympani at posterolateral aspect of basal turn of cochlea; Seen along posterior aspect of cochlear promontory
    - Sound waves enter vestibule through OW (1st window) & then scala vestibuli of cochlea perilymph
    - Waves transmit along helicotrema to scala tympani perilymph, & wave pressure let out into ST of RT through RW (2nd window)
    - Wave motion transmitted to endolymph of scala media of cochlea with basilar membrane vibration that stimulates hair cell receptors in organ of Corti
    - Hair cell movement generates electronic potentials converted to action potentials in cochlear nerve
    - **RW niche**: Triangular bony pouch defined by thin, overhanging bone that extends from cochlear promontory
      - Consists of **anterior pillar** (continues inferiorly as finiculus), **posterior pillar** (continues posteriorly as subiculum) & **tegmen** (thick bone at dorsolateral edge of cochlear promontory)
    - **RW chamber**: Between RW membrane & RW niche
    - **Air** within RW chamber becomes **continuous** posterolaterally with air in **ST**
    - **Fustis**: RW chamber floor, extending up to styloid eminence below
    - **Proctor's area concamerata**: Area between fustis & finiculus at medial wall of ME cavity, leading to subcochlear canaliculus
    - **Subcochlear canaliculus**: Anatomic **pneumatization** connecting RW to inferomedial petrous apex; variable
      - Coronal CT: Pneumatized temporal bone **below** cochlear promontory laterally & internal auditory canal medially

CORONAL GRAPHICS

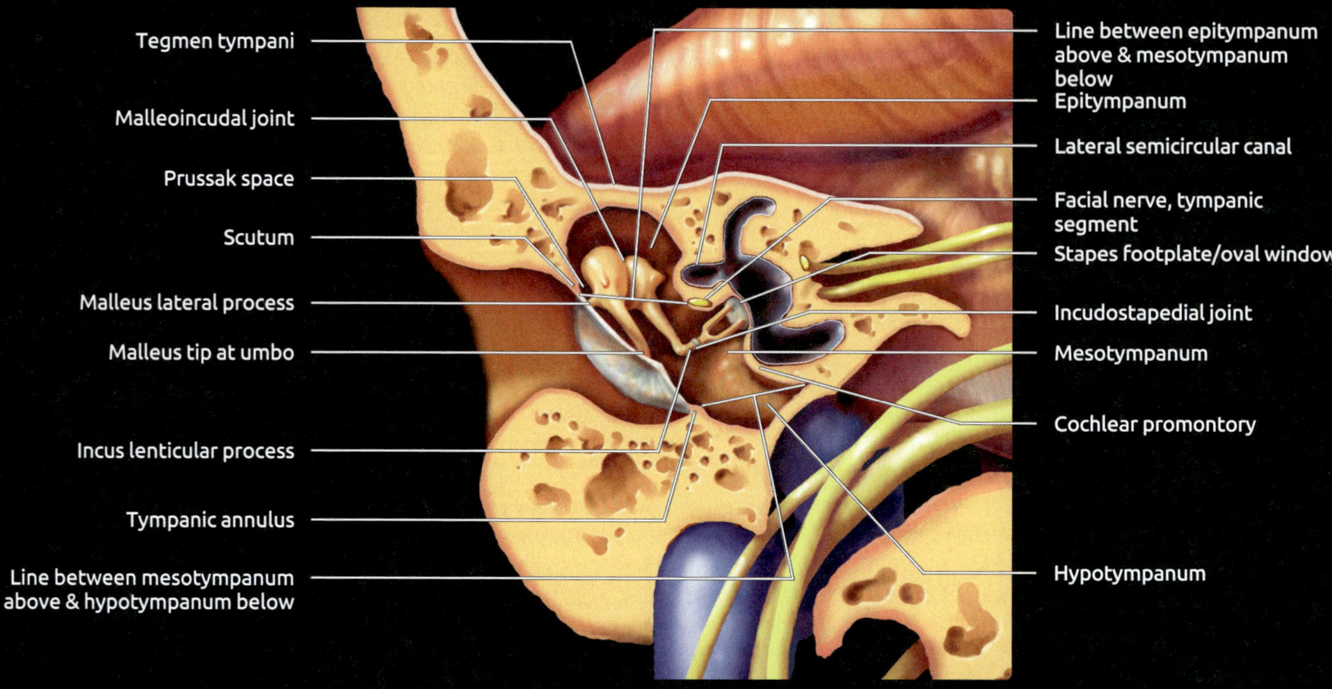

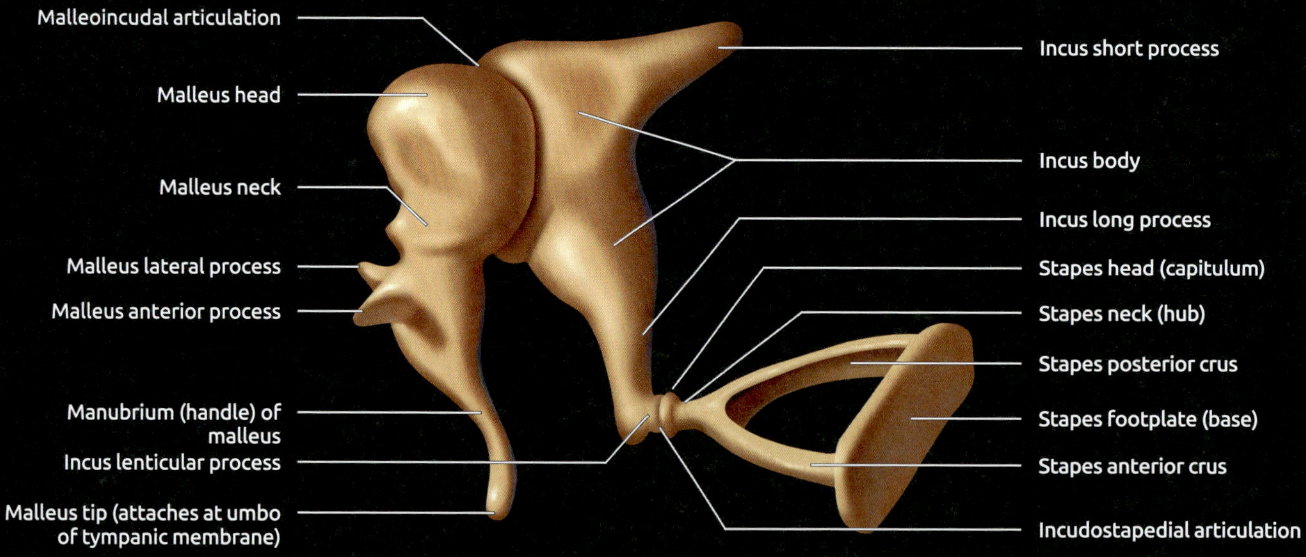

(Top) *Coronal graphic of the right temporal bone shows the middle ear (ME), which is divided into 3 components: Epitympanum, mesotympanum, & hypotympanum. Epitympanum is the ME cavity above a line drawn from the medial roof of EAC/scutal tip & tympanic segment of CNVII. Its roof is called the tegmen tympani. Mesotympanum extends from this line inferiorly to a line connecting the medial inferior margin of the external auditory canal (EAC)/tympanic annulus to the cochlear promontory base. Hypotympanum lies inferior to this line. Note the conductive chain from the tympanic membrane (TM) to the oval window. TM is attached superiorly to scutum & inferiorly to tympanic annulus. Two articulations between ossicles are malleoincudal & incudostapedial joints. Craniocaudally, ME medial wall structures include the tympanic segment of the facial nerve, oval & round windows, & cochlear promontory.* **(Bottom)** *Frontal graphic of right ME ossicles shows that the anterolateral malleus has a head, neck, & manubrium with lateral & anterior processes. The incus has a large body & short, long, & lenticular processes. The stapes has a head, neck, crura, & footplate.*

MIDDLE EAR: LATERAL & MEDIAL WALLS

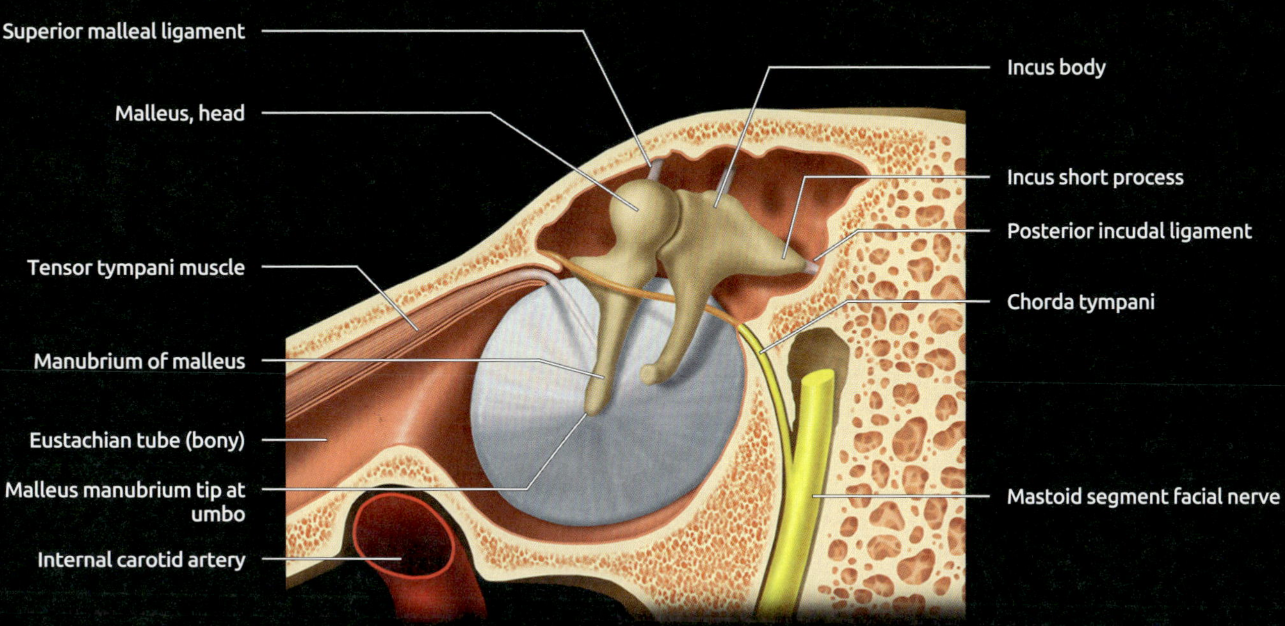

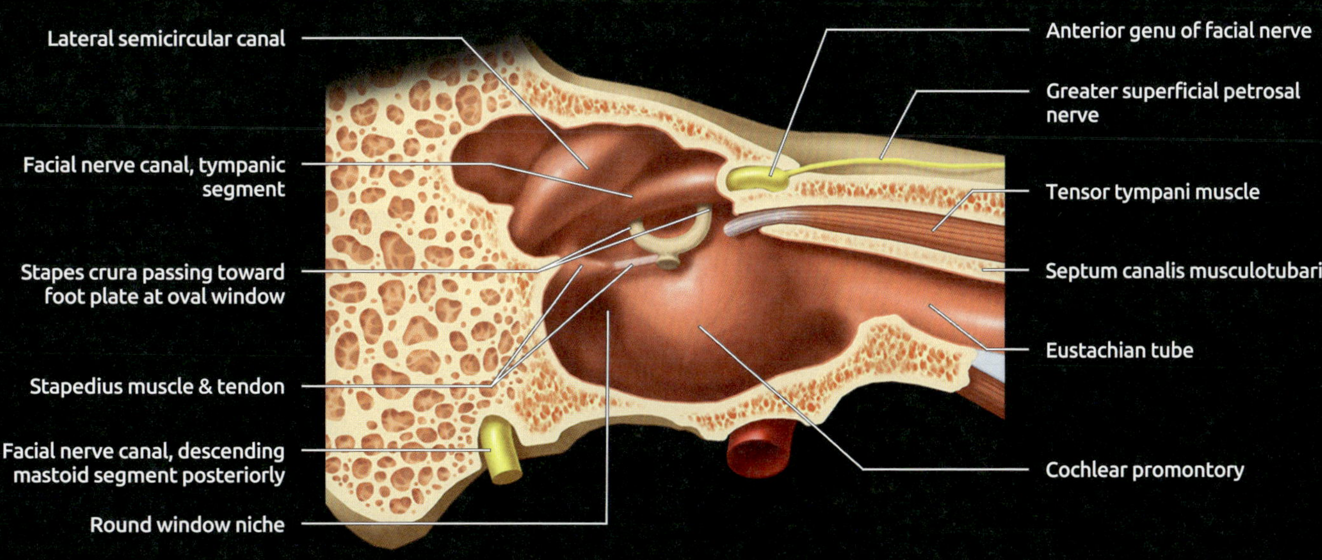

(Top) *Graphic shows internal view of lateral wall of ME cavity. TM is dominant structure along lateral wall. The central aspect of the TM is attached to the tip of manubrium of the malleus at the umbo. Note the relationship of the chorda tympani nerve as it leaves the mastoid segment of facial nerve, ascends through temporal bone, courses in ME cavity from posterior to anterior alongside the TM, & then between the malleus & incus on the medial side of neck of malleus.* **(Bottom)** *Sagittal graphic shows structures of the medial ME wall with craniocaudal orientation of the lateral semicircular canal (SCC), facial nerve, oval window (OW), & cochlear promontory. Stapes foot plate attaches to OW. The dominant feature of medial wall is the cochlear promontory bulging into the ME cavity. Round window (RW) niche lies posterior & inferior to the cochlear promontory. Part of the mesotympanum anterior to a frontal plane drawn through the anterior margin of EAC/tympanic annulus on axial images is called protympanum. It leads anteriorly to a semicanal for tensor tympani muscle above & eustachian tube below, separated by a thin, bony plate called septum canalis musculotubarii.*

CORONAL & AXIAL GRAPHICS

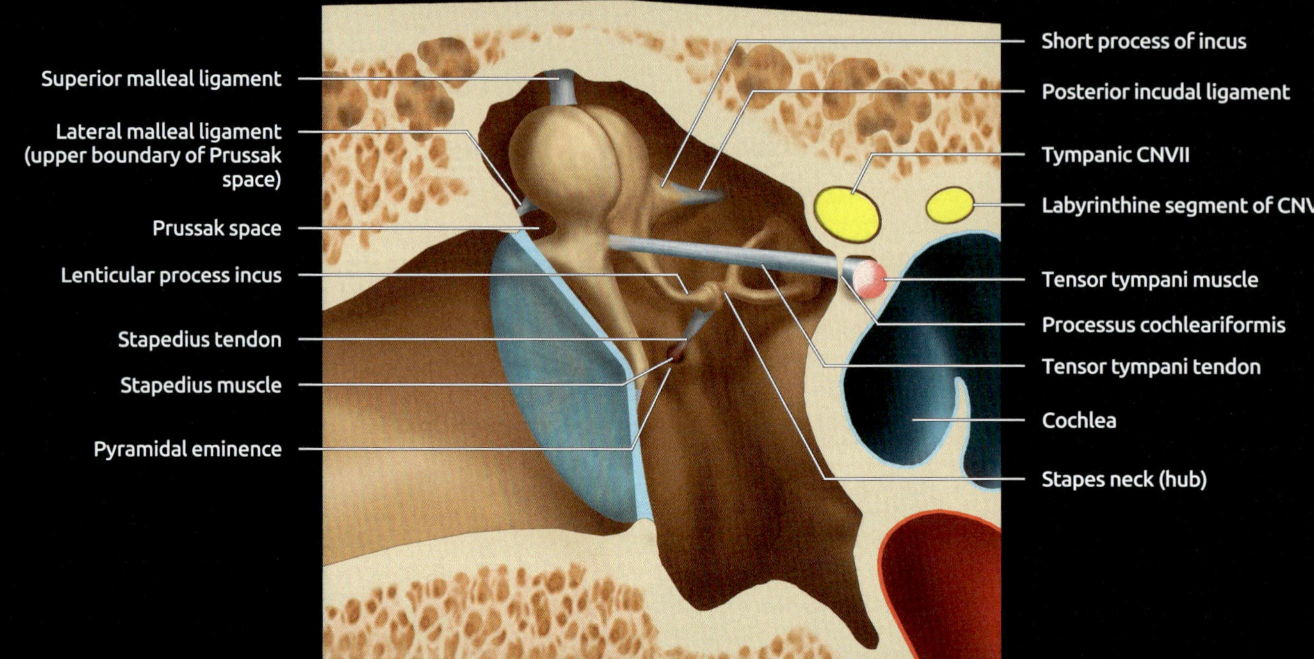

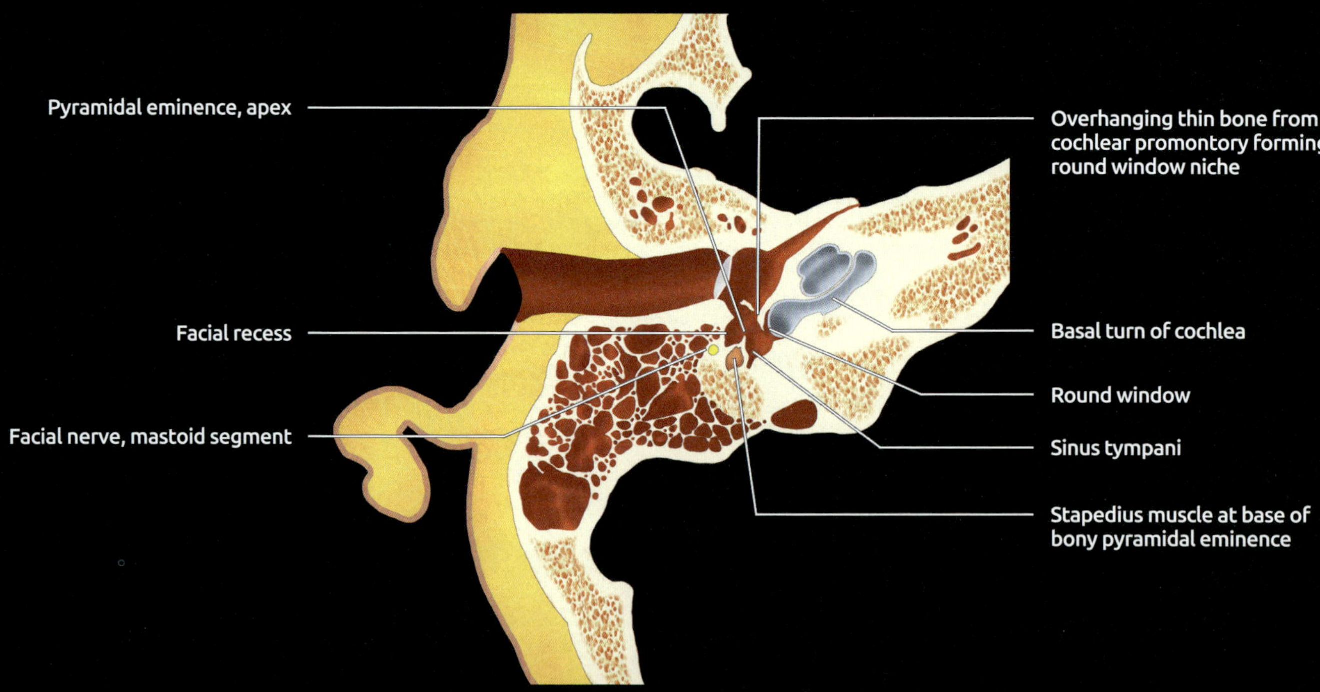

(Top) *Coronal graphic shows ME ligaments & tendons. Tensor tympani tendon turns 90° at the cochleariform process to cross the ME & attach to the upper aspect of manubrium (handle) of the malleus. Stapedius tendon emerges from the pyramidal eminence to attach to the neck of stapes. The 4 ossicle ligaments include the superior, lateral, & anterior (not shown) malleal ligaments, & the incudal ligament. Prussak space is the lowermost aspect of lateral epitympanic recess with its upper border being the lateral malleal ligament.* **(Bottom)** *Axial graphic shows the retrotympanum, which is the posterior aspect of mesotympanum, including its posterior wall. It has small, air-filled areas [called sinus tympani (ST)] & a facial (CNVII) recess with bony pyramidal eminence in between. A mnemonic to remember mediolateral orientation is that ST has an "m," hence, medial, & facial recess has an "l," hence, lateral. ST can be a blindspot at mastoidectomy where cholesteatoma may hide. RW niche is a bony pouch defined by thin, overhanging bone that extends from cochlear promontory. Air enclosed by RW niche becomes continuous posterolaterally with air in ST.*

EPITYMPANUM: AXIAL BONE CT

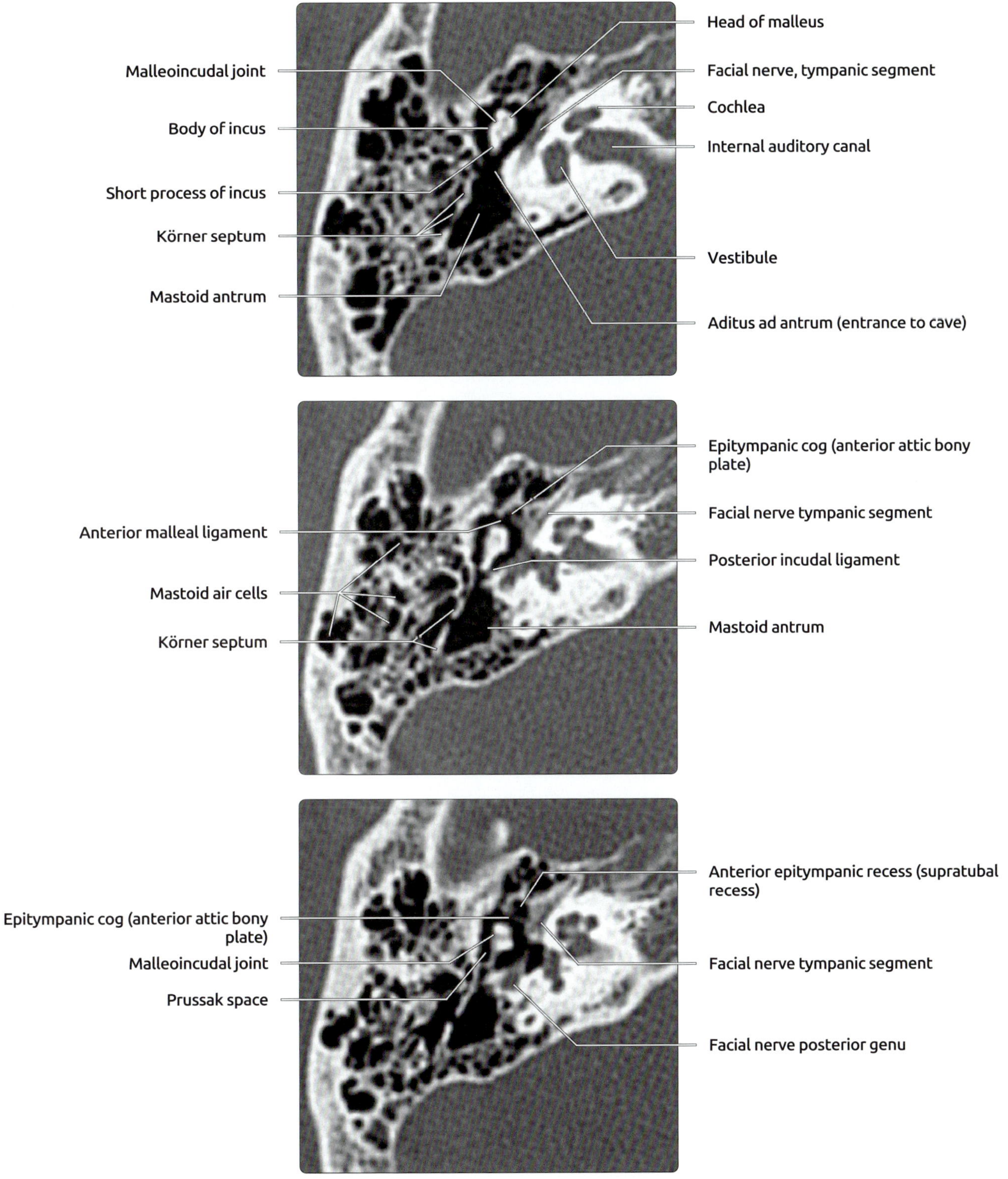

(Top) *First of 3 axial bone CT images through epitympanum from top to bottom shows the ice cream cone appearance of ME ossicles. Malleus head forms ice cream anteriorly. Cone is formed by body of incus anteriorly & short process of incus at tip of cone posteriorly. Aditus ad antrum ("entrance to cave") connects epitympanum of ME to mastoid antrum (cave). Körner septum (KS) (petrosquamous lamina) is a bony lamina dividing mastoid cavity at level of mastoid antrum into superficial mastoid air cells pneumatizing squamosal portion & a deeper petrosal portion. KS can be eroded by cholesteatoma.* **(Middle)** *Second bone CT shows the anterior malleal ligament & posterior incudal ligament. Epitympanic cog (middle portion of petrosquamous lamina) is a coronal bony septum suspended from the anterior aspect of the tegmen tympani. The cog can be a complete thin, bony plate (type I), small incomplete (type II), or nonvisualized on CT (type III).* **(Bottom)** *Third bone CT shows epitympanic cog partitioning anterior epitympanic recess [(AER)/supratubal recess)] from epitympanum. AER is bordered medially by geniculate fossa & anterior tympanic canal of facial nerve. Cholesteatoma may hide in AER.*

EPITYMPANUM: CORONAL BONE CT

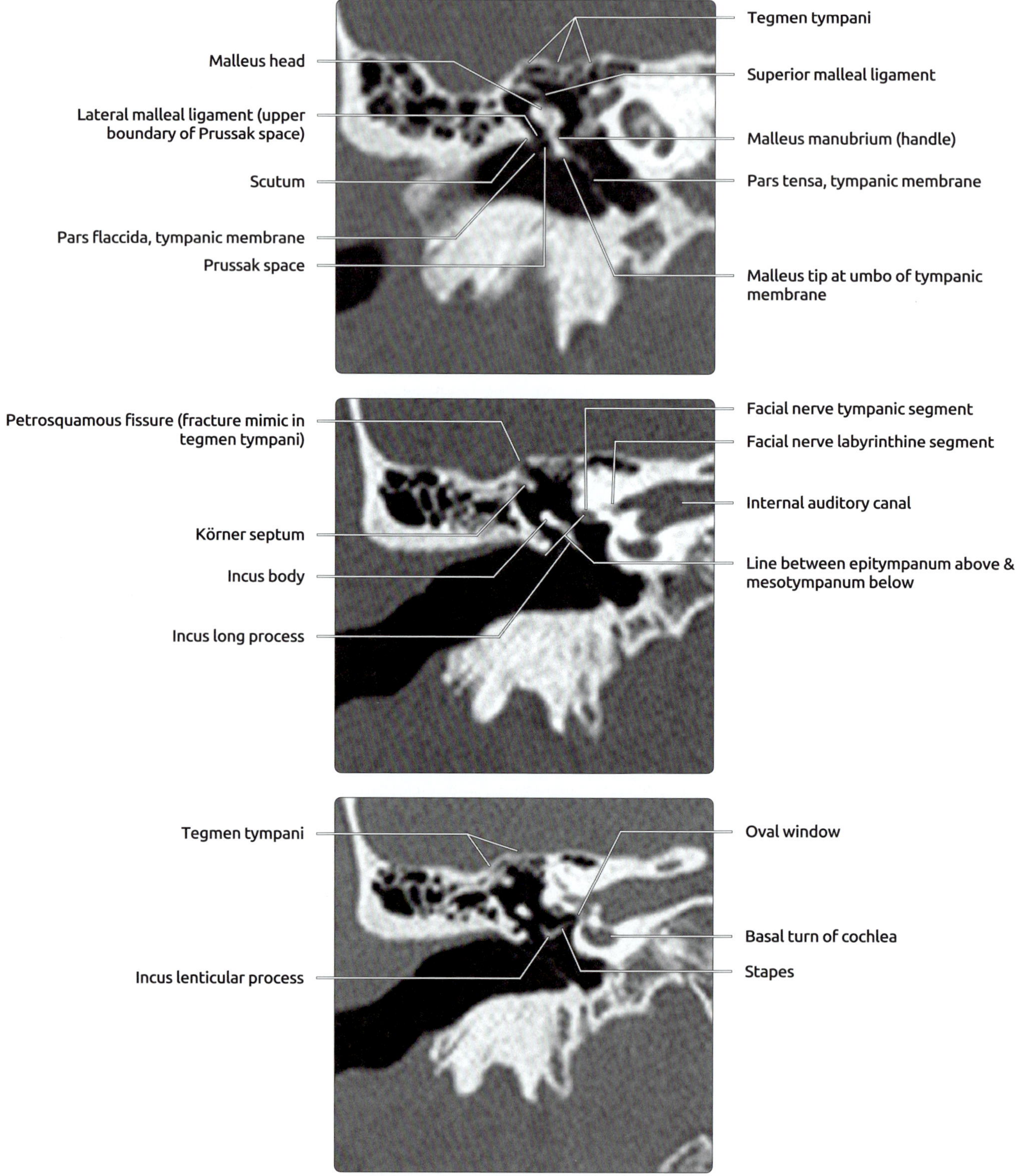

(Top) *First of 3 coronal bone CT images from anterior to posterior shows the superior & lateral malleal ligaments. Lateral malleal ligament forms the upper boundary of Prussak space (PS). PS is the lower aspect of lateral epitympanic recess extending from the level of scutum to the umbo of the TM. Scutum is the sharp, bony spur separating the superior aspect of the EAC from the ME. The umbo is the deepest point of concavity of the TM where the tip of the manubrium of malleus attaches. The lateral margin of PS is pars flaccida (upper part) of the TM. The medial margin of PS is formed by the manubrium (handle) of the malleus leading to the umbo. PS is the commonest site of acquired cholesteatoma formation.* **(Middle)** *Second bone CT shows the petrosquamous fissure as a small defect in the tegmen tympani (roof of epitympanum) continuous with the KS. The epitympanum is the ME cavity above a line drawn from the medial roof of the EAC/scutal tip & tympanic segment of facial nerve.* **(Bottom)** *Third bone CT shows the posterior aspect of tegmen tympani (roof of ME cavity). Note the posterior aspect of ME/mastoid roof above the mastoid cavity is called the tegmen mastoideum.*

MESOTYMPANUM: AXIAL & CORONAL BONE CT

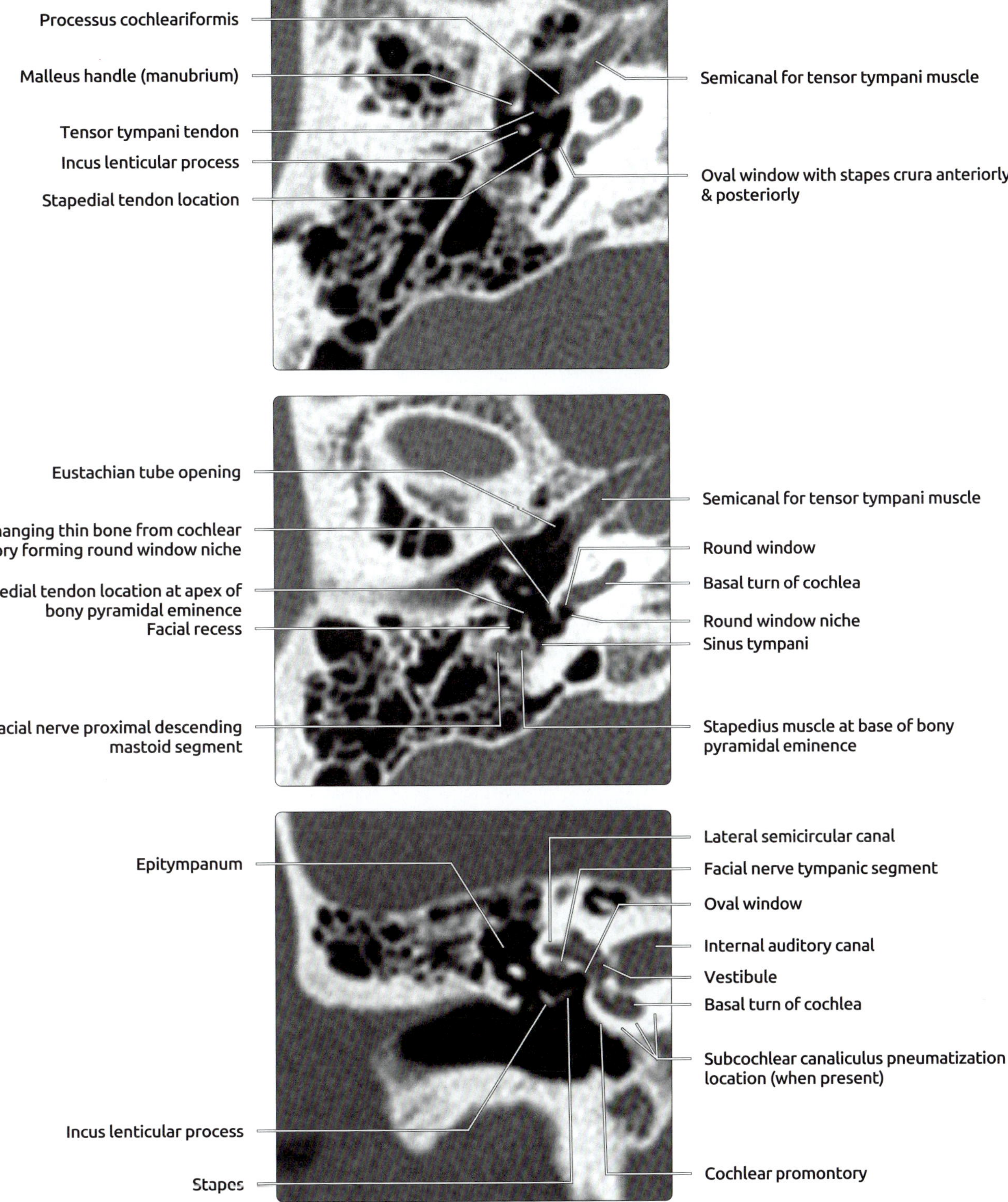

(Top) *First of 2 craniocaudal axial bone CT images of the mesotympanum shows the tensor tympani tendon curving around the pulley formed by processus cochleariformis (Pc) (cochleariform process) on its way towards its attachment at the upper aspect of the handle (manubrium) of malleus bone. Pc is a tiny, angulated, bony process above cochlear promontory. "Two parallel lines" in mesotympanum is important to assess for bony/ligamentous integrity with the anterior line formed by Pc/tensor tympani tendon/malleus handle & posterior line by incus & stapes bones.* **(Middle)** *Second bone CT shows the retrotympanum with small, air-filled ST & facial recess with the bony pyramidal eminence in between. RW niche is a triangular bony pouch defined by thin, overhanging bone that extends from cochlear promontory with air in RW chamber continuous posterolaterally with air in ST. Note the protympanum with eustachian tube below & semicanal for tensor tympani muscle above.* **(Bottom)** *Coronal bone CT shows duck/goose-shaped craniocaudal orientation of ME medial wall structures, which include lateral SCC, tympanic segment of CNVII, OW, & cochlear promontory.*

MIDDLE EAR LIGAMENTS & TENDONS

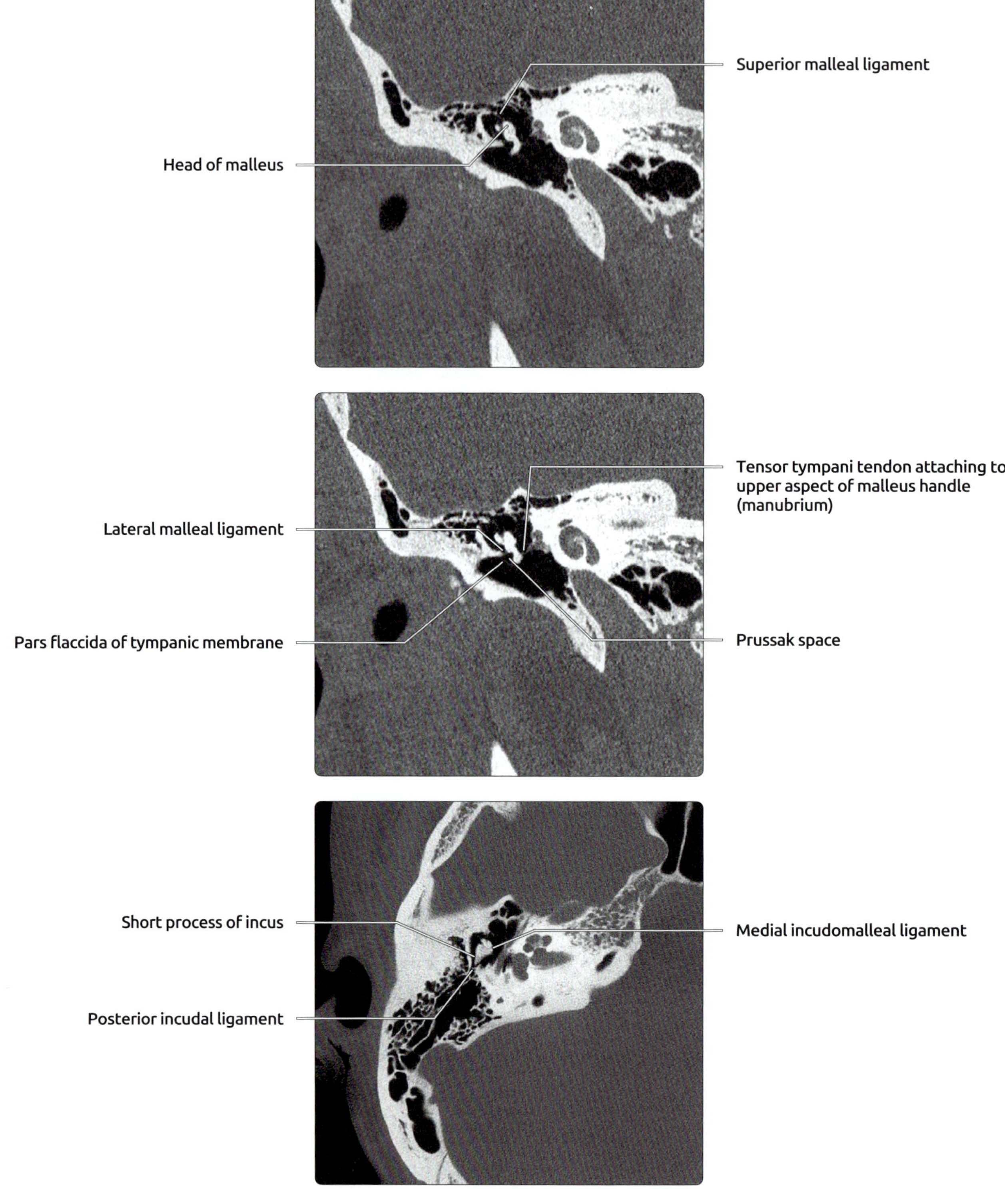

(Top) *Coronal photon-counting detector (PCD) CT through the malleus shows the superior malleal ligament extending from the malleus head to the epitympanic roof. A PCD CT scan of the temporal bone shows minute structures, such as ligaments & tendons, much better than conventional high-resolution CT scanners, which use energy-integrating detectors. ME ligaments include superior, lateral, & anterior malleal (malleolar) ligaments & the posterior incudal ligament. These ligaments are very thin, & "well seen" thickened ligaments could suggest tympanosclerosis. Do not confuse bony spurs from the ME walls with thickened ligaments.* **(Middle)** *Coronal PCD CT slightly posteriorly shows the lateral malleal ligament extending from the malleus head-neck junction to the tympanic annulus. It forms the upper boundary of PS.* **(Bottom)** *The 1st of 4 axial PCD CT images from top to bottom shows the posterior incudal ligament, which has medial & lateral parts. It connects the short process of incus to the margins of the fossa incudis. The fossa incudis is a small depression in the lower posterior epitympanic recess lodging the incus short process.*

MIDDLE EAR LIGAMENTS & TENDONS

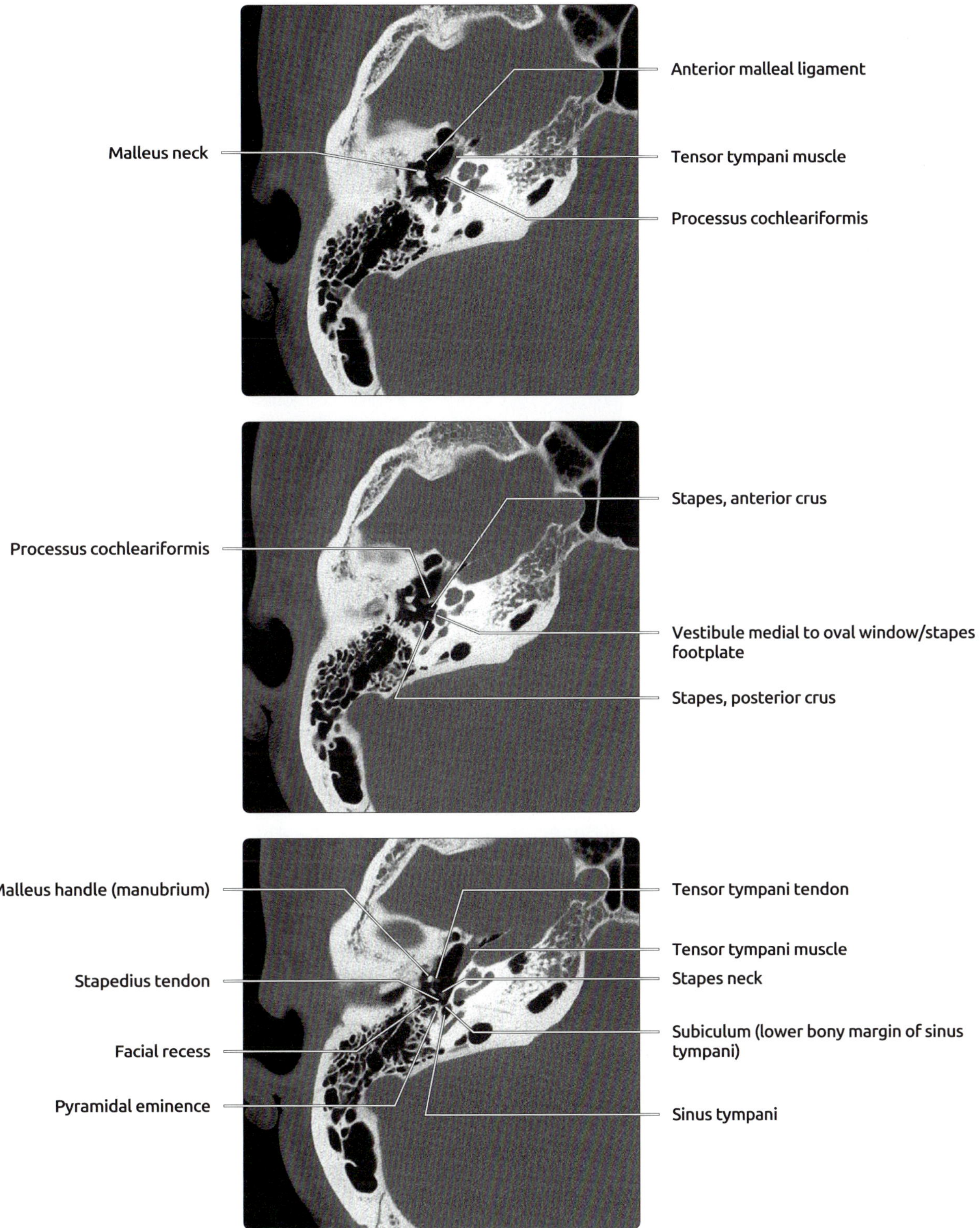

(Top) *Second PCD CT shows the anterior malleal ligament extending from the malleus neck (just above malleus anterior process) to the anterior tympanic wall near the petrotympanic fissure. The medial & lateral incudomalleal (malleoincudal) ligaments lie around the malleoincudal joint; the medial ligament is frequently seen on CT, but the lateral ligament is not readily seen.* **(Middle)** *Third PCD CT shows the thin stapes crura & footplate region. The annular ligament connects the stapes footplate to the OW & is difficult to see separately from the footplate. Note the Pc around which the tensor tympani tendon curves towards its attachment on the malleus handle. On routine conventional high-resolution temporal bone CT, the normal ME ligaments are usually equal to or slightly thicker than the tensor tympani tendon or anterior stapes crus, but could occasionally be double their thickness as normal variation.* **(Bottom)** *Final PCD CT shows the tensor tympani tendon attaching to the upper aspect of the manubrium (handle) of the malleus, & the stapedius tendon emerging from the tip of the pyramidal eminence on its way to the stapes neck attachment.*

TERMINOLOGY

Abbreviations

- Facial nerve (FN); greater superficial petrosal nerve (GSPN)

IMAGING ANATOMY

Overview

- **Internal auditory canal (IAC) segment**: Porus acusticus to IAC fundus; anterosuperior position above crista falciformis
- **Labyrinthine segment**: Connects fundal CNVII to geniculate ganglion (anterior genu)
- **Anterior genu**: Geniculate ganglion of FN resides here
  - **GSPN** originates at geniculate ganglion, where **nervus intermedius of Wrisberg (NIW)** joins FN
- **Tympanic segment**: Connects anterior to posterior genu
  - On coronal CT/MR, seen under lateral semicircular canal & above oval window in **medial wall of middle ear**
  - On more anterior coronal CT/MR, look for snake eyes (snail eyes) appearance of FN labyrinthine segment medially & tympanic segment laterally
- **Posterior genu**: Beyond this, FN dips down inferiorly as descending mastoid segment
- **Mastoid segment**: Inferiorly directed from posterior genu to exit mastoid temporal bone at **stylomastoid foramen**
  - Extracranial FN enters parotid gland
  - Gives off **nerve to stapedius** & **chorda tympani nerve (CTN)**
  - Runs in posterior wall of ME cavity with air-filled **facial recess** just anterior to FN upper mastoid segment
  - Bony **pyramidal eminence (PE)** with stapedius muscle at it base located just medial to FN upper mastoid segment
    - Do not confuse stapedius muscle for FN
  - Air-filled **sinus tympani** lies further medially in retrotympanum (RT) & connects to air underneath bony round window niche

Branches of Facial Nerve in Temporal Bone

- **GSPN**: Origin from geniculate ganglion (anterior genu)
  - Travels anteromedially through small hiatus in petrous temporal bone, then in middle cranial fossa floor between layers of dura mater underneath temporal lobe → **foramen lacerum**; at foramen lacerum, GSPN (parasympathetic via NIW) joined by **deep petrosal nerve (DPN)** (sympathetic fibers from internal carotid plexus) to form **vidian nerve**
  - Evaluate for GSPN schwannoma or perineural tumor spread in these locations
- **Nerve to stapedius**: Origin from upper aspect of descending mastoid segment of FN near PE
  - Motor innervation to stapedius muscle
- **CTN**: Origin from mastoid FN
  - From proximal, mid, or distal mastoid segment, or, rarely, even after exiting stylomastoid foramen
  - Ascends through **posterior canaliculus of CTN** in posterior wall of middle ear
    - Courses in middle ear cavity from posterior to anterior in substance of **tympanic membrane** between mucous & fibrous layers
    - Then between upper aspect of handle (manubrium) of malleus & long process of incus, on **medial** side of **upper** part of **handle of malleus**
    - Then travels through **anterior canaliculus of CTN** & exits temporal bone into masticator space (MS) through **petrotympanic fissure (Glaserian fissure)** posteromedial to TMJ; in MS, CTN joins lingual nerve (LN) 2 cm below skull base
  - **Chordal eminence**: Bony prominence on posterior wall of tympanic cavity formed by CTN posterior canaliculus
  - **Lateral RT** divided by chordal eminence into **facial recess** medially & **lateral tympanic sinus** laterally
    - **Styloid eminence** separates lateral RT superiorly from hypotympanum inferiorly
  - **Chordiculus**: Bony crest between chordal eminence inferolaterally & PE superomedially; origin of tympanic segment of CTN at lateral end of chordiculus

Anatomy Relationships

- **NIW** exits brainstem at pontomedullary junction between pons & inferior cerebellar peduncle lateral to motor root of FN & medial to CNVIII
- NIW then courses along with motor root of FN through cerebellopontine angle into anterosuperior IAC quadrant
- NIW **joins motor root of FN** near geniculate ganglion
- NIW: Somatic sensory, special sensory, & visceral motor (secretomotor) fibers from various brainstem nuclei
- **Superior salivatory nucleus (SSN)** in pons: **Parasympathetic** root through NIW → FN → **GSPN** (+ **DPN**, sympathetic) → **vidian nerve** → **pterygopalatine ganglion** in pterygopalatine fossa → **lacrimal gland** & **nasal** glands
- SSN in pons: **Parasympathetic** root through NIW → FN → **CTN** → **LN** (CNV3 branch) → **submandibular ganglion** suspended by roots from LN in sublingual space → **submandibular & sublingual salivary glands**
- **Nucleus of tractus solitarius (NTS)** in medulla/lower pons: **Geniculate ganglion** at anterior genu of CNVII in temporal bone contains pseudounipolar cell bodies
  - Central processes of cell bodies enter gustatory part of NTS, forming special visceral afferent root
  - Peripheral processes receive **taste** sensation from anterior 2/3rd of **tongue** (**CTN**) & palate (**GSPN**)
- **Mastoid canaliculus** with **Arnold nerve** [auricular branch of vagus (CNX)] extending laterally from lateral aspect of pars vascularis of jugular foramen toward **tympanomastoid fissure** first **connects to descending mastoid segment FN canal** several millimeters above stylomastoid foramen

CLINICAL IMPLICATIONS

Clinical Importance

- Enhancement of geniculate ganglion, tympanic & mastoid segments of CNVII normal on postcontrast T1W MR; can be asymmetric intensity of enhancement on right & left
  - Secondary to circumneural arteriovenous plexus
- **Cisternal**, **IAC**, **labyrinthine** & **parotid** segments **do not** normally **enhance** on MR
  - Faint enhancement may be seen depending on MR scanner, sequence, & type of contrast used
- Always check parotid in peripheral CNVII paralysis
- Focal dehiscence of undersurface of tympanic segment FN canal normal variant occurring in as much as 20- 25% of adults, most commonly just above oval window

GRAPHICS: SAGITTAL, CORONAL, & AXIAL

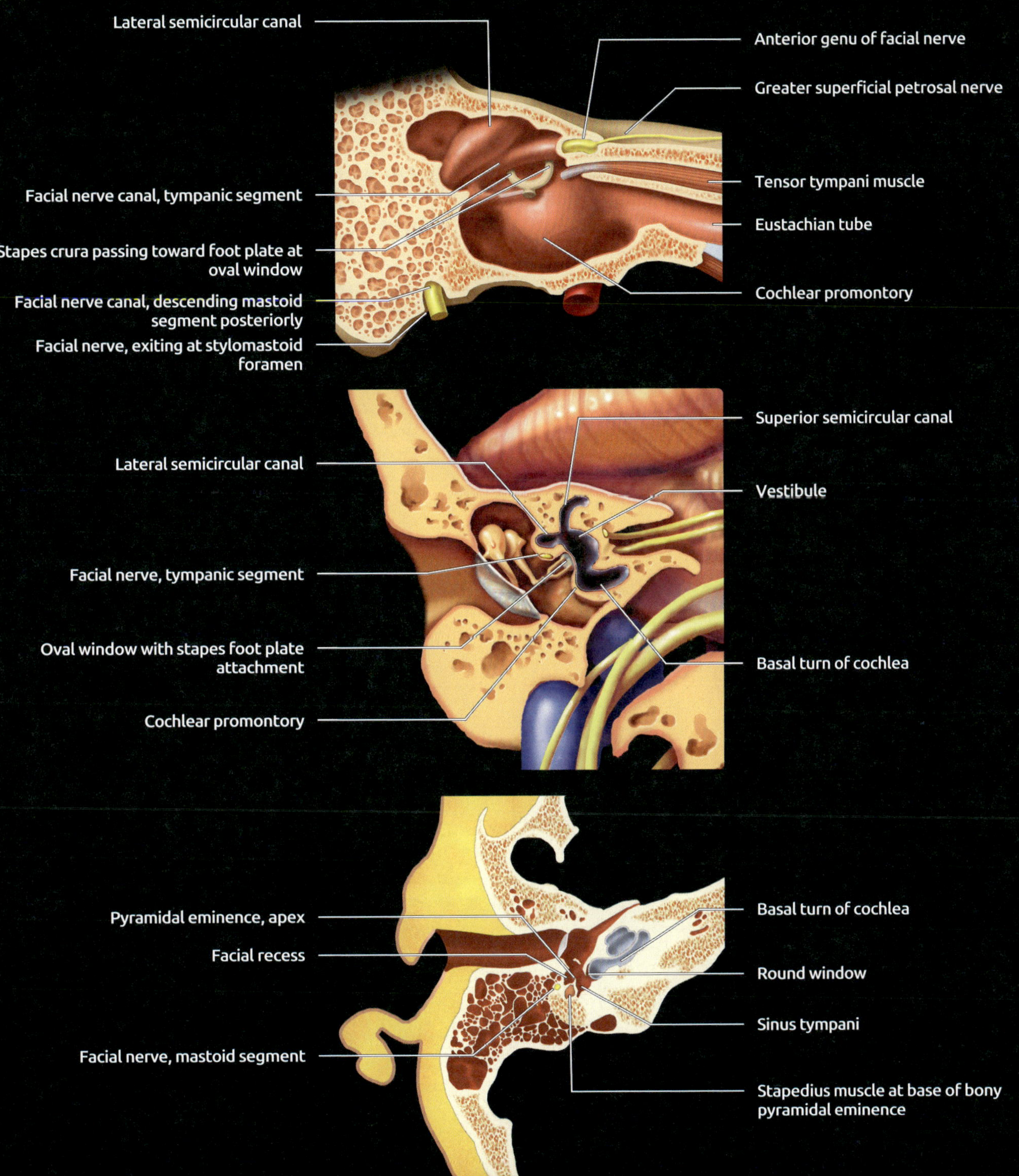

(Top) *Sagittal graphic shows the medial wall of the middle ear. Note craniocaudal orientation of the lateral semicircular canal (LSCC), facial nerve (tympanic segment), oval window (stapes footplate attaches to oval window), and cochlear promontory (bony bulge covering the basal turn of cochlea). Greater superficial petrosal nerve (GSPN) originates at geniculate ganglion in the anterior genu of the facial nerve, where the nervus intermedius of Wrisberg [(NIW) not shown] joins the facial nerve. Posteroinferiorly, the descending mastoid segment of the facial nerve exits the temporal bone at the stylomastoid foramen on its way to the parotid gland.* **(Middle)** *Coronal graphic shows craniocaudal orientation of LSCC, facial nerve canal (tympanic segment), oval window, & cochlear promontory, a very useful anatomic landmark for evaluating a coronal temporal bone CT. Superior & LSCCs, vestibule, & basal turn of cochlea together form a goose/duck-like appearance on coronal images.* **(Bottom)** *Axial graphic shows the posterior wall of the mesotympanum with small, air-filled areas (called sinus tympani) medially & facial (CNVII) recess laterally with the bony pyramidal eminence in between.*

CORONAL BONE CT

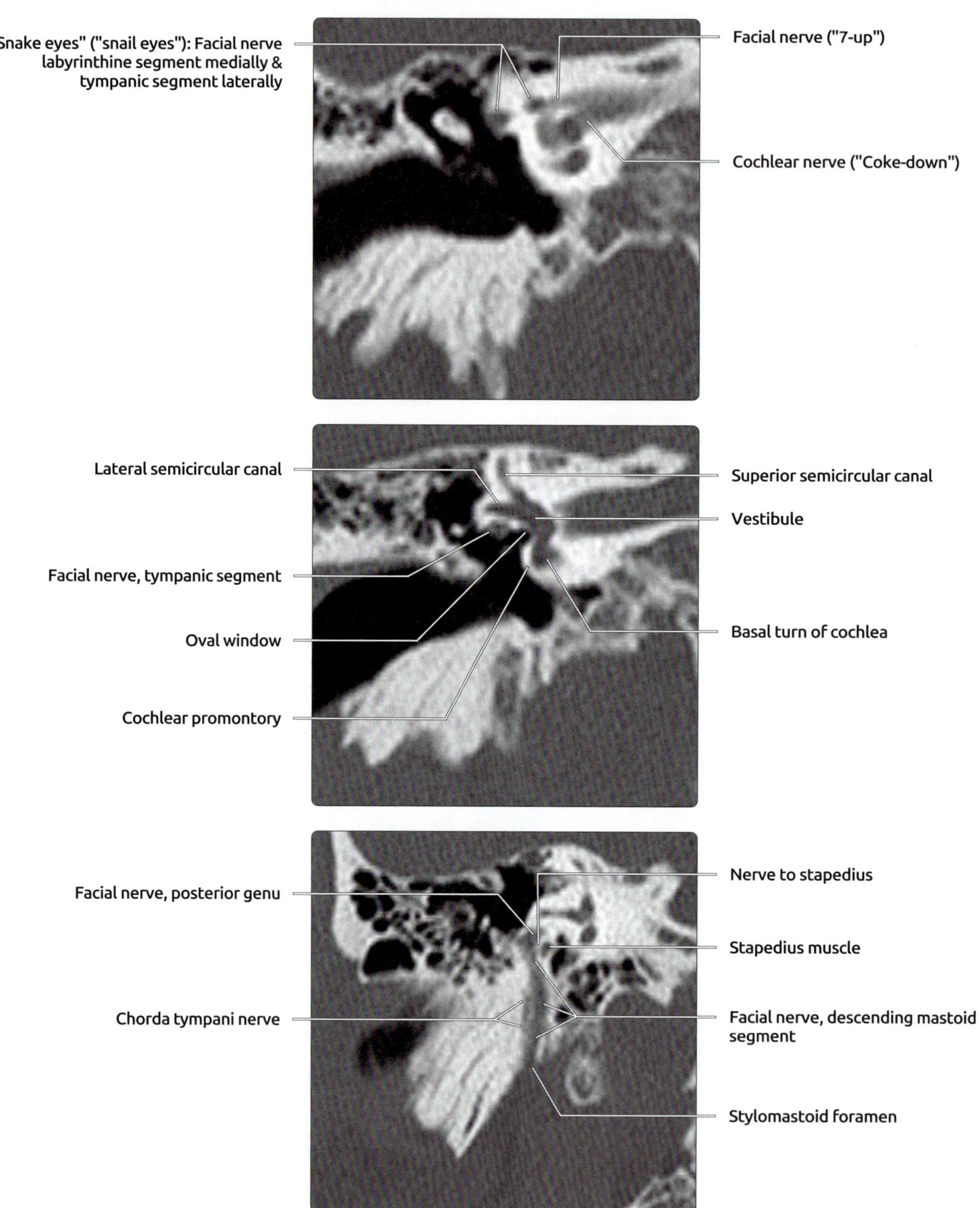

(Top) *First of 3 coronal reformatted bone CT images from anterior to posterior shows snake eyes (snail eyes) appearance of right facial nerve labyrinthine segment medially lying next to tympanic segment laterally. In the anterior aspect of the internal auditory canal (IAC)/petrous temporal bone, facial nerve (CNVII) lies above with cochlear nerve (CNVIII) lying below (mnemonic: "7-up"/"Coke-down"). The posterior aspect of IAC coronally will have the superior vestibular nerve above with inferior vestibular nerve lying below (both CNVIII); not shown.* **(Middle)** *CT shows characteristic craniocaudal orientation of the LSCC, facial nerve canal (tympanic segment), oval window, & cochlear promontory. Superior & LSCCs, vestibule, & basal turn of cochlea together form a goose/duck-like appearance. Focal dehiscence of undersurface of tympanic segment facial nerve canal is a normal variant occurring in as many as 20-25% of adults, most commonly just above oval window, but is important to mention in presurgical temporal bone CT reports to avoid nerve injury during middle ear surgery.* **(Bottom)** *CT shows the posterior genu & descending mastoid segment of the facial nerve with branches.*

AXIAL BONE CT

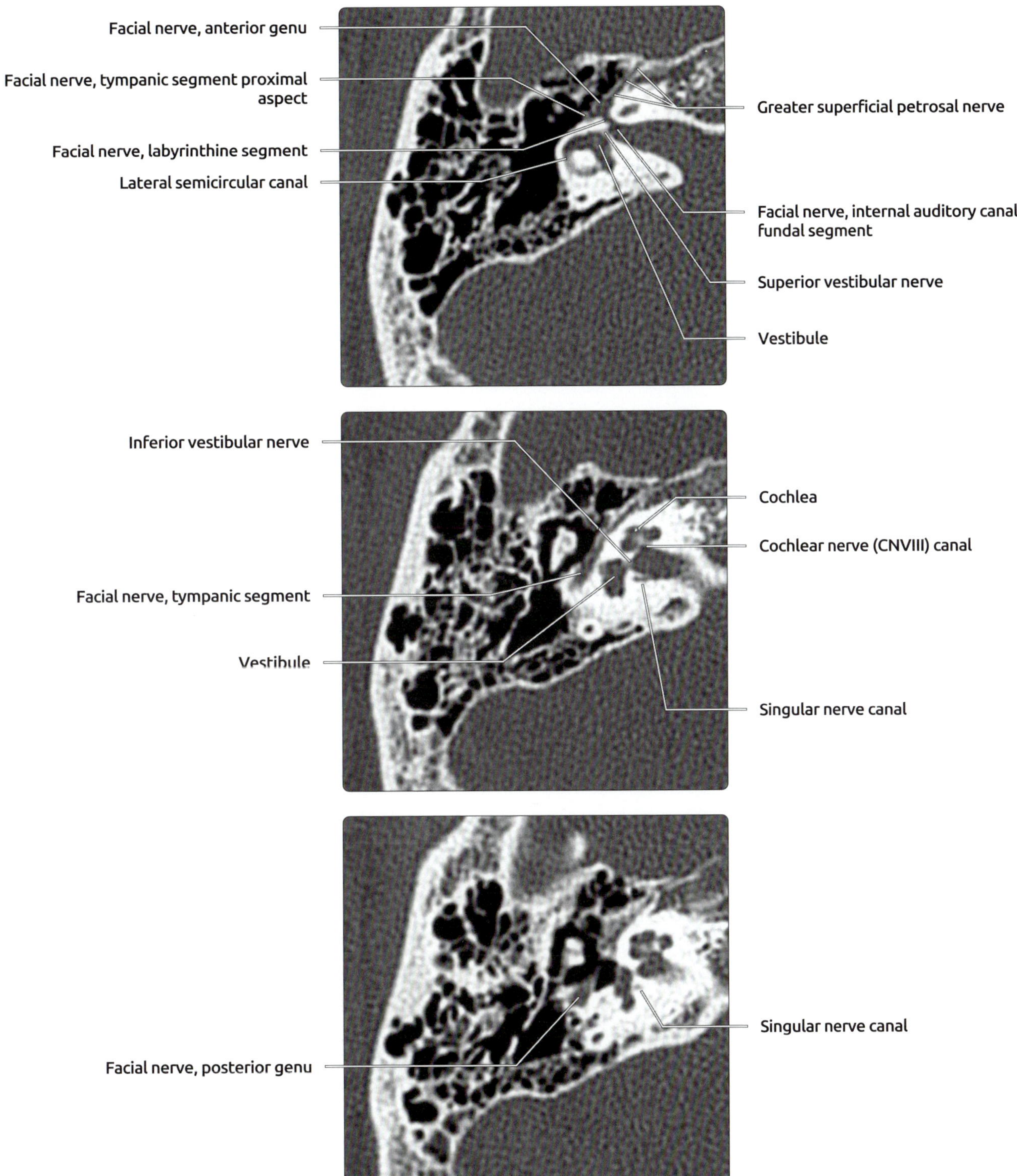

(Top) *First of 7 axial temporal bone CT images from top to bottom shows the right facial nerve IAC fundal segment continuing as the labyrinthine segment towards the anterior genu. GSPN originates at the geniculate ganglion in the anterior genu, where NIW joins the facial nerve. GSPN carries preganglionic parasympathetic fibers from superior salivatory nucleus (SSN) in lower dorsal pons (via NIW coming from cerebellopontine angle/IAC; then facial nerve geniculate ganglion in anterior genu; and then the vidian nerve) to supply lacrimal gland and nasal glands through the pterygopalatine ganglion in the pterygopalatine fossa. GSPN also carries sensory afferent taste fibers from the soft palate to nucleus of tractus solitarius (NTS) in medulla/lower pons. GSPN passes through a small hiatus in the petrous temporal bone & then in the middle cranial fossa floor between the 2 layers of dura mater underneath the temporal lobe. Also note the superior vestibular nerve.* **(Middle)** *Second bone CT shows the tympanic segment of the right facial nerve. Note the inferior vestibular nerve & singular nerve.* **(Bottom)** *Third bone CT shows the posterior genu of the right facial nerve.*

AXIAL BONE CT

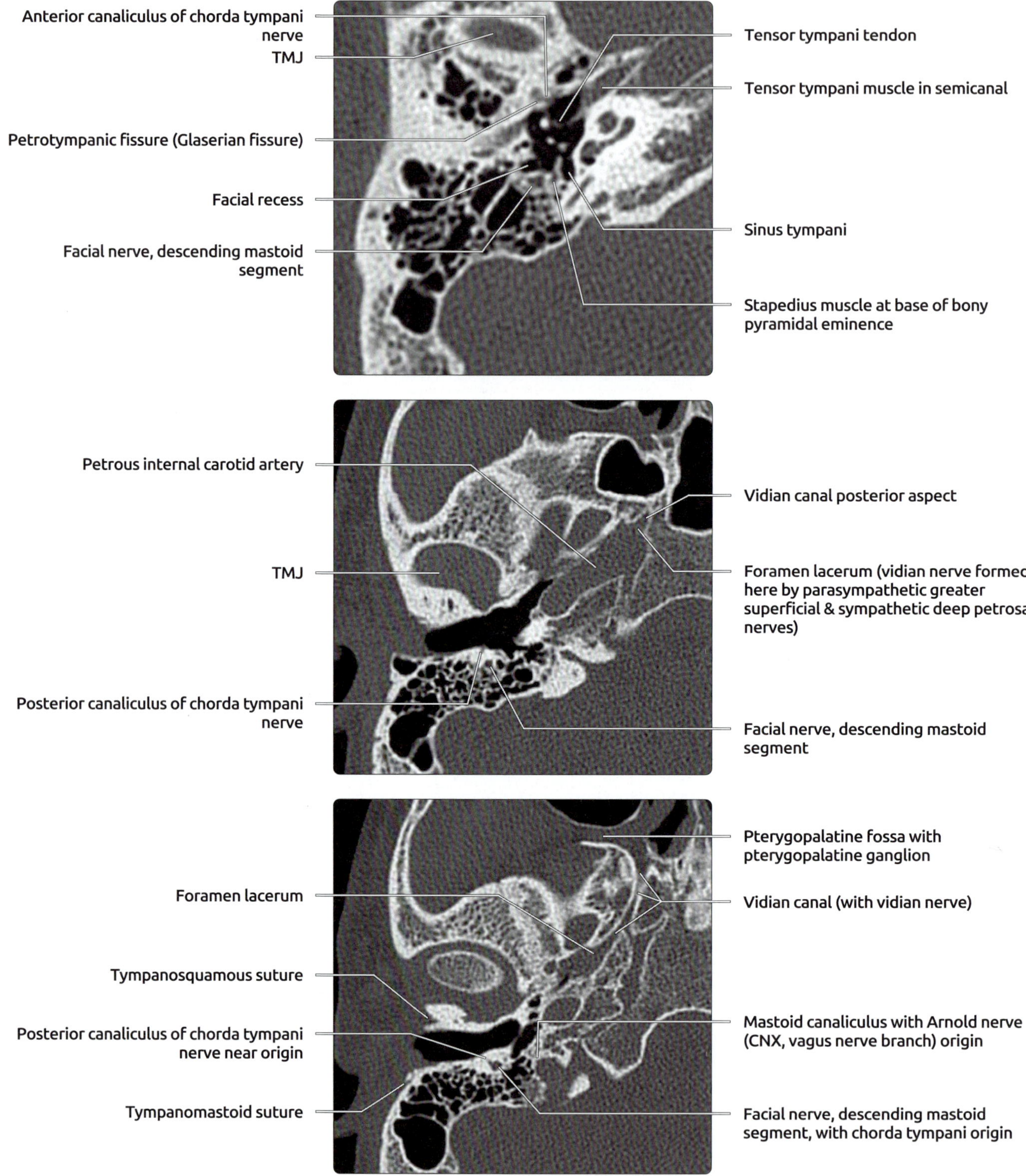

(Top) *Fourth bone CT shows the right facial nerve descending the mastoid segment, posteroinferior to posterior genu. Note the stapedius muscle; the tiny nerve to the stapedius arises from the proximal upper descending mastoid segment. Posterior mesotympanum (retrotympanum) has small, air-filled areas (called sinus tympani) medially & facial (CNVII) recess laterally with bony pyramidal eminence in between. Mnemonic for this mediolateral orientation is that sinus tympani has an "m," hence medial; & facial recess has an "l," hence lateral. Sinus tympani can be a blindspot at mastoidectomy where cholesteatoma may hide. Do not mistake the tensor tympani muscle for facial nerve tympanic segment. Chorda tympani nerve enters the anterior wall of the middle ear cavity at the anterior canaliculus of chorda tympani & continues into petrotympanic fissure (Glaserian fissure), which is medial to the TMJ.* **(Middle)** *Image shows descending mastoid segment & posterior canaliculus of the chorda tympani nerve. Note GSPN forming the vidian nerve at the foramen lacerum.* **(Bottom)** *Chorda tympani nerve origin from the descending mastoid segment of the right facial nerve is shown.*

AXIAL BONE CT, PHOTON-COUNTING DETECTOR CT, & GRAPHIC

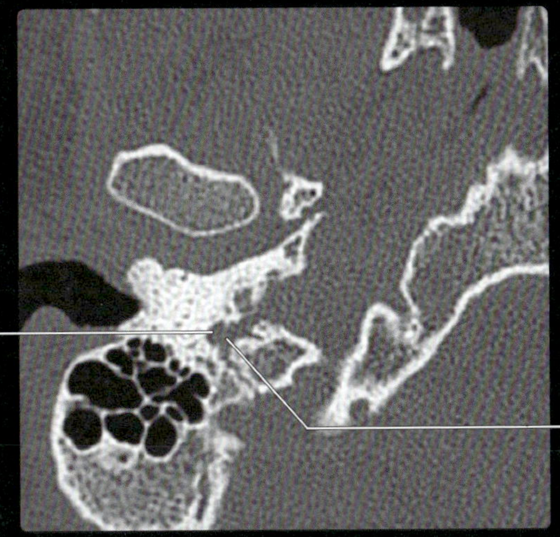

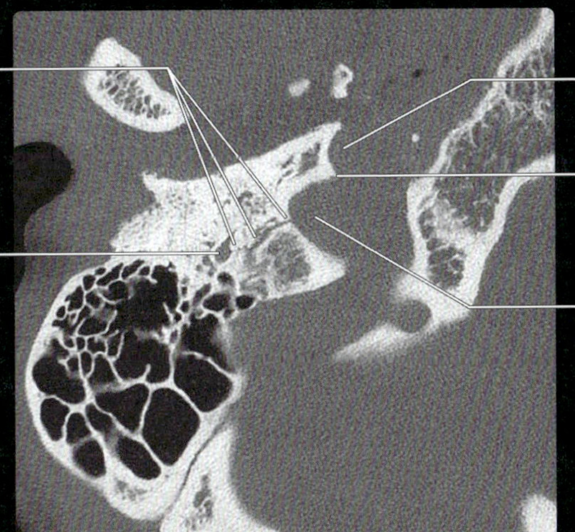

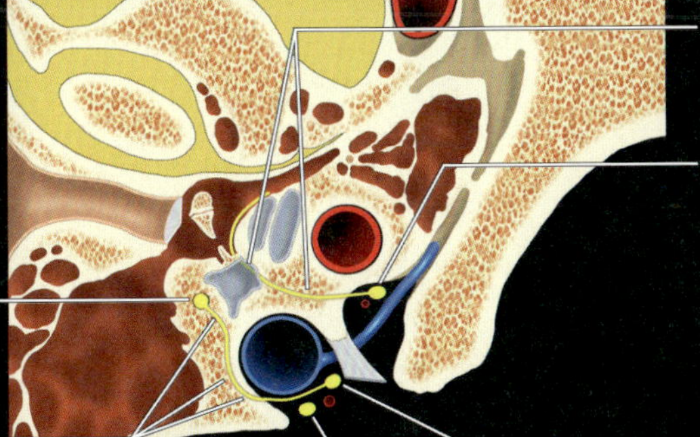
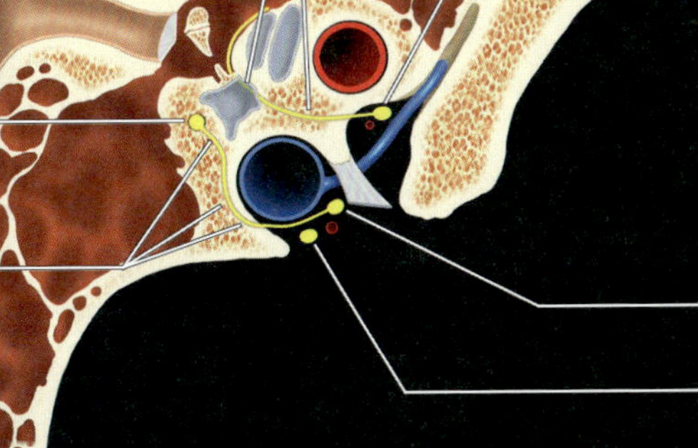

(Top) *Last of 7 axial bone CT images shows the right facial nerve exiting the mastoid temporal bone at the stylomastoid foramen on its way to ramify within the parotid gland. Facial nerve perineural tumor spread from parotid malignancy should always be carefully evaluated.* **(Middle)** *Axial photon-counting detector CT shows the mastoid canaliculus with the Arnold nerve (auricular branch of vagus [CNX]) originating from the lateral aspect of pars vascularis of the right jugular foramen. Mastoid canaliculus first connects laterally to the descending mastoid segment facial nerve canal a few millimeters above the stylomastoid foramen, then dips inferolaterally toward the tympanomastoid fissure (suture) at the posterior aspect of the external auditory canal (EAC). The Arnold nerve supplies part of the tympanic membrane & EAC & causes Arnold nerve cough reflex when mechanically stimulating the ear with a finger or ear bud.* **(Bottom)** *Axial graphic shows the right mastoid canaliculus with the Arnold nerve [auricular branch of vagus (CNX)] on its way from the lateral aspect of pars vascularis of the jugular foramen toward the descending mastoid segment facial nerve canal.*

CHORDA TYMPANI NERVE: SAGITTAL GRAPHIC, SAGITTAL BONE CT, & LONGITUDINAL OBLIQUE (STENVER) BONE CT REFORMATION

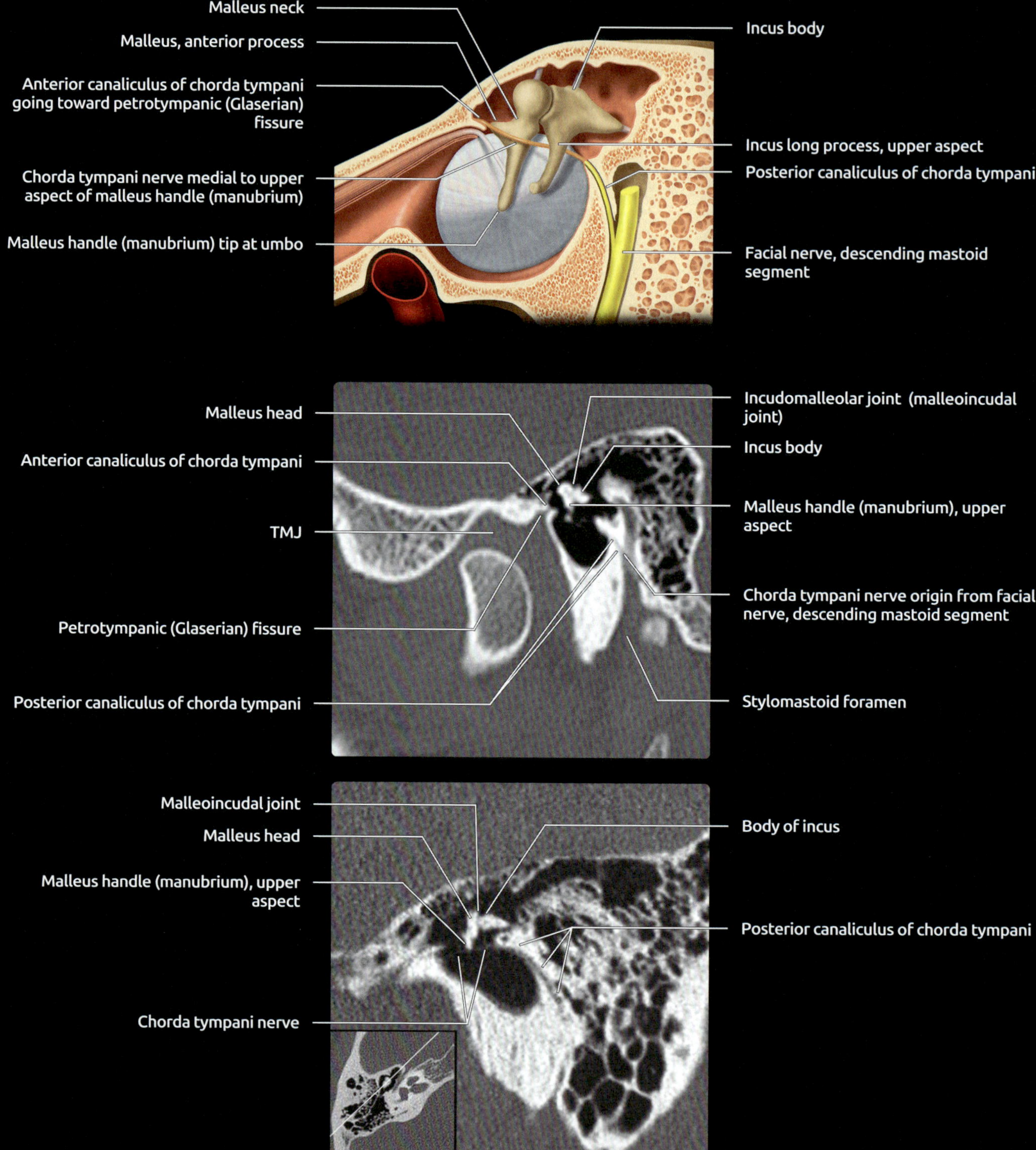

(Top) *Sagittal graphic shows an internal view of the lateral wall of the middle ear cavity. The chorda tympani nerve originates from the descending mastoid segment of the facial nerve, ascends through the posterior canaliculus of chorda tympani at the posterior wall of the middle ear, courses in the middle ear cavity from posterior to anterior in the substance of the tympanic membrane between mucous & fibrous layers, & then between the upper aspect of the handle (manubrium) of malleus & long process of incus, on the medial side of the upper part of the handle of malleus. It then travels through the anterior canaliculus of chorda tympani & exits the temporal bone into the masticator space through the petrotympanic fissure (Glaserian fissure), which is posteromedial to the TMJ, & joins the lingual nerve 2 cm below the skull base.* **(Middle)** *Straight parasagittal bone CT reconstruction perpendicular to the axial CT without any obliquity shows the course of the chorda tympani nerve.* **(Bottom)** *Longitudinal oblique (Stenver) bone CT of the right ear near the anterior margin of the petrous temporal bony pyramid shows the chorda tympani nerve canal & the nerve itself in the middle ear cavity.*

LONGITUDINAL OBLIQUE (STENVER) & TRANSVERSE OBLIQUE (PÖSCHL) BONE CT REFORMATIONS

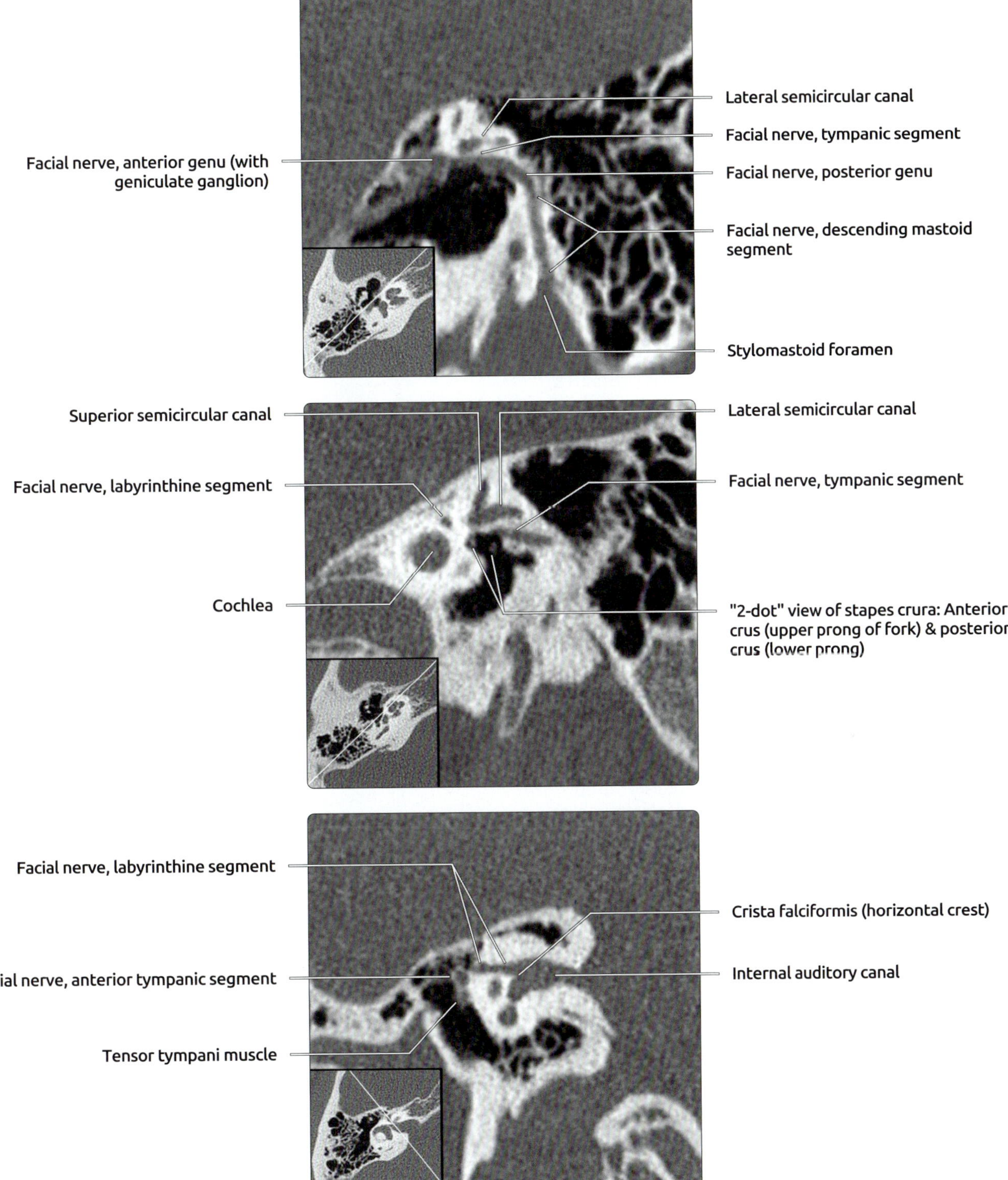

(Top) *Another longitudinal oblique (Stenver) bone CT more posteriorly shows the entire tympanic segment of the facial nerve. Note the anterior genu, tympanic segment, posterior genu, mastoid segment, & stylomastoid foramen, all seen on this single view. The tympanic segment passes beneath the LSCC.* **(Middle)** *Further posterior longitudinal oblique (Stenver view) bone CT shows the labyrinthine & tympanic segments of the right facial nerve canal. Note the "2-dot" view of crura of the stapes just before they meet the footplate of the stapes at the oval window.* **(Bottom)** *Transverse oblique (Pöschl) bone CT reformation of the right ear parallel to the long axis of the superior SCC is shown. The image toward the medial aspect of the petrous temporal bone shows the axis of the labyrinthine segment of the facial nerve. When CNVII pathology is present, it is very helpful to have multiple different views of its canal. Transverse oblique (Pöschl) view image set is made in a plane parallel to the axis created by a line through superior SCC, whereas the longitudinal oblique (Stenver) view image set is made in a plane perpendicular to the superior SCC axis.*

TERMINOLOGY

Definitions

- Inner ear: Cochlea, vestibule, semicircular canals (SCCs), associated interconnecting endolymphatic/perilymphatic compartments & surrounding bony otic capsule
- Inner ear houses sensorineural structures for sound detection (cochlea) & mechanoreceptors for spatial orientation & balance (vestibule & SCCs)

IMAGING ANATOMY

Overview

- **Inner ear**
  - Inner ear (a.k.a. labyrinth) given its complex & intercommunicating internal spaces
  - Architecturally complex bony compartment (bony labyrinth) that predominantly contains fluid
  - Internal fluid spaces further organized into distinct functional compartments: Membranous labyrinth & perilymphatic labyrinth
- **Bony labyrinth**
  - Essentially, otic capsule & internal osseous architecture
  - Hardest bone in body with trilamellar arrangement with islands of modified cartilage & high mineral content
  - Dense enchondral bone that surrounds cochlea, vestibule, SCCs, bony vestibular & cochlear aqueducts
  - **Vestibular aqueduct (VA)**: Along posterior aspect of petrous temporal bone; **endolymphatic duct (ELD)** & **endolymphatic sac (ELS)** located within bony VA
  - In **Ménière disease (MD)**, gap between vertical part of posterior SCC **(PSCC)** & posterior fossa may be narrower than normal on axial CT/3D T2 MR
    - **Gap** 2.9 mm in MD vs. 3.8 mm in controls
    - Endolymphatic hydrops in MD: Dilation (hydrops) of scala media of cochlea with displacement of Reissner membrane into scala vestibuli; saccular hydrops common but less frequent; utricular hydrops rare
    - Severe MD: Reissner membrane bulges into helicotrema; also bulges through saccule into SCCs (mainly lateral SCC) & onto stapes footplate
  - Perisaccular fibrosis, loss of epithelial integrity, atrophy of ELD, & narrowing/obstruction of ELD lumen with **narrowed bony VA**
    - **Resultant** posterior placement of PSCC with ↓ **gap**
  - **Cochlear aqueduct**: Small canal in bony labyrinth harboring **perilymphatic (periotic) duct** & draining perilymph into posterior cranial fossa subarachnoid space CSF
    - Seen parallel & inferior to internal auditory canal **(IAC)**
    - Arise superolaterally from **scala tympani** at basal turn of cochlea & run through otic capsule & petrous apex; difficult to see on CT
    - Funnel-shaped inferomedial end seen on CT opens at part of roof of **pars nervosa of jugular foramen** called **pyramidal fossa**
    - Pyramidal fossa lies superior to petrosal fossula (small depression on undersurface of petrous bone)
      - **Petrosal fossula**, which is part of pars nervosa of jugular foramen, lies in ridge between jugular foramen & external opening of carotid canal
      - Petrosal fossula houses inferior petrous ganglion of glossopharyngeal nerve (where Jacobson nerve originates) & gives rise to inferior tympanic canaliculus superiorly
- **Membranous labyrinth**
  - Consists of interconnecting, thin-walled, saccular & tubular structures that contain **endolymph**
  - Specific site in inner ear for specialized neural receptors for sound (cochlea) & balance (vestibule & SCCs)
  - In **cochlea**, membranous labyrinth represented by central tubular canal called **scala media (cochlear duct)**
    - Contains spiral **organ of Corti**
    - Very high endolymph **potassium (K+)** concentration creates environment allowing **high electric potential in scala media** of cochlea (+80 to +110 mV)
  - In **vestibule**, membranous labyrinth represented by sac-like components: **Utricle** postero**superiorly** & **saccule** antero**inferiorly**
    - Superior vestibular nerve innervates utricle & superior & lateral SCCs; inferior vestibular nerve innervates saccule & posterior SCC
    - Utricle & saccule each contain focal area **(macula)** of specialized mechanoreceptors with hair cells capable of detecting acceleration & gravitational pull
    - Macula of saccule lies in nearly vertical position & detects vertical linear acceleration
    - Macula of utricle lies in horizontal position & detects horizontal acceleration
    - Coordinated sensory perception of vertical & horizontal linear acceleration along vestibular nerve allow **linear acceleration** perception in any direction
    - Posterior area of utricle connected with SCCs
  - **Ductus reuniens**: Connects base of scala media of **cochlea** to anteroinferiorly situated saccule of **vestibule**
  - In each **SCC**, membranous labyrinth consists of tubular compartment called **semicircular duct**
    - Each semicircular duct contains dilated region **(ampulla)** that contains **crista**
    - Cristae: Mechanoreceptors containing hair cells capable of detecting **angular acceleration** in multiple directions
  - **ELD** & **ELS** represent posterior extensions of membranous labyrinth
    - **ELD** arises from crus communis at junction of posterior & superior SCC & extends posteriorly to intraosseous & then intradural (fovea area) **ELS**
      - Fovea: Cup-shaped area at posterior petrous bone
  - **Saccular duct** & **utricular duct** join in **endolymphatic sinus** at groove on posteromedial surface of vestibule
  - Proximal opening of utricular duct contains slit-shaped **utriculo-endolymphatic valve (Bast valve)** to control endolymph inflow from utricle towards ELD & ELS
  - Inferior portion of endolymphatic sinus connects to ELD
- **Perilymphatic labyrinth**
  - Fluid-filled space interposed between membranous labyrinth & inner periosteum of bony labyrinth
  - **Perilymph** composed of CSF-like fluid
  - **Cochlea** contains 2 distinct tubular components of perilymphatic labyrinth: **Scala tympani** & **scala vestibuli**

- Scala tympani at basal turn of cochlea communicate with subarachnoid space via **perilymphatic duct (periotic duct)** within bony cochlear aqueduct
  - **Helicotrema**: Connects scala tympani & scala vestibuli at apex of modiolus
    - Organ of Corti hair cells in scala media near helicotrema best detect low-frequency sounds
  - **Vestibule** contains **perilymphatic cistern** of perilymphatic labyrinth, round area containing perilymph surrounding utricle & saccule
  - Thin perilymphatic spaces are also identified in SCCs
  - Perilymphatic labyrinth includes **fissula ante fenestram** & **fossula post fenestram** (areas anterior & posterior to oval window where otospongiosis may occur)
- **4-hour delay post-IV contrast 3D inversion recovery MR**
  - Cochlear scala vestibuli, scala tympani, & perilymphatic cistern around vestibular saccule & utricle are **bright** due to **perilymphatic contrast** enhancement
  - **Endolymph**-filled cochlear scala media & vestibular saccule & utricle show **dark** signal as **IV contrast does not enter** it
  - **MD**: Larger dark signal of scala media & saccule/rarely utricle
    - With resultant narrowing of bright signal of scala vestibuli, scala tympani, & perilymphatic cistern around vestibular saccule & utricle

Anatomy Relationships

- **Cochlea** lies **anterior** to IAC
- **Vestibule** lies **lateral** to IAC
- SCCs bud out of vestibule
- **Osseous spiral lamina-basilar membrane complex** seen **within** each cochlear turn
- **Interscalar septum (ISS)** seen **separating** different cochlear turns
  - Unlike what its name sounds like, ISS **not between scala** of cochlea

Internal Contents

- **Cochlea**
  - Portion of inner ear responsible for hearing
  - Term derived from Greek word "kokhlos," meaning land snail
  - Essentially, partitioned tube arranged in spiral (snail-like) configuration, making ~ 2.5 turns around central perforated osseous structure called **modiolus**
  - Basilar turn bulges into medial wall of middle ear cavity, creating **cochlear promontory**
  - Basal turn merges with vestibule
  - **Modiolus**
    - Conical central bony axis of cochlea consisting of spongiform bone
    - Modiolus widest at its base: ~ 4 mm
    - Base directed towards IAC & perforated by branches of cochlear nerve
    - Cochlear nerve fibers traverse modiolus, branching & extending to spiral lamina
  - **Osseous spiral lamina**
    - Thin bony plate projecting outward as it spirals around modiolus from base to apex
    - Osseous spiral lamina readily identified on high-resolution CT and MR imaging
    - Provides supportive function & allows organized transmission of cochlear nerve fibers to each cochlear segment
    - Nerve fibers of cochlear nerve (both afferent & efferent) extend through medial aspects of spiral lamina
    - Thin bony plate tapers laterally; lateral margin connects to medial aspect of **basilar membrane**
    - Basilar membrane attaches laterally to **spiral ligament** at inner margin of otic capsule
    - **Osseous spiral lamina-basilar membrane complex** forms partition between 2 chambers: Scala media & posterior scala tympani
    - Thin (dark on high-resolution 3D T2 MR & bright on high-resolution temporal bone CT) transverse line **within each cochlear turn**
      - Between thinner bright T2 (perilymph-filled) scala vestibuli anteriorly & thicker bright (perilymph-filled) scala tympani posteriorly
      - Thickness of scala vestibuli & scala tympani reverses in incomplete partition type II (Mondini deformity)
    - Actually, basilar membrane (with organ of Corti on it) forms posterior wall of scala media, separating it from posteriorly situated scala tympani
      - Extremely thin scala media (endolymph-filled) cannot be distinguished separately on routine 3D T2 IAC protocol clinical MR; therefore, dark line appears to be in between scala vestibuli & scala tympani on 3D T2 images
      - Scala media lies in between scala vestibuli anteriorly & scala tympani posteriorly
  - **Spiral ganglion**
    - Spiral ganglion represents distinct population of primary sensory neurons critical to transmission of sound information to brain
    - Cells located in modiolus, arranged in spiral configuration, paralleling base of spiral lamina
    - Composed of bipolar cells
    - Each cell body emits peripheral axon extending towards organ of Corti & central axon that projects into auditory nerve
    - **Cochlear nerve fibers** traverse modiolus, branching onto **osseous spiral lamina-basal membrane complex,** & then innervate organ of Corti hair cells in posterior wall of scala media
  - **ISS**
    - Thin (dark on MR, bright bone on CT) lines separating basal, middle, & apical turns of cochlea
    - Membranous bony struts continuous with modiolus
    - ISS continuous, has 3 parts, & forms 3 interscalar ridges or notches (R1, R2, R3) along outer margin of cochlea
      - Important in incomplete partition type II (Mondini deformity) evaluation
  - **3 spiral chambers of cochlea**
    - **Scala media** (cochlear duct)
      - Separated from anterior scala vestibuli by **vestibular (Reissner) membrane**
      - Separated from posterior scala tympani by **basilar membrane**
      - Contains **organ of Corti** (hearing apparatus) & **endolymph**

- Smallest of 3 chambers & not identified on routine imaging
- Scala vestibuli
  - Anterior chamber containing **perilymph**
  - Scala vestibuli passes through basilar turn into perilymphatic space of vestibule posteromedially within inner ear
  - Sound vibration of stapes transmitted to **oval window** & into vestibule
  - Sound wave travels through perilymph through scala vestibuli to cochlear apex
  - At apex, scala vestibuli connected to scala tympani by small opening called **helicotrema**
- **Scala tympani**
  - Posterior chamber, containing **perilymph**
  - Allows sound waves to travel back from cochlear apex to **round window**
  - Round window opening covered by round window membrane 2-3 mm long & ~ 1.5 mm wide
  - Scala tympani intended chamber target for cochlear electrode placement through round window or cochleostomy just anterior to it
- **Cochlear nerve canal**
  - Opening to base of cochlea from IAC fundus

- **Vestibule**
  - Contains perilymph sleeve around vestibular membranous labyrinth
  - Utricle & saccule principal vestibular membranous labyrinth components
  - 3 recesses of vestibule: Elliptical recess close to ampullae of superior & lateral SCCs, cochlear recess near cochlea, & spherical recess adjacent to opening of scala vestibuli
  - SCCs arise from superior, posterior, & lateral margins of vestibule
- **SCCs**
  - Each bony SCC contains outer perilymphatic sleeve around semicircular duct
  - Superior SCC: Bony covering called **arcuate eminence**
    - **Subarcuate canal/petromastoid canal**: Inconsistent canal, underneath top of arc of superior SCC
    - Contains subarcuate artery & vein
    - Child < 5 years old = vessels surrounded by dura & CSF
    - Connects mastoid antrum to posterior fossa (infection rarely spread)
    - Usually involutes by 5 years, may persist in adult & mimic fracture
    - Size smaller than or equal to VA
  - Posterior SCC: Meets superior SCC at **crus communis**
    - VA connects to vestibular inner ear at crus communis
  - Lateral SCC: Projects laterally into middle ear cavity
    - Craniocaudal orientation of lateral SCC, facial nerve tympanic segment, & oval window on coronal CT helps simplify temporal bone CT anatomy interpretation
- **ELD & ELS**
  - Found within bony VA
    - VA connects crus communis to fovea (cup-shaped area along posterior temporal bone wall)
    - Axial temporal bone CT: VA width < 1 mm at midpoint, ± < 2 mm at opercular margin (Cincinnati criteria)
    - Transverse oblique reformat (Pöschl view) parallel to superior SCC plane: < 0.8-0.9 mm at midpoint
    - Literature variable; vertical & axial VA width > 1.5 mm at midpoint of labyrinth & operculum most accepted **for large VA** (classic Valvassori criteria)
  - ELD & ELS project from crus communis of vestibule posterolaterally to fovea along posterior wall of inner ear
    - ELD transition to ELS is defined by change in wall cell architecture (not visible with imaging)
    - ELD: Short proximal component connected to crus communis
    - ELS: Longer with both intraosseous & intradural (fovea area) components
- **Inner ear nerves**
  - Cochlear nerve: Afferent hearing fibers from bipolar spiral ganglion, which receives afferent information from organ of Corti, coalesce into cochlear nerve
  - Superior vestibular nerve: Afferent balance fibers from utricle, superior SCC, & lateral SCC coalesce at superior vestibular ganglion into superior vestibular nerve
  - Inferior vestibular nerve: Afferent balance fibers from saccule & posterior SCCs coalesce at inferior vestibular ganglion into inferior vestibular nerve

CLINICAL IMPLICATIONS

Function & Dysfunction

- **Anatomy of hearing**
  - Sound focused & amplified by **external ear**
  - **Tympanic membrane** transmits sound to **ossicles**
  - Movement of stapes → transmission of fluid waves via **oval window** through **vestibule** to cochlear recess
  - Cochlear recess fluid wave transmitted to **perilymph** of **scala vestibuli** (ascending spiral) **of cochlea**
  - Waves transmit along **helicotrema** to **scala tympani of cochlea perilymph** & wave pressure is let out into sinus tympani of retrotympanum through **round window**
  - Wave motion transmitted to **endolymph** of **scala media of cochlea** with **basilar membrane** vibration that stimulates hair cell receptors in **organ of Corti**
  - Hair cell movement generates electronic potentials converted to action potentials in **cochlear nerve**
    - High-frequency sounds converted at cochlear base
    - Low-frequency sounds converted at cochlear apex

EMBRYOLOGY

Embryologic Events

- Cochlea development between 3rd-8th fetal weeks
- Otic placode (3rd week) invaginates to becomes otic pit (4th week)
- Otic pit becomes otocyst (otic vesicle) at 5th
- Otocyst migrates to inner ear location during 5th
- Cochlear duct (scala media) forms (6th week)
- 2 1/2 turn cochlea forms (by end of 8th week)
- Fetus "hears" by 24th week when organ of Corti matures
- Inner ear forms separate from external & middle ear
- External auditory canal atresia usually has normal inner ear
- Injury to organ of Corti may occur long after cochlear formation: Profound sensorineural hearing loss patients often have normal cochlea on CT/MR

AXIAL 3D T2 MR

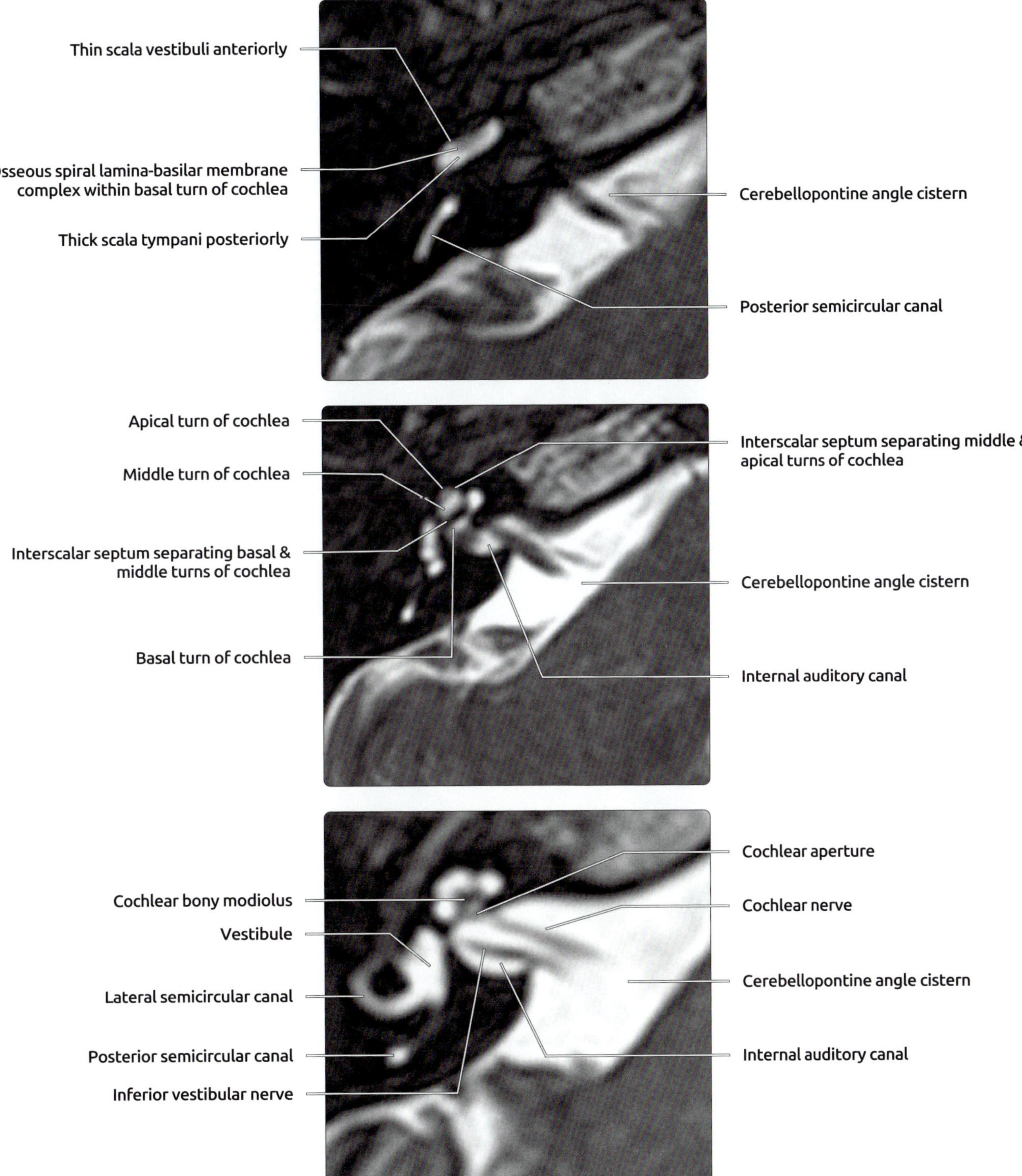

(Top) *First of 3 axial 3D T2 MR images from inferior to superior of the internal auditory canal (IAC) demonstrates the osseous spiral lamina-basilar membrane complex (OSL-BMC) seen within each cochlear turn & the interscalar septum (ISS) seen separating different cochlear turns. It also shows the thin, dark transverse line of the OSL-BMC between the thinner bright T2 (perilymph-filled) scala vestibuli anteriorly & thicker bright (perilymph-filled) scala tympani posteriorly within the basal turn of the cochlea. The basilar membrane (with the organ of Corti on it) forms the posterior wall of scala media, separating it from the posteriorly situated scala tympani. Extremely thin scala media (endolymph-filled) cannot be distinguished separately on routine 3D T2 IAC protocol clinical MR imaging; therefore, the dark line appears to be in between the scala vestibuli & scala tympani on 3D T2 MR.* **(Middle)** *Image shows the thin, dark lines of the ISS between the basal & middle turns of the cochlea & also between the middle & apical turns. The ISS is formed by membranous bony struts continuous with the modiolus.* **(Bottom)** *Third image shows cochlear aperture & the dark bony modiolus.*

GRAPHICS

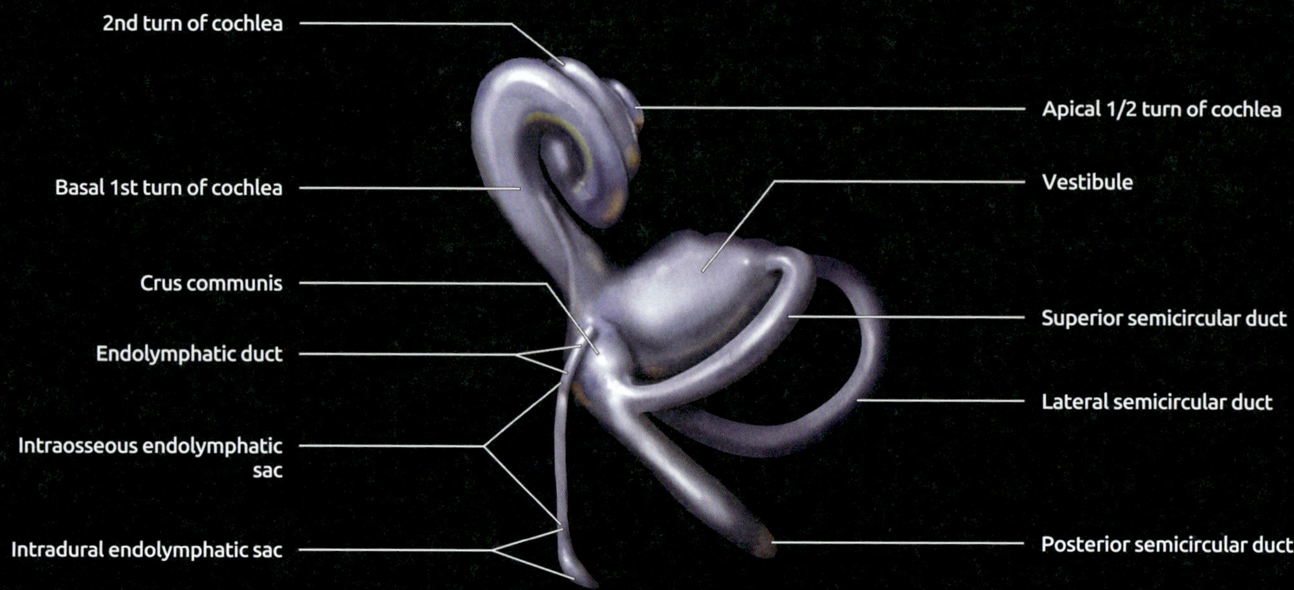

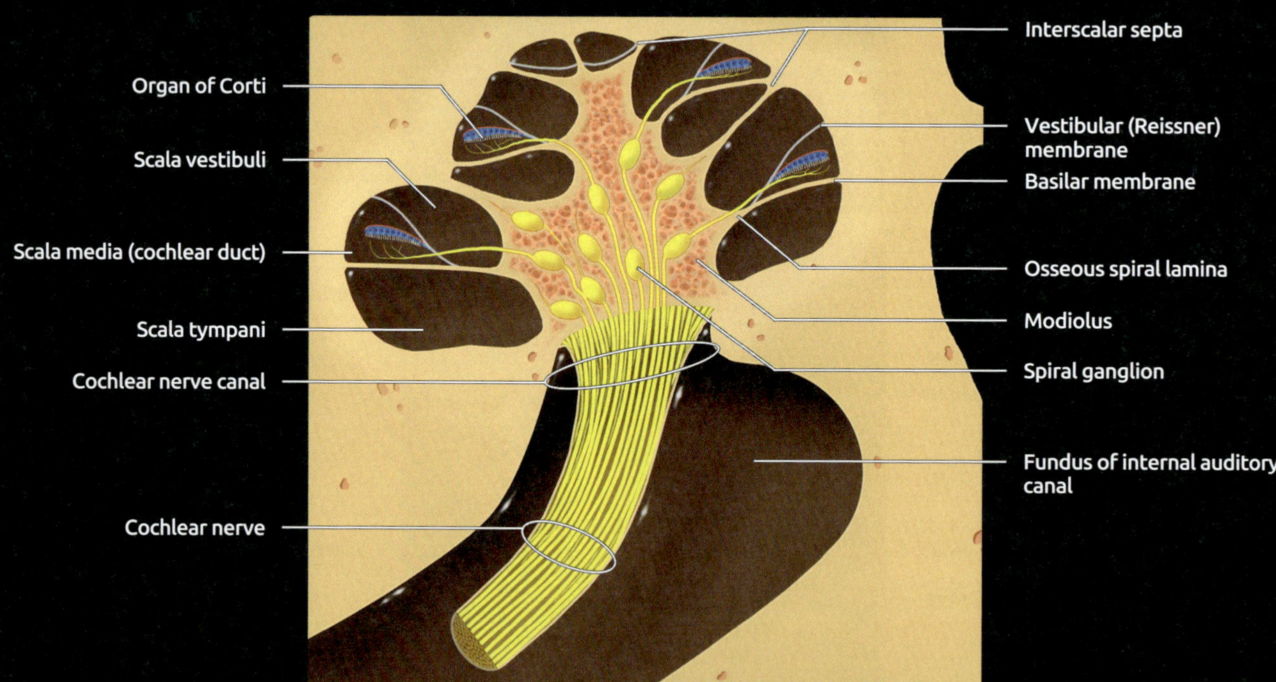

(Top) *Graphic shows fluid spaces of the inner ear viewed from above. The endolymph-filled structures include scala media of the cochlea, the vestibular utricle & saccule, semicircular ducts, & the endolymphatic duct & sac. The perilymph-filled areas are the scala tympani & scala vestibuli of the cochlea surrounding the utricle & saccule within the vestibule between semicircular ducts & the walls of the semicircular canals & surrounding the endolymphatic duct within the vestibular aqueduct (VA). Notice that the crus communis is the site of endolymphatic duct entry into the more central membranous labyrinth.* **(Bottom)** *Axial graphic of the cochlea shows the 3 scalar chambers: Scala media, scala vestibuli, & scala tympani. Note that the bipolar cell bodies of the spiral ganglia within the modiolus send distal fibers to the organ of Corti & proximal fibers into the cochlear nerve. The cochlear nerve passes through the cochlear nerve canal into the fundus of the IAC.*

AXIAL 3D T2 MR

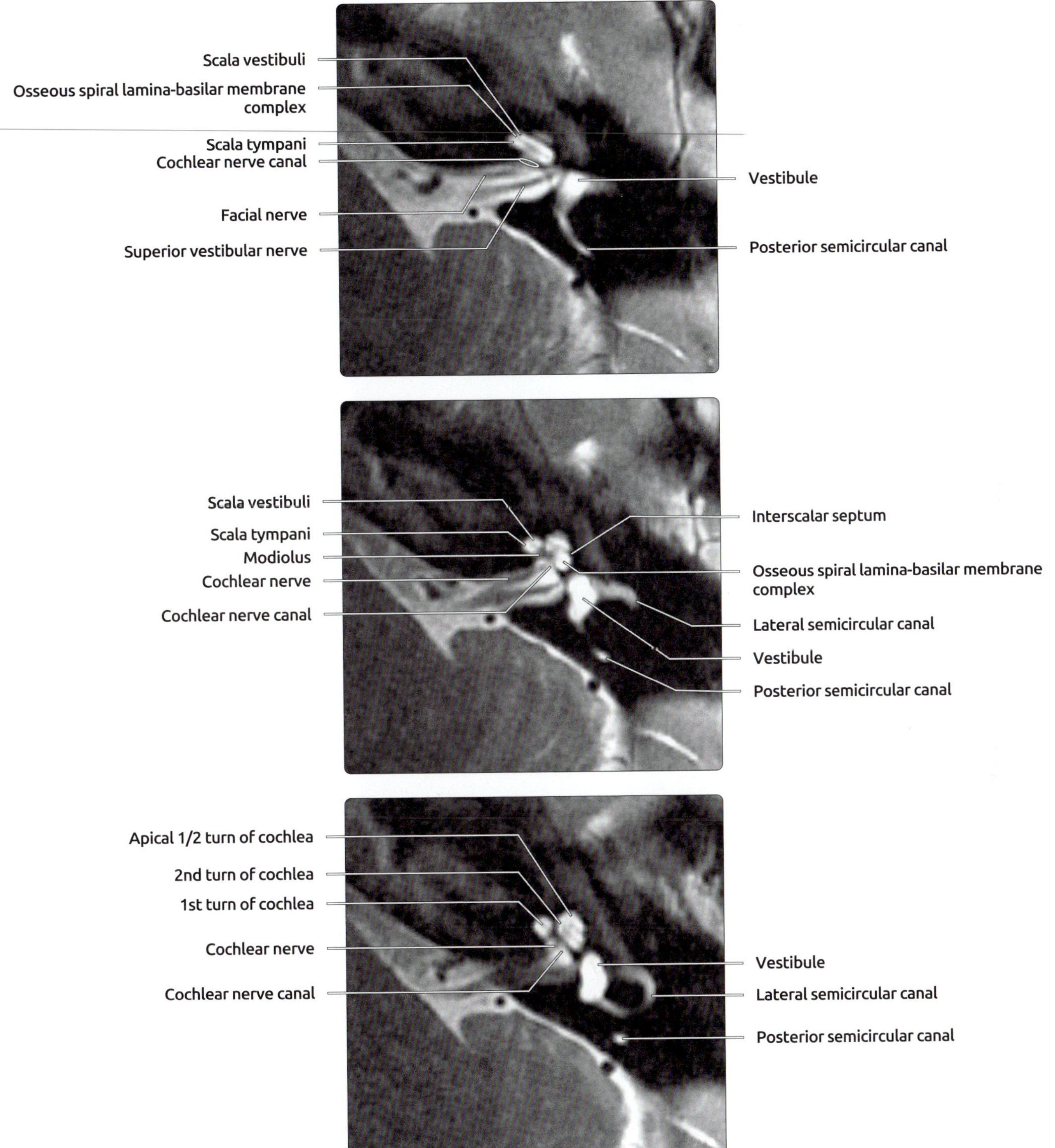

(Top) *First of 3 axial T2 MR images of the inner ear from superior to inferior reveals a high-signal membranous labyrinth within the low-signal bony labyrinth. The cochlea is divided by osseous spiral lamina into an anterior scala vestibuli & posterior scala tympani. Note that the scala vestibuli & tympani have equal transverse dimensions.* **(Middle)** *In this image through the midcochlea, the cochlear nerve is visible in the anteroinferior IAC. The cochlear nerve exits the fundus of the IAC to enter the cochlea through the CSF-filled cochlear nerve canal. The modiolus is visible as an intermediate-intensity structure at the cochlear base.* **(Bottom)** *The 1st & 2nd turns & the apical 1/2 turn of the cochlea are all visible on this image. Also note the cochlear nerve in the cochlear nerve canal on its way to the modiolus.*

LONGITUDINAL (STENVER) & TRANSVERSE (PÖSCHL) OBLIQUE CT REFORMATIONS

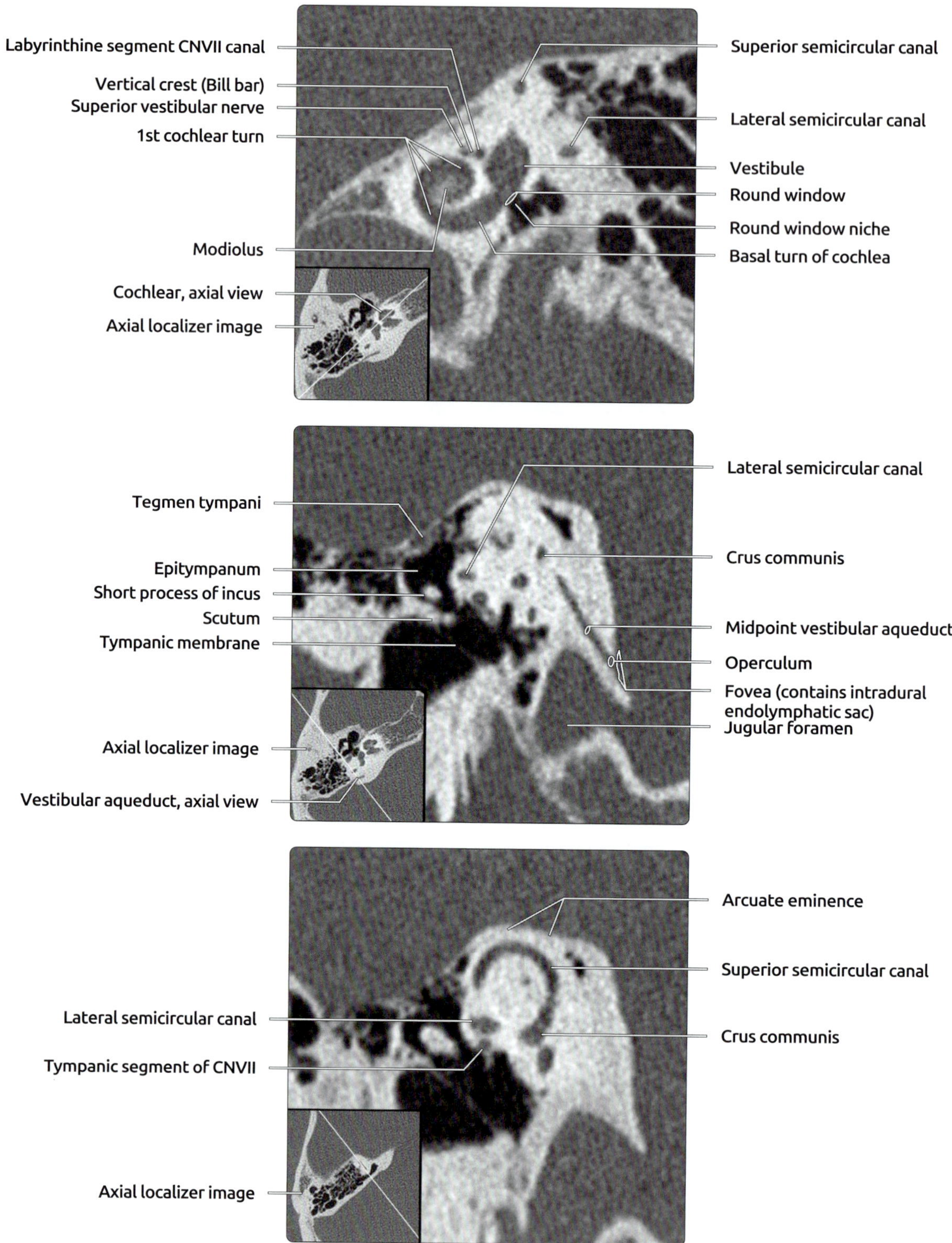

(Top) *Longitudinal oblique (Stenver) reformatted bone CT profiles the entire 1st turn of the cochlea. In the notch between the vestibule & the apical aspect of the 1st cochlear turn, note the superior vestibular nerve canal & the labyrinthine segment of the facial nerve (CNVII) canal. Such a view is helpful in evaluating cochlear implants.* **(Middle)** *Transverse oblique (Pöschl) bone CT of the right ear profiles the bony VA as it progresses from the fovea (bony cup in the posterior wall where the intradural endolymphatic sac resides) toward the crus communis of the more central inner ear. Normal VA measurements are < 1 mm at the midpoint & < 2 mm at the operculum.* **(Bottom)** *Transverse oblique (Pöschl) bone CT (1 mm) reformat created along the line of the superior semicircular canal demonstrates the entire span of this canal with the bony ridge above it (arcuate eminence). This view can be very helpful in delineating the extent of superior semicircular canal dehiscence when present.*

AXIAL BONE CT

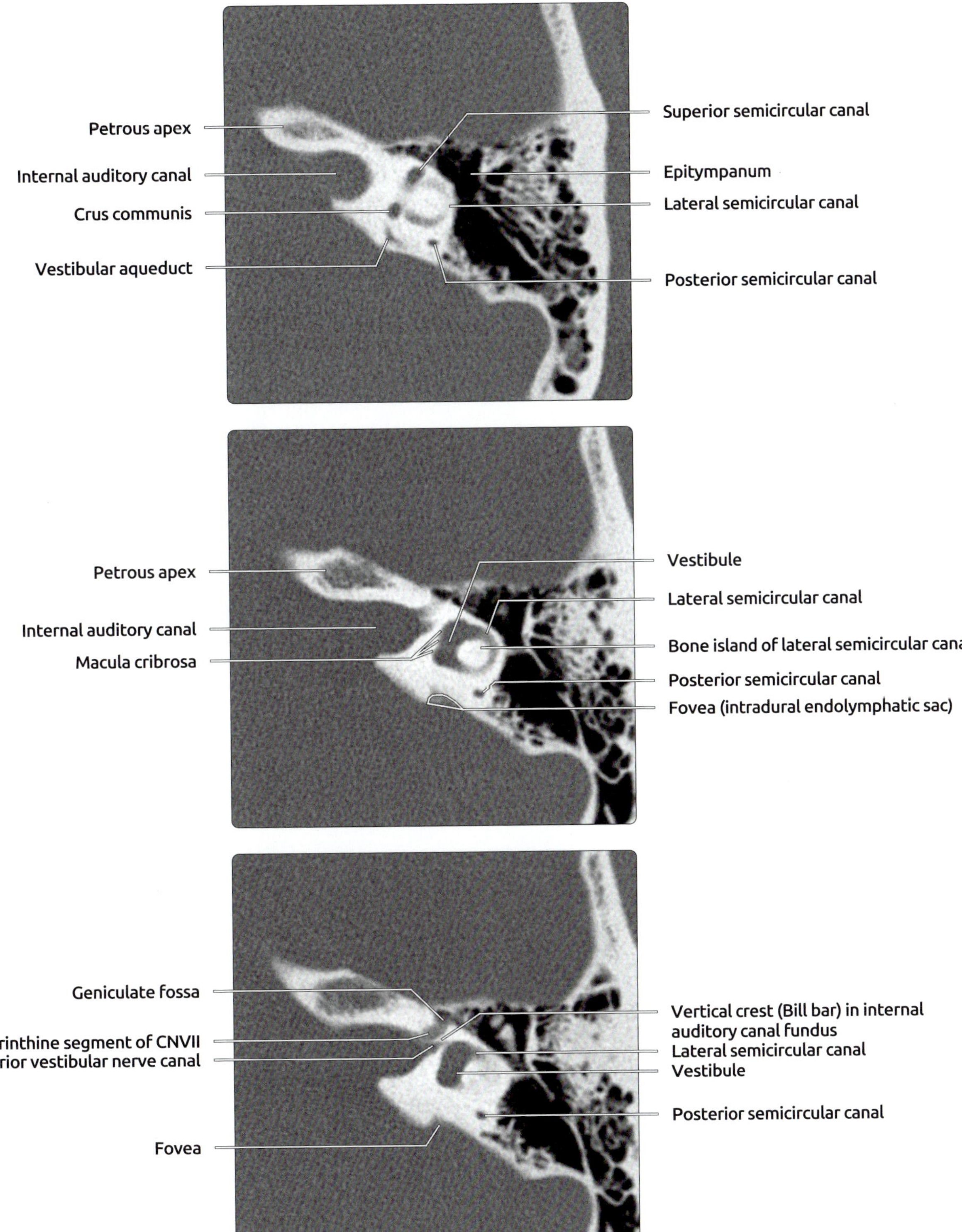

(Top) *Series of 6 axial CT images of the left temporal bone is presented from superior to inferior. At the level of lateral semicircular canal, the bony VA is seen turning anteriorly to connect with the more central inner ear at the crus communis.* **(Middle)** *At the level of the lateral semicircular canal, the fovea of the bony VA along the posterior wall of the temporal bone houses the intradural endolymphatic sac. Remember that bone CT permits visualization of the bony labyrinth, whereas MR shows the membranous labyrinth structures.* **(Bottom)** *Axial bone CT demonstrates the superior vestibular nerve canal as it pierces the macula cribrosa of the vestibule. Note that anterior to the superior nerve vestibular canal, the vertical crest in the IAC fundus & the labyrinthine segment of CNVII are visible. This anatomic distinction is the key to differentiate facial nerve schwannoma & superior vestibular nerve schwannoma, an important surgical distinction.*

AXIAL BONE CT

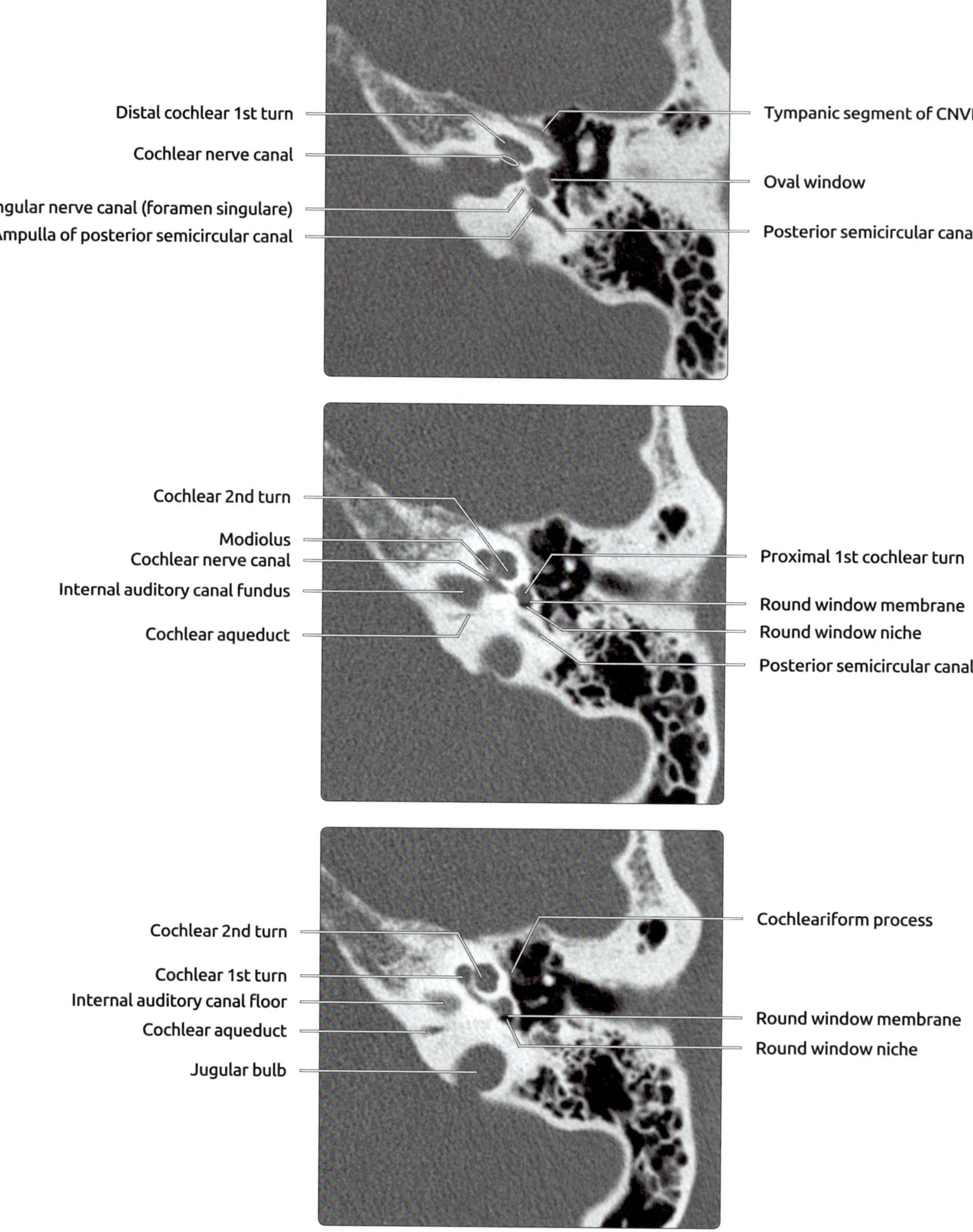

(Top) *Axial bone CT through the distal 1st turn of the cochlea shows the cochlear nerve canal connecting IAC fundus to the cochlea. A singular nerve canal is visible leaving the posterior wall of the IAC fundus & connecting to the ampulla of the posterior semicircular canal. It contains a singular nerve (posterior ampullary nerve), a branch of inferior vestibular nerve to the posterior semicircular canal. The posterior petrous bony wall is removed up to a singular canal only during retrosigmoid approach for IAC vestibular schwannoma surgery to prevent labyrinthine fenestration.* **(Middle)** *Axial bone CT through round window shows proximal cochlear aqueduct (CA) on its way to connect to proximal 1st turn of cochlea. CA contains perilymph & is a vestigial structure. CA connects the subarachnoid space with scala tympani of cochlea.* **(Bottom)** *Axial bone CT along the floor of IAC shows the entire proximal 1/2 of the 1st turn of cochlea. Round window membrane is visible between the 1st turn of the cochlea & the air-filled round window niche. Lower CA is seen along the posterior wall of the temporal bone inferior to IAC & anteromedial to the jugular bulb at the roof of pars nervosa of jugular foramen.*

ANATOMIC-PATHOLOGIC CORRELATION

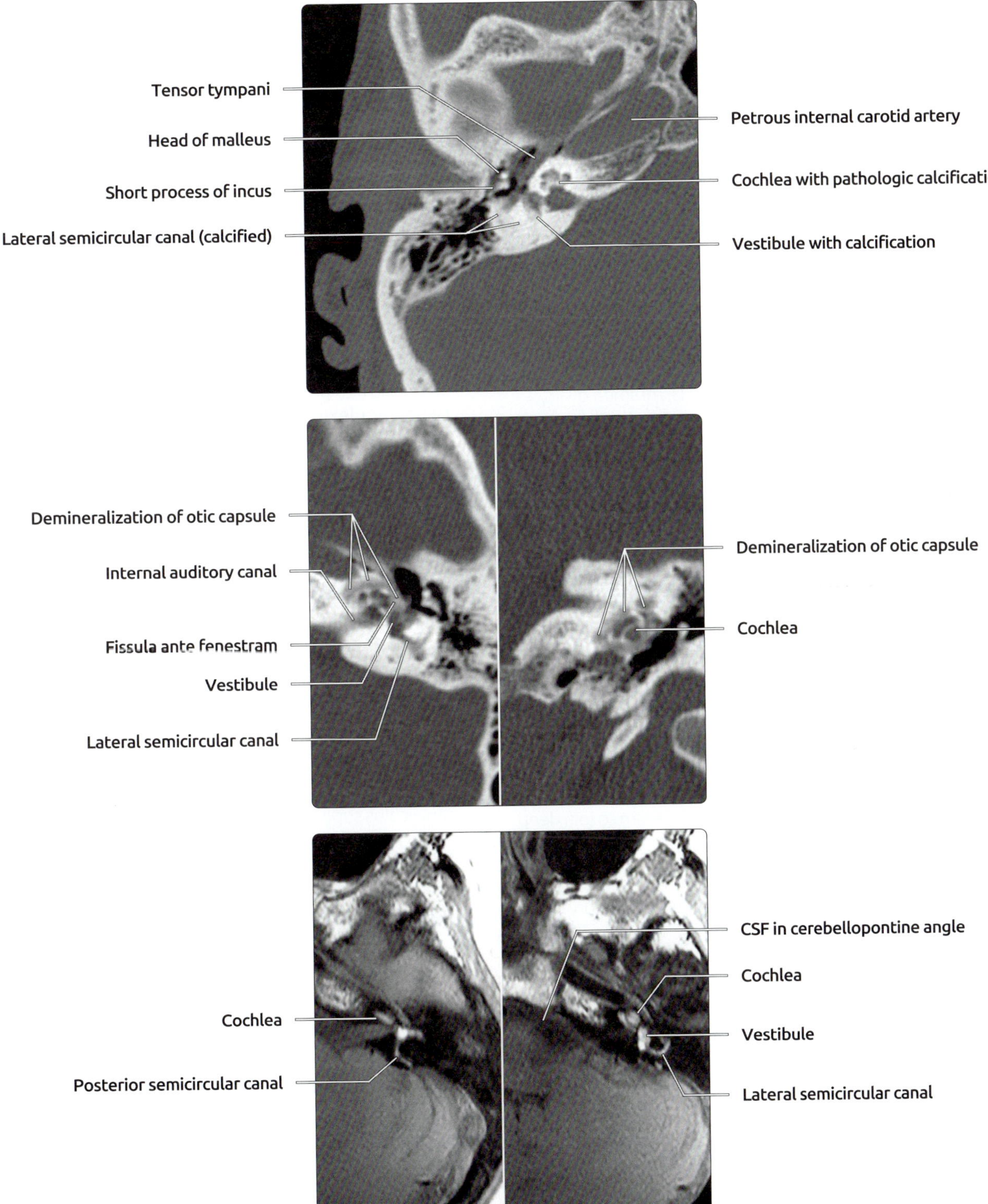

(Top) *Axial high-resolution CT scan through the temporal bone with labyrinthitis ossificans in a patient with a previous history of meningitis & subsequent hearing loss demonstrates relative hyperdensity in the cochlea, vestibule, & semicircular canals, compatible with calcification. Severe infection in the inner ear can result in granulation tissue, subsequent fibrosis, & ultimately progressive ossification & profound hearing loss.* **(Middle)** *Axial and coronal CT images of retrofenestral otosclerosis in a 50-year-old woman with bilateral mixed hearing loss shows fulminant fenestral & retrofenestral otosclerosis with extensive demineralization of the otic capsule. The architecture of inner ear compartments is preserved.* **(Bottom)** *Contiguous axial T1-weighted images through the left temporal bone in a patient with sudden loss of hearing in the left ear demonstrates diffuse hyperintensity throughout the membranous labyrinth. The signal characteristics of T1 hyperintensity in the absence of contrast & the abrupt onset of symptoms are compatible with labyrinthine hemorrhage. In general, fluid within the membranous labyrinth should follow CSF signal on all sequences.*

Minor Fissures and Sutures Around Temporal Bone

TERMINOLOGY

Abbreviations

- Greater superficial petrosal nerve (GSPN); facial nerve (FN)

IMAGING ANATOMY

Overview

- **Intrinsic channels**: Subarcuate canal, GSPN hiatus, singular canal, cochlear cleft, vestibular aqueduct, cochlear aqueduct, superior & inferior caroticotympanic nerve canals, inferior tympanic canaliculus, mastoid canaliculus, anterior & posterior canaliculi of chorda tympani
- **Intrinsic sutures (fissures)**: Petrotympanic (Glaserian) fissure, petrosquamous suture, tympanosquamous suture, tympanomastoid suture
- **Extrinsic sutures (fissures)**: Occipitomastoid suture, petrooccipital (petroclival) fissure, sphenopetrosal suture, sphenosquamosal suture
- **Extrinsic channels**: Eustachian tube (ET), foramen ovale, foramen spinosum, foramen lacerum, vidian canal, foramen of Vesalius, canaliculus innominatus

Subarcuate (Petromastoid) Canal

- Inconsistent canal underneath top of arc of superior semicircular canal (SCC)
- Contains subarcuate artery & vein
- Child < 5 years old, vessels surrounded by dura & CSF
- Connects mastoid antrum to posterior fossa (infection rarely spreads)
- Involutes by 5 years, may persist in adult & mimic fracture
- Size ≤ vestibular aqueduct

Greater Superficial Petrosal Nerve Hiatus

- Extends anteromedially from FN anterior genu
- GSPN then travels in middle cranial fossa (MCF) floor underneath temporal lobe between dura mater layers
- Then anteromedially towards foramen lacerum to join deep petrosal nerve & form vidian nerve

Singular Canal (Foramen Singulare)

- Extends from posteroinferior wall of internal auditory canal (IAC) fundus to ampulla of posterior SCC
- Contains singular nerve (posterior ampullary nerve), which is branch of inferior vestibular nerve to posterior SCC
- Important surgical landmark during retrosigmoid approach for IAC vestibular schwannoma surgery
  - Posterior IAC bony wall removed up to singular canal only to prevent labyrinthine fenestration

Cochlear Cleft

- Bilateral > unilateral developmental curvilinear C-shaped thin lucency adjacent to cochlea
  - Due to nonosseous otic capsule space
- Do not mistake for nodular lucency of otospongiosis in adjacent **fissula ante fenestram** (FAF)
  - FAF located immediately anterior to vestibule/oval window & posteromedial to processus cochleariformis

Vestibular Aqueduct

- Connects vestibule to posterior surface of petrous bone
- Connects crus communis (meeting point of posterior & superior SCC) to fovea (cup-shaped area along posterior temporal bone wall)
- Contains endolymphatic duct & endolymphatic sac distally

Cochlear Aqueduct

- Small canal in bony labyrinth harboring **perilymphatic** (periotic) duct; drains perilymph into posterior cranial fossa subarachnoid space CSF
- Seen parallel & inferior to IAC
- Arises from scala tympani at basal turn of cochlea & runs through otic capsule & petrous apex; difficult to see on CT
- Funnel-shaped inferomedial end opens at pyramidal fossa in roof of pars nervosa of jugular foramen (JF); seen on CT
- **Pyramidal fossa** lies superior to petrosal fossula (small depression on undersurface of petrous bone)

Superior & Inferior Caroticotympanic Nerve Canals

- Nerves arising from **carotid plexus** around internal carotid artery (ICA) to provide **sympathetic** nerve supply for **tympanic plexus** on middle ear (ME) medial wall cochlear promontory surface
- Seen extending laterally from ICA to ME cavity

Inferior Tympanic Canaliculus

- Seen extending laterally from **pars nervosa** of JF **between** petrous **ICA & internal jugular vein** (IJV)
- Contains **Jacobson nerve** (glossopharyngeal nerve, **CNIX** branch) & inferior tympanic artery
- Connects to ME to provide **parasympathetic** supply (from medullary **inferior salivatory nucleus**) to **tympanic plexus** over surface of cochlear promontory
- **Petrosal fossula** in pars nervosa of JF lies in ridge between JF & external opening of carotid canal
- Petrosal fossula houses inferior ganglion (petrosal ganglion) of glossopharyngeal nerve (where Jacobson nerve originates) & gives rise to inferior tympanic canaliculus superiorly

Mastoid Canaliculus

- Seen extending laterally from lateral aspect of **pars vascularis** of JF near **IJV**
- Contains **Arnold nerve** (auricular branch of vagus [**CNX**])
- First connects to descending mastoid FN canal several millimeters above stylomastoid foramen
- Then courses toward tympanomastoid fissure at posterior bony wall of external auditory canal (EAC) laterally

Anterior & Posterior Canaliculi of Chorda Tympani Nerve & Petrotympanic (Glaserian) Fissure

- Chorda tympani nerve (CTN) originates from FN descending mastoid segment; ascends through posterior canaliculus of CTN in posterior wall of ME
- Courses in ME cavity from posterior to anterior in substance of tympanic membrane between mucous & fibrous layers
- Then medial to upper aspect of handle (manubrium) of malleus, between it & long process of incus
- Then travels through anterior canaliculus of CTN & exits temporal bone into masticator space (MS) through petrotympanic fissure (Glaserian fissure)
  - Posteromedial to TMJ
- In MS, CTN joins lingual nerve (mandibular nerve, trigeminal nerve CNV3 branch) 2 cm below skull base

Petrosquamous Suture

- Small defect in tegmen tympani at top of **Körner septum** (KS) (petrosquamous lamina) on coronal CT
- Difficult to see on axial CT; may see as cleft oriented anteromedially from TMJ glenoid fossa
- KS: Continuation & persistence of petrosquamous suture
- KS: Bony lamina dividing mastoid cavity at mastoid antrum level into mastoid air cells pneumatizing superficial squamosal portion & deeper petrosal portion

Tympanosquamous Suture

- Anterior to bony EAC, continues medially into petrotympanic & petrosquamous sutures

Tympanomastoid Suture

- Posterior to bony EAC, inconstant
- Auricular branch of vagus (CNX) (**Arnold nerve**) passes through mastoid canaliculus, connects to descending FN canal, & emerges through tympanomastoid fissure
- Arnold nerve supplies part of tympanic membrane & EAC
- Arnold nerve cough reflex when mechanically stimulating ear with finger or ear bud

Occipitomastoid Suture

- Can be asymmetric or bifid and mimic fracture
- Anterior continuation of suture may give false appearance of temporal bone fracture fragment
- Scrolling through contiguous images helps to identify fragment as normal part of occipital bone rather than temporal bone fracture fragment

Petrooccipital (Petroclival) Fissure

- Fissure/synchondrosis/suture between petrous temporal bone laterally & occipital bone part of clivus medially
- Contains inferior petrosal sinus on its way to pars nervosa of JF & then connects to IJV in pars vascularis of JF
- Common site of origin of skull base chondrosarcoma

Sphenopetrosal Suture

- Between greater wing of sphenoid (GWS) & petrous apex
- Just posteromedial to foramen ovale on axial CT
- Lesser petrosal nerve occasionally exits floor of MCF through sphenopetrosal fissure

Sphenosquamosal Suture

- Between GWS & squamous temporal bone
- Just lateral to foramen spinosum on axial CT

Eustachian Tube

- Just posterolateral to sphenopetrosal suture on axial CT
- Do not confuse with suture when ET not air filled

Foramen Ovale

- Axial CT: Look for **ladies shoe** appearance of **foramen ovale** (front sole of shoe) **&** foramen **spinosum** (pointed heel of shoe) in GWS just anterolateral to petrous ICA canal
- Transmits mandibular nerve (CNV3, trigeminal nerve branch), accessory meningeal artery, emissary veins, lesser petrosal nerve, & sometimes nervus spinosus [meningeal branch from mandibular nerve (CNV3) main trunk]

Foramen Spinosum

- In GWS, posterolateral to foramen ovale, seen lateral to horizontal petrous ICA canal
- Transmits middle meningeal artery (MMA), middle meningeal vein, & nervus spinosus

Foramen Lacerum

- Cartilage-filled gap between sphenoid & temporal bones
- Not a foramen located in a single bone
- Floor anteroinferomedial to horizontal petrous ICA canal

Vidian (Pterygoid) Canal

- In sphenoid bone body/medial pterygoid junction
- Connects foramen lacerum posteriorly to pterygopalatine fossa (PPF) anteriorly
- Transmits vidian nerve, artery, & vein
- **Vidian nerve**: Superior salivatory nucleus (SSN) in pons → parasympathetic root through nervus intermedius of Wrisberg (NIW) → FN → GSPN (+ deep petrosal nerve from ICA sympathetic plexus) → **vidian nerve** → pterygopalatine ganglion in PPF → lacrimal gland & nasal glands

Foramen of Vesalius (Sphenoidal Emissary Foramen)

- Inconsistent canal in GWS, seen anterior to foramen ovale & lateral to vidian canal
- Transmits emissary vein connecting cavernous sinus (CS) superiorly near foramen rotundum to MS pterygoid venous plexus inferiorly
- Infection may spread from upper face/orbit/sinus to CS

Canaliculus Innominatus (Foramen Petrosum)

- a.k.a. foramen of Arnold (do not mistake this synonym for mastoid canaliculus with Arnold nerve)
- Inconsistent canal in GWS, seen in between & medial to foramen spinosum & foramen ovale
- Exit channel for **lesser petrosal nerve** from MCF (usually exits via foramen ovale)

Tympanic Plexus & Lesser Petrosal Nerve

- **Tympanic plexus**: Parasympathetic Jacobson nerve & sympathetic superior & inferior caroticotympanic nerves
  - Supplies mucosa of ME, ET, & mastoid air cells
  - **Branch to GSPN** via **opening anterior to oval window**
- **LPN**: Branch of **tympanic plexus** [continuation of tympanic branch (Jacobson nerve) of **glossopharyngeal nerve**]
  - Parasympathetic supply from medullary **inferior salivatory nucleus** to **otic ganglion (OG)**
  - LPN also receives parasympathetic contribution from pontine SSN via NIW/FN anterior genu-GSPN (CNVII branch) & Arnold nerve (CNX branch)
- LPN pass through **small canal** in petrous temporal bone **just below semicanal for tensor tympani**
- LPN runs past & receives **connecting branch from geniculate ganglion of FN**
- LPN exits petrous temporal bone anterior aspect via **small opening lateral to GSPN hiatus** to enter MCF floor
- LPN in **MCF floor** located between 2 layers of dura mater In between petrous branch of MMA medially & superior tympanic artery laterally
- LPN then passes forward almost parallel to GSPN & **exits MCF** skull base (GWS) to **join OG** via **foramen ovale** (or, occasionally, via **CI**, or via **sphenopetrosal fissure**)
  - In contrast, GSPN in MCF floor turns anteromedially toward foramen lacerum to form vidian nerve
- OG postganglionic secretomotor fibers supply **parotid gland** after joining **auriculotemporal nerve** (CNV3 branch)

AXIAL & CORONAL BONE CT

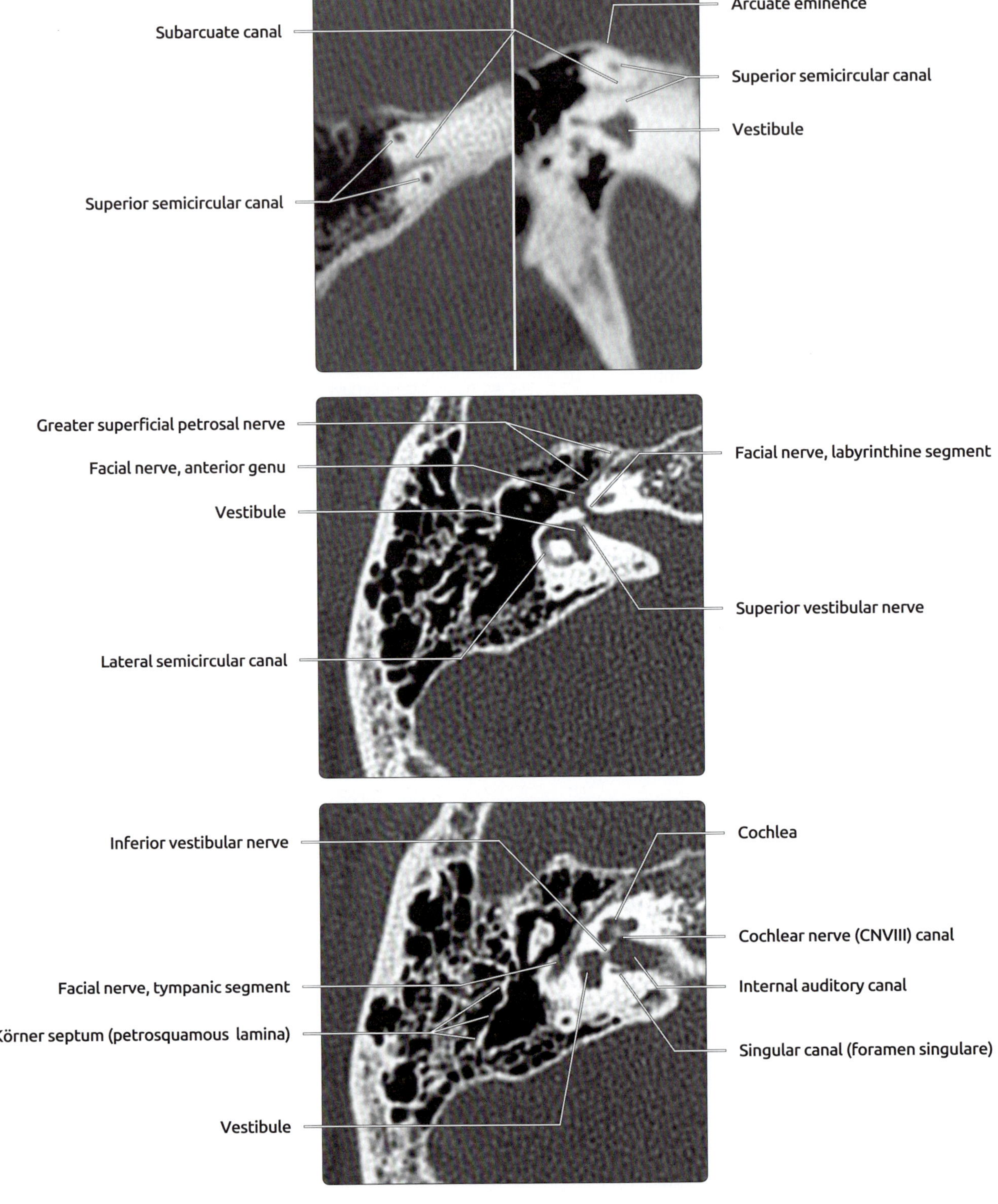

(Top) *Axial & coronal bone CT images show the subarcuate canal (petromastoid canal), an inconsistent canal underneath the top of the arc of the superior semicircular canal (SCC). The roof of the superior SCC is known as arcuate eminence, hence the name. Subarcuate canal connects mastoid antrum to posterior fossa (with infection rarely spread) & contains subarcuate artery & vein. Its size is smaller than or equal to the vestibular aqueduct. This canal & many of the other tiny fissures, foramina, & sutures in & around the temporal bone can be fracture mimics on CT scan.* **(Middle)** *First of 6 axial bone CT images from top to bottom shows the hiatus for greater superficial petrosal nerve (GSPN) in petrous temporal bone. GSPN then travels in middle cranial fossa floor underneath temporal lobe between dura mater layers, on its way towards foramen lacerum to join deep petrosal nerve & form vidian nerve. Also note the superior vestibular nerve.* **(Bottom)** *The cochlear, inferior vestibular & singular nerve (posterior ampullary nerve) canals, & Körner septum are shown. Singular canal extends from posteroinferior wall of internal auditory canal (IAC) fundus to posterior SCC ampulla.*

CORONAL & AXIAL BONE CT

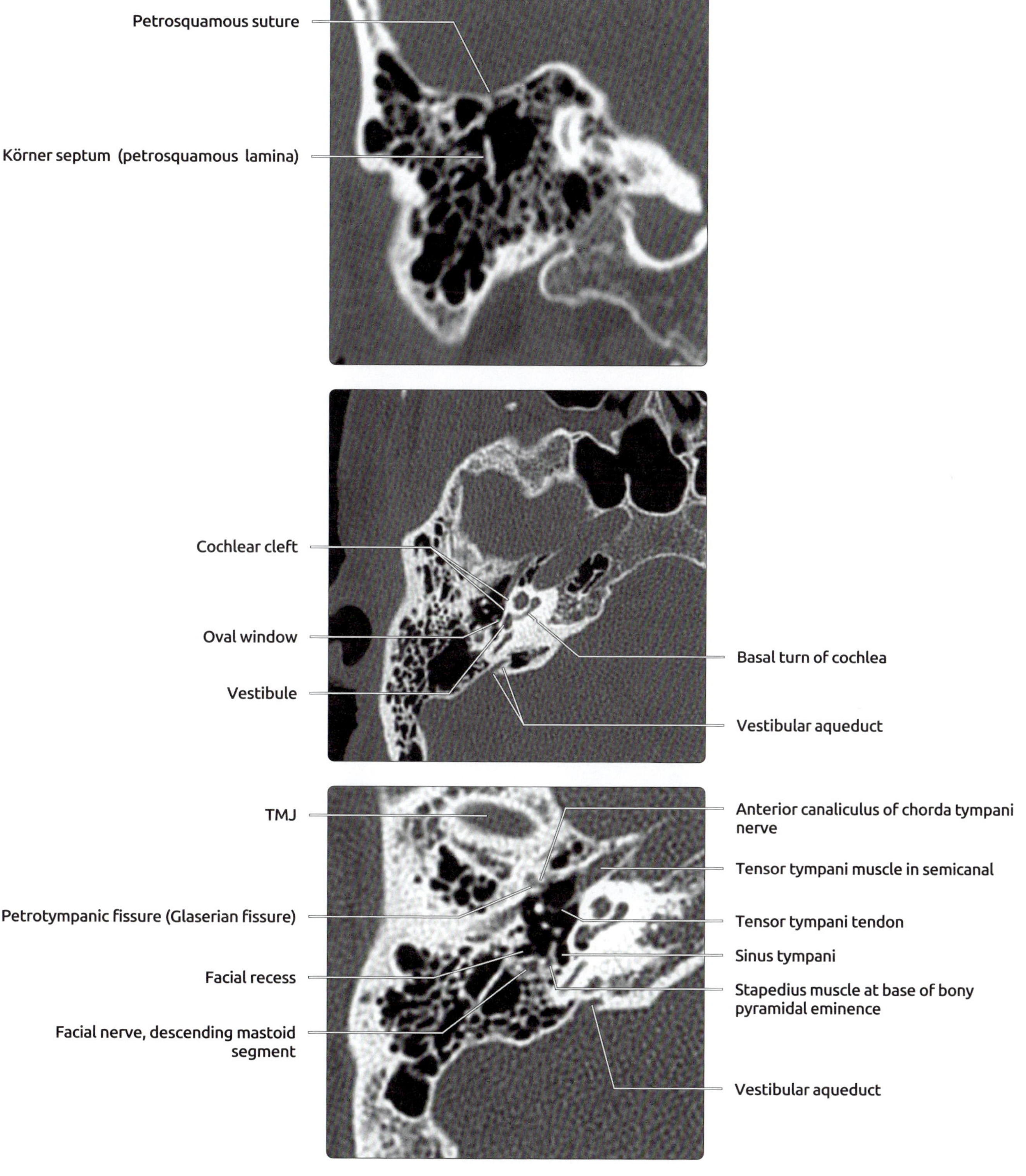

(Top) *Coronal bone CT shows the Körner septum (petrosquamous lamina) & the petrosquamous suture, which is a small defect in tegmen tympani at the top of the Körner septum on coronal CT; it is difficult to see on axial CT & may be seen as a cleft oriented anteromedially from the TMJ glenoid fossa. The Körner septum (petrosquamous lamina) represents the continuation & persistence of the petrosquamous suture.* **(Middle)** *Third axial bone CT shows the incidental anatomic variant of the cochlear cleft. Do not mistake this for fenestral otospongiosis, which will be seen as subtle nodular lucency at the fissula ante fenestram (in the bone anterior to the oval window/vestibule). Cochlear clefts are bilateral > unilateral, developmental, curvilinear C-shaped thin lucencies due to nonosseous otic capsule space adjacent to the cochlea. Also note the vestibular aqueduct extending from the vestibule to the posterior surface of the petrous temporal bone. It contains endolymphatic duct & larger endolymphatic sac at its end.* **(Bottom)** *Fourth axial bone CT shows the anterior canaliculus of chorda tympani & petrotympanic fissure (Glaserian fissure) posteromedial to the TMJ.*

AXIAL BONE CT & PHOTON-COUNTING DETECTOR CT

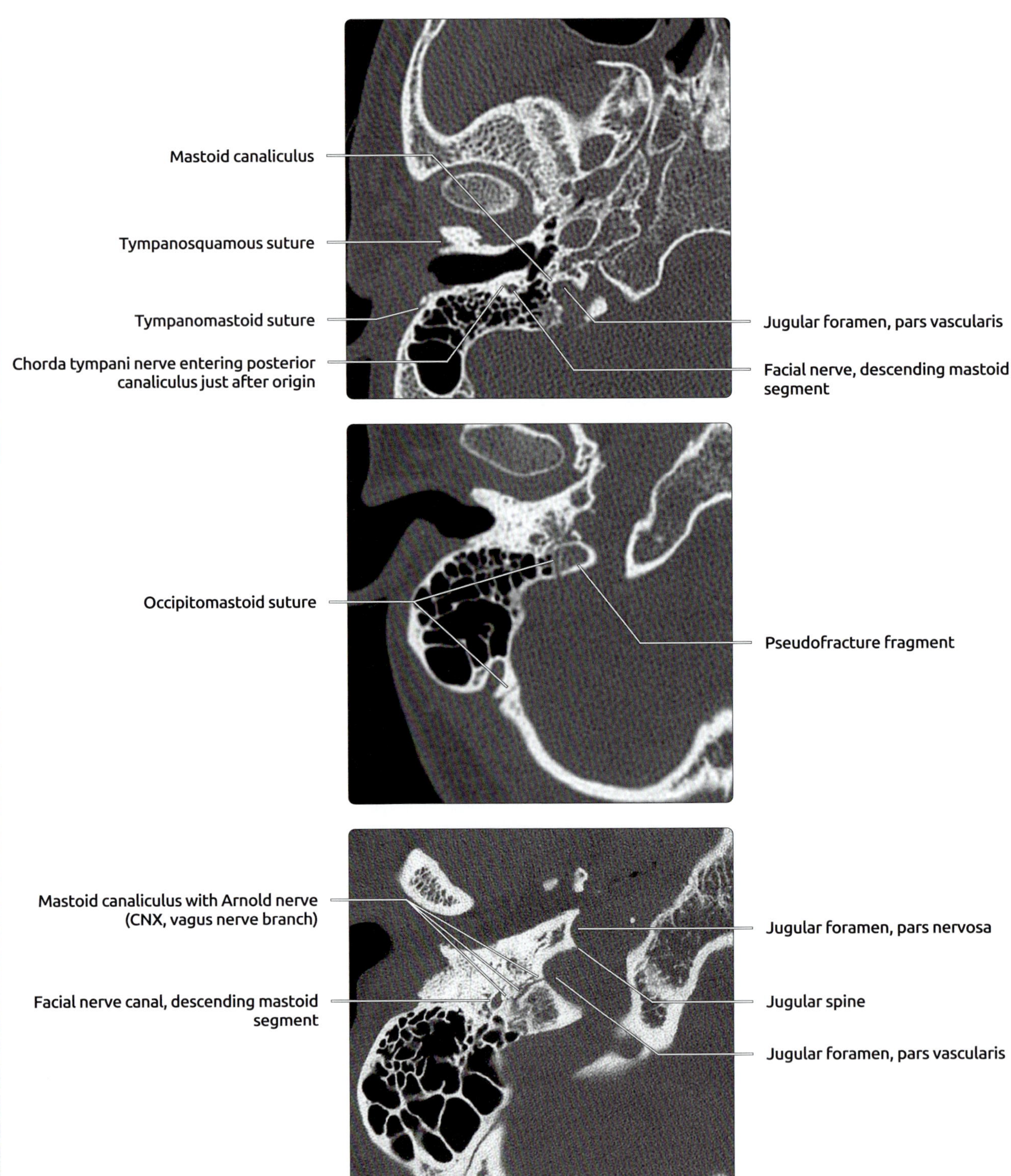

(Top) *Fifth axial bone CT shows the tympanosquamous & tympanomastoid sutures lying along the anterior & posterior bony walls of the external auditory canal (EAC), respectively. The tympanosquamous suture continues medially into the petrotympanic & petrosquamous sutures. An auricular branch of the vagus nerve (Arnold nerve) passes through the mastoid canaliculus, connects to the mastoid facial nerve canal, & emerges through the tympanomastoid fissure (suture). Arnold nerve supplies part of the tympanic membrane & EAC & causes the Arnold nerve cough reflex when mechanically stimulating the ear.* **(Middle)** *Final axial bone CT shows anterior continuation of the occipitomastoid suture, which may mimic a temporal bone fracture fragment. Scrolling through images identifies a fragment as normal occipital bone. Occipitomastoid suture can be asymmetric/bifid & mimic fracture.* **(Bottom)** *Axial photon-counting detector CT in another patient shows the mastoid canaliculus with Arnold nerve originating from the lateral aspect of pars vascularis of right jugular foramen & connecting laterally to the descending mastoid segment facial nerve canal on its way towards the tympanomastoid suture.*

JACOBSON, ARNOLD, & CAROTICOTYMPANIC NERVES: AXIAL GRAPHIC & BONE CT

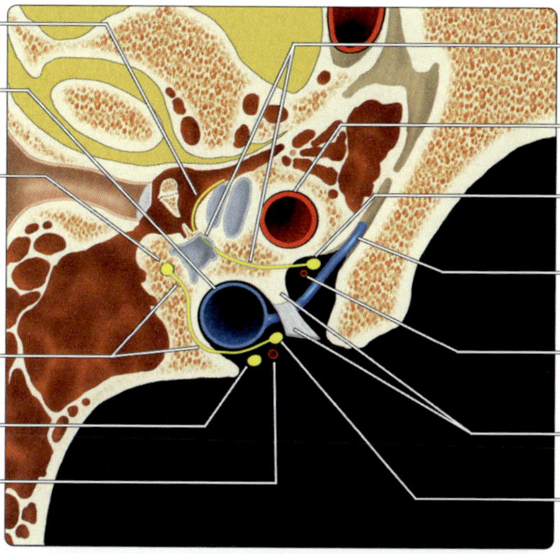

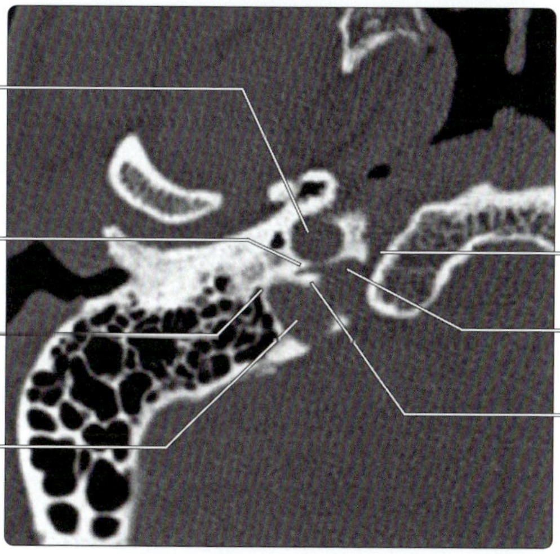

Tympanic plexus on cochlear promontory
Jugular bulb
Facial nerve, descending mastoid segment
Mastoid canaliculus with Arnold nerve (CNX, vagus nerve branch)
Spinal accessory nerve (CNXI)
Occipital artery, meningeal branch
Inferior tympanic canaliculus with Jacobson nerve (CNIX, glossopharyngeal nerve branch)
Internal carotid artery
Glossopharyngeal nerve (CNIX) in pars nervosa of jugular foramen
Inferior petrosal sinus in petrooccipital (petroclival) fissure
Ascending pharyngeal artery, meningeal branch
Jugular spine & fibrous septum
Vagus nerve (CNX) in pars vascularis of jugular foramen

Internal carotid artery
Inferior tympanic canaliculus with Jacobson nerve (CNIX branch)
Mastoid canaliculus with Arnold nerve (CNX branch)
Pars vascularis of jugular foramen with jugular bulb, CNX, & CNXI
Petrooccipital (petroclival) fissure with inferior petrosal sinus
Pars nervosa of jugular foramen with inferior petrosal sinus & CNIX
Jugular spine

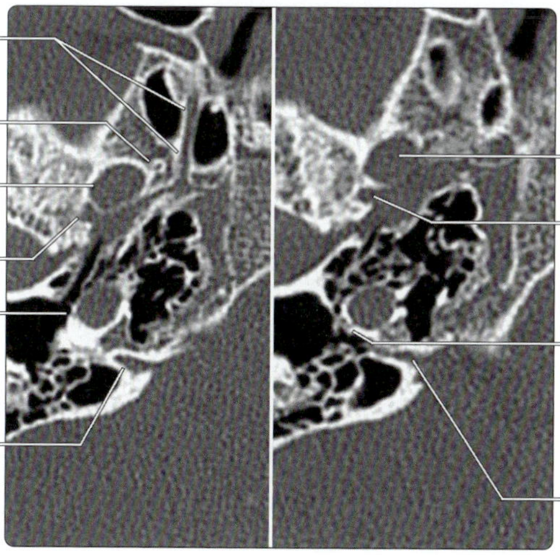

Vidian canal
Foramen of Vesalius
Foramen ovale
Foramen spinosum
Superior caroticotympanic nerve
Cochlear aqueduct
Foramen ovale
Foramen spinosum
Inferior caroticotympanic nerve
Cochlear aqueduct

(Top) *Axial graphic shows pars nervosa & pars vascularis of the jugular foramen separated by the jugular spine & fibrous septum. Note the inferior tympanic canaliculus (ITC) between the internal carotid artery & internal jugular vein, originating from the pars nervosa & connecting to the middle ear. The ITC contains the Jacobson nerve (CNIX branch, parasympathetic to tympanic plexus) & inferior tympanic artery. Also note the mastoid canaliculus with the Arnold nerve (auricular branch of vagus [CNX]) originating from lateral aspect of pars vascularis of jugular foramen. Mastoid canaliculus first connects laterally to descending mastoid segment of facial nerve canal a few millimeters above the stylomastoid foramen, & then dips inferolaterally towards the tympanomastoid fissure (suture) at posterior aspect of EAC.* **(Middle)** *Axial CT shows ITC & mastoid canaliculus.* **(Bottom)** *Axial CT images (1st just above 2nd, side by side) show superior & inferior caroticotympanic nerves (CTNs) arising from carotid plexus to provide sympathetic nerve supply for tympanic plexus on the middle ear medial wall cochlear promontory surface. Note foramen of Vesalius, vidian canal, & cochlear aqueduct.*

JACOBSON NERVE & ARNOLD NERVE: CORONAL GRAPHIC & BONE CT

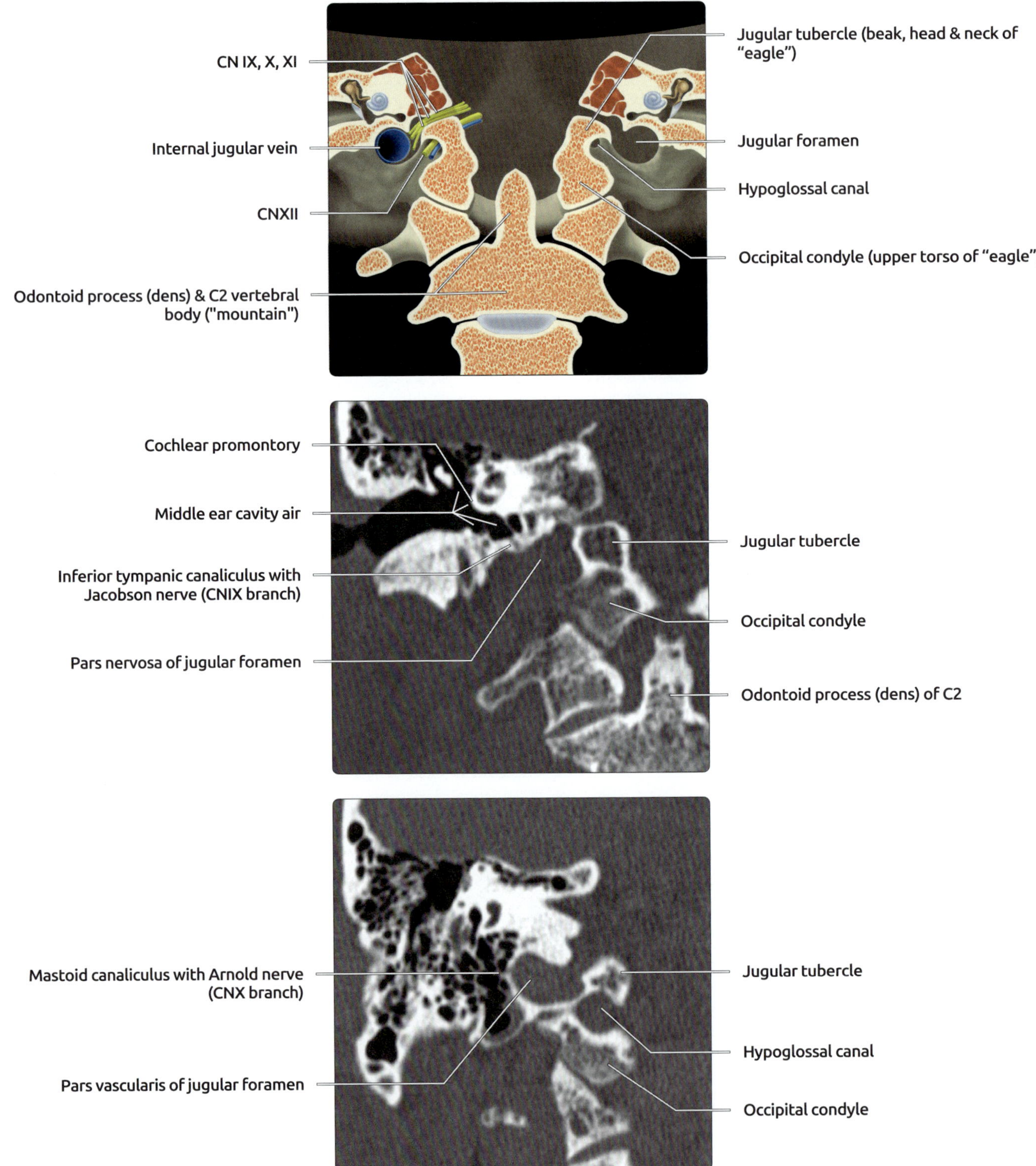

(Top) *Coronal graphic shows the appearance of a double eagle (jugular tubercle on the occipital condyle on both sides) sitting on a mountain top (C2 vertebra with odontoid process), which is very useful to identify the jugular foramen & hypoglossal canal on coronal CT/MR. The occipital condyle forms the upper torso of the eagle, & the jugular tubercle forms its beak, head, & neck. The jugular foramen with internal jugular vein, CNIX, X, & XI is seen superolateral to the beak & head of the eagle. Hypoglossal canal with veins & CNXII is seen underneath the beak & neck.* **(Middle)** *Coronal bone CT through the anterior aspect of the jugular foramen (pars nervosa) shows the ITC (with Jacobson nerve, CNIX branch) originating from the petrosal fossula [small depression under petrous bone lodging inferior (petrosal) ganglion of CNIX] at the roof of the pars nervosa & connecting to the middle ear cavity on its towards the tympanic plexus on the surface of the cochlear promontory.* **(Bottom)** *Coronal bone CT through the posterior aspect of the jugular foramen (pars vascularis) shows the mastoid canaliculus (with Arnold nerve, CNX branch) originating at the lateral aspect of the pars vascularis.*

CHORDA TYMPANI NERVE: SAGITTAL GRAPHIC & SAGITTAL & AXIAL BONE CT

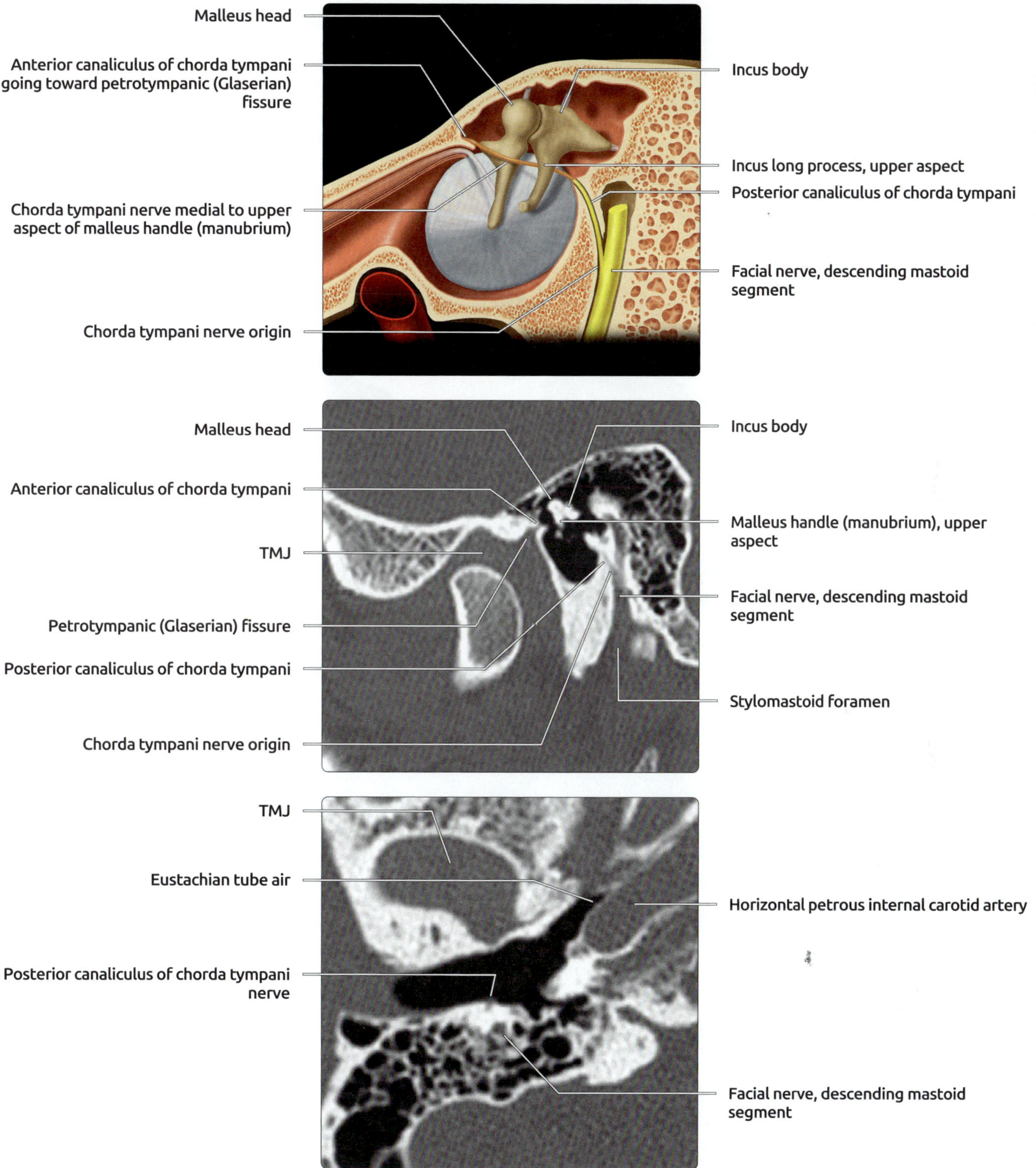

(Top) *Sagittal internal graphic of the lateral wall of the middle ear cavity shows the course of the chorda tympani nerve (CTN). The CTN originates from the descending mastoid segment of the facial nerve, which could be from the proximal, mid, or distal mastoid segment, or, rarely, even after exiting the stylomastoid foramen. It ascends through the posterior canaliculus of the CTN in the posterior wall of the middle ear, courses in the middle ear cavity from posterior to anterior in the substance of the tympanic membrane between mucous & fibrous layers, & then between the upper aspect of the handle (manubrium) of malleus & long process of incus, on the medial side of upper part of handle of malleus. It then travels through the anterior canaliculus of CTN and exits the temporal bone into the masticator space through the petrotympanic fissure (Glaserian fissure), which is posteromedial to TMJ, & joins the lingual nerve 2 cm below the skull base.* **(Middle)** *Straight parasagittal bone CT reformation perpendicular to the axial CT without any obliquity shows the course of the CTN.* **(Bottom)** *Axial bone CT shows the descending mastoid segment of the right facial nerve & posterior canaliculus of the CTN.*

OTHER SKULL BASE HOLES: AXIAL GRAPHIC & BONE CT

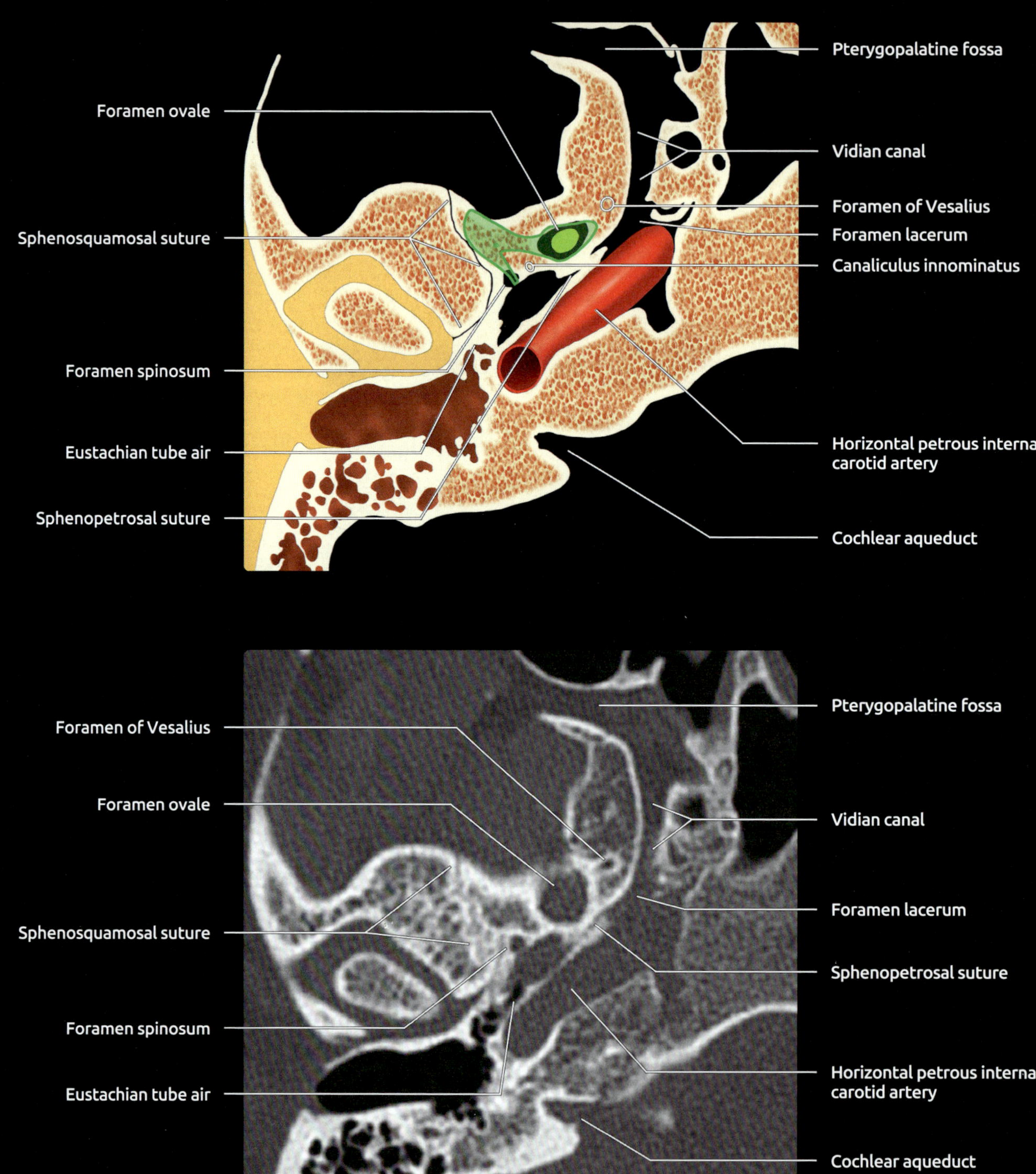

(Top) *Graphic shows identification pattern of skull base holes with the epicenter on the horizontal petrous ICA canal. Foramen lacerum is the cartilaginous floor anteroinferomedial to horizontal petrous ICA canal between sphenoid & temporal bones. Vidian canal connects foramen lacerum to pterygopalatine fossa anteriorly. Note the ladies shoe appearance of foramen ovale (FO) (front sole of shoe) & foramen spinosum (pointed heel of shoe) in greater wing of sphenoid (GWS) just anterolateral to petrous ICA. Sphenopetrosal suture (SPS) is seen just posteromedial to FO between GWS & petrous apex. Eustachian tube (ET) with air is seen just posterolateral to the SPS. Do not confuse ET with the SPS when ET is not air filled. Lesser petrosal nerve rarely exits through SPS. Sphenosquamosal suture is seen just lateral to foramen spinosum between GWS & squamous temporal bone. Foramen of Vesalius is seen lateral to vidian canal & anterior to FO, & canaliculus innominatus (foramen petrosum) is seen in between & medial to foramen spinosum & FO are only inconsistently present.* **(Bottom)** *Axial CT shows the anatomy of skull base holes. Note the inconsistent foramen of Vesalius.*

INCONSISTENT CANALS: AXIAL & CORONAL BONE CT

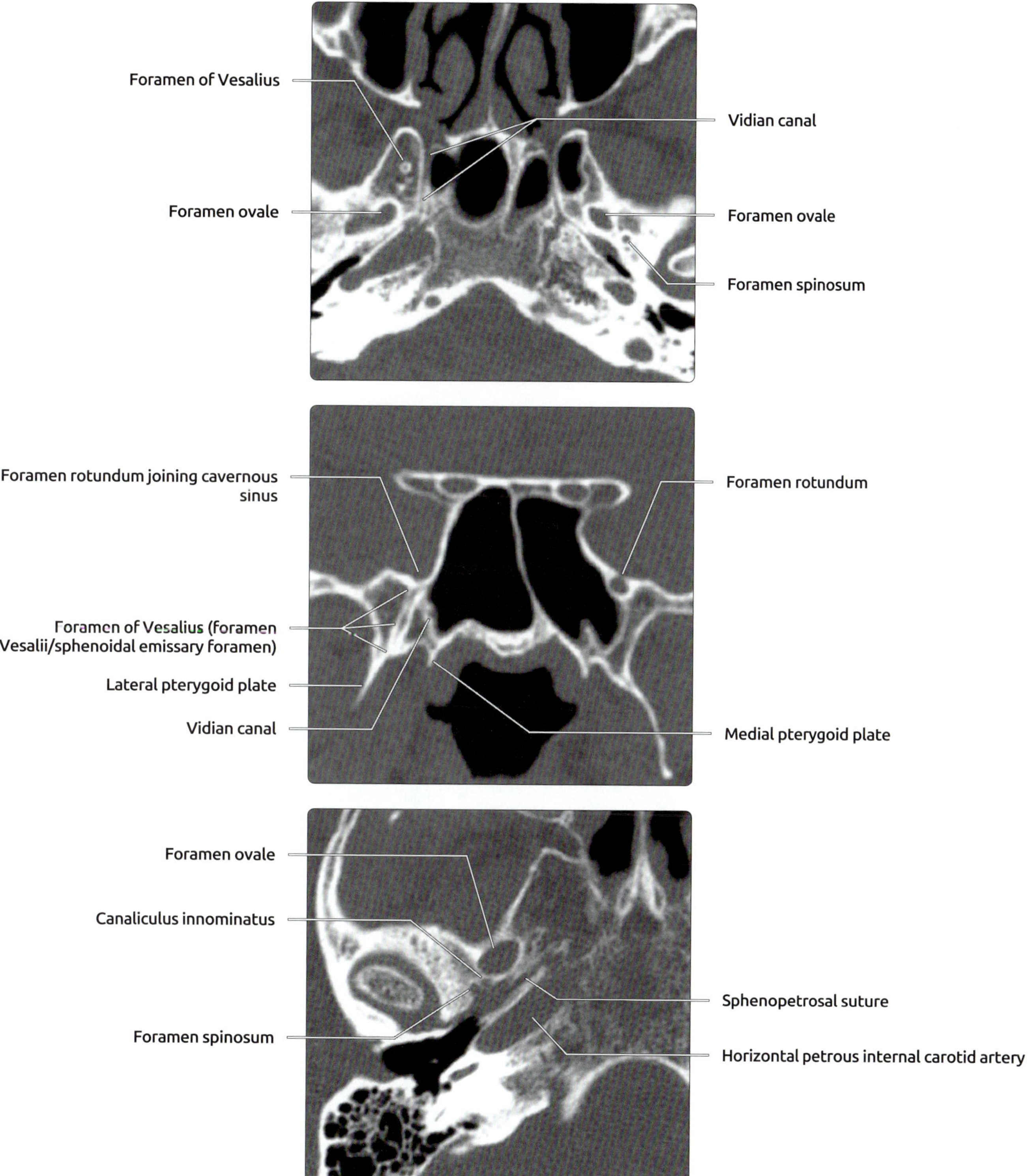

(Top) *Axial CT shows the inconsistently seen foramen of Vesalius (foramen Vesalii/sphenoidal emissary foramen) in the GWS, anterior to the FO & lateral to vidian canal. It contains an emissary vein connecting cavernous sinus superiorly near the foramen rotundum to the masticator space pterygoid venous plexus inferiorly; infection may spread from the upper face/orbit/sinus to cavernous sinus through this. Note that the foramen of Vesalius lies anterior to the FO inferiorly.* **(Middle)** *Coronal CT in the same patient shows foramen Vesalii passing from just underneath the foramen rotundum superiorly (near the cavernous sinus) to open into the masticator space inferiorly (near the pterygoid venous plexus) with its course just lateral to the vidian canal.* **(Bottom)** *Axial CT in another patient shows the inconsistent canaliculus innominatus (a.k.a. foramen of Arnold). The lesser petrosal nerve exits the middle cranial fossa floor (GWS) usually via the FO, but occasionally via canaliculus innominatus when present, or, rarely, via the sphenopetrosal fissure to eventually join the otic ganglion in the masticator space & provide parotid gland secretomotor supply via auriculotemporal nerve (CNV3 branch).*

TERMINOLOGY

Abbreviations

- Transverse oblique view (TOV); longitudinal oblique view (LOV)

Synonyms

- Pöschl view (TOV), Stenver view (LOV)

Definitions

- Longitudinal & transverse oblique terminology defined in relation to **long axis of pyramidal petrous temporal bone**
- **TOV (Pöschl)**: Image reformation series perpendicular to long axis of petrous pyramid
  - **Parallel to** line drawn between vertical components of **superior semicircular canal** (SCC) arch
- **LOV (Stenver)**: Image reformation series **parallel to long axis of petrous pyramid**
  - Perpendicular to line drawn between vertical components of superior SCC arch

IMAGING ANATOMY

Overview

- Standard temporal bone CT imaging on multislice CT produces axial data set
  - Coronal reformation data set: Standard additional plane in temporal bone imaging
  - TOV & LOV reformations: Variably created as additional planes available for viewing
- Many normal temporal bone structures **not** well seen in either axial or coronal imaging planes
  - Best examples include facial nerve canal, cochlea, round window, bony vestibular aqueduct (VA), superior & posterior SCCs, & cochlear nerve canal
  - Adding longitudinal & transverse oblique reformations to axial & coronal planes as 4-plane standard offering aids considerably in visibility of these structures
    - TOV & LOV CT reformations provide rich set of additional images that may profile some of these structures in unique & helpful ways
- Oblique view checklist in sequential CT scans
- **TOV (Pöschl view)**: Lateral to medial CT images
  - 1. Bony VA
  - 2. Incudostapedial articulation
  - 3. Oval & round window, "2-window" view
  - 4. Superior SCC & arcuate eminence
  - 5. Cochlear nerve canal
  - 6. Labyrinthine segment of facial nerve
- **LOV (Stenver view)**: Anterior to posterior CT images
  - 1. Malleoincudal joint & chorda tympani nerve
  - 2. Mastoid drainage pathway & eustachian tube
  - 3. Facial nerve canal: Geniculate ganglion, tympanic segment, posterior genu, & mastoid segment
  - 4. Stapes crura "2-dot" view
  - 5. Cochlear turns

Microanatomy Optimized in Transverse Oblique View (Pöschl View)

- **Bony VA**
  - Endolymphatic duct (ELD) & sac (ELS) located within bony VA
  - Connects crus communis (meeting point of posterior & superior SCCs to fovea)
  - Fovea: Cup-shaped area at posterior temporal bone margin
  - Operculum: Opening of VA into fovea
  - ELD: Short proximal part connected to crus communis
  - ELS: Longer distal part with both intraosseous & intradural (fovea area) components
  - Transverse oblique axis much more easily profiles VA from external aperture to crus communis than axial plane CT images
  - Axial temporal bone CT: VA width < 1 mm at midpoint, ± < 2 mm at opercular margin (Cincinnati criteria)
  - Transverse oblique reformat (Pöschl view) parallel to superior SCC plane: < 0.8-0.9 mm at midpoint
  - Literature variable; vertical & axial VA width > 1.5 mm at midpoint of labyrinth & operculum most accepted for **large VA** (classic Valvassori criteria)
  - Large VA has potential syndromic implications
- **"2-window"** view of **oval & round windows**
  - Shows oval & round window membranes clearly
  - When oval or round window atresia suspected, this view very helpful in confirming either diagnosis
  - Round window access assessment for cochlear implantation also assisted by this view
- **Superior SCC/arcuate eminence**
  - Coronal CT can diagnose canal dehiscence in most cases
  - Profile of superior SCC in TOV may help make diagnosis & guide type of surgical procedure

Microanatomy Optimized in Longitudinal Oblique View (Stenver View)

- **1st cochlear turn + round window niche/membrane**
  - Very useful for cochlear implant planning as it shows adequate access through round window/basal turn of cochlea; important if labyrinthine ossificans present
- **Facial nerve canal**
  - Geniculate ganglion, tympanic segment, posterior genu, & mastoid segment
  - Useful in assessing where along course of tympanic segment facial nerve injury may have occurred; traumatic injury or injury from cholesteatoma

ANATOMY IMAGING ISSUES

Imaging Approaches

- TOV & LOV image reconstruction easily learned & performed by CT technologist
  - Step 1: After axial acquisition, place line **parallel** to **superior SCC**
  - Step 2: Reformat 0.75-mm images in **TOV (Pöschl) plane** ~ 20 mm on either side of this line, making sure to extend laterally **covering middle ear structures**
  - Step 3: Place line **perpendicular to** initial TOV plane to create **LOV (Stenver) plane**
  - Step 4: Reformat 0.75-mm images in LOV plane to **cover petrous pyramid anterior & posterior margins**

Imaging Pitfalls

- Superior SCC anatomy complex in 3 dimensions; unfamiliarity can lead to confusion when viewing additional imaging planes, such as TOV & LOV

AXIAL CT PLANNING FOR TRANSVERSE (PÖSCHL) & LONGITUDINAL (STENVER) OBLIQUE REFORMATIONS

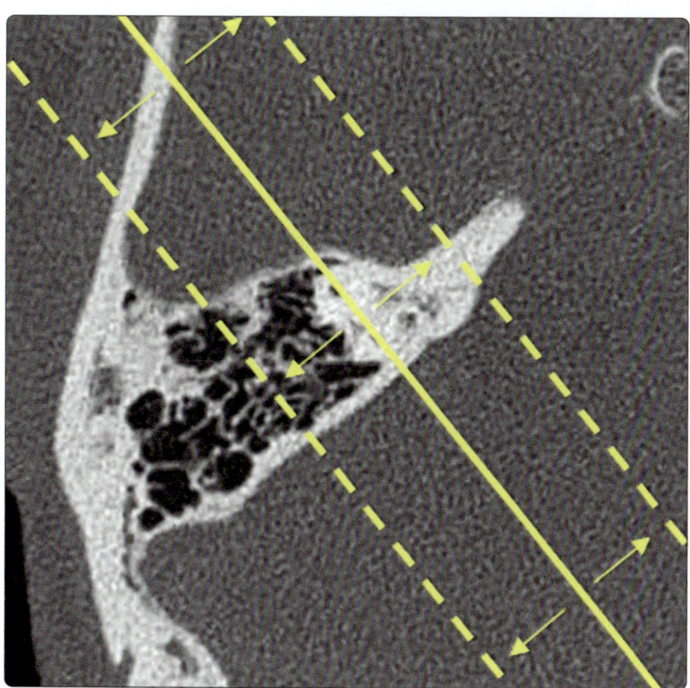

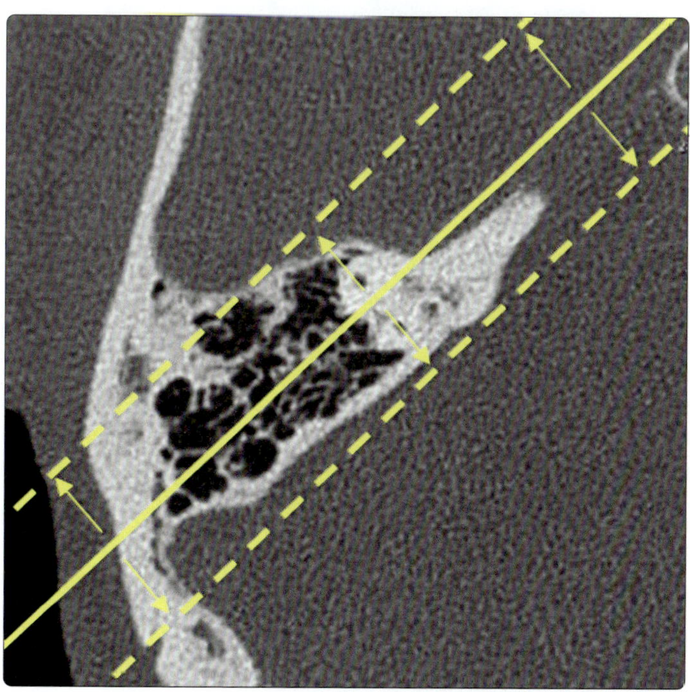

(Top) *Axial CT shows creation of transverse oblique (Pöschl) temporal bone reformations. Temporal bone oblique reformations can be a challenge for those unfamiliar with temporal bone anatomy, but can be easily learned & performed. Scroll through the axial image data set to the level of the superior semicircular canal. The transverse oblique reformation image set is made in a plane parallel to the axis created by the line through the superior semicircular canal. Be sure the data set extends laterally to cover the middle ear structures.* **(Bottom)** *Axial CT shows creation of longitudinal oblique (Stenver) temporal bone reformations. The longitudinal oblique reformation image set is made in a plane perpendicular to the axis created by the line through the superior semicircular canal. Be sure to cover the majority of the petrous pyramid, as shown.*

TRANSVERSE OBLIQUE (PÖSCHL) REFORMATIONS

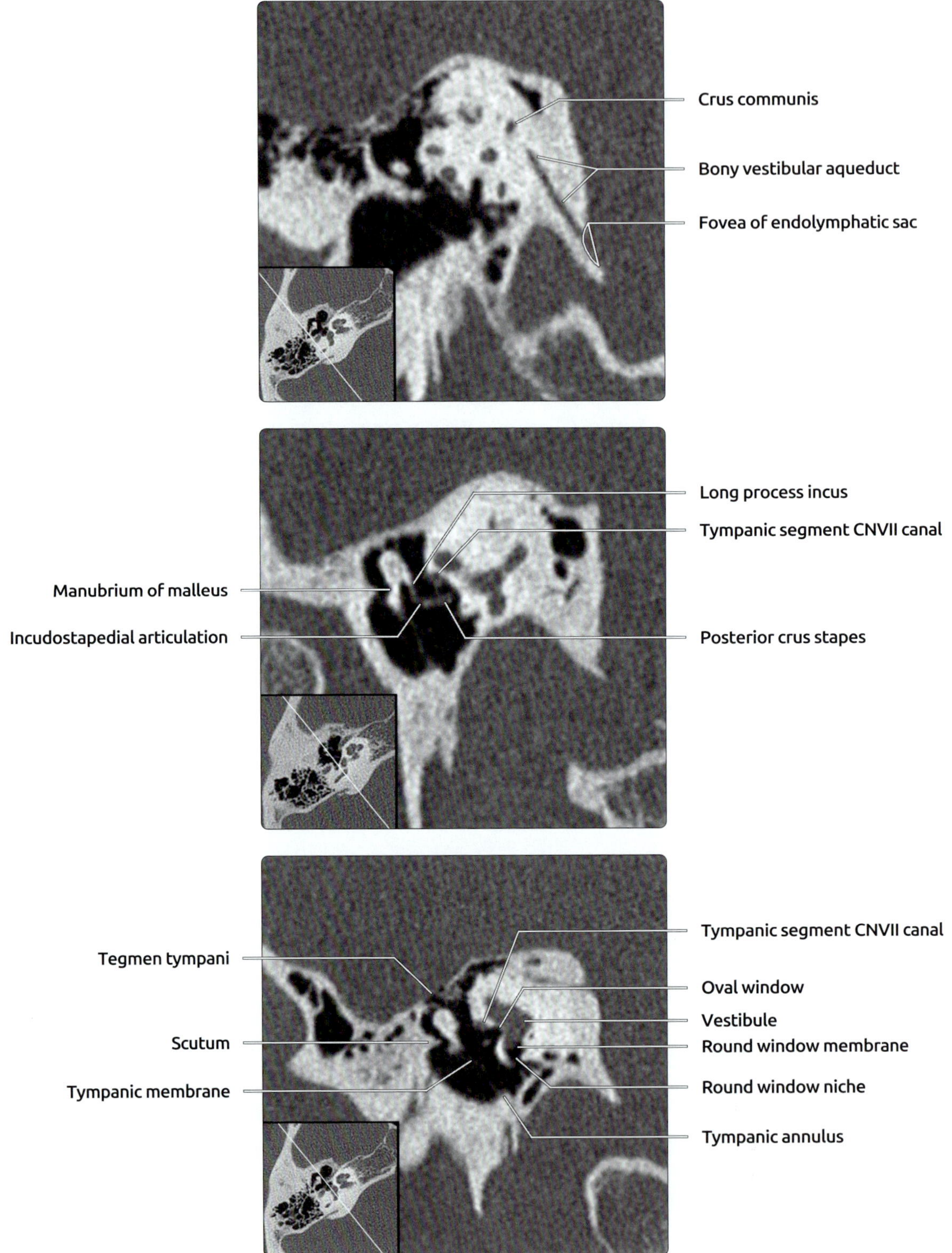

(Top) *First of 6 transverse oblique (Pöschl view) bone CT images of the right ear acquired parallel to the long axis of the superior semicircular canal is shown. The images are presented from the lateral to medial aspect perpendicular to the petrous temporal bony pyramid (from the lateral aspect of the middle ear towards the petrous apex). This reconstruction profiles the bony vestibular aqueduct as it progresses from the fovea of the endolymphatic sac toward the crus communis of the inner ear.* **(Middle)** *The 2nd image along the line of the posterior crus of the stapes permits identification of the incudostapedial articulation. The long process of the incus & manubrium of the malleus are also particularly well seen.* **(Bottom)** *This image shows the "2-window" view created by obtaining a transverse oblique reconstruction that passes through the axial view of the oval window (see inset). In this view, the oval window & round window niche & membrane are seen simultaneously. When cochlear implantation is anticipated, this view allows surgeons great confidence that they can access the basal turn of the cochlea through the round window niche with their cochlear implant.*

TRANSVERSE OBLIQUE (PÖSCHL) REFORMATIONS

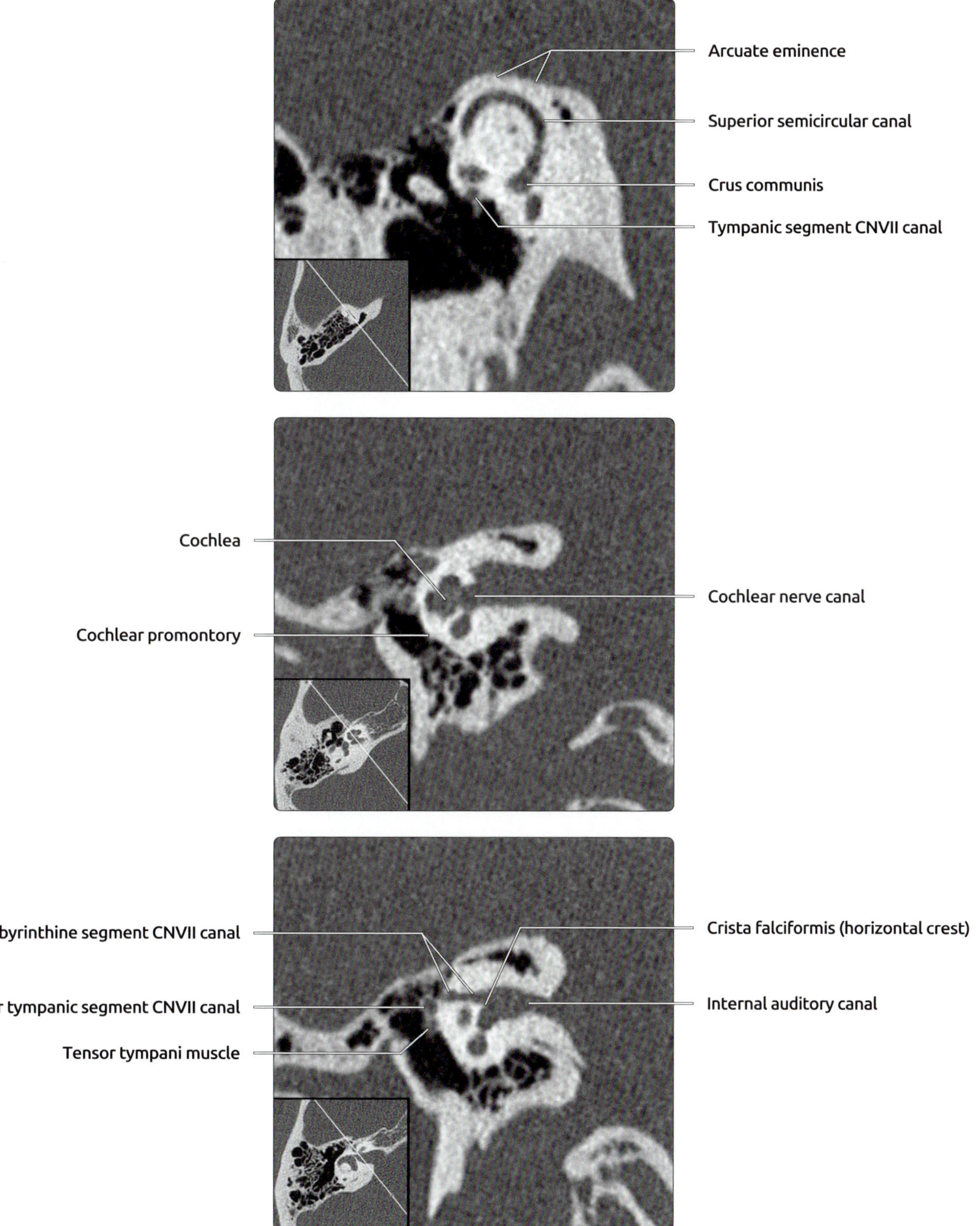

(Top) *Fourth of 6 transverse oblique (Pöschl view) CT reformatted images created along the line of the superior semicircular canal demonstrates the entire span of this canal with the bony ridge above it (arcuate eminence). This view can be very helpful in delineating the extent of superior semicircular canal dehiscence when present.* **(Middle)** *Fifth transverse oblique reformation along the line of the cochlear axis clearly delineates the length & dimension of the cochlear nerve canal as it connects the fundus of the internal auditory canal (IAC) to the cochlea. In congenital inner ear lesions where a "trapped/isolated cochlea" (cochlea & IAC have no connection; therefore, there is no cochlear nerve) is suspected, this view can help verify this imaging impression.* **(Bottom)** *The last & most medial image of the transverse oblique reformation series created along the axis of the labyrinthine segment of CNVII is shown. When CNVII pathology is present, it is very helpful to have multiple different views of its canal.*

LONGITUDINAL OBLIQUE (STENVER) REFORMATIONS

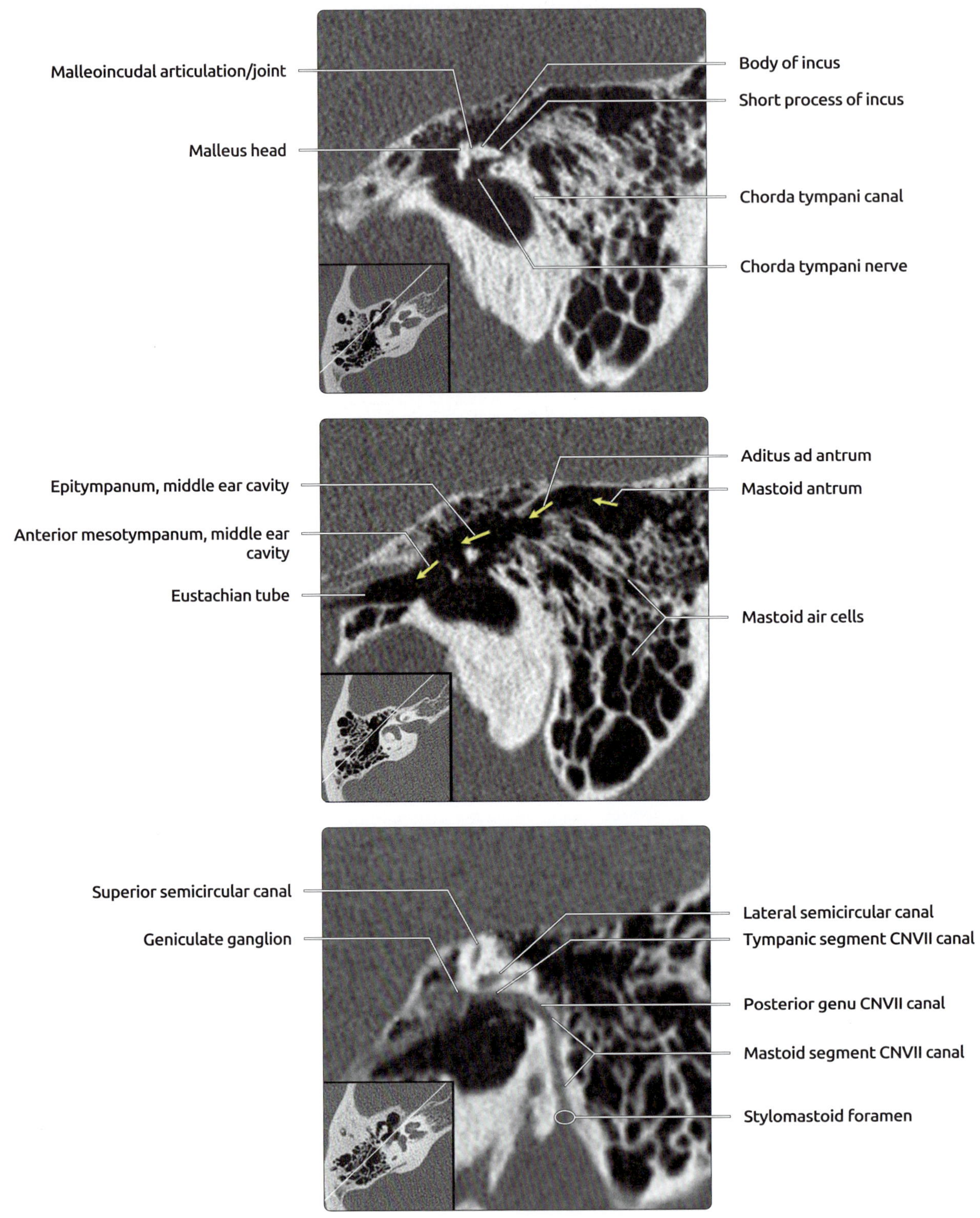

(Top) *First of 6 longitudinal oblique (Stenver view) bone CT images of the right ear presented from near the anterior margin of the petrous temporal bony pyramid & scrolling towards its posterior aspect profiles the malleoincudal articulation between the head of the malleus & the body of the incus. Also note the chorda tympani nerve canal (rising anteriorly & superiorly from the mastoid segment of facial nerve) as well as the nerve itself in the middle ear cavity.* **(Middle)** *Moving posteriorly, this image highlights the normal mastoid drainage route (yellow arrows). Fluid normally made by mastoid mucosal surfaces passes into the mastoid antrum, & from there, it reaches the middle ear cavity via the aditus ad antrum. The final common pathway exiting the middle ear cavity is the eustachian tube.* **(Bottom)** *The 3rd Stenver view image shows the tympanic segment of CNVII entirely on a carefully placed longitudinal oblique reformation. Note the geniculate ganglion, tympanic segment, posterior genu, mastoid segment, & stylomastoid foramen, all seen on this single view. The tympanic segment passes beneath the lateral semicircular canal.*

LONGITUDINAL OBLIQUE (STENVER) REFORMATIONS

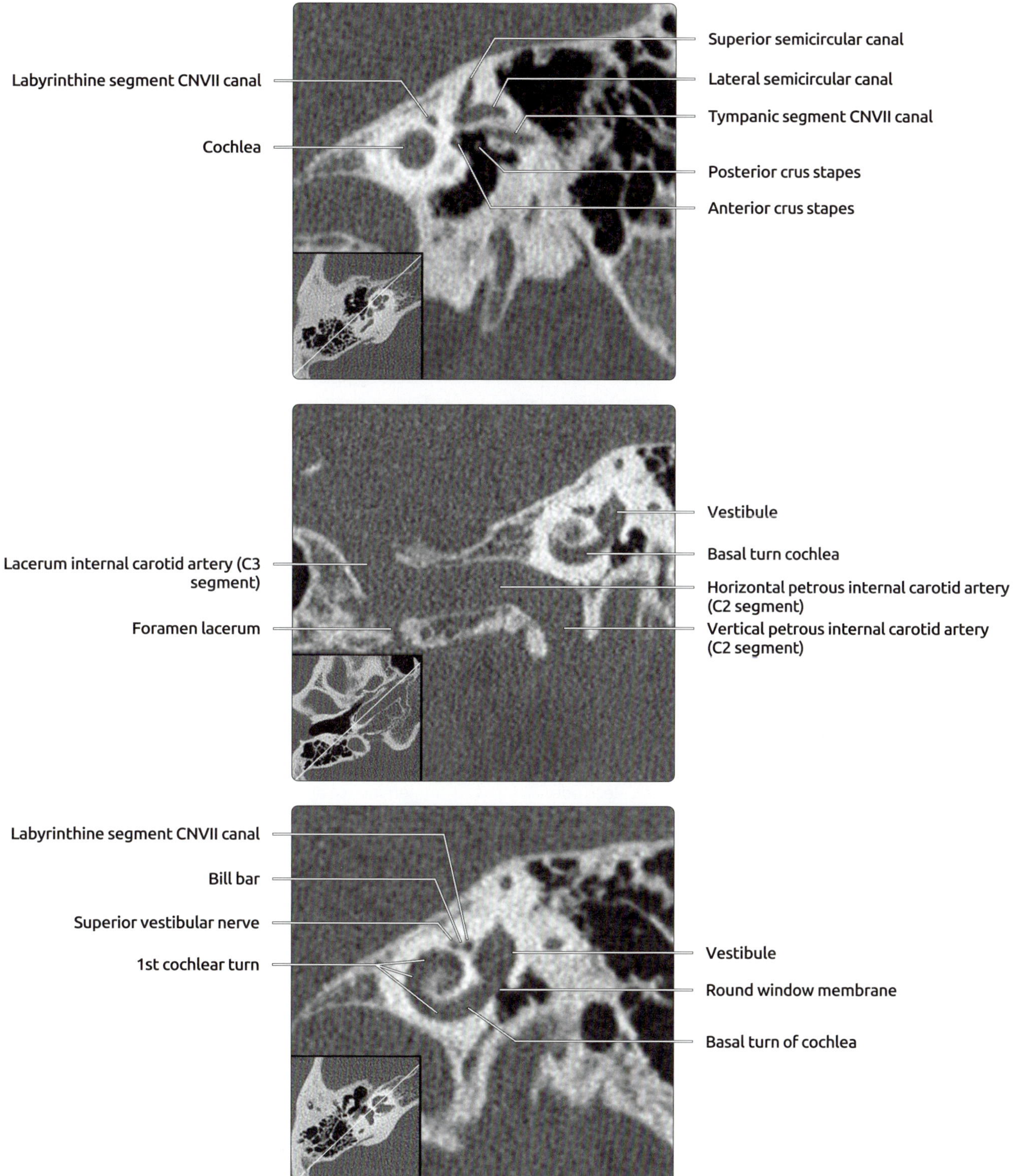

(Top) *The 4th of 6 longitudinal oblique CT Stenver view images of the right ear shows the "2-dot" view of crura of the stapes just before they meet the footplate of the stapes at the oval window. In patients with ossicular anomalies, this level of anatomic information about the stapes can be of great help.* **(Middle)** *More medially, the 5th image through the horizontal petrous ICA profiles the basal turn of the cochlea. Note the vertical & horizontal petrous ICA segments (C2 segment ICA) as well as the lacerum segment (proximal C3 segment ICA).* **(Bottom)** *The most posterior image of the 6 longitudinal oblique reformats profiles the entire 1st turn of the cochlea. In the notch between the vestibule & apical aspect of the 1st cochlear turn, note the superior vestibular nerve canal & the labyrinthine segment of the CNVII canal. Such a view could be helpful in evaluating cochlear implants.*

TERMINOLOGY

Abbreviations

- Photon-counting detector (PCD)

Definitions

- PCD CT uses semiconductor detector material that directly converts x-ray photons to electron-hole pair, which then gets converted to electronic signals at anode

TECHNOLOGY

Energy-Integrating Detector CT

- Use energy-integrating detector (EID) made of solid-state scintillator, such as gadolinium oxysulfide (Gd_2O_2S) or cadmium tungstate ($CdWO_4$)
- X-ray photon generate scintillation light on interaction with detector
- Scintillation light converted to electrical signal by photodiode
- Generated scintillation light intensity proportional to both energy of each x-ray photon and number of incident photons per unit time
- Electrical signal proportional to total amount of scintillation light generated in scintillator during measurement time
- Electrical signal generated by photodiode amplified and integrated; finally becomes output signal
- Separators between detectors limits spatial resolution in conventional EID CT

Photon-Counting Detector CT

- Use semiconductors, such as cadmium telluride (CdTe) or cadmium Zinc telluride (CdZnTe), as detector materials
- X-ray photon interaction with detector generates charge cloud of electron-hole pairs
- Electric field applied across PCD pulls electron to pixel electrodes (anode electrode:anode pixel), generating pulse
- Spatial resolution depends on size of pixel electrode, reduction in its size improves spatial resolution
- Concept of "multiple detector rows" cannot apply to PCD as they have no separators
- Application-specific integrated circuits (ASIC): Electronic circuits connected to anode, shape electric pulses and count signals according to their energy values
- PCD classifies incident photons into 2-8 energy bins based on their energy by comparing all pulses with several thresholds

Advantages of PCD CT

- High spatial resolution; slice thickness can be up to 0.2 mm
- Simultaneous multienergy acquisition; can aid in material decomposition
- Energy binning aid in low electronic noise, K-edge imaging, and metal artifact reduction
- Uniform photon weighting and improved contrast-to-noise ratio with iodinated contrast material
- Radiation dose reduction

Disadvantages of PCD CT

- Cross talk: Charge sharing, K-escape, and Compton scattering can take place in PCD to generate inaccurate signals
- Pulse pile-up: If detector signal processing is relatively slow, pulse pile-up occurs and some of generated electric pulses overlap

ANATOMIC IMAGING ISSUES

Imaging Recommendations

- Noncontrast PCD CT with 0.2-mm slice thickness
- Multiplanar reformats of right and left temporal bone in axial, coronal, Pöschl, and Stenver planes
- CECT when infection or tumor suspected

Imaging Quality

- Higher signal-to-noise ratio (SNR) than EID CT
- Provides sharper images than EID CT, improving visualization of small critical structures
- Can achieve 21% noise reduction and up to 30% radiation dose reduction
- Very high spatial resolution significantly improves ability to assess complex anatomy of temporal bone
- Thinner slices reduce partial volume averaging, further improving assessment of small critical structures of temporal bone

CLINICAL APPLICATIONS

Better Visualization of Anatomy and Subtle Pathology

- **Ossicles and ossicular alignment**
  - Stapes superstructure very well visualized on PCD CT when compared to EID CT
  - Incudomalleolar and incudostapedial joints
- **Middle ear tendons and ligaments**
  - Tensor tympani tendon curving around processus cochleariformis, turning laterally across middle ear and attaching to upper part of malleus handle (manubrium)
  - Stapedius tendon emerging from apex of pyramidal eminence and its attachment to neck of stapes
  - Superior, anterior, and lateral malleolar ligaments and posterior incudal ligament
- **Minor fissures and sutures around temporal bone**
  - **Intrinsic channels**: Subarcuate canal, greater superficial petrosal nerve hiatus, singular canal, cochlear cleft, vestibular aqueduct, cochlear aqueduct, superior and inferior caroticotympanic nerve canals, inferior tympanic canaliculus, mastoid canaliculus, anterior and posterior canaliculi of chorda tympani
  - **Intrinsic sutures (fissures)**: Petrotympanic (Glaserian) fissure, petrosquamous suture, tympanosquamous suture, tympanomastoid suture
  - **Extrinsic sutures (fissures)**: Occipitomastoid suture, petrooccipital (petroclival) fissure, sphenopetrosal suture, sphenosquamosal suture
- **Ossicular anomalies**
  - Ossicular chain discontinuity, ossicular fixation
- **Oval window or round window aplasia or dysplasia**
- **Early fenestral otospongiosis**
  - Radiolucent focus at anterior margin of oval window margin ≈ fissula ante fenestram
- **Semicircular canal dehiscence**
- **Temporal bone fractures**
- **Postoperative temporal bone with ossicular prosthesis**

GRAPHICS

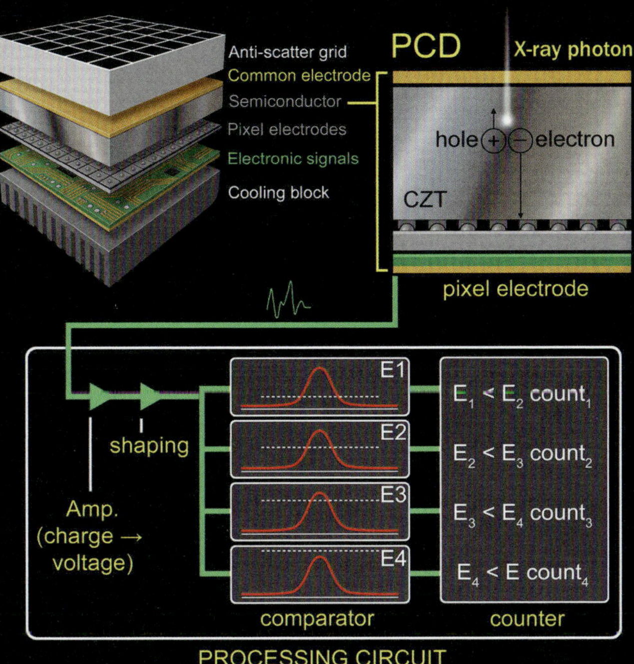

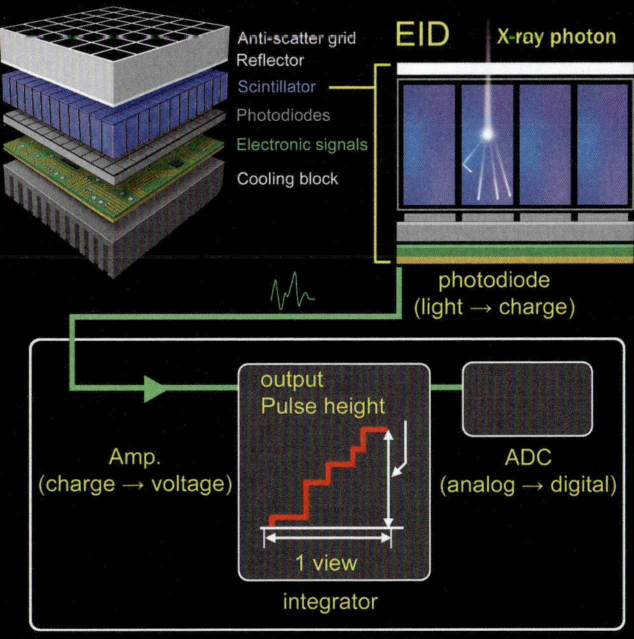

(Top) *Graphic shows a photon-counting detector (PCD) CT mechanism. Semiconductor materials, such as cadmium telluride (CdTe) or cadmium zinc telluride (CdZnTe), are used as detectors that generate a charge cloud of electron-hole pairs. The voltage across the PCD pulls the electrons toward the pixel electrode, which then generates an electrical pulse.* **(Bottom)** *Graphic shows an energy-integrating detector (EID) CT mechanism. A solid-state scintillator, such as gadolinium oxysulfide (lGd2O2S) or cadmium tungstate (CdWO4), are used as detector materials, which generate scintillation light when x-ray photon interacts with it. Thus, generated light is converted to an electrical signal via photodiode.*

AXIAL NECT

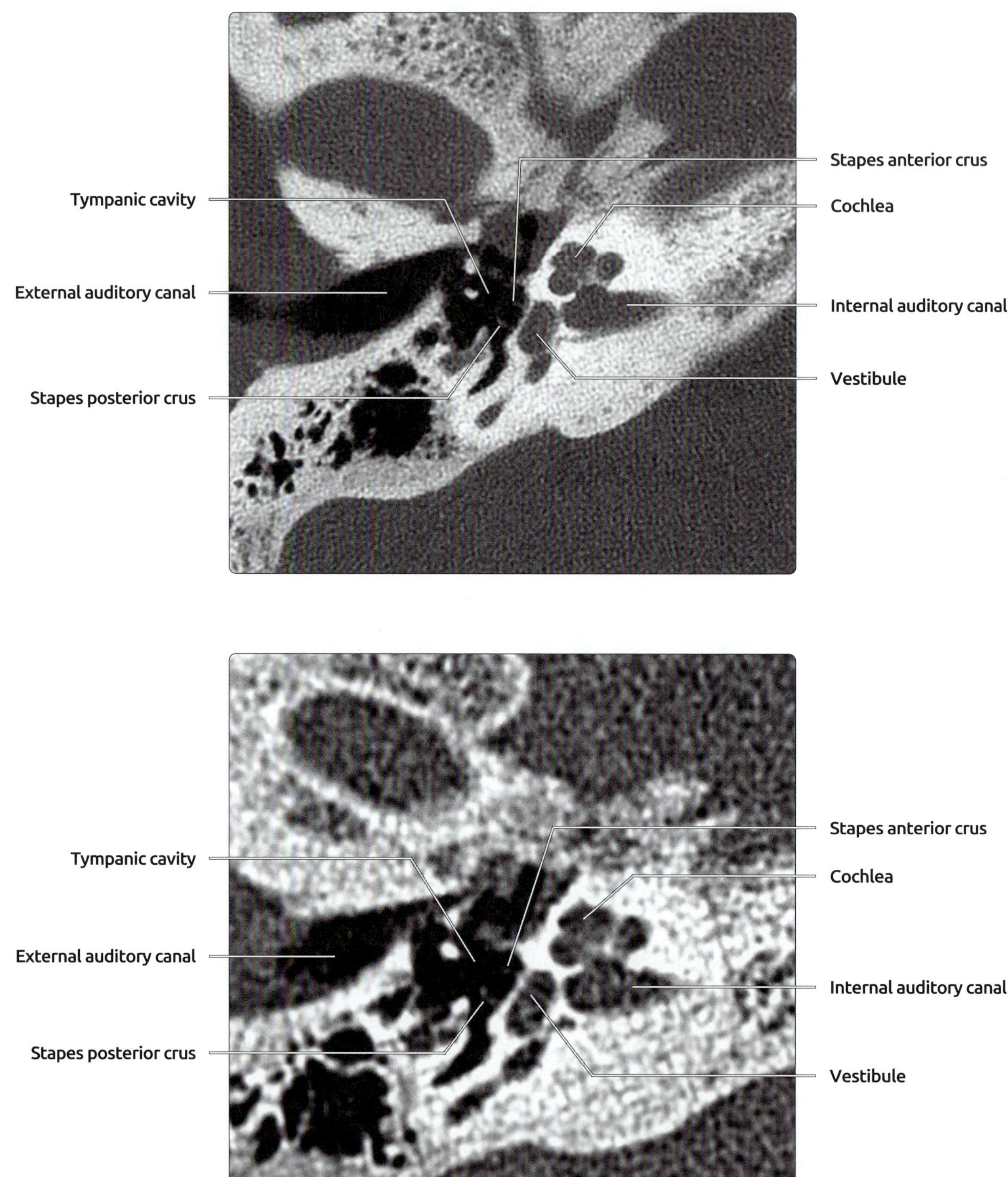

(Top) *Axial reformat of a PCD CT of the right temporal bone clearly depicts the anterior and posterior crura of stapes.* **(Bottom)** *Axial reformat of an EID CT of the right temporal bone in the same patient faintly depicts the anterior and posterior crura of stapes. Stapes superstructure consists of the head, neck, anterior and posterior crura, and tympanic portion of the foot plate, which are derived from the 2nd branchial arch. The vestibular portion of the stapes footplate and annular ligament are otic capsule derived.*

CORONAL NECT

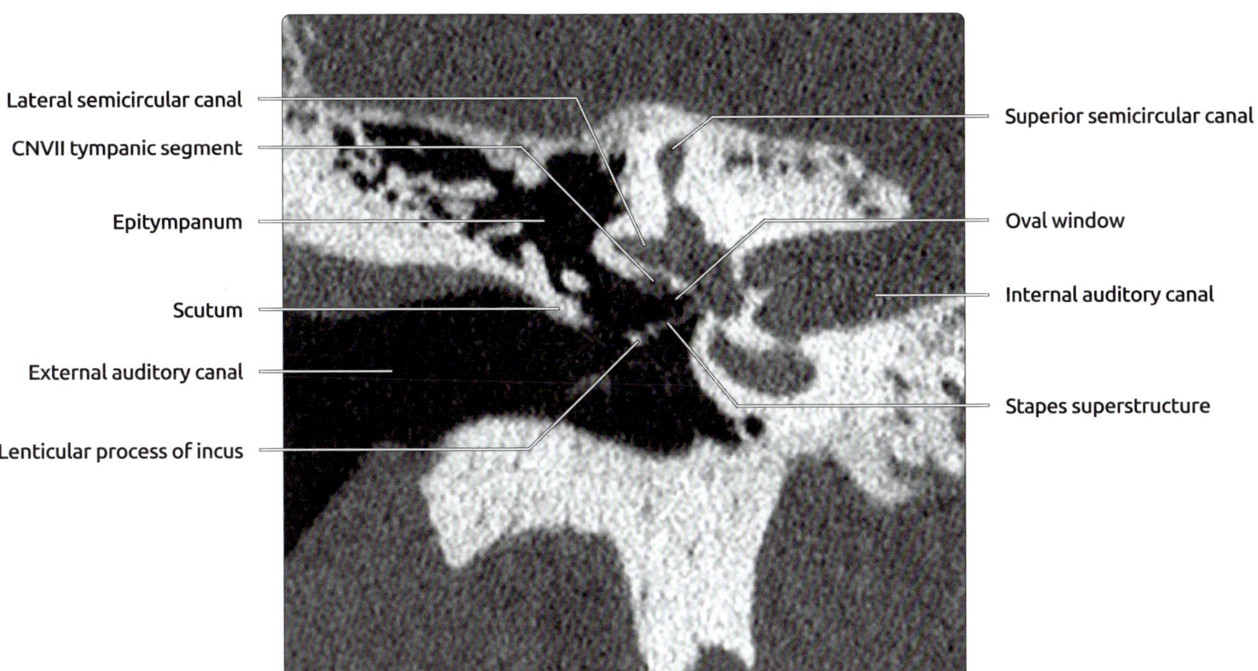

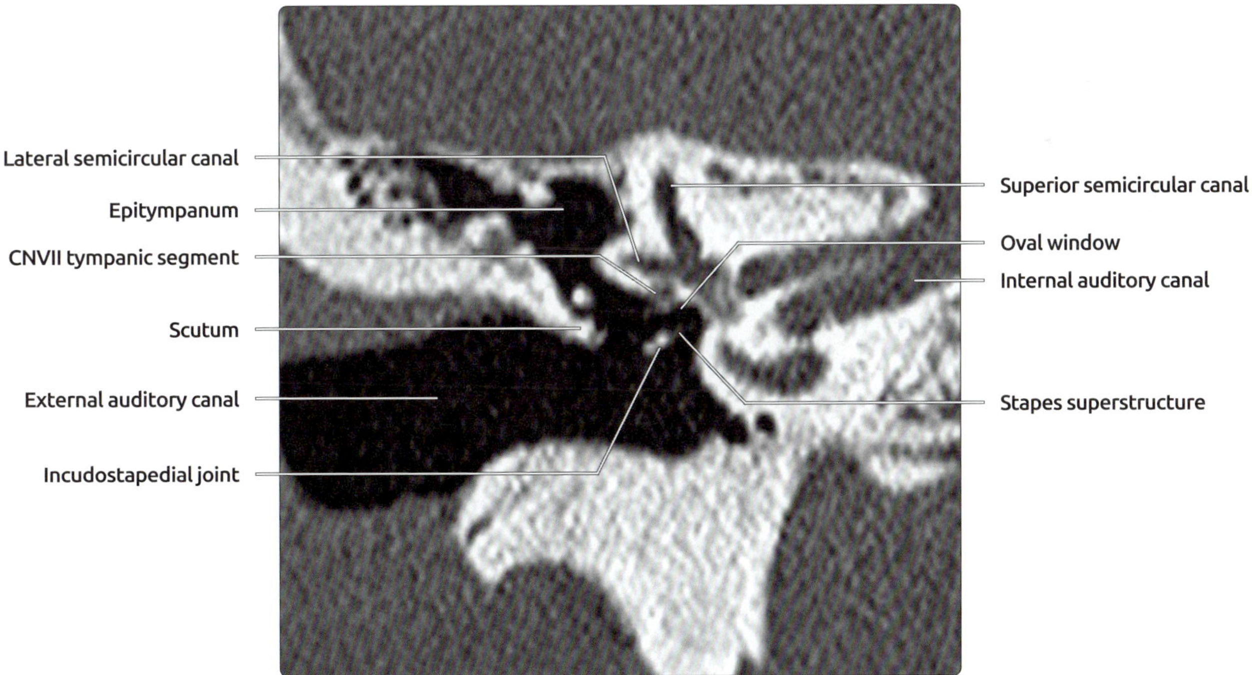

(Top) *Coronal reformat of a PCD CT of the right temporal bone shows articulation of the lenticular process of the incus with the head of the stapes. Stapes superstructure consists of the head, neck, and anterior and posterior crura of the stapes along with the tympanic portion of the foot plate. The stapes foot plate occupies the oval window and is circumferentially attached by an annular ligament.* **(Bottom)** *Coronal reformat of an EID CT of the right temporal bone in the same patient shows the incudostapedial joint and faint visualization of stapes superstructure in the oval window region. The oval window is located just inferomedial to the tympanic segment of CNVII.*

CORONAL NECT

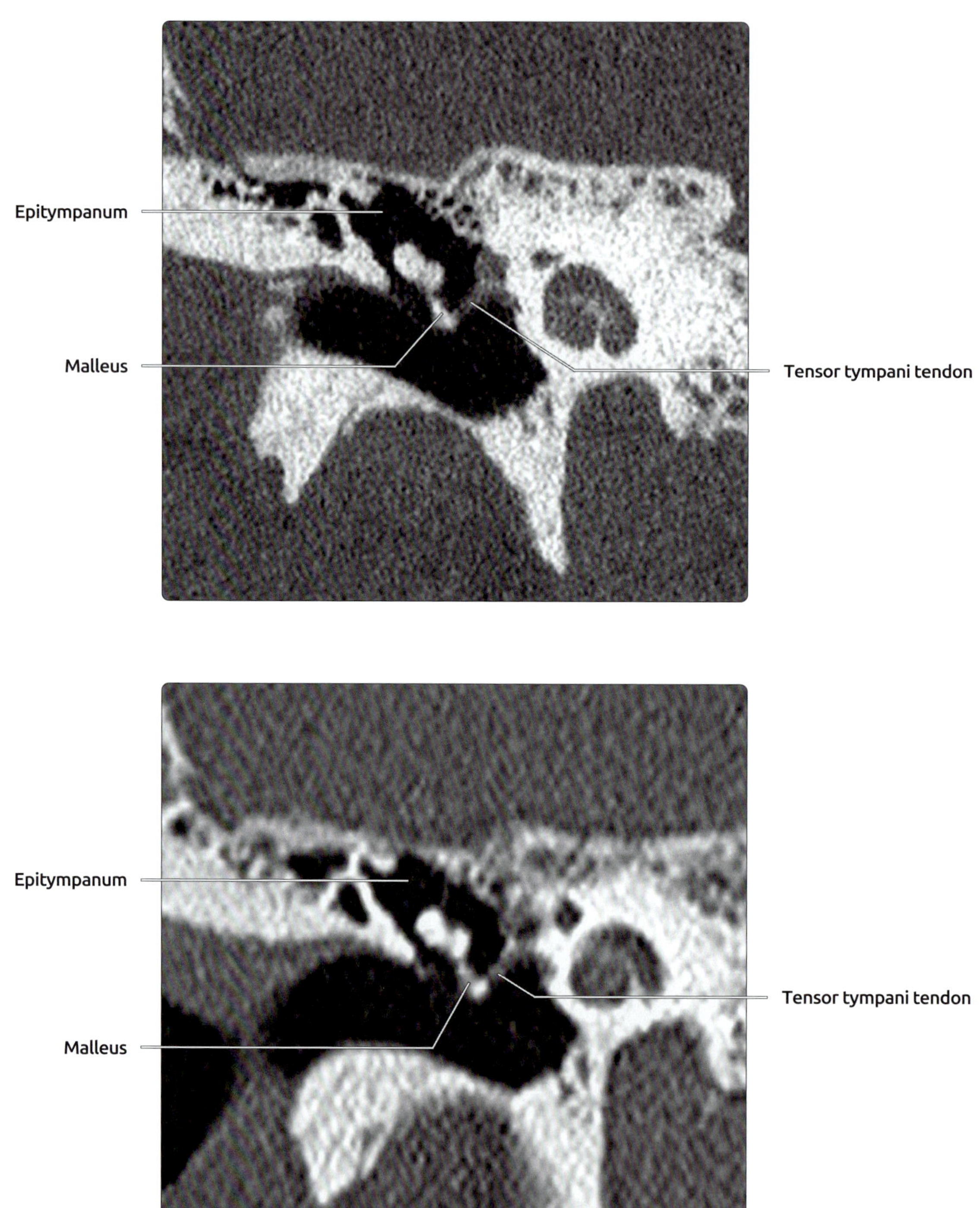

(Top) *Coronal reformat of a PCD CT of the right temporal bone shows the tensor tympani muscle tendon inserting onto the upper part of the malleus handle (manubrium). Note significant improvement in spatial resolution and decreased noise in this image.* **(Bottom)** *Coronal reformat of an EID CT of the right temporal bone in the same patient shows the tensor tympani muscle tendon inserting onto the upper part of the malleus handle (manubrium). The tensor tympani muscle originates from the semicanal of the tensor tympani along the cartilaginous margin of the eustachian tube and is innervated by a nerve to the medial pterygoid branch of the mandibular nerve (CNV3) via the nonrelaying motor root to the otic ganglion.*

AXIAL NECT

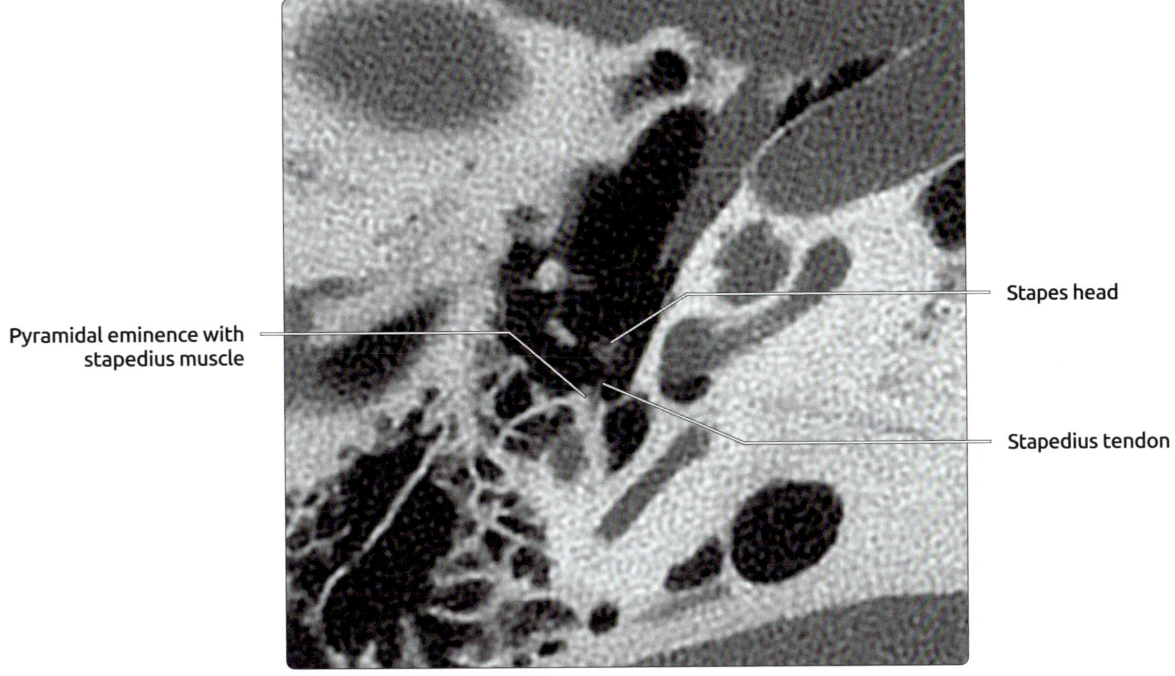

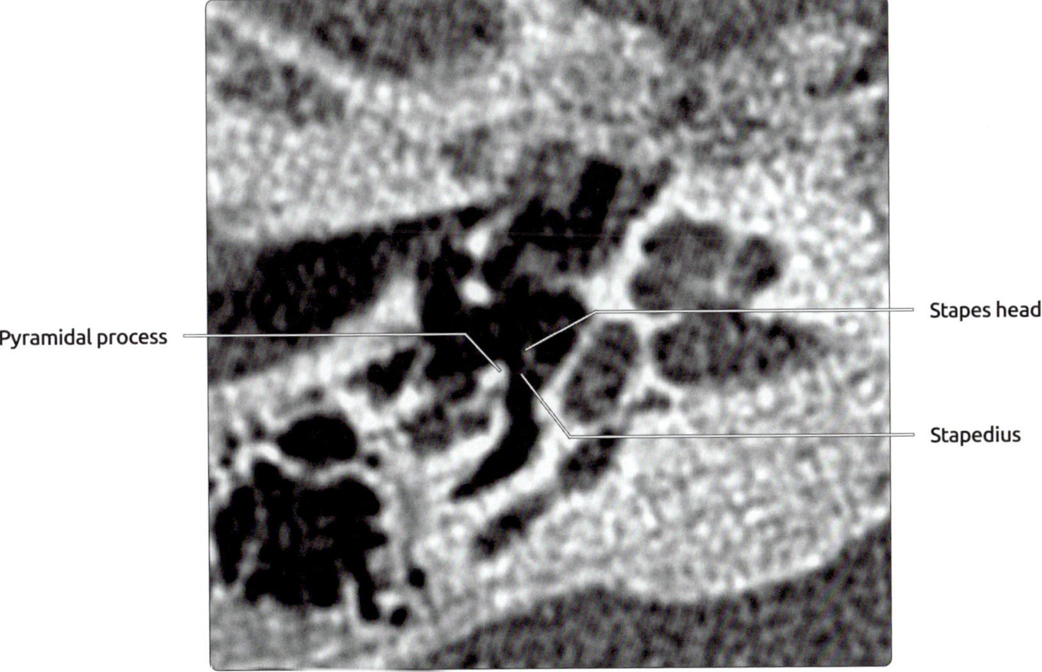

(Top) *Axial reformat of a PCD CT of the right temporal bone shows the stapedius muscle emerging from the pyramidal eminence and inserting onto the neck of the stapes. The stapedius originates from fasciculi of the posterior belly of the digastric muscle and is innervated by CNVII mastoid segment.* **(Bottom)** *Axial reformat of an EID CT of the right temporal bone in the same patient shows pyramidal eminence and faint visualization of the stapes. The stapedius muscle is not well visualized on this CT due to poor resolution and high noise levels.*

AXIAL NECT

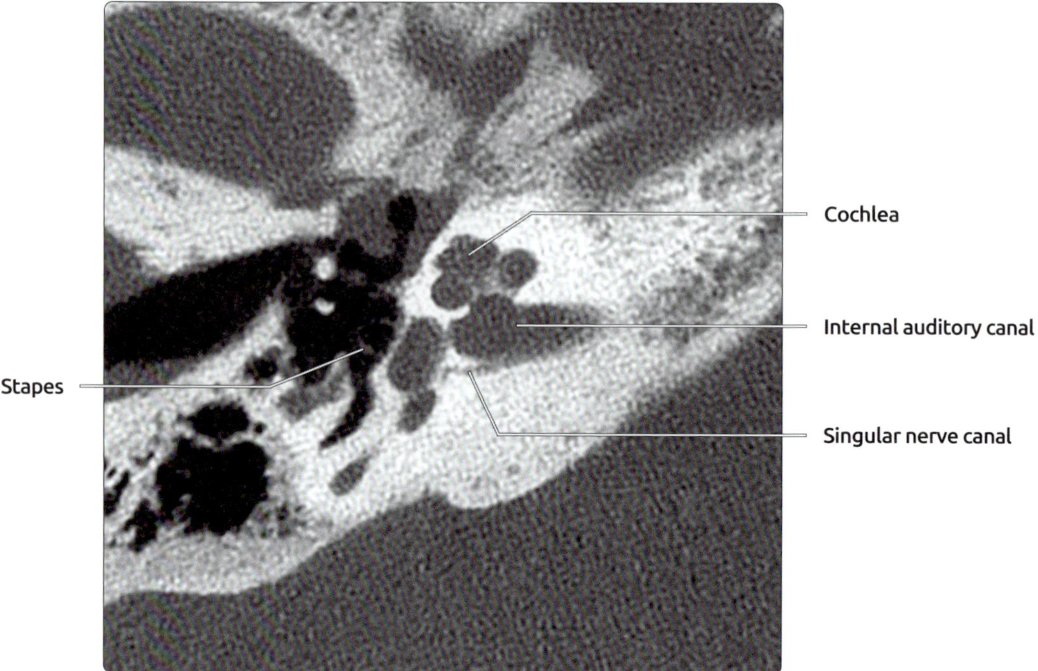

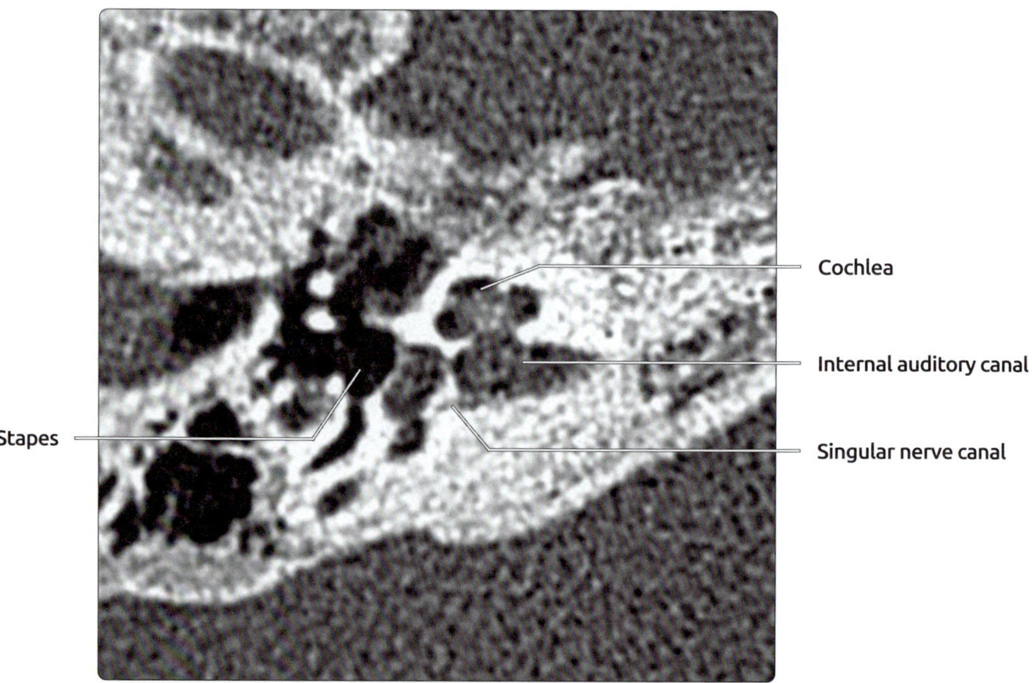

(Top) *Axial reformat of a PCD CT of the right temporal bone shows a singular nerve canal (foramen singulare) coursing from the internal auditory canal to the ampulla of the posterior semicircular canal.* **(Bottom)** *Axial reformat of an EID CT in the right temporal bone in the same patient faintly depicts a singular nerve canal coursing from the internal auditory canal to the saccule. A singular nerve (posterior ampullary nerve) is a branch of the inferior vestibular nerve, which supplies the saccule and posterior ampullary crest.*

AXIAL NECT

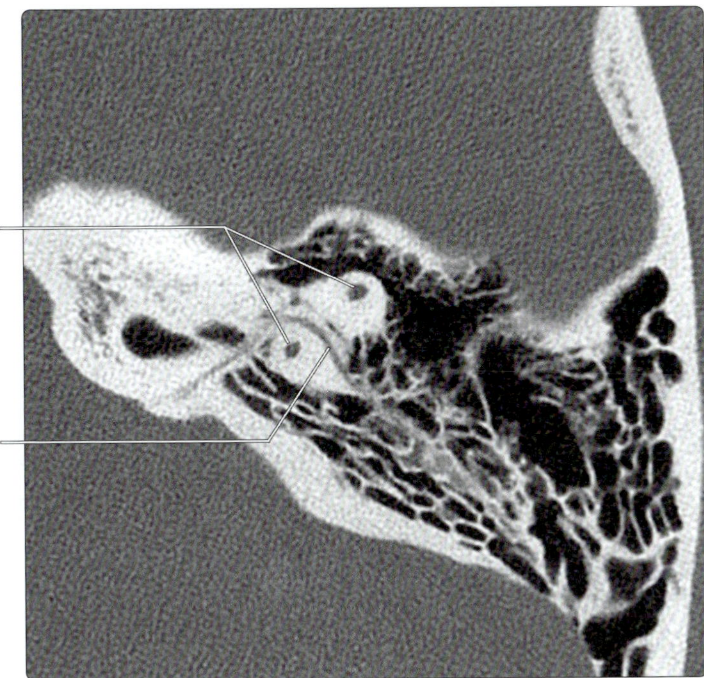

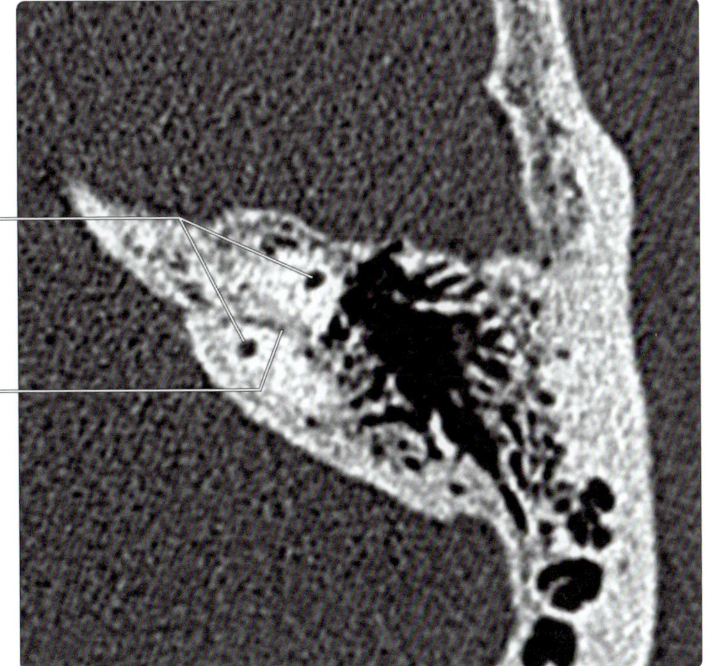

(Top) *Axial reformat of a PDC CT of the left temporal bone shows the subarcuate (petromastoid) canal coursing underneath the arc of the superior semicircular canal.* **(Bottom)** *Axial reformat of an EID CT in the left temporal bone in the same patient faintly depicts the subarcuate canal underneath the arch of the superior semicircular canal. The bony arcuate eminence forms the roof of the superior semicircular canal, hence the name for the subarcuate canal lying below it. The subarcuate canal transmits the subarcuate artery and vein in children < 5 years old. It usually involutes by 5 years of age, although sometimes it can persists in adults.*

TERMINOLOGY

Abbreviations

- Petrous apex (PA); internal carotid artery (ICA); internal auditory canal (IAC); petrooccipital fissure (POF)

Definitions

- Petrous bone: Pyramid-shaped medial portion of temporal bone (T-bone); contains inner ear, IAC, labyrinthine segment, anterior genu of facial nerve canal, & PA
- PA: Part of petrous bone **anteromedial to inner & IAC**

IMAGING ANATOMY

Overview

- Important unique location of PA intimately related to important anatomic structures, including POF, clivus, Meckel cave, cavernous sinus (CS), & jugular foramen
- Normal imaging appearance on CT or MR highly dependent on presence of marrow space vs. pneumatized air cells within PA
- **Bone & bone marrow of PA**
  - Most commonly, PA composed of rim of cortical bone & intrinsic trabecular bone containing bone marrow
  - PA marrow signal on MR characterized by T1 hyperintensity due to marrow fat
  - Abnormal marrow signal can be related to number of causes, ranging from benign (red marrow conversion) to malignant (myeloma, metastatic disease)
- **Pneumatization of PA**
  - Occurs in 9-30% when epithelial-lined air cells develop as medial communications from mastoid air cells
  - Highly variable in extent & can be asymmetric in 5%
  - Air cells of PA susceptible to similar pathologic processes that occur in mastoid, including obstruction, opacification, inflammation, & infection
  - Metastasis more common in nonpneumatized fatty marrow-filled PA

Extent

- PA anatomic subunit of petrous bone, anteromedial to inner ear
- PA shaped like triangular pyramid with 3 distinct sides, directed medially toward central skull base
- Base formed at junction with lateral portion of petrous bone & merges with squamous & mastoid segments of T-bone
- Along superior margin of PA, narrow ridge (**petrous ridge**) that extends from apical tip to lateral petrous bone
- Petrous ridge formed by fusion of 2 sloped surfaces (2 sides of triangular pyramid): Ventral slope & dorsal slope
- Ventral slope forms posterior wall of middle cranial fossa
- Posterior slope forms anterior wall of posterior fossa
- 3rd (inferior) side roughly horizontal, is best identified viewing extracranial surface of skull from below, & forms part of skull base

Anatomy Relationships

- **Petrous ICA canal**
  - ICA enters base of petrous bone (petrous segment)
  - ICA travels vertically for ~ 8 mm → turn horizontally (posterior genu) at level of cochlea → travels anteromedially towards apex through carotid canal
  - ICA emerges from endocranial carotid canal through irregular bony opening, just above horizontal layer of cartilage that bridges foramen lacerum → turns upward (anterior genu), becoming short lacerum segment
  - Sympathetic fibers travel along periphery of ICA through carotid canal
  - Petrous ICA gives rise to 2 branches: **Caroticotympanic artery** & **vidian artery** (artery of pterygoid canal)
- **Foramen lacerum**
  - Foramen lacerum represents gap between osseous PA (T-bone) & clivus (sphenoid bone)
  - In dried skull, best identified along extracranial aspect of skull base as irregular quadrangular or triangular space continuous superiorly into intracranial compartment, hence term foramen
  - In vivo, foramen lacerum not open; rather, inferior extracranial margin covered by horizontal plate of fibrocartilage forming floor of lacerum segment of ICA
  - On axial imaging, foramen lacerum anteromedial to POF & forms posterior margin of vidian canal
  - Important pathway for spread of disease from nasopharynx to central skull base & intracranial compartment
- **Eustachian tube (ET)**
  - Thin tubular canal that extends medially from middle ear cavity along anterolateral inferior portion of PA & squamous portion of T-bone
  - Separated from **semicanal for tensor tympani** above ET by thin, bony plate called **septum canalis musculotubarii**
  - Tensor tympani muscle & ET cross anteriorly & medially from middle ear to nasopharynx, passing through small gap (**petrosphenoid fissure**) between greater wing of sphenoid & anterior margin of PA
  - As ET passes through this gap, lies medial to foramen spinosum, posterior to foramen ovale, & immediately anterior to horizontal petrous ICA canal
  - At this location, ET transitions from bony canal from middle ear to cartilaginous canal that extends to torus tubarius of nasopharynx
  - Anterior cartilaginous component often collapsed at imaging & seen only as soft tissue density or signal; occasionally, it contains air or fluid
- **POF (a.k.a. petroclival fissure)**
  - POF oblique junction between petrous T-bone & basilar occipital bone
  - Joins posterior aspect of foramen lacerum
  - Clinical relevance: Cartilage occupying POF site of origin for majority of skull base chondrosarcomas
- **Trigeminal nerve & Meckel cave**
  - **Trigeminal impression**: Shallow groove along petrous ridge superiorly & anteriorly near tip of apex
  - **Porus trigeminus** represents small opening formed by trigeminal impression of PA below & tentorial insertion & superior petrosal sinus along ridge above
  - Trigeminal nerve passes through porus trigeminus into **Meckel cave** cistern
  - Meckel cave variable in size, houses trigeminal ganglion
  - Meckel cave formed by meningeal layer of dura lined by arachnoid; pia covers CNV in trigeminal cave
  - Lateral wall relatively thick, consisting of 2 layers of dura

- Meckel cave filled with CSF (90%) & continuous with prepontine subarachnoid space
- Meckel cave inferior & posterior to CS
- **Dorello canal & CNVI**
  - Small gap separates medial & superior PA tip from clivus
  - Small ligament, **petrosphenoid ligament of Gruber**, crosses from PA tip to base of posterior clinoid process, creating small bridge or roof over gap
    - This gap or space, called **Dorello canal**, contains venous tissue at confluence of posterior CS & petrosal sinuses
  - CNVI passes from prepontine cistern through Dorello canal to enter CS
  - CNVI palsy & ophthalmoplegia most common symptom related to PA mass
  - Dorsal meningeal artery pass through Dorello canal
- **Petrolingual ligament (PLL)**
  - Extends form PA to lingula of sphenoid bone
  - PLL invariably surrounds dorsal & lateral walls of lacerum segment of ICA
  - PLL oriented in sagittal plane just medial to trigeminal ganglion in Meckel cave
  - Important **surgical landmark** that marks point at which **ICA lacerum** segment transitions **to cavernous segment**
  - Marks inferior & posterior margin of CS
- **CS**
  - CS, superior petrosal sinus, & inferior petrosal sinus converge at petroclival junction
  - Margins of CS roof partially determined by petroclinoid dural folds
    - **Anterior petroclinoid fold**: Anterior extension of tentorial edge from PA to anterior clinoid process
      - Forms lateral margin of CS roof separating roof from CS lateral wall
    - **Posterior petroclinoid fold** extends from tentorial edge at PA to posterior clinoid process
    - **Interclinoid fold** extends from anterior to posterior clinoid process
    - These dural folds form **oculomotor triangle**, central portion of CS roof through which CNIII (oculomotor nerve) & cistern pass
  - Lateral wall of CS extends from superior orbital fissure to PA, just medial to trigeminal impression
    - Posteroinferior part of lateral wall of CS contiguous with upper margin of PLL
- **Nasopharynx**
  - Nasopharyngeal mucosa & superior constrictor muscle anchored to skull base by pharyngobasilar fascia
  - Pharyngobasilar fascia attached to clivus, inferior PA, POF, & foramen lacerum
  - **ET** passes from skull base through **sinus of Morgagni** (gap in fascia & superior constrictor muscle) & terminates in lateral wall of nasopharynx at torus tubarius
  - **Levator veli palatini** muscle originates from PA undersurface & also passes through sinus of Morgagni
  - Tumor & infection can spread from nasopharynx to skull base via ET, sinus of Morgagni, foramen ovale, or direct invasion
  - Foramen lacerum also potential pathway of invasion of nasopharyngeal lesion to skull base & CS
  - Vidian canal, tiny, inconsistent palatovaginal canal, & vomerovaginal canal can transmit disease from nasopharyngeal skull base to pterygopalatine fossa
- **Jugular foramen**
  - Inferolateral petrous bone forms lateral border of jugular foramen
- **IAC**
  - Narrow passage along posterior & lateral margin of PA
  - Transmits CNVII & CNVIII
- **Greater superficial petrosal nerve**
  - Passes from geniculate ganglion through facial hiatus into epidural space along ventral surface of PA
  - Parasympathetic fibers join sympathetic fibers from ICA to become vidian nerve within vidian canal

ANATOMY IMAGING ISSUES

Imaging Recommendations

- T-bone CT excellent for defining osseous destruction & normal-variant asymmetric PA aeration
- CTA useful for evaluation of petrous ICA
- MR of skull base with T1 noncontrast & nonfat-saturated images combined with contrast-enhanced fat-saturated images allows comprehensive evaluation of soft tissue, marrow space, CS, & cranial nerves

CLINICAL IMPLICATIONS

Clinical Importance

- PA not visible by direct examination; therefore, evaluation of anatomy & pathology requires cross-sectional imaging
- Most common symptom related to PA mass: CNVI palsy
- **Triad of Gradenigo syndrome**
  - Otorrhea & ear pain: Suppurative otitis media
  - Diplopia: CNVI palsy in/around PA, including Dorello canal from apical petrositis
  - Facial pain: Retroorbital/trigeminal nerve distribution pain due to adjacent trigeminal nerve/Meckel cave inflammation

Normal Findings/Variants Mimicking Petrous Apex Mass

- **PA trapped fluid**: Nonexpansile
  - CT: Opacified air cells; **cortex & trabeculae intact**
  - T1W MR: Low/intermediate signal or minimally hyperintense (rarely bright); T2W MR hyperintense
  - T1 C+ MR: No enhancement of lesion or meninges
- **PA asymmetric marrow**: Nonexpansile
  - CT: Fat density of nonpneumatized PA marrow
  - T1W MR: Hyperintense; T2W MR intermediate to hyperintense signal; **suppresses** on fat-saturated MR
- **PA cephalocele**: Expansile
  - Congenitally deficient dura or CSF pulsations producing erosion of thin bone over pneumatized PA
  - May be rare cause of CSF otorrhea, meningitis, or trigeminal neuralgia
  - Associations: Idiopathic intracranial hypertension (pseudotumor cerebri), NF1, Usher syndrome
  - CT: Sharply marginated PA lucency; cisternography contrast enters lesion
  - MR: CSF-like on all sequences; peripheral enhancement of venous plexus around Gasserian ganglion

NORMAL PETROUS APEX ANATOMY

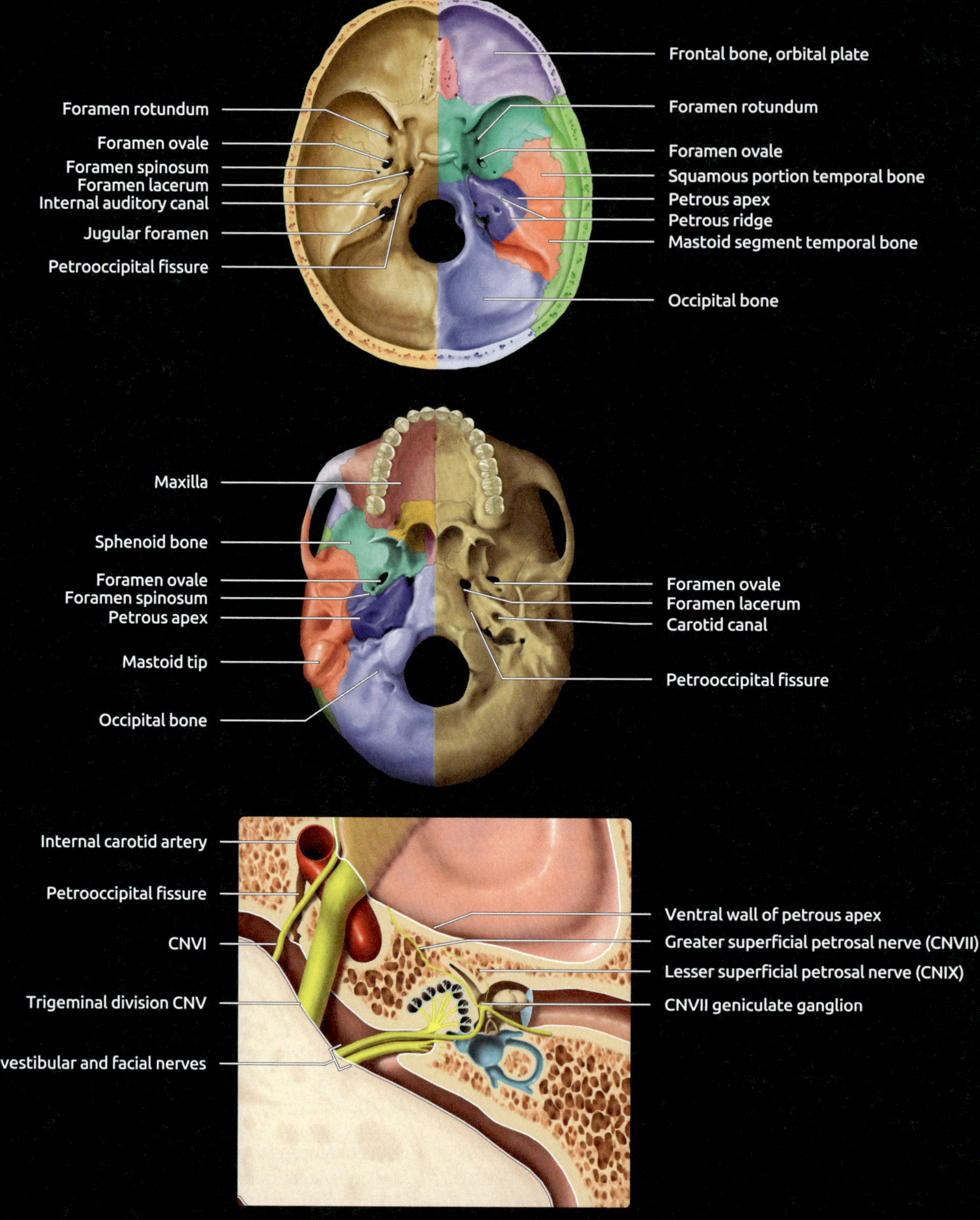

(Top) *Graphic of the skull base from above shows petrous apex (PA) in blue represents pyramidal-shaped medial extension of temporal bone. Petrous ridge is formed by junction of ventral & dorsal slopes. Ventral slope forms posterior margin of middle cranial fossa; dorsal slope forms anterior margin of posterior fossa. Note relationship of PA with sphenoid bone, foramen lacerum, jugular foramen, & clivus.* **(Middle)** *External/extracranial view of skull base shows undersurface of PA (blue). Note relationship of PA with irregular, oblique petrooccipital fissure (POF) that separates PA from occipital bone. Foramen lacerum represents a gap between PA & clivus. In a dried skull, this is an opening that communicates with intracranial compartment. In vivo, this opening is covered by fibrocartilage.* **(Bottom)** *Axial graphic shows PA below surface of petrous ridge. Petrous carotid is located along anterior margin. CNVI & CNV course over the anterior superior margin near medial tip. Internal auditory canal & inner ear are at posterior margin. Greater superficial petrosal nerve carries parasympathetic fibers from facial nerve geniculate ganglion through facial hiatus along epidural surface of PA to vidian canal.*

NORMAL ANATOMY OF PETROUS APEX: AXIAL CT

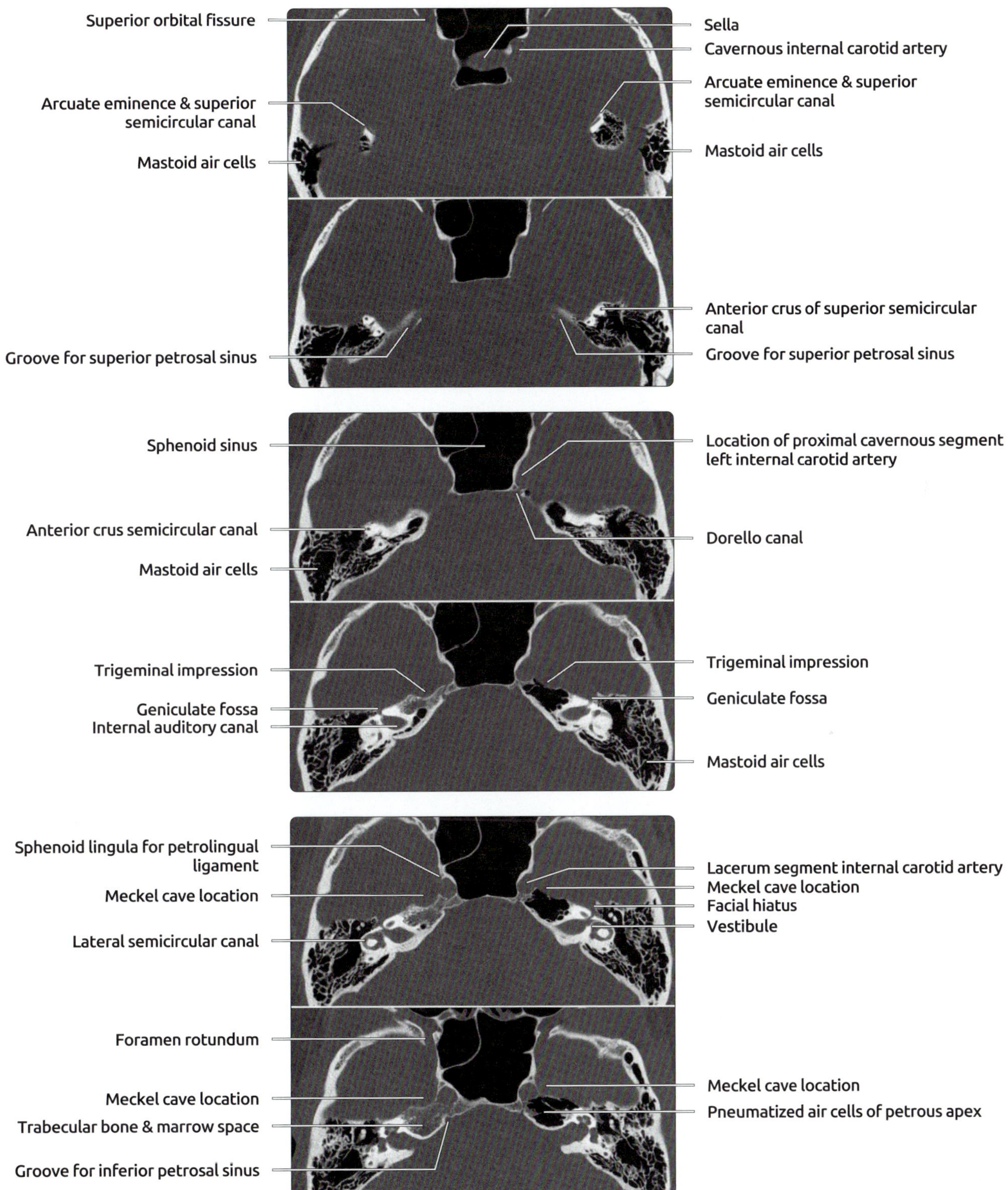

(Top) *Axial CT images show the petrous ridge through the skull base. Superior semicircular canal projects superiorly from the vestibule of the inner ear, & overlying bone often produces small elevation, arcuate eminence. The superior petrosal sinus lies within the groove along the attachment of the tentorium cerebelli of the petrous ridge.* **(Middle)** *Axial upper temporal bone CT images show extensive pneumatization of mastoid air cells bilaterally. Pneumatization extends into PAs bilaterally but asymmetrically. Along superior aspect of the petroclival junction there is a small "canal," the Dorello canal, bounded by PA (inferolateral), clivus (inferomedial), & petrosphenoidal ligament of Gruber (superiorly). CNVI passes from prepontine cistern through the Dorello canal into the cavernous sinus. Note trigeminal impression near PA tip.* **(Bottom)** *Axial CT images through the inner ear level show asymmetric pneumatization of PAs. Note the relationship of PA to lacerum segment of internal carotid artery (ICA) medially as well as its relationship to Meckel cave. Facial hiatus represents a small opening from geniculate ganglion to ventral face of PA & transmits greater superficial petrosal nerve.*

NORMAL ANATOMY OF PETROUS APEX: AXIAL CT

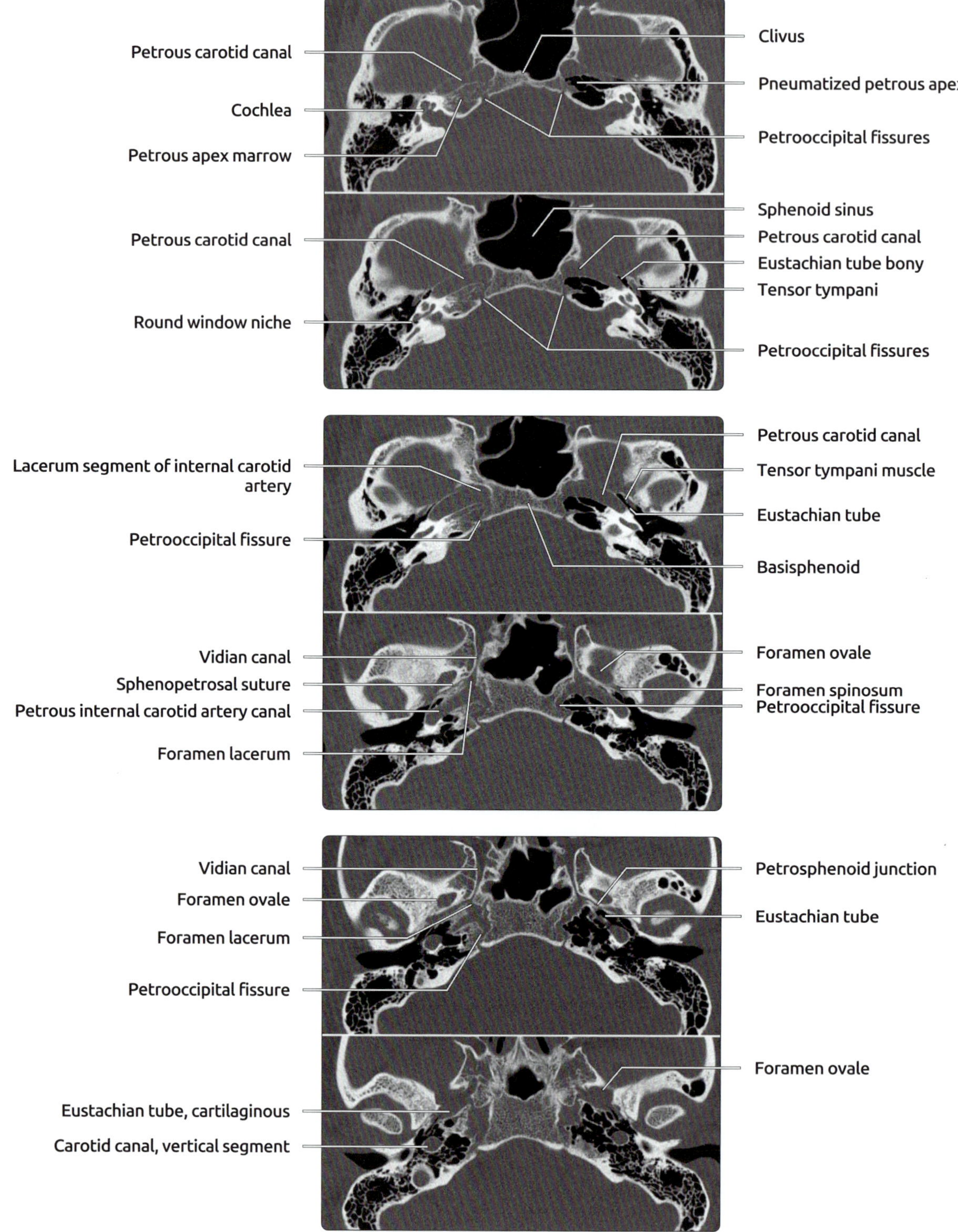

(Top) *Descending axial CT images through PAs are shown. POFs are identified bilaterally. At this level, POFs are mostly fused solid with a small groove posteriorly for inferior petrosal sinus. Anterior genu of the petrous ICA turns upward to become lacerum segment. Note the intimate relationship of the anterior genus to the sphenoid sinus.* **(Middle)** *Selected descending axial CT images through the temporal bone again show asymmetry in PAs. The horizontal carotid canal passes obliquely through the petrous bone, from lateral to medial, & the medial opening is just superior to foramen lacerum.* **(Bottom)** *Axial CT images through the central skull base at the level of the inferior aspect of PA demonstrate funnel-shaped vidian canals that transmit vidian nerves through sphenoid bone from foramen lacerum region to pterygopalatine fossa. Note cartilaginous POF appears to merge anteriorly with cartilaginous-filled foramen lacerum. The foramen lacerum is a bony gap that is covered by cartilage, & this cartilaginous plate serves as the floor of the medial carotid canal. As the horizontal petrous portion of ICA reaches this point, it turns upward, & the short vertical segment is called the lacerum segment.*

NORMAL PETROUS APEX: CECT

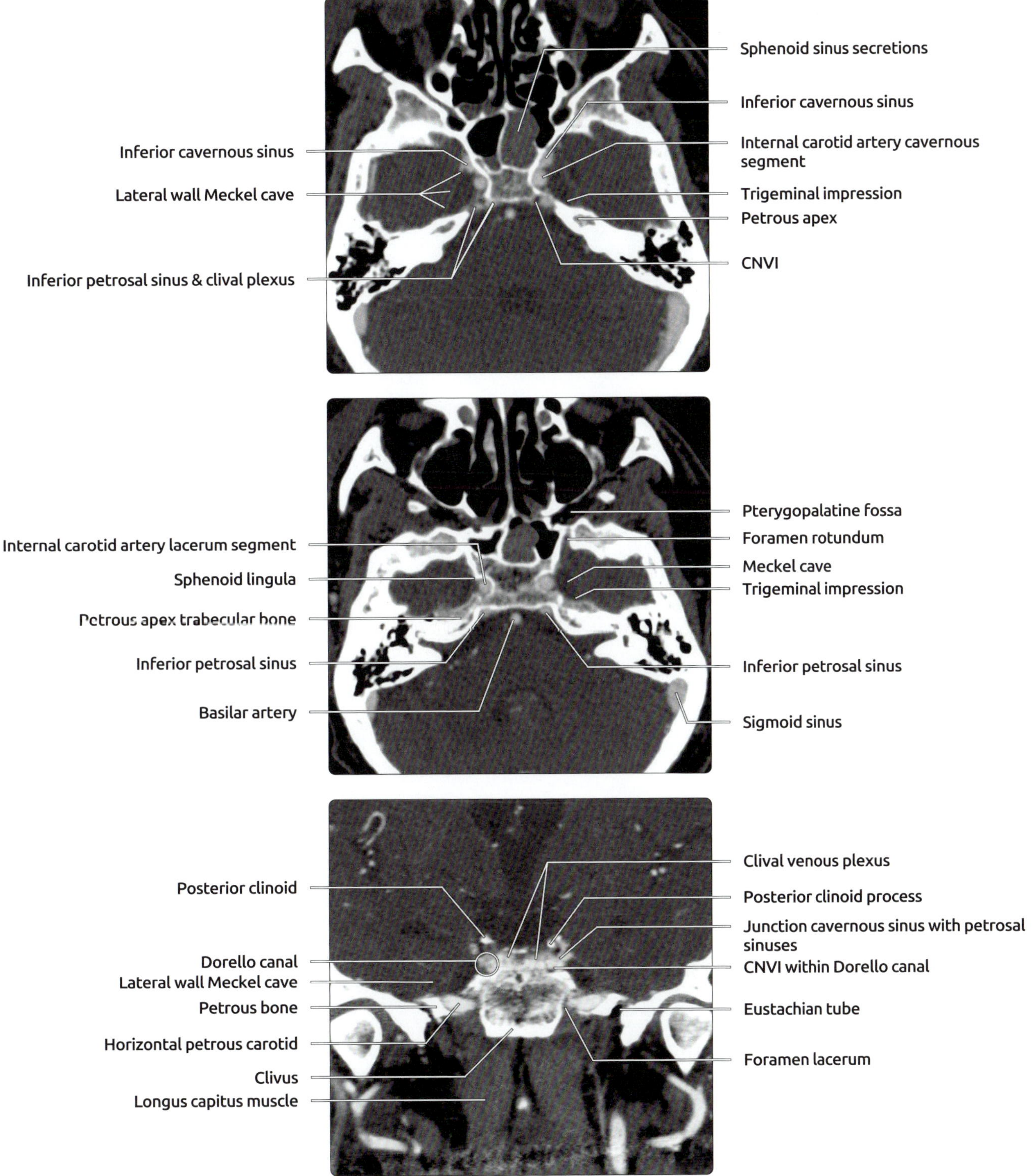

(Top) *Axial source image from a CTA demonstrates opacification of the ICAs (lacerum segments) bilaterally. There is also venous opacification of cavernous sinuses & inferior petrosal sinuses bilaterally. CNVI can be seen passing through the venous plexus within the Dorello canal bilaterally en route to the cavernous sinus.* **(Middle)** *Axial CTA through the skull base shows the relationship of the lacerum segment ICA to trigeminal impression & lower Meckel cave. Intraarterial contrast is identified within ICAs bilaterally as well as the basilar artery. There is also contrast in inferior petrosal sinuses bilaterally. In this case, there is symmetric lack of pneumatization of PAs.* **(Bottom)** *Coronal CECT through the clivus demonstrates the relationship of Meckel cave to the distal horizontal petrous ICA. CNVI can be visualized passing through the region of the Dorello canal. It is seen as a nonenhancing filling defect within enhancing venous plexus at the junction of the cavernous sinus & petrosal sinuses. The foramen lacerum is a triangular opening in the inferior skull base between the inferior tip of the PA & clivus. Cartilage bridges the gap horizontally & forms the floor of the lacerum segment of the ICA.*

NORMAL PETROUS APEX: T1 MR CISTERNOGRAM

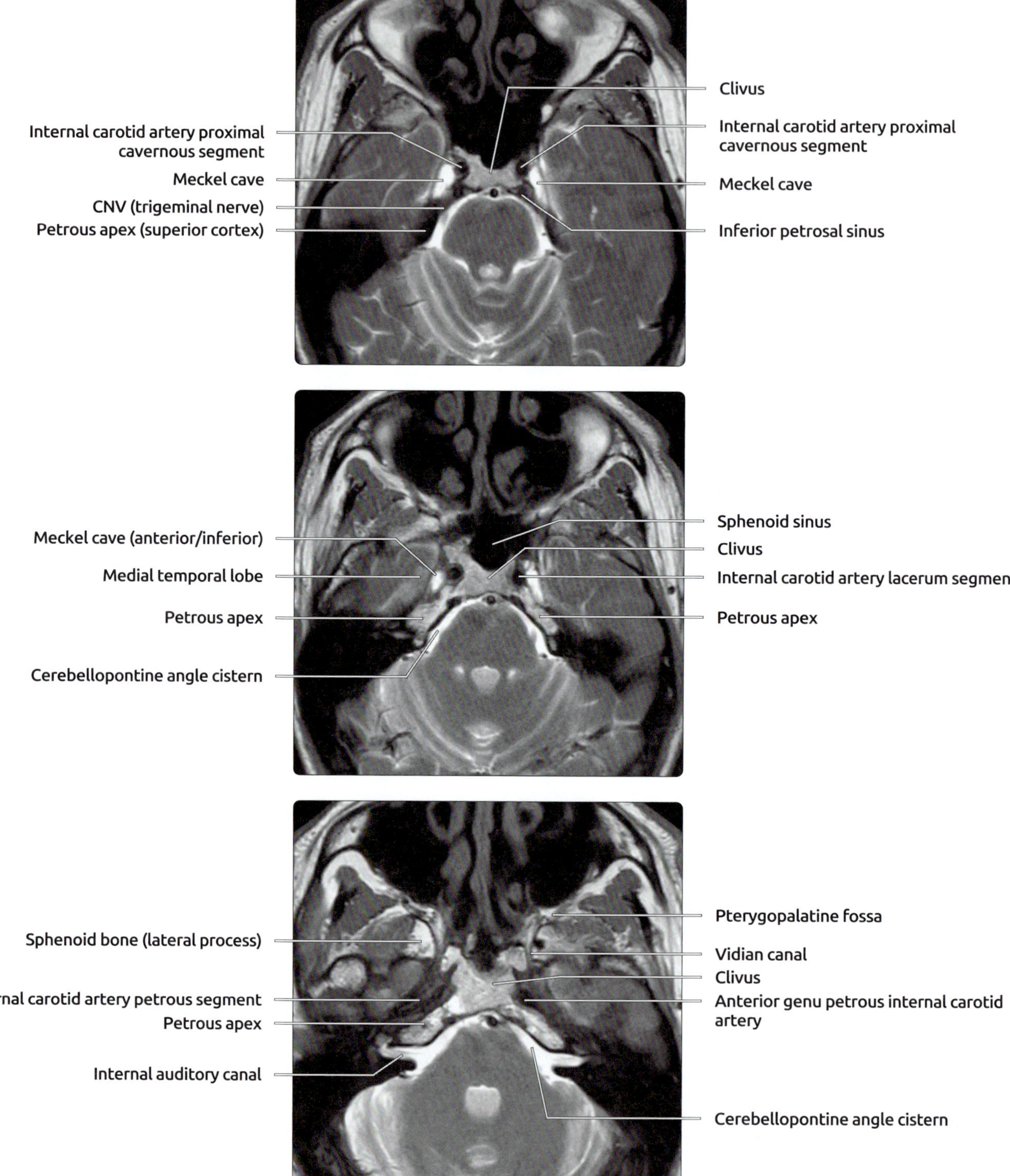

(Top) *Axial T1W MR performed following intrathecal gadolinium (off-label use) in a patient undergoing MR cisternogram is shown. Increased signal is identified within the CSF spaces, including prepontine cistern & Meckel cave, due to presence of gadolinium. At this axial level, CNV (trigeminal nerve) is passing over the superior cortical rim of the PA along the trigeminal impression. The upper clivus (basisphenoid) is relatively hyperintense due to marrow fat. With this technique, normal venous structures are relatively hypointense & do not enhance.* **(Middle)** *Axial T1W MR performed following intrathecal gadolinium (off-label use) is shown. This axial slice is below that of the previous image. The PAs are relatively hyperintense due to presence of marrow fat that is contiguous with marrow fat of the clivus.* **(Bottom)** *Axial T1 C+ MR through the internal auditory canal demonstrates hyperintensity of the CSF in canals secondary to intrathecal gadolinium. The petrous ICAs are partially visualized as hypointense flow voids. The vidian canal contains fat & the vidian nerve & is contiguous anteriorly with the pterygopalatine fossa.*

ANATOMIC-PATHOLOGIC CORRELATION: PETROOCCIPITAL FISSURE CHONDROSARCOMA

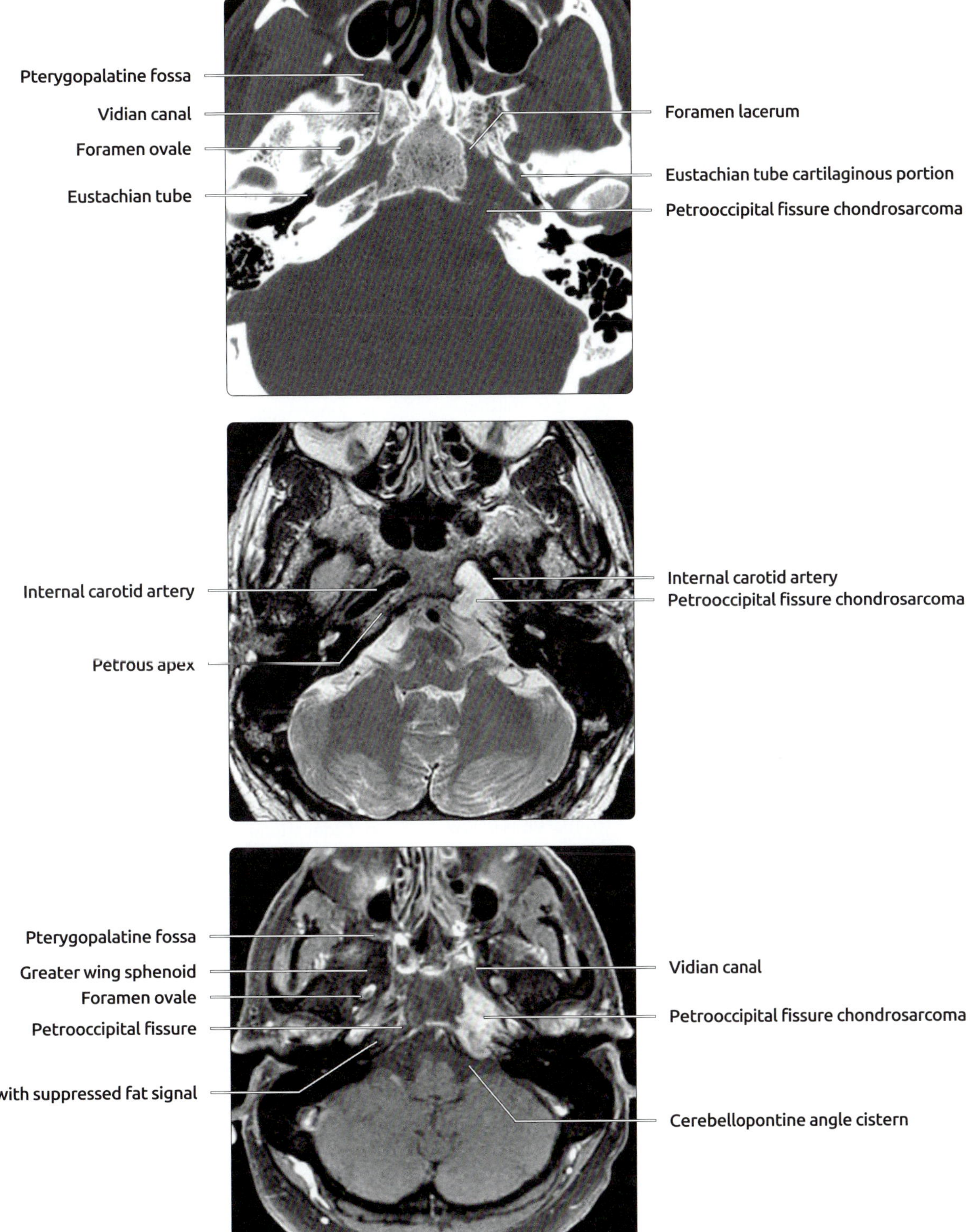

(Top) *POF chondrosarcoma is shown. Axial bone CT through the PAs demonstrates a lytic, destructive lesion involving the left PA. Note the medial aspect of the lesion involves the POF, a clue to the diagnosis in this case of POF chondrosarcoma. While some chondrosarcomas will demonstrate chondroid calcifications, many lesions in this location are predominantly lytic without calcified matrix.* **(Middle)** *Axial T2 MR through the central skull base demonstrates a lobulated, hyperintense lesion arising from the POF. This is path-proven chondrosarcoma. The lesion pushes the petrous ICA anterolaterally. While the lesion appears to have cystic qualities with similar signal to CSF on T2W images, the lesion is actually solid & demonstrates avid enhancement.* **(Bottom)** *Axial contrast-enhanced MR with fat-saturated technique allows suppression of any high signal related to fat & allows better detection of enhancing lesions that might occur in bone marrow. This chondrosarcoma demonstrates robust enhancement at the POF & PA. The lesion is expansile, causing bone destruction & marrow replacement.*

TERMINOLOGY

Abbreviations

- Cerebellopontine angle (CPA); internal auditory canal (IAC); internal acoustic meatus (IAM); anterior inferior cerebellar artery (AICA); superior vestibular nerve (SVN); inferior vestibular nerve (IVN)

Definitions

- **CPA-IAC cistern**: CSF space in CPA & IAC containing CNVII, CNVIII, & AICA loop
- **Porus acusticus**: Large opening at medial aspect of IAC connecting it to CPA cistern
- **IAC fundus**: Lateral CSF-filled cap of IAC cistern containing distal CNVII & CNVIII [SVN, IVN, & cochlear nerve (CN)]
- **Macula cribrosa**: Perforated bone between IAC & vestibule
- **CN canal (CNC)**: Bony opening connecting IAC fundus to cochlea
- **Cochlear aperture (CA)**, a.k.a. **modiolar base** or **cochlear fossette**: Bony opening at base of modiolus transmitting blood vessels & nerve fibers from spiral ganglion to CN
- CNC, CA, & modiolar base terms interchangeably used
- CNC (CA) width: Narrowest diameter between IAC fundus & modiolus on axial images
- **CNC/CA hypoplasia**: Width < **1.4 mm**
- **Isolated cochlea**: CNC (CA) absent & filled with bone
- **Narrow IAC**: < 2.5 mm at midpoint of IAC

IMAGING ANATOMY

Internal Contents

- **CNVII & CNVIII position in IAC**
  - Anteriorly: **"7up (CNVII)/Coke (CN VIII) down"**
  - Posteriorly: Vestibular nerves; SVN up, IVN down
  - **Crista falciformis** (horizontal crest): Horizontal bony projection from IAC fundus
    - Separates facial nerve/SVN above from CN/IVN below
  - **Bill bar** (vertical crest): Vertical bony ridge in superior portion of IAC fundus
    - Separates facial nerve anteriorly from SVN posteriorly
- **Vestibulocochlear nerve (CNVIII)**: CPA-IAC cistern
  - Components: SVN, IVN, & CN
    - Vestibular (balance) & cochlear (hearing) portions
  - Vestibular nerve sensory ganglion (**Scarpa ganglion**) situated at lateral aspect of IAC
  - **CN portion, CNVIII course**
    - Leaves **spiral ganglion** as auditory axons
    - Travels as **CN** in anterior-inferior quadrant of IAC
    - Joins SVN & IVN at porus acusticus to **become CNVIII bundle in CPA cistern**
    - Crosses CPA cistern as posterior nerve bundle to enter brainstem at pontomedullary junction
    - Enters brainstem & bifurcates to synapse with both dorsal & ventral cochlear nuclei
    - Normal **CN larger** than either SVN or IVN in 90%
    - Normal **CN** almost similar size of facial nerve, or larger than facial nerve in 64%
    - CN deficiency: CN hypoplasia or absence (aplasia)
    - CN size correlates with spiral ganglion cell population, but thin CN may still transmit impulses for hearing
- **Facial nerve (CNVII): CPA-IAC cistern**
  - Root exit zone in pontomedullary junction
  - Travels anterior to CNVIII in CPA cistern
  - Anterosuperior in IAC cistern
- **Nervus intermedius of Wrisberg (NIW/intermediate nerve/glossopalatine nerve)**
  - NIW exits brainstem at pontomedullary junction between pons & inferior cerebellar peduncle lateral to motor root of facial nerve & medial to vestibulocochlear nerve
  - NIW then courses along with motor root of facial nerve through CPA into anterosuperior IAC quadrant
  - NIW joins motor root of facial nerve (CNVII) near geniculate ganglion in temporal bone
  - NIW: Somatic sensory, special sensory, & visceral motor (secretomotor) fibers from various brainstem nuclei
  - **Superior salivatory nucleus** in pons: **Parasympathetic** root through NIW → facial nerve → **greater superficial petrosal nerve (GSPN)** → vidian nerve → pterygopalatine ganglion → **nasal** & **lacrimal glands**
  - Superior salivatory nucleus in pons: Parasympathetic root through NIW → facial nerve → **chorda tympani** nerve → lingual nerve → submandibular ganglion → **submandibular & sublingual salivary glands**
  - **Nucleus of tractus solitarius (NTS)** in medulla/lower pons: **Geniculate ganglion** at anterior genu of CNVII in temporal bone contains pseudounipolar cell bodies
    - Central processes of cell bodies enter gustatory part of NTS, forming special visceral afferent root
    - Peripheral processes receive **taste** sensation from anterior 2/3 of tongue through **chorda tympani** & palate through **GSPN**
  - **Main sensory nucleus of CNV** in pons: General somatic afferents **sensation** from **lateral pinna, posterior external auditory canal, & mastoid** through **geniculate ganglion**
- **Vestibular schwannoma (VS) anatomic origin**
  - Older studies suggested predominantly IVN origin of VS
  - Later studies found equal SVN & IVN origins of VS
  - VS classically thought to arise at glial-Schwann cell junction (Obersteiner-Redlich zone)
  - Later histologic studies of small VS have shown their origin from cells laterally in IAC within or near Scarpa ganglion rather than central glial-Schwann cell junction
  - Some authors suggested VS origin from Schwann cells in axonal sheaths anywhere from glial-Schwann junction to nerve termination in vestibule laterally
  - **NIW (intermediate nerve)** could be origin of some VS & CNVII schwannomas
  - **Intermediate nerve schwannoma**: VS originating medial to IAC with more cystic components, larger size, rapid growth in cistern medially towards pons, & earlier cerebellar, trigeminal, facial, & CN dysfunction
- **AICA loop**
  - Arises from basilar artery then rises into IAC
  - Continues in IAC as **internal auditory artery** (IAA)
  - May mimic cranial nerve on high-resolution T2 MR
  - IAA supplies 3 branches to inner ear
- **Other structures in CPA cistern**
  - **Flocculus** of cerebellum in posteromedial CPA
  - **Choroid plexus** passes from 4th ventricle though foramen of Luschka into CPA cistern

GRAPHICS

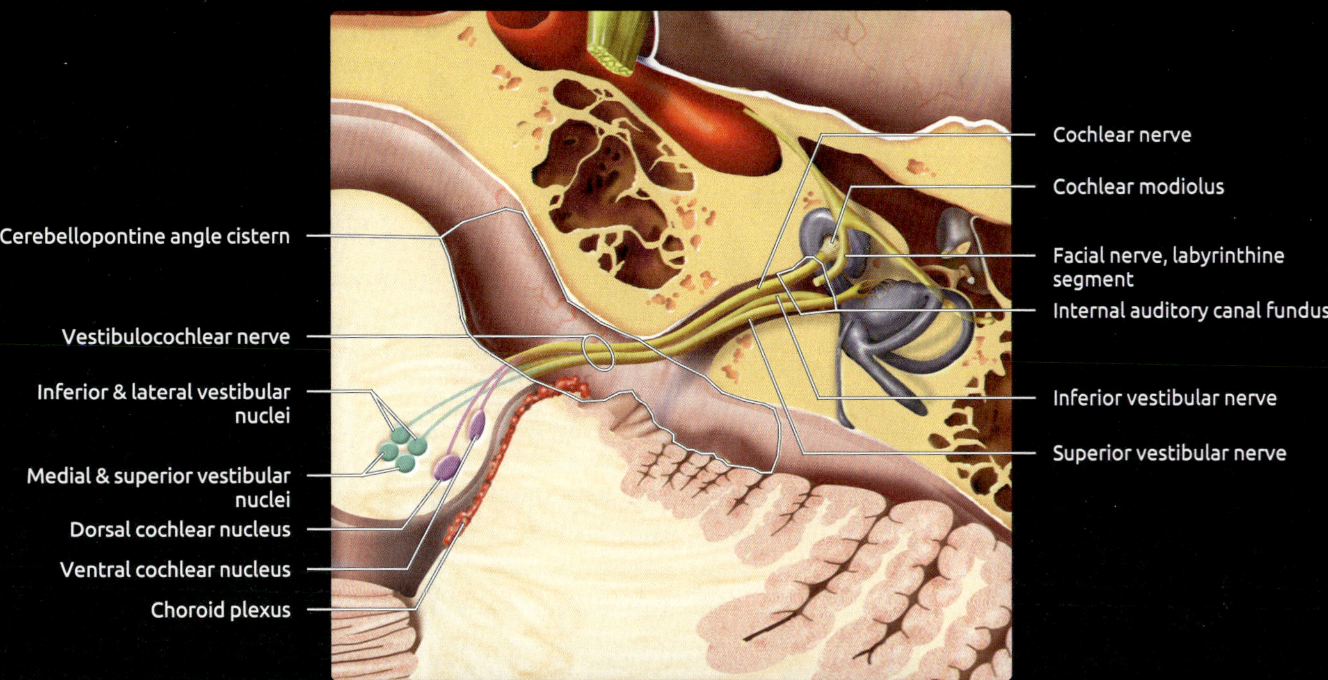

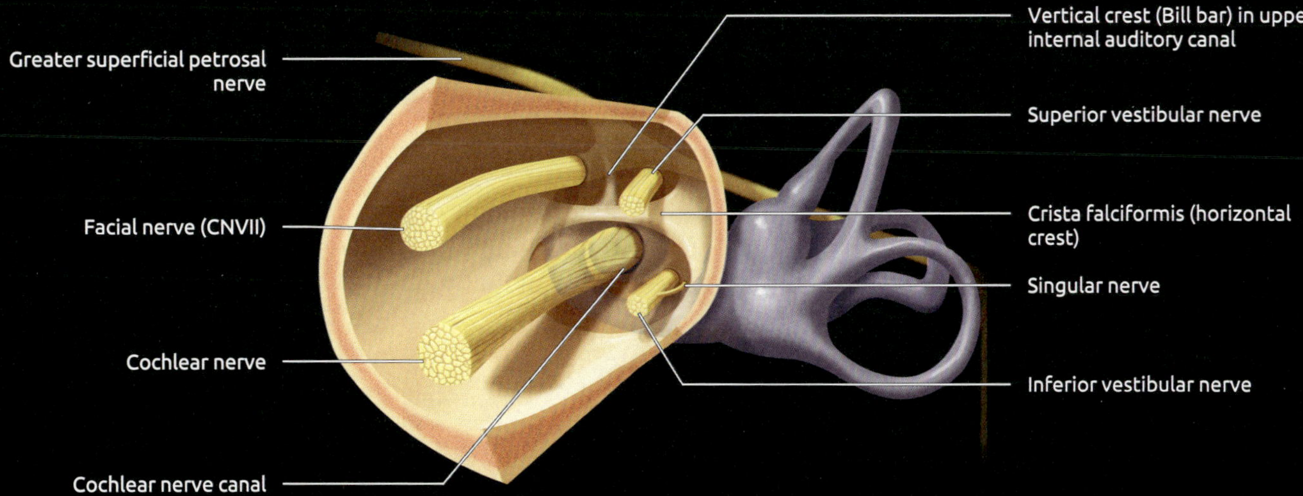

(Top) *Graphic shows the cerebellopontine angle-internal auditory canal (CPA-IAC) cisterns & inner ear. The inferior & superior vestibular nerves begin in cell bodies in the vestibular ganglion, from there coursing centrally to 4 vestibular nuclei. Cochlear component of CNVIII begins in bipolar cell bodies in spiral ganglion of modiolus. Central fibers run in cochlear nerve to dorsal & ventral cochlear nuclei near inferior cerebellar peduncle. Facial nerve lies in anterosuperior IAC, & the nervus intermedius of Wrisberg (not shown) courses along with the motor root of facial nerve in CPA, joining it near the geniculate ganglion in temporal bone.* **(Bottom)** *Graphic depicts fundus of the IAC. Note horizontal crista falciformis separates the facial nerve & superior vestibular nerve above from cochlear nerve & inferior vestibular nerve below, while the vertical crest (Bill bar) separates the facial nerve from the superior vestibular nerve. Sagittal oblique high-resolution T2 imaging has become critically important in work-up of cochlear implant candidates because it is now possible to determine if a cochlear nerve is present with this type of imaging. No cochlear nerve significantly diminishes cochlear implant outcome.*

AXIAL GRAPHIC & CORONAL T2 MR

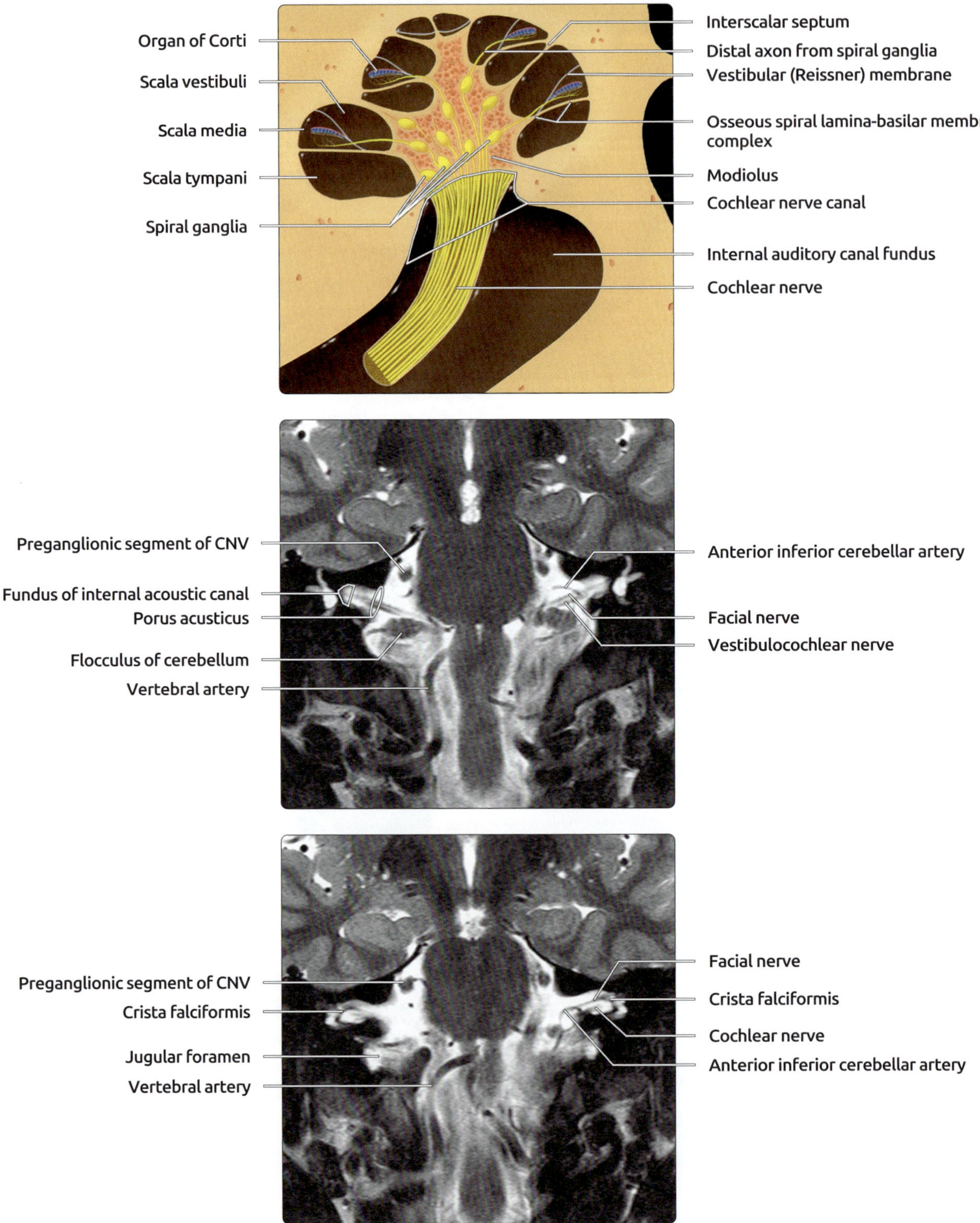

(Top) *Axial graphic of the cochlea shows the bony modiolus, cochlear nerve canal, & cochlear nerve in IAC fundus. CT & MR imaging identifies the scala tympani & vestibuli but not the scala media. Note that the interscalar septum separates the cochlear turns (unlike what its name sounds like, interscalar septa are not between the scala of cochlea). The spiral ganglion are a group of bipolar neuron cell bodies of the cochlear nerve. Cochlear nerve fibers traverse the modiolus, branching onto the osseous spiral lamina-basal membrane complex, & then innervate the organ of Corti hair cells in the scala media.* **(Middle)** *First of 2 coronal T2 MR images presented from posterior to anterior through the CPA & IAC cisterns shows important regional structures, including the preganglionic segment of CNV, anterior inferior cerebellar artery loop, flocculus of cerebellum, & vertebral artery.* **(Bottom)** *This image shows the crista falciformis in the fundus of the IAC. The facial nerve & superior vestibular nerve are above & the cochlear nerve & inferior vestibular nerve are below the crista falciformis.*

AXIAL BONE CT

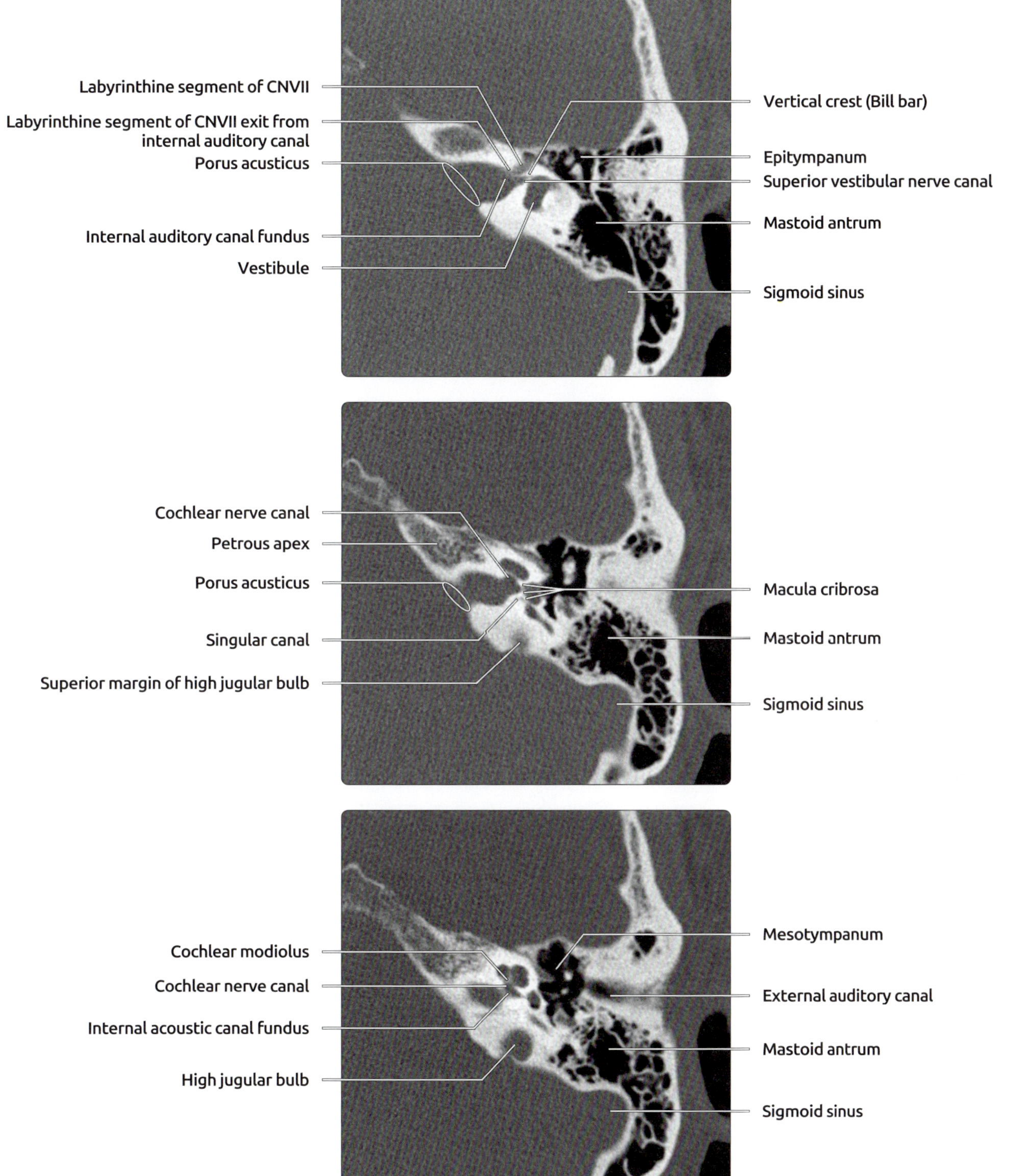

(Top) *First of 3 axial bone CT images of the left ear through the IAC presented from superior to inferior shows the labyrinthine segment of the facial nerve exiting the anterosuperior fundus of the IAC. Note also that the vertical crest separates the anterior labyrinthine segment of CNVII from the posterior superior vestibular nerve canal in the upper aspect of the IAC.* **(Middle)** *This image shows the cochlear nerve canal connecting the anteroinferior fundus of the IAC to the cochlea. The cochlear nerve accesses the modiolus of the cochlea through the cochlear nerve canal. Note the posterolateral fundal bony wall abutting the medial vestibule. Multiple branches of vestibular nerves pass through this wall (the macula cribrosa) to the vestibule & semicircular canals. A singular canal extends from the posteroinferior wall of IAC fundus to the ampulla of the posterior semicircular canal & contains the singular nerve (posterior ampullary nerve), a branch of inferior vestibular nerve, to the posterior semicircular canal.* **(Bottom)** *Last image shows the cochlear modiolus as a high-density structure at the cochlear base near the cochlear nerve canal. High-riding jugular bulb projects above the level of IAC floor.*

SAGITTAL T2 MR

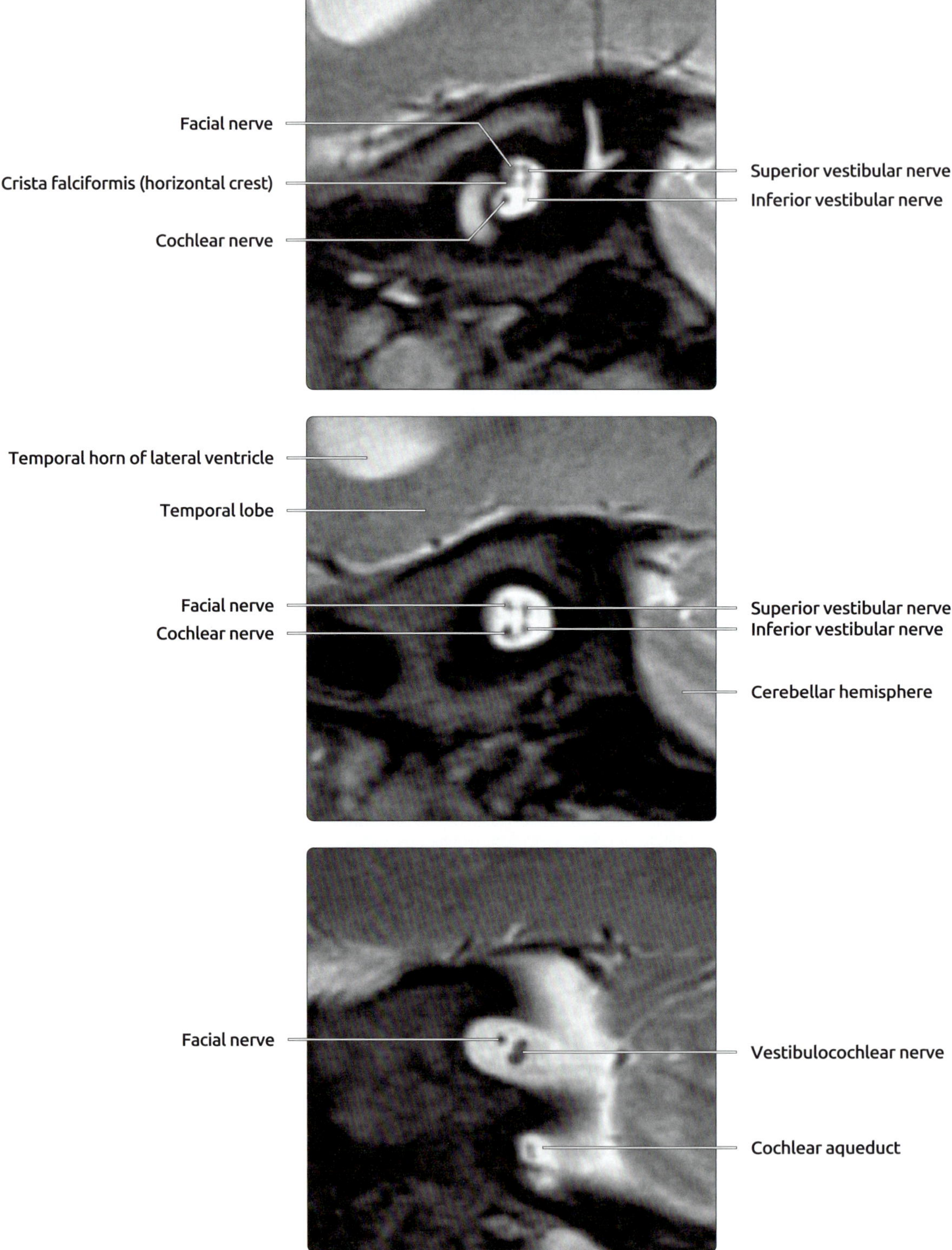

(Top) *First of 3 oblique sagittal high-resolution T2 MR images presented from lateral to medial shows the IAC fundus filled with high-signal CSF. The horizontal low-signal line in the fundus is the crista falciformis. The facial nerve is anterosuperior, whereas the cochlear nerve is anteroinferior. A good mnemonic for the anatomic arrangement of nerves in the anterior aspect of the IAC is "7-up (CNVII)/Coke (CNVIII) down." Vestibular nerves lie posteriorly in the IAC with the superior vestibular nerve (SVN) up & inferior vestibular nerve (IVN) down.* **(Middle)** *In this image through the mid-IAC, the 4 discrete nerves are well seen. Notice that the anteroinferior cochlear nerve is normally slightly larger than the other 3 nerves in the IAC.* **(Bottom)** *At the level of the porus acusticus, the facial nerve is visible just anterior to the vestibulocochlear nerve. The overall appearance of these 2 nerves is that of a ball (facial nerve) in a catcher's mitt (vestibulocochlear nerve). The vestibulocochlear nerve contains the cochlear, inferior, & superior vestibular nerves.*

AXIAL T2 MR

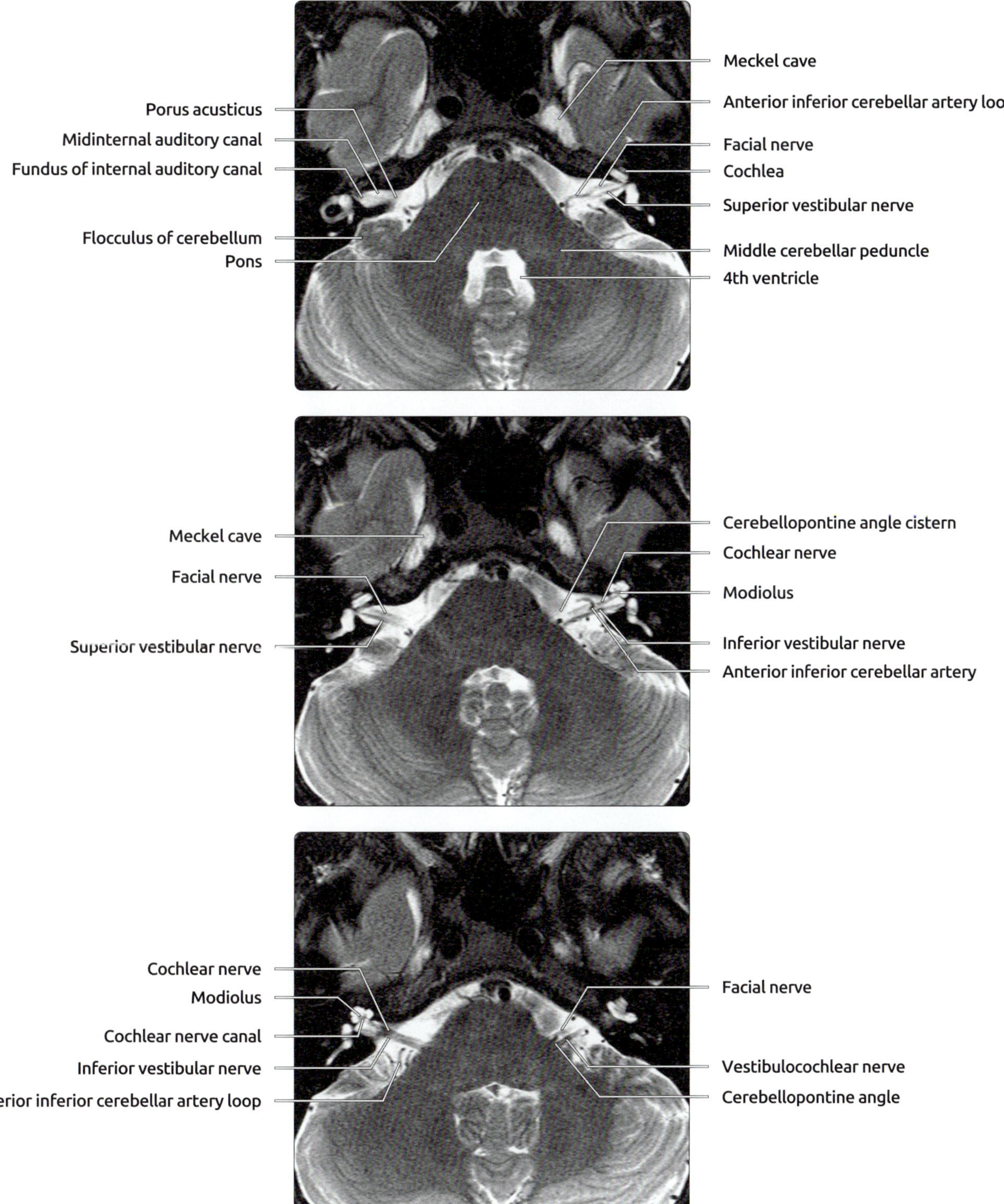

(Top) *First of 3 axial T2 MR images presented from superior to inferior reveals the porus acusticus, midportion, & fundus of the IAC on the right. On the left, the anterior inferior cerebellar artery is seen looping through the CPA cistern. Also note the facial nerve & superior vestibular nerve on the left within the IAC.* **(Middle)** *In this image, the facial nerve & superior vestibular nerve are seen in the right IAC, & the cochlear nerve & inferior vestibular nerve are visible on the left.* **(Bottom)** *In this image, the cochlear nerve is seen in the right IAC exiting through the cochlear nerve canal to reach the modiolus of the cochlea. On the left, the CPA is seen with the vestibulocochlear nerve emerging from the brainstem at this point.*

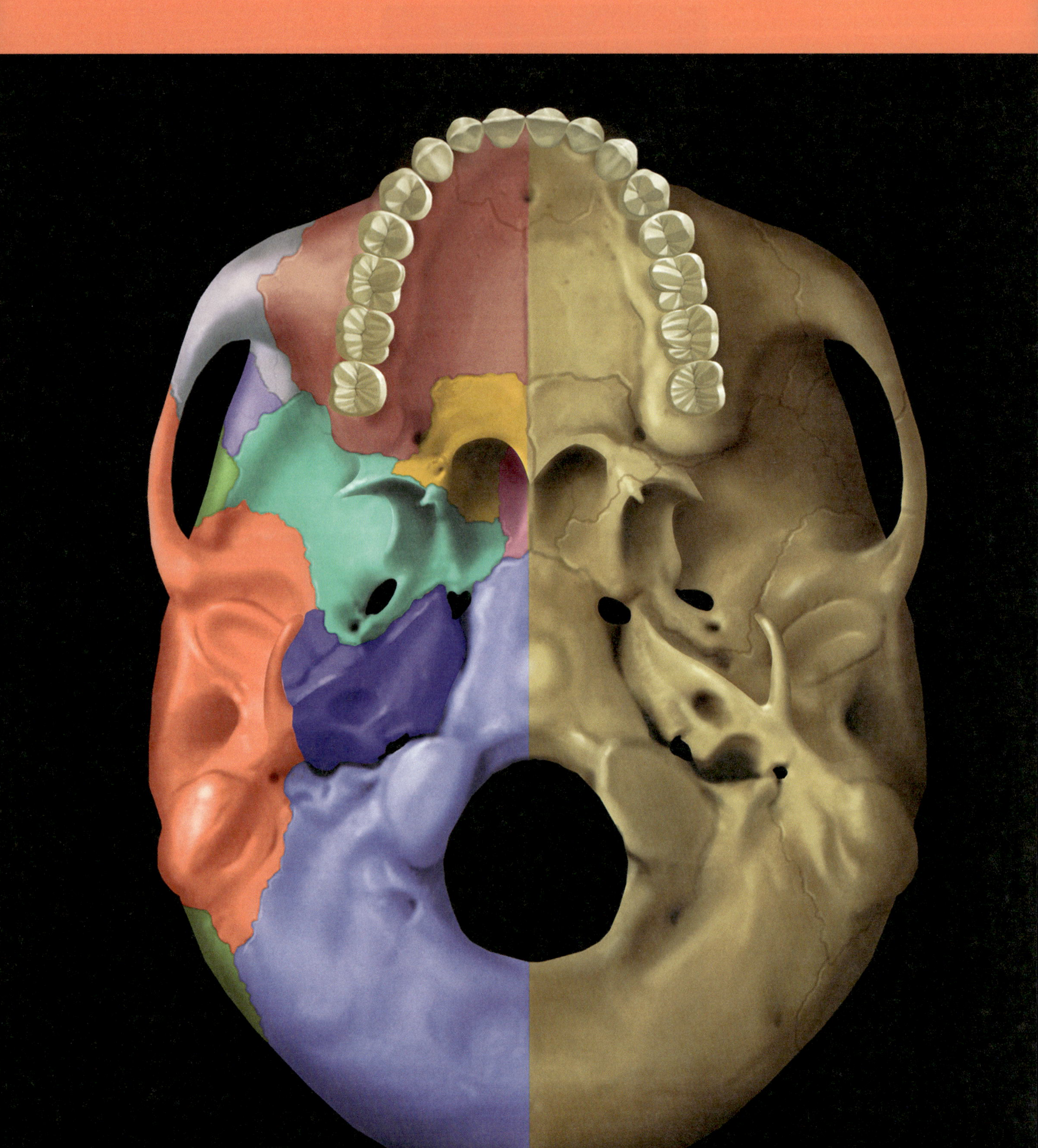

SECTION 5

Skull Base

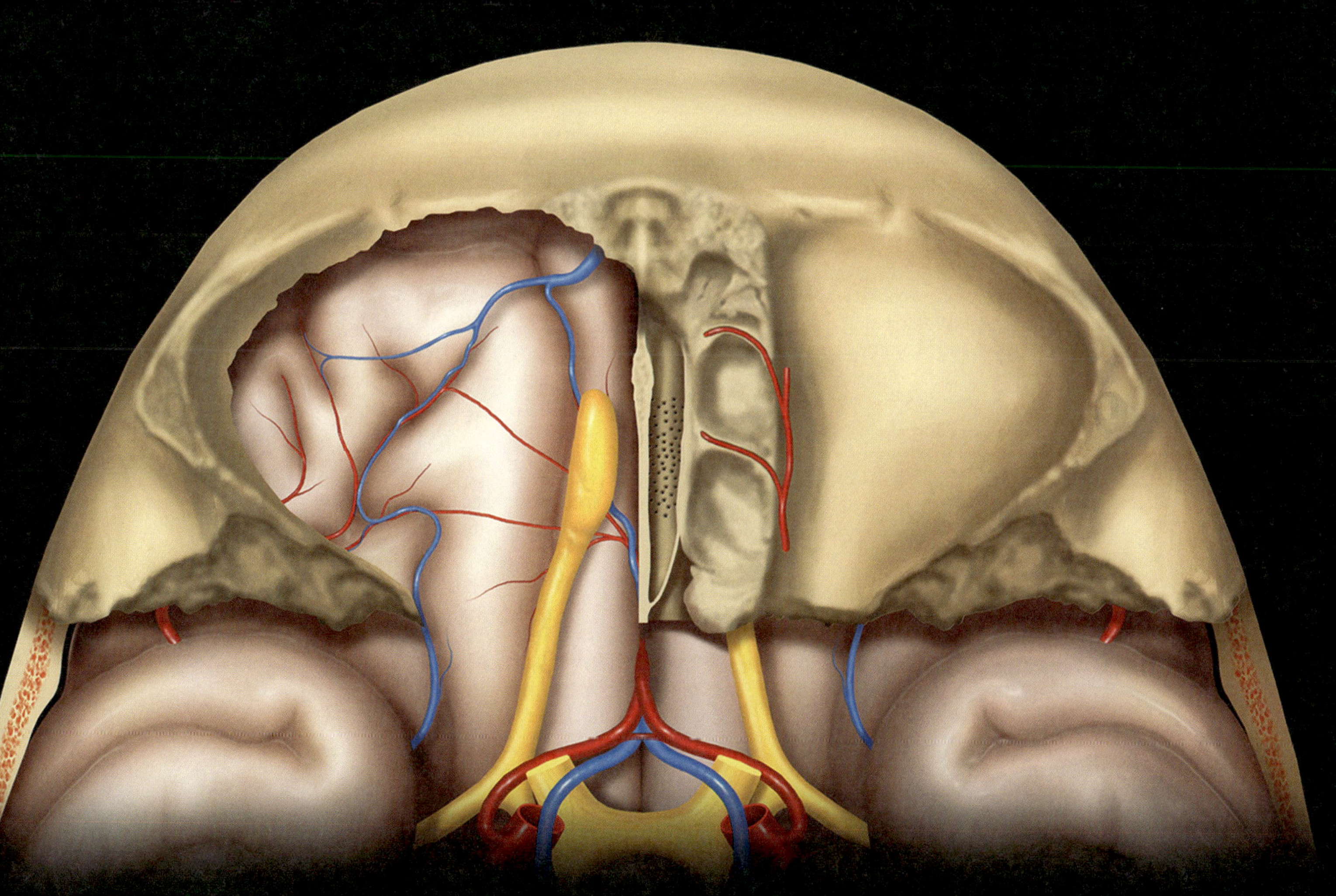

TERMINOLOGY

Abbreviations

- Skull base (SB)

Definitions

- SB: Complex osseous foundation of cranial vault; separates intracranial structures from sinuses, orbits, and suprahyoid neck (SHN)
- Transmits critical neurovascular structures between cranial vault and SHN, orbits, sinuses

IMAGING ANATOMY

Overview

- **5 bones** make up base of skull
  - **Paired bones**: Frontal and temporal bones
  - **Unpaired bones**: Ethmoid, sphenoid, and occipital bones
- **2 surfaces**
  - **Endocranial surface**: Brain, pituitary, cisterns, cranial nerves (CN), and intracranial vascular structures, including cavernous sinuses
  - **Exocranial surface**: Extracranial head and neck
    - Anterior portion: Nasal cavity, frontal and ethmoid sinuses, orbits
    - Central portion: Nasopharyngeal mucosal space, masticator, parotid and parapharyngeal spaces
    - Posterior portion: Nasopharyngeal mucosal space, carotid, retropharyngeal, perivertebral spaces
- **3 regions**
  - **Anterior (ASB), central (CSB), and posterior (PSB)**
  - **ASB**
    - Anterolateral boundary: Frontal bones
    - Inferior relationships: Nasal vault, ethmoid and frontal sinuses; orbit and orbital canals
    - Superior relationships: Frontal lobes, CNI
    - ASB-CSB boundary: Lesser wing of sphenoid (sphenoid ridge) and planum sphenoidale
  - **CSB**
    - Inferior relationships: Roof of pharyngeal mucosal space, masticator, parotid and parapharyngeal spaces
    - Superior relationships: Temporal lobes, pituitary, cavernous sinus, Meckel cave, CNI-IV, CNVI, CNV1-3
    - CSB-PSB boundary: Dorsum sella and posterior clinoid processes medially, petrous ridges laterally
  - **PSB**
    - Inferior relationships: Posterior pharyngeal mucosal space, carotid, retropharyngeal, perivertebral spaces
    - Superior relationships: Brainstem, cerebellum, CNVII-VIII, CNIX-XII, transverse-sigmoid sinuses
    - Posterior boundary: Occipital bone

Internal Contents

- **ASB**
  - Contents: Frontal, ethmoid bones, lesser wing and planum sphenoidale of sphenoid bone
  - Foramina and structures transmitted
    - **Cribriform plate**: CNI, ethmoid arteries
    - **Optic canal**: CNII, ophthalmic artery
- **CSB**
  - Contents: Body and greater wing of sphenoid bone and anterior temporal bones
  - Foramina and structures transmitted
    - **Superior orbital fissure**: CNIII, CNIV, CNV1, CNVI, and superior ophthalmic vein
    - **Inferior orbital fissure**: Infraorbital artery, vein, nerve
    - **Carotid canal**: Internal carotid artery (ICA), sympathetic plexus
    - **Foramen rotundum**: CNV2, artery of foramen rotundum, and emissary veins
    - **Foramen ovale**: CNV3, lesser petrosal nerve, accessory meningeal branch maxillary artery, and emissary vein
    - **Foramen spinosum**: Middle meningeal artery and vein, meningeal branch of mandibular nerve
    - **Foramen lacerum**: Not true foramen; cartilaginous floor of anteromedial horizontal petrous ICA canal
    - **Vidian canal**: Vidian artery and nerve
- **PSB**
  - Contents: Occipital and posterior temporal bones
  - Foramina and structures transmitted
    - **Internal acoustic meatus**: CNVII, CNVIII, labyrinthine artery
    - **Hypoglossal canal**: CNXII
    - **Foramen magnum**: Spinal portion CNXI, vertebral arteries, and medulla oblongata
    - **Jugular foramen**
      - **Pars nervosa**: CNIX, Jacobson nerve, and inferior petrosal sinus
      - **Pars vascularis**: CNX, Arnold nerve, CNXI, jugular bulb, and posterior meningeal artery

ANATOMY IMAGING ISSUES

Questions

- Imaging of SB best done with focused MR and bone CT
  - MR requires T1, T2, T1 C+ FS and DWI for full evaluation
  - Bone CT defines bone changes
- SHN spaces/structures abut SB, allowing extracranial tumor to access intracranial area via perineural tumor
  - Masticator space: CNV3
  - Parotid space: CNVII
  - Orbit: CNV1, CNIII, CNIV, and CNVI
  - Sinus and nose, pterygopalatine fossa: CNV2

Imaging Recommendations

- **Bone CT**
  - Axial thin slices with coronal reformations
  - Edge-enhancing algorithm and wide window settings (> 2,000 HU) necessary to evaluate bony anatomy
  - Narrow windows (200-400 HU) and smoothing algorithm to inspect regional soft tissues
  - If MR available, contrast unnecessary
- **MR**: Thin slices (≤ 4 mm), axial and coronal, T1, T2, and T1 C+ FS, axial DWI
  - Precontrast T1 images use native fatty marrow for "contrast"
  - Use MRA and MRV for arteries and veins

Imaging Pitfalls

- Prominent foramen cecum, accessory foramina can be normal variants
- MR flow in jugular foramen may mimic mass

GRAPHIC

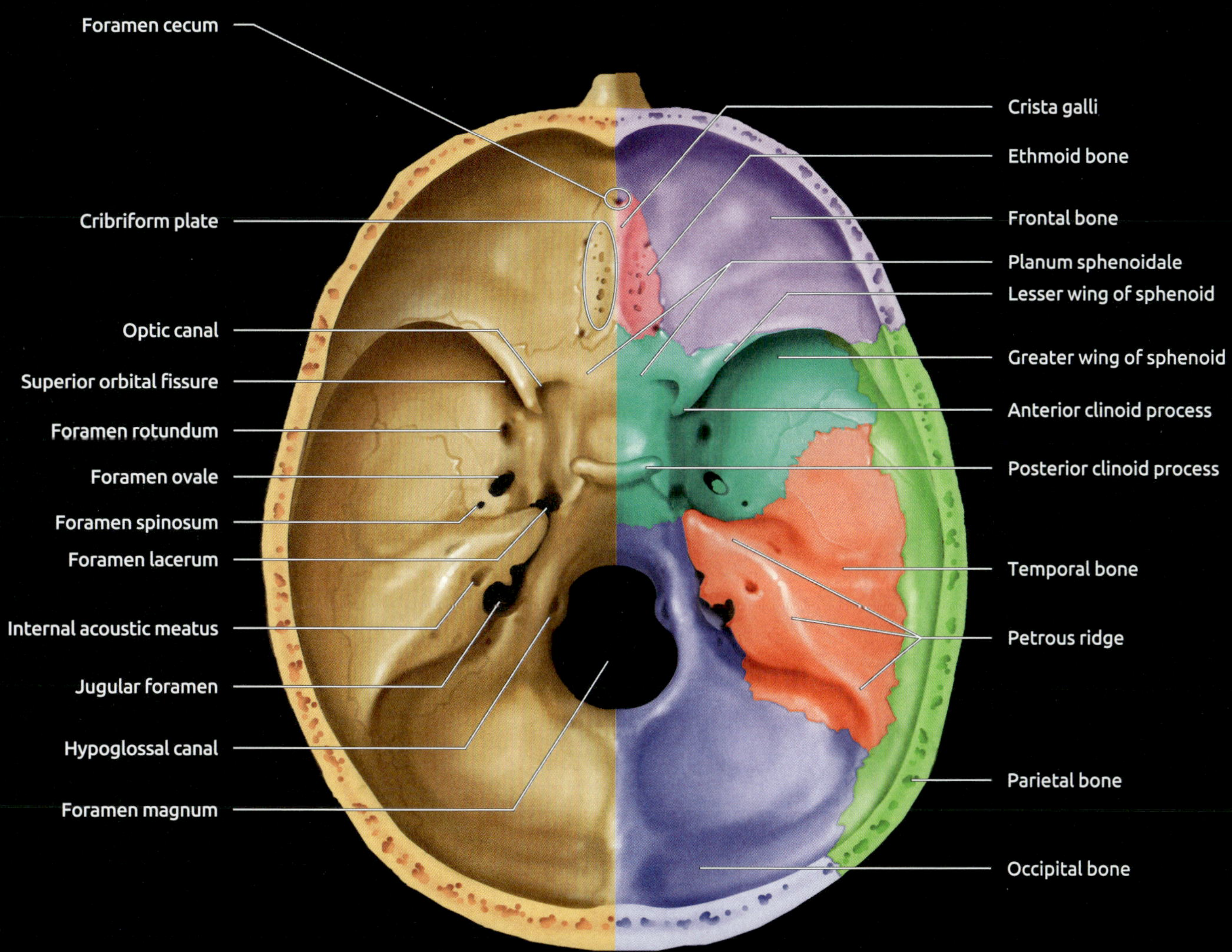

Graphic of the endocranial skull base viewed from above is shown. Osseous landmarks are labeled on the right. Important foramina are labeled on the left. The skull base is formed by the frontal, ethmoid, sphenoid, temporal, and occipital bones. The frontal, parietal, and occipital bones form the lateral vault of the cranium. The skull base is an undulating surface with grooves formed by the brain above and rough bony structures providing dural attachments. The lesser wing of the sphenoid and planum sphenoidale form the anterior-central skull base border, while the petrous ridge and dorsum sella form the central-posterior skull base border. The majority of important foramina are in the central skull base (sphenoid bone).

GRAPHICS

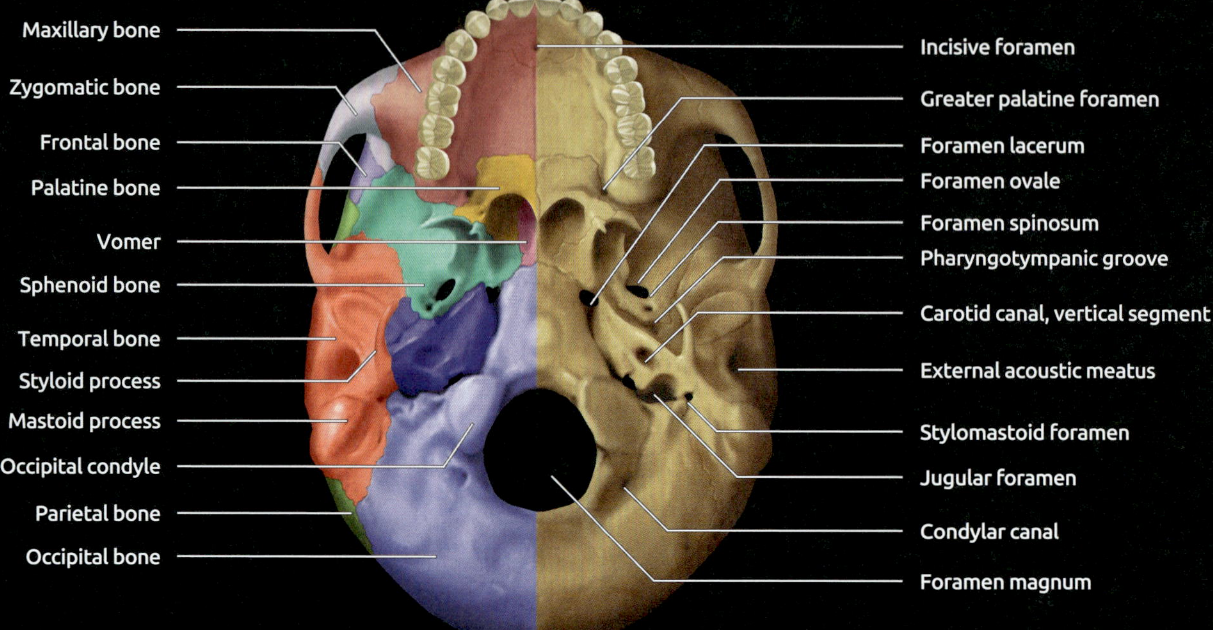

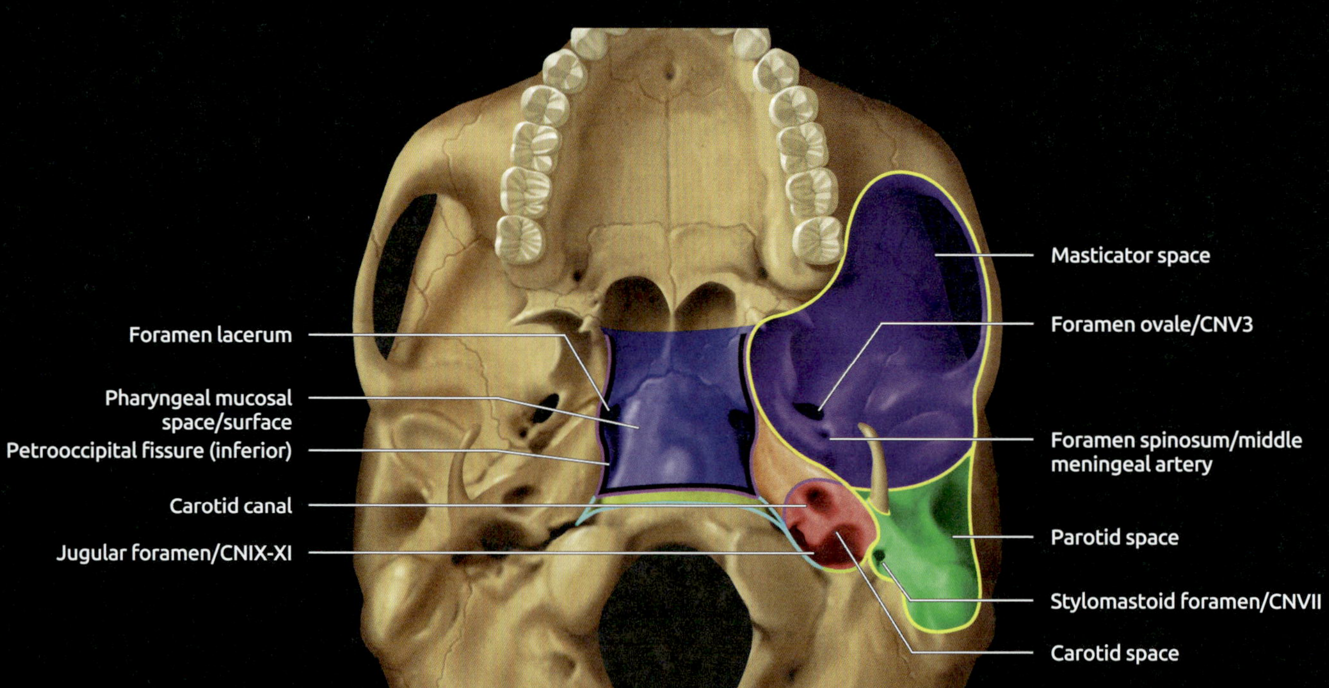

(Top) *Graphic of the skull base viewed from below shows the complexity of the exocranial skull base with bony landmarks labeled on the left and foramina labeled on the right. Note that in addition to the frontal, sphenoid, temporal, and occipital bones, the undersurface of the skull base is formed by the maxilla, vomer, palatine, and zygomatic bones. The ethmoid bone is not part of the exocranial skull base.* **(Bottom)** *Graphic of the skull base viewed from below shows the relationships to the suprahyoid neck spaces and structures. Four spaces have key interactions with the skull base: Masticator, parotid, carotid, and pharyngeal mucosal spaces. Parotid space (green) malignancy can follow CNVII into the stylomastoid foramen. Masticator space (purple) receives CNV3, while CNIX-XII enter the carotid space (red). The pharyngeal mucosal space abuts the foramen lacerum, which is covered by fibrocartilage.*

AXIAL BONE CT

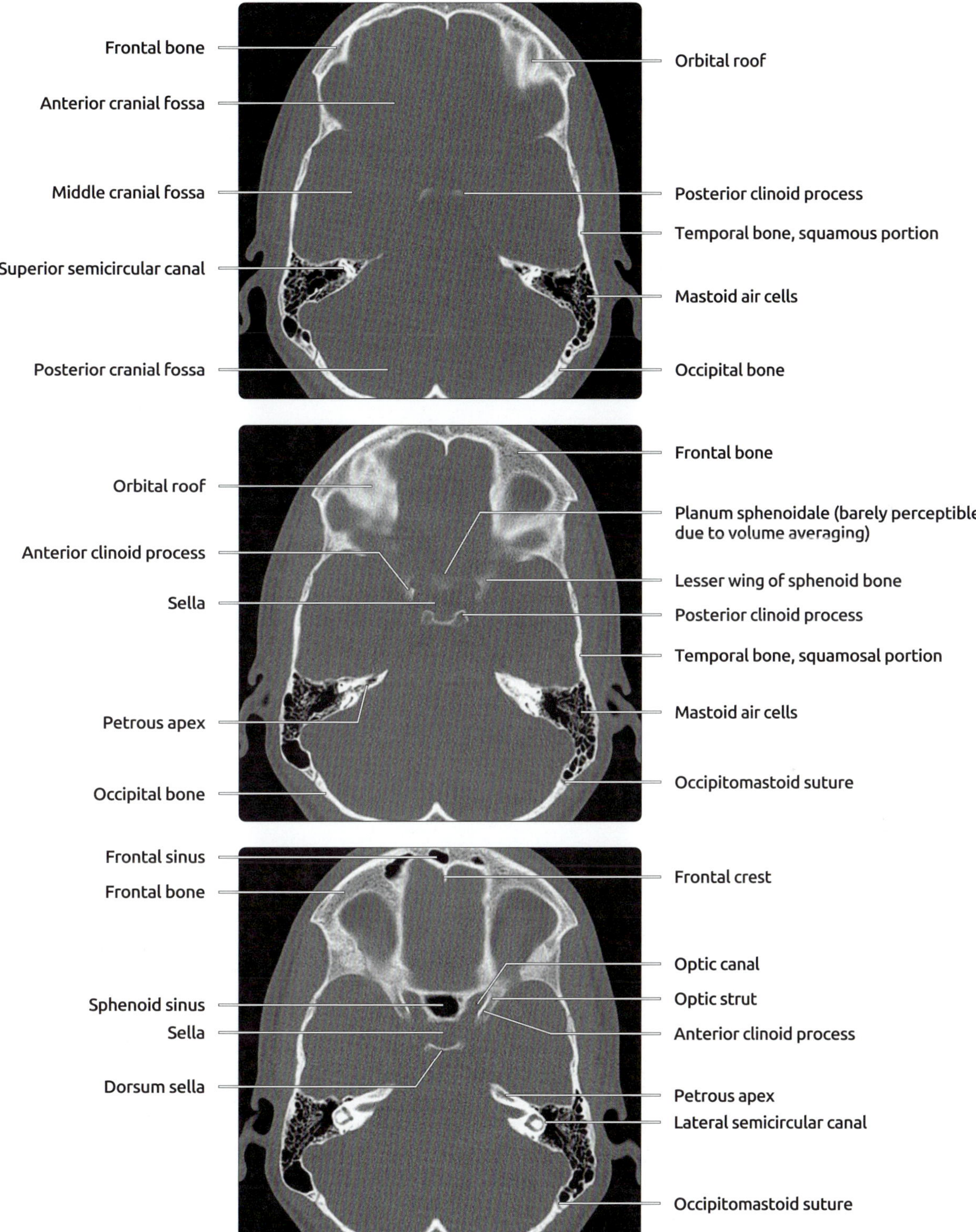

(Top) *First of 12 axial bone CT images of the skull base presented from superior to inferior is shown. At the level of the orbital roof, the brain within the anterior, middle, and posterior fossae is cradled above respective regions of the skull base: Anterior, central, and posterior.* **(Middle)** *At the level of the upper sella, the lesser wings of the sphenoid and planum sphenoidale, which demarcate the anterior-central skull base border, are barely visible. More posterior, the petrous apices divide the central skull base from the posterior skull base. The posterior skull base houses the cerebellum, covered superiorly by the tentorium cerebelli, which attaches to the posterior clinoid processes.* **(Bottom)** *At the level of the anterior clinoid, the optic canals pass through the sphenoid bone, bounded by the anterior clinoid process laterally and the sphenoid sinus medially. The dorsum sella marks the anteromedial border of the posterior skull base.*

AXIAL BONE CT

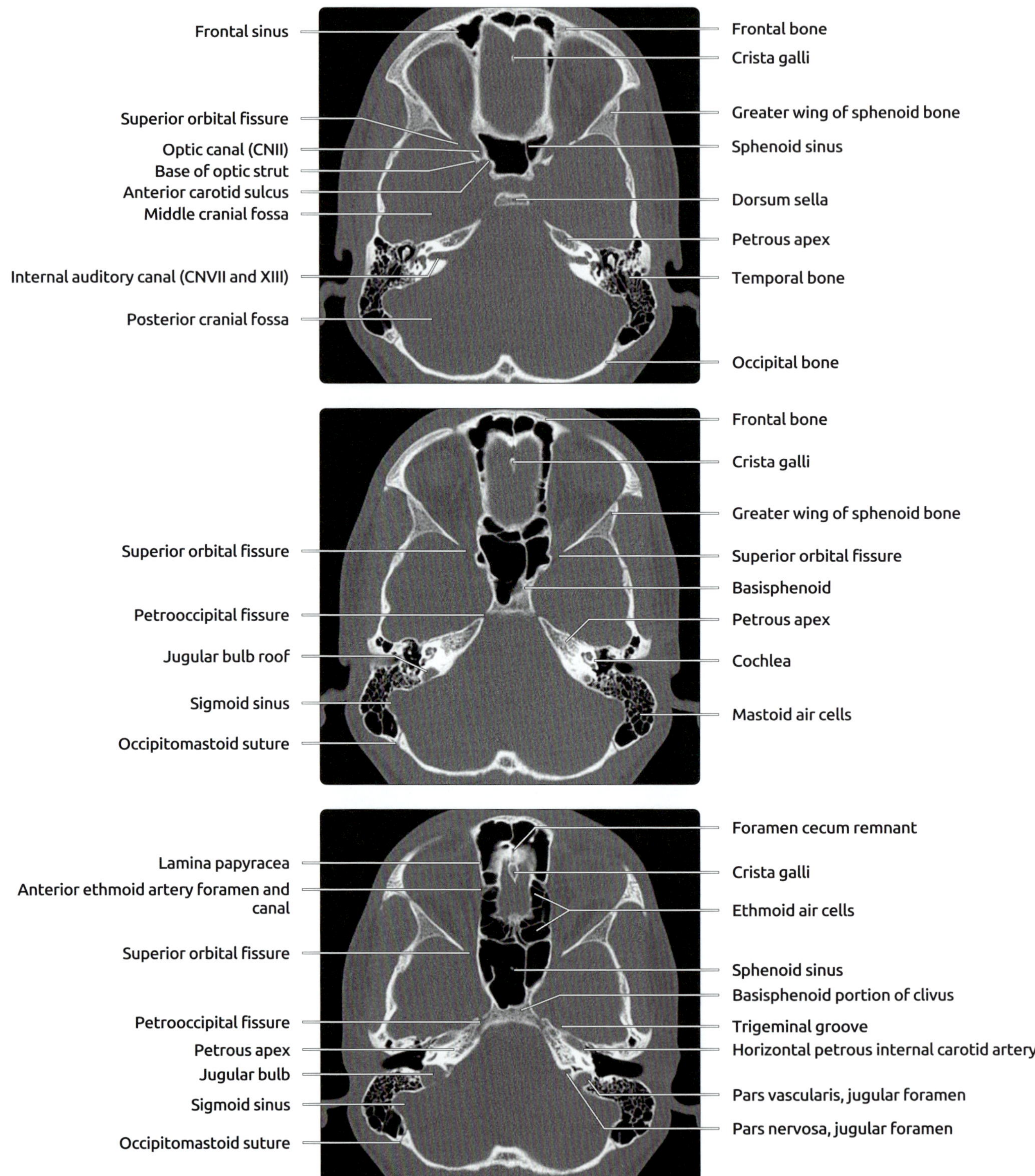

(Top) *In this image, the crista galli superior tip is just visible. The optic canal transmits CNII and the ophthalmic artery to the orbit, while the superior orbital fissure transmits CNIII, CNIV, CNV1, CNVI, and the superior ophthalmic vein. Notice the close approximation of the optic canal and superior orbital fissure, separated only by a thin, often pneumatized, optic strut. The internal auditory canal is on the medial wall of the temporal bone.* **(Middle)** *Crista galli provides attachment for the falx cerebri and divides the anterior aspect of the anterior skull base into 2 symmetric halves. Ethmoid air cells extend superior to the cribriform plate. The sphenoid sinus is immediately below the sella and medial to the superior orbital fissure. The superior margin of the petrooccipital fissure is visible at the medial tip of the petrous apex, where the petrosphenoid ligament (Gruber ligament) can be found. This short ligament spans the petrous ridge to the clivus. Below the ligament is the Dorello canal containing dural venous structures and CNVI.* **(Bottom)** *At the anterior base of the crista galli is foramen cecum remnant. The petrooccipital fissure is the most common location for skull base chondrosarcoma.*

AXIAL BONE CT

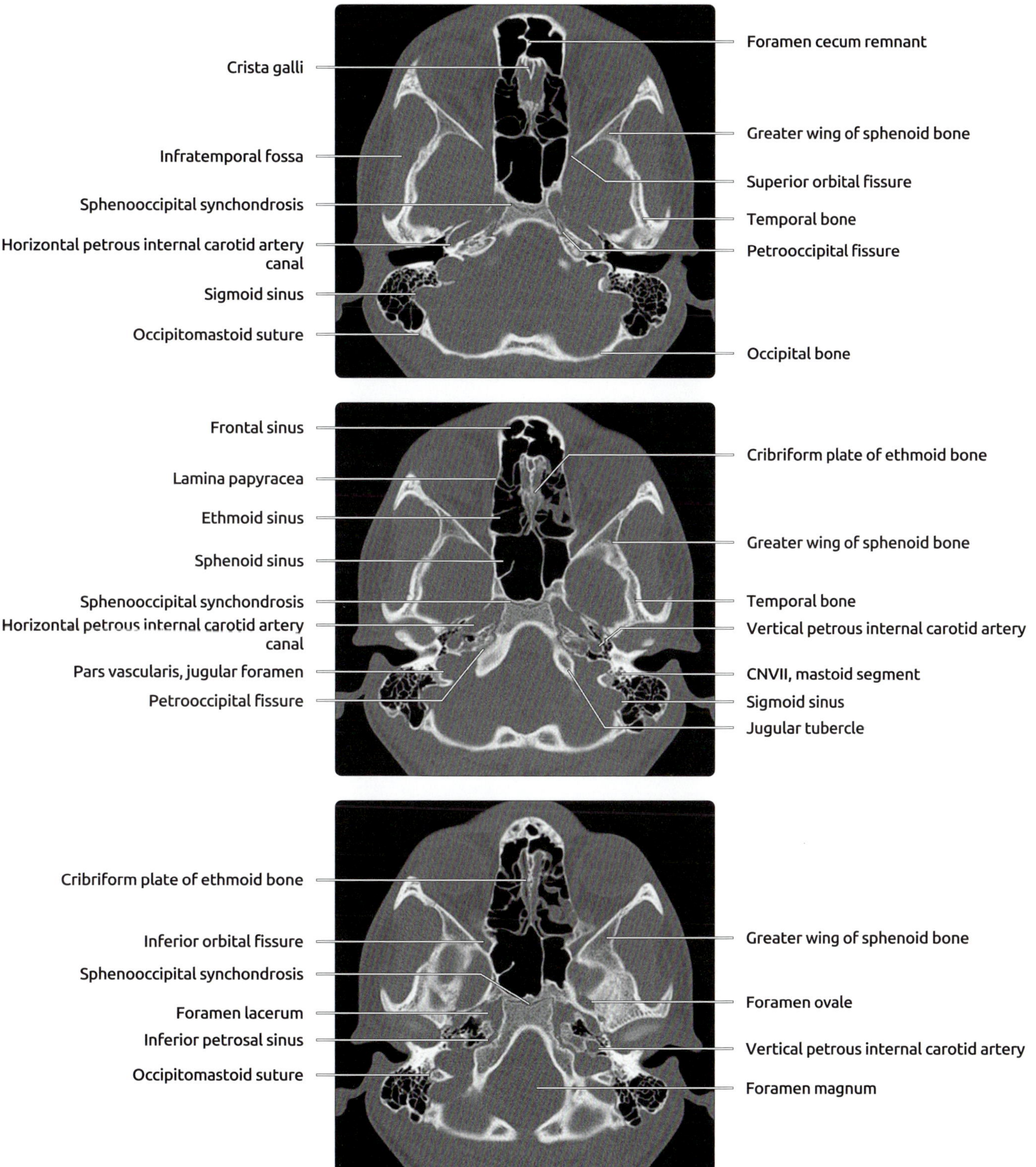

(Top) *At the level of the upper clivus, the sphenooccipital synchondrosis is visible, delineating the more anterior basisphenoid from the more posterior basiocciput. Posterolaterally, the petrooccipital fissure is seen separating the more medial occipital bone from the more lateral temporal bone.* **(Middle)** *At the level of the cribriform plate of the ethmoid bone, the frontal, ethmoid, and sphenoid sinuses are all visible. Also note the vertical and horizontal segments of the petrous internal carotid arteries.* **(Bottom)** *The inferior orbital fissure is bounded by the sphenoid sinus posteromedially and the greater wing of the sphenoid bone laterally. It contains the infraorbital artery, vein, and nerve. The foramen lacerum is occupied by cartilage and is contiguous posteriorly with the petrooccipital fissure. Inferiorly and posteriorly, the petrooccipital fissure contains the inferior petrosal sinus.*

AXIAL BONE CT

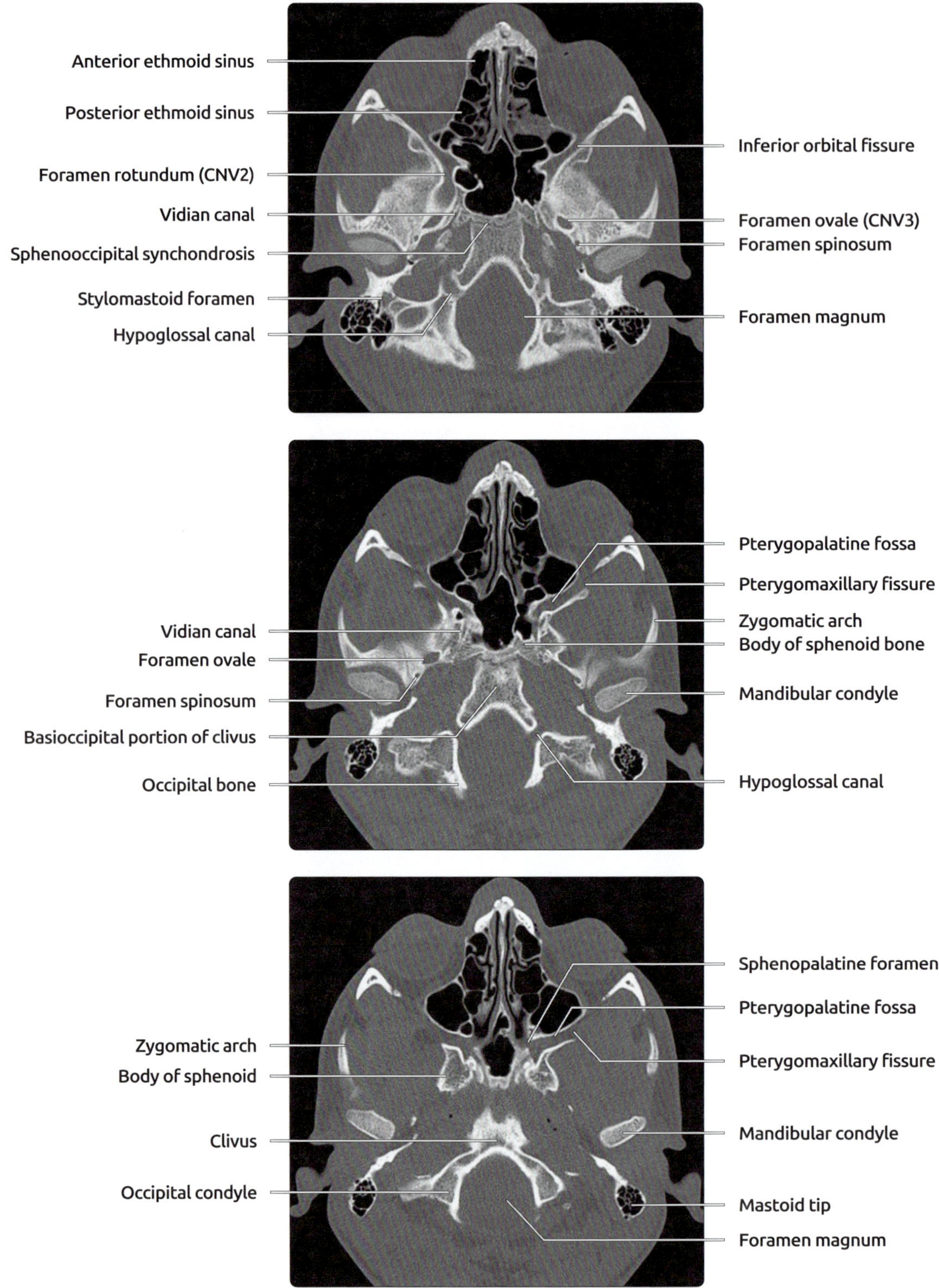

(Top) *At the level of inferior orbital fissure and foramen rotundum, the vidian canal is also seen. The foramen rotundum provides a conduit for CNV2 to access the confluence of the medial inferior orbital fissure and the superior pterygopalatine fossa. CNV3 traverses sphenoid bone via the foramen ovale. The hypoglossal canal is seen in the inferior occipital bone.* **(Middle)** *This image is at the level of the hypoglossal canal in the low occipital bone. Anteriorly, the pterygomaxillary fissure is the lateral opening of the pterygopalatine fossa.* **(Bottom)** *At the inferior margin of the foramen magnum, the mastoid tips are still visible. The pterygopalatine fossa is well seen, connecting medially with the nasal cavity via the sphenopalatine foramen and laterally with the masticator space through the pterygomaxillary fissure. The foramen rotundum and vidian canals also lead into the pterygopalatine fossa.*

3D-VRT BONE CT

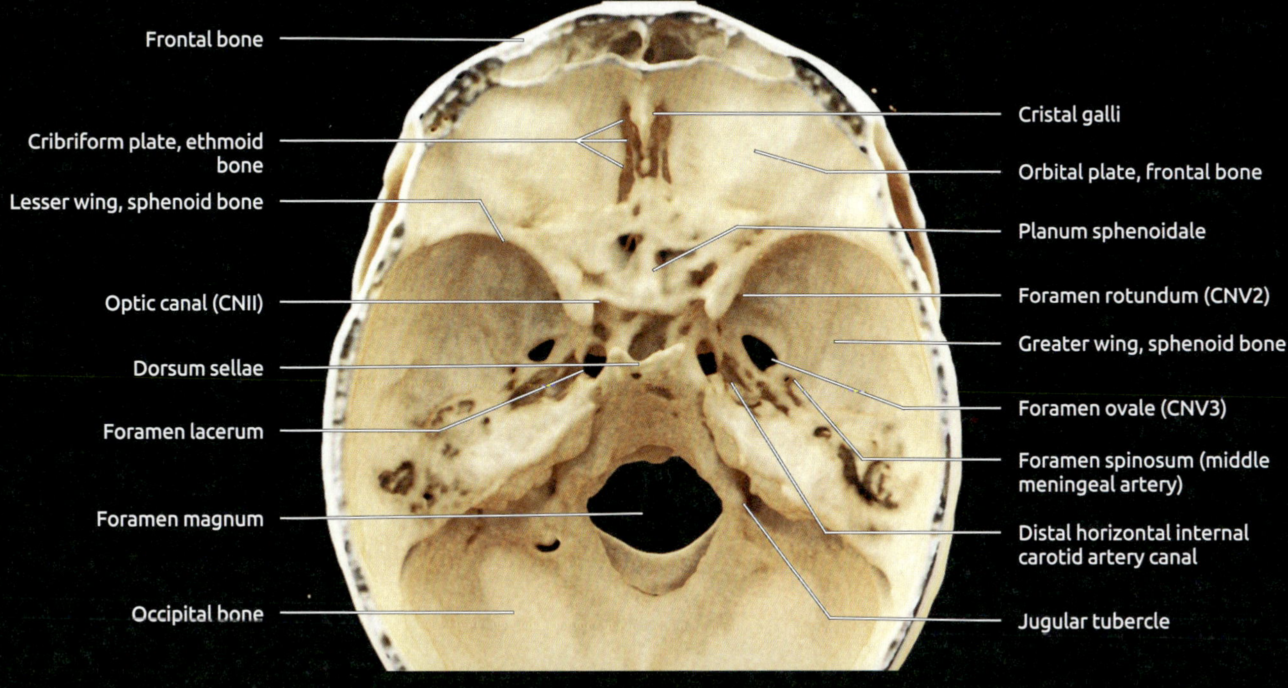

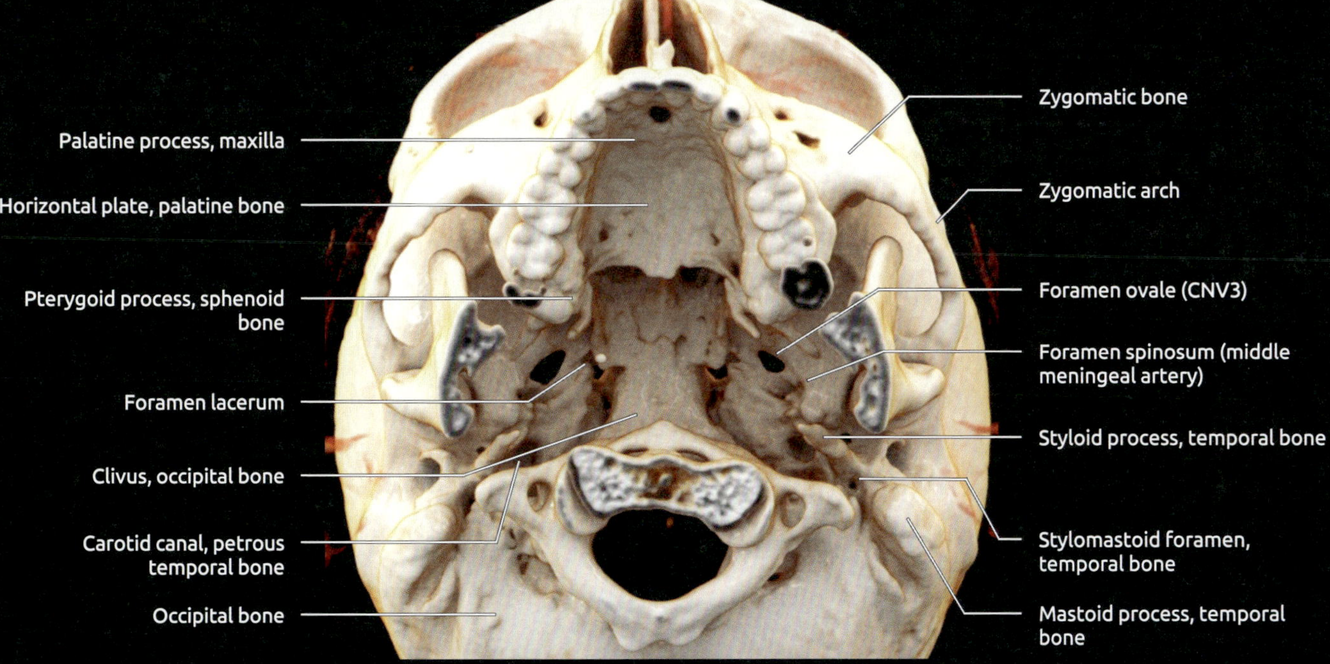

(Top) *PCD 3D-cinematic rendering CT scan of the osseous skull base from above is shown. The anterior skull base is bounded by frontal bones anteriorly and the lesser wing of the sphenoid and planum sphenoidale posteriorly. The central skull base, with its multitude of fissures and foramina, is made up of sphenoid bone and anterior temporal bone. It is bounded anteriorly by the lesser wing of the sphenoid and posterior planum sphenoidale and posteriorly by the dorsum sellae and petrous ridge. The posterior skull base extends from the dorsum sellae medially and petrous ridges laterally to the occiput posteriorly.* **(Bottom)** *PCD 3D-cinematic rendering CT scan of the osseous skull base from below highlights sphenoid bone with the foramen ovale and spinosum as well as the mastoid and styloid processes. Notice the frontal bone is not seen, but instead, maxillary, palatine, and zygomatic bones are present anteriorly.*

SAGITTAL BONE CT AND T1 MR

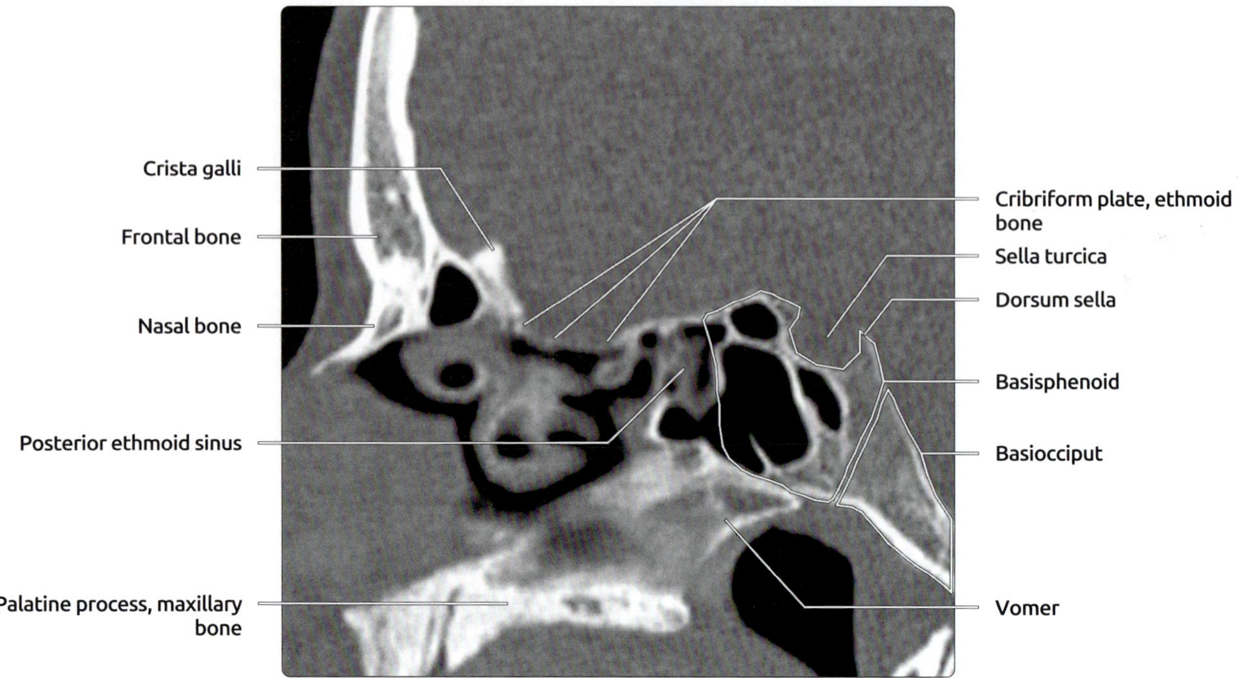

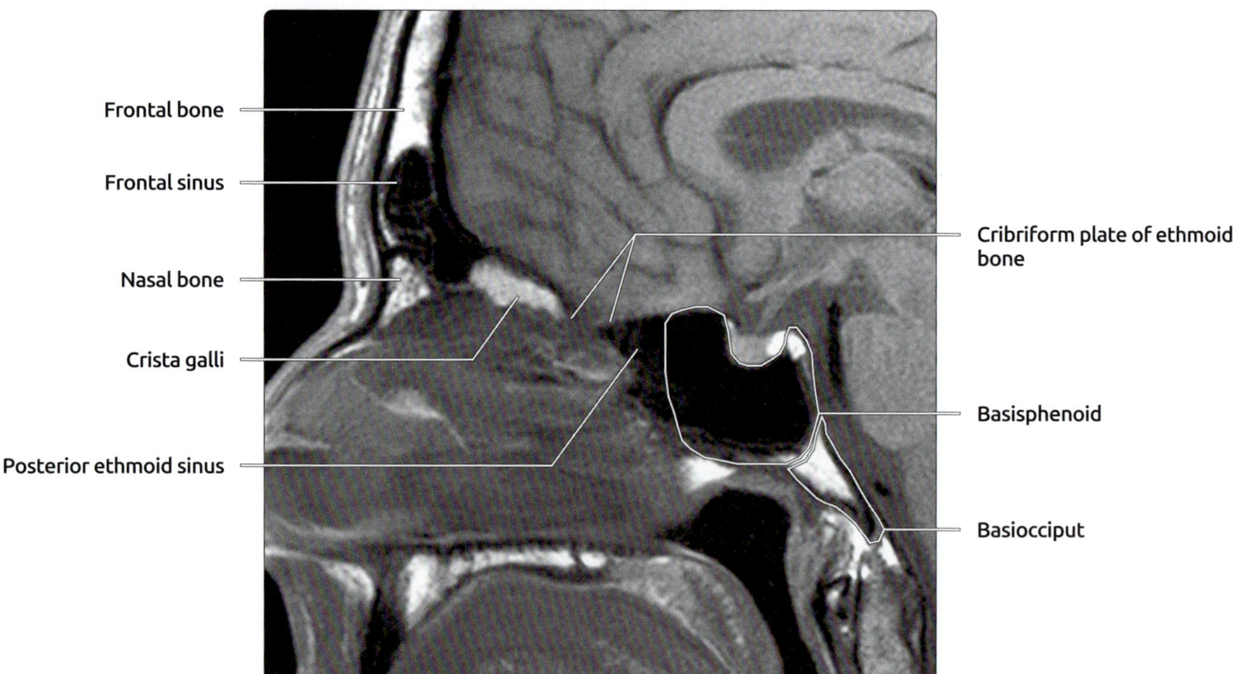

(Top) *Paramedian sagittal bone CT through the anterior skull base shows the intimate relationship of the skull base to the paranasal sinuses. From anterior to posterior, note the frontal and nasal bones, crista galli, cribriform plate basisphenoid, and basiocciput. The sella is entirely embedded in the sphenoid bone.* **(Bottom)** *Paramedial sagittal T1 MR through the skull base shows the anterior, central, and posterior skull bases. The anterior skull base in this image is made up of the frontal bone, crista galli, and cribriform plate of ethmoid bone. The crista galli is high signal secondary to fatty marrow. The central skull base in the midline is often called the basisphenoid. It is made up of the sphenoid bone-sinus and cradles the pituitary gland. The sphenooccipital synchondrosis separates the basisphenoid from the basiocciput of the posterior skull base.*

AXIAL T1 MR

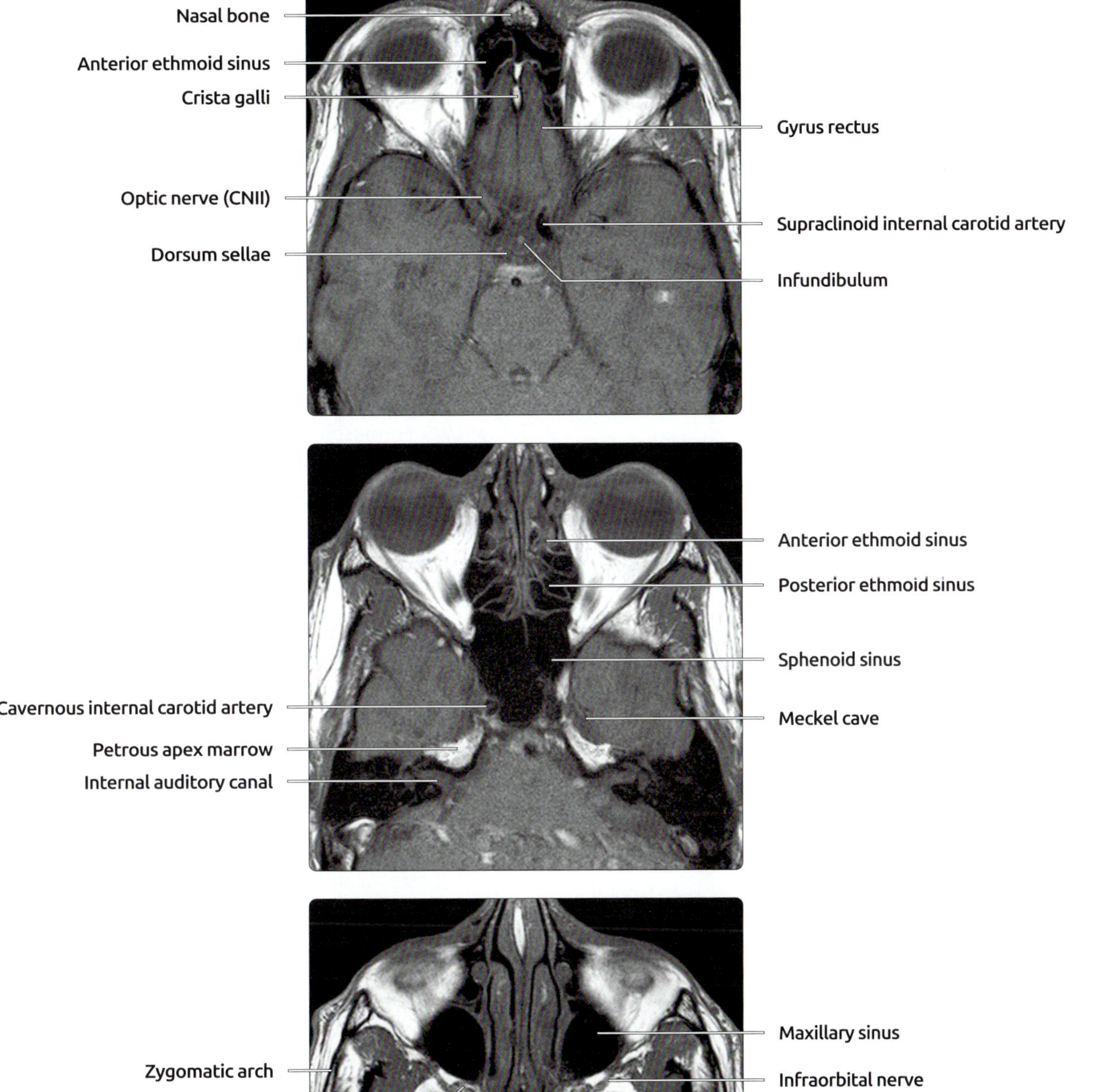

(Top) *First of 3 axial T1 MR images through the skull base from superior to inferior shows the high-signal fatty marrow in the crista galli. Adjacent to this are gyri recti of the frontal lobes.* **(Middle)** *Image through the cavernous sinus reveals the ethmoid sinuses in the ethmoid bones of the anterior skull base and the sphenoid sinus in the sphenoid bone of the central skull base. The petrous apex fatty marrow is high signal with Meckel cave seen on its anterior margin.* **(Bottom)** *At the level of the pterygopalatine fossa, the infraorbital nerve can be seen exiting anterolaterally. The vidian canal, another sphenoid bone structure, is visible connecting to the medial pterygopalatine fossa. Middle meningeal artery and CNV3 are noted passing through the foramen spinosum and ovale, respectively. More posterolaterally, the carotid canal and jugular foramen can be seen.*

TERMINOLOGY

Abbreviations

- Anterior skull base (ASB)

Definitions

- Skull base anterior to lesser wing of sphenoid (LWS) and planum sphenoidale

IMAGING ANATOMY

Overview

- ASB is floor of anterior cranial fossa and roof of nose, ethmoid sinuses, and orbits
  - Forms broad, relatively flat floor of anterior cranial fossa that predominantly houses frontal lobes of brain
- Bones forming ASB
  - Ethmoid: Cribriform plate and ethmoid sinus roof centrally
  - Frontal: Orbital plate laterally
  - Sphenoid: Planum sphenoidale and lesser wing posteriorly
- Boundaries of ASB
  - Anterolaterally: Frontal bone
  - Posteriorly: LWS and planum sphenoidale
- Relationships of ASB
  - Superior: Frontal lobes, CNI
    - Inferior frontal lobe gyri include gyrus rectus medial to olfactory sulcus, medial orbital gyrus, anterior and posterior orbital gyri, and lateral orbital gyri
  - Inferior: Nasal vault and ethmoid sinus medially, orbit laterally
  - Anterior: Frontal sinuses
  - Posterior: Posterior margins of ASB critically associated with optic nerve canal, superior orbital fissure, and sella

Bony Landmarks of Anterior Skull Base

- **Frontal crest**: Anterior midline ridge between frontal bones; falx cerebri attaches here
- **Crista galli**: Midline upward triangular process of ethmoid bone; anteroinferior falx cerebri attaches here
  - Crista galli is pneumatized (contains mucosal lined air cell) in 10-15% of adults
  - Origin of pneumatization is extension of left or right frontal air cell, not ethmoid sinus
- **Cribriform plate (lamina cribrosa)**: Horizontal, perforated, bony plate of superomedial ethmoid
  - Forms part of nasal cavity roof
  - Forms floor of olfactory fossa (groove)
  - Shape and depth of olfactory fossa is variable and depends on length of lateral lamella of cribriform plate
    - Keros classification of olfactory fossa depth
      - Type I: < 3 mm
      - Type II: 4-7 mm
      - Type III: 8-16 mm
- **Ethmoid roof (fovea ethmoidalis)**: Horizontal or downward-sloping projection from medial margin of orbital plate
  - Ethmoid roof actually extension of orbital plate of frontal bone
  - Medially, roof fuses with lateral lamella of cribriform plate
  - Ethmoid roof forms superior bony margin of ethmoid sinus air cells, separating ethmoid sinuses from anterior cranial fossa
  - Appearance asymmetric > 50% of time
- **Perpendicular plate of ethmoid**: Midline sagittally oriented bony plate that extends below level of cribriform plate and forms superior portion of bony nasal septum
  - Appears contiguous with crista galli above
  - Fuses with vomer by 2 years of age
- **Anterior clinoid process**: Medial aspect of LWS; free edge of tentorium cerebelli attaches here
  - Attaches to body of sphenoid by 2 roots
    - Superior root forms roof of optic canal and merges with planum sphenoidale
    - Inferior root is optic strut and forms lateral and inferior margin of optic canal
    - Variant: Posterior inferior root attaches to sphenoid bone, creating complete bony ring around cavernous internal carotid artery
- **LWS**: Forms sphenoid ridge; separates anterior from central skull base (CSB); forms superior boundary of optic nerve canal
  - Medially, LWS forms superior boundary of optic nerve canal
  - Laterally, LWS forms part of lateral superior margin of superior orbital fissure
- **Planum sphenoidale**: Superomedial plate of sphenoid bone, posterior to cribriform plate, anterior to tuberculum sellae
- **Chiasmatic sulcus (prechiasmatic sulcus)**: Horizontal groove or shelf of variable depth and width just dorsal and slightly inferior to posterior lip (limbus sphenoidale) of planum sphenoidale and just anterior to upper lip of tuberculum sella
  - Some authors would consider part of CSB
  - Optic chiasm does not sit in sulcus; rather, chiasm is posterior and superior to sulcus itself

Foramina and Fissures of Anterior Skull Base

- **Foramen cecum**
  - Transmits: Variably transmits small emissary vein from nasal mucosa to superior sagittal sinus
  - Location: In margin between posterior aspect of frontal bone and anterior aspect of ethmoid
  - Relationships: Small midline pit found immediately anterior to crista galli
- **Anterior ethmoidal artery foramen, canal, and sulcus**
  - Transmits: Anterior ethmoidal artery, vein, nerve
    - Anterior ethmoidal artery arises from distal ophthalmic artery and passes anteromedially from orbit to olfactory fossa
      - Anterior ethmoidal artery foramen: Small, funnel-shaped opening/notch along lamina papyracea of orbit
      - Anterior ethmoidal groove or canal: Small groove/channel through ethmoid sinus roof or sinus proper; connects anterior ethmoid foramen to ethmoid artery sulcus
      - Anterior ethmoidal artery sulcus: Small slit that opens along lateral lamella of olfactory groove, just lateral to cribriform plate

- Location: Thin passageway between orbit to olfactory groove
- Relationships: Canal may pass through roof of ethmoid sinus or be "exposed," passing through anterior ethmoid sinus proper
  - If ethmoid artery canal passes through ethmoid sinus proper, it is vulnerable to injury during trauma or surgery
- **Posterior ethmoidal foramen, canal, and sulcus**
  - Transmits: Posterior ethmoidal artery, vein, nerve
  - Location: Passes from posterior orbit, through ethmoid roof, to lateral olfactory groove
  - Relationships: Medial sulcus just posterior to cribriform plate, at seam between cribriform plate and planum sphenoidale
- **Foramina of cribriform plate**
  - Transmits: Afferent fibers from nasal mucosa to olfactory bulbs (CNI)
  - Location: ~ 20 perforations within cephalad ethmoid bone plate
  - Relationships: Medial aspect of ethmoid, supports olfactory bulbs
- **Optic nerve canal**
  - Dural-lined canal through LWS
  - Transmits optic nerve and ophthalmic artery from intracranial compartment to orbital apex
  - Anterior root of lesser wing forms roof of optic nerve canal
  - Inferior root of lesser wing forms optic strut, which is variably pneumatized pillar that forms inferolateral border of optic nerve canal and separates canal from superior orbital fissure
- **Superior orbital fissure**
  - Oblong defect in posterior orbital apex that provides communication from orbit to cavernous sinus
  - Superior margin formed by LWS
  - Medial margin formed by optic strut
  - Inferior margin formed by greater wing of sphenoid
  - Transmits superior ophthalmic vein and nerves: Nasociliary, frontal, lacrimal, abducens, trochlear, superior and inferior branches of oculomotor
- **Hyrtl canal**
  - Thin channel lateral to superior orbital fissure
  - Within greater wing of sphenoid
  - Potential middle meningeal artery to ophthalmic artery connection

Development of Anterior Skull Base

- **Overview**
  - Skull base originates largely from cartilaginous precursors
    - Minimal contribution from membranous bone
  - > 100 ossification centers in skull base development
  - Ossifies posterior to anterior and lateral to medial
  - Ossification orderly and constant in first 2 years
    - Does not correspond to exact age, however
- **Birth**: ASB develops primarily from cartilage with limited ossification at birth
  - Early ethmoid air cells may be seen, but unossified crista galli is faint
- **1 month**: Ossification begins from ethmoidal labyrinth and turbinates; proceeds medially
- **3 months**: Roof of nasal cavity and tip of crista galli begin to ossify
  - Ethmoid air cells still inferior to cribriform plate
- **6 months**: Nasal roof well ossified; > 90% of infants have partial ossification nasal roof on every coronal CT
  - Perpendicular plate of ethmoid begins to ossify
  - Ethmoid sinus extends above cribriform plate plane
- **12 months**: Crista galli well ossified; > 70% have ossified posterior cribriform plate
- **18 months**: Ethmoid air cells now extend above plane of cribriform plate, and orbital plates of frontal bones help form early fovea ethmoidalis
- **24 months**: Fovea ethmoidalis achieves more mature appearance; perpendicular plate of ethmoid begins to fuse with ossified vomer, most patients still have gap between nasal and ethmoid bones
- **> 24 months**
  - ASB nearly completely ossified; small gaps persist in nasal roof until early 3rd year
  - Foramen cecum ossifies as late as 5 years
  - Majority of cribriform plate and at least some of crista galli should be ossified

ANATOMY IMAGING ISSUES

Questions

- Pediatric
  - ASB ossification constant but variable in first 5 years
  - Understanding of normal development will avoid confusion or misdiagnoses
  - Anterior neuropore closes in 4th gestational week
- Adult: Understanding critical relationships to ASB necessary to fully evaluate region
  - Intracranial: Dura, inferior frontal lobe, olfactory bulb, tuberculum sella, cavernous sinus
  - Extracranial: Nasal vault, frontal, ethmoid, sphenoid sinuses, orbit and orbital apex, optic nerve canal, superior orbital fissure

Imaging Recommendations

- MR to search for anterior neuropore anomalies
- MR and CT complementary in evaluation of ASB abnormalities

Imaging Approaches

- Bone CT viewed at wide windows (> 2,000 HU)
- Reformat at least 2 orthogonal planes
- High-resolution techniques necessary to evaluate microanatomy of ASB

Imaging Pitfalls

- Pediatric
  - Apparent small gaps in ASB > age 3 are normal
  - Do not confuse nonossified foramen cecum for anterior neuropore anomaly
- Adult
  - Beware: Fatty marrow in crista galli or ossified falx cerebri is not pathology

GRAPHICS

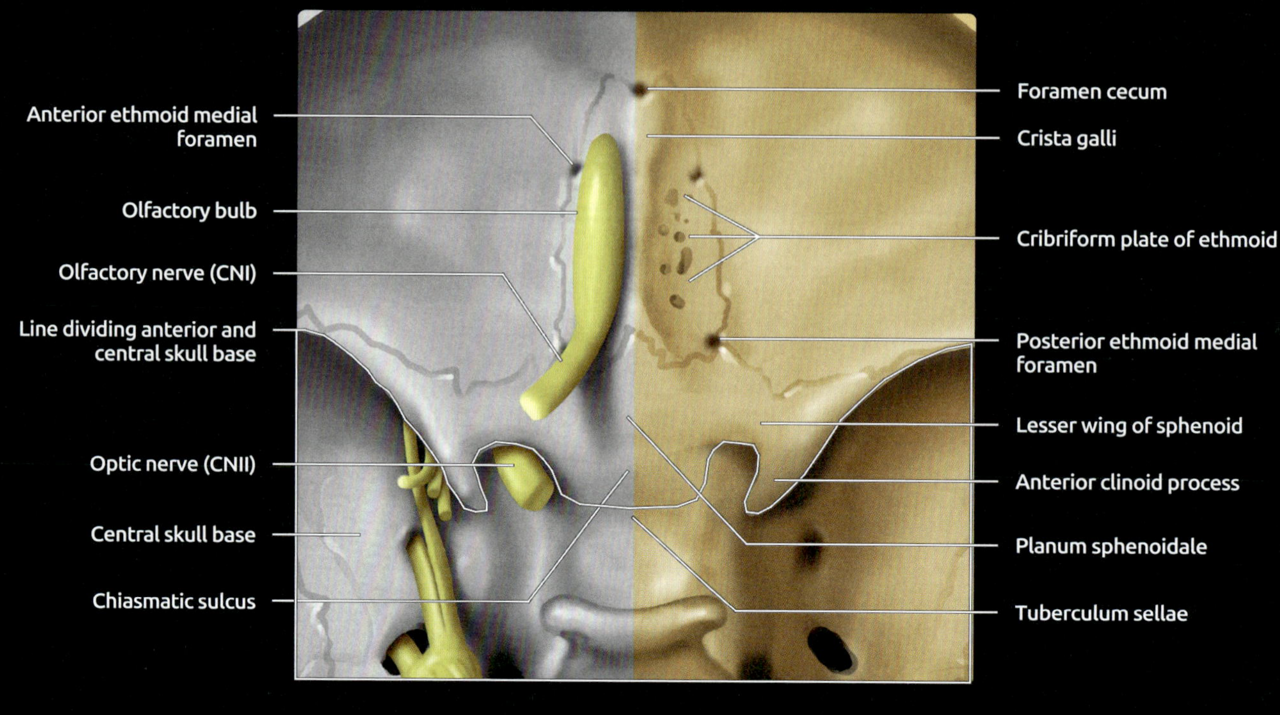

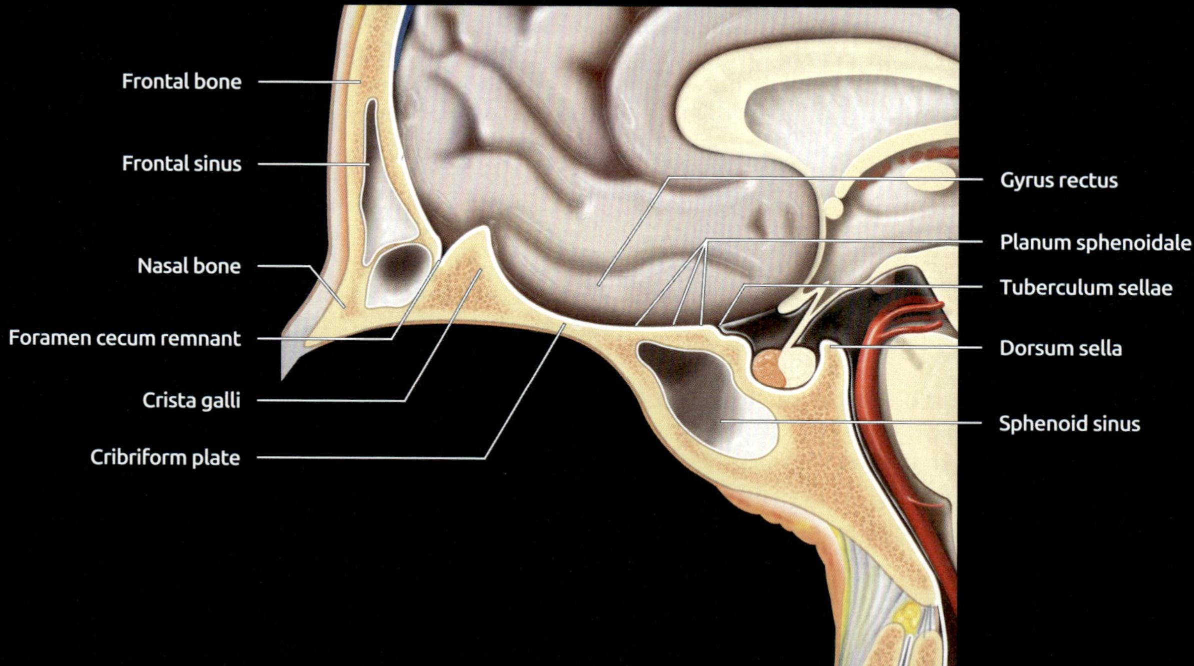

(Top) *Graphic of the anterior skull base (ASB) seen from above shows olfactory bulb of CNI lying on the cribriform plate. Neural structures have been removed on the right, allowing visualization of numerous perforations in the cribriform plate, through which afferent fibers from olfactory mucosa pass to form the olfactory bulb. Note the foramen cecum, a small pit anterior to the crista galli, bounded anteriorly by the frontal bone and posteriorly by the ethmoid bone. The posterior margin of the ASB is formed by the lesser wing of sphenoid (LWS) and planum sphenoidale.* **(Bottom)** *Sagittal graphic of the ASB shows midline vertical crista galli. Anterior to the crista galli is the foramen cecum remnant, and posterolateral to the crista galli is the horizontal cribriform plate. The planum sphenoidale is the posteromedial ASB.*

GRAPHICS

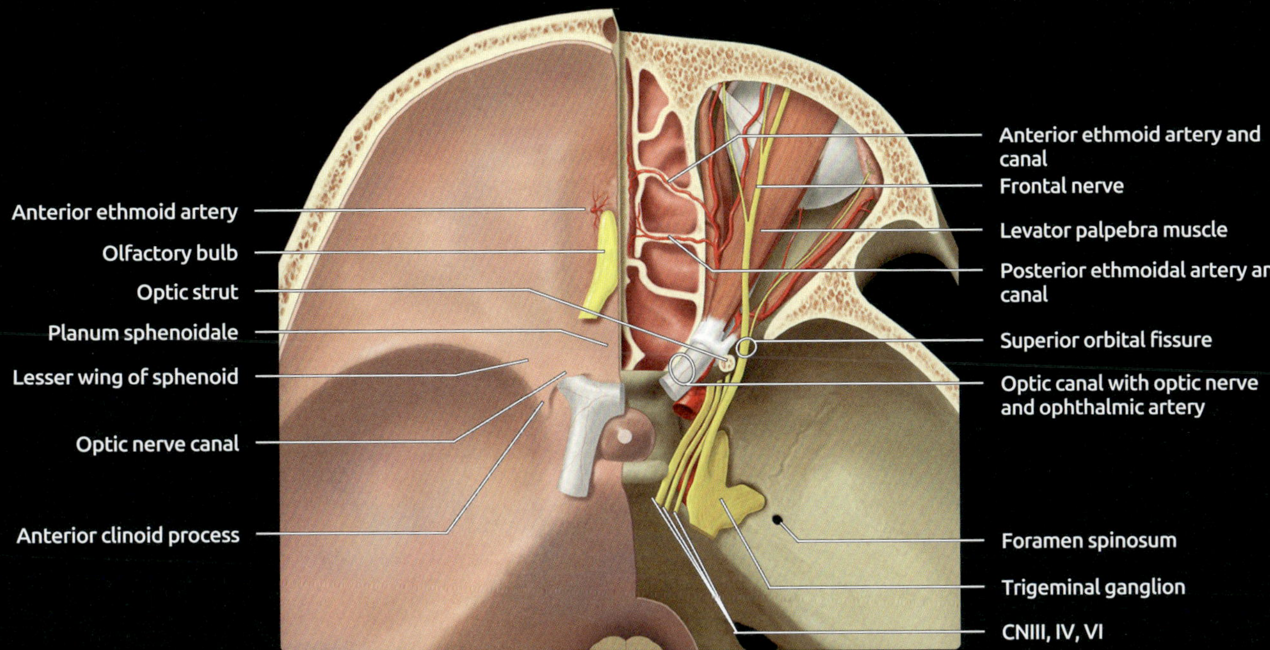

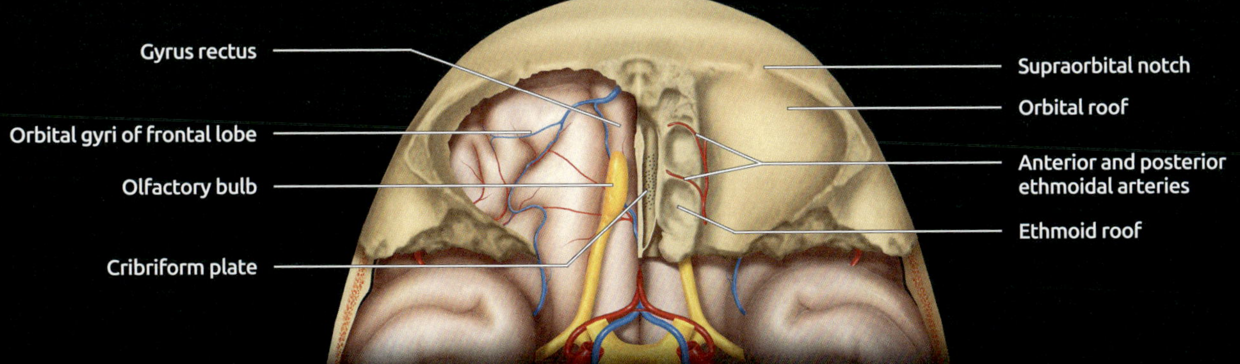

(Top) *Graphic shows a partially dissected ASB. Notice the expansive dural covering that can give rise to meningiomas in a variety of anterior locations. On the right side, the cribriform plate, the ethmoid roof, orbital plate of the frontal bone, LWS, and anterior clinoid process have been resected. This exposes the ethmoid air cells, the superior orbit, the optic nerve canal, and the superior orbital fissure. The optic strut, often pneumatized, separates the optic nerve canal medially from the superior orbital fissure laterally. The cavernous sinus has also been dissected, exposing CNIII, CNIV, and CNVI.* **(Bottom)** *Graphic shows the anatomic relationships of the ASB from below. On the left side, there has been dissection of ASB, revealing the inferior frontal lobe (the orbital gyri), rectus gyrus, and the olfactory nerve. On the right side, the cribriform plate, ethmoid roof, and orbital roof are seen from below.*

GRAPHICS

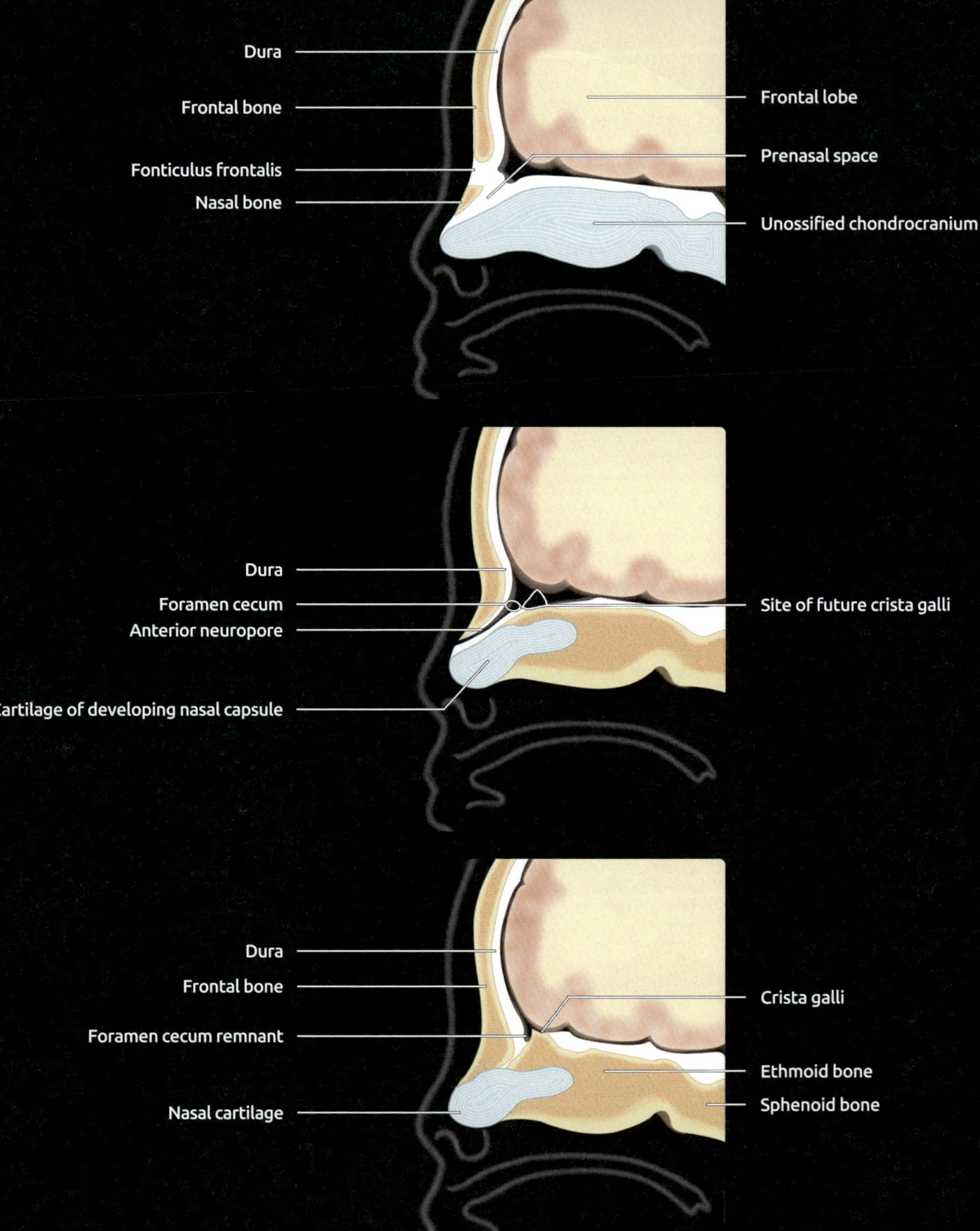

(Top) *Sagittal graphic shows normal ASB development. The fonticulus frontalis, a small ASB fontanelle, is the normal cartilaginous gap between developing, partially ossified frontal and nasal bones. The prenasal space is also present as a dura-filled space between developing nasal bones and cartilage of developing nasal capsule. Both sites can become the location of a cephalocele.* **(Middle)** *Sagittal graphic shows the ASB slightly later in development. The fonticulus frontalis has closed, and ossification of the chondrocranium has proceeded from posterior to anterior. The prenasal space has now encased in bone and becomes foramen cecum. A normal stalk of dura extends through foramen cecum to skin (anterior neuropore).* **(Bottom)** *Sagittal graphic shows the ASB even later in development. Anterior neuropore has regressed. Foramen cecum will completely fuse by age 5.*

AXIAL BONE CT

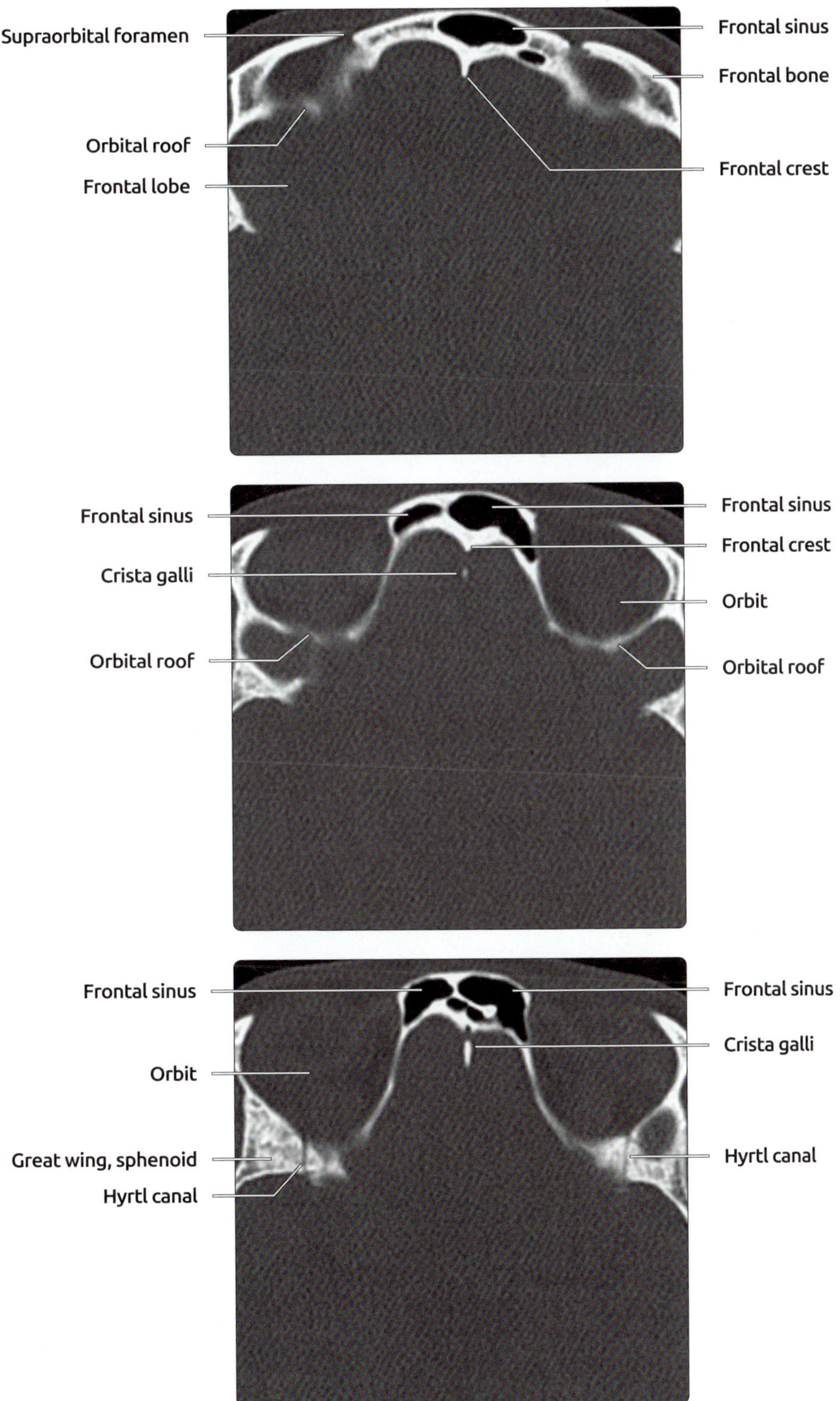

(Top) *First of 9 axial bone CT images of the ASB from superior to inferior is shown. The orbital roof is formed by the orbital plate frontal bone and the LWS bone. The frontal crest gives attachment to the falx cerebri. The supraorbital foramen transmits the supraorbital nerve, artery, and vein.* **(Middle)** *More inferiorly, the cephalad tip of the crista galli is seen in the midline where it and the frontal crest give attachment to the falx cerebri.* **(Bottom)** *In this image, the crista galli is visualized. Note the variable Hyrtl canal within the greater wing of the sphenoid bone, which is visualized bilaterally. The Hyrtl canal is a potential middle meningeal artery to ophthalmic artery connection via the anastomosis of the orbital branch of middle meningeal artery and lacrimal branch of the ophthalmic artery.*

AXIAL BONE CT

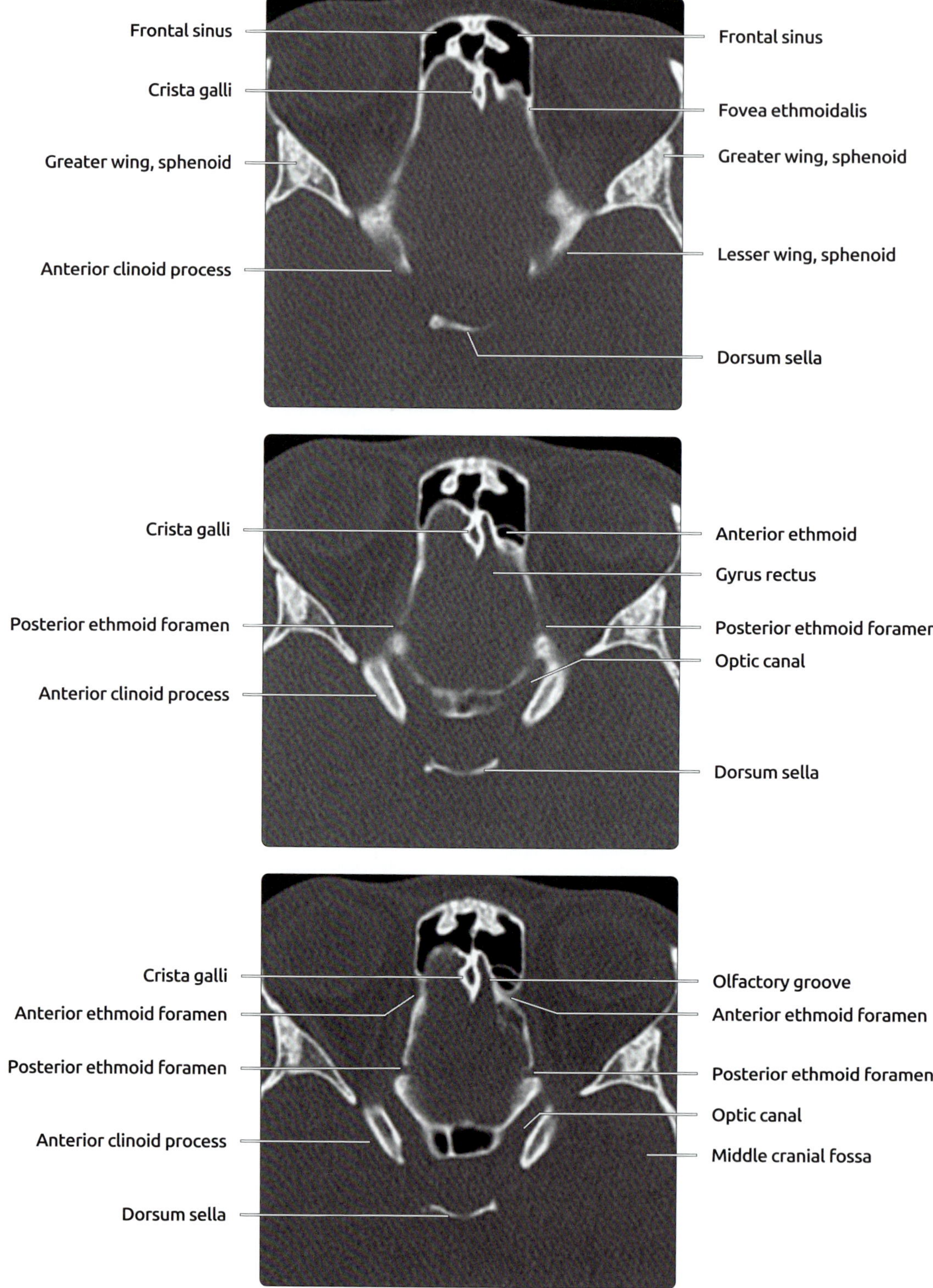

(Top) *At this level, the base of the crista galli is visible. The medial end of the LWS bone forms the anterior clinoid process, which acts as an attachment for tentorium cerebelli.* **(Middle)** *In this image, the posterior ethmoid foramen is visualized that passes from the posterior orbit, through the ethmoid roof, to the lateral olfactory groove. It transmits the posterior ethmoidal artery, vein, and nerve.* **(Bottom)** *In this image, the anterior and posterior ethmoid foramina are visible. The anterior ethmoidal foramen are seen bilaterally along the lateral wall of the ethmoid sinuses. This foramen contains the anterior ethmoidal artery, vein, and nerve.*

AXIAL BONE CT

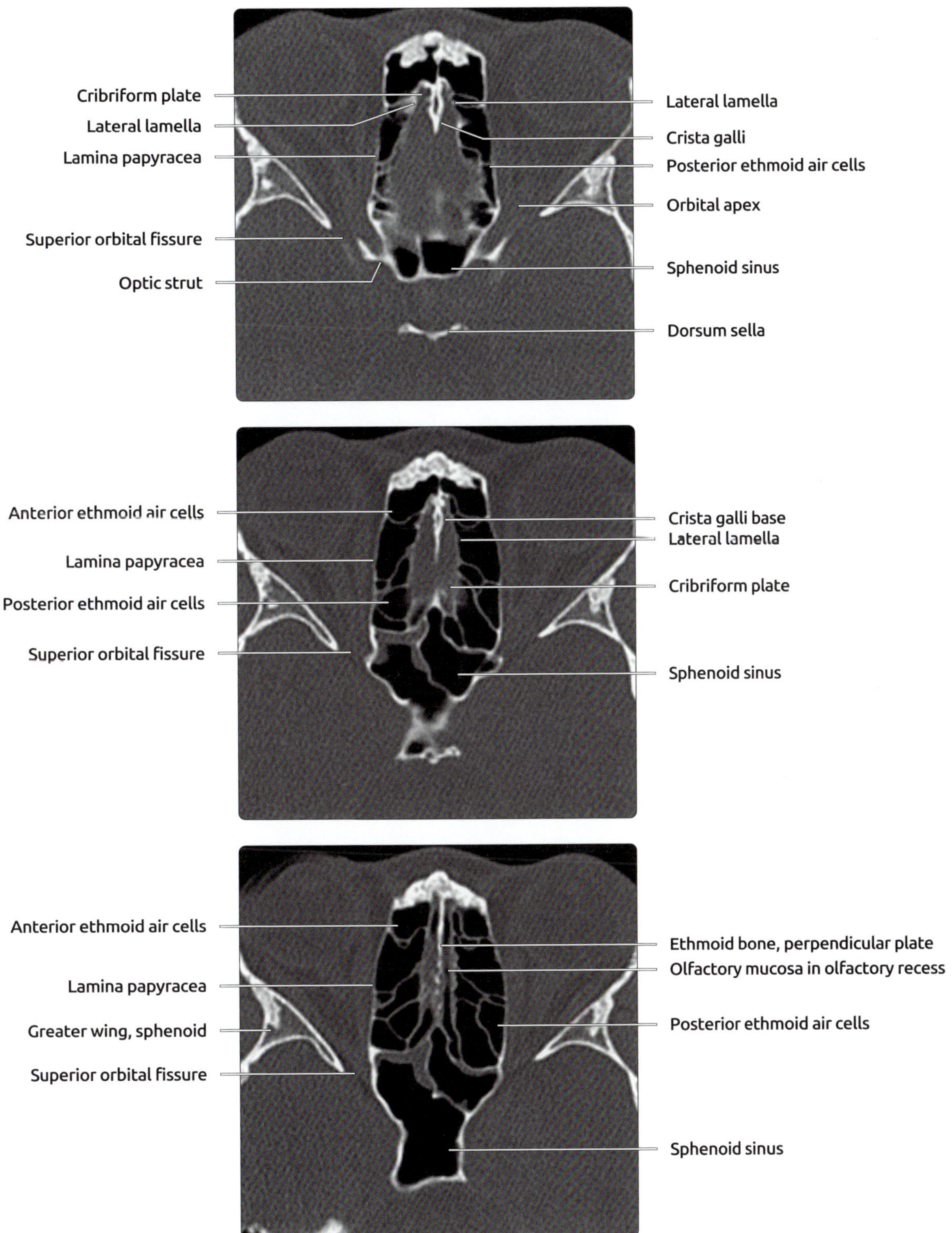

(Top) *In this image through the cribriform plate, the perforated bone is visible. Notice the lateral lamella represents the vertical bony wall of the ethmoid sinus that projects inferiorly from the fovea ethmoidalis (ethmoid sinus roof) down to the cribriform plate. This is far better seen on coronal sinus CT. Notice the cribriform plate is inferomedial to the ethmoid sinuses themselves. The ethmoid air cells are laterally bounded by the lamina papyracea, the paper-thin medial wall of the orbit.* **(Middle)** *The cribriform plate has a variable relationship to the roof of the ethmoid sinuses (fovea ethmoidalis). The more inferior to the fovea ethmoidalis the cribriform plate is found, the larger the dimension of the lateral lamella, the deeper the olfactory groove, and the more easily a sinus surgery complication may occur.* **(Bottom)** *This image is just below the cribriform plate. The perpendicular plate of the ethmoid bone if visible as is the olfactory mucosa in the olfactory recess of the nasal cavity. The olfactory mucosa is the site of origin of esthesioneuroblastoma.*

CORONAL BONE CT

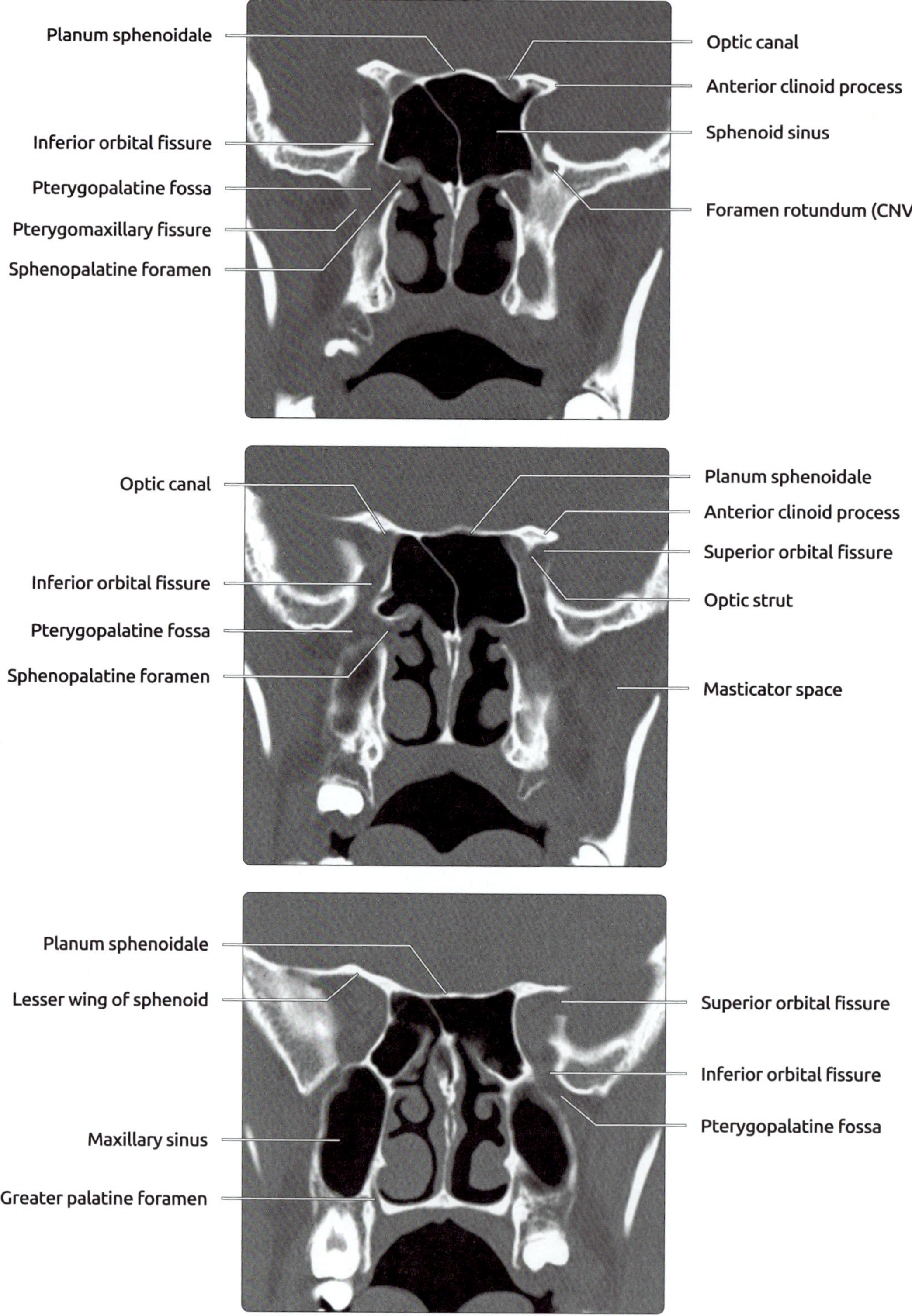

(Top) *First of 6 coronal sinus bone CT images presented from posterior to anterior shows the transition from central skull base to ASB. Notice the optic canal medial to the anterior clinoid processes. The inferior orbital fissure is seen inferolateral to the optic canal. The planum sphenoidale is the posterior sphenoid sinus roof.* **(Middle)** *Inferior to the planum sphenoidale and lateral to the sphenoid sinus is the complex anatomy of the orbital apex. The most superomedial structure of the orbital apex is the optic canal, divided from the superior orbital fissure by a small bony spur called the optic strut. The inferior orbital fissure communicates inferiorly with the pterygopalatine fossa.* **(Bottom)** *At the level of the orbital apex, the LWS is visible as the posterior orbital roof. The planum sphenoidale is the anterior roof of the sphenoid bone.*

CORONAL BONE CT

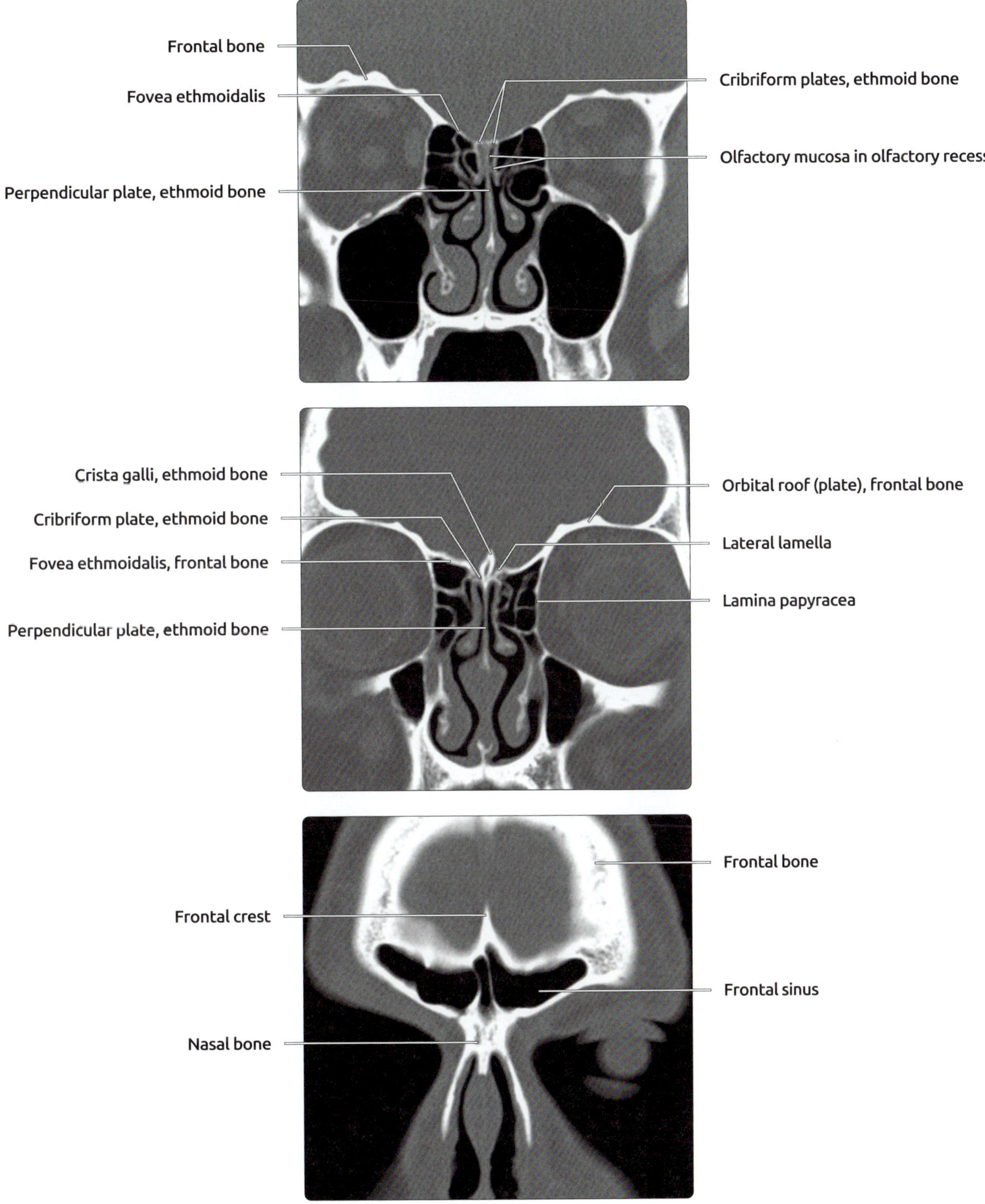

(Top) *At the level of the posterior cribriform plate, the fovea ethmoidalis is seen sloping gradually toward the midline. In the midline, the cribriform plates themselves are visible.* **(Middle)** *At the level of the crista galli, it is possible to see the multiple pieces of the ethmoid bone. The crista galli is the most cephalad portion of the ethmoid bone, extending directly inferiorly into the perpendicular plate of the ethmoid bone. Just lateral to the base of the crista galli are the cribriform plates, lateral lamellae, and fovea ethmoidalis portions of the frontal bone.* **(Bottom)** *In this image through the frontal bone and sinus, note the anteroinferior nasal bone. Do not confuse the more anterosuperior frontal crest (part of frontal bones) with crista galli (part of ethmoid), not seen on this image.*

AXIAL BONE CT, DEVELOPMENT

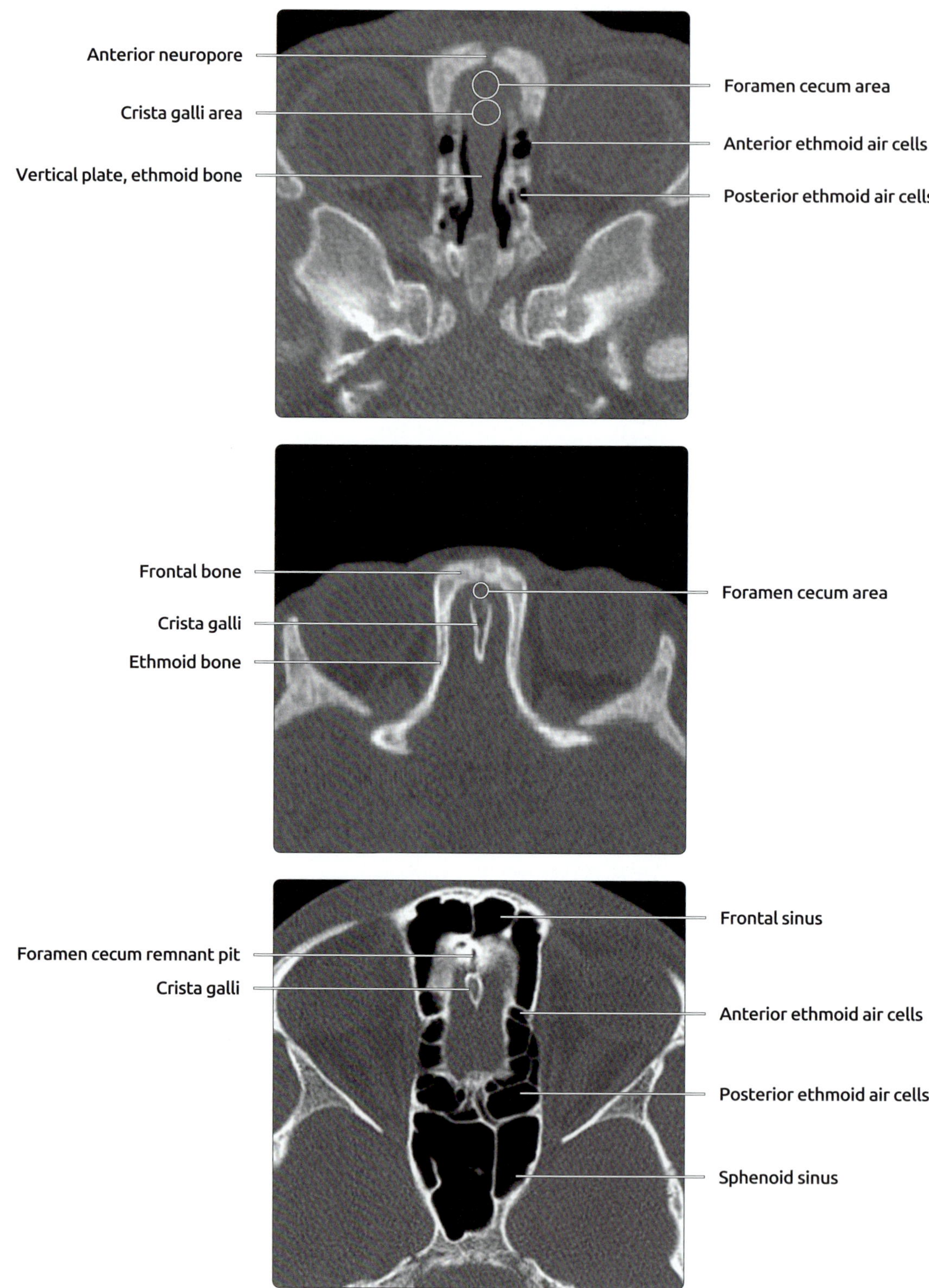

(Top) *Axial bone CT through the ASB in a newborn is shown. The unossified gap between the nasal and frontal bones normally contains dura at this age and represents the regressing anterior neuropore. The area of the foramen cecum, crista galli, cribriform plate, and perpendicular plate of the ethmoid bone are all normally unossified in the newborn.* **(Middle)** *Axial bone CT through the ASB at 12 months of age is shown. The crista galli is now well ossified. The foramen cecum area is still not ossified. The foramen cecum is still open, but the margins cannot be defined.* **(Bottom)** *Axial bone CT through the ASB in an adult is shown. The ethmoid air cells now extend far above the horizontal plane of the cribriform plate. The crista galli is thickened and heavily ossified. Although closed, the foramen cecum still demonstrates a small remnant pit.*

CORONAL BONE CT, DEVELOPMENT

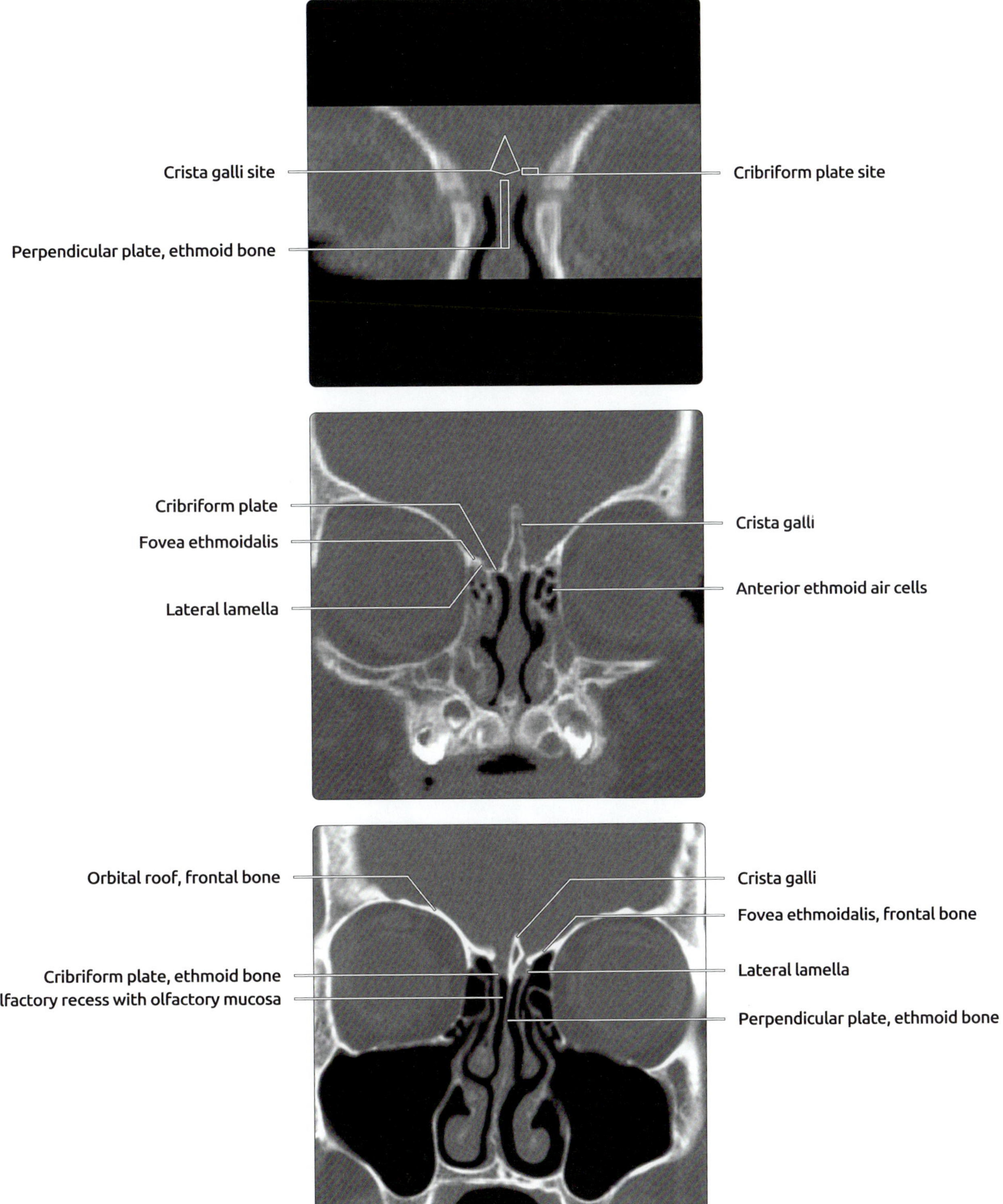

(Top) *Coronal bone CT through the ASB in a newborn is shown. The ASB is largely unossified, including crista galli, cribriform plate, and perpendicular plate of ethmoid bone. There is a large gap between the orbital plates of frontal bones. Ethmoid air cells are not yet developed.* **(Middle)** *Coronal bone CT through the ASB at 12 months of age is shown. The ethmoid bone is now mostly ossified, particularly the crista galli and posterior cribriform plate. Until 2-3 years of age, unossified gaps in the anterior cribriform plate and foramen cecum (not shown) can be normal. Note that the developing lateral lamella and fovea ethmoidalis are small.* **(Bottom)** *Coronal bone CT through the ASB in an adult is shown. The ASB is completely ossified. Ethmoid air cells extend superolateral to the plane of the cribriform plate. The fovea ethmoidalis is connected to the cribriform plate by the lateral lamella.*

CORONAL T2 MR, DEVELOPMENT

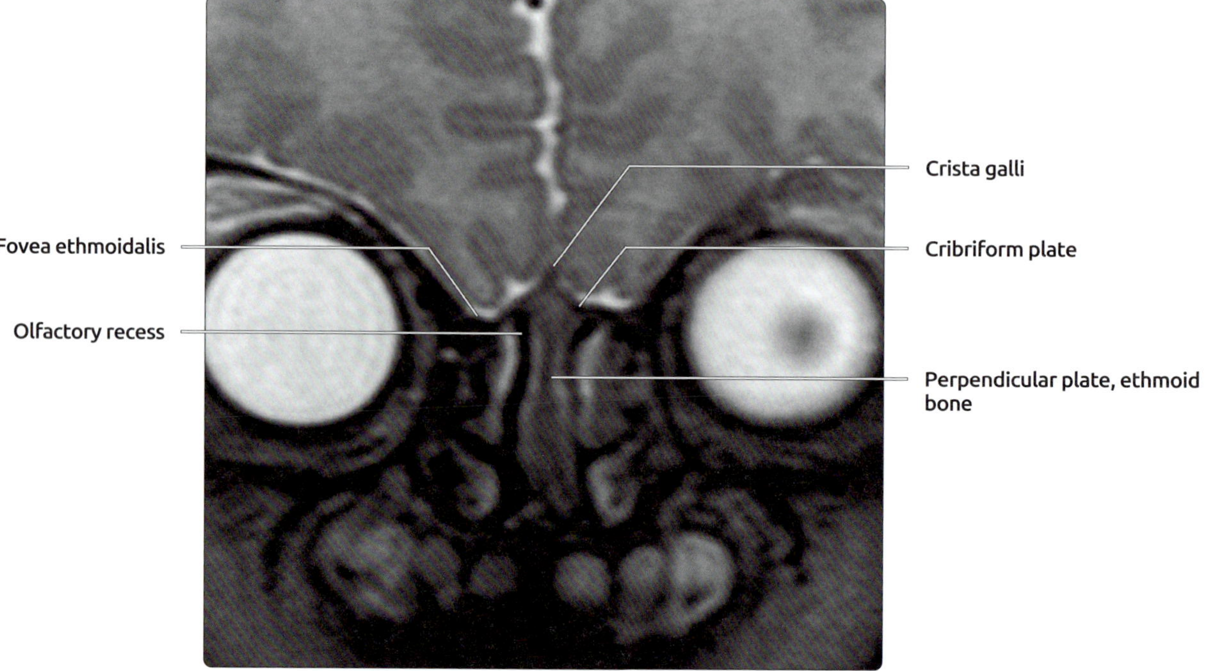

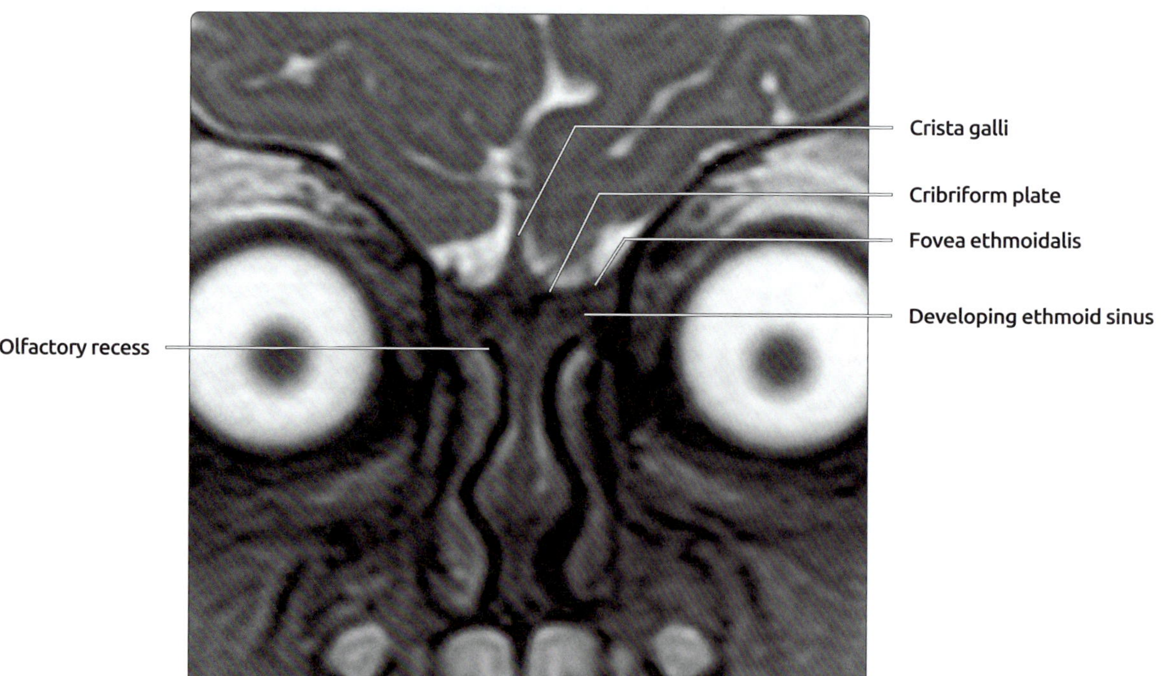

(Top) *Coronal T2 MR through the ASB in a newborn is shown. The ASB is poorly ossified at birth. The cartilaginous crista galli and cribriform plate have intermediate signal intensity.* **(Bottom)** *Coronal T2 MR through the ASB at 6 months of age is shown. Notice the distance between the cribriform plate/fovea ethmoidalis and the olfactory recess of the nose is enlarging with the development of ethmoid sinuses.*

CORONAL T2 MR, DEVELOPMENT

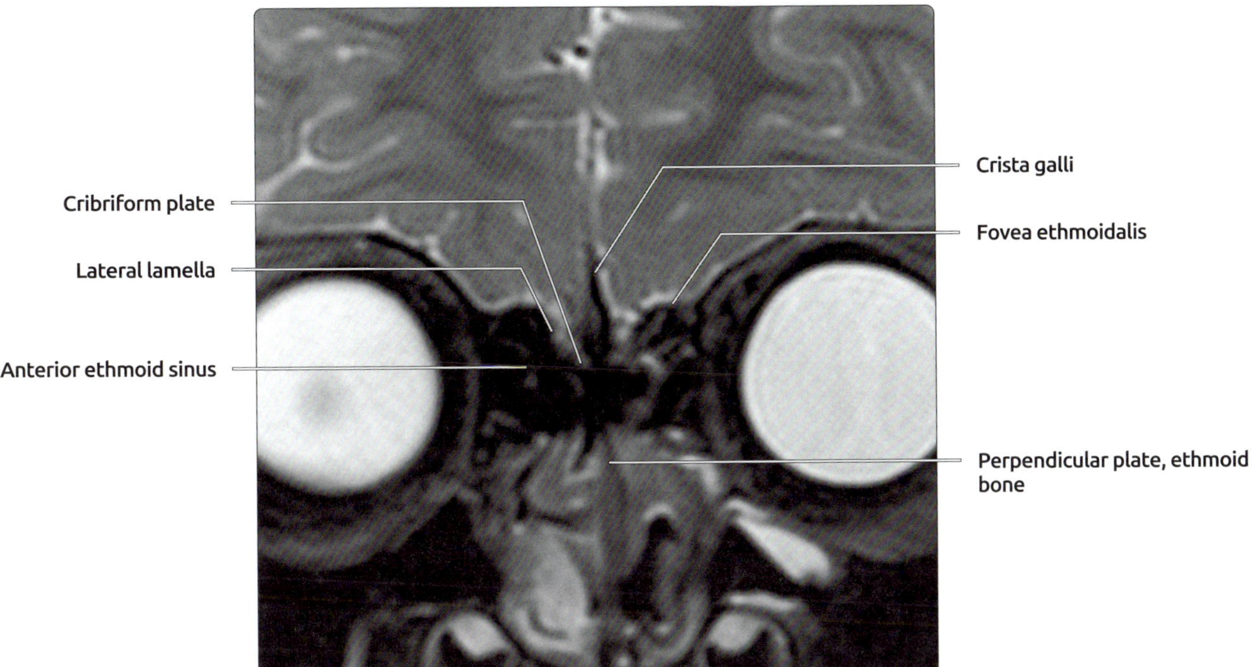

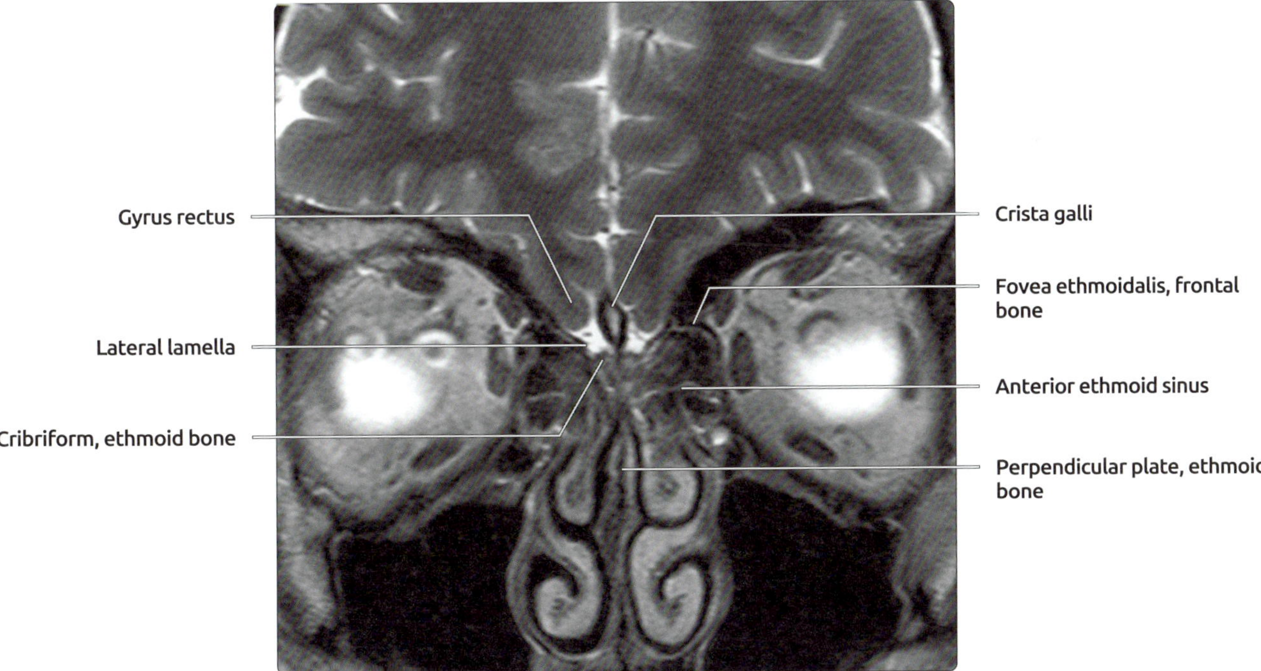

(Top) *Coronal T2 MR through the ASB at 12 months of age is shown. The crista galli, cribriform plate, lateral lamella, and fovea ethmoidalis are largely ossified at this age. As a result, the ASB appears as low signal intensity form cortical bone. Notice the ethmoid sinus aeration now projects cephalad to the level of the crista galli base. The lateral lamella connects the fovea ethmoidalis to the lateral cribriform plate.* **(Bottom)** *Coronal T2 MR through the ASB in an adult is shown. By adulthood, there is a significant amount of high-signal fat in the well-ossified crista galli. Gyri recti appear to extend far more inferiorly than in childhood because the ethmoid air cells have enlarged superiorly.*

SAGITTAL T1 MR, DEVELOPMENT

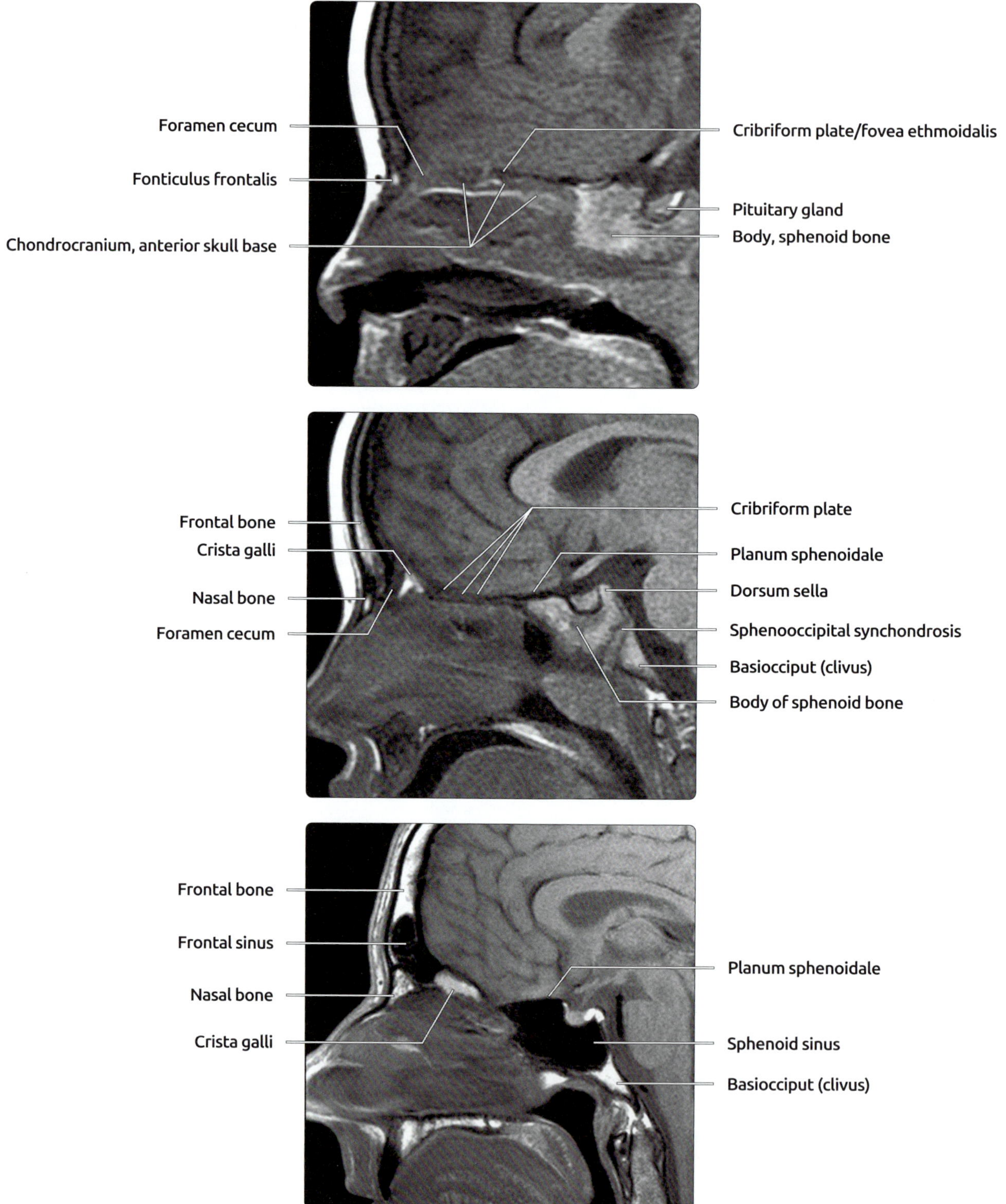

(Top) *Sagittal T1 MR of the ASB at 6 months of age is shown. The area of cribriform plate/fovea ethmoidalis has begun to ossify, hence the low-signal line. Foramen cecum margins are difficult to discern as a result of absent ossification in the area.* **(Middle)** *Sagittal T1 MR of the ASB at 18 months of age is shown. There is rapid ossification of this area in the 1st year of life. Note high-signal fatty marrow in crista galli. The foramen cecum is visible anterior to the crista galli, normally containing a thin dural stalk that will obliterate by 5 years of age.* **(Bottom)** *Sagittal T1 MR of the ASB in an adult is shown. Crista galli is readily visible due to its fatty marrow. Foramen cecum is not seen because it is now fused. The frontal bone is distinguishable from the nasal bone anteriorly.*

SAGITTAL T2 MR, DEVELOPMENT

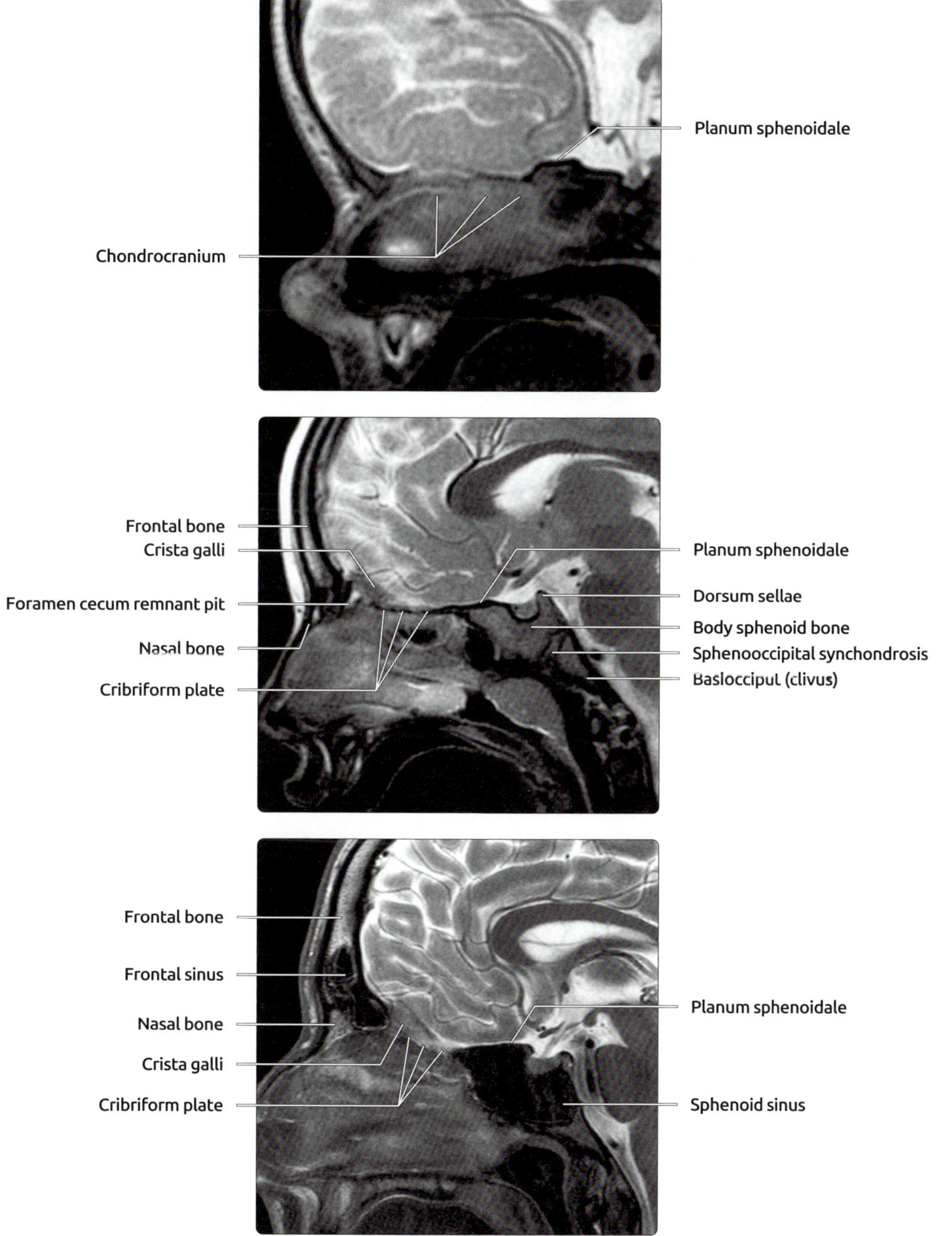

(Top) *Sagittal T2 MR of the ASB in a newborn is shown. The chondrocranium is mostly intermediate signal intensity. Large "gaps" of the ASB are seen because there is little ossification, particularly anteriorly.* **(Middle)** *Sagittal T2 MR of the ASB at 18 months of age is shown. As ASB progressively ossifies, crista galli becomes more conspicuous. The frontal and sphenoid bones are higher signal due to fatty marrow. Both the sphenoid and frontal sinuses continue to pneumatize well into the teenage years. Cribriform plate ossification is signaled by a dark line anterior to the planum sphenoidale.* **(Bottom)** *Sagittal T2 MR of the ASB in an adult is shown. The crista galli is fully ossified and filled with high-signal fatty marrow. The foramen cecum is fused and therefore not visible. The sphenoid sinus is fully pneumatized.*

TERMINOLOGY

Abbreviations

- Anterior, central, posterior skull base (ASB, CSB, PSB)
- Greater, lesser wings of sphenoid (GWS, LWS)

Definitions

- CSB: Skull base posterior to LWS/planum sphenoidale & anterior to petrous ridge/dorsum sella

IMAGING ANATOMY

Overview

- CSB is floor of middle cranial fossa & roof of sphenoid sinus
- Bones forming CSB
  - Sphenoid bone, basisphenoid, & GWS
  - Temporal bone anterior to petrous ridge
- Boundaries of CSB
  - Anteriorly boundary: Planum sphenoidale posterior margin (limbus sphenoid) medially & LWS laterally
  - Posterior boundary: Dorsum sella medially & petrous ridges laterally
  - Lateral boundary: Squamous temporal bone & GWS
- Relationships of CSB
  - Superior: Pituitary, cavernous sinus, Meckel cave, CNI-IV, CNVI, CNV1-3, temporal lobe
  - Inferior: Anterior roof of pharyngeal mucosal space, masticator, parotid & parapharyngeal spaces

Bony Landmarks of Central Skull Base

- **Sella turcica**: Contains pituitary gland
- **Anterior clinoid processes**: Extend posteromedially off LWS
- **Posterior clinoid processes**: Extend posterolaterally off dorsum sellae; attachment for tentorium cerebelli
- **Chiasmatic sulcus**: Shallow groove between posterior margin of planum sphenoidale and tuberculum sella
- **Tuberculum sellae**: Anterosuperior margin of sella turcica

Foramina and Fissures of Central Skull Base

- **Optic canal**
  - Transmits: CNII with dura, arachnoid & pia, CSF & ophthalmic artery
  - Formed by LWS, superomedial to superior orbital fissure
- **Superior orbital fissure (SOF)**
  - Transmits: CNIII, CNIV, CNV1, & CNVI, superior ophthalmic vein
  - Formed by cleft between LWS & GWS
  - SOF is separated from optic canal by optic strut, variably pneumatized extension from sphenoid body
- **Inferior orbital fissure**
  - Transmits: Infraorbital artery, vein, & nerve (CNV2)
  - Formed by cleft between body of maxilla & GWS
- **Carotid canal**
  - Transmits: Internal carotid artery & sympathetic plexus
  - Formed by GWS & temporal bone
- **Foramen rotundum**
  - Transmits: CNV2, artery of foramen rotundum, & emissary veins
  - Within sphenoid bone; superolateral to vidian canal
  - Provides direct connection to pterygopalatine fossa
- **Foramen ovale**
  - Transmits: CNV3, lesser petrosal nerve, accessory meningeal branch of maxillary artery, & emissary vein
  - Within GWS, connection to masticator space
- **Foramen spinosum**
  - Transmits: Middle meningeal artery & vein, meningeal branch of CNV3
  - Within GWS, posterolateral to foramen ovale
- **Foramen lacerum**
  - Not true foramen, between temporal & sphenoid bones
  - Cartilaginous floor of medial part of horizontal petrous internal carotid artery canal
- **Vidian canal**
  - Transmits: Vidian artery and nerve
  - Inferomedial to foramen rotundum

Development of Central Skull Base

- CSB formed by > 25 ossification centers
- Ossification occurs from posterior to anterior
- **Important ossification centers**: Orbitosphenoids, alisphenoids, pre- and postsphenoid, basiocciput
  - **Orbitosphenoids** → LWS, **alisphenoids** → GWS
  - **Presphenoid** and **postsphenoid** fuse at ~ 3 months
  - **Postsphenoid** and **basiocciput** fuse → clivus
- **Sphenooccipital synchondrosis**
  - Between postsphenoid and basiocciput
  - Open until 14 years, fuses by ~ 16 years in girls & ~ 18 years in boys

Variant Anatomy

- **Palatovaginal canal**
  - Inferomedial to vidian canal
- **Vomerovaginal canal**
  - Variable, may communicate with palatovaginal canal
- **Persistent craniopharyngeal canal**
  - Vertical cleft in sphenoid body
  - Extends from floor of sella turcica to nasopharynx
- **Extensive pneumatization of sphenoid sinus**
- **Canaliculus innominatus**
  - Medial between foramen ovale & foramen spinosum
- **Foramen of Vesalius**
  - Anteromedial to foramen ovale, transmits emissary vein from cavernous sinus to pterygoid plexus
- **Canalis basilaris medianus**
  - Well-corticated channel along midline basiocciput
- **Fossa navicularis magna**
  - Osseous defect along anterior aspect of clivus
- **Sternberg canal**
  - Osseous defect between sphenoid body & lesser wing
  - Medial to SOF & foramen rotundum

ANATOMY IMAGING ISSUES

Imaging Pitfalls

- Beware sphenoid MR signal changes
  - Sphenoid sinus: Low-signal cartilage until 2 years → high-signal fat until 6 years → low-signal air (adult)
  - Clivus low signal until 25 years, then high-signal fat
  - "Don't touch me" lesion: Arrested pneumatization of sphenoid, persistent atypical fatty marrow
- Do not confuse pneumatized clinoid processes with vascular flow voids on MR

GRAPHICS

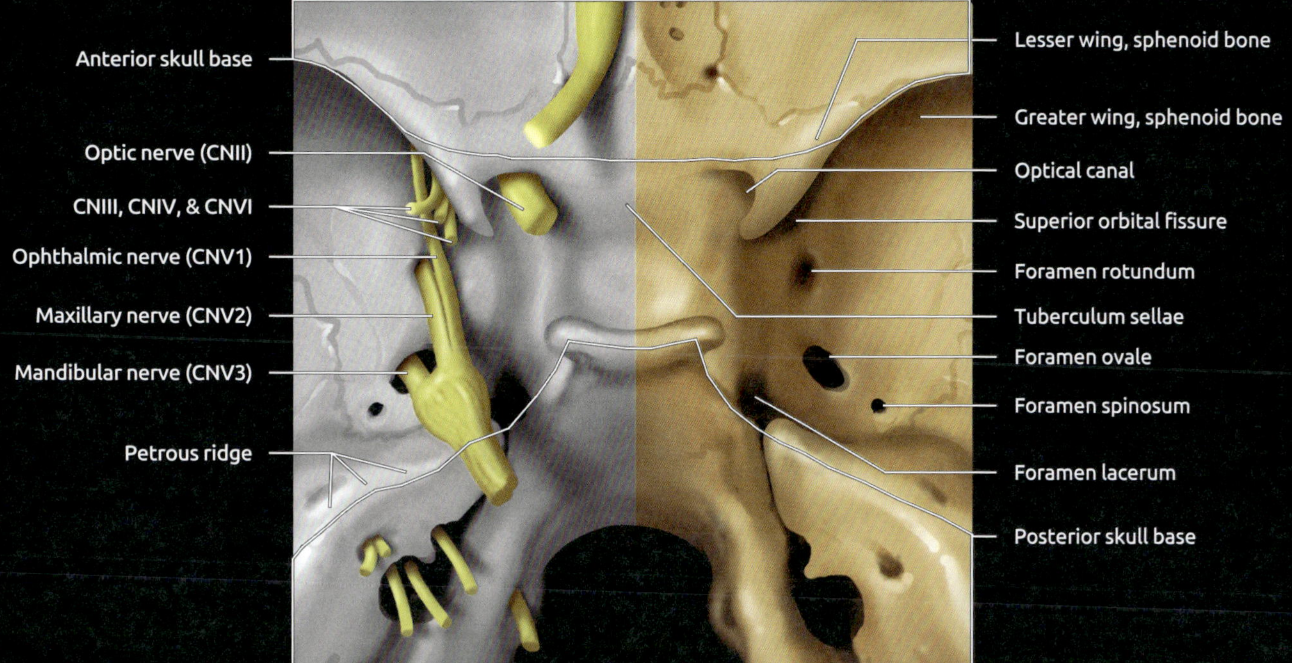

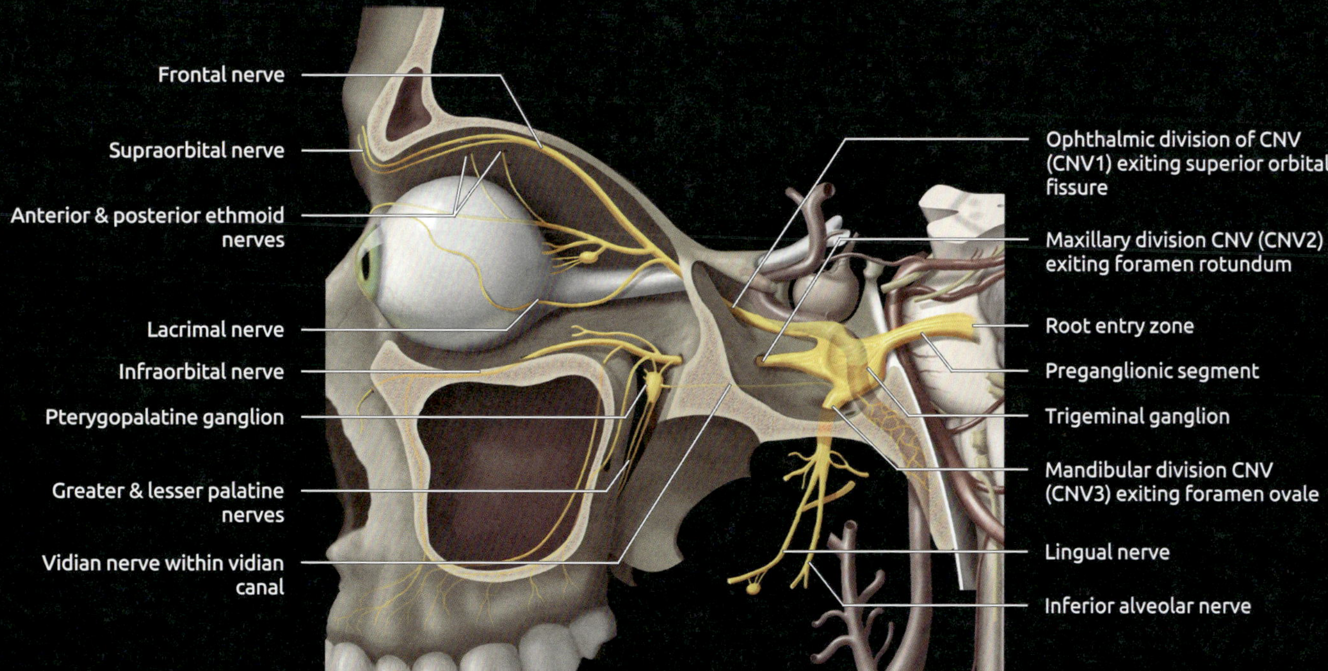

(Top) *Graphic of the central skull base (CSB) from above shows important nerves on the left. The numerous fissures & foramina of CSB are shown on the right. Greater wing of sphenoid forms anterior wall of middle cranial fossa. The posterior limit of the CSB is the dorsum sella medially & petrous ridge laterally.* **(Bottom)** *Sagittal graphic through the central & anterior skull base depicts the trigeminal nerve branches & exiting foramina. Ophthalmic division of CNV exits into orbit via the superior orbital fissure. Maxillary division of CNV exits via foramen rotundum to become infraorbital nerve as well as give rise to the greater & lesser palatine nerves inferiorly to provide sensation for the hard & soft palates. Mandibular division of CNV exits through foramen ovale, then divides into 2 main trunks, lingual & inferior alveolar nerves. Note the vidian nerve in vidian canal.*

GRAPHICS

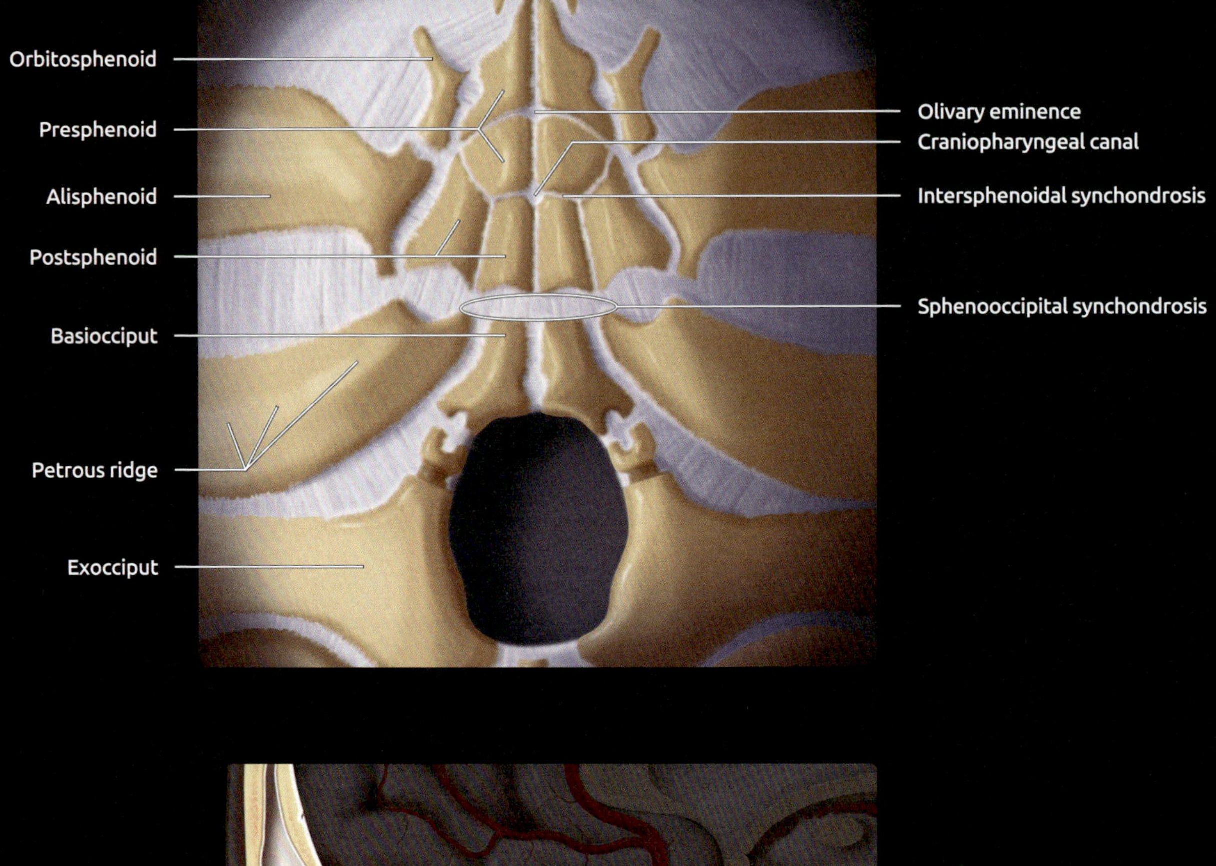

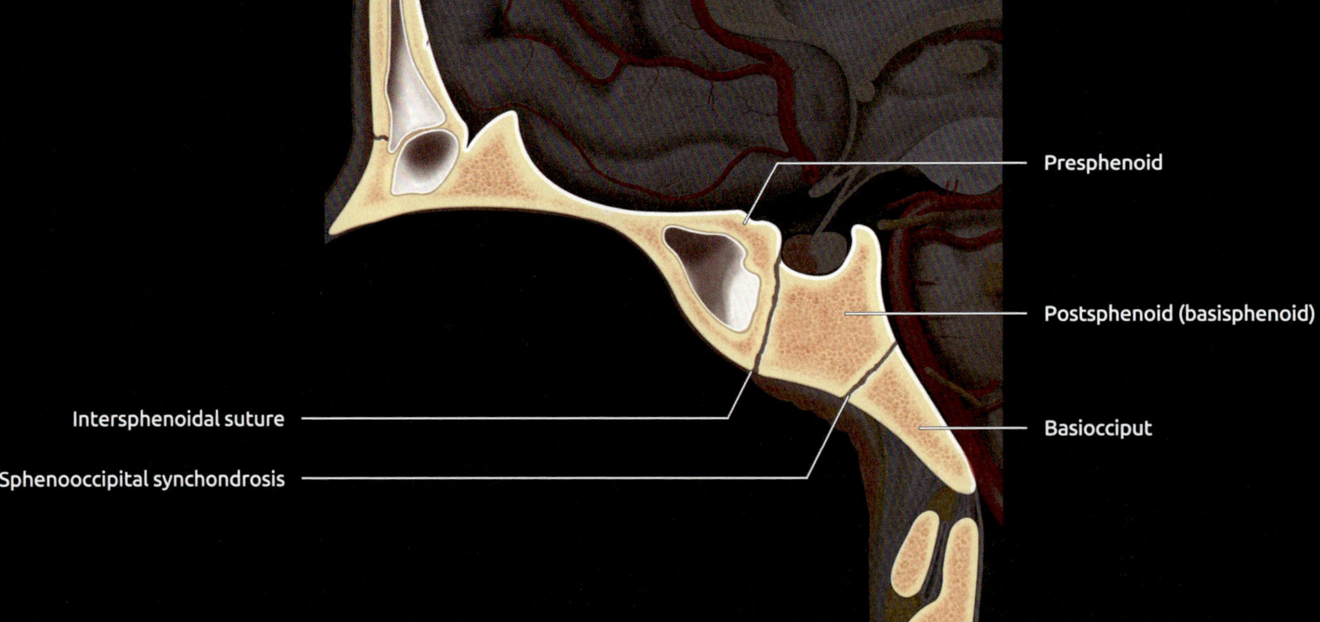

(Top) *Graphic of CSB from above shows its many ossification centers. Between the ossification centers of presphenoid is a cartilaginous gap called the olivary eminence, which is obliterated shortly after birth. A persistent cleft, called the craniopharyngeal canal, can also be variably seen in intersphenoid synchondrosis. Do not confuse these variants with pathology.* **(Bottom)** *Lateral graphic of CSB shows major ossification centers & the location of sutures. Intersphenoidal suture closes at ~ 3 months age. At ~ 2 years of age, the presphenoid begins to demineralize & become pneumatized. Pneumatization progresses posteriorly into postsphenoid until ~ 5-7 years of age. Sphenooccipital synchondrosis is one of the last sutures to fuse at ~ 16 years of age. It is the suture most responsible for growth of the skull base.*

AXIAL BONE CT

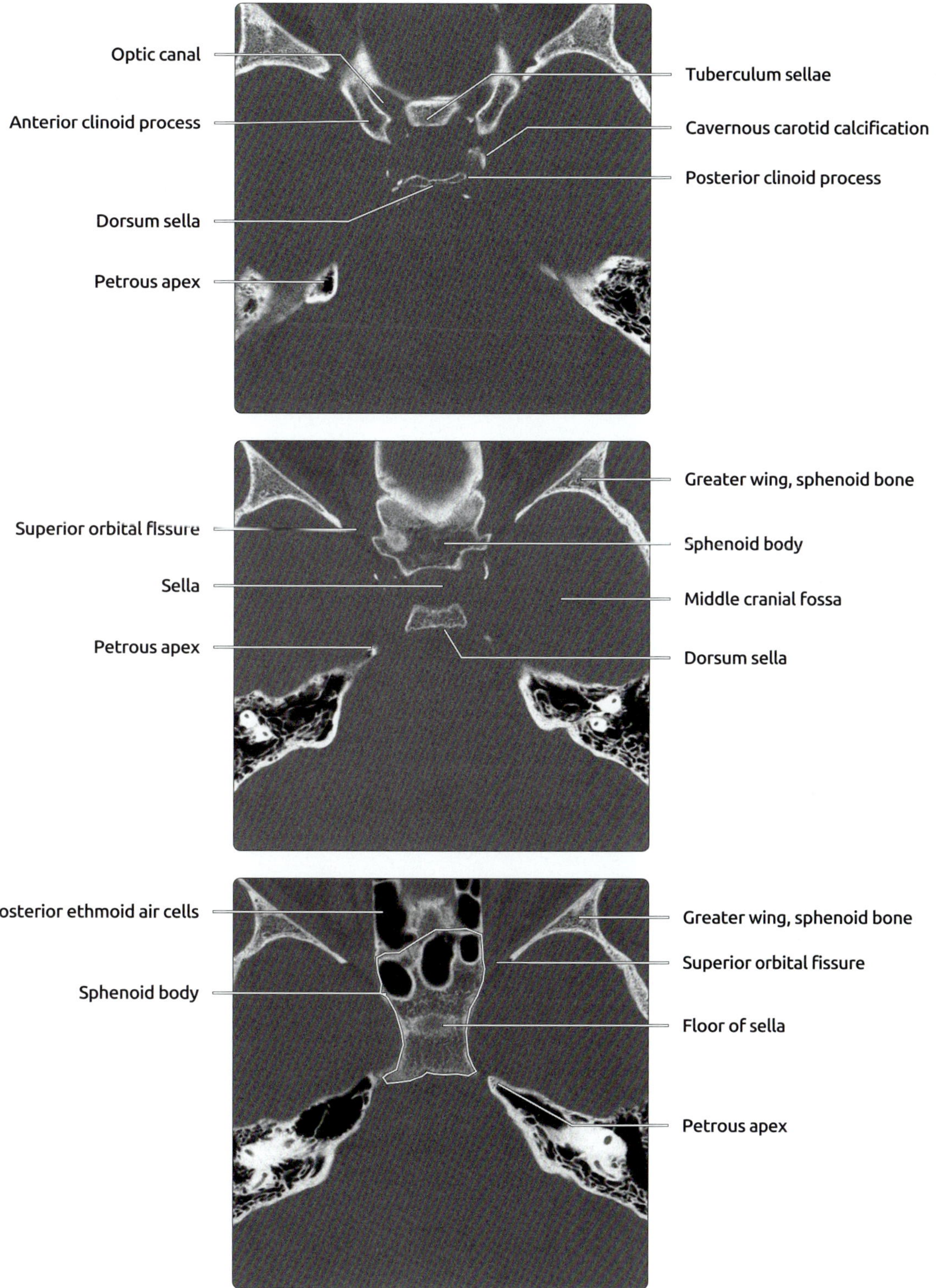

(Top) *First of 9 axial bone CT images of the CSB presented from superior to inferior is shown. Note that the posterior clinoids merge with the dorsum sella. The optic canal is bound by the sphenoid sinus medially and the anterior clinoid process laterally. Inferolateral to optic canal is the superior orbital fissure.* **(Middle)** *At the level of the sella turcica, the superior orbital fissure is seen as the medial opening of the orbit into the middle cranial fossa. It lies below the optic canal, between the greater wing of the sphenoid and the sphenoid body. The sella turcica is bound by the dorsum sella posteriorly.* **(Bottom)** *In this image, the body of the sphenoid bone is seen to be made up of the sphenoid sinus, sella turcica, and dorsum sella. Anterior to the sphenoid bone is the ethmoid bone.*

AXIAL BONE CT

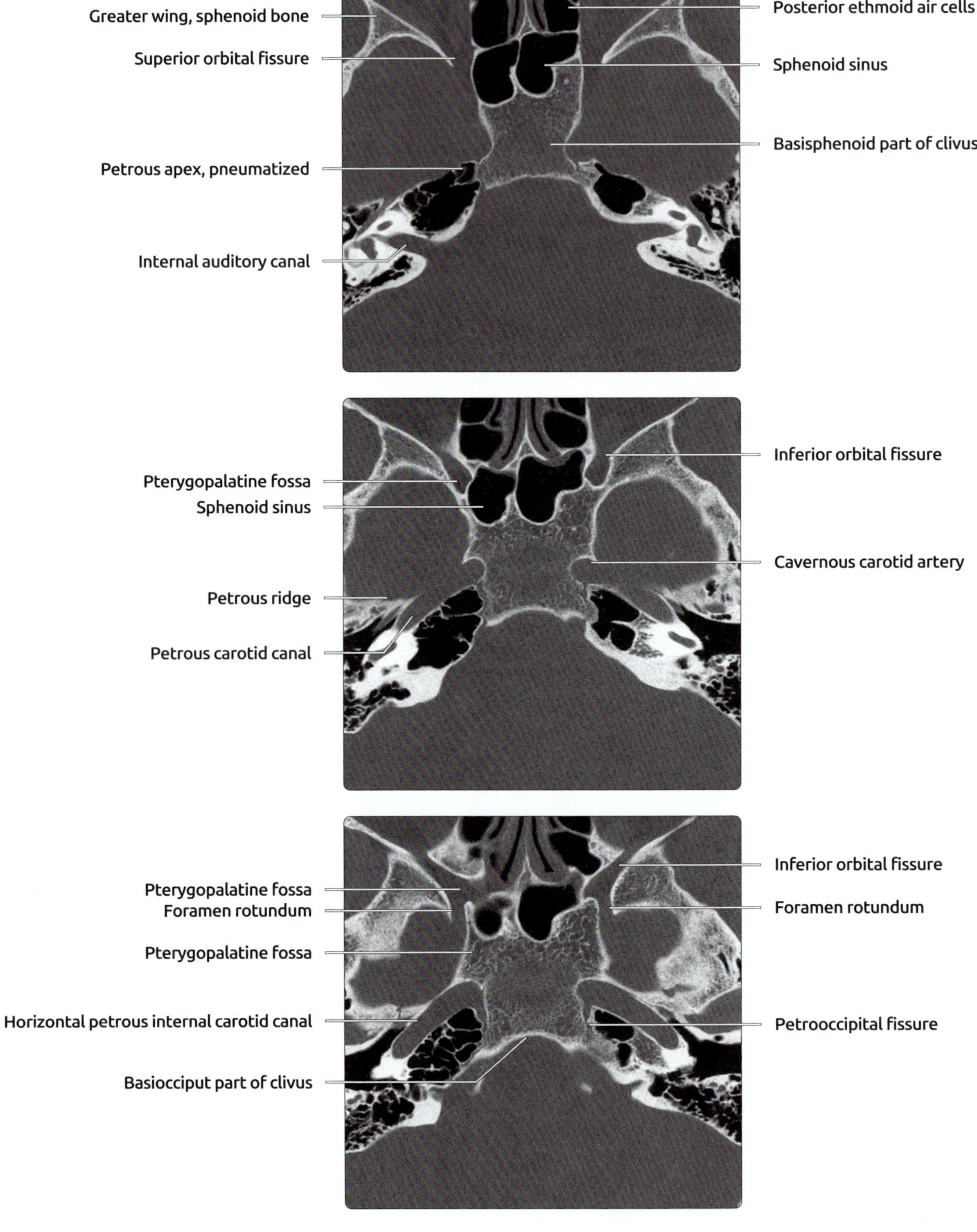

(Top) *In this image, the clivus can be seen forming the medial posterior boundary of CSB, while the petrous ridge defines its lateral posterior margin.* **(Middle)** *This image shows the inferior orbital fissure along the floor of the orbit inferior to the superior orbital fissure. It is bounded superiorly by the greater wing of sphenoid, inferiorly by the maxilla and orbital process of palatine bone, and laterally by the zygomatic bone.* **(Bottom)** *At the level of the foramen rotundum, both pterygopalatine fossae are clearly visible. The maxillary division of the trigeminal nerve (CNV2) exits the skull base through the foramen rotundum & continues as the infraorbital nerve into orbit via the inferior orbital fissure. Malignant tumors of the skin of the cheek, orbit, & sinonasal area may all use CNV2 as a perineural route to gain intracranial access. Note the foramen rotundum empties anteriorly into the pterygopalatine fossa, which connects laterally with the masticator space through the pterygomaxillary fissure.*

AXIAL BONE CT

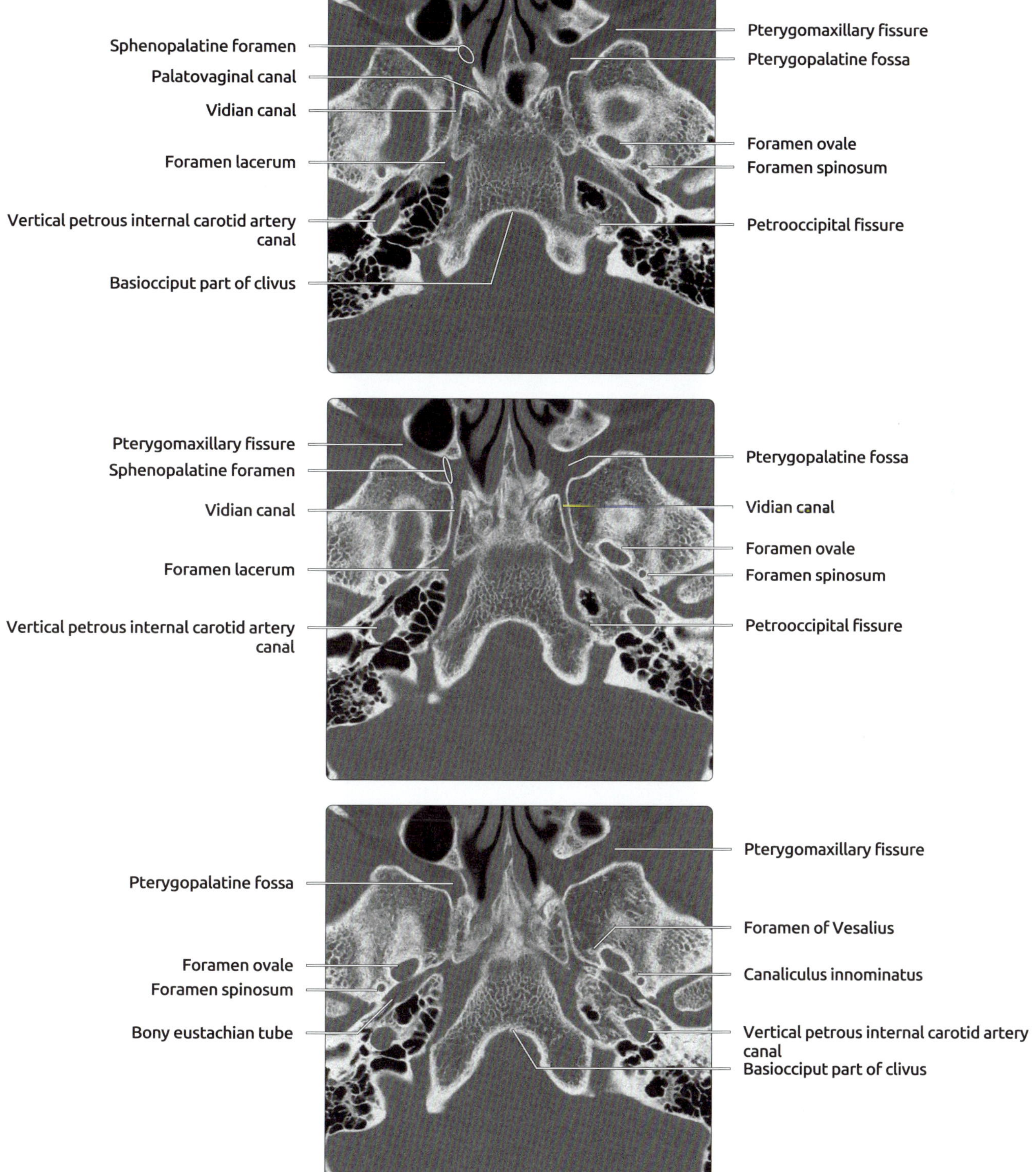

(Top) *In this image, the vidian canal is visible connecting the pterygopalatine fossa anteriorly to the carotid canal floor (foramen lacerum) posteriorly. A malignant tumor that has accessed the pterygopalatine fossa may reach the carotid canal of the skull base via perineural spread on the vidian nerve in the vidian canal. There is a medial connection between the pterygopalatine fossa & nose, the sphenopalatine foramen. Juvenile angiofibroma begins along the nasal margin of this foramen.* **(Middle)** *In this image, note that the foramen ovale is located in the greater wing of the sphenoid bone. Extracranial perineural malignancy on CNV3 enters the intracranial area via the foramen ovale.* **(Bottom)** *In this image, note the foramen spinosum is posterolateral to the foramen ovale in the greater wing of the sphenoid bone. The middle meningeal artery passes intracranially via the foramen spinosum. The inconstant foramen of Vesalius is anteromedial to the foramen ovale. The inconstant canaliculus innominatus is between the foramen ovale and foramen spinosum.*

CORONAL BONE CT

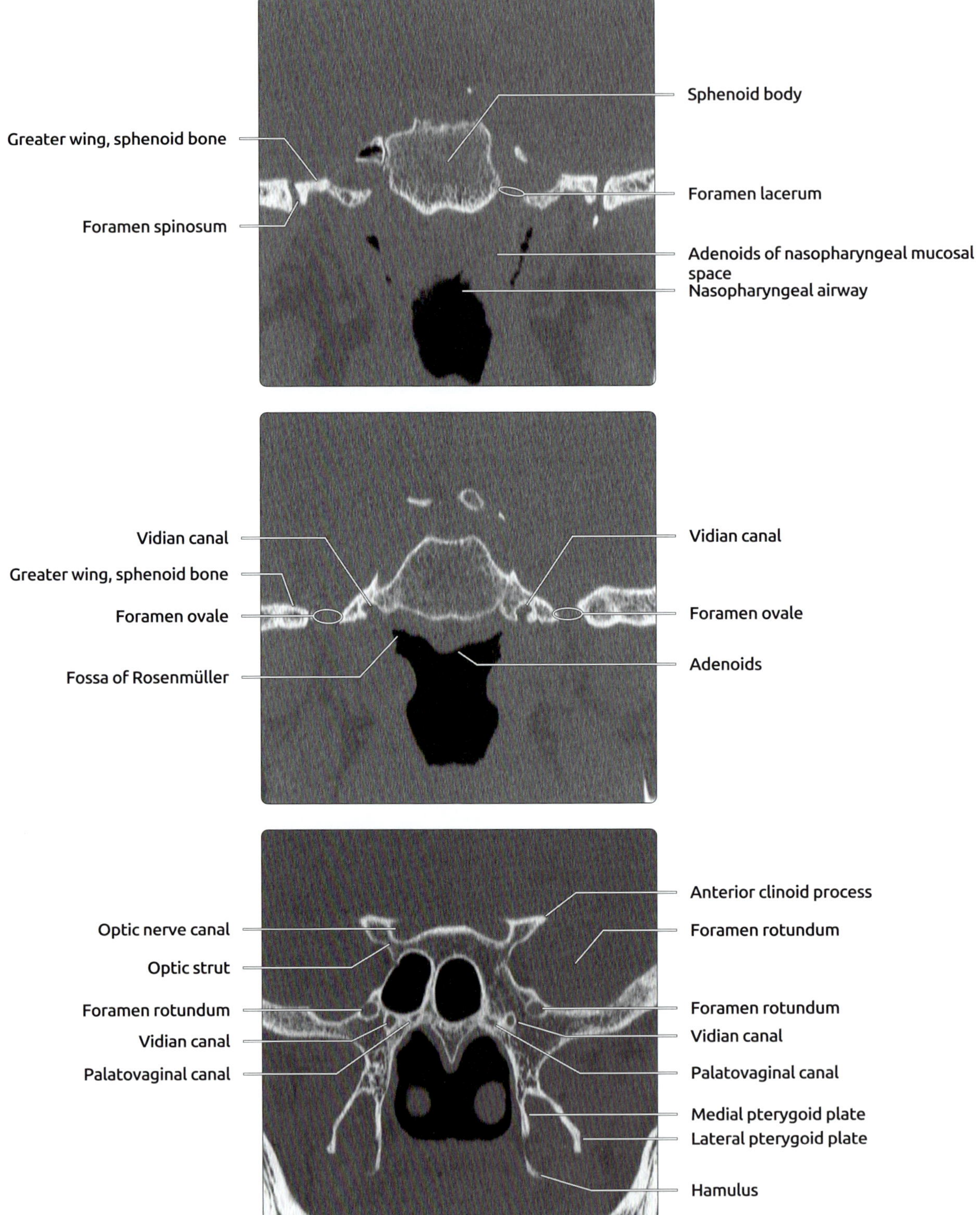

(Top) *First of 3 coronal bone CT images of the CSB presented from posterior to anterior is shown. The foramen lacerum is seen as a large defect between the greater wing of the sphenoid bone and the sphenoid body. The foramen lacerum is not a true foramen; it represents the cartilaginous floor of the anteromedial horizontal segment of the petrous internal carotid artery canal.* **(Middle)** *In this image, the foramen ovale is evident lateral to the vidian canal and anterolateral to the foramen lacerum. It transmits CNV3 from the middle cranial fossa to the masticator space.* **(Bottom)** *More anteriorly, the foramen rotundum and vidian canal are both seen running in the transverse plane. Both the foramen rotundum and vidian canal open into the pterygopalatine fossa. Also note the pterygoid plates inferiorly.*

AXIAL T1 C+ MR

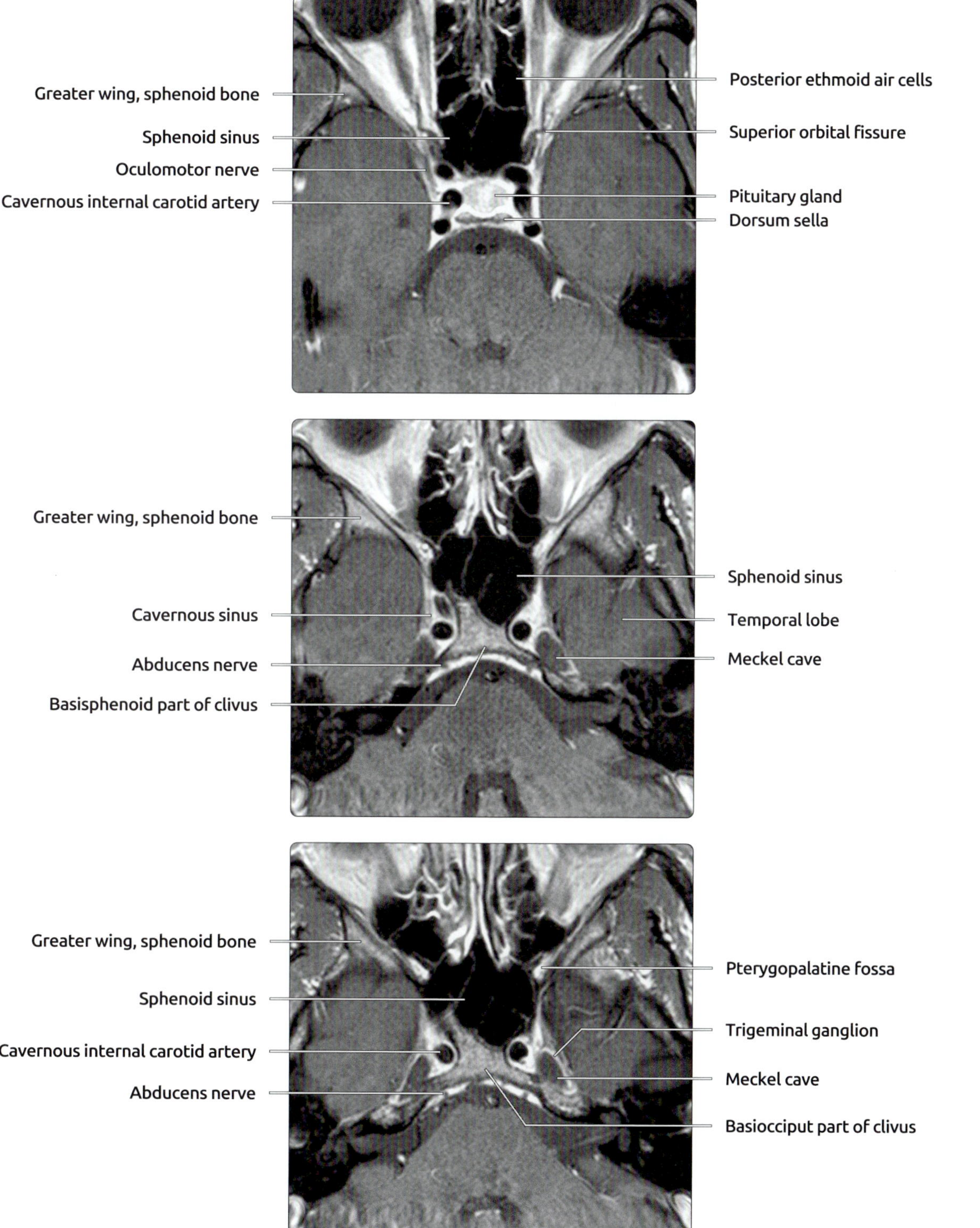

(Top) *First of 6 axial T1 C+ MR images of the CSB presented from superior to inferior is shown. The enhancing venous plexus of the cavernous sinus is seen surrounding the cavernous internal carotid artery. Medially, the enhancing pituitary gland in the sella turcica is bound by the dorsum sella posteriorly and the sphenoid sinus anteriorly.* **(Middle)** *In this image, the upper basisphenoid part of the clivus is seen. Cerebrospinal fluid-filled Meckel cave is seen along the posterior border of the cavernous sinus.* **(Bottom)** *In this image, the basiocciput part of the clivus is visible. The upper clivus above the fused sphenooccipital synchondrosis is part of the sphenoid bone, while the lower clivus is part of the occipital bone. Notice the marrow space of the clivus enhances.*

AXIAL T1 C+ MR

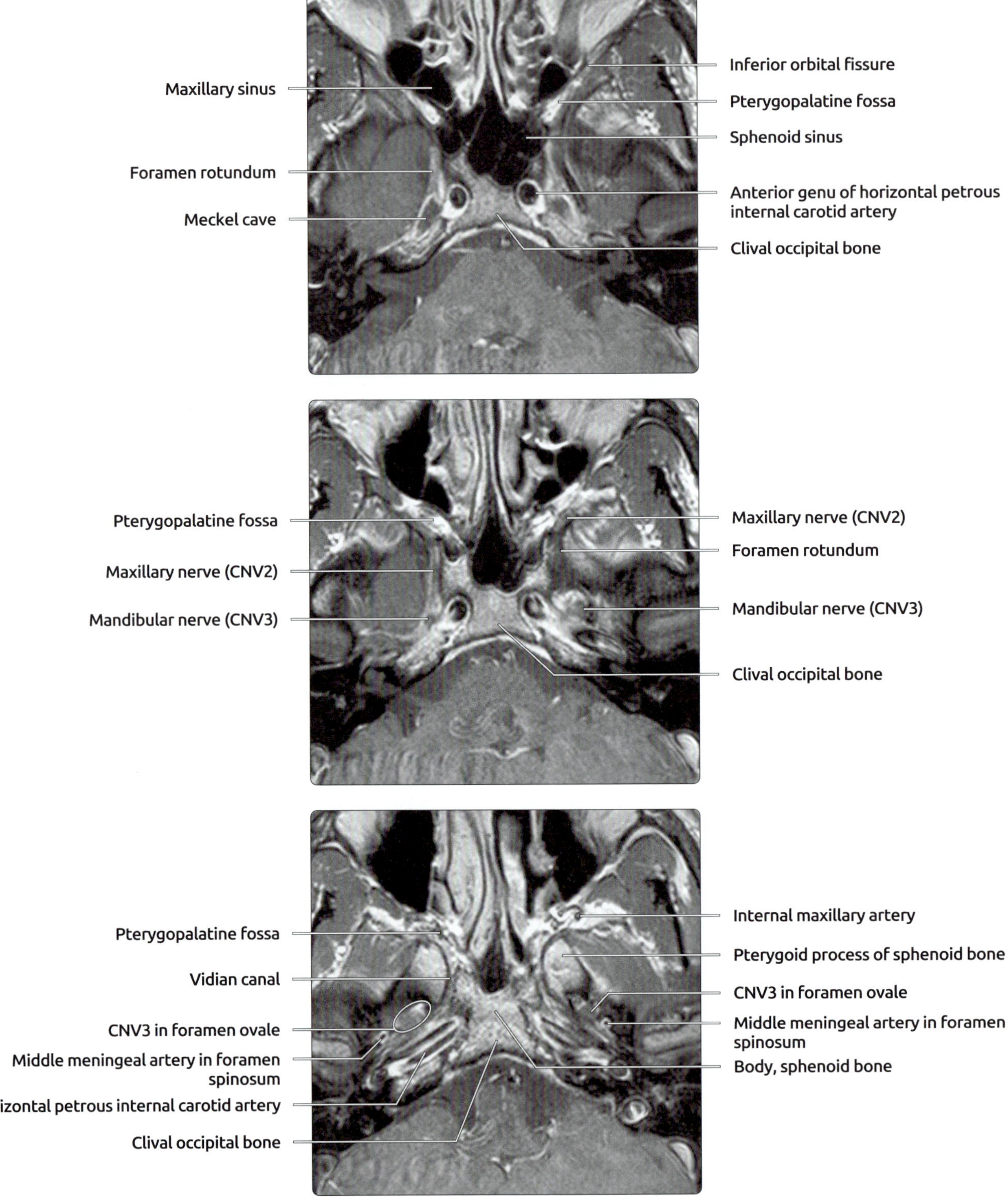

(Top) *Image through the superior pterygopalatine fossa shows its anterolateral connection to the inferior orbital fissure. The anteriorly projecting foramen rotundum can also be seen. The sphenoid bone is partially pneumatized (sphenoid sinus).* **(Middle)** *In this image, the maxillary nerve (CNV2) is seen as a linear low-intensity structure in the foramen rotundum on the right. On the left, this same nerve can be seen exiting the foramen rotundum into the pterygopalatine fossa.* **(Bottom)** *At the level of the foramen ovale, the mandibular nerve (CNV3) is seen bilaterally. Also note the middle meningeal artery passing through the foramen spinosum. The vidian canal is clearly visible medial to the foramen ovale. The clival occipital bone should be distinguished from the body of the sphenoid bone even though the sphenooccipital fissure cannot be discerned.*

SAGITTAL T1 & T2 MR, DEVELOPMENT

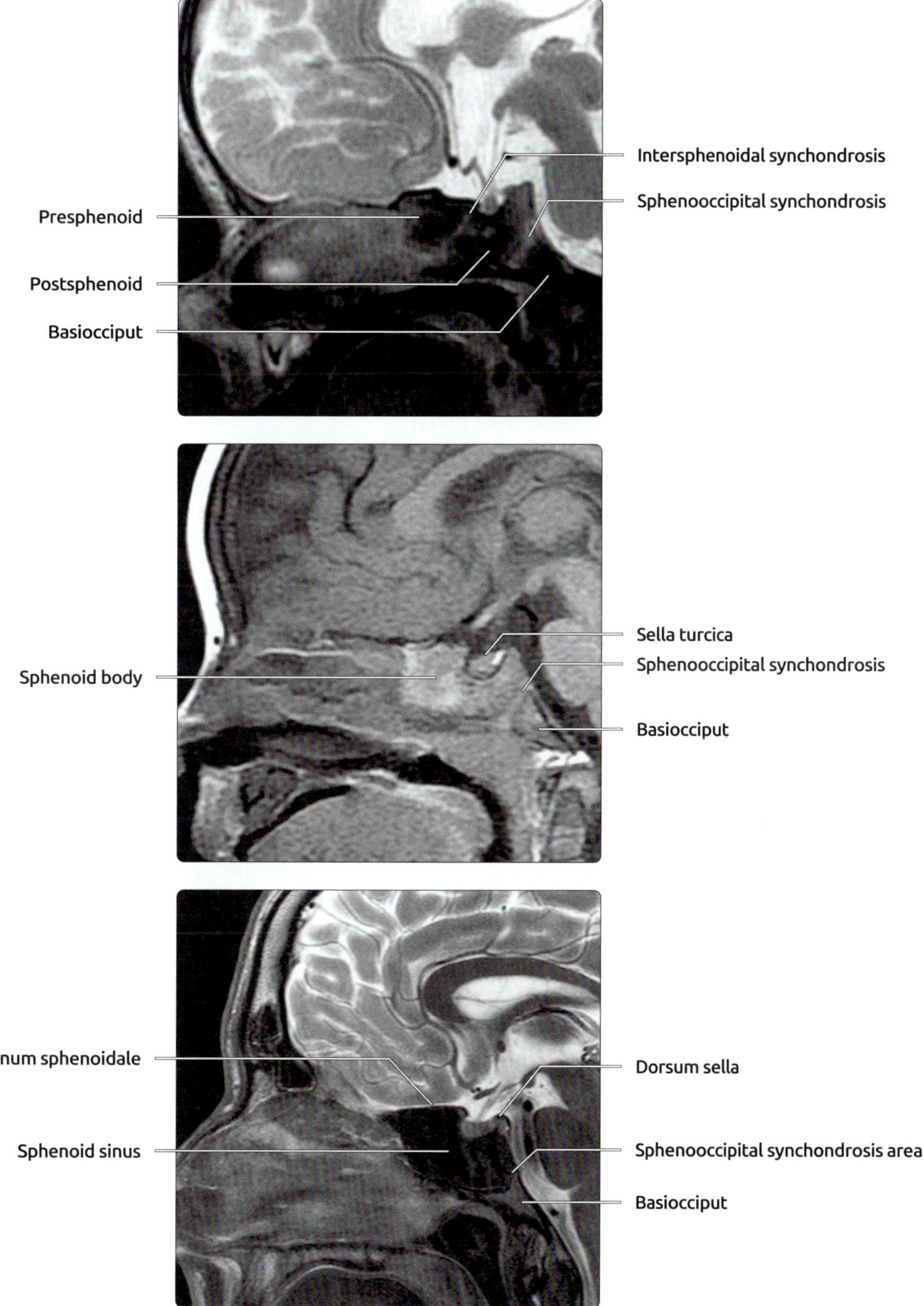

(Top) *Sagittal T2 MR of the CSB in a newborn shows the important synchondroses of this area. The intersphenoidal suture separates presphenoid from postsphenoid while the sphenooccipital synchondrosis separates postsphenoid from basiocciput.* **(Middle)** *Sagittal T1 MR shows the CSB at 6 months. The intersphenoidal suture closes at ~ 3 months of age, resulting in formation of the sphenoid body from the presphenoid and postsphenoid. There is normal high-signal fat within what used to be presphenoid. The sphenooccipital synchondrosis will remain open until adolescence.* **(Bottom)** *Sagittal T2 MR shows the CSB in an adult. Typically, pneumatization extends throughout the entire sphenoid body up to the fused sphenooccipital synchondrosis. The sphenooccipital synchondrosis is one of last sutures of the skull base to close. It fuses completely by ~ 16-18 years of age.*

TERMINOLOGY

Abbreviations

- Posterior skull base (PSB)

Definitions

- Skull base (SB) posterior to dorsum sella and petrous ridges

IMAGING ANATOMY

Overview

- PSB made up of posterior temporal bones and occipital bone
  - Transmits CNVII-XII, medulla oblongata, and jugular vein
- Bones of PSB
  - Temporal bones posterior to petrous ridges
  - **Occipital bone** (3 parts)
    - **Basilar part** (basiocciput): Quadrilateral part anterior to foramen magnum
    - **Condylar part** (exoccipital): Occipital condyles lateral to foramen magnum
    - **Squamous part**: Large bony plate posterosuperior to foramen magnum
- Boundaries of PSB
  - Anterior boundary: Dorsum sella, clivus
  - Posterior boundary: Occipital bone
  - Lateral boundary: Petrous and mastoid segments of temporal bone, occipital condyles
- Relationships of PSB
  - Inferior relationships: Posterior roof of pharyngeal mucosal space, carotid, parotid, retropharyngeal, perivertebral spaces
  - Superior relationships: Brainstem, cerebellum, CNVII-VIII, CNIX-XII, transverse-sigmoid sinuses

Bony Landmarks of Posterior Skull Base

- **Petrous ridge of temporal bone**
  - Divides central SB from PSB
  - Attachment for fixed edge of tentorium cerebelli
- **Jugular tubercle**
  - Roof of hypoglossal canal seen well on coronal imaging
  - "Eagle's head" on coronal images: Jugular tubercle

Foramina and Fissures of Posterior Skull Base

- **Internal acoustic meatus**
  - Transmits: CNVII-VIII, labyrinthine artery
  - Opening in posterior wall temporal bone superior to jugular foramen
  - Porus acusticus: Internal opening of internal acoustic meatus
- **Jugular foramen**
  - 2 parts: Pars nervosa and pars vascularis partially divided by jugular spine
  - Between temporal and occipital bones
  - Carotid space extends directly up to jugular foramen
  - **Pars nervosa**
    - Transmits CNIX, Jacobson nerve, and inferior petrosal sinus
    - Anteromedial but contiguous with pars vascularis
  - **Pars vascularis**
    - Transmits CNX, Arnold nerve, CNXI, jugular bulb, and posterior meningeal artery
    - Larger than pars nervosa
- **Groove for sigmoid sinus**
  - Groove in medial mastoid temporal bone
- **Hypoglossal canal**
  - Transmits CNXII, meningeal branch of ascending pharyngeal artery, venous plexus
  - Formed in condylar occipital bone
  - Inferomedial to jugular foramen
- **Foramen magnum**
  - Transmits CNXI (cephalad component), vertebral arteries, and medulla oblongata
- **Stylomastoid foramen**
  - Transmits CNVII
  - Between mastoid tip and styloid process, extends directly into parotid space, fat pad surrounding exiting CNVII

Development of Posterior Skull Base

- Occipital bone: 4 major ossification centers around foramen magnum
  - **Supraoccipital**, **basioccipital**, and paired **exoccipital**
- PSB is nearly completely ossified by birth
- **Sutures of PSB** remain unfused until 2nd decade
  - Intraoccipital sutures fuse between 8-16 years
  - Petrooccipital and occipitomastoid sutures are among last to close (15-17 years)
- **Kerckring ossicle**
  - Small, ovoid ossicle at posterior margin of foramen magnum
  - Kerckring-supraoccipital suture fuses by 1 year

Variant Anatomy of Posterior Skull Base

- **Posterior condylar canal**
  - Inconstant canal for emissary vein and meningeal branch of occipital artery
  - One of largest emissary foramina of SB
- **Asymmetric petrous apices**
  - Can contain high-signal fat or low-signal air
- **Mastoid foramen**
  - Variably transmits emissary vein from sigmoid sinus
- **Persistent Kerckring ossicle**
- **Jugular foramina asymmetry**
  - Right usually larger than left

ANATOMY IMAGING ISSUES

Questions

- PSB is largely ossified at birth, but PSB sutures are last in SB to fuse
- PSB is intimately related to carotid and parotid spaces

Imaging Recommendations

- Bone CT with edge enhancement algorithm and wide windows (> 2,000 HU)
- Use coronal imaging to examine normal "double eagles" of hypoglossal canal and jugular foramen area

Imaging Pitfalls

- Watch for asymmetric petrous apex air &/or fat
- Beware of jugular foramen pseudolesion from MR flow phenomenon
- Beware of open synchondroses/suture as pseudofracture

GRAPHICS

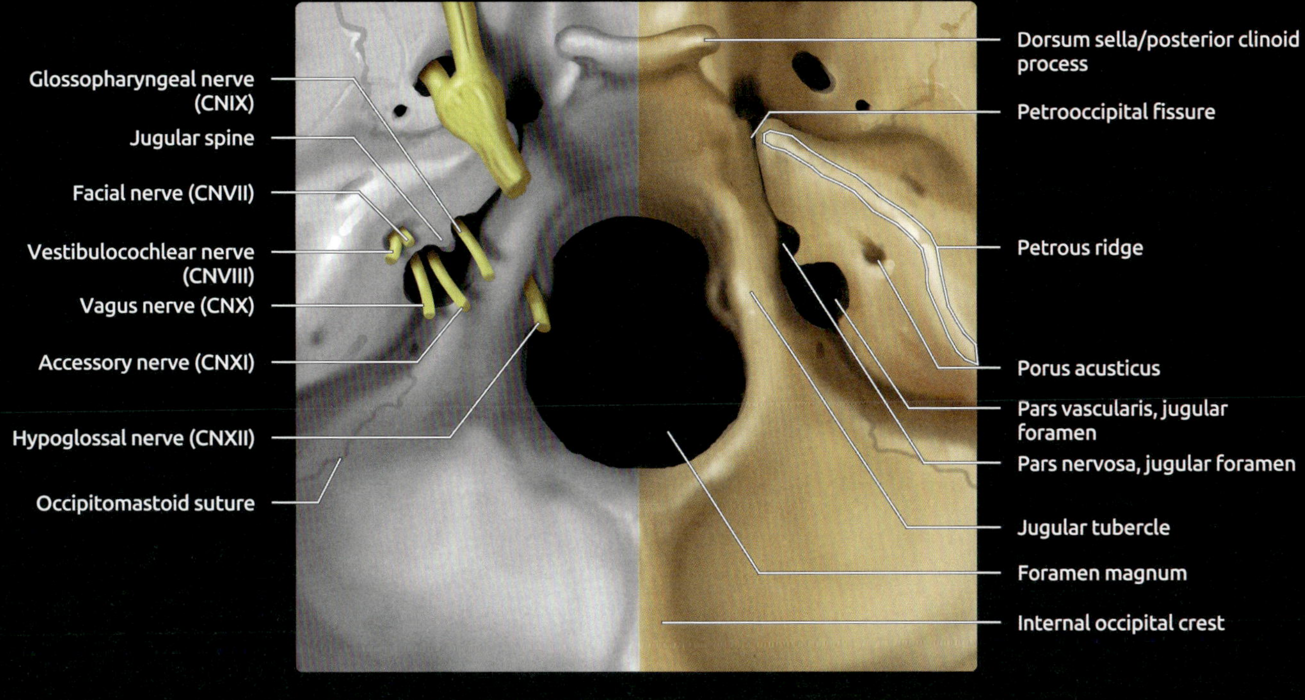

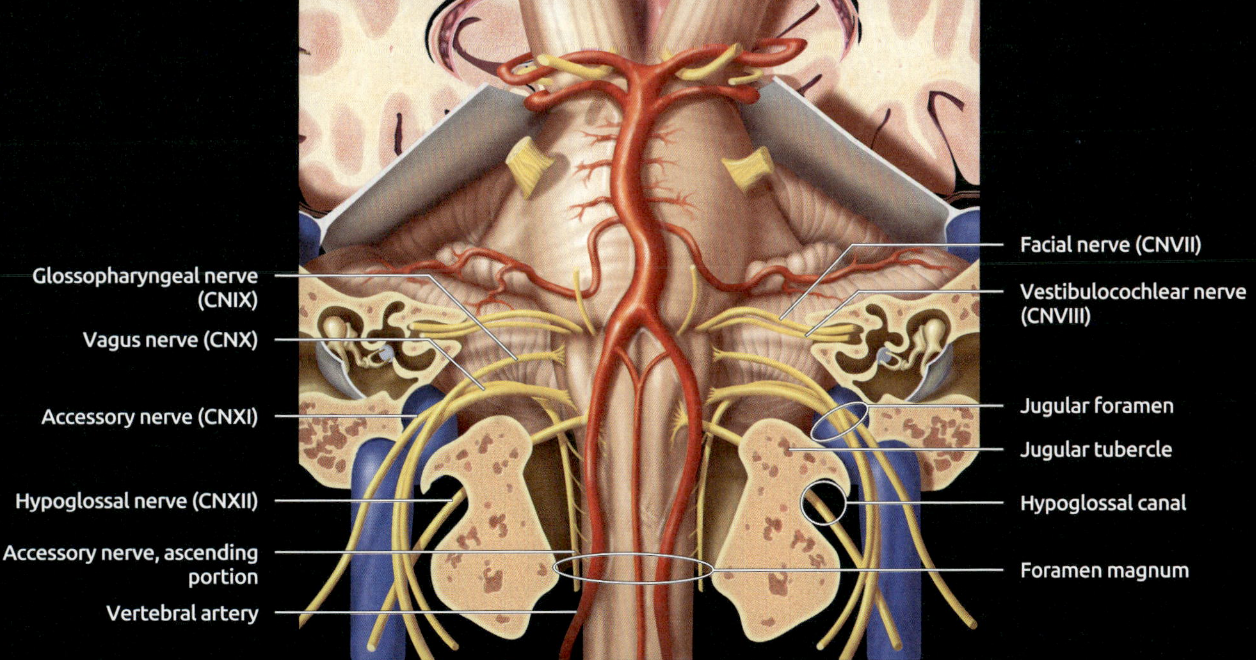

(Top) *Graphic of the posterior skull base as seen from above is shown. Neural structures are shown on the left, and bony landmarks are shown on the right. The anterior boundary of the posterior skull base is the clivus medially and the petrous ridge laterally. The major foramina are the foramen magnum, porus acusticus, jugular foramen, and hypoglossal canal. Notice that the jugular foramen connects anteriorly with the petrooccipital fissure.* **(Bottom)** *Coronal graphic of the posterior skull base viewed from the front shows the classic double eagle appearance in the area of the hypoglossal canal. The jugular tubercle (eagle's head and beak) separates the inferomedial hypoglossal canal from the jugular foramen. The hypoglossal nerve is found in the hypoglossal canal, while CNIX-XI traverse the skull base in the jugular foramen.*

GRAPHIC AND MR VENOGRAM

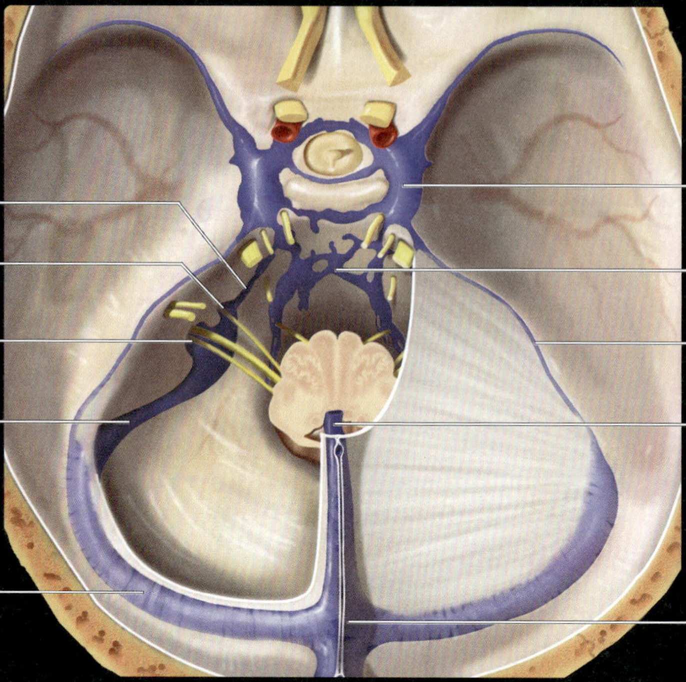

Inferior petrosal sinus
Pars nervosa, jugular foramen
Pars vascularis, jugular foramen
Sigmoid sinus
Transverse sinus
Cavernous sinus
Clival venous plexus
Superior petrosal sinus
Straight sinus
Sinus confluence (torcular Herophili)

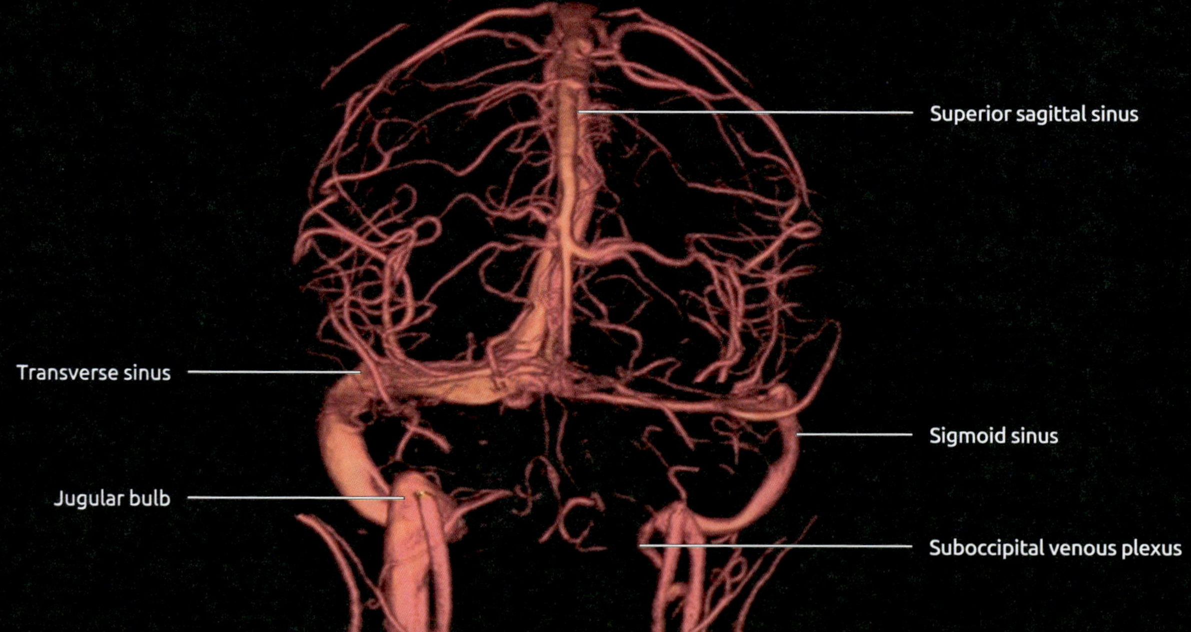

(Top) *Graphic shows the major dural venous sinuses and the jugular foramen from the top down. The midbrain and pons as well as the left 1/2 of the tentorium cerebelli have been removed. Notice the transverse sinus is in the wall of the occipital bone, while the sigmoid sinus is in the medial wall of the temporal bone. The 2 portions of the jugular foramen are also visible. The anterior pars nervosa receives the glossopharyngeal nerve (CNIX), while the pars vascularis has the vagus (CNX) and accessory (CNXI) nerves passing through it.* **(Bottom)** *3D volume-rendered view of MR venogram shows the transverse sinuses feeding through the sigmoid sinuses into the jugular foramen. The jugular bulb connects inferiorly with the internal jugular vein of the carotid space. Asymmetry of the transverse sinuses is normal with the right often being dominant.*

AXIAL BONE CT

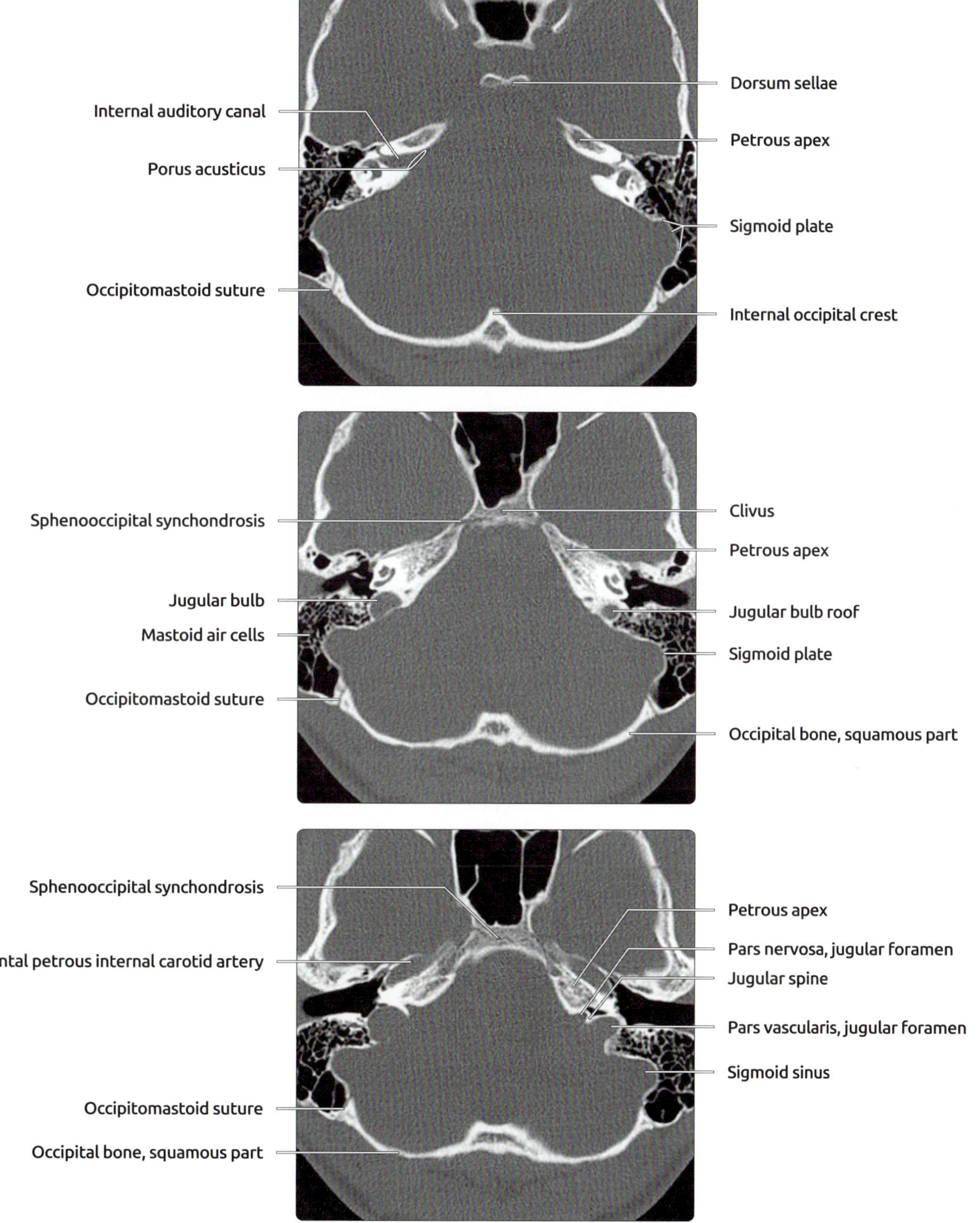

(Top) *First of 9 axial bone CT images, presented from superior to inferior, shows the dorsum sella and the petrous temporal bone as the anterior margin of the posterior skull base. Posteriorly, the midline is demarcated by the bony internal occipital crest, which provides attachment for the falx cerebelli. Porus acusticus is the most superior foramen of the posterior skull base and transmits CNVII and CNVIII.* **(Middle)** *At the level of the midcochlea, the posterior cranial fossa is completely divided from middle cranial fossa by the clivus and petrous temporal bone. Laterally, the sigmoid plate separates the mastoid air cells from the sigmoid sinus. The jugular bulbs are visible bilaterally.* **(Bottom)** *At the level of the midjugular foramen, note the smaller anteromedial pars nervosa (CNIX, Jacobsen nerve, inferior petrosal sinus) and the larger pars vascularis (jugular bulb, Arnold nerve, CNX, and CNXI).*

AXIAL BONE CT

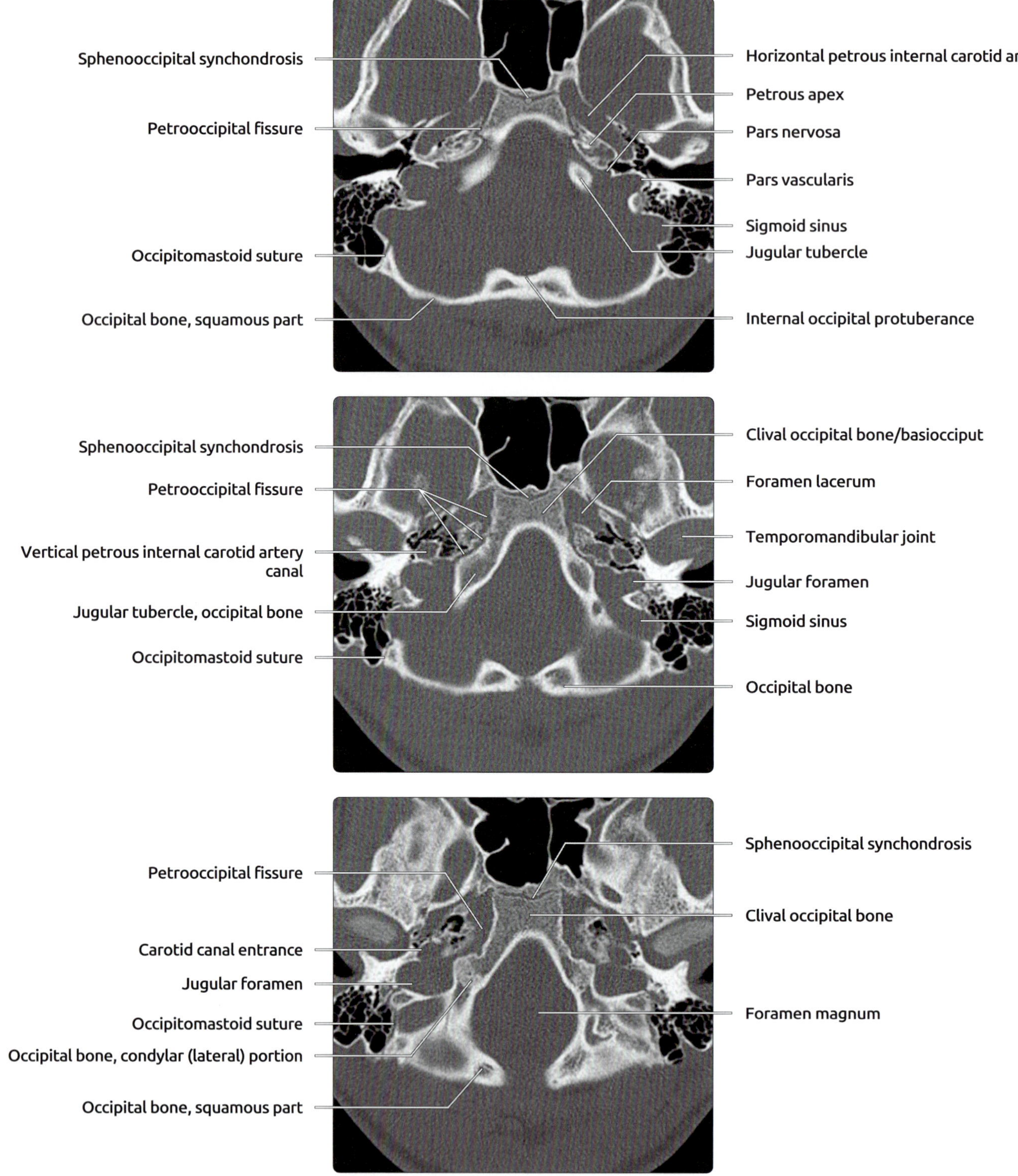

(Top) *Image of the posterior skull base shows the sphenooccipital synchondrosis, the petrooccipital fissure, and the occipitomastoid suture all in the same plane. The sphenooccipital synchondrosis has not yet fused in this young adolescent.* **(Middle)** *Image through the jugular tubercle of the clivus is made up almost completely of anterior occipital bone. The upper 1/3 of the clivus is above the sphenooccipital synchondrosis and is therefore part of the sphenoid bone.* **(Bottom)** *In this image, the lower clivus (below the sphenooccipital synchondrosis) is clearly made up of occipital bone. The petrooccipital fissure separates the temporal bone from the occipital bone. The occipitomastoid suture separates the mastoid sinus from the squamosal portion of the occipital bone.*

AXIAL BONE CT

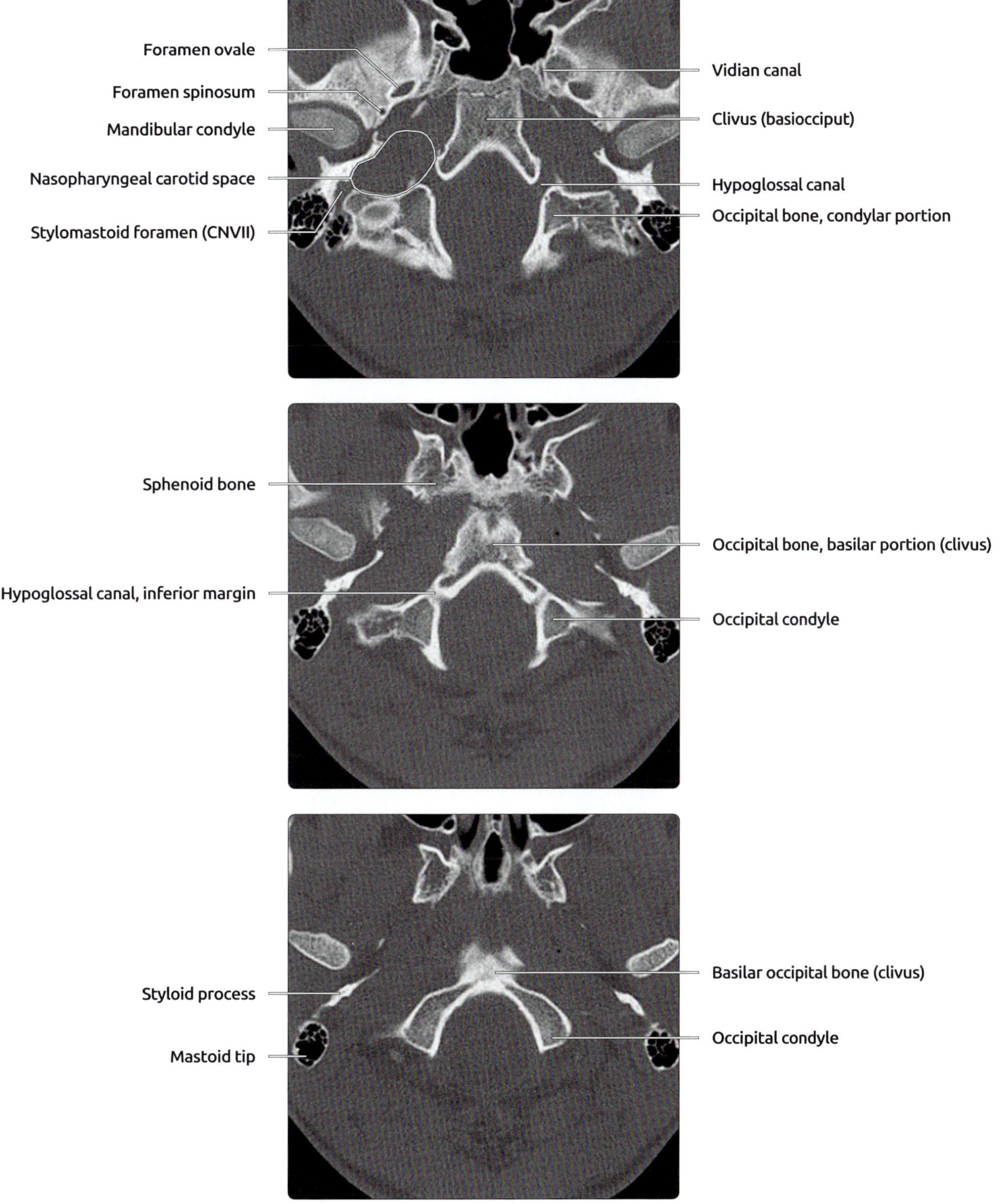

(Top) *This image passes directly through the hypoglossal canal and stylomastoid foramen. This canal transmits only the hypoglossal nerve. Notice that as soon as the nerve exits the hypoglossal canal, it immediately enters the nasopharyngeal carotid space to join the glossopharyngeal (CNIX), vagus (CNX), and accessory (CNXI) cranial nerves.* **(Middle)** *In this image, the inferior margin of the hypoglossal canal runs within the occipital bone, between the basilar (clival) and condylar portions. The inferior surface of the condylar occipital bone is comprised of the occipital condyles.* **(Bottom)** *In this image through the occipital condyle, the inferiormost junction of the basilar (clival) occipital bone and the condylar occipital bone is visible. The occipital condyles rest the cranium upon the lateral masses of atlas (C1 vertebral body).*

CORONAL BONE CT

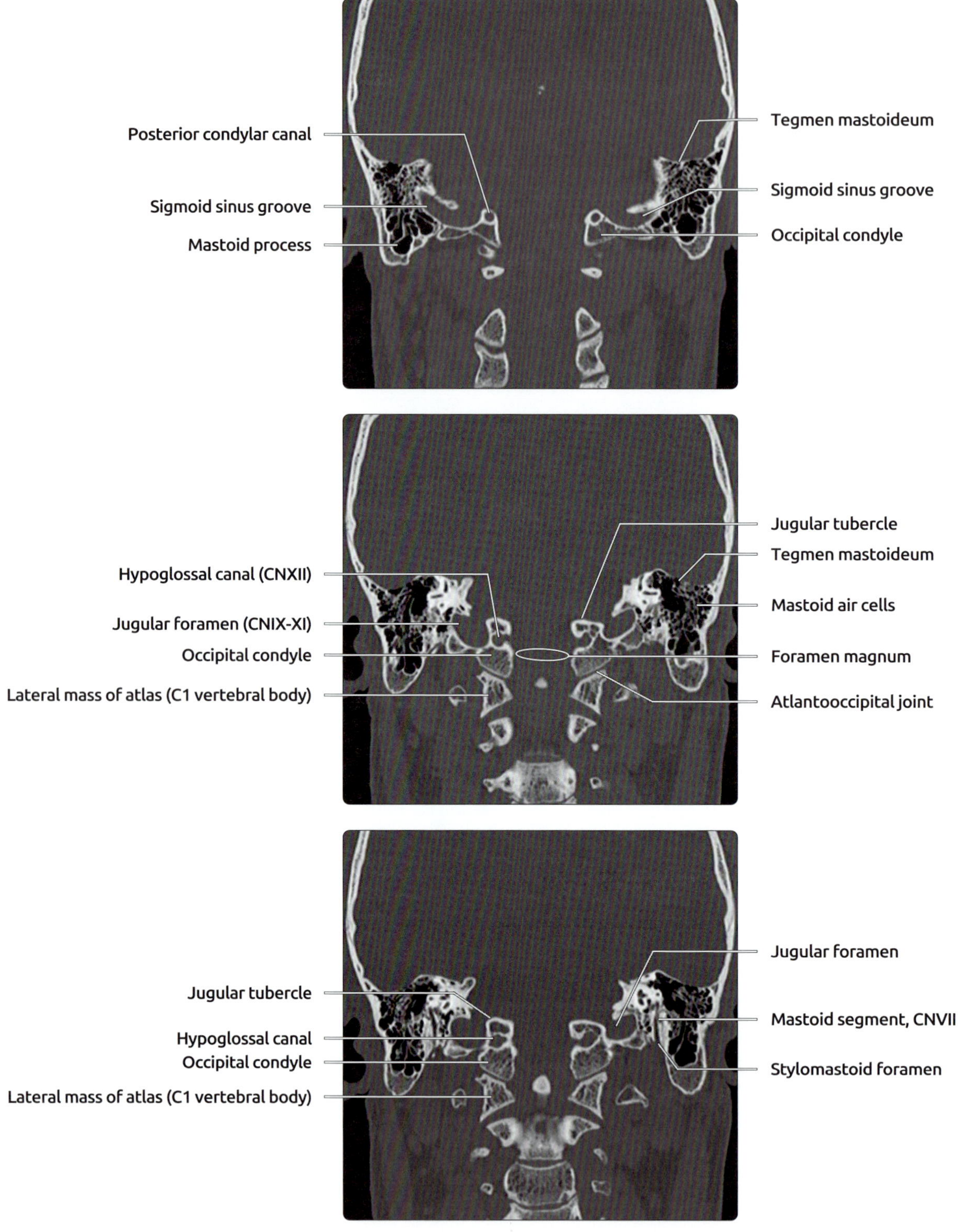

(Top) *First of 6 coronal bone CT images of the posterior skull base, presented from posterior to anterior, is shown. The groove for the sigmoid sinus is seen along the medial mastoid temporal bone. Note the posterior condylar canal, an inconstant canal for supracondylar emissary vein and a meningeal branch of the occipital artery.* **(Middle)** *In this image through the proximal hypoglossal canal and jugular foramen, the foramen magnum is outlined. The jugular tubercle is medial to the jugular fossa and superior to the hypoglossal canal. Jugular foramina are often asymmetric in size with the right often larger than left, as seen in this image.* **(Bottom)** *Coronal image through the midsegment of the hypoglossal canal is shown. The hypoglossal canal passes through the condylar (lateral) portion of the occipital bone. Note the mastoid (descending) portion of the intratemporal facial nerve canal and the stylomastoid foramen.*

CORONAL BONE CT

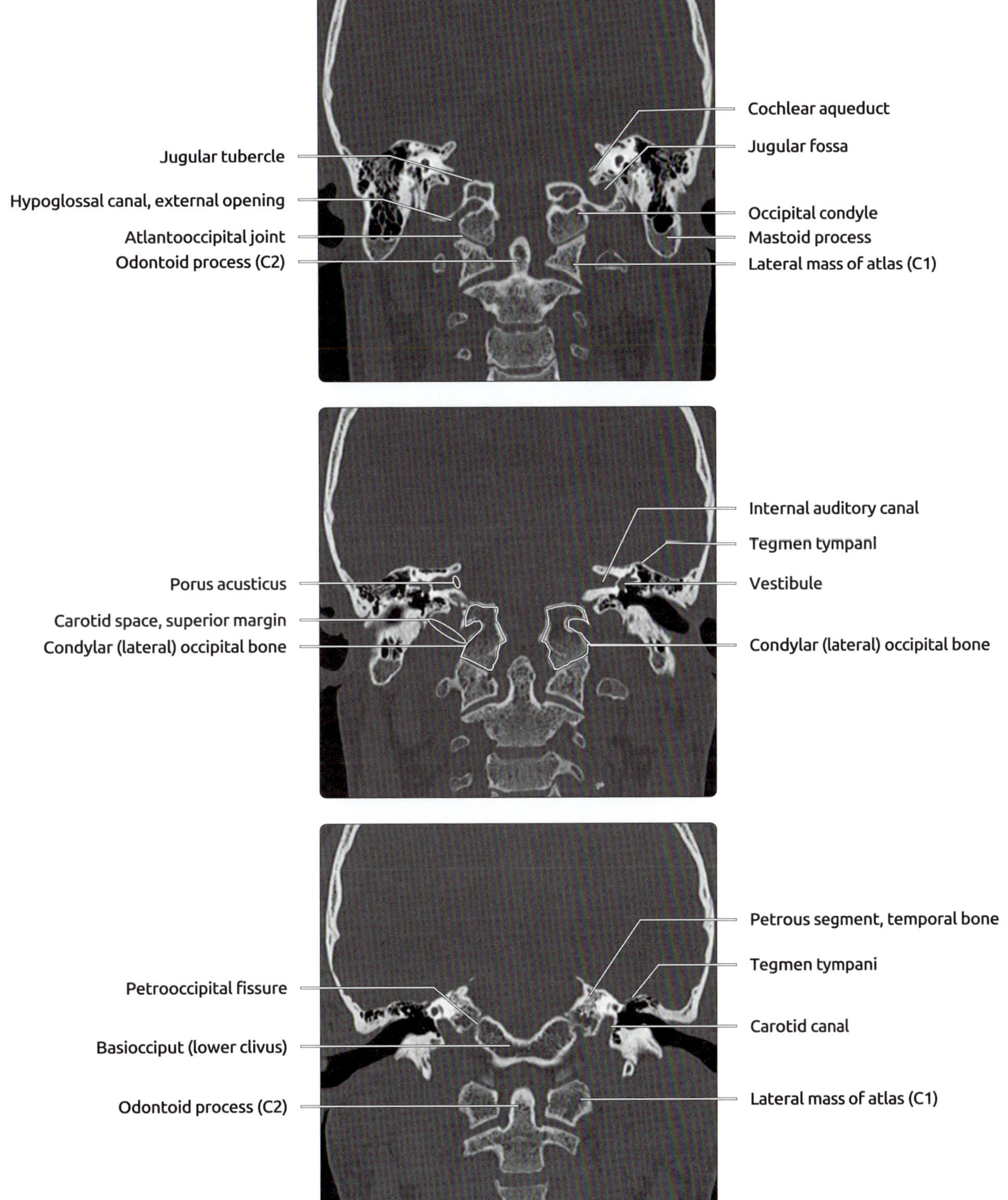

(Top) *In this image of the skull base, the cochlear aqueduct is visible opening at the roof (pyramidal fossa) of the jugular foramen pars nervosa. The hypoglossal canal opens into the carotid space.* **(Middle)** *In this image through the midinternal auditory canal, the condylar part of the occipital bone is outlined. This image shows the classic "double eagle" of the posterior skull base with the "beak" of the jugular tubercle separating the jugular foramen from the hypoglossal canal. Lesions of the hypoglossal canal affect the undersurface of the "beak," while lesions of the jugular foramen affect the superior surface of the "beak."* **(Bottom)** *In this image, the petrooccipital fissure is seen between the basiocciput and the temporal bone. The basiocciput is a large quadrilateral portion of the occipital bone that extends anterosuperiorly from the anterior margin of the foramen magnum to reach the sphenoid bone about 2/3 of the way up the clivus.*

AXIAL T1 C+ FS MR

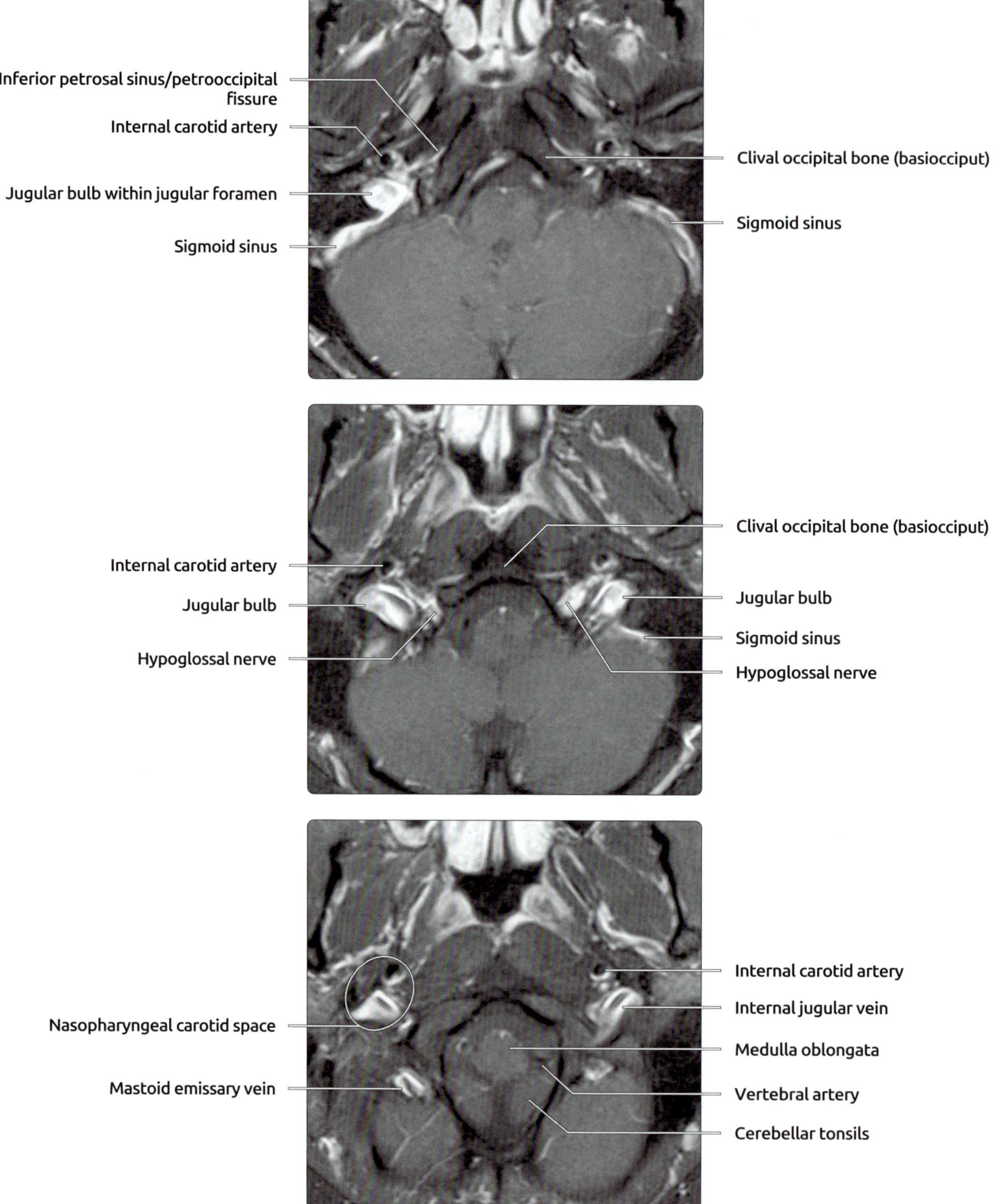

(Top) *First of 3 axial T1 C+ FS MR images of the posterior skull base, presented from superior to inferior, is shown. On the patient's right, the high-signal enhancing sigmoid sinus can be seen connecting anteromedially with the jugular bulb.* **(Middle)** *At the level of the hypoglossal canals, the hypoglossal nerves can be seen as linear, low-intensity structures surrounded by the enhancing high-signal basiocciput venous plexus. The complex signal seen in both jugular bulbs should not be mistaken for a lesion.* **(Bottom)** *At the level of the foramen magnum, the internal jugular vein and internal carotid artery of the carotid space are visible. The vertebral arteries, medulla oblongata, and inferior cerebellar tonsils are normally seen at this level.*

CORONAL T1 C+ MR

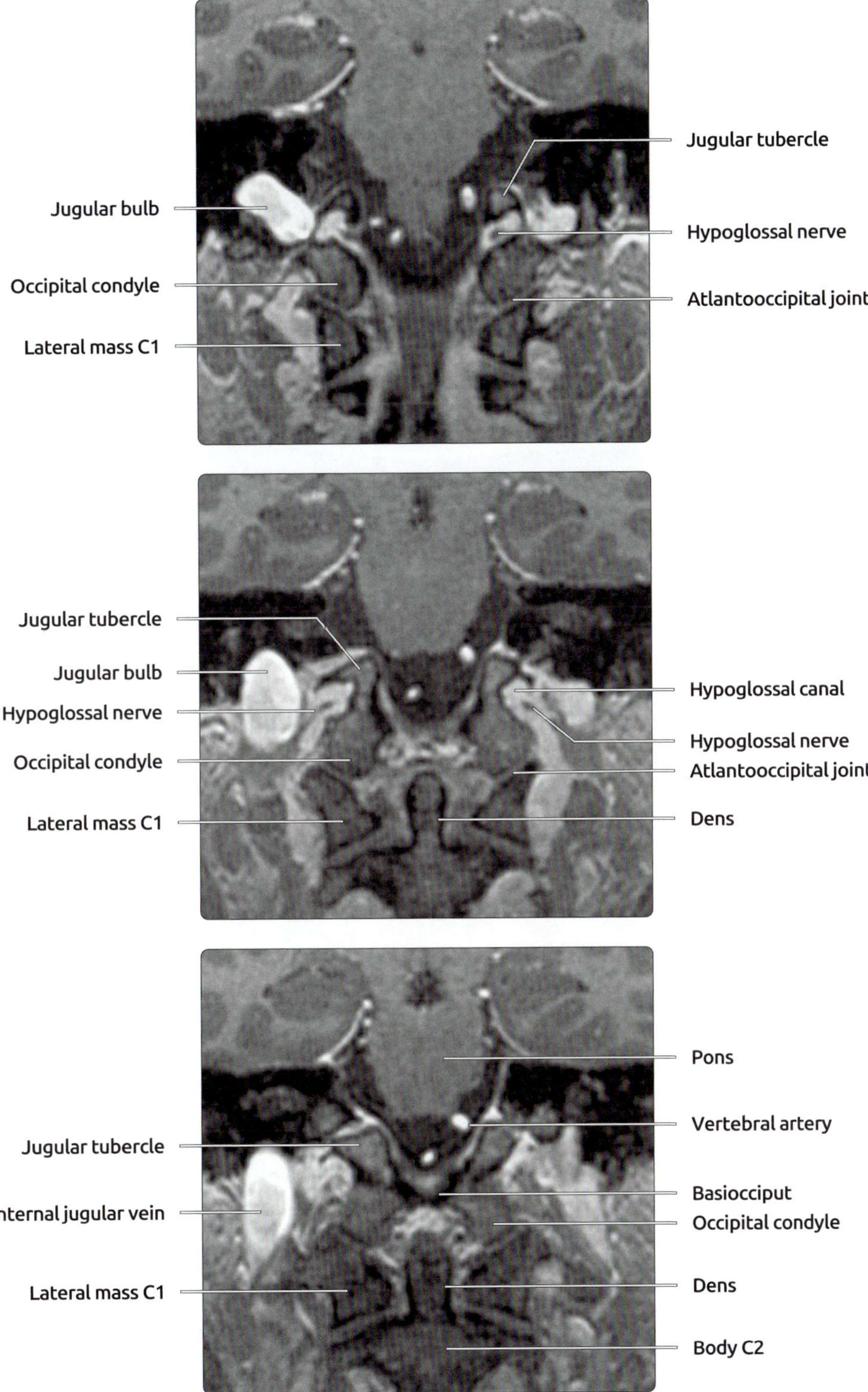

(Top) *First of 3 coronal T1 C+ MR images of the posterior skull base, presented from posterior to anterior, shows the jugular bulb within the jugular foramen. The low-signal hypoglossal nerve is seen just below the "eagle's head" in the hypoglossal canal. The high-signal perineural basiocciput venous plexus is visible surrounding the hypoglossal nerve.* **(Middle)** *In this image, the classic "double eagle heads" are visible (jugular tubercles) with the hypoglossal nerve seen exiting the inferior hypoglossal canal. As in this case, the jugular bulbs are often asymmetric in size.* **(Bottom)** *In this image, the anterior jugular tubercle can be seen meeting the inferior basiocciput. The jugular bulb has connected inferiorly with the internal jugular vein. The internal jugular vein is within the nasopharyngeal carotid space.*

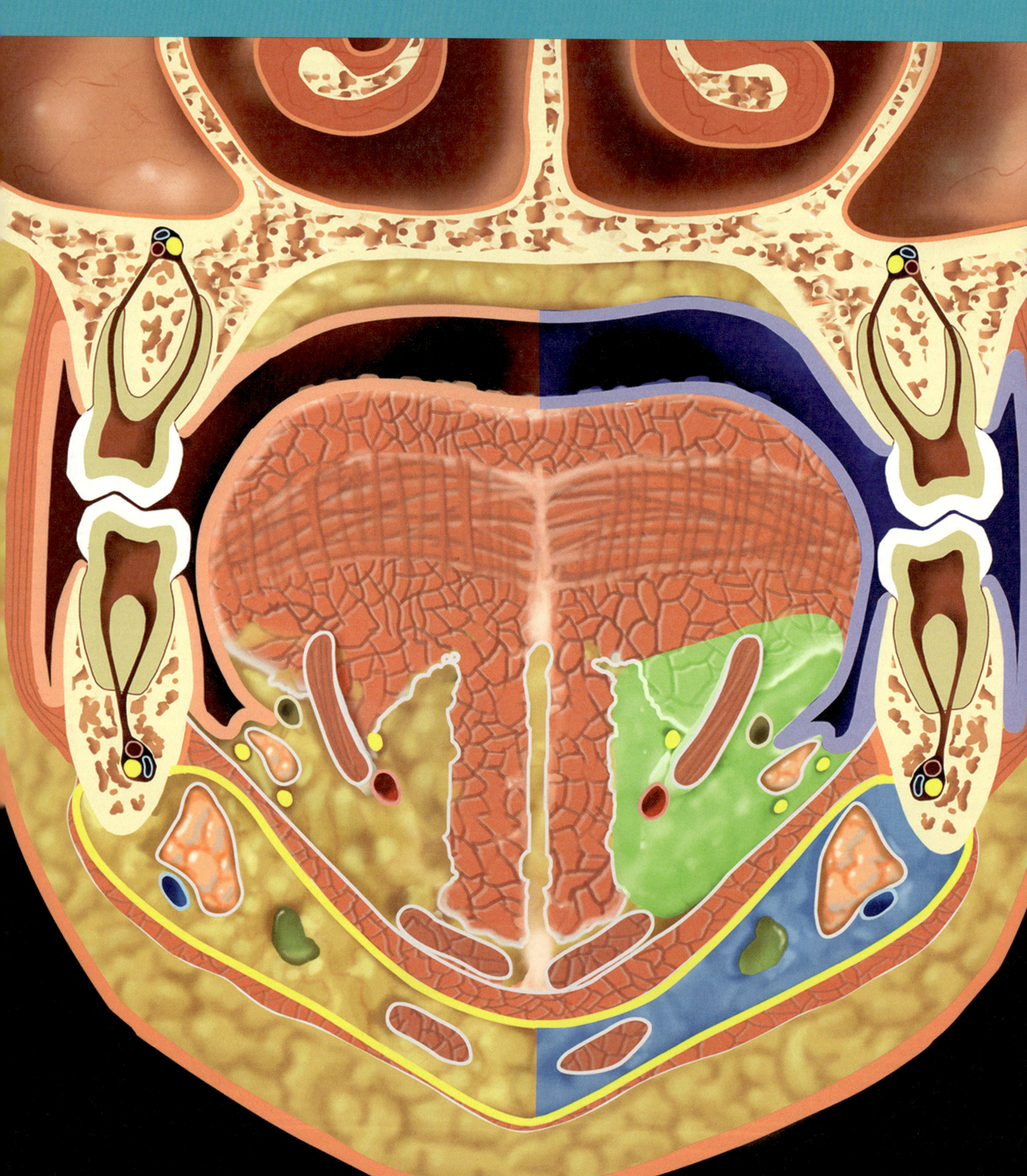

SECTION 6
Oral Cavity

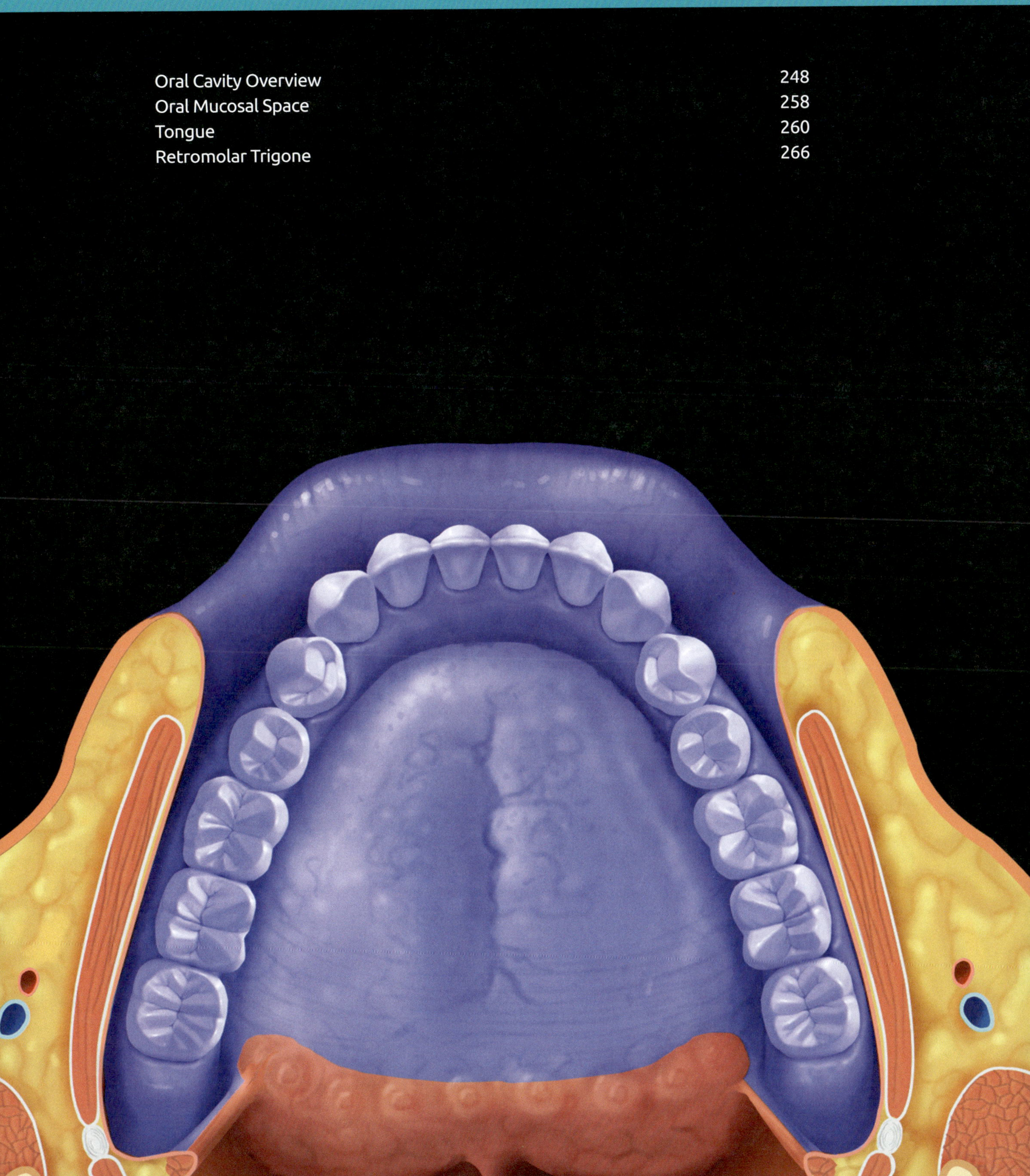

TERMINOLOGY

Definitions

- Oral cavity (OC): Area of suprahyoid neck below sinonasal region and anterior to oropharynx

IMAGING ANATOMY

Overview

- OC separated from oropharynx posteriorly by soft palate, anterior tonsillar pillars, and circumvallate papillae
- Suggested approach to OC imaging anatomy: Consider as 4 distinct regions
  - **Oral mucosal space/surface (OMS): Cavity** includes a central part **OC proper** and lateral **vestibules** on either side
  - **Sublingual space (SLS)**: Non-fascial-lined area superomedial to mylohyoid muscle
  - **Submandibular space (SMS)**: Located inferolateral to mylohyoid muscle
  - **Root of tongue (ROT)**: Made up of genioglossus-geniohyoid complex and lingual septum

Anatomy Relationships

- **OMS** regional relationships
  - **OC proper**: Bounded by alveolar arches and communicates posteriorly with oropharynx
    - Roof formed by hard palate and maxillary alveolar ridge
    - Floor formed by mucosa of floor of mouth (FOM)
    - Contains anterior 2/3 of tongue (mobile tongue)
  - **Oral vestibule**: Lined laterally by **buccal mucosa** with **buccal space** (cheek) lying further lateral to oral vestibule
    - Lined superiorly by reflection of buccal mucosa onto maxilla: Upper (superior) **gingivobuccal sulcus (GBS)**
    - Lined inferiorly by reflection of buccal mucosa onto mandible: Lower (inferior) GBS
    - Lined medially by **gingival mucosa**
  - Posterior: Soft palate/uvula, anterior tonsillar pillars, and lingual tonsil (base of tongue)
  - Anterior: **Vermilion (red part of lips)** covered by specialized stratified squamous epithelium, continuous with oral mucosa of gingivolabial groove
    - **Vermilion border**: Rim of paler skin at vermilion-skin junction
    - **Oral commissure**: Location where lateral aspects of vermilion of upper and lower lips join at angle of mouth
- **SLS** relationships
  - Situated below FOM mucosa and superomedial to mylohyoid muscle; lateral to paramidline extrinsic ROT muscles (genioglossus-geniohyoid)
  - FOM: Variable definition: Some define FOM as inferior recess of OC, beneath oral tongue, limited to squamous epithelial mucosa, and amenable to clinical visual inspection
    - Some define FOM as region of OC beneath oral tongue, including mucosa and SLS
  - Both SLSs communicate anteriorly beneath frenulum
    - Form **"horizontal horseshoe"** below oral tongue
  - Posteriorly, SLS empties into posterosuperior aspect of SMS and inferior parapharyngeal space (PPS)
  - No fascia separates posterior SLS from SMS and inferior PPS
    - Direct communication allows spread of purulent exudate (e.g., from odontogenic abscess) among these 3 spaces
- **SMS** relationships
  - **"Vertical horseshoe"** space between hyoid bone below and mylohyoid muscle sling above
  - SMS communicates posteriorly with **inferior PPS** and **posterior SLS**
  - SMS continues inferiorly as **anterior cervical space**
- **ROT** relationships
  - Inferiorly, ROT ends at hyoid and mylohyoid sling
  - Anteriorly, ends at mandibular symphysis (genioglossus/geniohyoid muscles origin on genial tubercles)

Internal Contents

- **Oral tongue**
  - Anterior 2/3 of tongue in OC proper
    - Base of tongue: Posterior 1/3 of tongue, including lingual tonsil, considered part of oropharynx
  - **Intrinsic tongue muscles**: Represent major tissue of oral tongue
  - **Extrinsic tongue muscles**
    - Genioglossus, hyoglossus, styloglossus, palatoglossus
    - Anchor main body of oral tongue to osseous structures and fibrous connective tissue to affect tongue movement and alter shape of tongue
- **Mylohyoid muscle**
  - Separates lower OC into SMS and SLS, except along free posterior margin
  - Arises from **mylohyoid line** of mandible
  - **Mylohyoid boutonniere: Cleft** at junction of anterior 1/3 and posterior 2/3 of mylohyoid muscle
    - May be prominent with fat ± vessels ± accessory salivary tissue
  - Uncinate process of submandibular gland "hooks" superiorly around posterior free edge of mylohyoid
- **OMS**
  - Squamous epithelial lining of OC, including tongue, buccal, gingival, palatal, and lingual surfaces
    - Buccal mucosa attached tightly to inner fascia of buccinator muscle, limiting variegation or "wrinkling" of mucosa when mouth is closed
  - Submucosal **minor salivary glands** throughout OC
    - Most common locations at inner surface of lip, buccal mucosa, and palate
  - **Retromolar trigone (RMT)**: Small, triangular region of mucosa behind last molar tooth on mandibular ramus
    - Covers anterior surface of lower ascending ramus of mandible
    - Anatomic crossroads of OC, oropharynx, soft palate, buccal space, FOM, masticator space, and PPS
    - Extends superiorly up to maxillary tuberosity near 3rd molar
- **Pterygomandibular raphe**
  - Fibrous band extending from posterior mandibular mylohyoid line to medial pterygoid plate hamulus

- Buccinator and superior pharyngeal constrictor meet at pterygomandibular raphe
- Lies beneath mucosa of **RMT**
- Perifascial route of spread for squamous cell carcinoma
- **SLS**
  - Lingual nerve: V3 sensory fibers combined with CNVII chorda tympani nerve (taste to anterior 2/3 of tongue) via submandibular ganglion
  - Distal glossopharyngeal nerve (CNIX; motor to stylopharyngeus muscle) and CNXII (motor to tongue)
  - Deep lingual artery and veins
  - Sublingual glands and Wharton ducts
  - Hyoglossus muscle anterior margin projects into posterior SLS
  - Deep portion of submandibular gland and submandibular gland duct
  - Deep lingual lymph nodes
  - **Lateral compartment** contents
    - Superolateral: Lingual nerve
    - Middle: Sublingual salivary gland, submandibular duct, and deep part of submandibular salivary gland
    - Inferomedial: Hypoglossal nerve
    - Submandibular duct and lingual nerve cross each other at anterior border of hyoglossus
  - **Medial compartment** contents
    - Superior: Glossopharyngeal nerve
    - Inferior: Lingual artery
- **SMS**
  - Large superficial portion of submandibular gland
  - Submental (level IA) and submandibular (level IB) lymph node groups
  - Facial vein and artery
  - Inferior loop of CNXII
  - Anterior belly of digastric muscles

Fascia

- SLS **not** lined by fascia
- SMS lined by superficial layer of deep cervical fascia
  - Deeper slip of fascia runs along external surface of mylohyoid muscle, and more shallow slip parallels deep margin of platysma
  - No fascia separates posterior SMS and SLS from inferior PPS

ANATOMY IMAGING ISSUES

Imaging Recommendations

- Multidetector CT (MDCT), including dynamic maneuvers
- MR with dynamic maneuvers better for small OC lesions
  - Especially with submucosal fibrosis, postsurgical cases, RMT malignancy, and dental hardware streak artifacts

Imaging Pitfalls

- Small gingival, buccal, and RMT lesions usually difficult to detect on CT/MR
  - Due to apposition of mucosal surfaces of lips and cheeks to gingival surfaces (gum margins) of mandibular and maxillary alveolus
- Small oral tongue lesions also difficult to detect on CT/MR
  - Due to apposition of tongue to hard palate and lingual surfaces of maxillary and mandibular alveolus
- Dynamic maneuvers extremely helpful to detect these small lesions
- Dynamic maneuvers also better to evaluate OC tumor depth of invasion (DOI) and tumor thickness (TT)

Dynamic Maneuvers

- **Puffed cheek maneuver**
  - Blowing mouth uniformly through pursed lips; moving tongue away from hard palate and teeth during scan
  - Air distending oral vestibule separates buccal (cheek) and labial (lip) mucosa from gingival (gum) mucosa
  - Buccinator muscle better seen to evaluate invasion
  - Small tumors of **anterior** tongue, buccal mucosa, anterior part of superior/inferior GBS and angle of mouth better seen
  - Better evaluation of lesions in presence of dental hardware artifacts
  - Limited utility in presence of severe submucosal fibrosis and in postsurgical cases where large flaps/grafts prevent proper OC air distention
  - Limited utility in evaluation of posterior GBS and RMT lesions
  - Make sure not to overdo/perform Valsalva maneuver; breathe through nose during puffed cheek maneuver to avoid Valsalva
    - Valsalva could distend and better show posterior oral tongue, RMT, and posterior GBS lesions
    - But Valsalva may elevate and posteriorly displace tongue, partially obscuring and producing pseudolesions of posterior OC and oropharynx
- **Water distention of OC**
  - Holding water in mouth during scan
  - Helpful to detect **anterior** OC lesions like puffed cheek technique
  - Water distends dependent **posterior** aspects of tongue, buccal/gingival mucosa, superior and inferior GBS, RMT, and pterygomandibular raphe/medial pterygoid muscle region adequately that are not well evaluated with puffed cheek technique
  - Water distention better delineates OC lesions in patients with **severe submucosal fibrosis** (especially chronic tobacco chewers) and **postoperative fibrosis** that prevent proper OC air distention
  - Water distention cannot be done by patients with orocutaneous fistula and difficult with large flap reconstruction and edentulous patients
- **Tongue protrusion maneuver**
  - Protruding tongue to maximum extent against FOM during scan
  - Small lateral and ventral anterior oral tongue or tongue tip (apex) lesion detection
  - Limited use in large tongue lesions or isolated FOM/base of tongue lesions
  - Motion artifacts common
- **Open-mouth maneuver**
  - Holding mouth open during scan
  - Small hard/soft palate, upper alveolus, RMT, GBS lesions better seen
  - Also useful to detect oropharynx lesions obscured by dental artifact
  - Motion artifacts common; device, such as syringe, may be placed between teeth to avoid motion

GRAPHICS

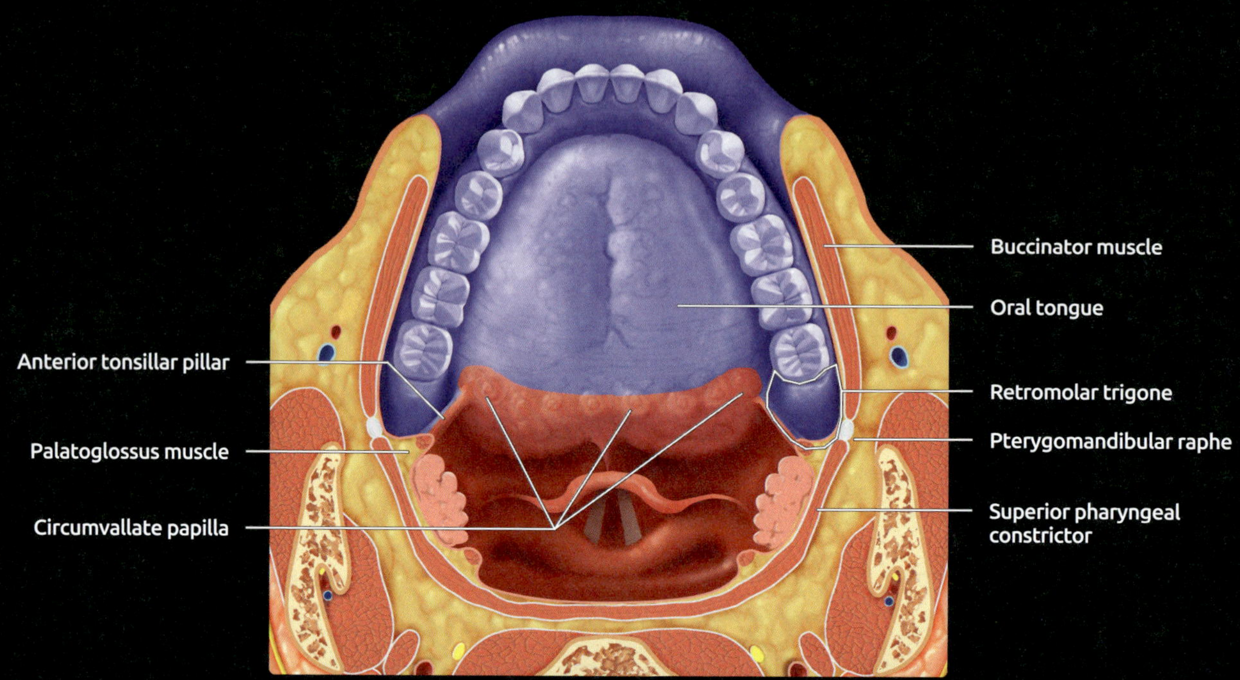

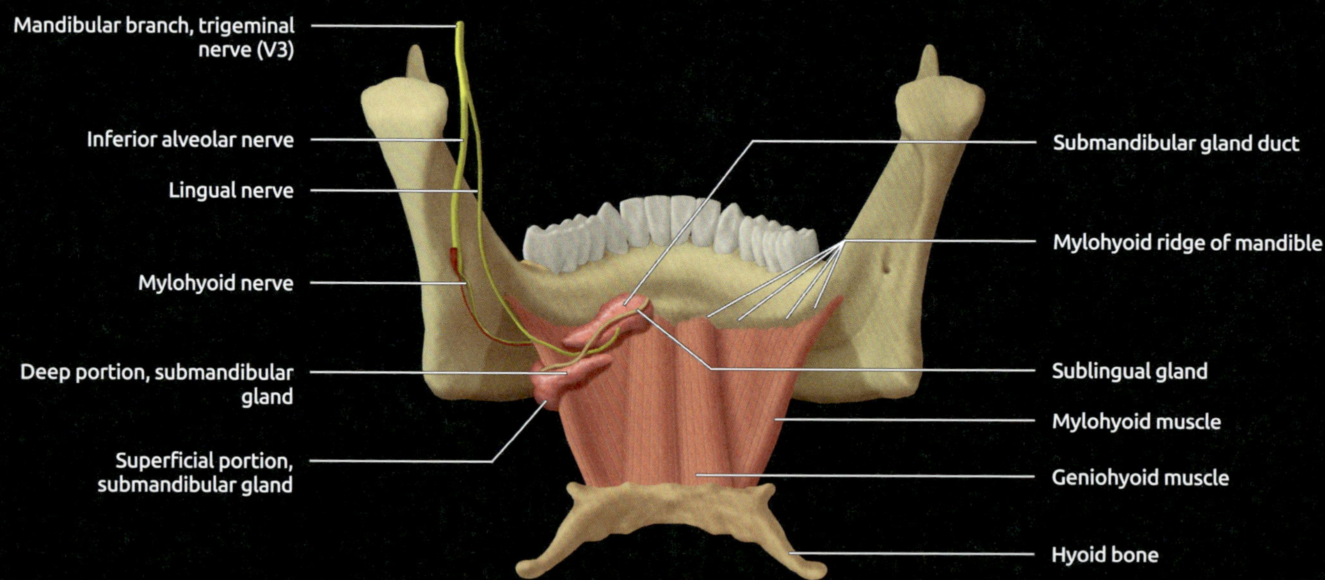

(Top) *Graphic from above shows the oral mucosal space/surface shaded in blue. Notice the circumvallate papilla, a superficial line of taste buds, divides the anterior oral cavity from the posterior oropharynx. The lingual tonsil is part of the oropharynx, not the oral cavity. The pterygomandibular raphe connects the posterior margin of the buccinator muscle to the anterior margin of the superior pharyngeal constrictor muscle. It also represents a key route of perifascial spread of squamous cell carcinoma of the retromolar trigone.* **(Bottom)** *Graphic shows the floor of the mouth from above. The mylohyoid muscle sling is the principal structure of the floor of the mouth. This muscle attaches to the hyoid bone inferiorly and the mylohyoid ridge of the medial mandibular cortex. Superomedial to the mylohyoid muscle is the sublingual space, while the submandibular space is inferolateral to this muscle.*

GRAPHICS

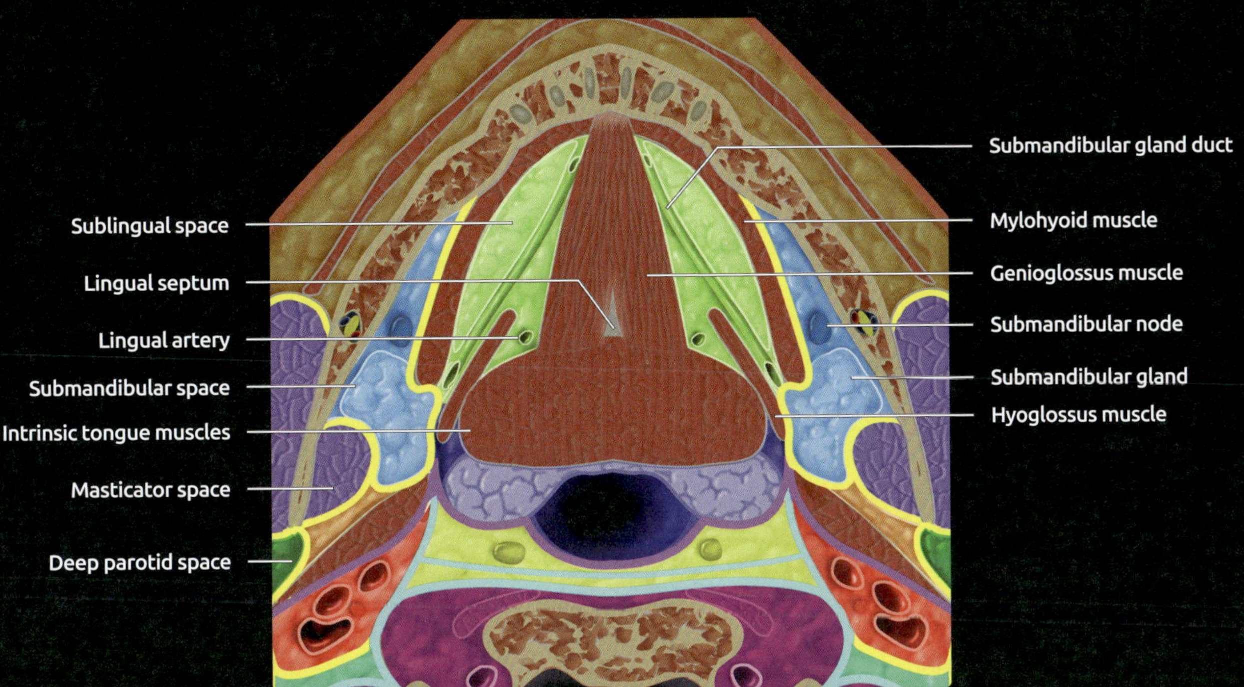

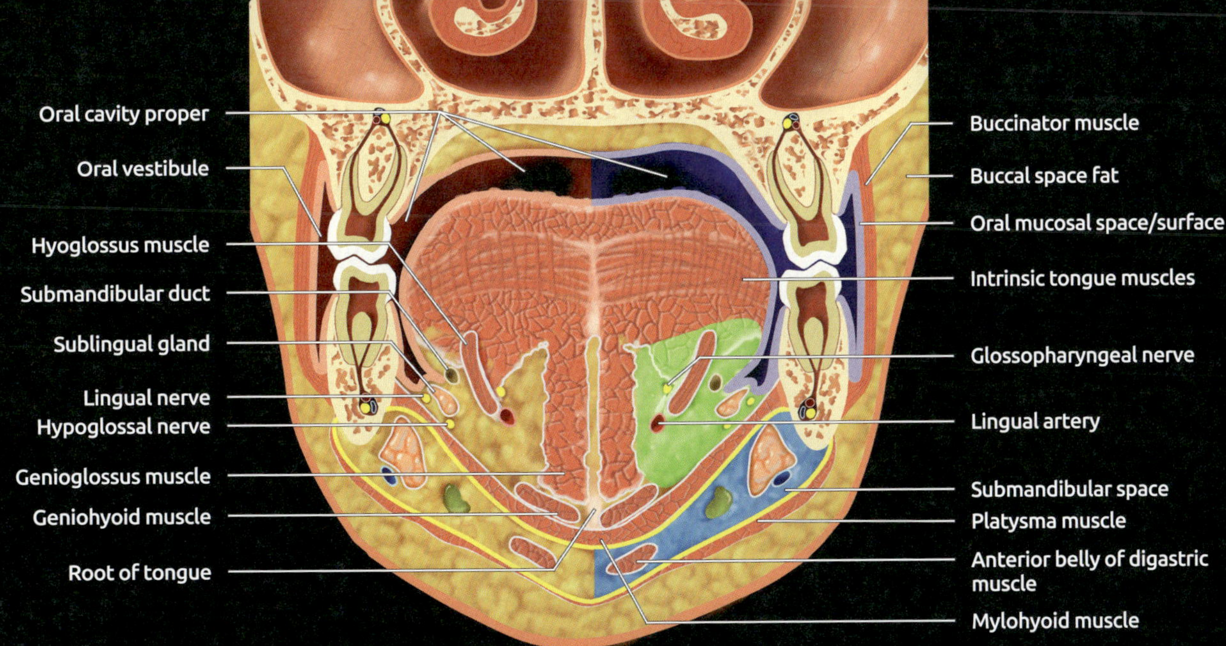

(Top) *Axial graphic through the oral cavity shows the superficial layer of the deep cervical fascia (yellow line) circumscribing masticator and parotid spaces posteriorly and defining the deep margin of the submandibular space anteriorly, colored in blue. Note the principal occupants of the submandibular space are the submandibular gland and nodes. The green sublingual space has many structures within it, including the sublingual gland, submandibular duct, and anterior margin of the hyoglossus, to name a few.* **(Bottom)** *Coronal graphic shows the mylohyoid muscle stretched from side to side from the mylohyoid ridges. Mylohyoid muscle separates the sublingual space (green) from the submandibular space (blue). Sublingual space contains the lingual nerve and artery, submandibular duct, CNIX and CNXII, and sublingual gland. Genioglossus and geniohyoid complex with the lower lingual septum forms the root of the tongue. Oral cavity air space consists of central oral cavity proper and lateral oral vestibules on either side. Air distending the central oral cavity proper outlines the oral tongue. Air in the lateral oral vestibules on either side separates buccal from gingival mucosal margins.*

AXIAL CECT

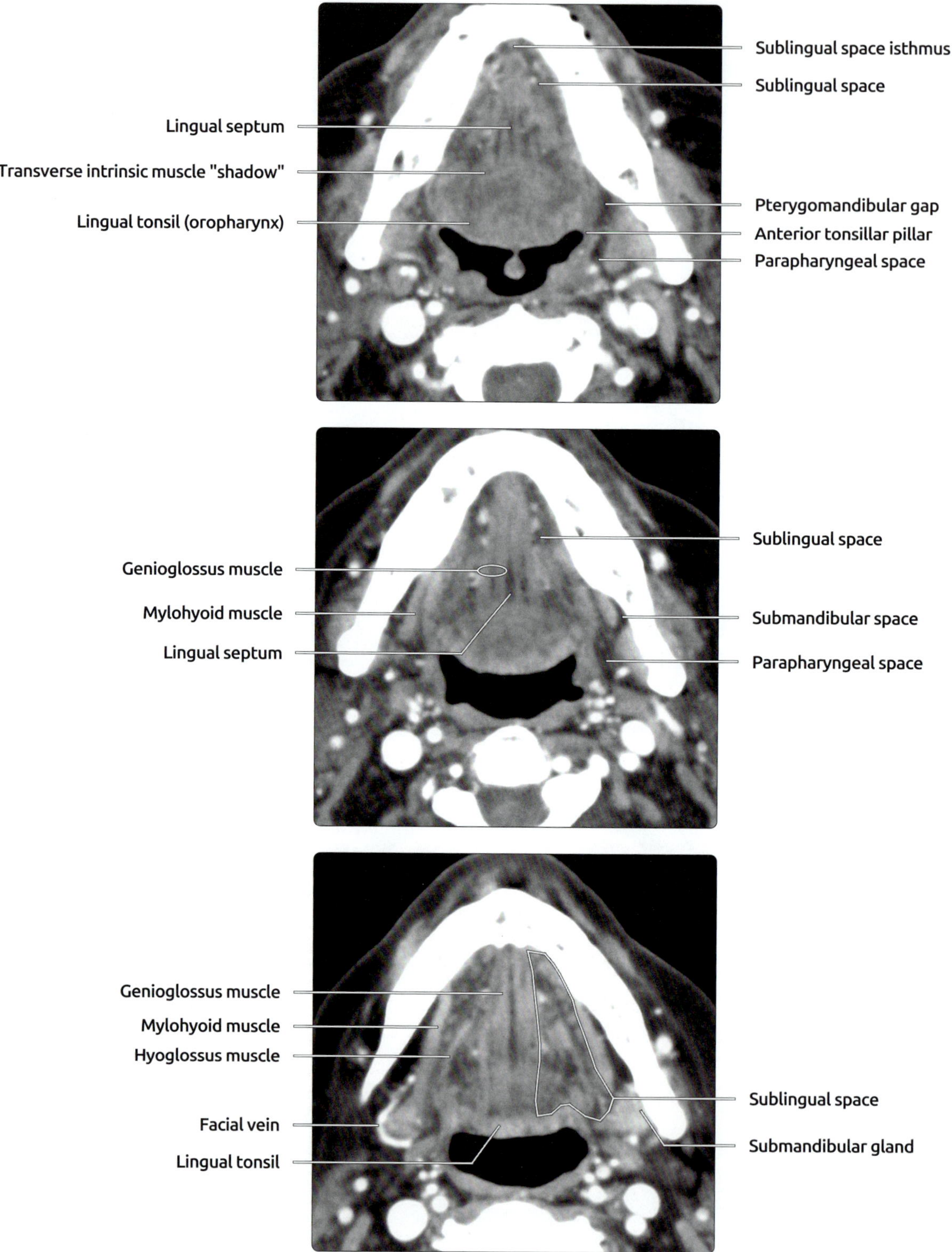

(Top) *First of 6 axial CECT images of the oral cavity presented from superior to inferior is shown. On the most cephalad image, the parapharyngeal space can be seen emptying anteriorly into the submandibular space via the pterygomandibular gap.* **(Middle)** *The large paired genioglossus muscles are seen on either side of the lingual septum. The cephalad submandibular space fat is just coming into view.* **(Bottom)** *The sublingual space is lateral to the genioglossus muscle, superomedial to the mylohyoid muscle, and anterior to the lingual tonsil. On the patient's right, the facial vein curves around the lateral margin of the submandibular gland.*

AXIAL CECT

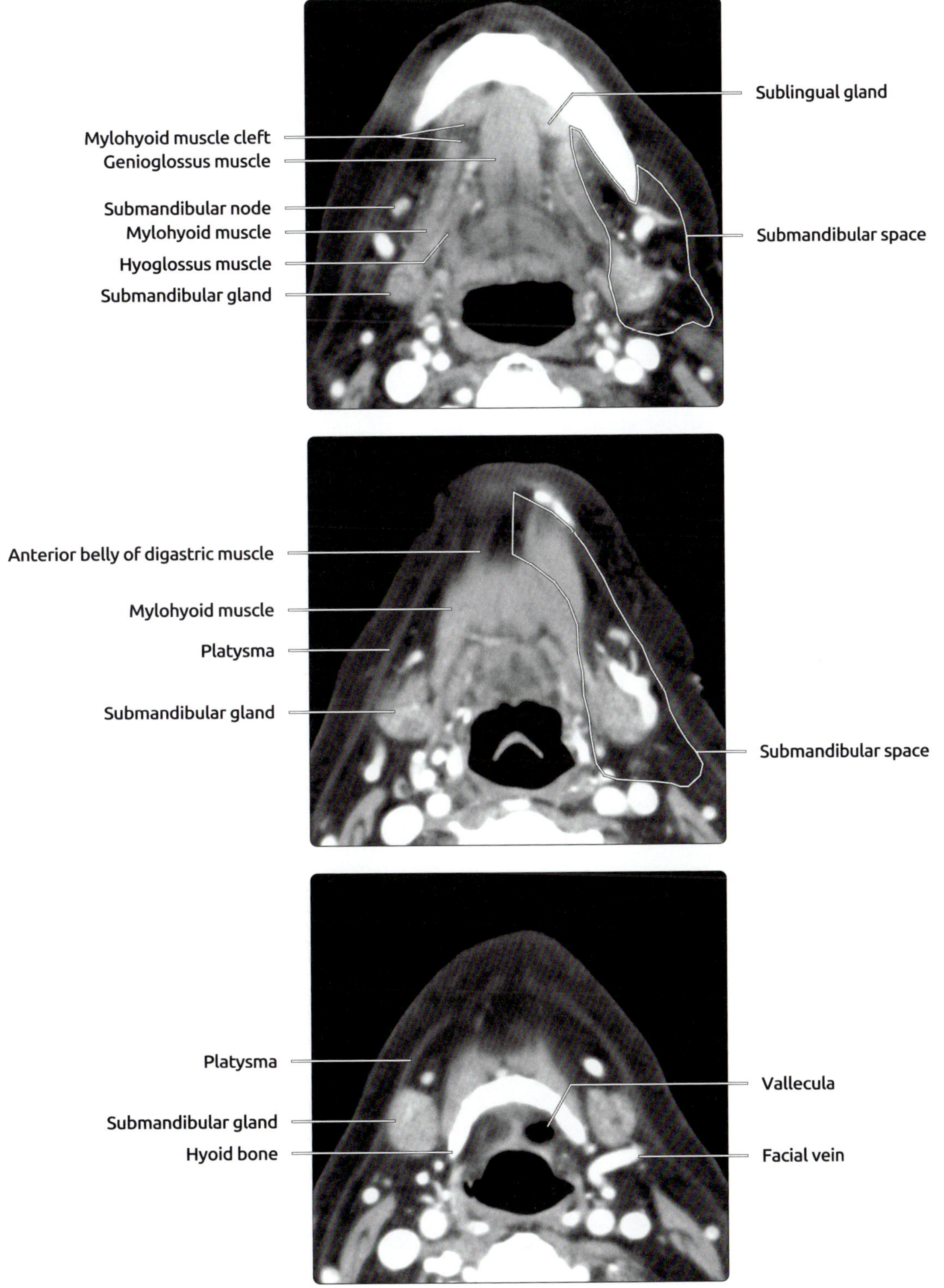

(Top) *The complex shape of the submandibular space is outlined on the patient's left. Notice the mylohyoid muscle gap anteriorly on the right. This is a normal variant and can be large and fat filled, as in this image.* **(Middle)** *The left 1/2 of the more inferior submandibular space is outlined. The submandibular gland and anterior belly of the digastric muscles are seen as normal occupants of this space. Remember, there is no vertical fascia dividing the 2 sides of the submandibular space.* **(Bottom)** *The platysma muscle represents the superficial border of the submandibular space. The anterior cervical space connects to the submandibular space in the infrahyoid neck.*

AXIAL T2 MR

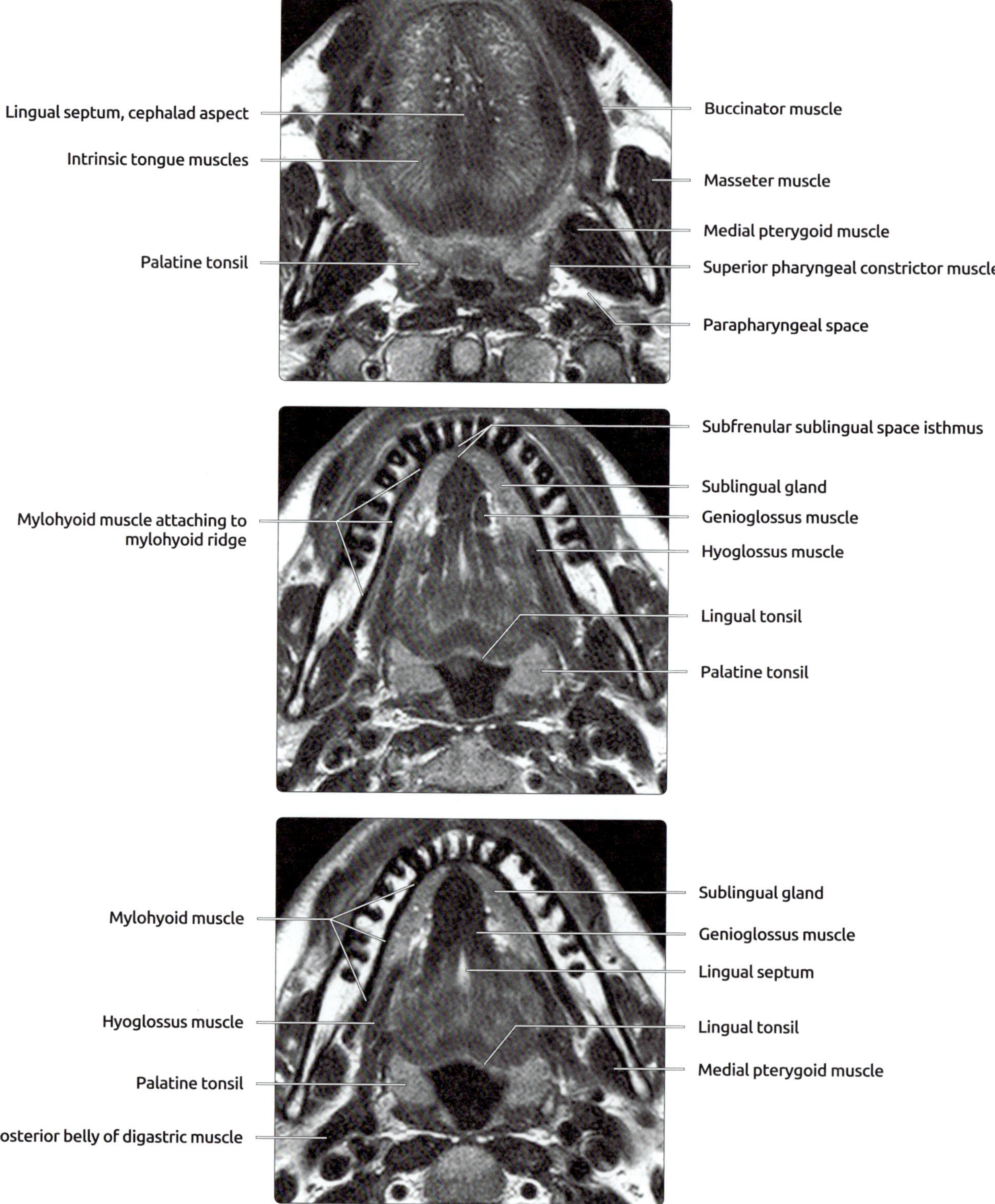

(Top) *First of 6 axial T2 MR images through the oral cavity presented from superior to inferior is shown. This 1st image reveals the cephalad surface of the oral tongue.* **(Middle)** *In this image, the mylohyoid muscle can be seen attaching to the mylohyoid ridge bilaterally. The sublingual space communicates anteriorly in the subfrenular isthmus.* **(Bottom)** *In this image, the hyoglossus muscle is seen projecting into the posterior aspect of the sublingual space.*

AXIAL T2 MR

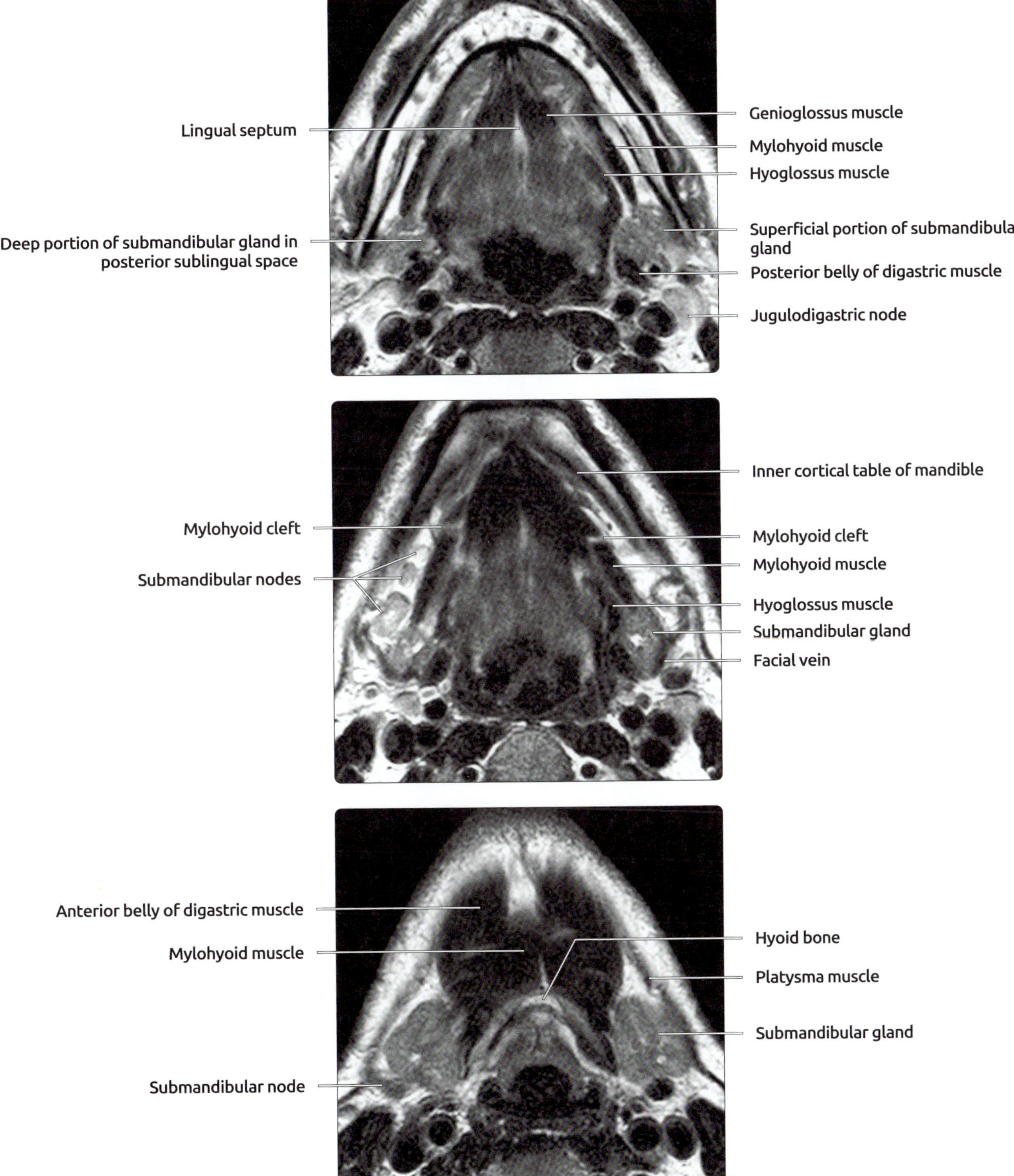

(Top) *In the lower oral cavity, the submandibular gland becomes visible. Notice the deep portion "plugs" the back of the sublingual space (visible on the left). The larger, superficial submandibular gland is in the submandibular space proper.* **(Middle)** *At the level of the inferior body of the mandible, the fatty gap in the mylohyoid muscle is visible. Also notice the multiple reactive submandibular nodes on the left.* **(Bottom)** *At the level of the hyoid bone, the bulk of the anterior bellies of the digastric muscles are visible. The platysma is seen as the superficial margin of the submandibular space.*

CORONAL T1 MR

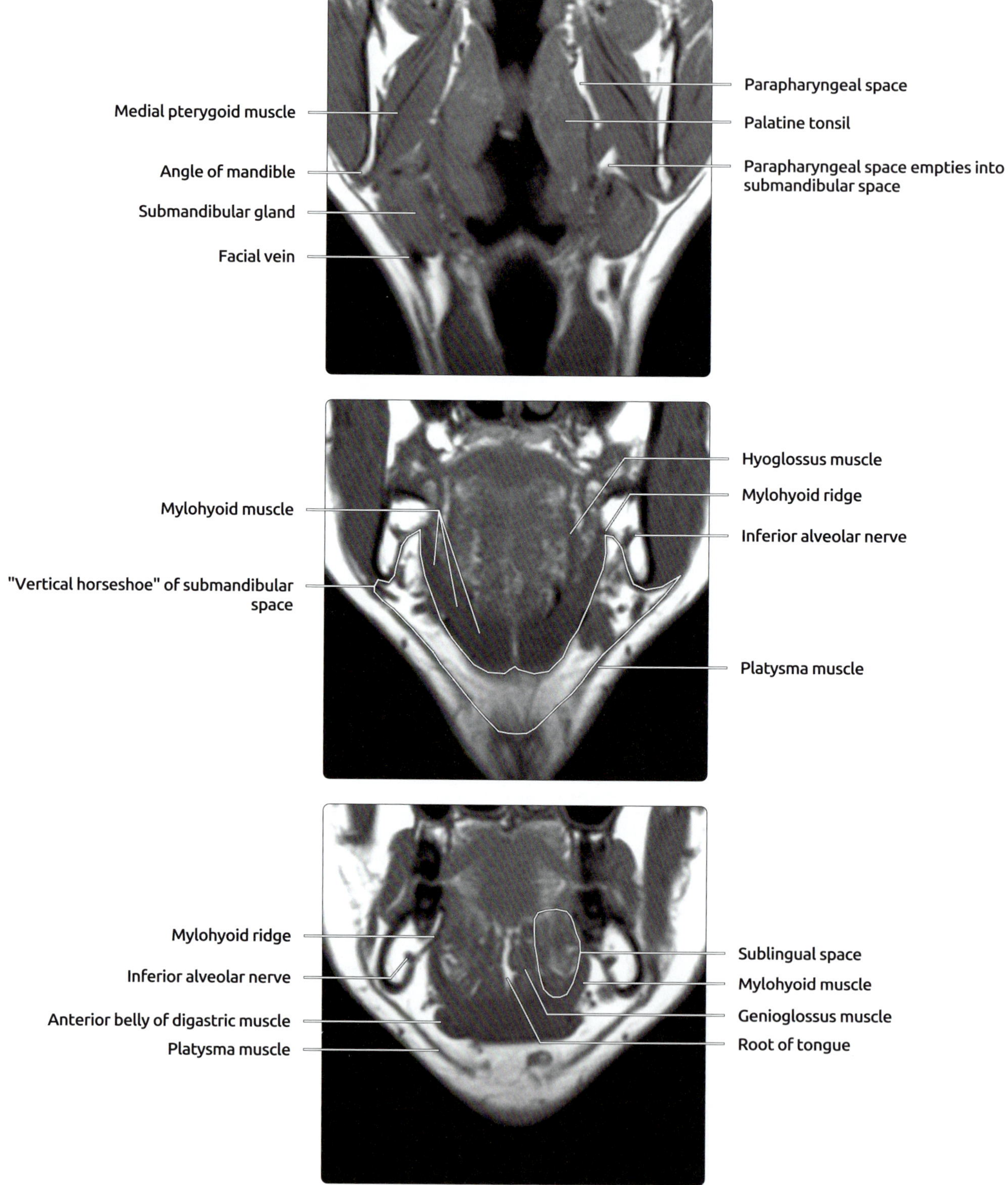

(Top) *First of 3 coronal T1 MR images through the oral cavity presented from posterior to anterior is shown. In this most posterior image, the parapharyngeal space can be seen "emptying" inferiorly into the posterior submandibular space on the right.* **(Middle)** *This more anterior view delineates the "vertical horseshoe" of the submandibular space, bounded superficially by the platysma and superomedially by the mylohyoid muscle.* **(Bottom)** *The sublingual space becomes more obvious in the anterior oral cavity. Notice it is a potential space drawn in on the right, lateral to the genioglossus muscle and superomedial to the mylohyoid muscle.*

PUFFED CHEEK MANEUVER

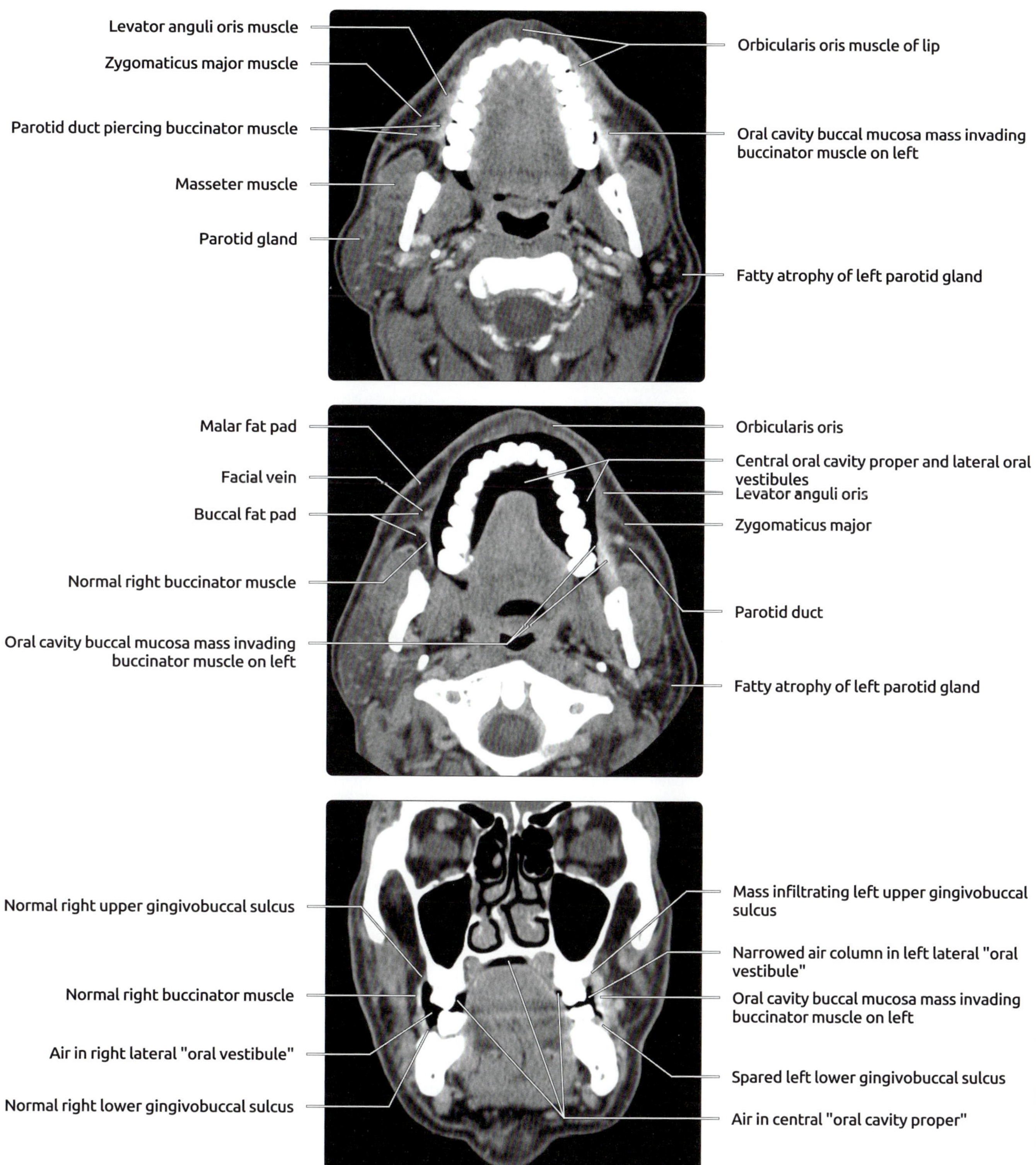

(Top) *Axial CECT in a patient with left buccal mucosal squamous cell carcinoma shows subtle thickening of the left posterior buccal region, which is very difficult to recognize. Parotid duct pierces the buccinator muscle opposite the maxillary 2nd molar tooth. Buccinator muscle lies just lateral (superficial) to buccal mucosa lining the oral cavity. Orbicularis oris (Oo) muscle makes up the bulk of the lip, and the levator anguli oris (LAO) muscle attaches at the modiolus of angle of the mouth just posterior to Oo. Zygomaticus major (ZMj) muscle inserts at modiolus deep to LAO insertion, at the anterior margin of buccinator muscle.* **(Middle)** *Puffed cheek technique CECT in the same patient better delineates the buccal mucosal mass lesion invading the buccinator muscle, including where the parotid duct pierces buccinator. Note left parotid gland fatty atrophy. Note air distending the central "oral cavity proper" outlining the oral tongue. Air in the lateral "oral vestibules" on either side separates buccal mucosal margin from maxillary/mandibular dental alveolar gingival margin.* **(Bottom)** *Coronal puffed cheek CECT shows that the mass extends into the left superior gingivobuccal sulcus.*

TERMINOLOGY

Abbreviations

- Oral mucosal space/surface (OMS)

Definitions

- Mucosal surface of oral cavity (OC) extending from vermilion border of lips anteriorly to hard/soft palate junction above & to line of circumvallate papillae below posteriorly
- Located anterior to mucosal surface of oropharynx
- Cavity of OMS: Central **OC proper** & lateral **oral vestibules** on either side
- OMS, sublingual space (SLS), root of tongue (ROT), & submandibular space (SMS) form 4 distinct regions of broader classification of OC overview

IMAGING ANATOMY

Extent

- Anterior: **Vermilion (red part of lips)** covered by specialized stratified squamous epithelium, continuous with oral mucosa of gingivolabial groove
  - **Vermilion border**: Pale skin rim at vermilion-skin junction
  - **Oral commissure**: Location where lateral aspects of vermilion of upper & lower lips join at angle of mouth
- Posterior extent of OMS
  - Posterosuperior extent: Junction of hard & soft palate
  - Posteroinferior extent: Junction of anterior 2/3 & posterior 1/3 of tongue at circumvallate papillae
    - Anterior 2/3 of tongue: **Oral tongue**; in **OMS**
    - Posterior 1/3 of tongue: **Lingual tonsil**; in **oropharynx**
- **OC proper**: Bounded by alveolar arches & communicates posteriorly with oropharynx
  - Roof formed by hard palate & maxillary alveolar ridge
  - Floor formed by mucosa of floor of mouth (FOM)
  - Contains anterior 2/3 of tongue (mobile tongue)
- **Oral vestibule**: Laterally lined by buccal mucosa with buccal space (cheek) lying further lateral to oral vestibule
  - Superiorly lined by reflection of buccal mucosa onto maxilla: Upper (superior) gingivobuccal sulcus (GBS)
  - Inferiorly lined by reflection of buccal mucosa onto mandible: Lower (inferior) GBS
  - Medially lined by gingival mucosa

Anatomy Relationships

- Roof: Mucosa underneath hard palate & maxilla (palatine process & alveolus of maxilla & palatine bone)
  - Nasal floor & maxillary sinuses lie above OMS roof
- Floor: Formed by mucosa of FOM
  - SLSs, SMS below SLSs separated by mylohyoid muscle, & ROT between SLS of either side lie below OMS floor

Internal Contents

- OMS divided into 8 specific areas
  - **Mucosal lip**
    - Lip begins at vermilion border junction with skin
    - Includes only vermilion surface or portion of lip that makes contact with opposing lip
  - **Upper alveolar ridge mucosal surface**
    - Mucosa overlying medial lingual & lateral buccal aspects of gums on alveolar process of maxilla
    - Extends from line of attachment of mucosa in upper GBS to junction of hard palate on either side
    - Posterior margin at upper end of pterygopalatine arch
  - **Hard palate mucosal surface**
    - Semilunar mucosal area between upper alveolar ridge & mucous membrane covering palatine process of maxilla & palatine bones
    - Extends from inner surface of superior alveolar ridge to posterior edge of palatine bone
  - **Lower alveolar ridge mucosal surface**
    - Mucosa overlying medial lingual & lateral buccal aspects of gums on alveolar process of mandible
    - Extends from line of attachment of mucosa in lower GBS to line of free mucosa of FOM on either side
    - Posteriorly extends to ascending ramus of mandible
  - **FOM mucosal surface**
    - Semilunar mucosal surface overlying mylohyoid & hyoglossus muscles
    - Extends from inner surface of lower alveolar ridge to undersurface of tongue
    - Posterior boundary at base of anterior pillar of tonsil
    - Divided into 2 sides by tongue **frenulum**
    - Contains ostia of submandibular & sublingual salivary glands
  - **Retromolar trigone (RMT)** mucosal surface
    - Mucosa overlying ascending ramus of mandible
    - Extends from level of posterior surface of last mandibular molar tooth to apex superiorly, adjacent to tuberosity of maxilla
  - **Buccal mucosa**
    - Mucosa lining inner surface of cheeks & lips
    - Extends from line of contact of opposing lips to line of attachment of mucosa of alveolar ridge (upper & lower) & pterygomandibular raphe
  - **Anterior 2/3 of tongue (oral tongue) mucosal surface**
    - Mucosal surface overlying oral tongue
    - Extends anteriorly from line of circumvallate papillae (anterior edge of lingual tonsil) to undersurface of tongue at junction of FOM mucosal surface
    - Composed of 4 areas, including tongue tip, lateral borders, dorsum, & undersurface (nonvillous oral tongue ventral surface)
- Contents of OMS
  - **Minor salivary glands** (MSG)
    - Concentrated in buccal, palatal, & lingual submucosa

CLINICAL IMPLICATIONS

Clinical Importance

- Primary malignancies arising from OMS include squamous cell carcinoma (SCCa) (majority) & MSG malignancy (rare)
- **Depth of invasion (DOI)** measured from **"plumb line" joining normal** OMS component (e.g., tongue) **tissue along borders of all** flat, exophytic or ulcerated **tumors** to deepest point of tumor invasion
- Different from **tumor thickness (TT)**: Distance from **actual tumor surface** (different for flat, exophytic, & ulcerated tumors) to deepest point of tumor invasion
- CT/MR with **dynamic maneuvers**, such as **puffed cheek**, water distention, etc., helps detect small OMS lesions

GRAPHICS

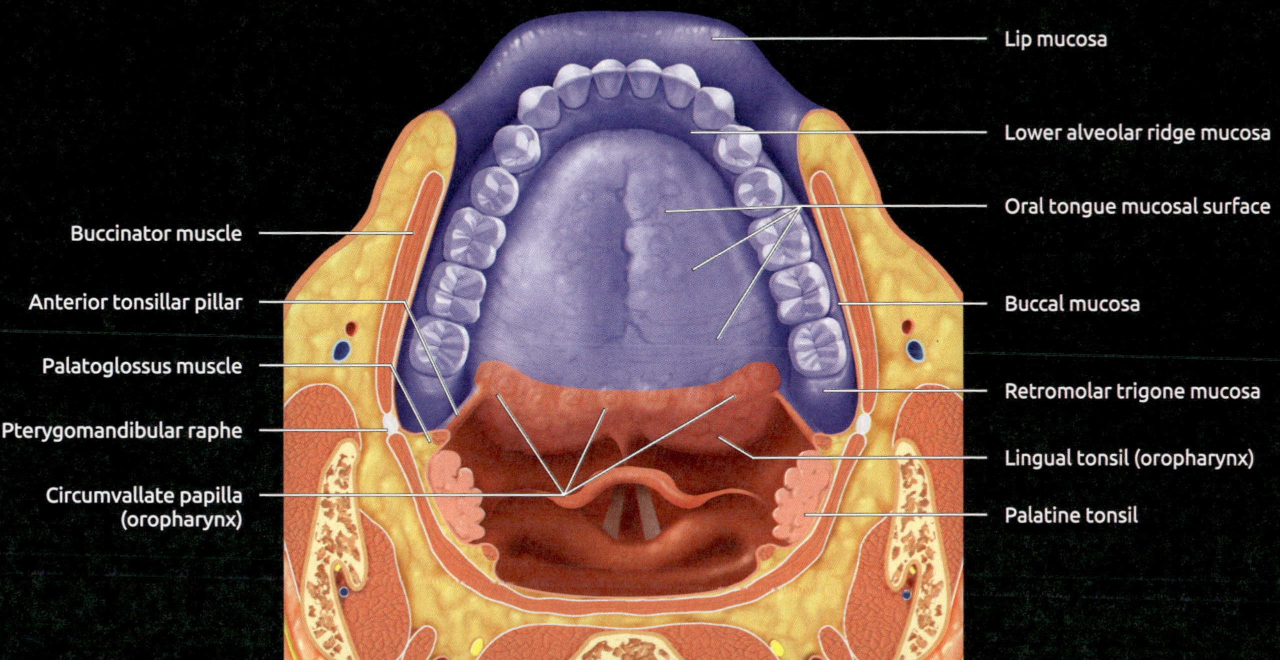

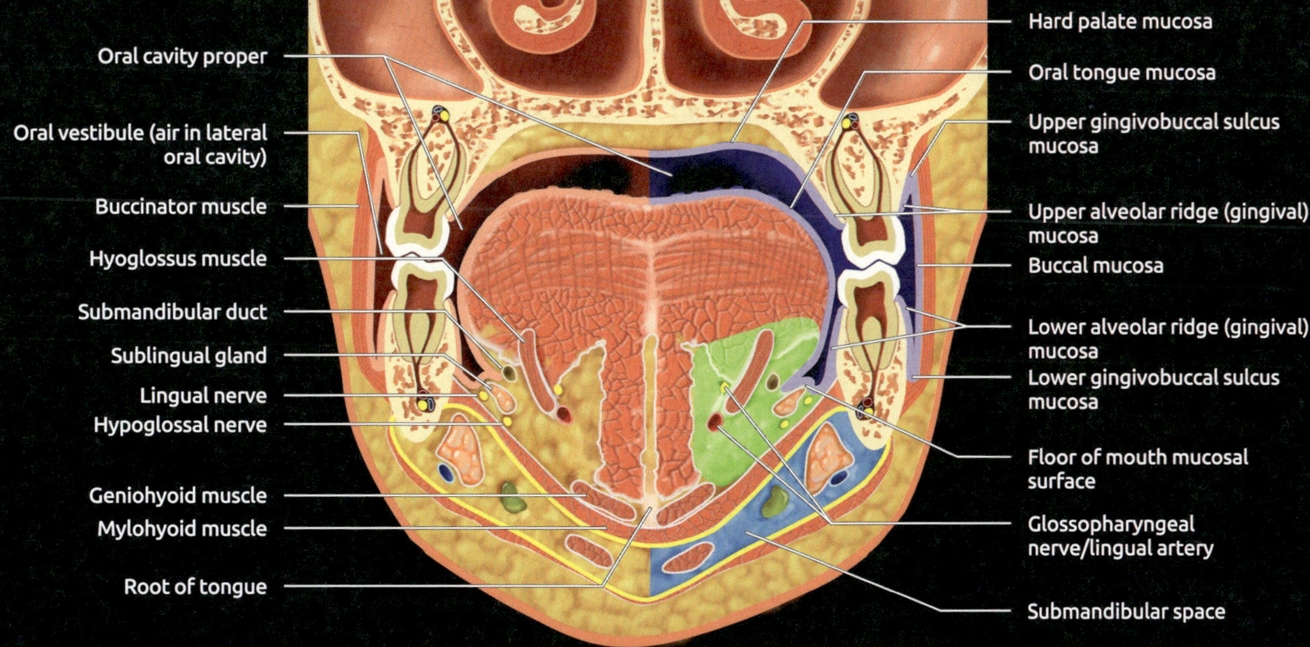

(Top) *Axial graphic through the oral cavity and oropharynx is shown. The area in blue delineates the oral mucosal space/surface (OMS). Notice the posterior oropharynx contains the lingual and palatine tonsils. The circumvallate papilla are a superficial line of taste buds that separate the anterior oral cavity from the posterior oropharynx.* **(Bottom)** *Coronal graphic of oral cavity highlights OMS in blue. The hard palate, oral tongue, upper and lower alveolar ridge, and buccal and floor of mouth mucosal surfaces are seen. Also notice that the 4 main areas of the oral cavity are all present: (1) OMS (blue), (2) sublingual space (green), (3) submandibular space (light blue), and (4) root of tongue. Cavity of OMS consists of central "oral cavity proper" and lateral "oral vestibules" on either side. Air distending the central "oral cavity proper" outlines the oral tongue. Air in the lateral "oral vestibules" on either side separates buccal mucosal margin from maxillary/mandibular dental alveolar gingival margin. CT/MR with dynamic maneuvers, such as puffed cheek, water distention, tongue protrusion, or open-mouth maneuvers, helps detect small OMS lesions by separating opposed mucosal surfaces.*

TERMINOLOGY

Abbreviations

- Oral mucosal space/surface (OMS); floor of mouth (FOM); base of tongue (BOT); root of tongue (ROT)

Definitions

- **Oral tongue**: Anterior 2/3 of tongue, not including tongue base **(part of OMS)**
  - By imaging, includes freely mobile portion of tongue anterior to lingual tonsil
- **FOM**: Variable definition; some define FOM as inferior recess of oral cavity, beneath oral tongue, limited to squamous epithelial mucosa & seen on visual inspection
  - Extending from inner aspect of lower alveolar ridge to undersurface of anterior oral tongue
  - Some define FOM as region of oral cavity beneath oral tongue, including mucosa **& sublingual space** (SLS)
  - Be aware, some authors have historically used term FOM to refer to mylohyoid muscle sling
- **BOT**: Posterior 1/3 of tongue (**part of oropharynx**)
  - By imaging, includes **lingual tonsil**
- **ROT**: Undersurface of oral tongue beneath its junction with anterior FOM & mandible
  - By imaging, includes lingual septum, inferior portion of genioglossus muscles, & geniohyoid muscles

IMAGING ANATOMY

Anatomy Relationships

- **SLS**
  - Nonfascia-lined potential space containing lingual nerve, CNIX, CNXII, lingual artery & vein, sublingual glands/ducts, submandibular gland deep portion, submandibular duct, & anterior hyoglossus muscle
  - SLS situated below FOM mucosa & superomedial to mylohyoid muscle; lateral to extrinsic tongue muscles (genioglossus-geniohyoid)
  - Connects to opposite SLS beneath **frenulum** anteriorly

Internal Contents

- **Oral tongue** consists of 4 anatomic regions: Tip, lateral borders, dorsum, & undersurface (nonvillous surface)
- **Extrinsic tongue muscles**: Move tongue body, alter shape
  - **Genioglossus**: Large, fan-shaped muscle lying parallel to median plane in sagittal plane
  - Origin from superior **genial tubercle** behind symphysis menti of mandible
  - Superior fibers insert along entire length of undersurface of tongue & intermediate fibers into posterior tongue
  - Inferior fibers attach to upper anterior hyoid body by thin aponeurosis
    - Few fasciculi pass between hyoglossus & chondroglossus to merge with middle constrictor
  - Protrudes tongue (safety muscle; if paralyzed, tongue falls back into airway of oropharynx); nerve: CNXII
  - Geniohyoid arises just below it & inserts into hyoid
  - **Hyoglossus**: Thin & quadrilateral-shaped muscle
  - Origin from body & greater cornu of hyoid bone
  - Passes vertically upward to insert into side of tongue between styloglossus laterally & inferior longitudinal muscle medially
  - Depresses tongue; nerve: CNXII
  - **Chondroglossus**: Some describe it as part of hyoglossus
  - Genioglossus inferior fibers separate it from hyoglossus
  - Origin from medial side & base of lesser cornu & adjacent body of hyoid; occasionally, cartilago triticea
  - **Styloglossus**: Origin from styloid process & stylomandibular ligament; passes anteroinferiorly **between internal & external carotid arteries**
  - Divides into longitudinal part, **blending** with **inferior longitudinal muscle** in front of hyoglossus, & oblique part decussating with **hyoglossus** at side of tongue
  - Retracts tongue upward & backward; nerve: CNXII
  - **Palatoglossus**: Origin from undersurface of palatine aponeurosis; inserts into side & dorsum of tongue
  - Forms palatoglossal arch (anterior tonsillar pillar); nerve: CNX, pharyngeal plexus branch
- **Intrinsic tongue muscles**: Alters shape of tongue during deglutition & speech; complicated bundles of interlacing fibers innervated by CNXII
  - **Superior longitudinal muscle**: Origin from median fibrous septum near epiglottis; inserts into tongue edges
    - Elevates apex & sides of tongue, shortening & making its dorsum concave
  - **Inferior longitudinal muscle**: Origin from ROT & inserts into its apex, seen between genioglossus & hyoglossus; anteriorly blends with styloglossus
    - Depresses apex & sides of tongue, shortening & making its dorsum convex
  - **Transverse muscle**: Origin from fibrous lingual septum; runs transversely to insert in submucosal fibrous tissue at lateral tongue margins, blending with palatopharyngeus
    - Makes tongue narrow & elongated (sticks out tongue)
  - **Vertical muscle**: Origin from submucosal fibrous layer of dorsum of tongue; inserts into its inferior surface borders, found at borders of anterior tongue
    - Makes tongue broad & flattened
- **Innervation of tongue**
  - Sensory supply (touch, pain, temperature, & **taste**): Anterior 2/3: Lingual nerve (taste fibers are from chorda tympani branch of CNVII); posterior 1/3: CNIX
  - **Hypoglossal nerve** (CNXII): Emerges from upper carotid space; receives fibers from 1st & 2nd cervical nerves; loops inferiorly to level of hyoid bone & rises anteriorly
    - Enter posterior SLS just lateral to hyoglossus; runs in SLS on lateral surface of genioglossus
    - Innervates extrinsic & intrinsic tongue muscles
- **Vasculature of tongue**
  - Lingual artery: 2nd branch of external carotid artery
    - Divides in SLS into sublingual & deep lingual branches
  - Lingual vein: Parallels lingual artery; drains into internal jugular or facial veins
- **Lymphatics of tongue**
  - **Tip of tongue** drains bilaterally to submental nodes
  - **Anterior 2/3 of remaining lateral tongue** drains unilaterally to submandibular nodes of either side
    - Central lymphatics here drain bilaterally to deep cervical or submandibular nodes
  - **Posterior tongue** drains to upper deep cervical nodes, including jugulodigastric nodes (level II)
  - Finally, all drain into **juguloomohyoid** nodes (level III) known as **lymph nodes of tongue**

GRAPHICS

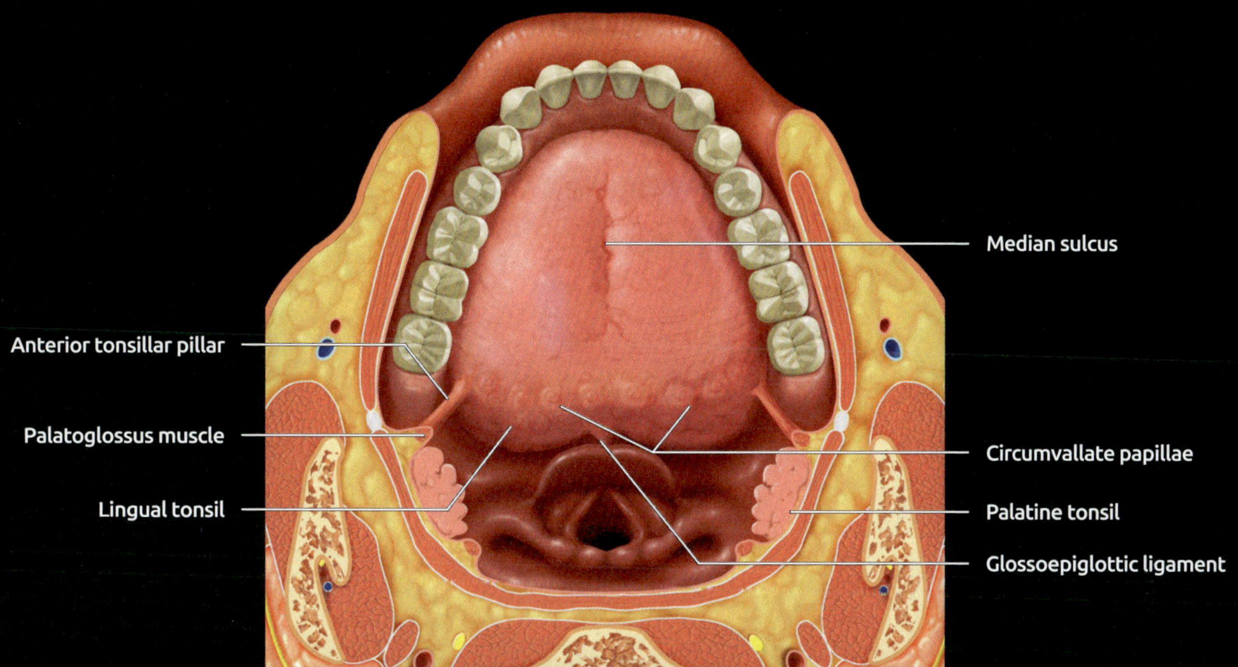

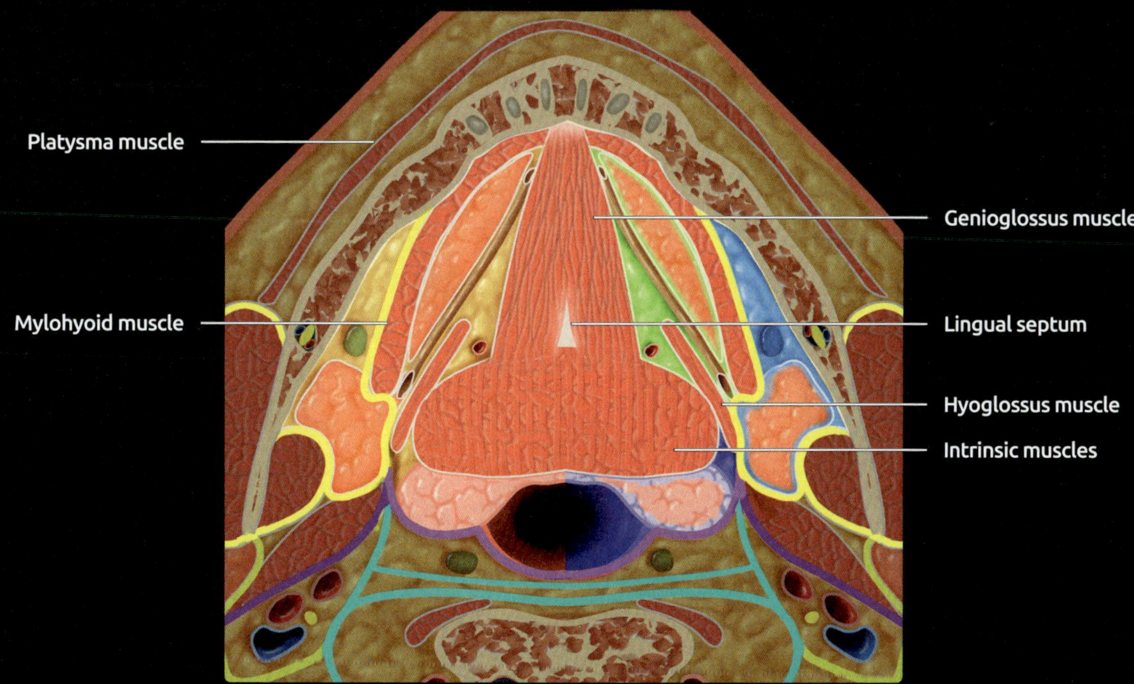

(Top) *Axial graphic of the surface of the oral tongue is shown. The oral tongue sits anterior to the oropharyngeal lingual tonsil. The line of the circumvallate papillae delineates the mucosal surface transition to the more anterior oral cavity.* **(Bottom)** *In this axial graphic through the deep portion of the oral tongue, it is possible to see the large, bilateral paramedian genioglossus muscles bordering the midline lingual septum and extending down into the root of tongue. The genioglossus muscles rise to mingle with the complex tangle of intrinsic tongue muscles. The hyoglossus muscles are also seen rising from the hyoid bone below into the posterior sublingual space.*

GRAPHICS

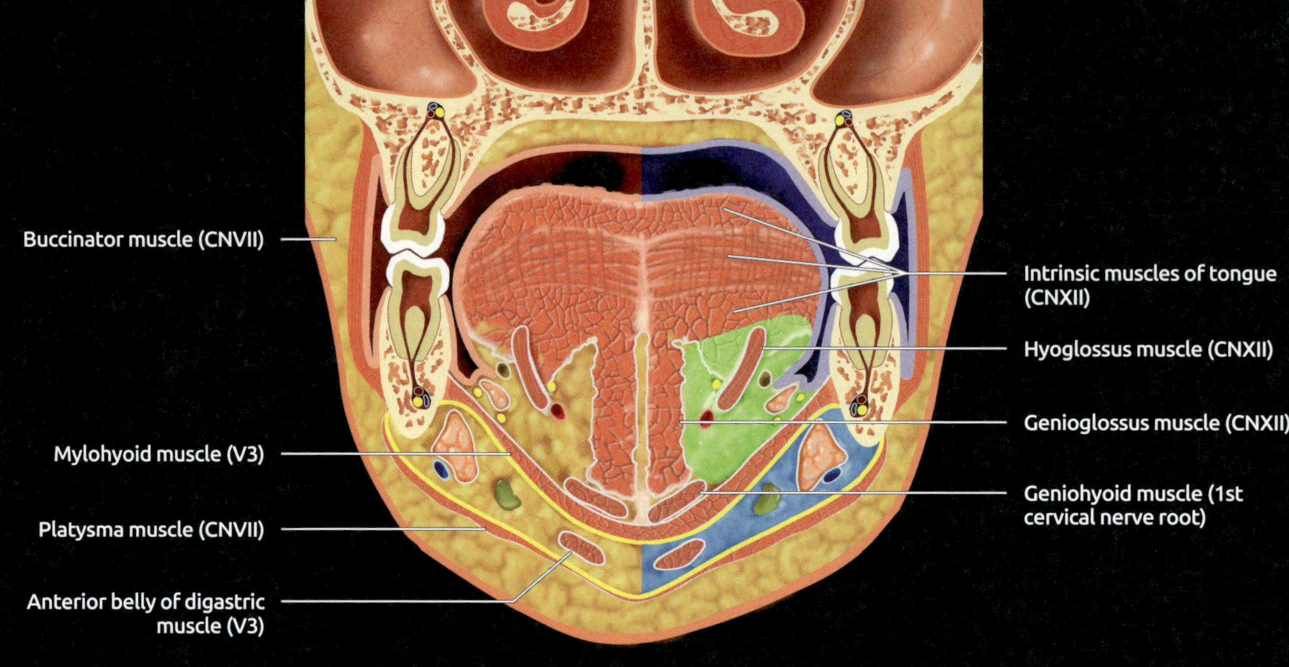

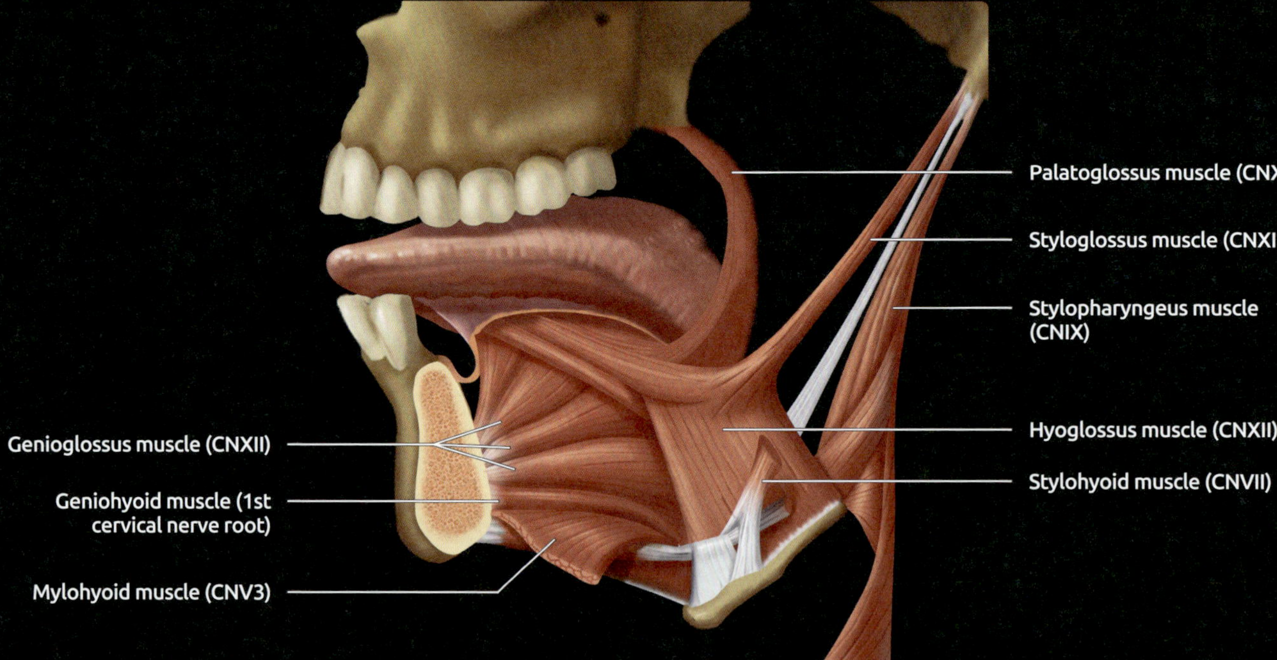

(Top) *Coronal graphic through the oral cavity highlights all major muscles with their innervations indicated in parentheses. Note all intrinsic and extrinsic (genioglossus, hyoglossus, styloglossus, palatoglossus) tongue muscles are innervated by CNXII except palatoglossus. The buccinator and platysma, both muscles of facial expression, are innervated by CNVII.* **(Bottom)** *Sagittal graphic shows muscles of the tongue area. Each muscle is labeled with its innervating nerve in parentheses. Pay attention to the fan-shaped genioglossus, which represents much of the deep tongue extrinsic musculature extending from the oral tongue into the root of the tongue. Note the hyoglossus muscle projecting upward from the hyoid bone like 2 big arms into the oral tongue's posterior sublingual space. The geniohyoid muscle is not considered part of the extrinsic muscles of the tongue but instead is the suprahyoid neck muscle innervated by the CNXII branch with the 1st cervical nerve root in it.*

SAGITTAL AND CORONAL T1 MR AND AXIAL NECT

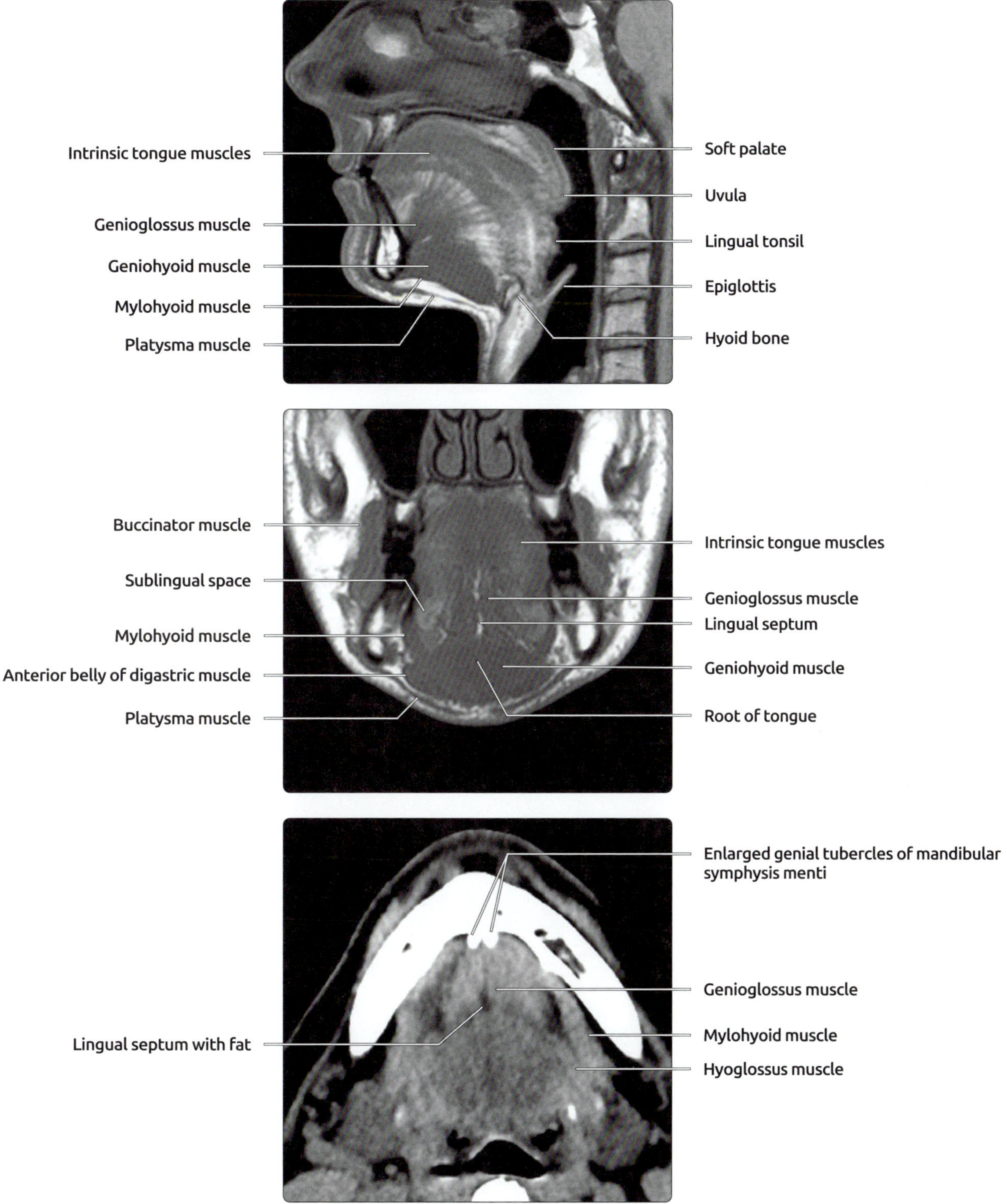

(Top) *Sagittal T1 MR shows the full extent of the genioglossus muscle extending cephalad in a fan shape from its attachment to the posteroinferior mandible. Notice that it is difficult to distinguish the mylohyoid, geniohyoid, and inferior genioglossus muscles.* **(Middle)** *On this coronal T1 MR, 4 stacked muscles can be identified from inferior to superior, namely, the anterior belly of the digastric, mylohyoid, geniohyoid, and genioglossus muscles. The stacked muscles are difficult to differentiate completely from each other. Note the T1-hyperintense fat in the thin midline lingual septum. Sublingual spaces lie lateral to the genioglossus muscles and superolateral to the mylohyoid muscle.* **(Bottom)** *Axial NECT shows the unusually enlarged genial tubercles of the mandible (normal variant). Genioglossus and geniohyoid muscles originate from genial tubercles. The genioglossus dilates the upper airway, modulated by changes in airway pressure during breathing and also by changes in the posture of the jaw and head. Attachment to genial tubercles prevents the tongue from falling back and obstructing the airway; it also aids in jaw thrust/chin lift maneuvers during airway resuscitation.*

AXIAL T2 MR

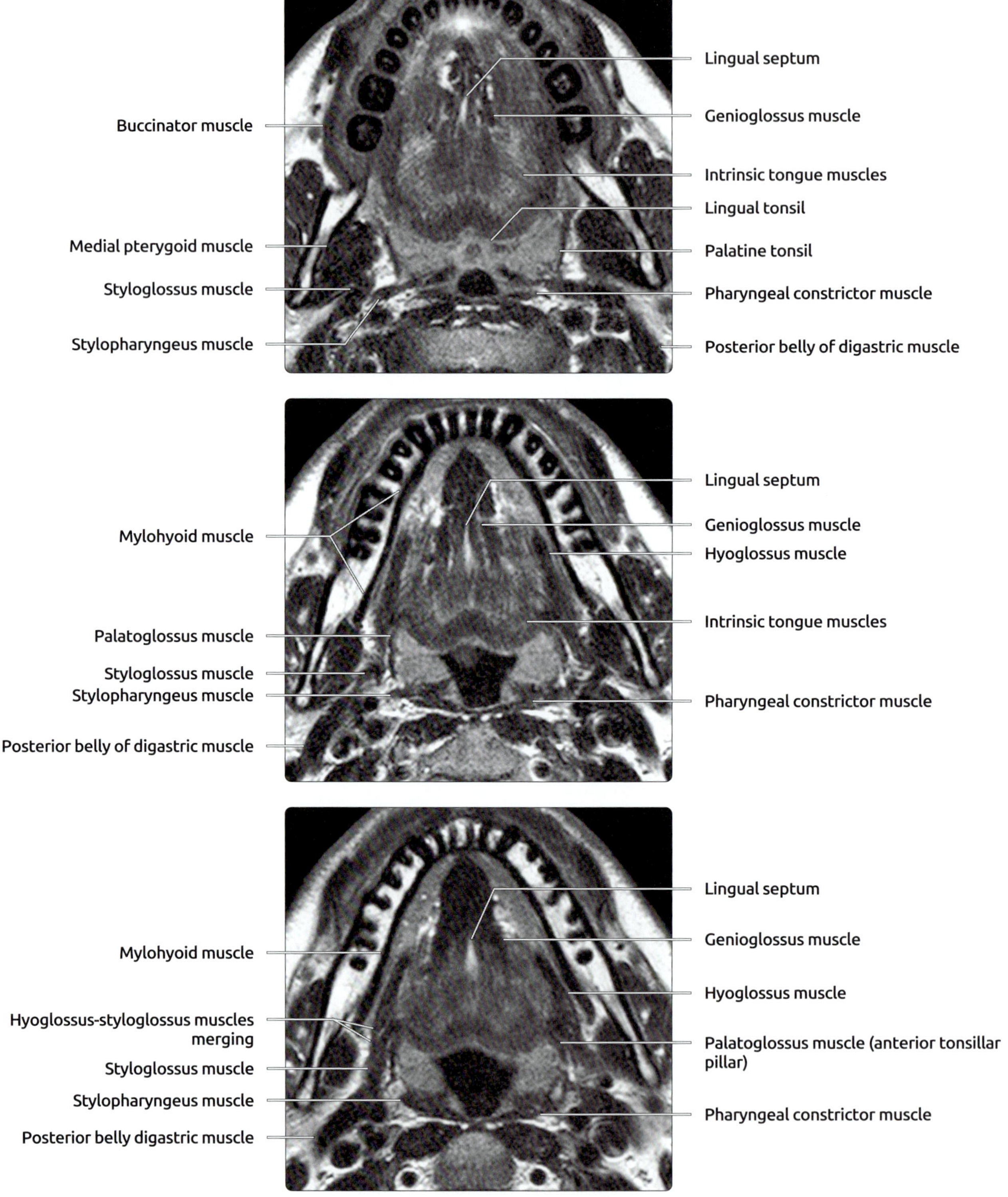

(Top) *First of 6 axial T2 MR images of the oral tongue from superior to inferior is shown. In this most superior MR, the superior aspect of the oral tongue is seen. The intrinsic muscles, especially the transverse group, are well seen with just the top of the genioglossus muscle visible. The styloglossus muscle is seen in its expected location just medial to the medial pterygoid muscle. The stylopharyngeus is identified melding with the pharyngeal constrictor muscle.* **(Middle)** *Inferior T2 MR shows the hyoglossus upper margin rising into the posterior sublingual space. The genioglossus is now readily apparent on either side of the fibrofatty lingual septum.* **(Bottom)** *T2 MR shows the styloglossus merging with the hyoglossus. The styloglossus muscle divides into a longitudinal part, blending with the inferior longitudinal muscle of the tongue in front of the hyoglossus, and an oblique part merging and decussating with the hyoglossus muscle at the side of the tongue. Palatoglossus is now visible along the anterior margin of the palatine tonsil, creating the fold of tissue called the "anterior tonsillar pillar." "Posterior tonsil pillar" is the fold of tissue just behind the tonsils created by palatopharyngeus muscle.*

AXIAL T2 MR

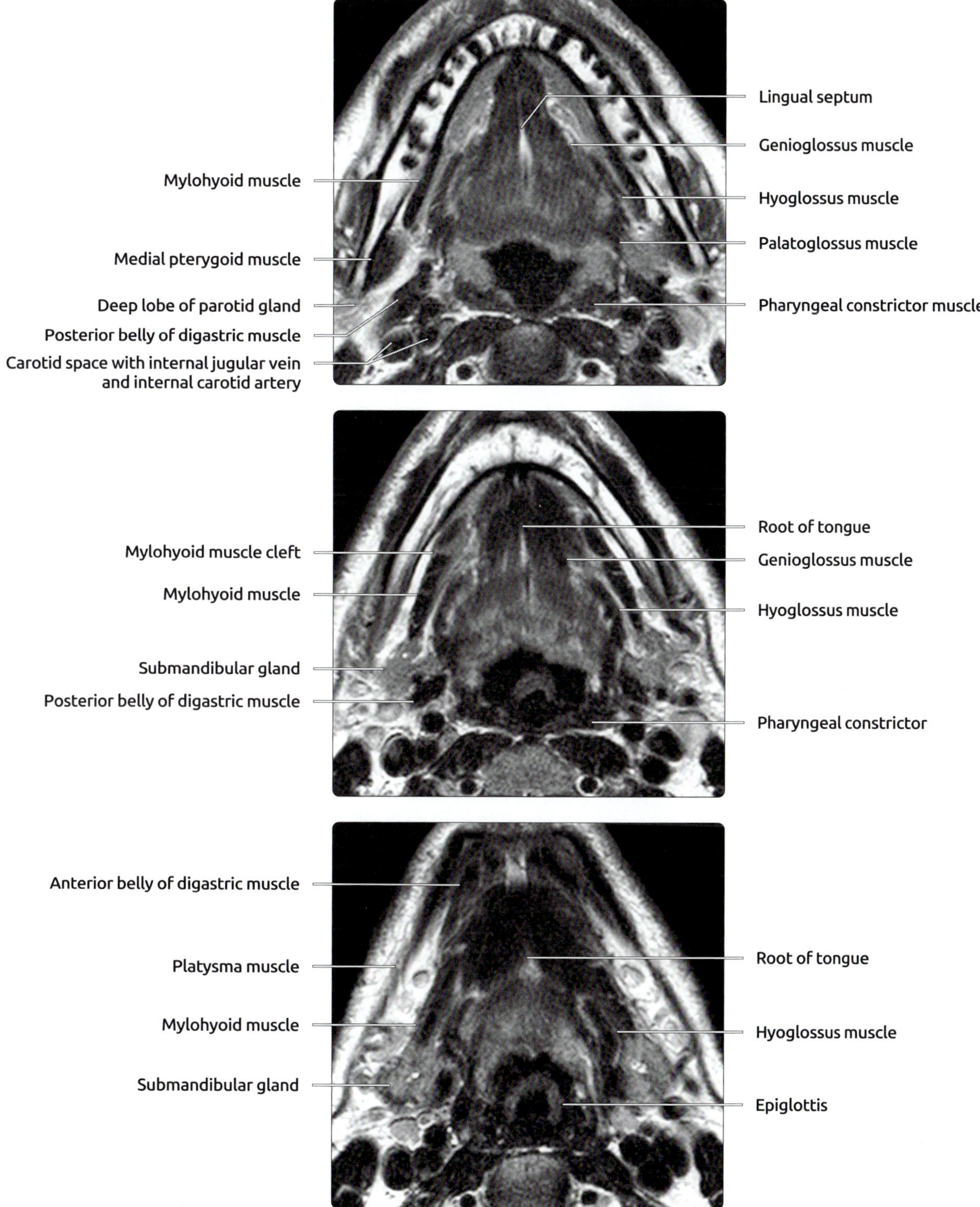

(Top) *At the level of the mandibular teeth roots, the posterior belly of the digastric (PBD) muscle is seen passing deep to the most inferior aspect of the medial pterygoid muscle on the patient's right. The PBD is larger and more inferior than the styloglossus muscle. The PBD separates the posteromedial carotid space from the anterolateral deep lobe of the parotid gland in relation to it and aids in localizing the site of origin of mass lesions from these spaces on CT/MR.* **(Middle)** *This T2 MR shows the mylohyoid muscle has left the mylohyoid ridge of the mandible. A prominent mylohyoid muscle cleft is present on the patient's right. The area of the root of the tongue is labeled.* **(Bottom)** *The most inferior T2 MR shows the convergence of the anteroinferior genioglossus muscle with the geniohyoid muscle to form the area of the root of the tongue. The origins of the hyoglossus muscles are also seen rising off the hyoid bone. The free margin of the epiglottis is visible within the pharyngeal airway.*

TERMINOLOGY

Abbreviations

- Retromolar trigone (RMT)

Definitions

- **RMT**: Small triangular subsite of oral cavity composed of mucosa posterior to last mandibular molar tooth
  - Covers anterior surface of lower ascending ramus of mandible & extends superiorly up to maxillary tuberosity
- **Pterygomandibular raphe (PMR)**: Thick fascial band that extends between posterior border of mandibular mylohyoid ridge & hamulus of medial pterygoid (MP) plate
  - Fascial band represents thickening of **middle layer** of deep cervical fascia (**ML-DCF**)
  - Condensed between posterior margin of buccinator muscle & anterior margin of superior constrictor muscle

IMAGING ANATOMY

Overview

- PMR lies posteriorly beneath mucosa of RMT
- RMT squamous cell carcinoma (SCCa) can involve PMR early
- PMR: Both inferior & superior routes of SCCa spread

Extent

- RMT extent
  - Cephalad tip (apex of trigone): Continuous with maxillary tuberosity behind **last maxillary molar tooth**
  - Base of mucosal trigone: Posterior margin of **last mandibular molar tooth**
  - Bounded laterally by **gingivobuccal sulcus** & medially by **anterior tonsillar pillar**
    - Anterior tonsillar pillar: Palatoglossal arch formed by palatoglossus muscle

Anatomy Relationships

- RMT seen on few contiguous axial CT scan sections
  - Oblique CT reformats help to evaluate entire superoinferior extent of RMT
- PMR located at line of junction between buccinator (posterior margin) muscle & superior constrictor muscle (anterior margin)
  - PMR represents junction of oral cavity anteriorly & oropharynx posteriorly
  - Focally thickened ML-DCF runs along superficial margin of buccinator muscle & along deep & lateral margins of superior constrictor muscle
- **Lingual nerve** (CNV3, mandibular nerve branch) comes in **direct contact with mandible medial to 3rd molar tooth close to RMT** on its way to lateral sublingual space
- Lingual nerve branches out from mandibular nerve posterior division 1 cm below skull; first runs between tensor veli palatini and lateral pterygoid (LP), then between LP & MP, and then anteroinferiorly between MP and mandibular ramus before it reaches medial to mandibular 3rd molar tooth location

Internal Contents

- Gingiva/mucosa of RMT
- Mucosa covering RMT rigid & tightly adherent to underlying alveolar bone
  - Facilitates early infiltration of mandible by RMT SCCa

ANATOMY IMAGING ISSUES

Questions

- RMT SCCa can spread in multiple directions
  - Posterior spread of SCCa
    - Posterolaterally along gingivobuccal sulcus to buccal fat & masticator space, &, rarely, perineural CNV3
    - Posteromedially to tongue
    - Posteriorly to anterior tonsillar pillar/oropharynx
  - Anterior spread of SCCa
    - Along alveolar ridge & anterolaterally to buccinator muscle & cheek
  - Inferior spread of SCCa
    - Direct spread into mandible may extend anteriorly via perineural spread along inferior alveolar nerve
    - Caudal spread along PMR reaches posterior mylohyoid line of mandible & thereby posterior margin of mylohyoid muscle
  - Superior spread of SCCa
    - Cephalad spread along PMR to inferior margin of MP plate at hamulus; maxillary tuberosity may be involved at apex of RMT

Imaging Recommendations

- Tiny RMT lesions may be missed due to opposition of mucosal surfaces on CT/MR
  - Loss of adjacent fat planes act as diagnostic clue
- **Puffed-cheek technique** may help to detect small lesions
  - Also helps evaluate adjacent gingivobuccal sulcus
- CECT provides both soft tissue & bone information
  - May be severely degraded by dental amalgam artifact
  - Bone window critical for bony invasion of mandible or secondary involvement of pterygoid plates
- MR less affected by dental amalgam artifact in most cases
  - Reserve for invasive RMT SCCa
  - Axial T2 & T1 fat-saturated enhanced MR sequences best for evaluation of cephalad PMR

Imaging Pitfalls

- Dental amalgam artifact on CECT may obscure RMT SCCa primary site ± spread along PMR in cephalad direction

CLINICAL IMPLICATIONS

Clinical Importance

- Most RMT tumors are SCCas; sometimes minor salivary gland tumors
- SCCa of RMT may spread along PMR
  - Cephalad spread along PMR takes tumor up to inferolateral pterygoid plate-anteromedial masticator space (especially MP, producing trismus)
    - Tumor seen at level of inferior pterygoid plate involving posterior buccinator muscle & anterior superior constrictor muscle
    - Enlarging tumor involves maxillary sinus, buccal & masticator spaces
  - Caudal spread along PMR takes tumor inferiorly to posterior margin of mylohyoid muscle
    - Enlarging tumor in this location involves floor of mouth of oral cavity
- Look for perineural spread along lingual nerve as it comes in close relation to medial aspect of RMT

GRAPHICS

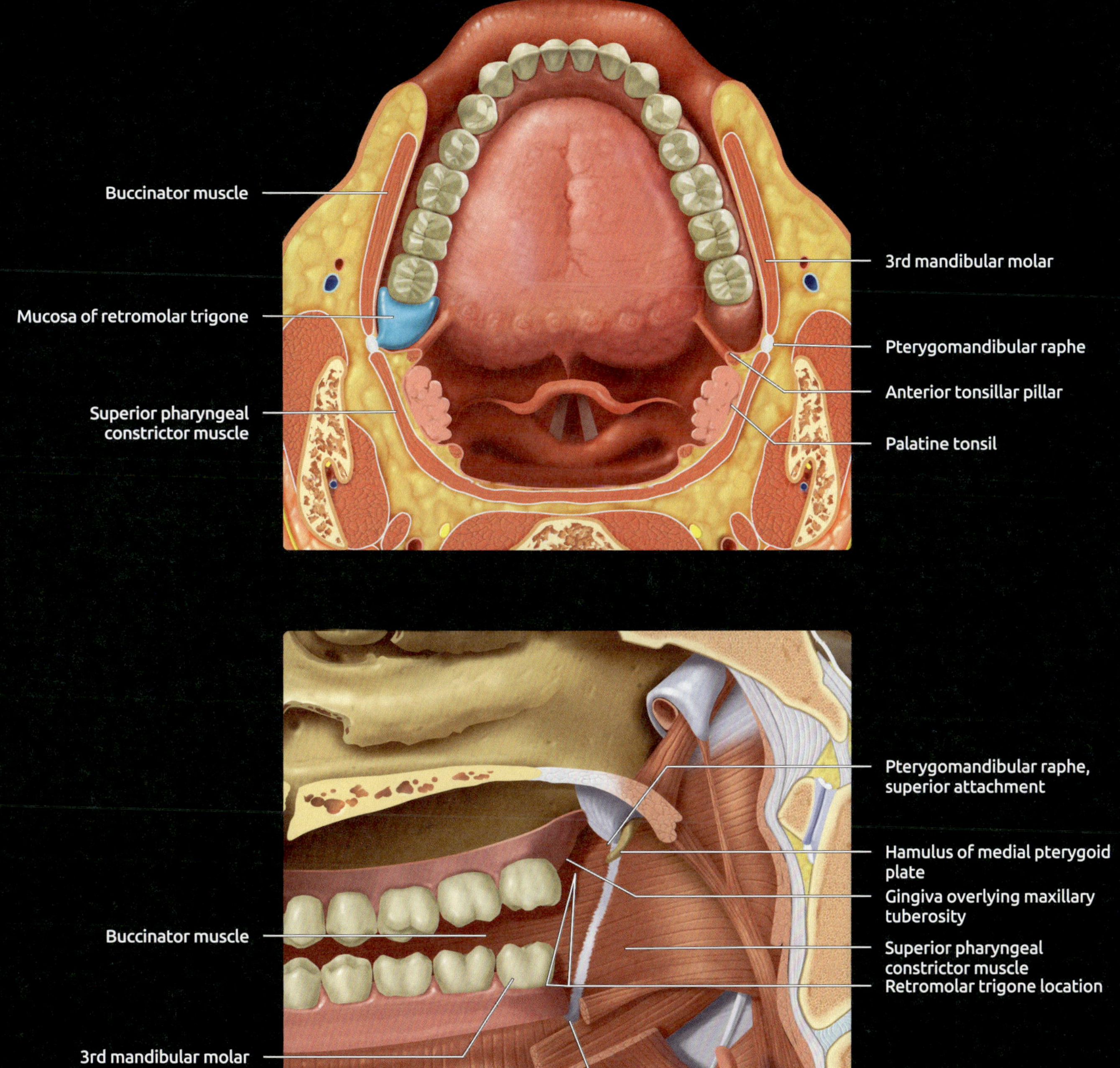

(Top) *Axial graphic highlights the retromolar trigone (RMT) (shaded in blue on the left) and the pterygomandibular raphe (PMR). Notice that the mucosal surface of RMT is found directly behind the mandibular 3rd molar. Its proximity to the PMR (fascial band connecting the buccinator and superior pharyngeal constrictor muscles) is important when squamous cell carcinoma occurs here because of this tumor's propensity for spreading on this fascia.* **(Bottom)** *Sagittal graphic viewed from inside the mouth delineates the full extent of the PMR. Note the cephalad PMR attachment to the hamulus of the medial pterygoid plate and its inferior attachment to the posterior aspect of the mylohyoid ridge on the inner mandibular cortex. PMR "connects" the buccinator muscle to the superior pharyngeal constrictor muscle. Buccinator muscle occupies the interval between the maxilla and mandible with origins from alveolar margins of both. Note that the cephalad apex of the RMT reaches up to maxillary tuberosity. Maxillary tuberosity is the most posterior aspect of the maxilla with its posterior border curving upward. The 3rd maxillary molar tooth lies just in front and within the maxillary tuberosity.*

AXIAL T2 MR

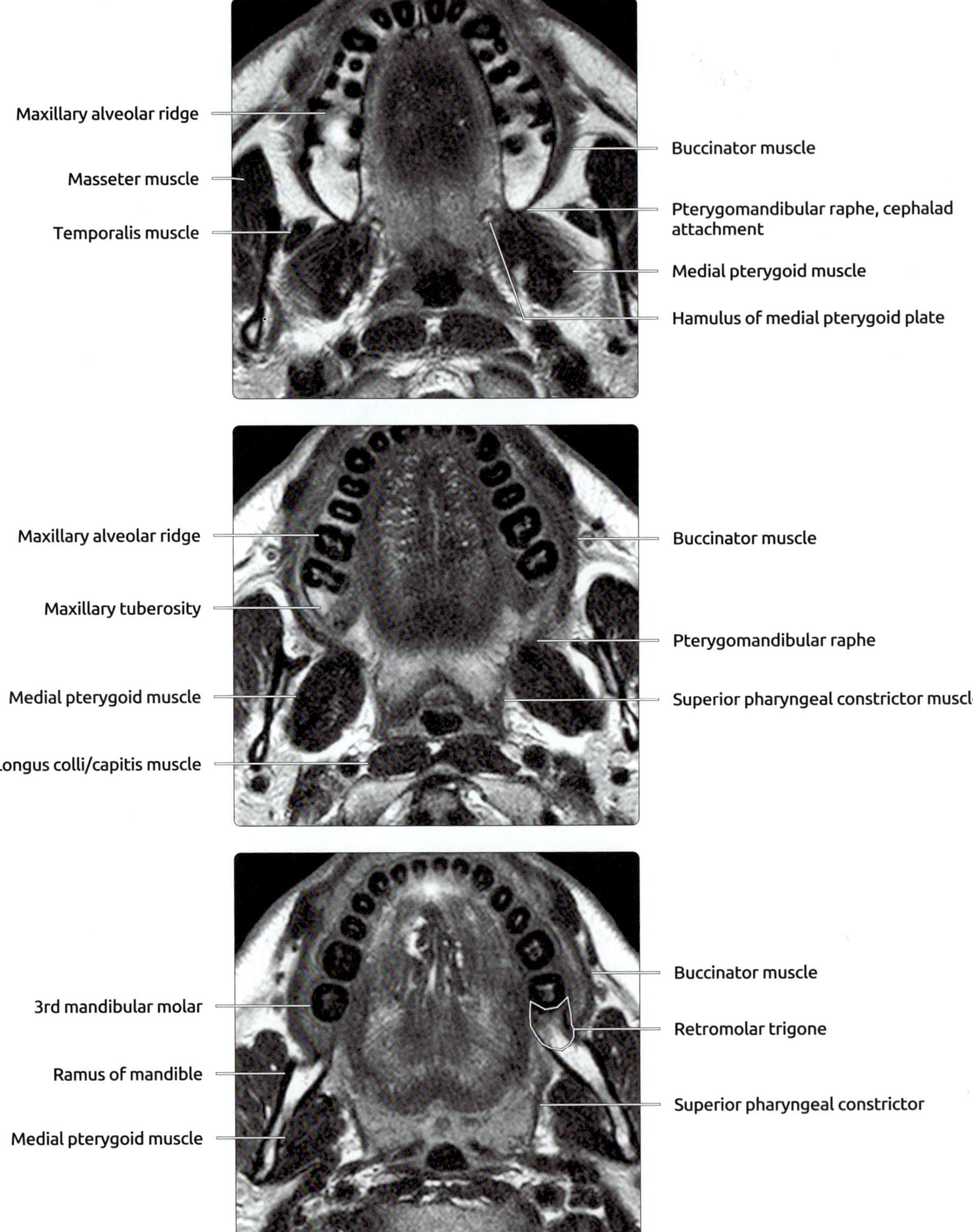

(Top) *First of 3 axial T2 MR images presented from superior to inferior is shown. This most superior image shows the point of attachment of the PMR to the hamulus of the medial pterygoid plate. A tendon of the tensor veli palatini muscle passes along the hamulus and is covered with a bursa, reducing friction on the hamular process by the tendon during motion. Inflammation of this bursa (hamular bursitis) can cause referred pain in the orofacial region. Local erythema, mucosal ulceration, and palpable hypertrophy of the hamulus may be associated.* **(Middle)** *On this most inferior image, the buccinator can be seen meeting the superior pharyngeal constrictor muscle at the PMR. The raphe itself is difficult to visualize. Note that the superior apex of the triangular RMT extends up to the maxillary tuberosity.* **(Bottom)** *At the level of the mandibular alveolar ridge, the area of the RMT can be outlined. Notice it is found directly behind the mandibular 3rd molar tooth. The buccinator is seen along its lateral margin, while the superior pharyngeal constrictor can be seen approaching its medial margin. Squamous cell carcinoma of the RMT often spreads cephalad along this raphe.*

AXIAL CECT

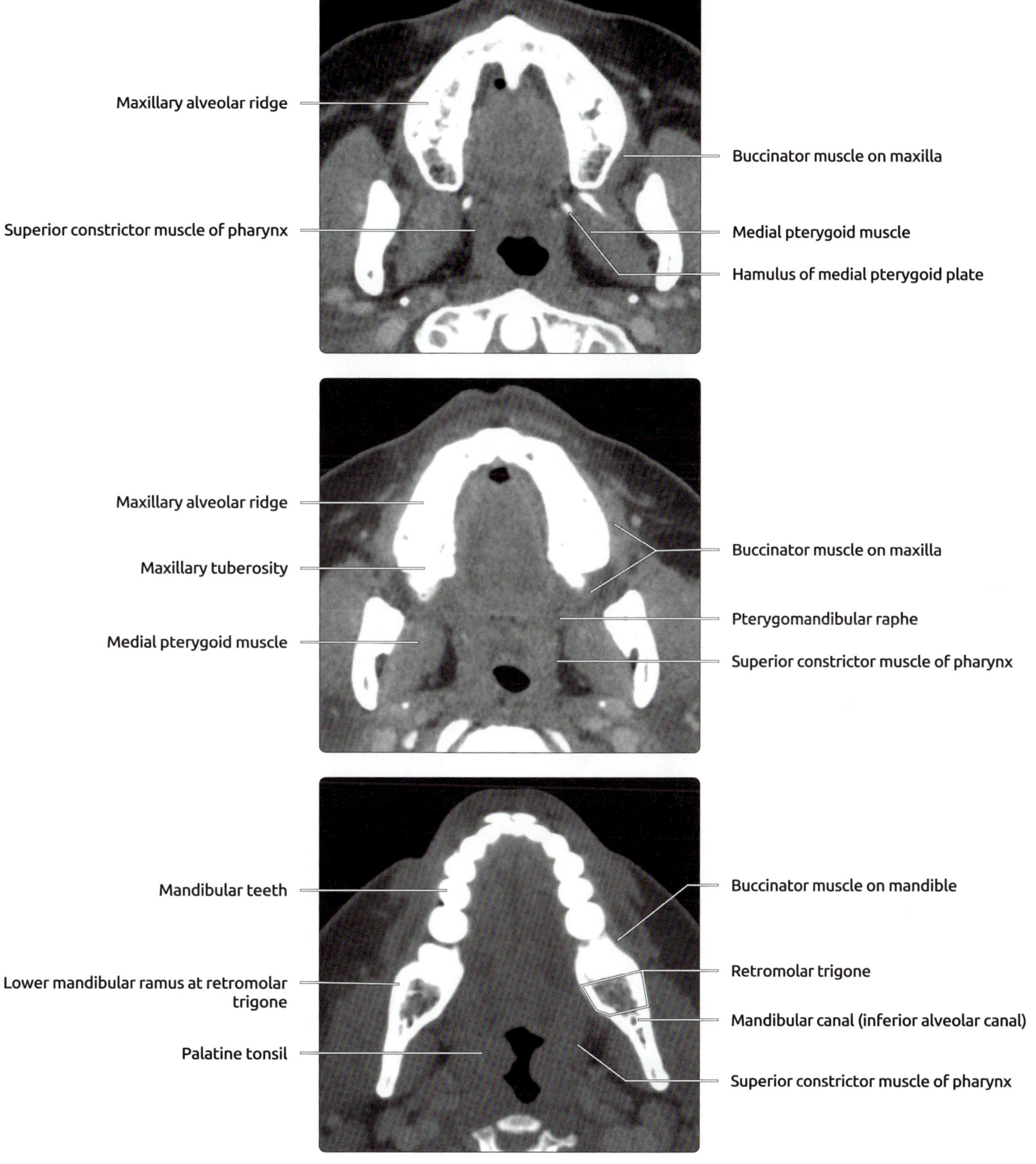

(Top) *First of 3 axial CECT images through the oropharynx-oral cavity presented from superior to inferior is shown. On this most inferior image, the hamulus of the medial pterygoid plate is seen, which provides the superior attachment to PMR and acts as a pulley to the tendon of the tensor veli palatini muscle (with a bursa in between).* **(Middle)** *Slightly lower image shows the buccinator muscle and the superior constrictor muscle meeting at the PMR. The superior constrictor muscle cannot be differentiated from the oropharyngeal palatine (faucial) tonsil on CT scan.* **(Bottom)** *The most inferior image at the mandibular alveolus level shows the RMT outlined on the patient's left. The RMT is found directly behind the last mandibular molar tooth. Squamous cell carcinoma can spread up the PMR from this location. The mandibular canal with the inferior alveolar nerve is located in close vicinity of the RMT, a potential route for perineural tumor (PNT) spread. Note that the lingual nerve (CNV3, mandibular nerve branch) comes in direct contact with the mandible medial to the 3rd molar tooth close to the RMT on its way to lateral sublingual space, which is another potential route for PNT spread.*

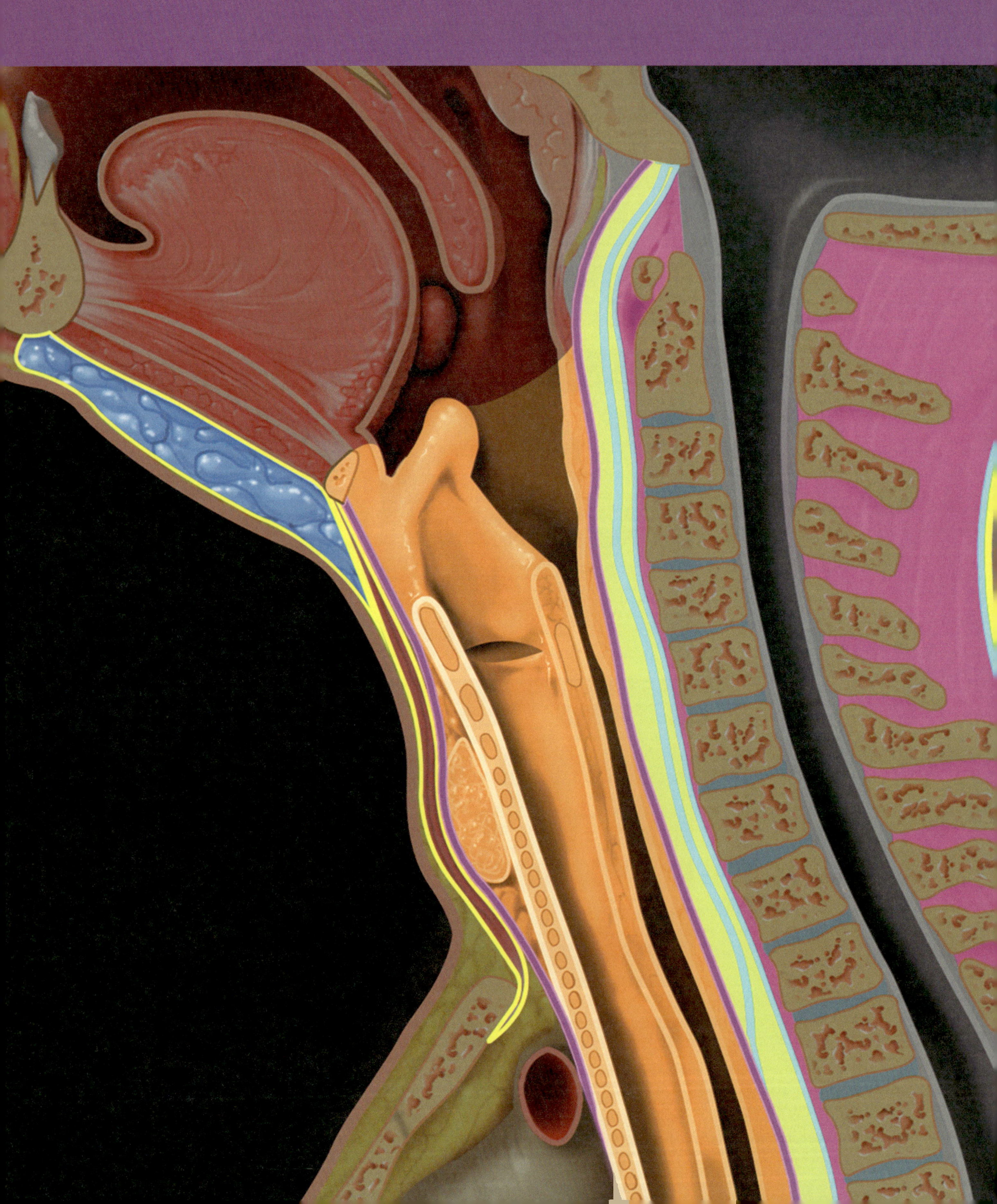

SECTION 7

Suprahyoid and Infrahyoid Neck

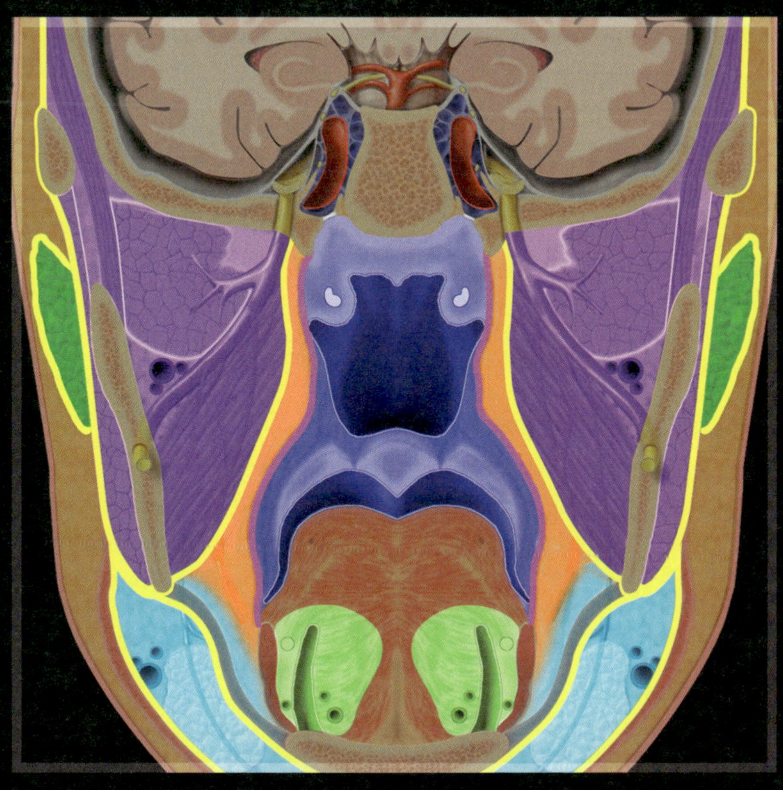

TERMINOLOGY

Abbreviations

- Suprahyoid neck (SHN); infrahyoid neck (IHN)

Definitions

- SHN: Spaces from skull base to hyoid bone (excluding orbit, sinuses, & oral cavity): Pharyngeal mucosal (PMS), parapharyngeal (PPS), masticator (MS), parotid (PS), carotid (CS), buccal (BS), retropharyngeal (RPS), perivertebral (PVS), submandibular (SMS), & sublingual (SLS) spaces
- IHN: Spaces below level of hyoid bone, some continue into mediastinum: Visceral space (VS), posterior cervical space (PCS), anterior cervical space (ACS), CS, RPS, & PVS

IMAGING ANATOMY

Overview

- **Key** to understanding SHN & IHN spaces is **fascia**
- 3 layers of deep cervical fascia cleave neck into spaces
  - **Superficial layer of deep cervical fascia (SL-DCF)**
    - SHN: Around MS & PS; part of carotid sheath
    - IHN: **Investing layer** around all neck structures, splits to enclose sternocleidomastoid & trapezius muscles
    - Coverage of strap muscles by SL-DCF controversial, many consider it covered by middle layer of DCF (ML-DCF)
  - **ML-DCF**
    - SHN: ML-DCF defines PMS deep margin; contributes to carotid sheath
    - IHN: Circumscribes VS; part of carotid sheath
  - **Deep layer, deep cervical fascia (DL-DCF)**
    - SHN & IHN: Surrounds PVS
    - SHN & IHN: Contributes to carotid sheath
    - SHN & IHN: **Alar fascia**: Slip of DL-DCF within RPS separating "true" RPS from danger space (DS)

Spaces of Suprahyoid & Infrahyoid Neck

- **PPS**
  - Location: Bilateral **prestyloid** fat-filled spaces in SHN from skull base to posterosuperior SMS
    - PMS medially; MS & PS laterally
  - Contents: Fat & pharyngeal venous plexus
  - Importance: Displacement pattern defines mass origin
- **PMS**
  - Location: SHN space medial to PPS, anterior to RPS
  - Contents: Mucosa, minor salivary glands, PMS lymphatic ring, constrictor muscles
    - Nasopharyngeal, oropharyngeal, & hypopharyngeal mucosal surfaces
    - PMS of nasopharynx: Torus tubarius, adenoids, superior constrictor, & levator veli palatini muscles
    - PMS of oropharynx: Anterior & posterior tonsillar pillars, palatine & lingual tonsils, soft palate
  - Fascia: ML-DCF on nonairway side of PMS
  - Importance: Squamous cell carcinoma (SCCa) & NHL
- **MS**
  - Location: Anterolateral to PPS in SHN
  - Contents: Ramus & posterior body of mandible, CNV3, masseter, medial & lateral pterygoid & temporalis muscles, pterygoid venous plexus
  - Fascia: MS surrounded by SL-DCF
  - Importance: Perineural tumor on CNV3; sarcoma
- **PS**
  - Location: Lateral to PPS in SHN
  - Contents: Parotid gland, extracranial CNVII, nodes, retromandibular vein, external carotid artery
  - Fascia: PS surrounded by SL-DCF
  - Importance: Parotid nodes; perineural tumor on CNVII
- **CS**
  - Location: **Poststyloid** posterior to PPS in SHN; lateral to VS & RPS in IHN
    - Begins at inferior jugular foramen & carotid canal of skull base; extends to aortic arch
  - Contents: CNIX-XII, internal jugular vein, carotid artery
  - Fascia: All 3 layers, deep cervical fascia
  - Importance: CNX & carotid here; SCCa nodes along superficial margin
- **RPS**
  - Location: Posterior to PMS in SHN & VS in IHN
    - Begins at clivus; traverses SHN-IHN to T3 (variable C6-T6) level where alar fascia fuse to ML-DCF
  - Contents: Nodes & fat in SHN; no nodes in IHN
  - Fascia: Anterior fascia ML-DCF, posterior fascia DL-DCF
  - Alar fascia divides RPS into "true" RPS & DS
  - Importance: Fascial "trapdoor", usually at T3 level, serves as infection conduit from RPS along DS to mediastinum
- **DS**: Posterior to RPS in SHN & IHN; continues inferiorly into mediastinum & to level of diaphragm
- **PVS**
  - Location: Behind RPS & around spine in SHN & IHN
    - Defined from skull base above to clavicle below
  - Contents: Prevertebral & paraspinal components
    - Prevertebral: Vertebral body, prevertebral & scalene muscles, veins, arteries, brachial plexus, phrenic nerve
    - Paraspinal: Posterior elements of vertebra, levator scapulae, & paraspinal muscles
  - Fascia: Surrounded by DL-DCF
    - DL-DCF slip divides PVS into prevertebral & paraspinal
  - Importance: PVS malignancy may be epidural
- **VS**
  - Location: IHN only; extends into mediastinum
  - Contents: Thyroid & parathyroids, paratracheal nodes, esophagus, trachea, recurrent laryngeal nerve
  - Fascia: VS surrounded by ML-DCF
  - Importance: Trachea & esophagus traverse VS
- **PCS**
  - Location: SHN PCS begins at mastoid tip, extends to clavicle; most PCS volume in IHN
  - Contents: Fat, CNXI, spinal accessory nodes
  - Fascia: Between SL- & DL-DCF
  - Importance: Spinal accessory nodal diseases

Key Spatial Relationships

- **SHN spaces surrounding PPS**
  - PMS medially: PMS mass displaces PPS laterally
  - MS anterolaterally: MS mass displaces PPS posteromedially
  - PS laterally: PS mass displaces PPS medially
  - CS posteriorly: CS mass displaces PPS anteriorly
  - Lateral RPS posteromedially: Lateral RPS nodal mass displaces PPS anterolaterally

GRAPHICS

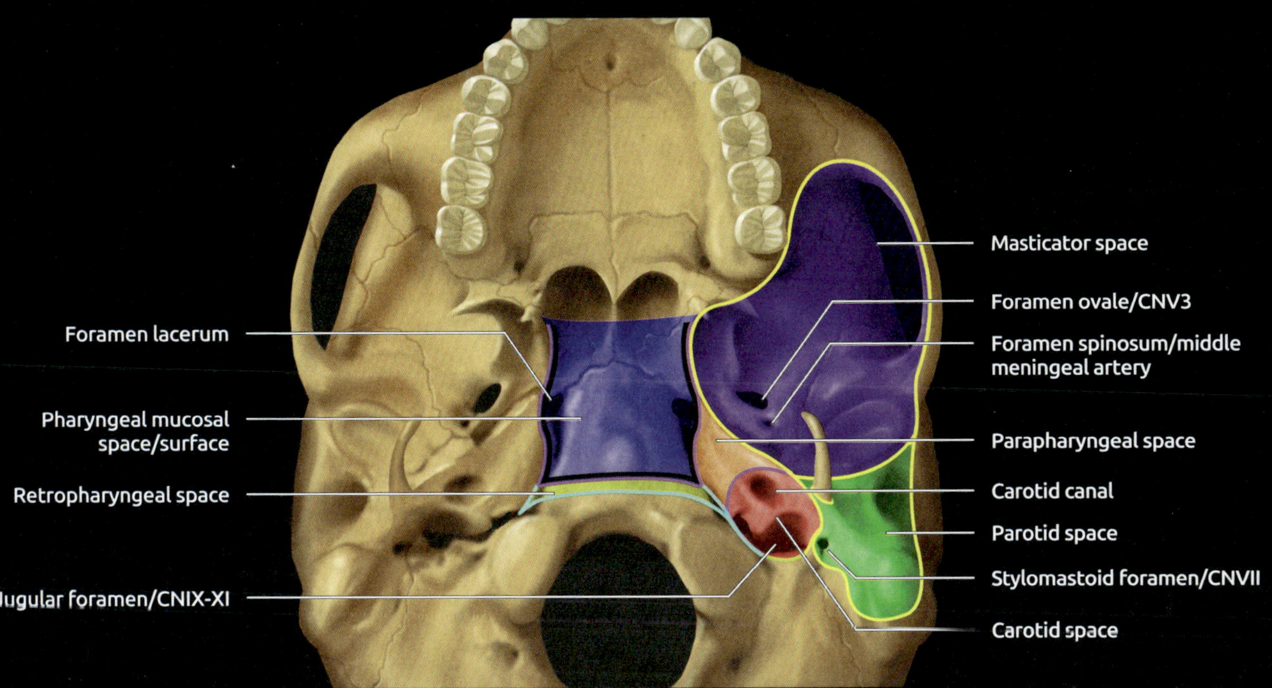

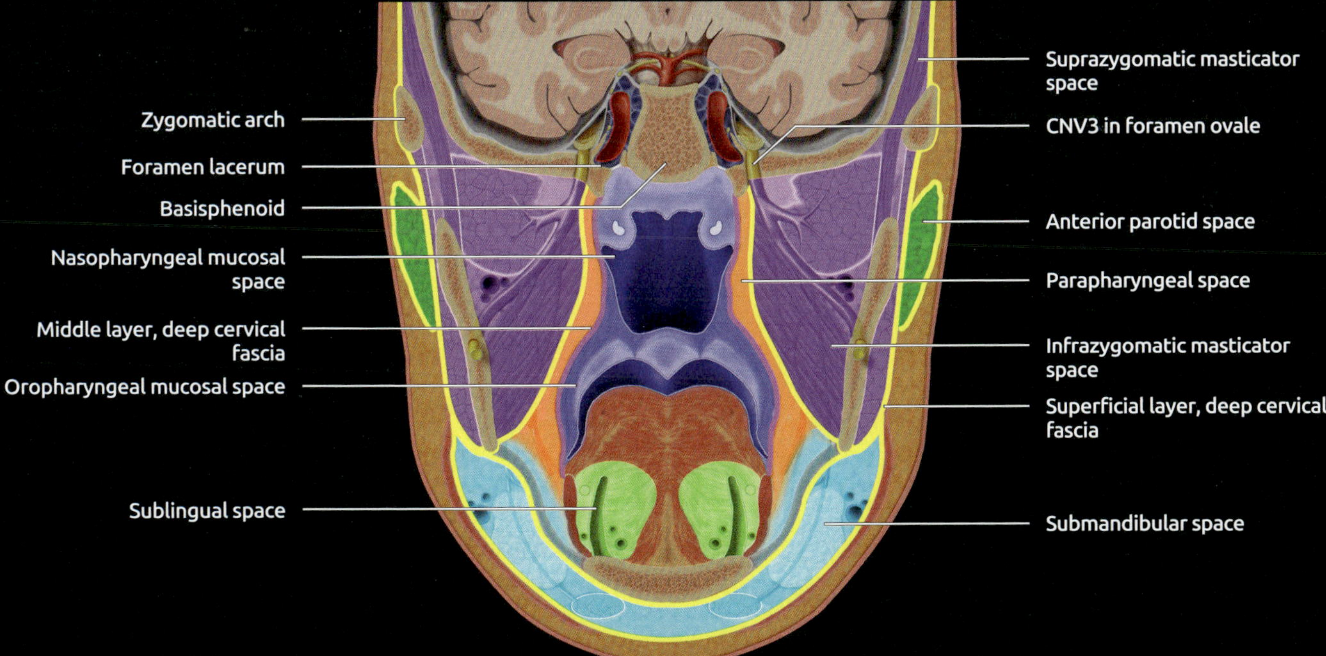

(Top) *Graphic of skull base from below shows spaces of suprahyoid neck with relationship to skull base. Four spaces have key interactions with skull base: Masticator (MS), parotid (PS), carotid (CS), and pharyngeal mucosal spaces (PMS). PS (green) malignancy can follow CNVII into stylomastoid foramen. MS (purple) receives CNV3 while CNIX-XII enter the CS (red). The PMS abuts the foramen lacerum, which is covered by fibrocartilage in life. Also note that the superficial layer of deep cervical fascia (SL-DCF) (yellow line) surrounds the MS and PS, and middle layer is on nonairway side of PMS (pink line).* **(Bottom)** *Coronal graphic shows suprahyoid neck spaces as they interact with the skull base. The MS has the largest area of abutment with the skull base, including CNV3. The PMS abuts the basisphenoid and foramen lacerum.*

GRAPHICS

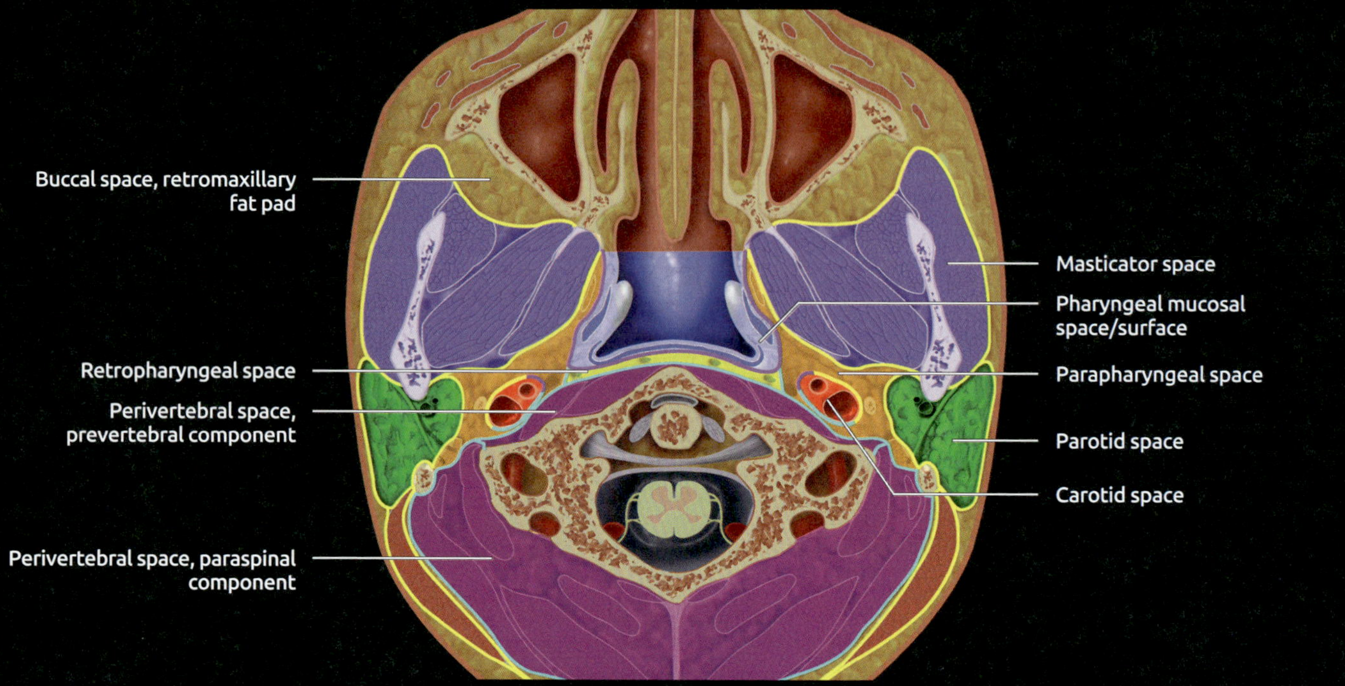

Buccal space, retromaxillary fat pad
Masticator space
Pharyngeal mucosal space/surface
Retropharyngeal space
Parapharyngeal space
Perivertebral space, prevertebral component
Parotid space
Carotid space
Perivertebral space, paraspinal component

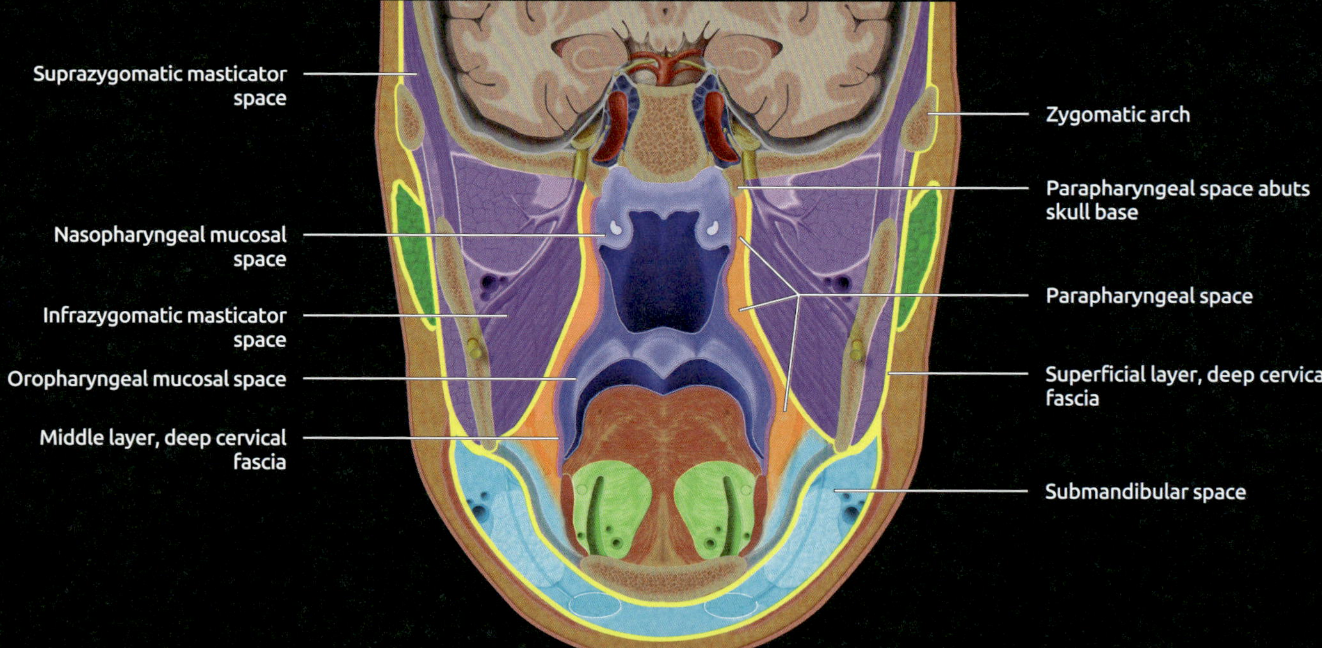

(Top) *Axial graphic depicts the spaces of the suprahyoid neck. Surrounding the paired, fat-filled parapharyngeal spaces (PPSs) are the 4 critical paired spaces of this region: The PMS, MS, PS, and CS. The retropharyngeal and perivertebral spaces are the midline nonpaired spaces. A PMS mass pushes the PPS laterally; MS mass pushes PPS posteromedially; PS mass pushes PPS medially; CS mass pushes PPS anteriorly.* **(Bottom)** *Coronal graphic shows the PPS. The PPSs are paired, fat-filled spaces in the more lateral aspect of the suprahyoid neck. This space abuts the skull base between the MS and PMS. There are no important structures at the point of intersection between the PPS and the skull base. Inferiorly, the PPS communicates with the posterosuperior aspect of the submandibular space (SMS).*

GRAPHICS

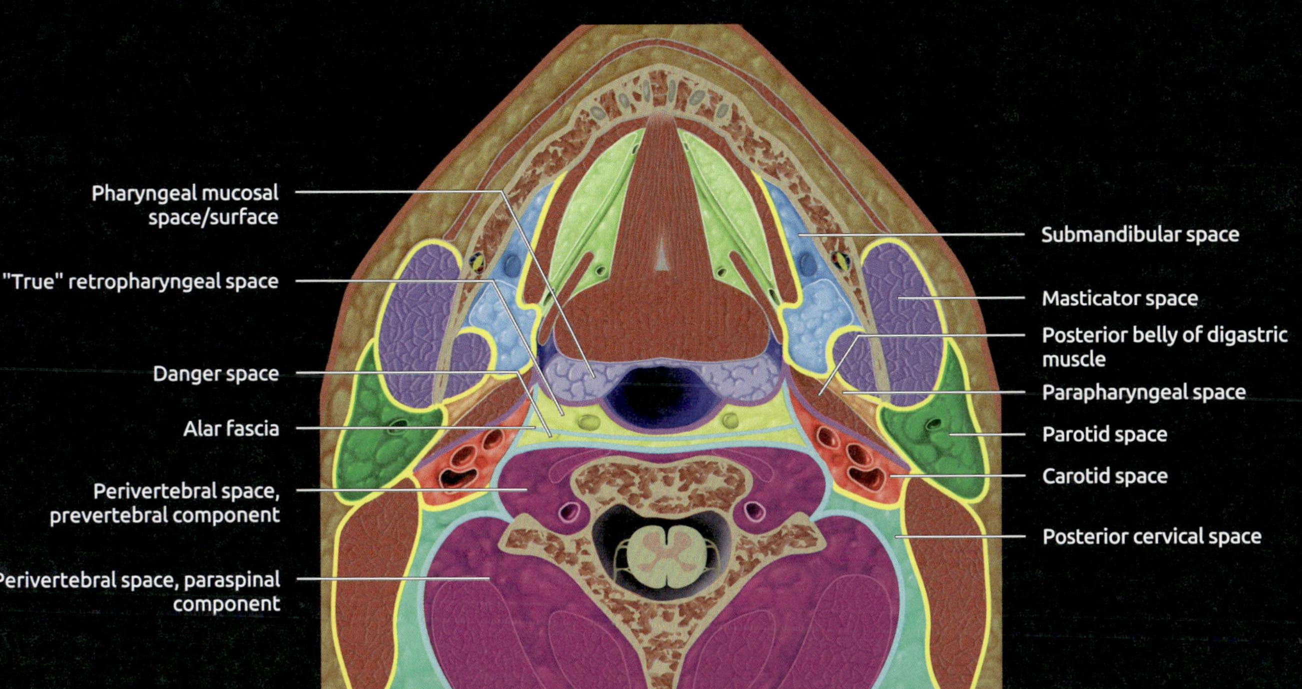

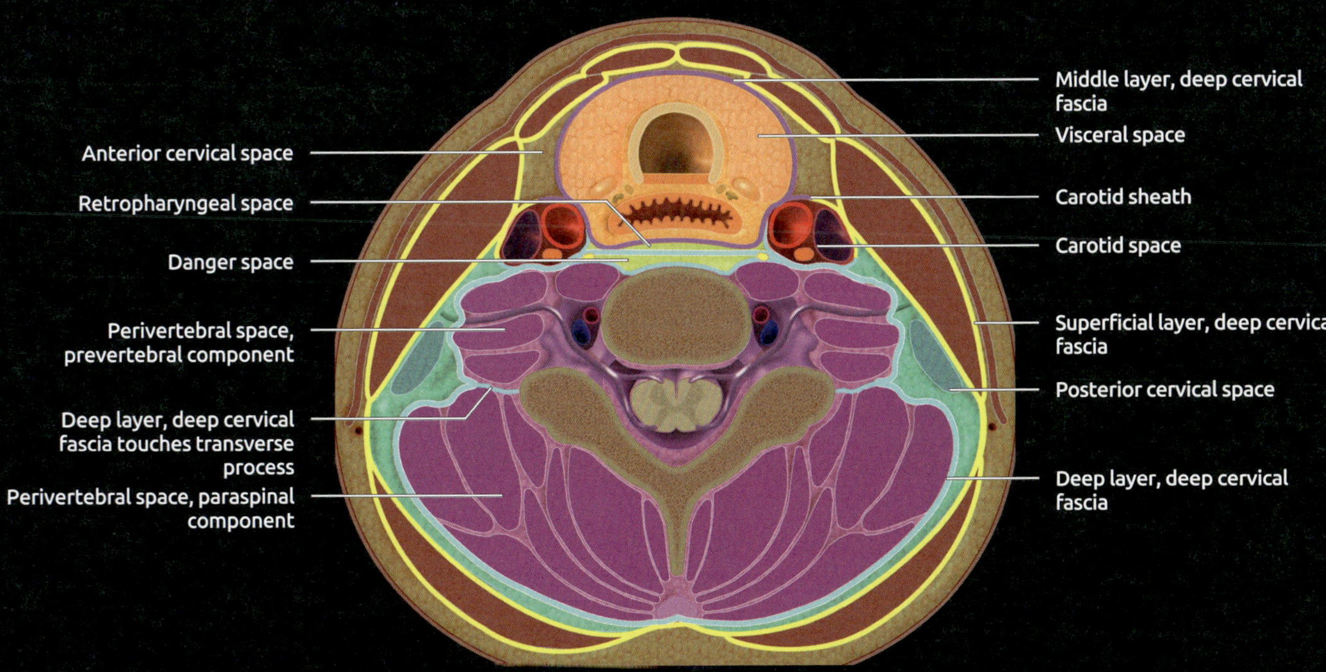

(Top) *Axial graphic shows suprahyoid neck spaces at the level of the oropharynx. Superficial (yellow line), middle (pink line), and deep (turquoise line) layers of deep cervical fascia (DCF) outline suprahyoid neck spaces. Alar fascia slip of the deep layer of DCF (DL-DCF) separates the anterior true retropharyngeal space and posterior danger space.* **(Bottom)** *Axial graphic depicts fascia and spaces of the infrahyoid neck. The 3 layers of DCF are present in the suprahyoid and infrahyoid neck. The carotid sheath is made up of all 3 layers of DCF (tricolor line around CS). The SL-DCF is also called the investing layer. Coverage of strap muscles by SL-DCF is controversial in literature with many considering it to be covered by the middle layer of DCF (ML-DCF). SL-DCF surrounds trapezius and sternomastoid muscles, attaches to external occipital protuberance and superior nuchal line of skull superiorly, hyoid bone anteriorly, scapular spine and acromion, clavicle, sternal manubrium inferiorly, and nuchal ligament posteriorly. Notice the deep layer completely encircling the perivertebral space, diving in laterally to divide it into prevertebral and paraspinal components.*

GRAPHICS

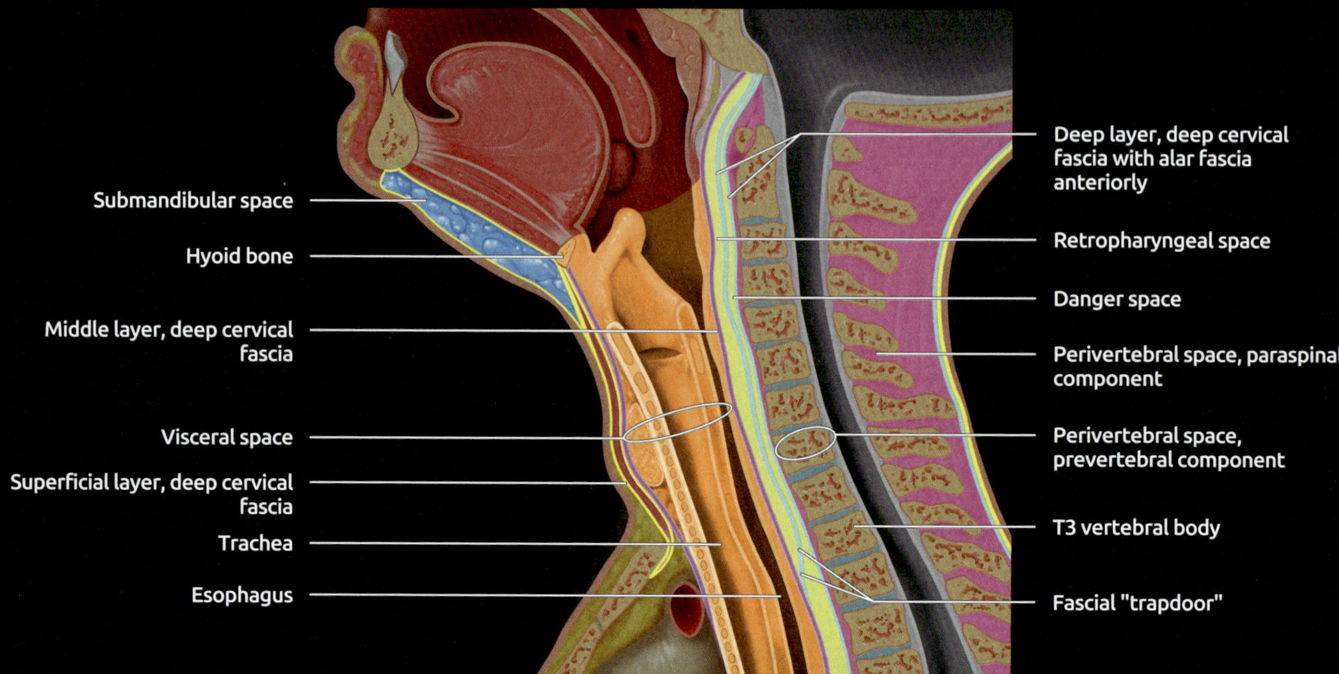

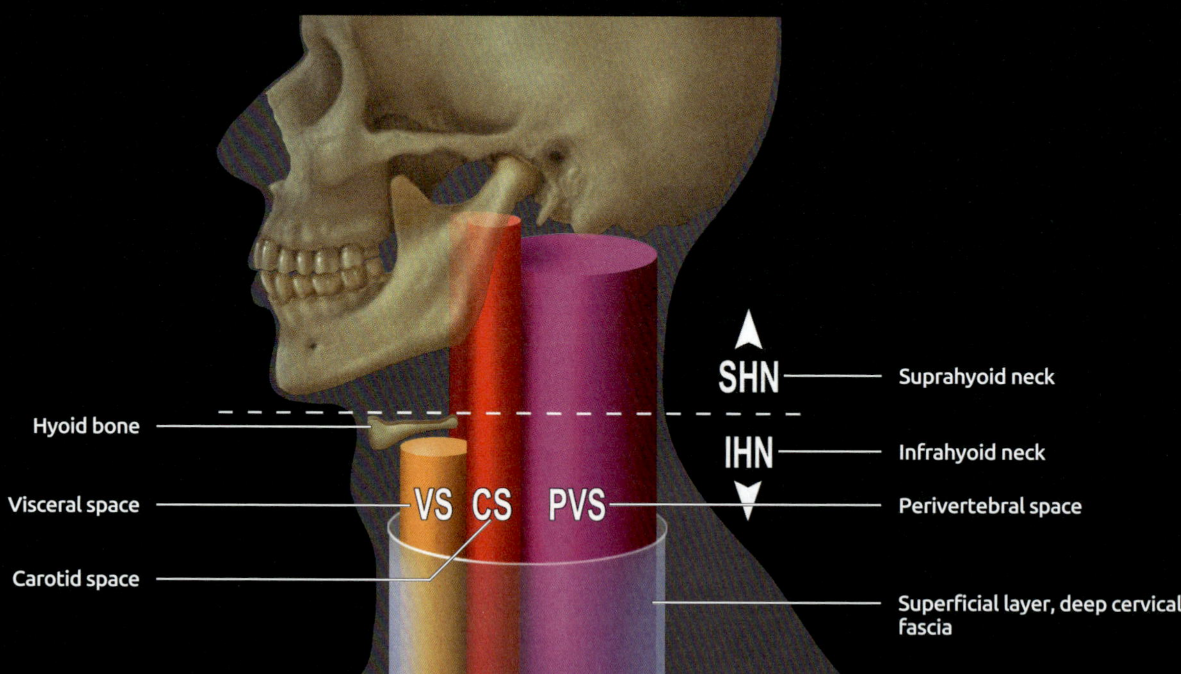

(Top) *Sagittal graphic depicting longitudinal spatial relationships of the infrahyoid neck is shown. Anteriorly, the visceral space is seen surrounded by ML-DCF. Just anterior to the vertebral column, the true retropharyngeal (posterior) and danger (anterior) spaces formed by alar fascia slip of DL-DCF in between run inferiorly towards the mediastinum. Notice the fascial "trapdoor" found at the approximate level of the T3 vertebral body that serves as a conduit from the retropharyngeal to the danger space. Retropharyngeal space infection or tumor may access the mediastinum via this route of spread.* **(Bottom)** *Lateral graphic of the extracranial head and neck show the spaces as "tubes" as they traverse the area. This is particularly true of the CSs, which reach from the skull base to the aortic arch. Both the visceral and perivertebral spaces continue inferiorly into the thorax.*

AXIAL CECT OF SUPRAHYOID NECK

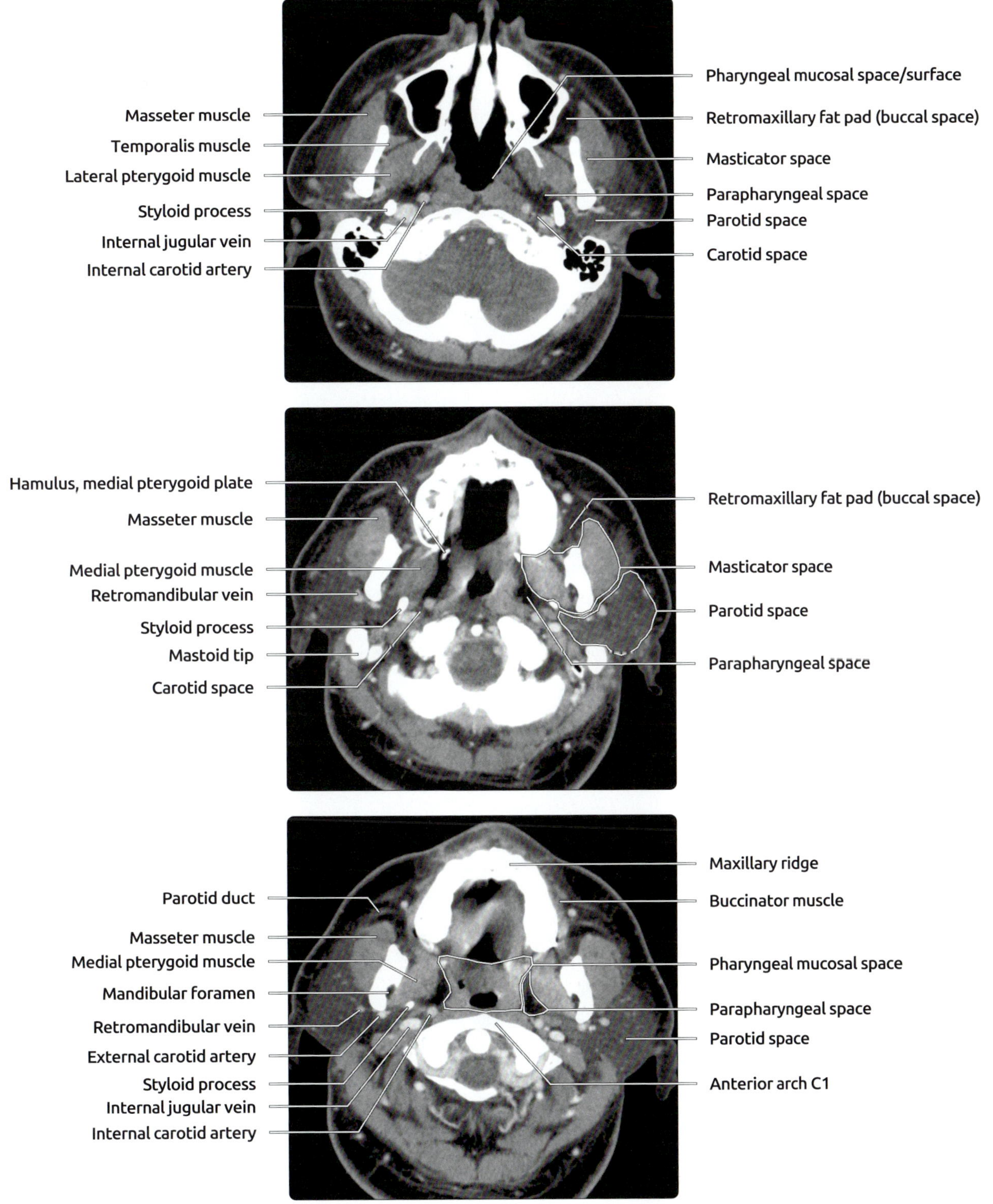

(Top) *First of 12 axial CECT images of both the suprahyoid and infrahyoid aspect of the extracranial head and neck presented from superior to inferior is shown. This image at the level of the nasopharynx shows the 4 key spaces surrounding the PPS: PMS, MS, PS, and CS.* **(Middle)** *In this image at level of inferior maxillary sinus, the styloid process is seen anterolateral to the CS. The superficial layer of deep cervical fascia defines the MS and PS. The more anterior buccal space (BS) has no fascial definition.* **(Bottom)** *At the level of the maxillary ridge, the area of the PMS is outlined between the paired, fat-filled PPSs. Posterior to the PMS are the tightly packed retropharyngeal and perivertebral spaces.*

AXIAL CECT OF SUPRAHYOID NECK

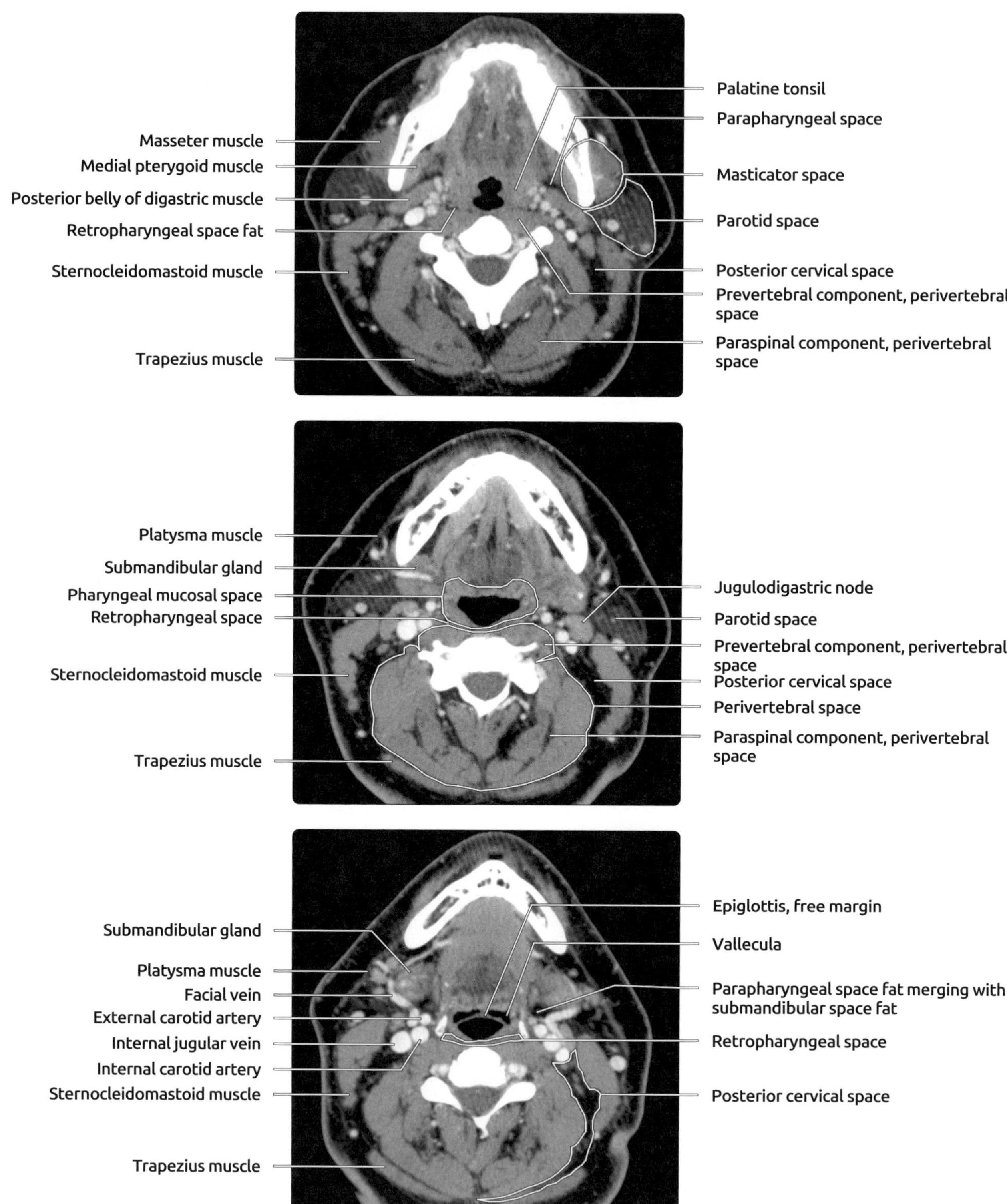

(Top) *In this image at the level of the mandibular body, the posterior belly of the digastric muscle can be seen dividing the parotid tail from the CS. The direction of displacement of this muscle can define whether a lesion is in the PS (posteromedial displacement) or in the CS (anterolateral displacement).* **(Middle)** *In this image through the low oropharynx, the PMS has been outlined anterior to the perivertebral space. The space between them is the retropharyngeal space that includes an anterior true retropharyngeal space in front of alar fascia and a posterior danger space behind it. The very thin alar fascia that separates these compartments of the retropharyngeal space is not usually visualized and may be identified in patients with retropharyngeal space edema in situations like postradiation therapy.* **(Bottom)** *At the level of the free margin of the epiglottis, the retropharyngeal space is outlined behind the PMS. The posterior cervical space contains fat, accessory cranial nerve (CNXI), and the spinal accessory nodal chain (level V nodes). Note that the inferior aspect of PPS fat merges with that of posterosuperior SMS.*

AXIAL CECT OF INFRAHYOID NECK

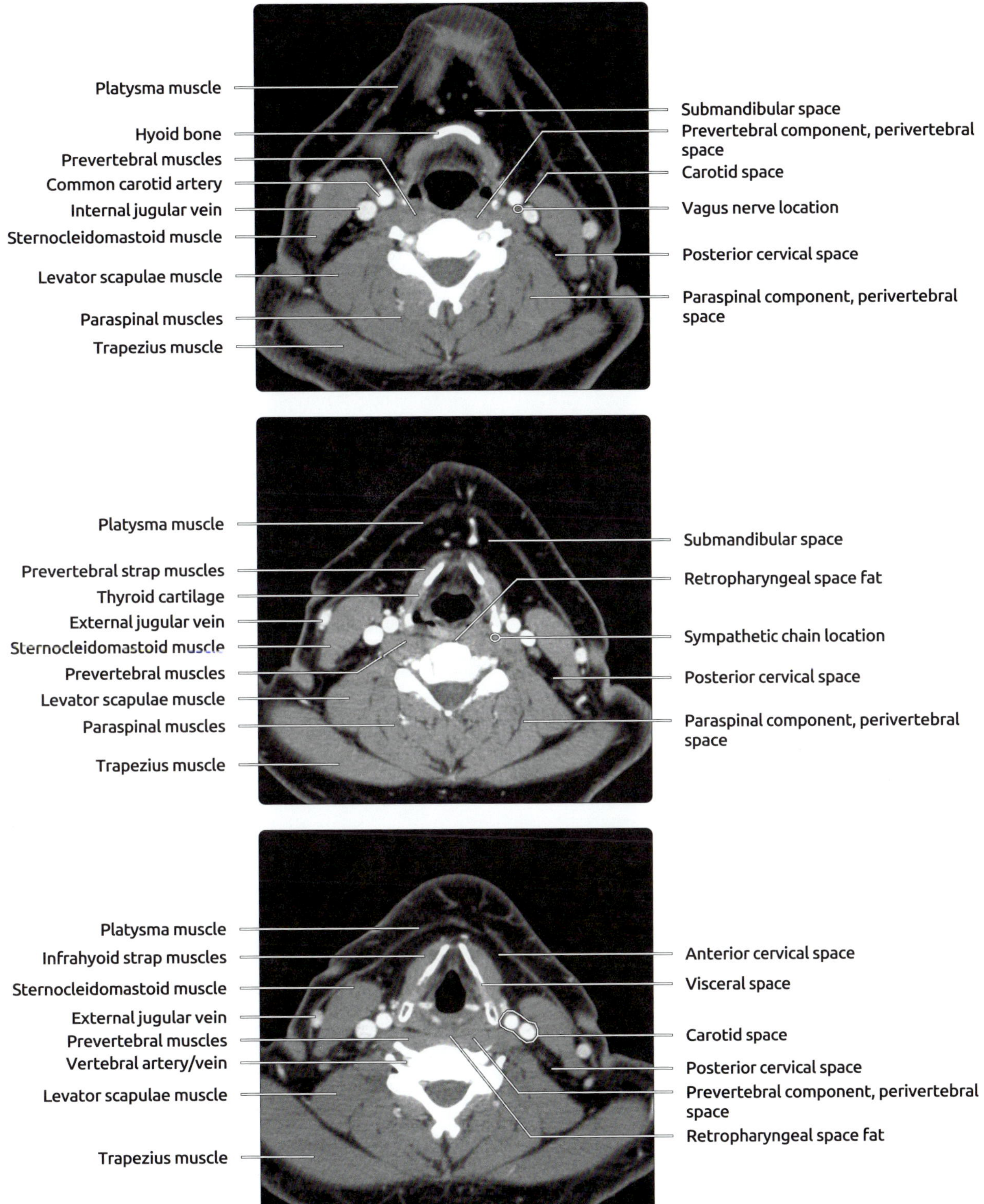

(Top) *Axial CECT at the level of the hyoid bone shows that the CS now contains the common carotid artery, internal jugular vein, and vagus nerve only. The large, fat-filled SMS is seen anteriorly.* **(Middle)** *In this image at the level of the supraglottis of the larynx, the large sternocleidomastoid and trapezius muscles are seen in the lateral neck. Both muscles are innervated by the accessory cranial nerve.* **(Bottom)** *In this image at the level of the glottis of the larynx, the visceral space contains the hypopharynx, larynx, and infrahyoid strap muscles. Just behind the hypopharynx is the retropharyngeal space, the SMS that contains only fat in the infrahyoid neck. Notice that the inferior extension of the SMS into the infrahyoid neck is the anterior cervical space (ACS).*

AXIAL CECT OF INFRAHYOID NECK

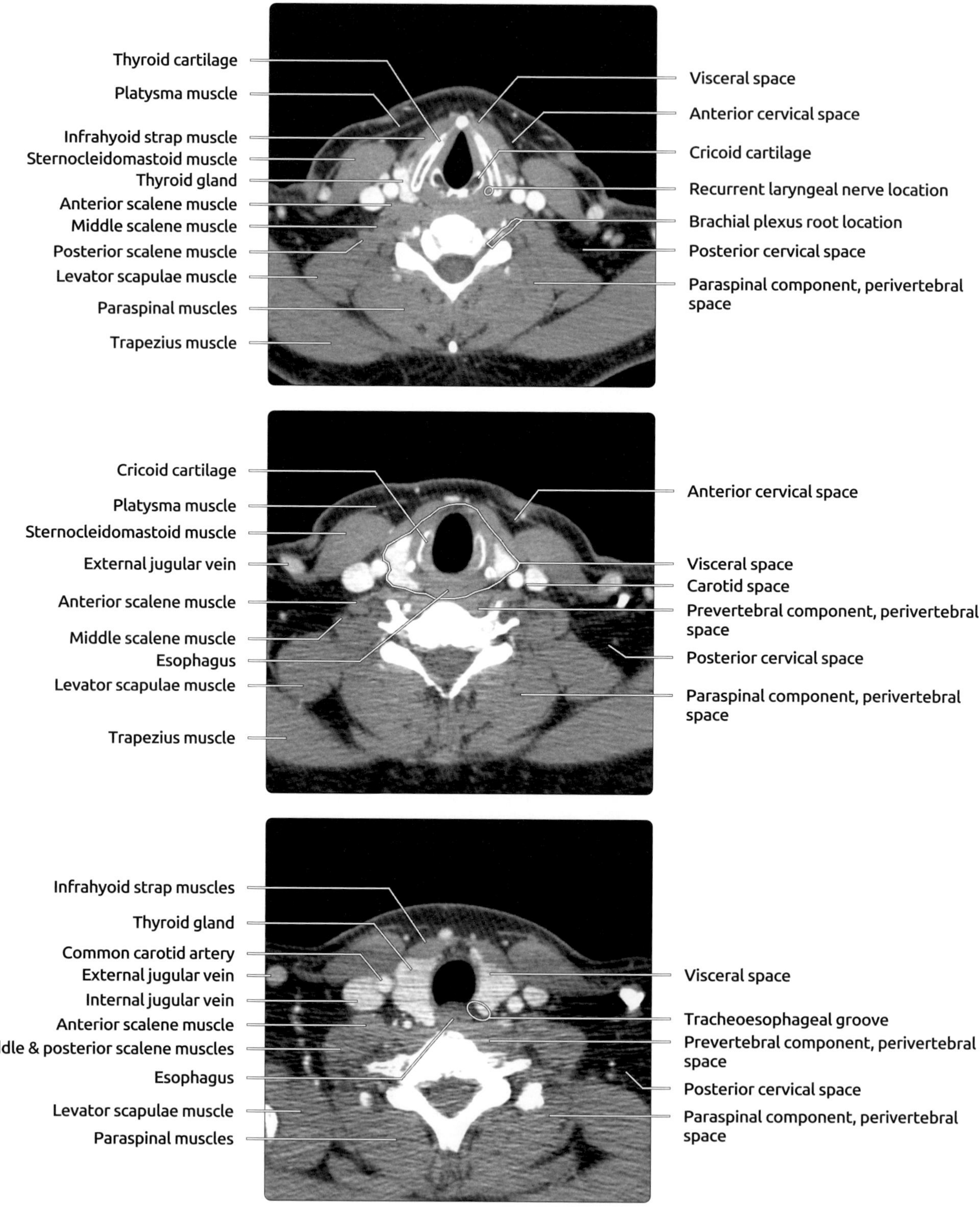

(Top) *At the cricoid cartilage level, the visceral space now contains the upper thyroid gland. The low-density brachial plexus root projects anterolaterally from the neural foramen to pass between the anterior and middle scalene muscles in the prevertebral component of perivertebral space.* **(Middle)** *In this image, the visceral space contains the high-density thyroid gland, the upper cervical esophagus, and the cricoid cartilage. The ML-DCF circumscribes the visceral space.* **(Bottom)** *At the level of the upper cervical trachea, the visceral space is filled with the thyroid gland, parathyroid glands (not visible), trachea, and cervical esophagus. The area of tracheoesophageal groove contains the recurrent laryngeal nerve and the paratracheal nodal chain. It is via the paratracheal nodal chain that differentiated thyroid carcinoma accesses the mediastinum.*

AXIAL CECT OF CERVICOTHORACIC JUNCTION

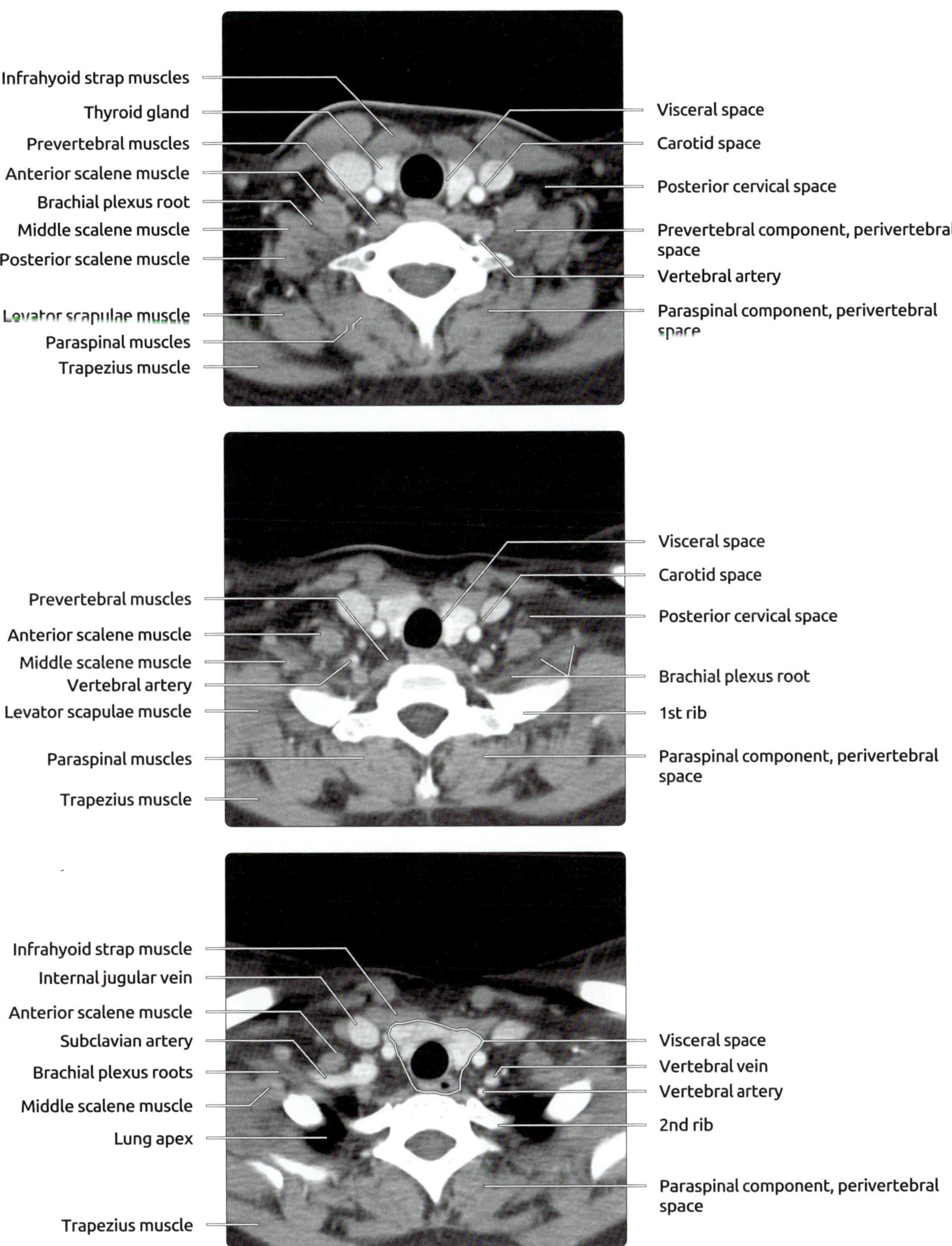

(Top) *First of 3 axial CECT images through the lower cervical neck and cervicothoracic junction presented from superior to inferior shows the anterior, middle, and posterior scalene muscles in the prevertebral component of the perivertebral space. Notice the brachial plexus roots between the anterior and middle scalene muscles.* **(Middle)** *At the level of the 1st thoracic vertebral body and 1st rib, the anterior scalene is clearly visible anterior to the roots of the brachial plexus. The visceral space contains the thyroid gland, parathyroid glands (not visible on CT), the cervical esophagus, and trachea.* **(Bottom)** *In this image at the level of the lung apices, the visceral space is outlined by the ML-DCF. The right subclavian artery passes between the anterior and middle scalene muscles along with the brachial plexus roots.*

AXIAL T1 MR

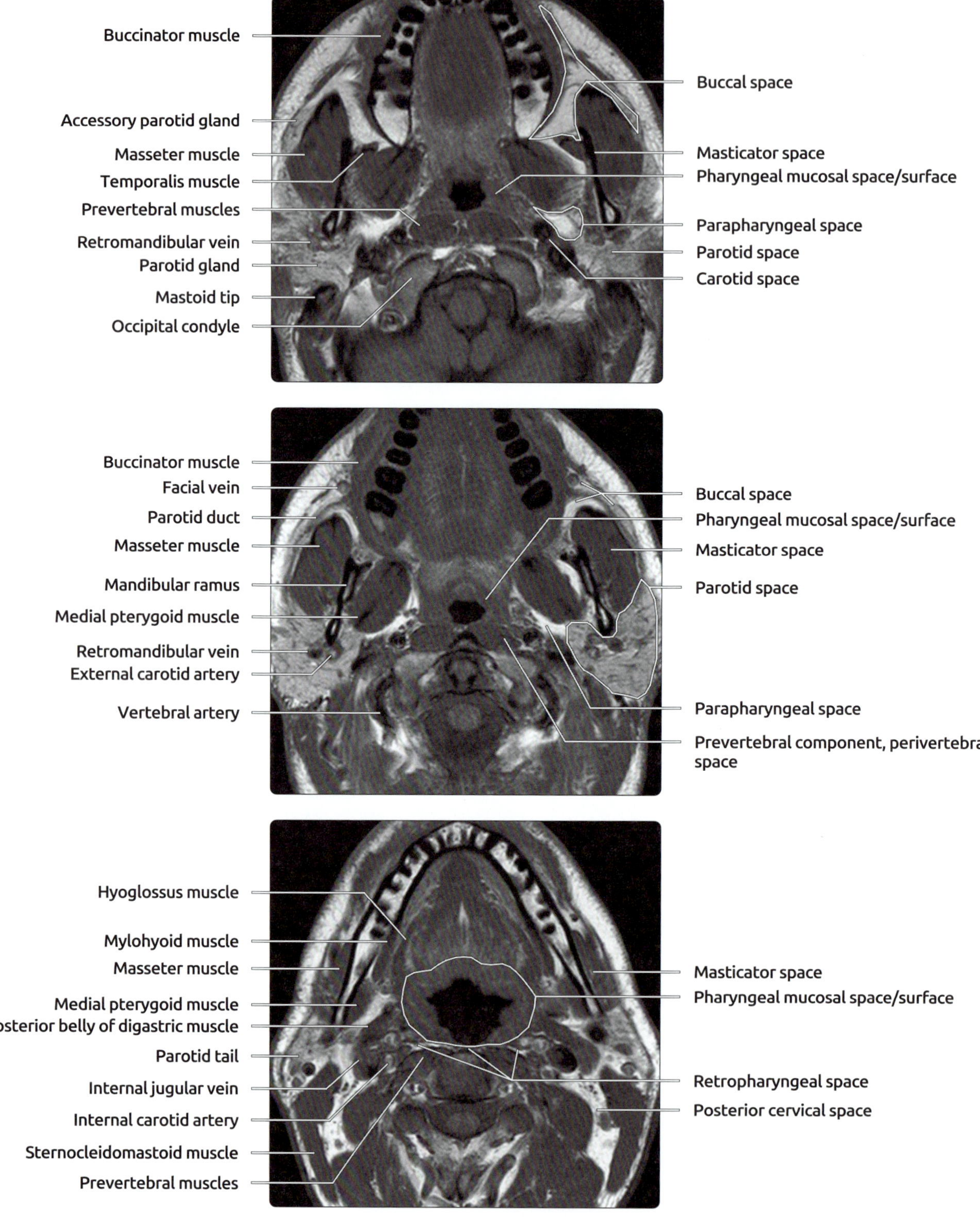

(Top) *First of 6 axial T1 MR images of the suprahyoid and infrahyoid neck from superior to inferior is shown. In this image, the BS is outlined on the left. The BS is bounded medially by the buccinator muscle, posteriorly by MS, laterally by PS, and anteriorly by superficial muscles of facial expression and investing fascia. Inferiorly, it blends imperceptibly with the SMS. The BS does not have complete fascial coverings separating it from adjacent spaces, allowing disease to spread easily. The BS contents are fat, minor salivary glands, parotid duct, lymph nodes, facial veins, facial, angular, and buccal arteries, and buccal branches of facial and mandibular nerves. The PPS is seen as a fat-filled region bordered by the PMS, MS, PS, and CS.* **(Middle)** *In this image at the mandibular teeth level, the PS is seen posterior to the MS. Both are surrounded by the SL-DCF.* **(Bottom)** *In this image, the PMS is made up of the anterior lingual and lateral palatine tonsils. The fat stripe behind the PMS is the retropharyngeal space; behind that is the prevertebral component of the perivertebral space. The posterior belly of digastric muscle separates the CS from the PS.*

AXIAL T1 MR

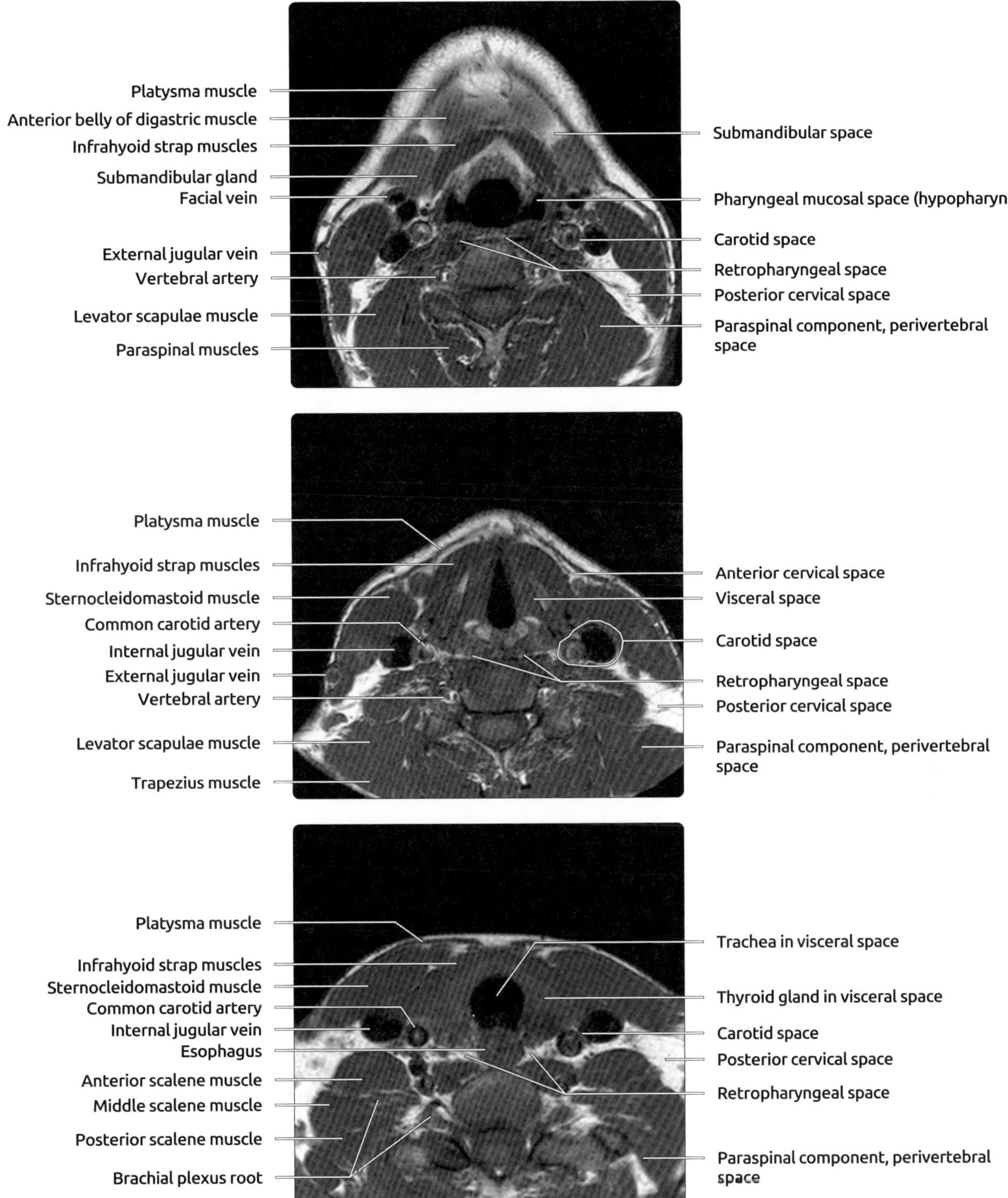

(Top) *In this image, the visceral space of the infrahyoid neck is visible. The ML-DCF circumscribes the visceral space. The visceral space at this level contains the infrahyoid strap muscles, pyriform sinuses, and epiglottis.* **(Middle)** *At the level of true vocal cords, both the anterior and posterior cervical spaces are seen. Note the anterior cervical space is a direct extension of the SMS into the infrahyoid neck. The CS is surrounded by the carotid sheath. The common carotid artery, internal jugular vein, and vagus nerve are found in the infrahyoid CS.* **(Bottom)** *At the level of the upper trachea, the thyroid gland is now the largest structure in the visceral space. The parathyroid glands, cervical trachea and esophagus, paratracheal nodes, and recurrent laryngeal nerve are all in the visceral space.*

AXIAL T2 MR

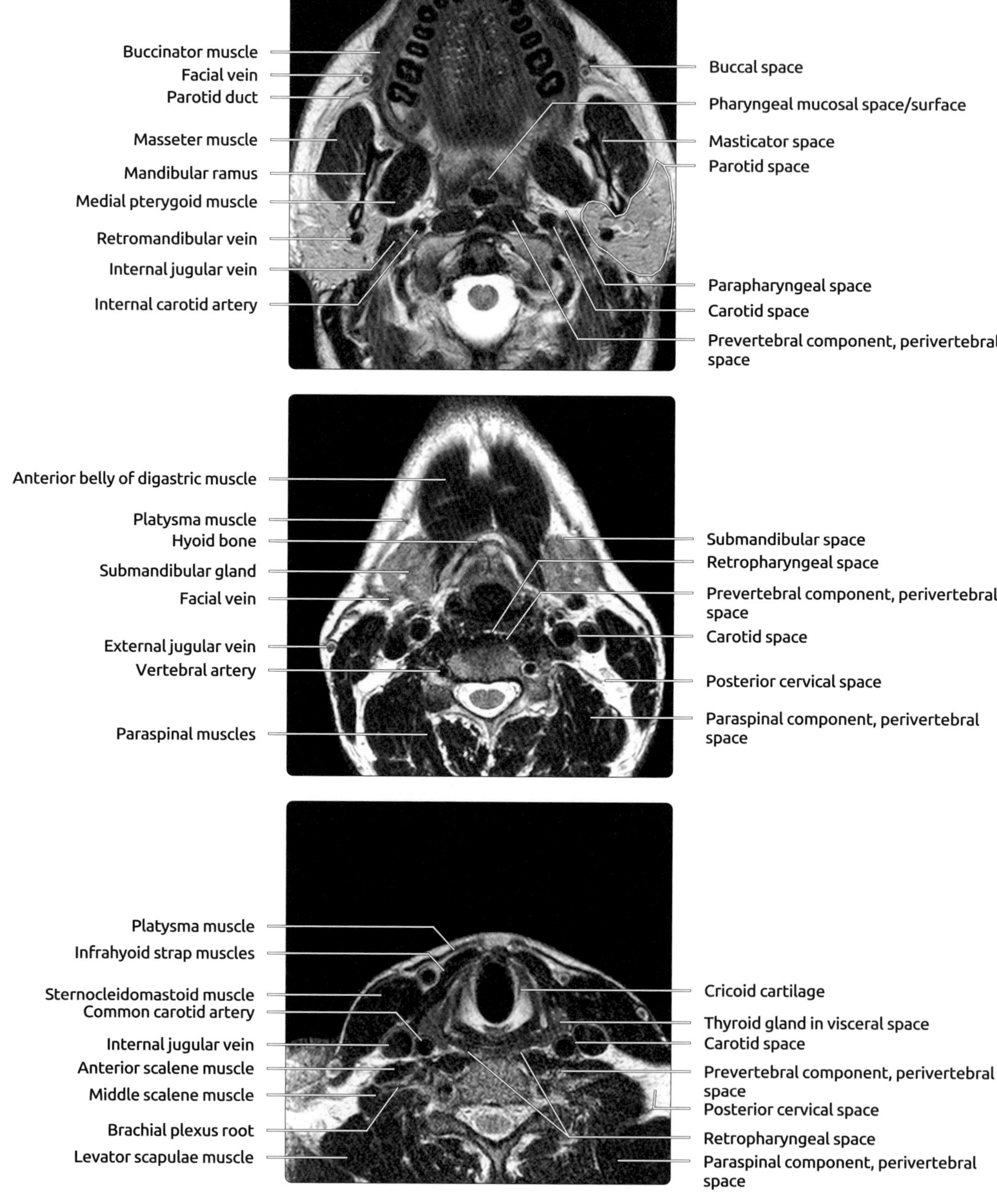

(Top) *First of 3 axial T2 MR images of the neck at the level of the maxillary alveolar ridge shows the 4 key spaces surrounding the fat-filled PPS. These important 4 spaces are the PMS, MS, PS, and CS. The PS and MS are circumscribed by a SL-DCF.* **(Middle)** *In this image at the level of hyoid bone, the large submandibular glands are visible in the SMS deep to the platysma muscle.* **(Bottom)** *At the level of the cricoid cartilage, the prevertebral and paraspinal components of the perivertebral space can be seen. The brachial plexus roots exit the prevertebral component between the anterior and middle scalene muscles to enter the posterior CS fat on their way to the axilla.*

CORONAL T1 MR

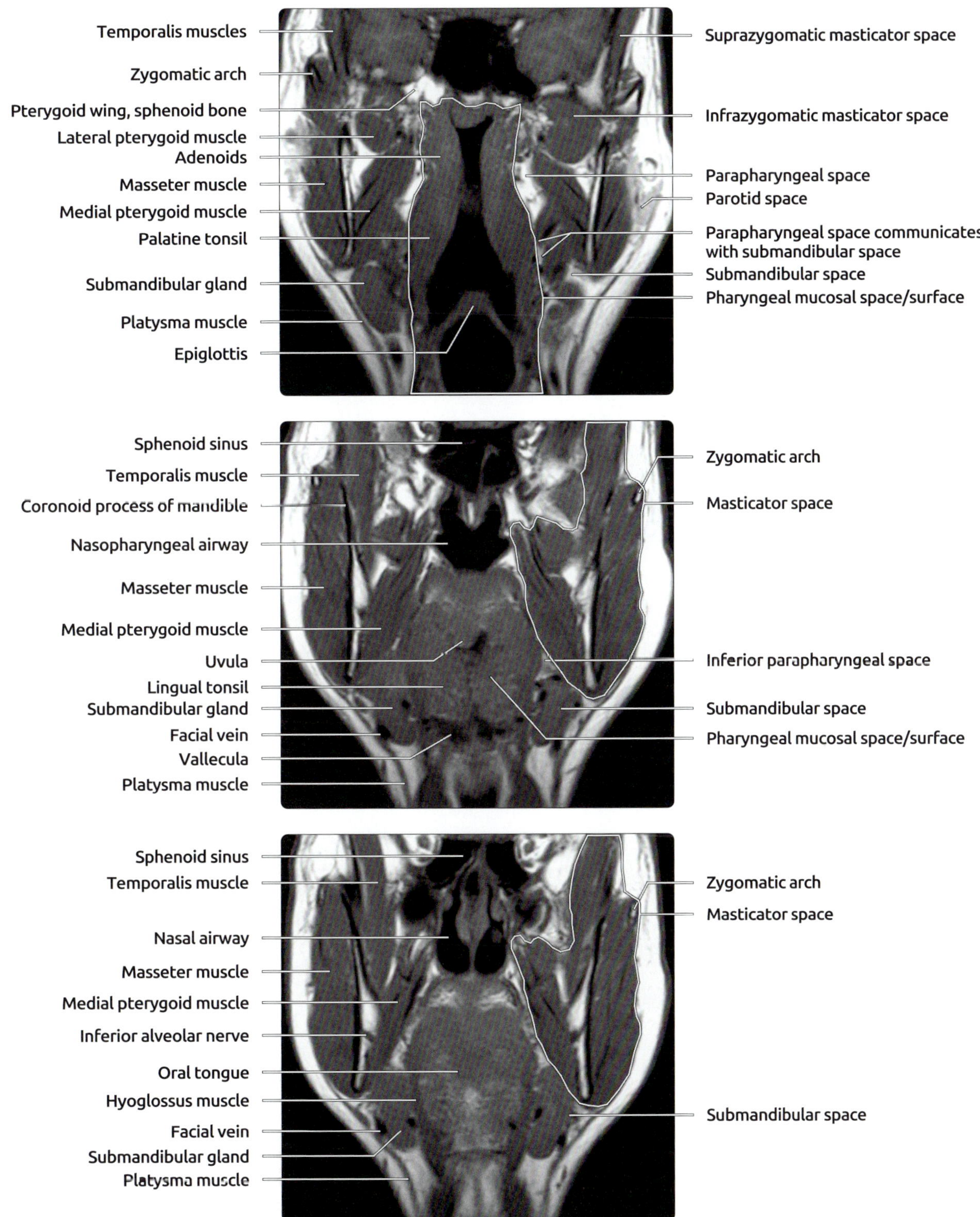

(Top) *First of 3 coronal T1 MR images presented from posterior to anterior shows the PMS extending from the nasopharynx to hypopharynx. It is from the PMS that the most common malignancies of the head and neck arise: Squamous cell carcinoma from the mucosa, non-Hodgkin lymphoma (NHL) from the tonsils, and minor salivary gland malignancy from the minor salivary glands.* **(Middle)** *In this image, the MS has been outlined. Remember this space has a suprazygomatic and an infrazygomatic component. Since there is no "horizontal fascia" between the zygomatic arch, diseases may spread within the MS between the suprazygomatic and infrazygomatic components.* **(Bottom)** *In this image through the posterior nose, 3 of the major muscles of mastication are visible: The masseter, medial pterygoid, and temporalis muscles.*

TRANSVERSE ULTRASOUND

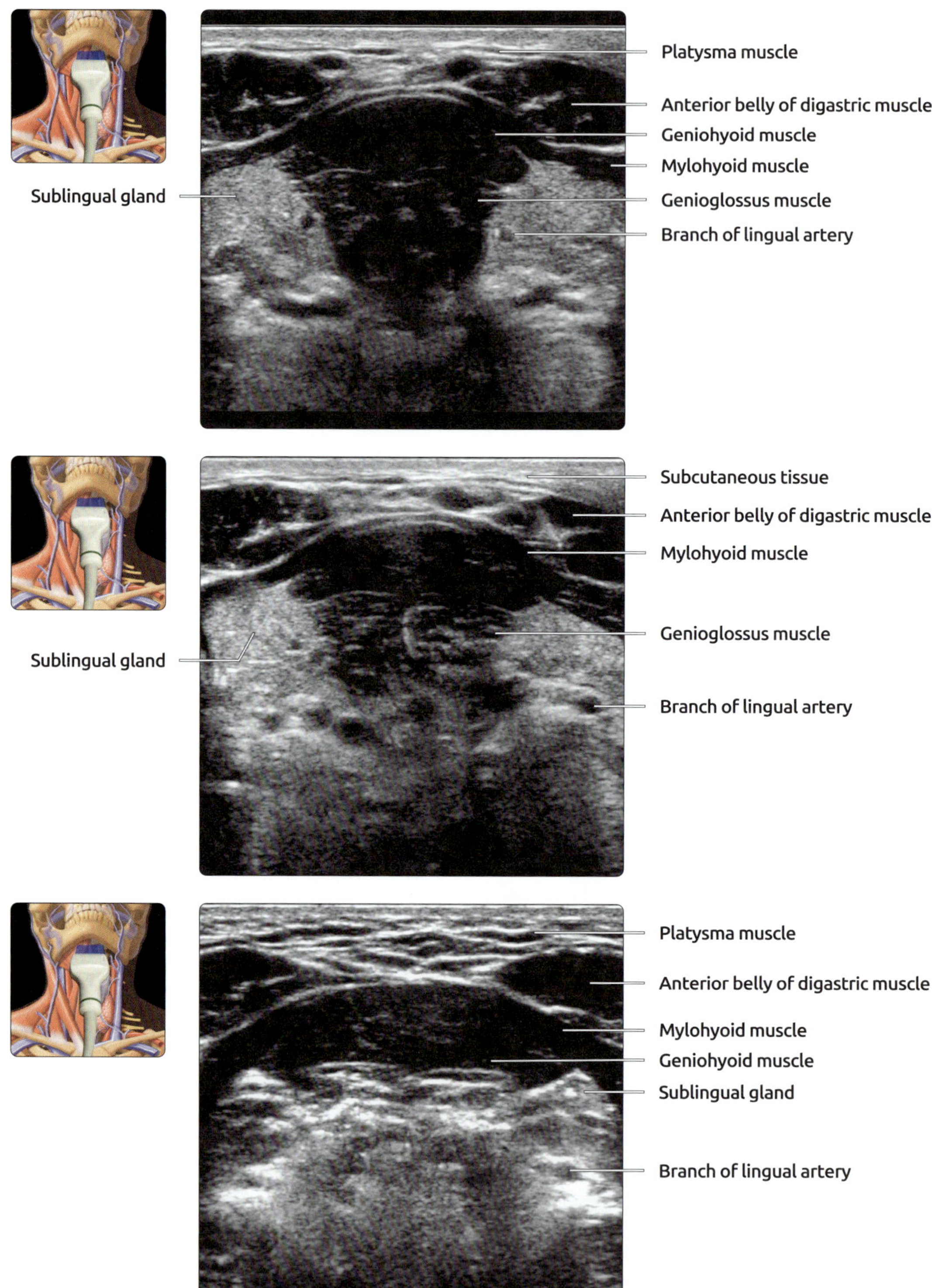

(Top) *Anterior transverse grayscale ultrasound of the submental and sublingual region is shown. The mylohyoid muscle is the landmark for division of the sublingual space (deep to the mylohyoid plane) and SMS (superficial to the muscle plane). The sublingual gland appears as a homogeneous, hyperechoic structure lateral to the geniohyoid/genioglossus muscle. Branches of the lingual artery can be easily picked up on a transverse plane. The submandibular duct sits alongside the lingual vessels, and a submandibular calculus may impact at this site.* **(Middle)** *Slightly more posterior transverse grayscale ultrasound allows the clear depiction of extrinsic muscles of the tongue at the root.* **(Bottom)** *Transverse grayscale ultrasound shows the submental region in a more posterior location.*

POWER DOPPLER ULTRASOUND AND TRANSVERSE ULTRASOUNDS

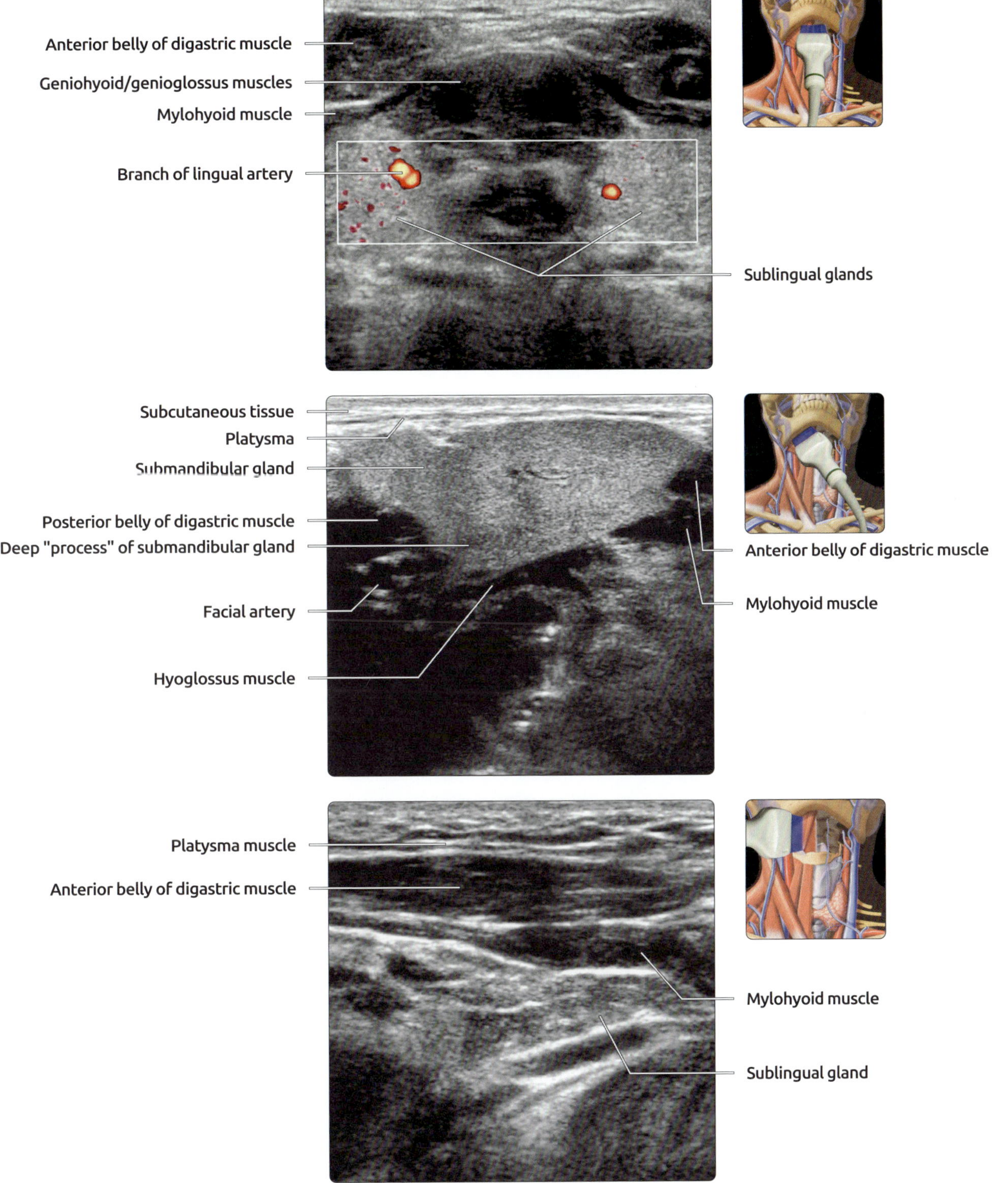

(Top) *Power Doppler ultrasound of the submental region shows the presence of color flow within the branches of the lingual artery. The use of Doppler examination aids in differentiation from the dilated submandibular duct.* **(Middle)** *Transverse grayscale ultrasound of the submandibular region taken more laterally shows the submandibular gland. The submandibular gland is the key structure in this region and is easily recognized by its homogeneous echotexture. The gland sits astride the mylohyoid and posterior belly of the digastric muscles.* **(Bottom)** *Parasagittal longitudinal grayscale ultrasound shows the submental region. The sublingual gland is visualized within the sublingual space (deep to the mylohyoid muscle) underneath the anterior belly of the digastric and mylohyoid muscles.*

TRANSVERSE ULTRASOUND

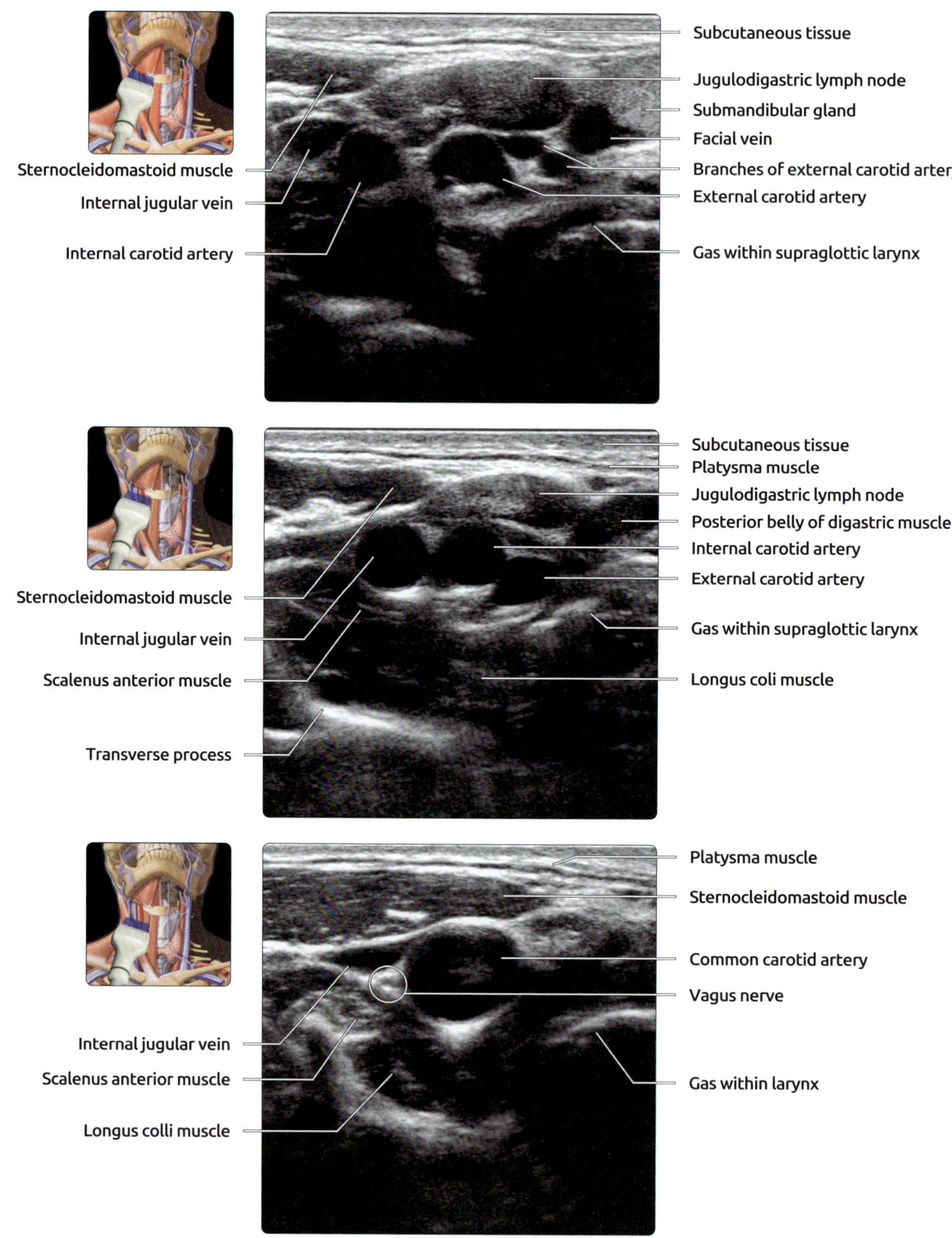

(Top) *First image in a series of consecutive transverse grayscale ultrasound images of the upper cervical level clearly identifies key vascular landmarks, including the internal and external carotid arteries and the internal jugular vein. The uppermost and largest deep cervical lymph node (i.e., the jugulodigastric lymph node) is consistently seen in the upper cervical level superficial to the carotid artery. It is usually elliptical, hypoechoic, and demonstrates echogenic hilum.* **(Middle)** *Second image shows the carotid bifurcation in the transverse plane. The external carotid artery is usually more medial and smaller than the internal carotid artery.* **(Bottom)** *Third image below the level of carotid bifurcation clearly shows the common carotid artery, internal jugular vein, and vagus nerve to be major structures within the carotid sheath.*

TRANSVERSE ULTRASOUND

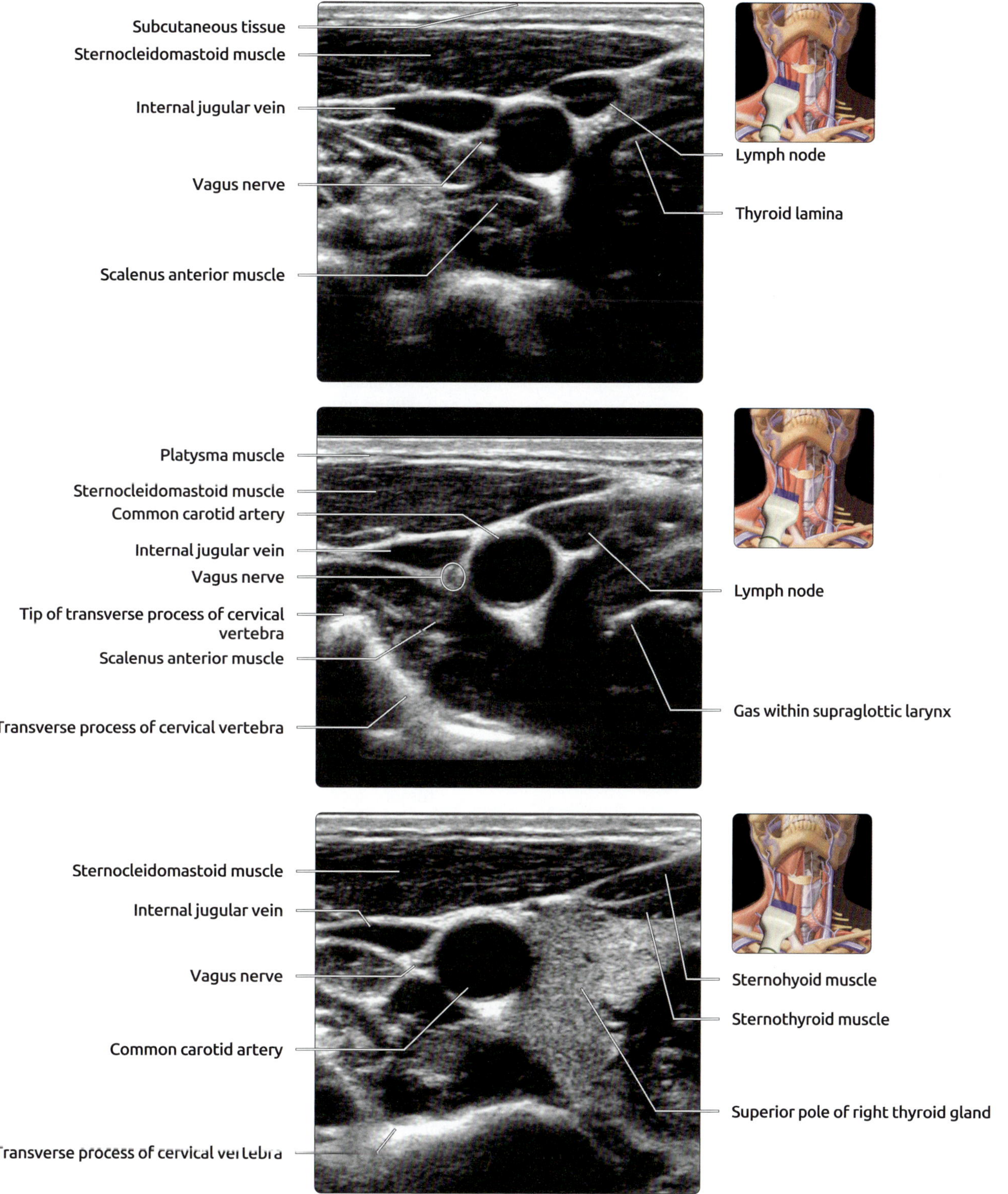

(Top) *First image in a series of consecutive transverse grayscale ultrasound images shows the midcervical level. Deep cervical lymph nodes are commonly found along and anterior to the major vessels of the carotid sheath. These are commonly hypoechoic and elliptical with a normal echogenic hilum and hilar vascularity.* **(Middle)** *Second ultrasound shows the midcervical level in the transverse plane. At this level, the common carotid artery, internal jugular vein, and vagus nerve are the main structures within the carotid sheath. The vagus nerve is usually located between the common carotid artery and the internal jugular vein and appears as a small, round, hypoechoic nodule with a central echogenic dot.* **(Bottom)** *Third ultrasound shows the midcervical level. The cricoid cartilage may not be routinely seen on ultrasound, but visualization of the superior pole of the thyroid gland approximately coincides with this level.*

TERMINOLOGY

Abbreviations

- Parapharyngeal space (PPS)

Synonyms

- Some authors define PPS more broadly, separating it into prestyloid and poststyloid components
- In this text, **PPS** is preferred over prestyloid PPS and **carotid space** (CS) over poststyloid PPS

Definitions

- **PPS**: Central, fat-filled space in lateral suprahyoid neck (SHN) with important adjacent spaces
  - Surrounding important spaces include pharyngeal mucosal space (PMS), masticator space (MS), parotid space (PS), and CS

IMAGING ANATOMY

Overview

- PPS has limited contents with few lesions originating in PPS
  - Diseases of PPS usually arise in adjacent spaces (PMS, MS, PS, CS), extending secondarily into PPS
- Conspicuity of PPS on CT and MR and its direction of displacement by lesions of surrounding spaces makes it important
  - **PPS displacement pattern helps define actual space of origin**
    - PMS lesion pushes PPS laterally
    - MS lesion pushes PPS posteriorly
    - PS lesion pushes PPS medially
    - CS lesion pushes PPS anteriorly
    - Lateral retropharyngeal space mass (nodal) pushes PPS anterolaterally
  - Combining center of mass lesion with displacement direction of PPS yields strong impression of "space of origin" of SHN mass lesion

Extent

- Crescent-shaped, fat-filled space in craniocaudal dimension extends from skull base above to superior cornu of hyoid bone inferiorly

Anatomy Relationships

- As fatty tube separating different SHN spaces, PPS functions as "elevator shaft" for spread of infection and tumor from these adjacent spaces between skull base to hyoid bone
- Inferiorly, there is **no fascia** separating inferior PPS from submandibular space (SMS) with open communication between inferior PPS and posterior SMS
- Superiorly, PPS interacts with skull base in bland triangular area on inferior surface of petrous apex
  - **No exiting skull base foramina** are found in this area
- Surrounding spaces include
  - PMS medially
  - MS anterolaterally
  - PS laterally
  - CS posteriorly
  - Retropharyngeal posteromedially

Internal Contents

- PPS has **no** mucosa, muscle, bone, nodes, or major salivary gland tissue within its boundaries
  - Very few pathologies primarily begin in PPS
- **Critical PPS contents**
  - **Fat**: Key constituent making PPS easily identifiable even with larger SHN mass lesions
  - Minor salivary glands (ectopic, rare)
  - Internal maxillary artery
  - Ascending pharyngeal artery
  - Pterygoid venous plexus (small portion, mostly MS)
  - Small branches of mandibular division of trigeminal nerve

Fascial Margins of Parapharyngeal Space

- Fascial margins of PPS are complex; made up of different layers of deep cervical fascia
  - Medial fascial margin of PPS
    - Made up of middle layer, deep cervical fascia as it curves around lateral margin of PMS
  - Lateral fascial margin of PPS
    - Formed by medial slip of superficial layer of deep cervical fascia along deep border of MS and PS
  - Posterior fascial margin of PPS
    - Formed by deep layer of deep cervical fascia on anterolateral margin of retropharyngeal space and anterior part of carotid sheath (made up of components of all 3 layers of deep cervical fascia)

ANATOMY IMAGING ISSUES

Questions

- Because of limited normal anatomic contents of PPS, few lesions primarily arise in PPS
  - Rare lesions found in PPS include benign mixed tumor (from minor salivary gland rests in PPS), nerve sheath tumors, lipomatous tumors, vascular lesions, atypical 2nd branchial cleft cyst, and, very rarely, ectopic thyroid
  - To call primary PPS lesion, it must be completely surrounded by PPS fat
  - In most cases where lesion thought to be primary to PPS, careful observation will find connection to surrounding space (usually PS)
- **PPS fat displacement: Key imaging relationship** used in evaluation of SHN lesions

Imaging Recommendations

- MR better delineates skull base, meningeal, and perineural lesions
  - T1 C+ FS MR may make PPS fat difficult to see

Imaging Pitfalls

- Remember, most PPS lesions arise from adjacent SHN spaces

CLINICAL IMPLICATIONS

Clinical Importance

- Since PPS empties inferiorly into SMS, PPS lesion may present as "angle of mandible" mass
- However, most lesions within PPS cannot be evaluated by physical examination

GRAPHICS

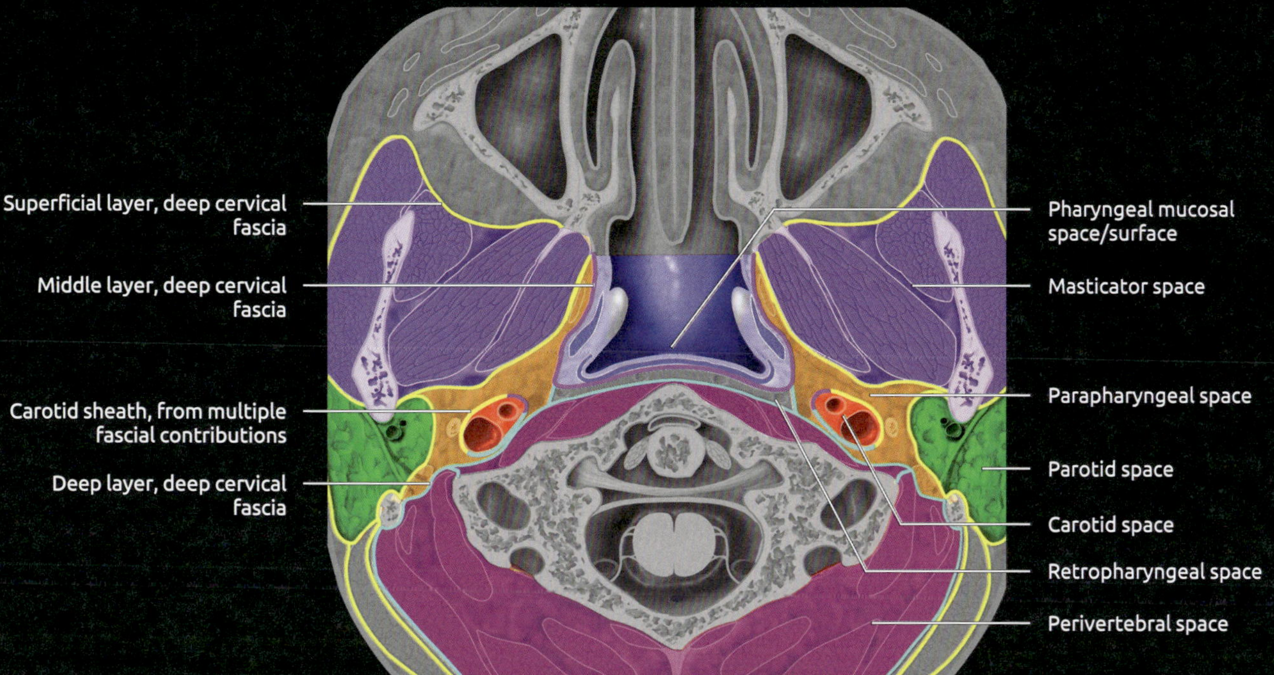

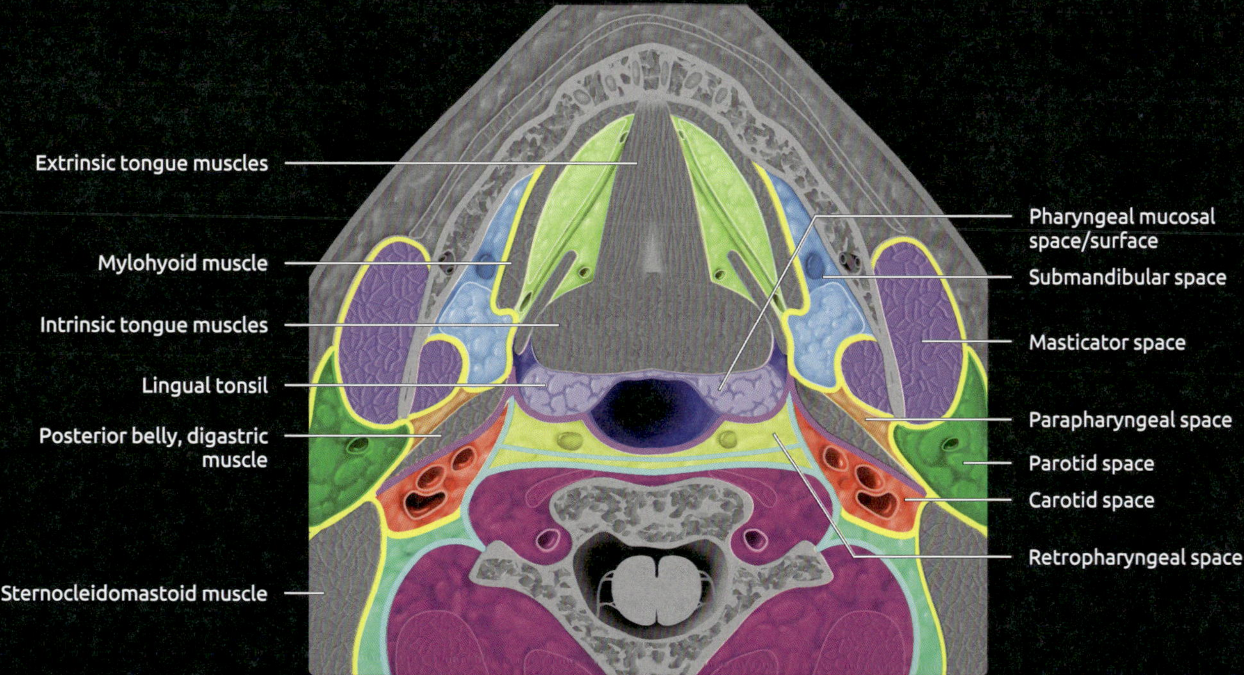

(Top) *Axial graphic of the normal parapharyngeal space at the level of the nasopharynx demonstrates the complex fascial margins and the fat-only contents. The surrounding pharyngeal mucosal, masticator, parotid, and carotid spaces, when affected by mass lesions, push into the parapharyngeal space. The resulting displacement pattern of the parapharyngeal space may be helpful in defining the space of origin of a mass in the suprahyoid neck.* **(Bottom)** *Axial graphic at the level of the low oropharynx shows the slip of parapharyngeal space fat is just anterolateral to the posterior belly of the digastric muscle. Inferior to this level, the parapharyngeal space communicates anteriorly with the submandibular space. Yellow lines represent the superficial layer, pink lines the middle layer, and aquamarine lines the deep layer of the deep cervical fascia.*

GRAPHICS

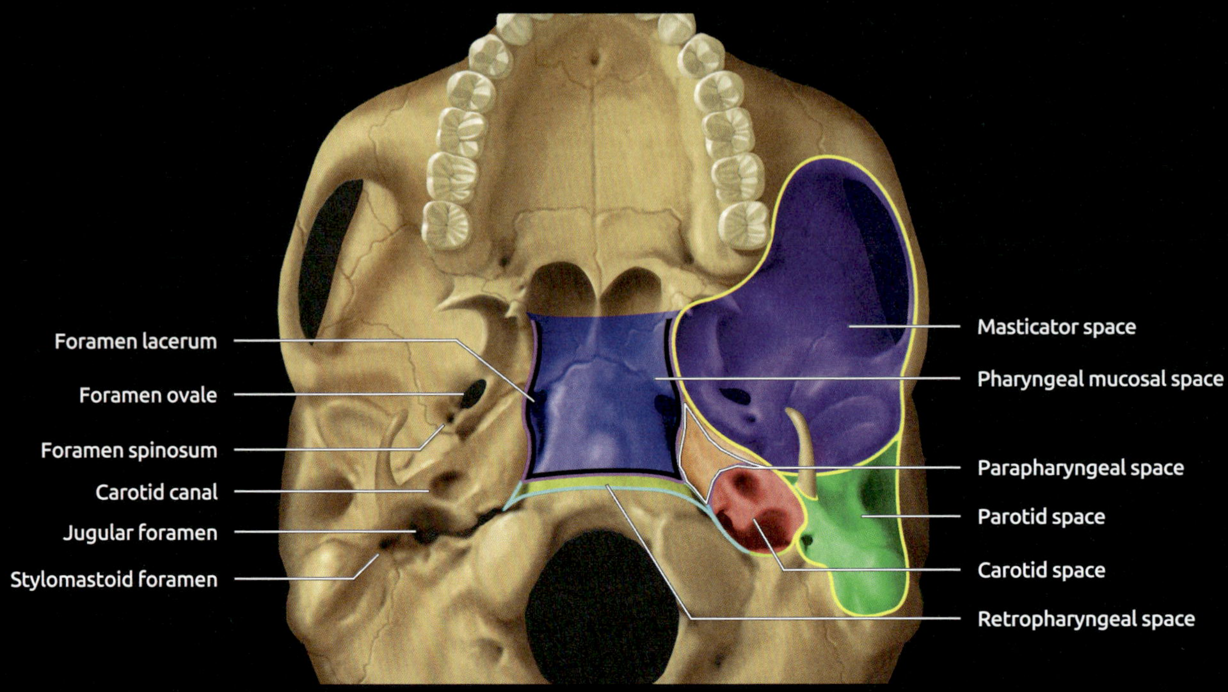

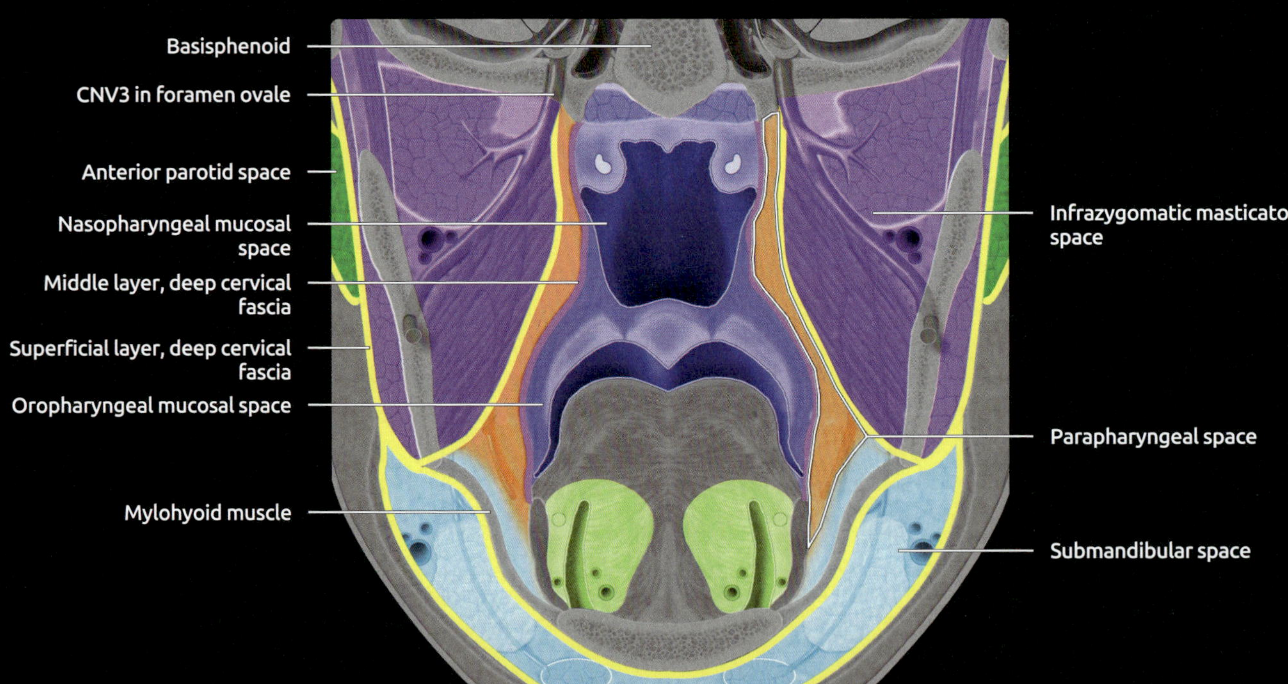

(Top) *Axial graphic shows the suprahyoid neck spaces interacting with the skull base, highlighting the parapharyngeal space. Notice that the parapharyngeal space abuts the inferior surface of the skull base in an area with no critical structures.* **(Bottom)** *Coronal graphic shows the suprahyoid neck spaces as they interact with the skull base superiorly and submandibular space inferiorly. The parapharyngeal space interacts with no critical structures as it abuts the skull base. Inferiorly, it "empties" into the posterior submandibular space along the posterior margin of the mylohyoid muscle. As a consequence of this anatomic arrangement, it is possible for an infection or a malignant tumor that breaks into the parapharyngeal space to present inferiorly as an "angle of mandible" mass.*

AXIAL CECT

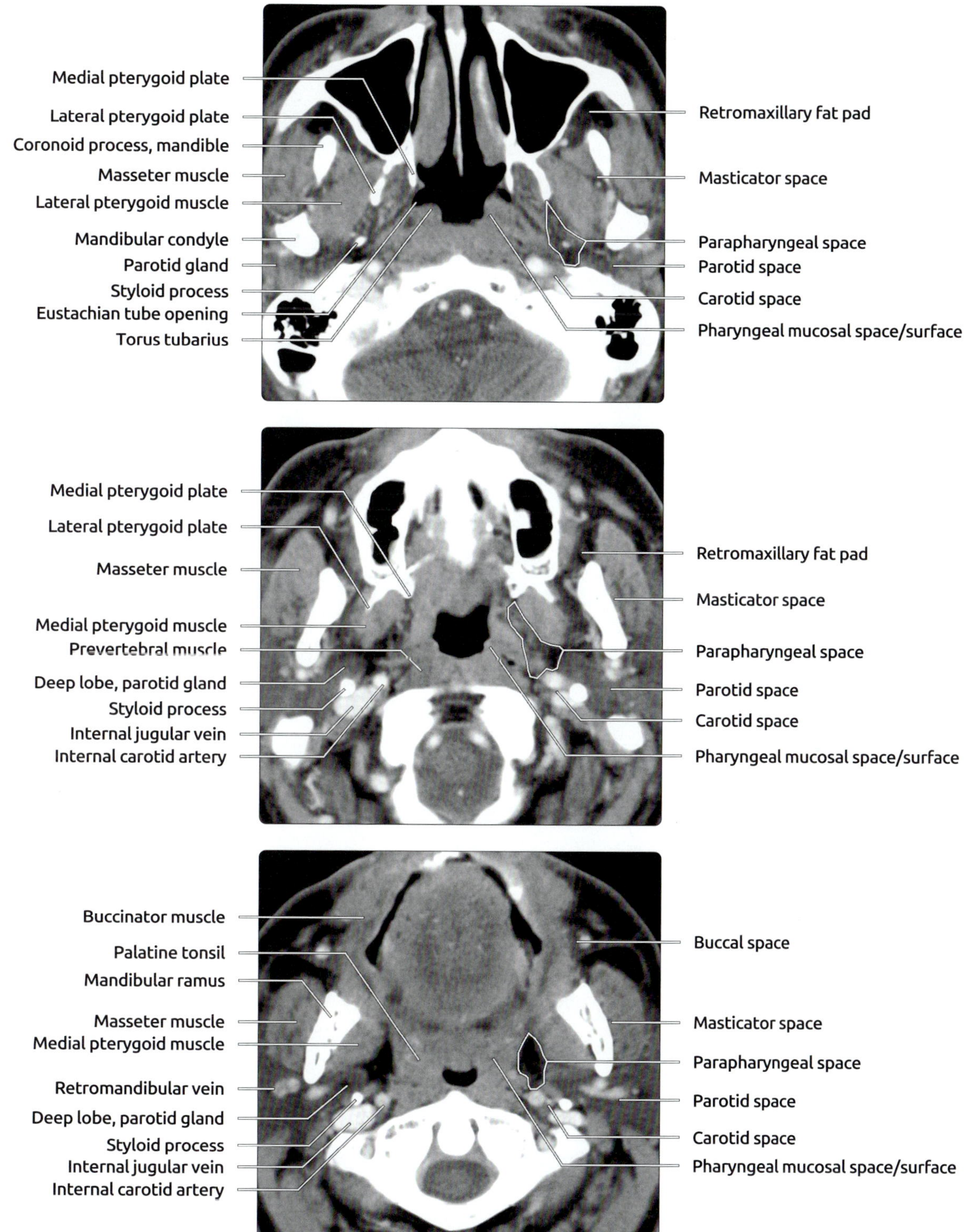

(Top) *First of 6 axial CECT images of the suprahyoid neck, presented from superior to inferior, shows the superior end of the parapharyngeal space just before it abuts the skull base. Notice the 4 major spaces surrounding the parapharyngeal space, the pharyngeal mucosal, masticator, parotid, and carotid spaces.* **(Middle)** *In this image at the level of the inferior maxillary sinus, the complex shape of the parapharyngeal space is visible. Notice the lateral margin of the parapharyngeal space is formed by the deep lobe of the parotid gland.* **(Bottom)** *In this midoropharynx image, the parapharyngeal space has the palatine tonsil on its entire medial border. It is easy to see that a squamous cell carcinoma of the palatine tonsil that is deeply invasive would immediately enter the parapharyngeal space fat, pushing it from medial to lateral.*

AXIAL CECT

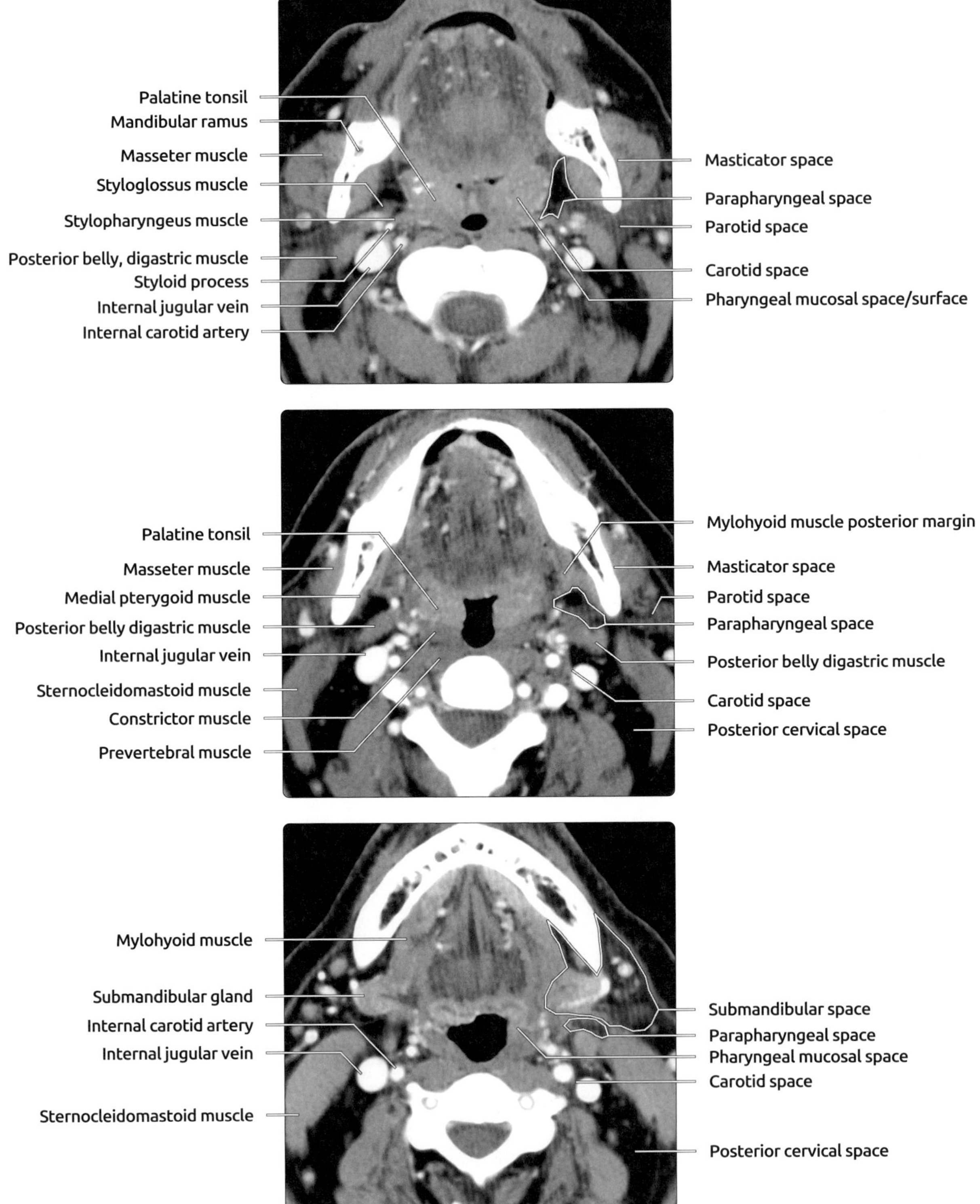

(Top) *In this image, the parapharyngeal space points anteriorly toward the submandibular space. On more inferior images, it will communicate with the posterosuperior submandibular space in this area. Notice the stylopharyngeus and styloglossus muscle on the posterior margin of the parapharyngeal space.* **(Middle)** *At the level of the mandibular body, the parapharyngeal space is seen entering the superior submandibular space just anterior to the posterior belly of the digastric muscles and just posterior to the mylohyoid muscle.* **(Bottom)** *In this image through the superior submandibular space, it is possible to see the most inferior parapharyngeal space merging with the submandibular space. Remember there is no fascia separating the inferior parapharyngeal, posterior submandibular, and sublingual spaces at the posterior margin of the mylohyoid muscle.*

AXIAL T1 MR

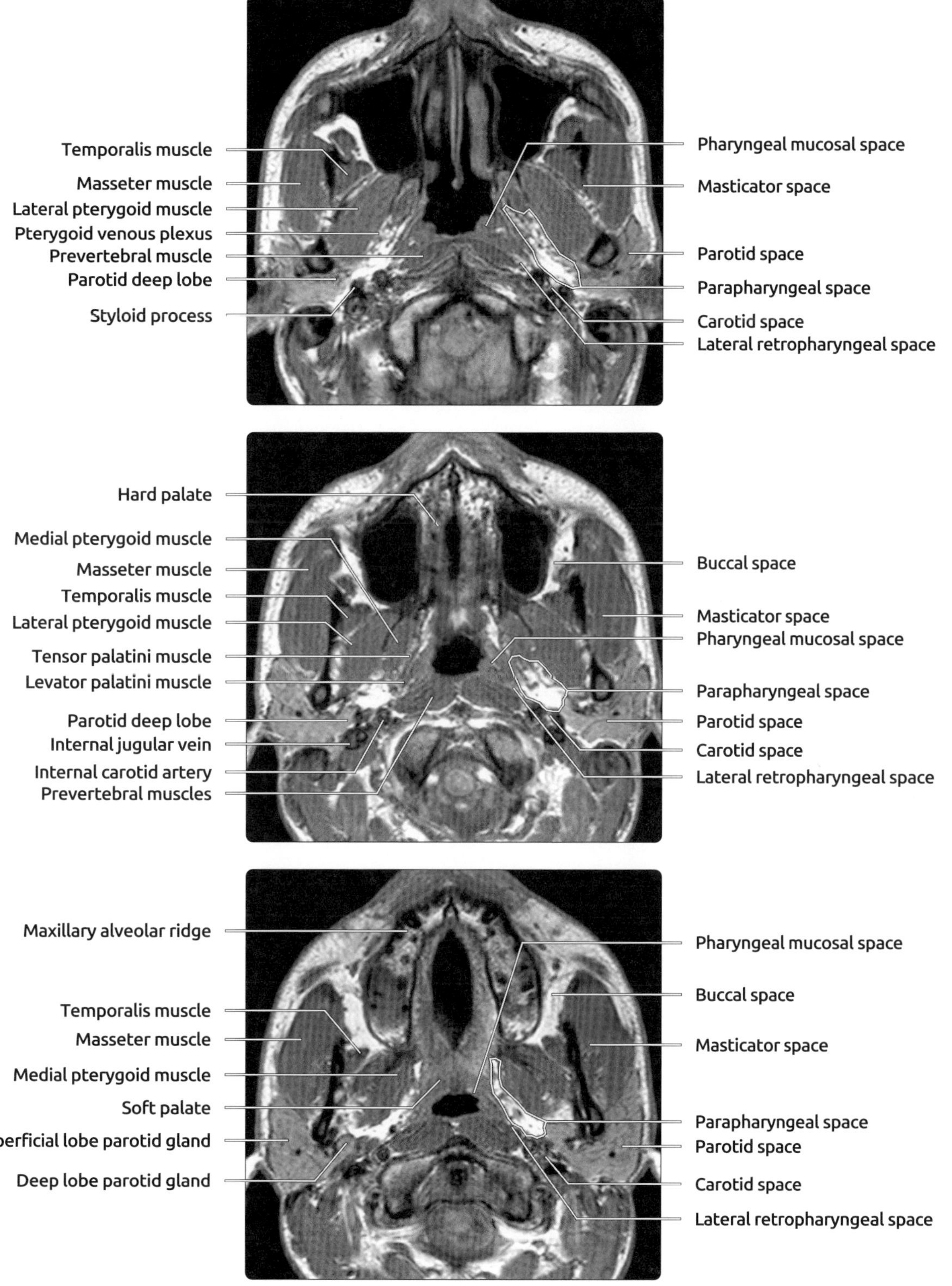

(Top) *First of 6 axial T1 MR images of the suprahyoid neck, presented from superior to inferior, shows the parapharyngeal space at the level of the nasopharynx. Here, the surrounding spaces include the pharyngeal mucosal, masticator, parotid, and carotid spaces. Notice the lateral retropharyngeal space is on the posteromedial aspect of the parapharyngeal space.* **(Middle)** *In this image at the level of the hard palate, the posterior margins of the tensor and levator palatini muscles are visible along the anteromedial margin of the parapharyngeal space on the right.* **(Bottom)** *At the level of the maxillary alveolar ridge, the parapharyngeal space on the left is surrounded in clockwise order by the medial pterygoid muscle, deep lobe of parotid, internal carotid artery, lateral pharynx, and soft palate.*

AXIAL T1 MR

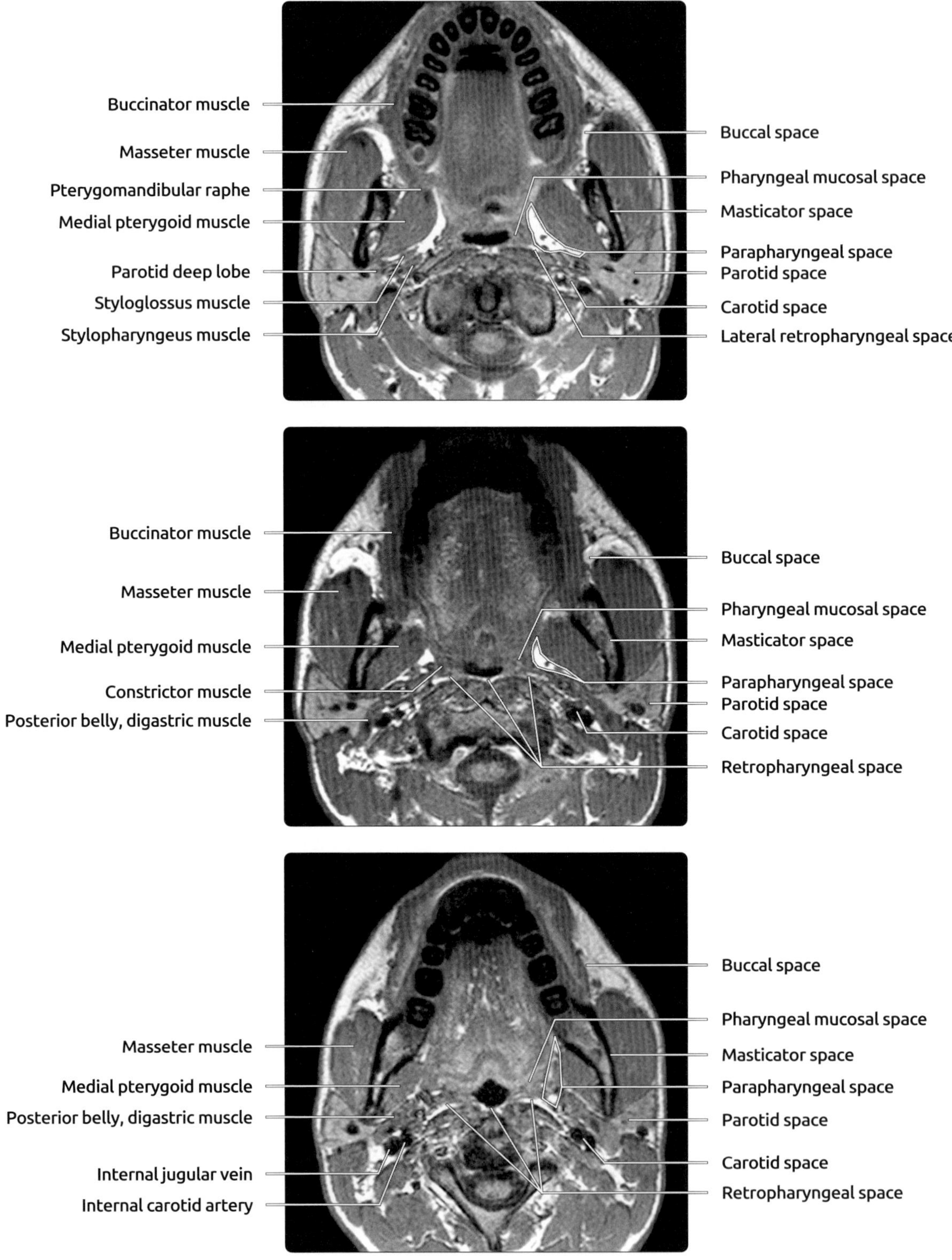

(Top) *In this image at the level of the maxillary teeth, the parapharyngeal space takes on a crescentic shape as it bends around the medial pterygoid muscle of the masticator space. The pharyngeal mucosal space makes up the medial border of the parapharyngeal space. Posteromedially, the lateral retropharyngeal space is found, while the carotid space makes up the posterolateral border of the parapharyngeal space. The deep lobe of the parotid gland makes up the lateral margin of the parapharyngeal space.* **(Middle)** *In this image at the level of the midoropharynx, the parapharyngeal space becomes smaller along its inferior margin.* **(Bottom)** *In this image at the level of the mandibular teeth, the parapharyngeal space is visible "pointing" anteriorly where it joins the posterosuperior margin of the submandibular space. Parapharyngeal abscess and tumor may access the submandibular space via this route.*

CORONAL T1 MR

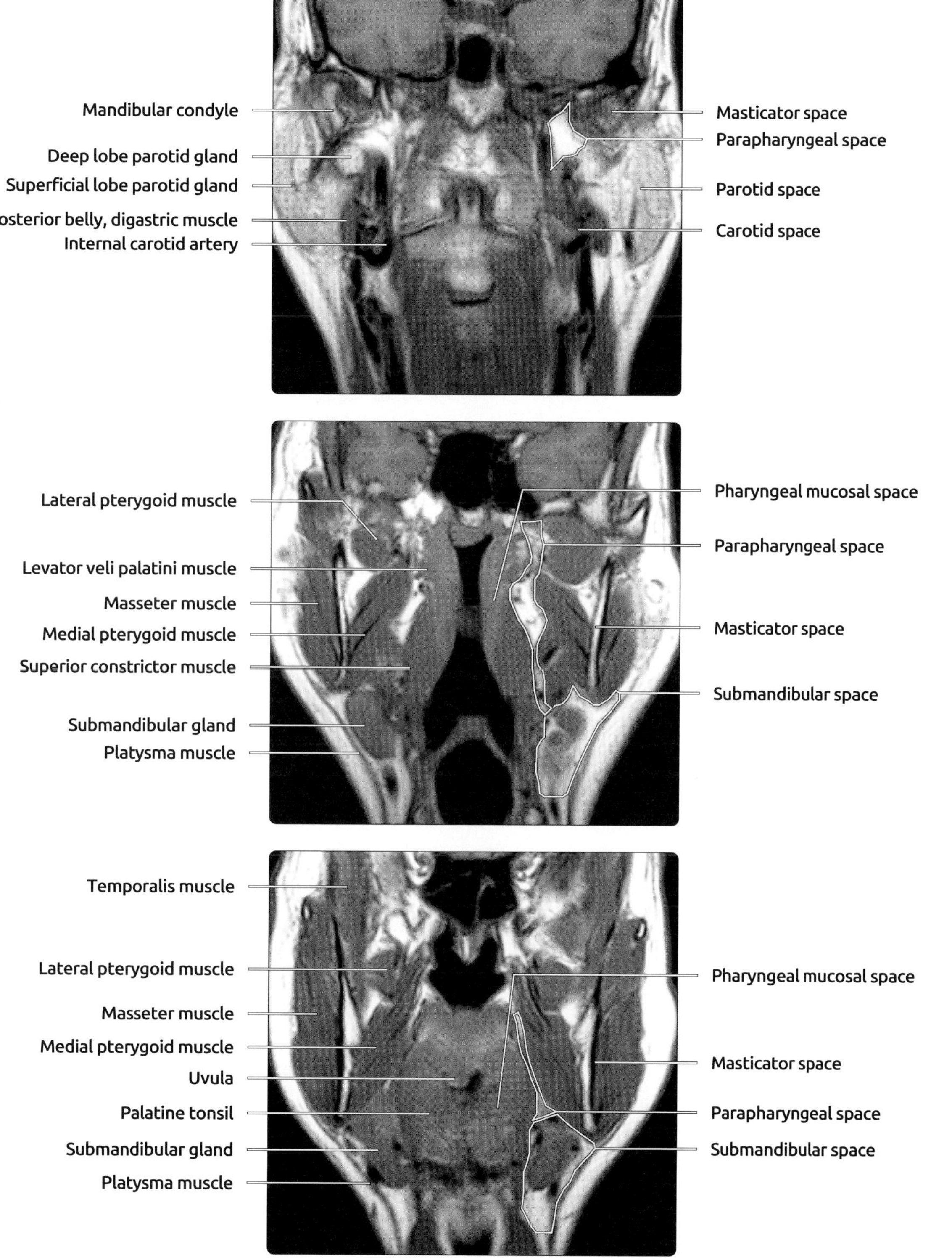

(Top) *First of 3 coronal T1 MR images of the suprahyoid neck, presented from posterior to anterior, is shown. In this image through the mandibular condyles, the posterior parapharyngeal space is seen medial to the deep lobe of the parotid gland.* **(Middle)** *In this image, the parapharyngeal space is visible from its superior aspect of skull base abutment to its inferior aspect merging with the submandibular space. Note the site of abutment with the skull base contains no vital structures. Remember that there is no fascia present between the inferior parapharyngeal space and the posterior submandibular space.* **(Bottom)** *In this image through the anterior parapharyngeal space, the connection between the parapharyngeal space and submandibular space is seen. Submandibular space disease, especially abscess, may, at times, spread superiorly into the parapharyngeal space via this connection.*

TERMINOLOGY

Abbreviations

- Pharyngeal mucosal space (PMS)

Synonyms

- Pharyngeal mucosal surface

Definitions

- **PMS**: Nasopharyngeal, oropharyngeal, & hypopharyngeal surface structures on airway side of middle layer of deep cervical fascia (ML-DCF)

IMAGING ANATOMY

Overview

- PMS: Conceptual construct to complete map of spaces of suprahyoid neck
- **No fascia on surface of PMS**
  - PMS not true fascia-enclosed space

Extent

- PMS: Continuous mucosal sheet defined from nasopharynx to hypopharynx (includes soft palate)
- Nasopharyngeal, oropharyngeal, & hypopharyngeal mucosal space components

Anatomy Relationships

- Airway side of PMS: No fascial border
- Posterior to PMS: Retropharyngeal space
- Lateral to PMS: Parapharyngeal space (PPS)
- Skull base relationship to PMS
  - Broad area of attachment to skull base
  - Attachment area includes posterior basisphenoid (sphenoid sinus floor), anterior basiocciput (anterior clivus)
  - Also includes **foramen lacerum**
    - Cartilaginous floor of anterior horizontal petrous internal carotid artery
    - Represents route for nasopharyngeal carcinoma to access intracranial structures

Internal Contents

- **Mucosal surface of pharynx**
- **PMS lymphatic ring**: Lymphatic ring of tissue of PMS that declines in size with advancing age
  - Synonym: Waldeyer ring
  - Nasopharynx: **Adenoids**
  - Oropharynx, lateral wall: **Palatine (faucial) tonsil**
  - Oropharynx, base of tongue: **Lingual tonsil**
  - Glossotonsillar sulcus: Cleft between lower palatine tonsil & lingual tonsil
- **Minor salivary glands**
  - Soft palate mucosa has highest concentration
- **Pharyngobasilar fascia**
  - Tough aponeurosis that connects superior constrictor muscle to skull base
  - Posterosuperior margin notch = **sinus of Morgagni**
    - Levator palatini muscle & eustachian tube pass through this notch on way from skull base to PMS
    - May be route of tumor spread laterally from PMS
- **PMS muscles**
  - Superior, middle, & inferior constrictor muscles
  - Salpingopharyngeus muscle
  - Levator palatini muscle, distal end
- **Torus tubarius**: Cartilaginous end of eustachian tube
- **Lateral pharyngeal recess**: Fossa of Rosenmüller, cleft posteromedial to torus tubarius

Fascia of Pharyngeal Mucosal Space

- **ML-DCF** represents deep margin of PMS
  - In nasopharynx, ML-DCF encircles lateral & posterior margins of pharyngobasilar fascia
  - In oropharynx, ML-DCF on deep margin of superior & middle constrictor muscles
  - In hypopharynx, ML-DCF on deep margin of inferior constrictor muscle

ANATOMY IMAGING ISSUES

Questions

- What imaging findings define lesion as primary to PMS
  - Lesion designated primary to PMS when
    - Lesion center **medial to PPS**
    - PMS mass **pushes PPS fat from medial to lateral**
    - PMS mass **disrupts normal PMS mucosal & submucosal architecture**

Imaging Recommendations

- CECT or MR can both successfully image PMS
- If skull base invasion or perineural tumor suspected, T1 C+ fat-saturated MR best
- Bone CT may then be added to delineate skull base bone changes & tumor matrix

Imaging Approaches

- If malignant tumor of PMS suspected, remember to stage primary tumor & cervical nodes in neck

Imaging Pitfalls

- Most common error in interpreting images of PMS: Labeling normal asymmetry as tumor
- Lateral pharyngeal recess (fossa of Rosenmüller) notoriously asymmetric & may have fluid within it
- Variable amounts of lymphoid tissue or lymphoid hypertrophy in Waldeyer ring can mimic tumor
- Retropharyngeal course of carotid may cause asymmetry of posterior pharynx

CLINICAL IMPLICATIONS

Clinical Importance

- Referring doctor sees PMS surface directly or on endoscopy
  - Use clinical impressions as part of imaging report
- Most common PMS lesion: Squamous cell carcinoma (SCCa)
  - Become familiar with routes of spread of SCCa by specific primary tumor site
  - Become familiar with staging criteria for each specific primary tumor site
- **Differential diagnosis of PMS mass**
  - From mucosa: SCCa
  - From lymphoid tissue: Non-Hodgkin lymphoma
  - From minor salivary glands: Minor salivary gland malignancies (uncommon)

GRAPHICS

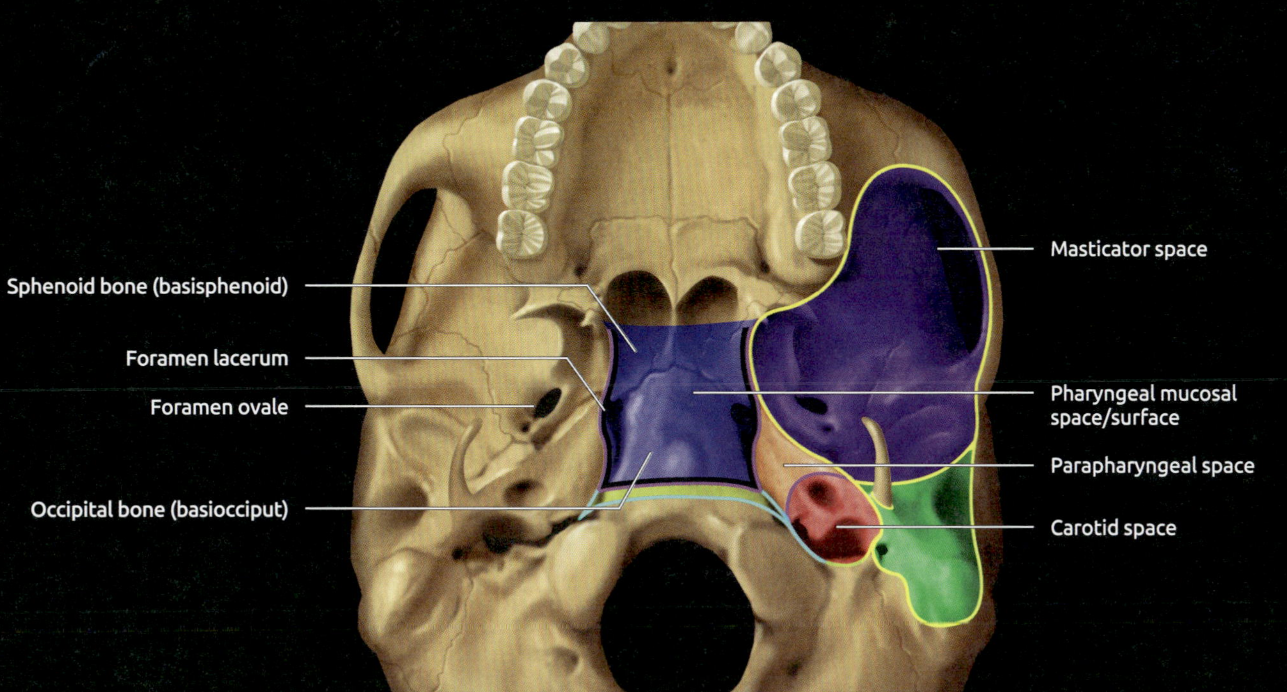

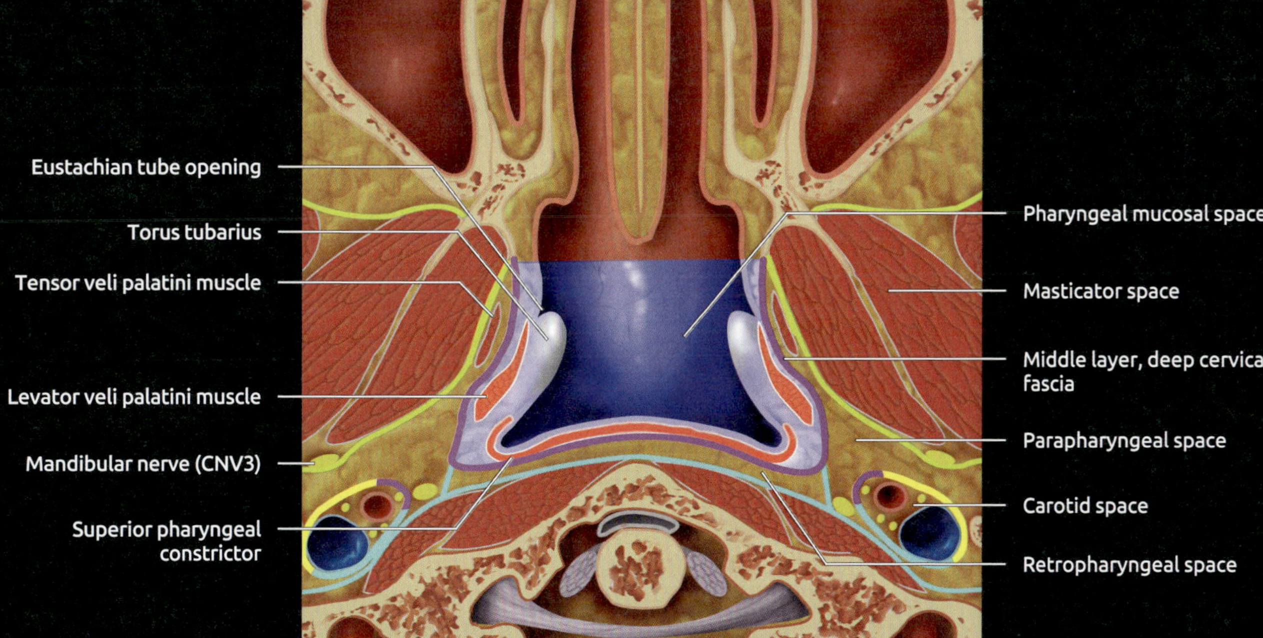

(Top) *Graphic of the skull base from below shows the relationships of the spaces of the suprahyoid neck and the skull base with an emphasis on the pharyngeal mucosal space. Notice the pharyngeal mucosal space abuts a broad area of the sphenoid and occipital bones. The foramen lacerum, the cartilaginous floor to the anteromedial horizontal petrous internal carotid artery canal, is within this abutment area. Malignant tumors of the nasopharyngeal mucosal space can access the intracranial compartment via the foramen lacerum.* **(Bottom)** *Axial graphic of the nasopharyngeal mucosal space (in blue) shows the superior pharyngeal constrictor and levator veli palatini muscles are within the space. The middle layer of the deep cervical fascia provides a deep margin to the space. In the upper nasopharynx, the pharyngobasilar fascia spans the gap from the superior margin of the superior pharyngeal constrictor muscle to the skull base. The retropharyngeal space is posterior, and the parapharyngeal space is lateral to the pharyngeal mucosal space.*

GRAPHICS

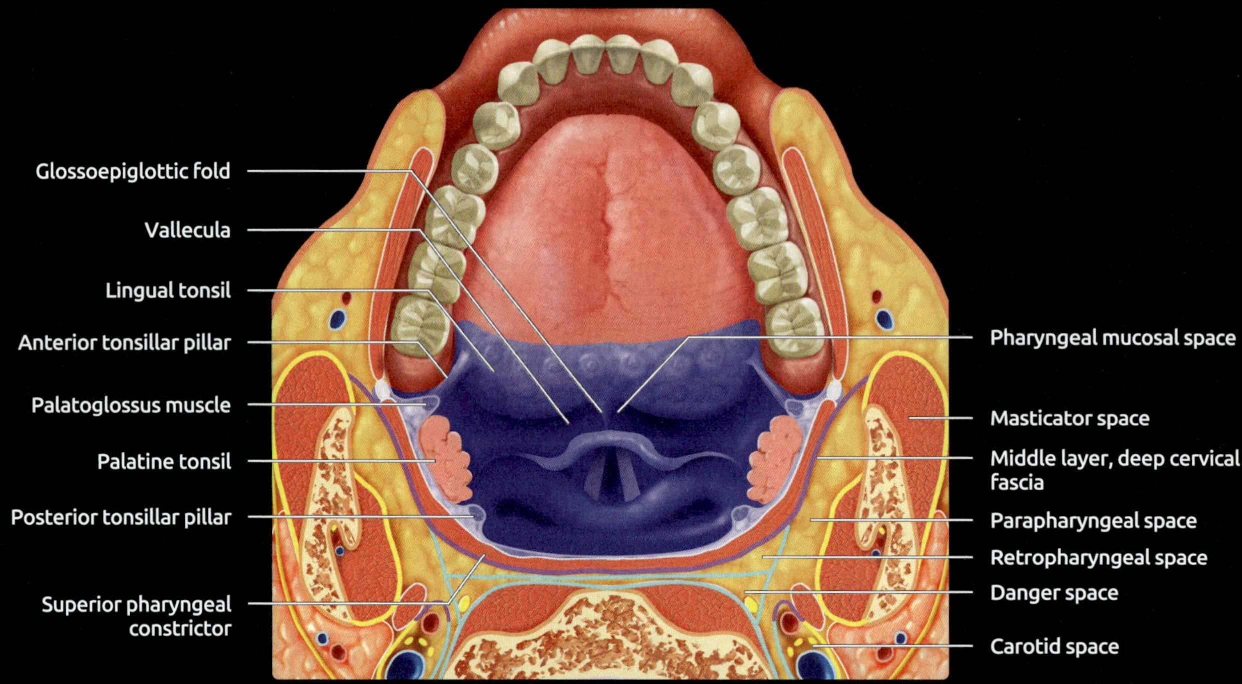

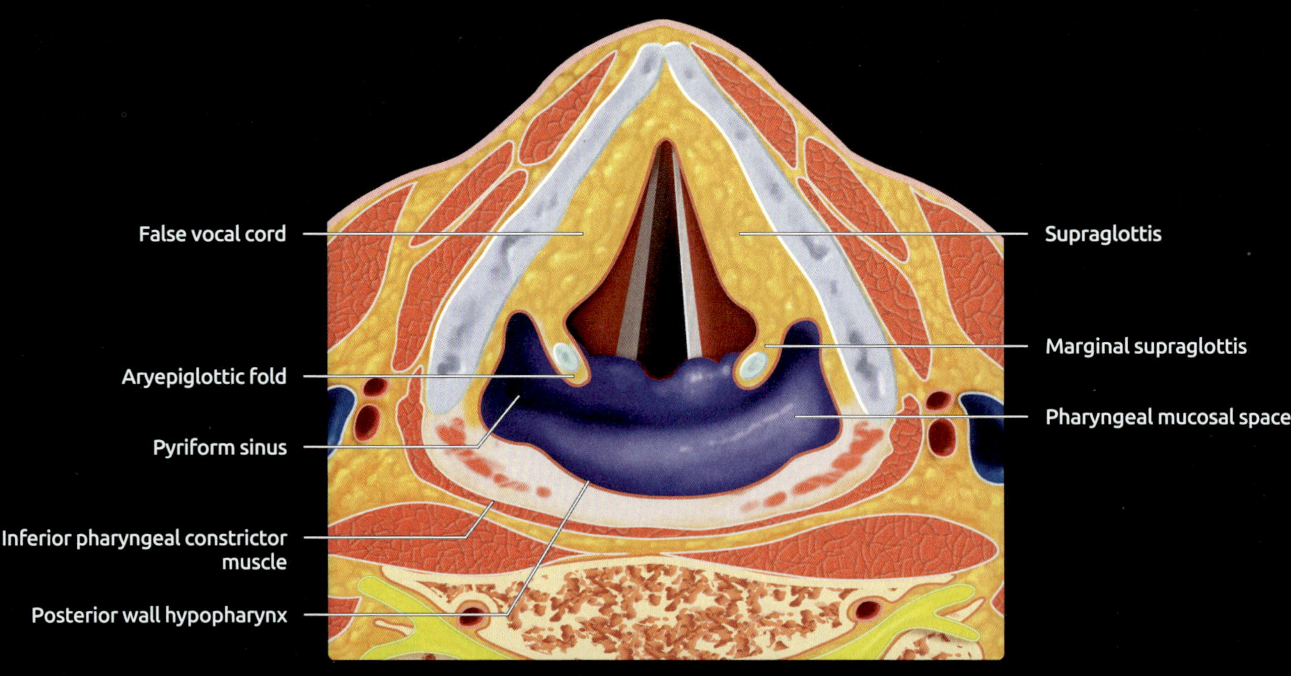

(Top) *Axial graphic of the oropharyngeal mucosal space (in blue) viewed from above reveals the superior pharyngeal constrictor; the tonsillar pillars along with the palatine and lingual tonsils are all occupants of this space. The middle layer of the deep cervical fascia provides a deep margin to the space. The retropharyngeal space is behind, and the parapharyngeal space is lateral to, the pharyngeal mucosal space.* **(Bottom)** *Axial graphic of the hypopharyngeal aspect of the pharyngeal mucosal space is shown. At the level of the supraglottis, the hypopharynx is made up of the pyriform sinus and posterior wall. Notice that the posterior wall of the aryepiglottic fold is in the hypopharynx, while the anterior wall is in the supraglottic larynx. For this reason, this area is commonly referred to as the "marginal supraglottis."*

GRAPHICS

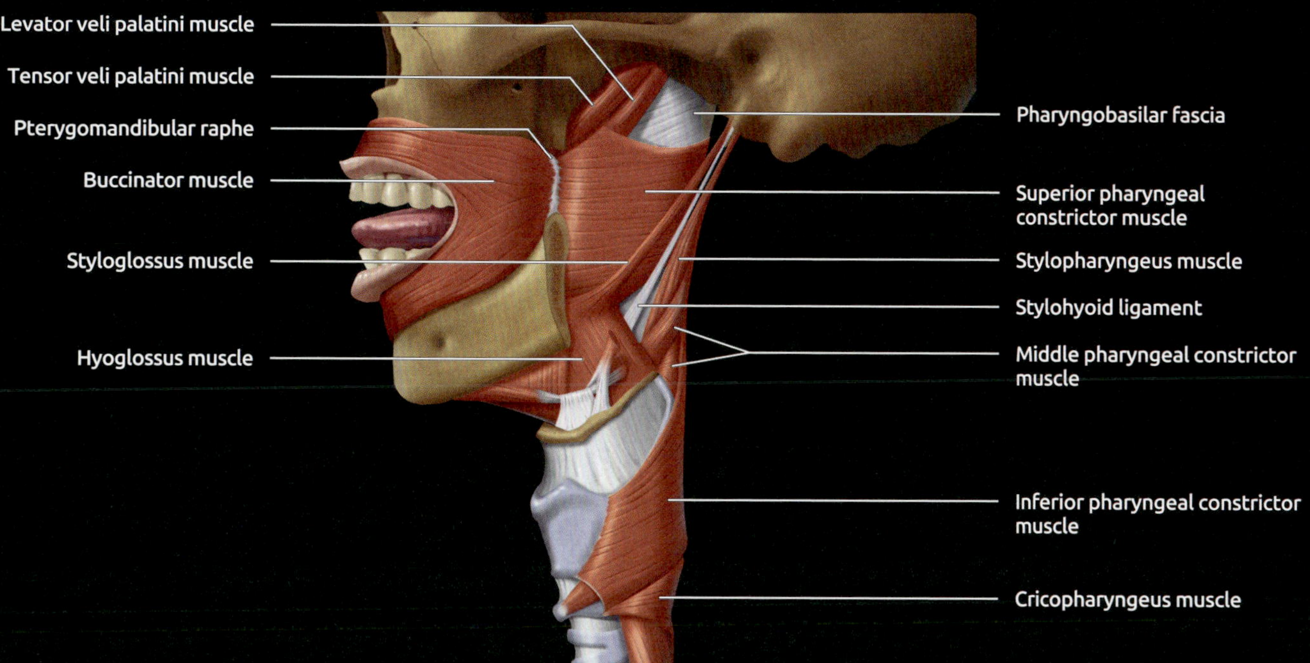

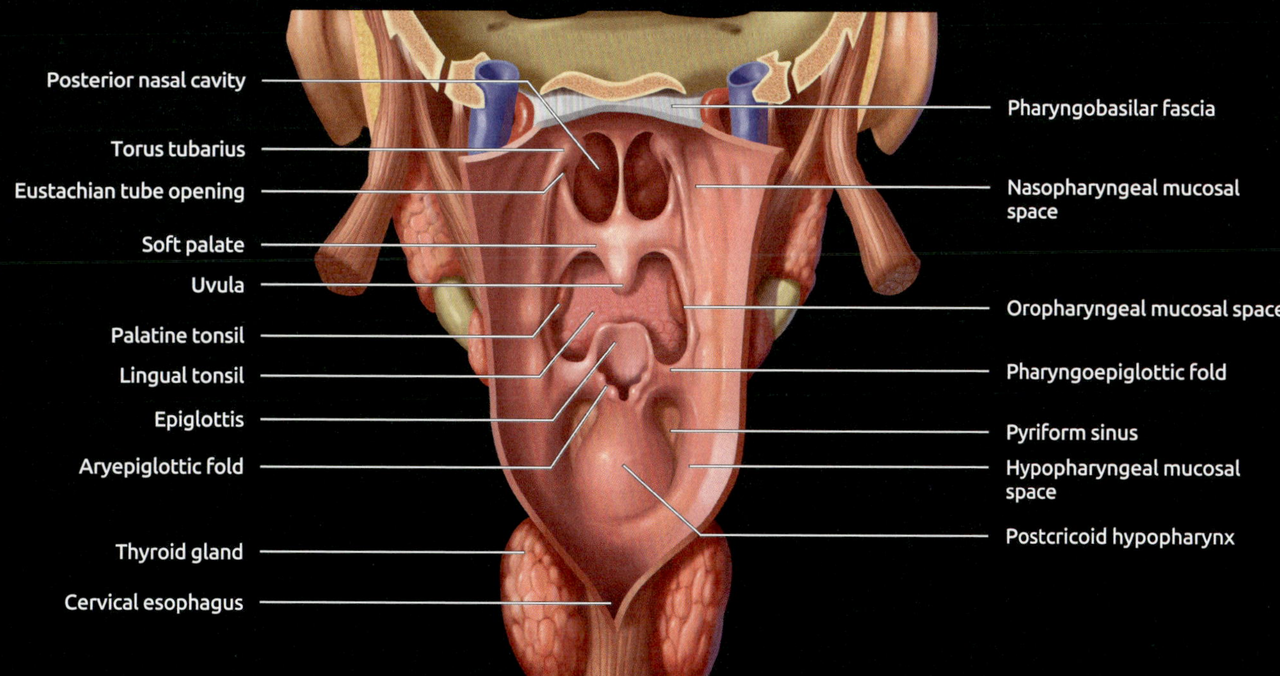

(Top) *Lateral graphic shows the major muscles of the pharyngeal mucosal space. Notice the superior, middle, and inferior pharyngeal constrictor muscles are in the posterior wall of the pharyngeal mucosal space from the nasopharynx through the oropharynx to the hypopharynx. The pharyngobasilar fascia attaches the superior pharyngeal constrictor to the skull base. The distal end of the levator veli palatini muscle is on the airway side of the middle layer of deep cervical fascia, making it a part of the pharyngeal mucosal space.* **(Bottom)** *Graphic of the pharyngeal mucosal space/surface seen from behind shows this space can be divided into nasopharyngeal, oropharyngeal, and hypopharyngeal areas. The lymphatic ring of the pharyngeal mucosal space contains the nasopharyngeal adenoids and the oropharyngeal palatine and lingual tonsils.*

GENERIC PHARYNGEAL MUCOSAL SPACE MASS

Levator veli palatini muscle
Torus tubarius
Lateral pharyngeal recess
Superior constrictor muscle
Pharyngeal mucosal space mass
Parapharyngeal space

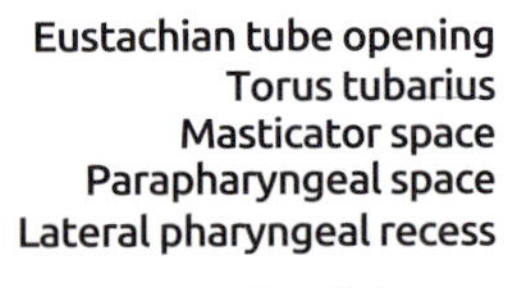

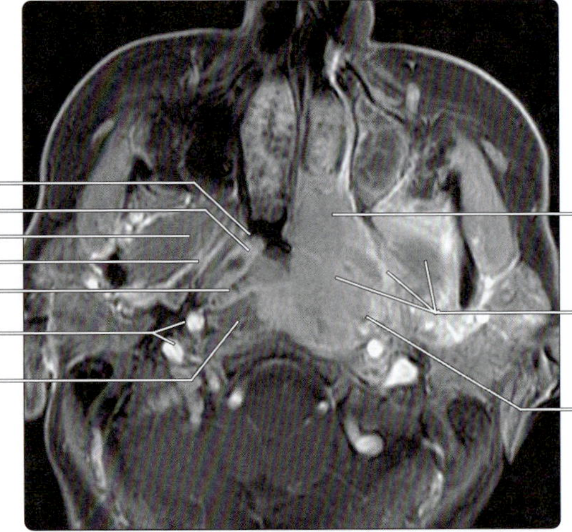

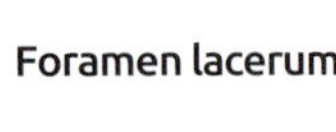

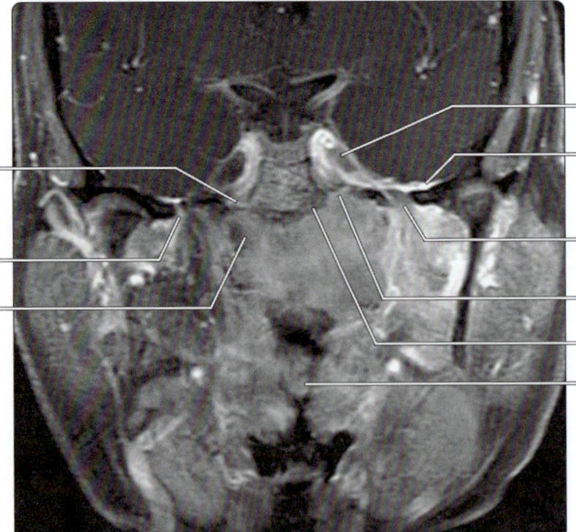

(Top) *Axial graphic of a generic pharyngeal mucosal space mass demonstrates the disruption of the normal architecture of the surface of the pharynx with bulging of the mass into the pharyngeal airway. Also notice the deep margin of the mass is displacing the parapharyngeal space fat from medial to lateral.* **(Middle)** *In this example of nasopharyngeal carcinoma, normal anatomy is labeled on the unaffected side for reference. The mass is centered in the area of the lateral pharyngeal recess and invades the prevertebral musculature. Tumor extends laterally across the parapharyngeal space into the masticator space. The posterolateral portion of the tumor is in close proximity to the carotid space.* **(Bottom)** *The normal anatomy is indicated on the same patient's right side. Note that the medial aspect of the normal torus tubarius is the location of the lateral pharyngeal recess, not visible due to mucosal apposition, but directly inferior to foramen lacerum. Tumor is invading the foramen lacerum with abnormal marrow signal and subtle contour deformity of the clivus. The lateral tumor component has invaded foramen ovale, involving the dura and Meckel cave.*

BARIUM SWALLOW

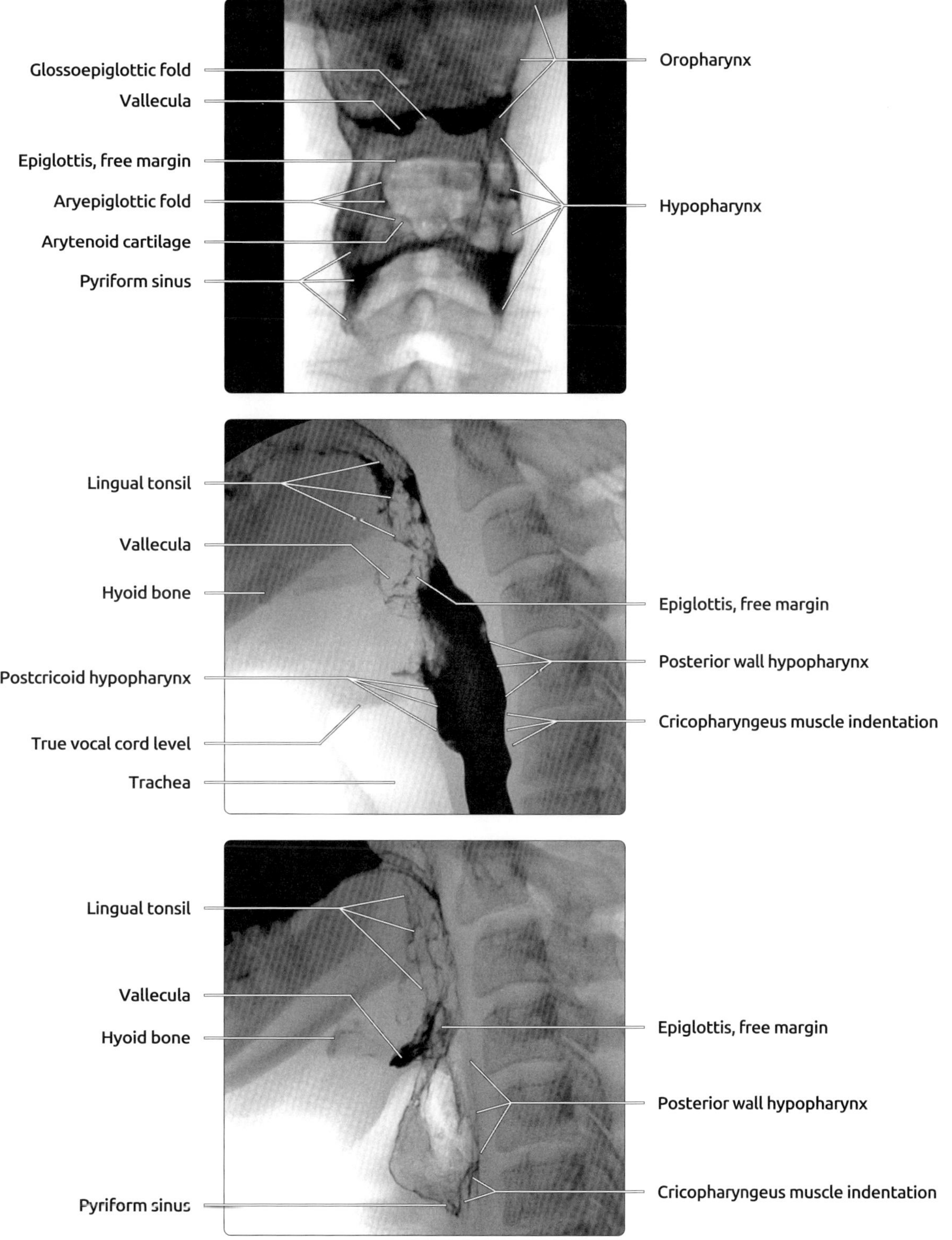

(Top) *AP barium swallow image focused on the low oropharyngeal and hypopharyngeal mucosal space surfaces is shown. Notice the hypopharynx extends from the level of the vallecula and glossoepiglottic fold superiorly to the inferior margin of the pyriform sinus.* **(Middle)** *In this lateral view of a barium swallow, the irregular surface of the lingual tonsil is recognized along the posterior margin of the tongue. The postcricoid area and the posterior wall of the hypopharynx make up 2 of the 3 major subsites within the hypopharynx. The 3rd subsite is the pyriform sinus.* **(Bottom)** *In this lateral barium swallow image, the indentation of the cricopharyngeus muscle is particularly well seen. Remember, the inferior margin of the vallecula marks the transition from oropharynx to hypopharynx.*

AXIAL T1 MR

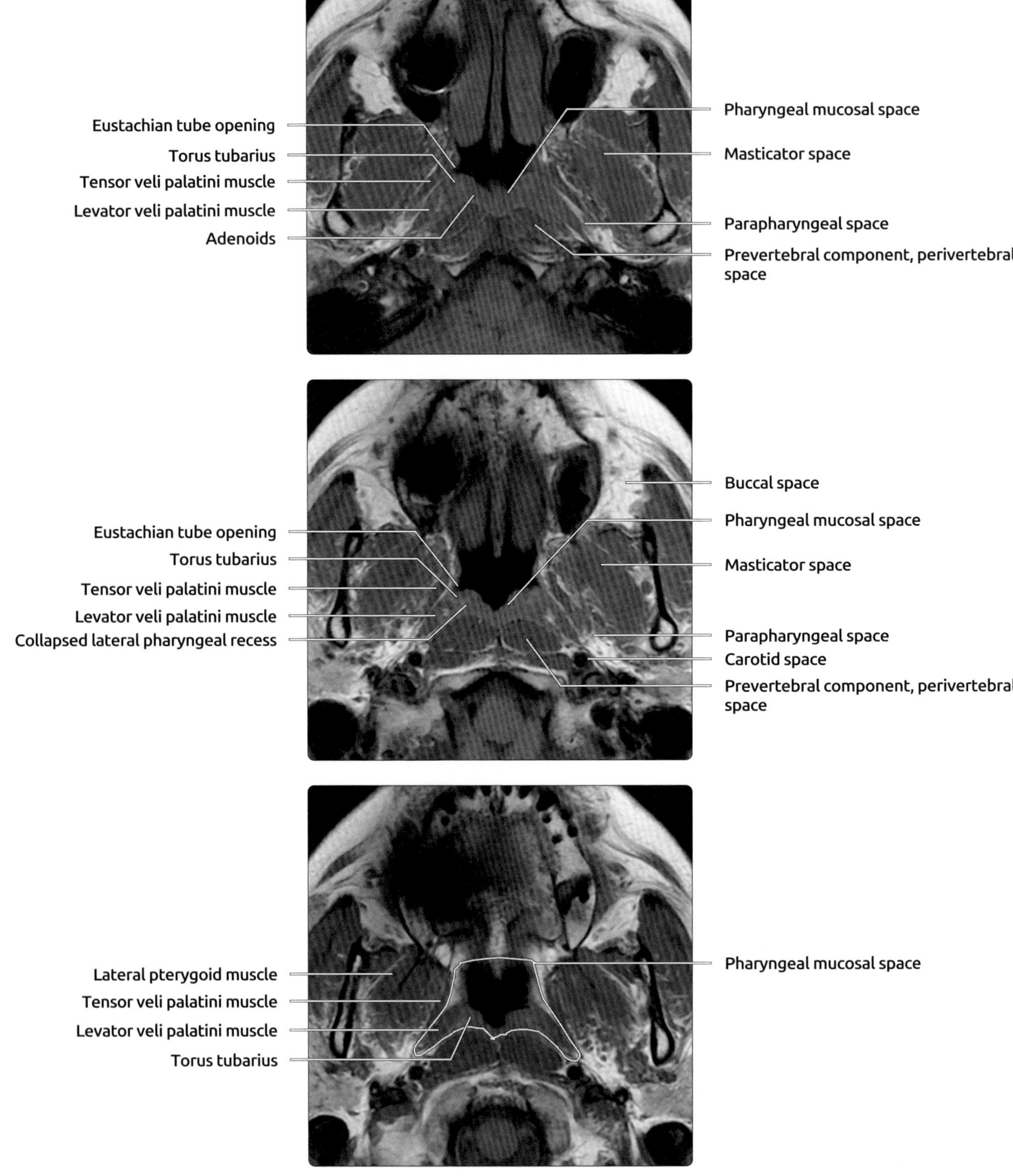

(Top) *First of 6 axial T1 MR images presented from superior to inferior shows the pharyngeal mucosal space at the level of the nasopharynx. Notice the torus tubarius (distal cartilaginous eustachian tube) and nasopharyngeal adenoids. The lateral pharyngeal recess is collapsed and therefore not visible.* **(Middle)** *In this image, the levator veli palatini muscle is transitioning to the pharyngeal mucosal space through the sinus of Morgagni, a gap in the pharyngobasilar fascia that also transmits the distal cartilaginous eustachian tube (torus tubarius). The tensor veli palatini does not enter the pharyngeal mucosal space. The lateral pharyngeal recess is collapsed and therefore not visible.* **(Bottom)** *At the inferior aspect of the torus tubarius, the lateral and posterior margins of the pharyngeal mucosal space are likely transitioning from the pharyngobasilar fascia to the middle layer of deep cervical fascia.*

AXIAL T1 MR

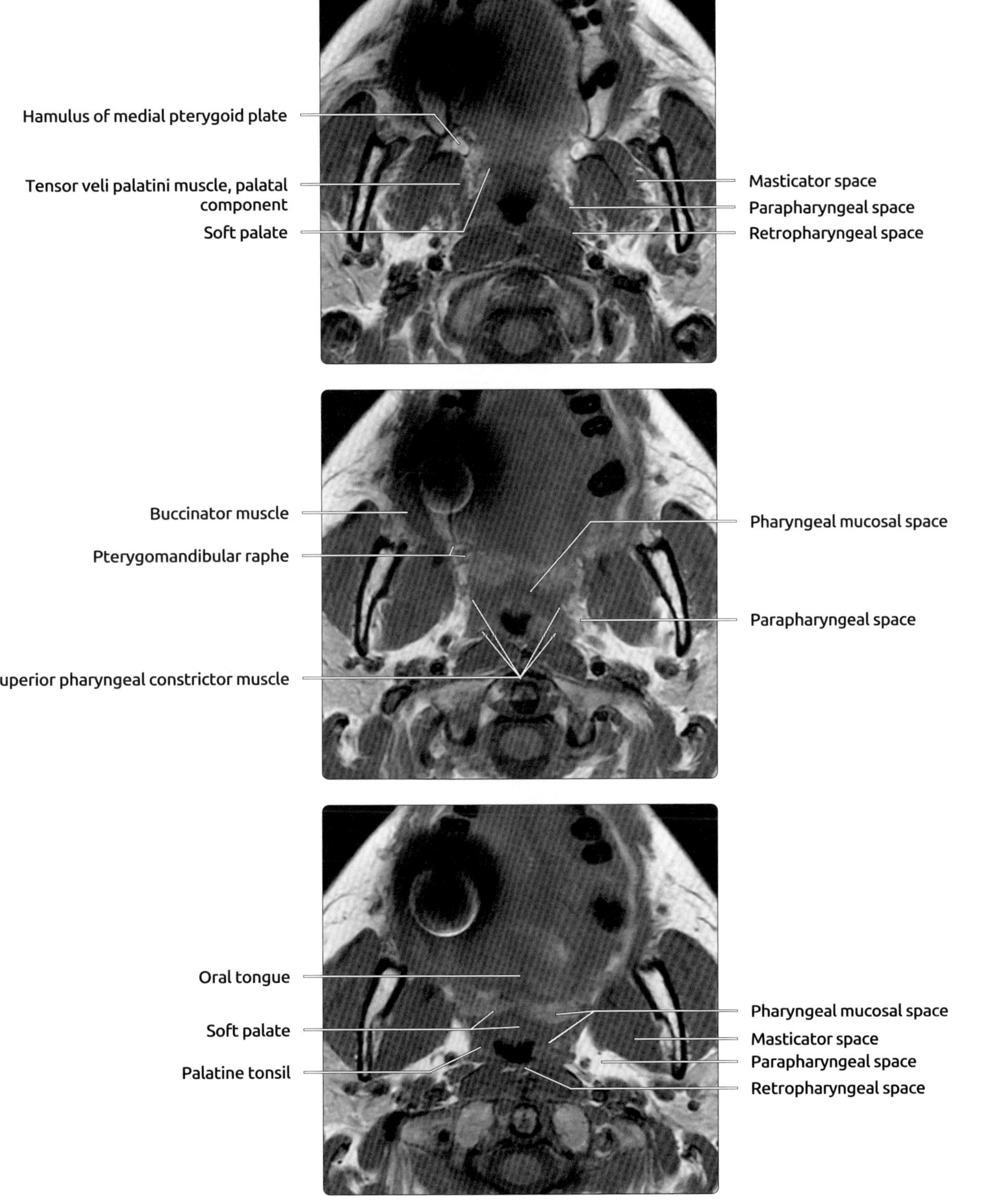

(Top) *At the level of the maxillary alveolar ridge, the tensor veli palatini muscle is seen posterior to the hamulus of the medial pterygoid plate, about to attach to the anterolateral soft palate. Notice that posterior to the pharyngeal mucosal space, the thin fat stripe of the retropharyngeal space is just visible in front of the prevertebral component of the perivertebral space.* **(Middle)** *At the level of the maxillary teeth, the pharyngeal mucosal space of the superior oropharynx is seen. The superior pharyngeal constrictor muscle is present along the margins of the pharyngeal mucosal space just inside the middle layer of deep cervical fascia, which cannot be seen with imaging.* **(Bottom)** *Note the superior margin of the palatine tonsil at its junction with the soft palate. Note the superior margin of the palatine tonsil along with the soft palate itself. The most posterior portion of the soft palate, including the uvula, may be opposing the dorsum of the oral tongue in the supine patient.*

AXIAL T2 MR

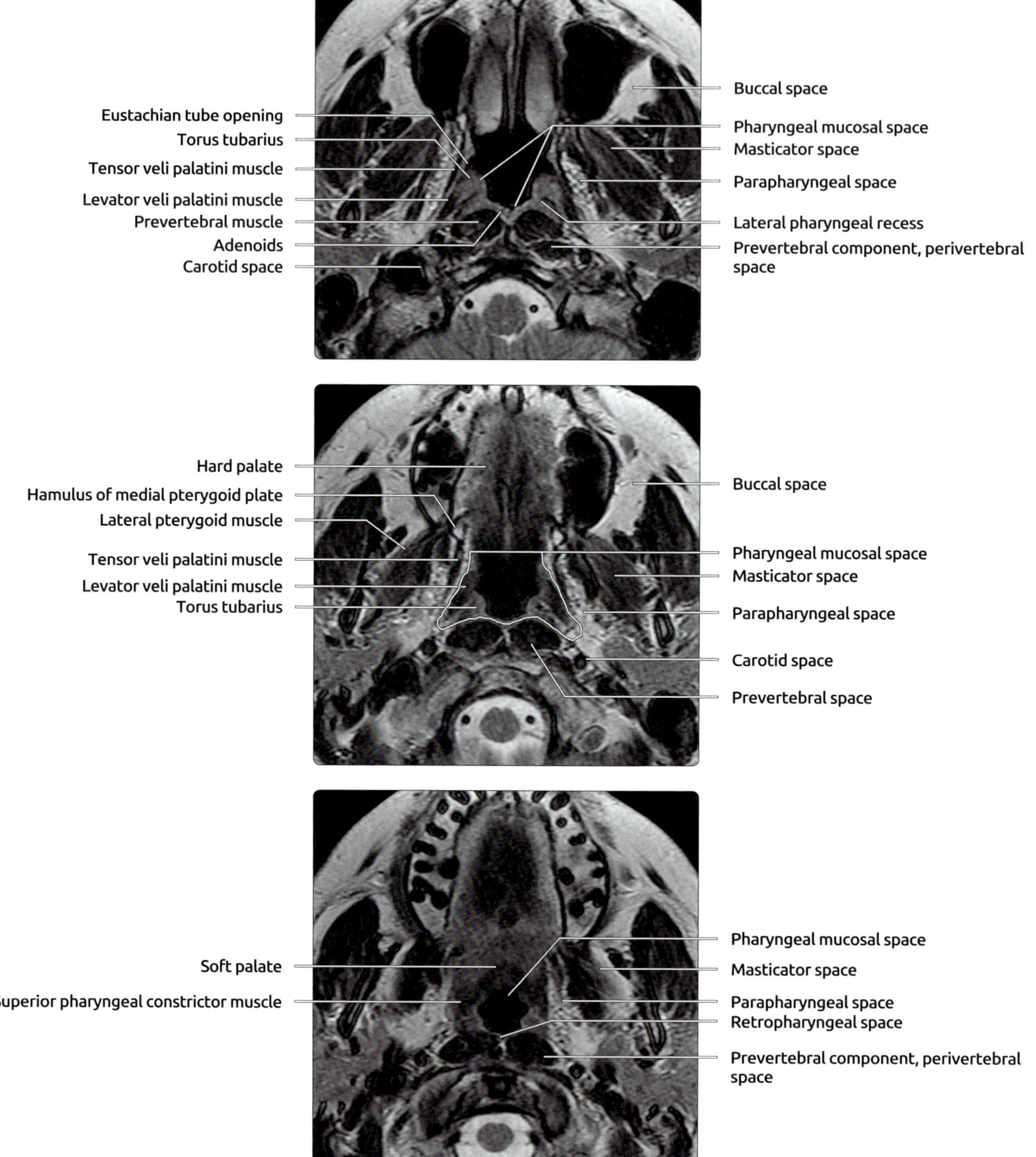

(Top) *First of 9 T2 MR images from superior to inferior shows the pharyngeal mucosal space at the level of the nasopharynx. The lateral pharyngeal recess is collapsed and therefore not visible.* **(Middle)** *In this image, the levator veli palatini muscle is transitioning to the pharyngeal mucosal space through the sinus of Morgagni, a gap in the pharyngobasilar fascia that also transmits the distal cartilaginous eustachian tube (torus tubarius). The tensor veli palatini does not enter the pharyngeal mucosal space. The lateral and posterior portions of the outline of the pharyngeal mucosal space correspond to the pharyngobasilar fascia.* **(Bottom)** *At the level of the soft palate, below the pharyngobasilar fascia, the boundary of the pharyngeal mucosal space is now the middle layer of deep cervical fascia (not visible) surrounding the superior pharyngeal constrictor muscle. The retropharyngeal space is very thin at this level.*

AXIAL T2 MR

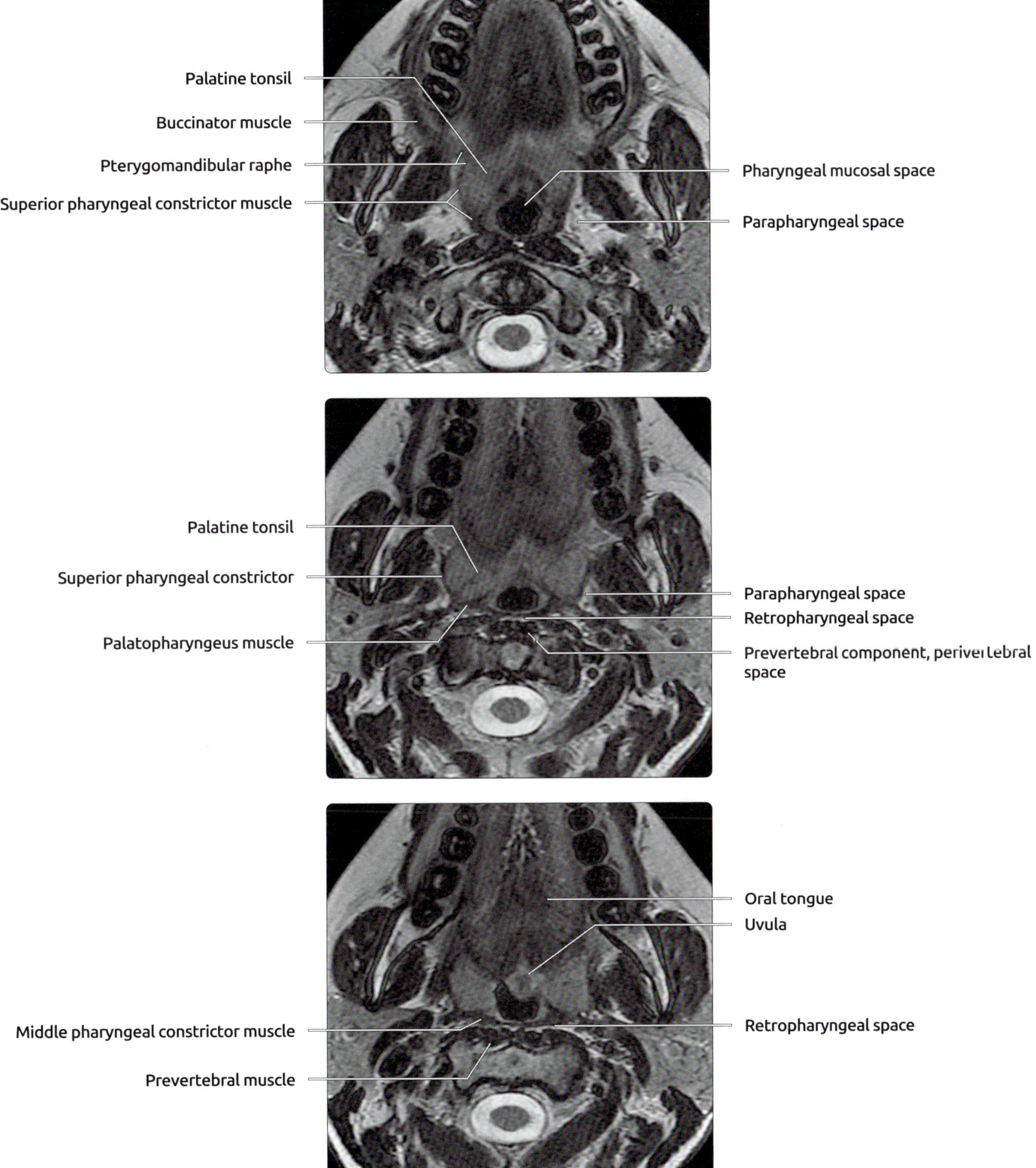

(Top) *At the level of the superior oropharynx, the superior aspect of the palatine tonsil is visible just posterolateral to the soft palate. The posterior margin of the buccinator muscle and anterior margin of the superior pharyngeal constrictor muscle meet at the pterygomandibular raphe.* **(Middle)** *In this image through the midoropharynx, the palatopharyngeus muscle may be seen along the posterior margin of the palatine tonsil. The retropharyngeal space fat is posterior to the pharyngeal mucosal space, and the parapharyngeal spaces are lateral.* **(Bottom)** *At the level of the mandibular teeth, the middle pharyngeal constrictor muscle is visible along the posterolateral aspects of the palatine tonsils. The most posterior portion of the soft palate, including the uvula, may be opposing the dorsum of the oral tongue in the supine patient.*

AXIAL T2 MR

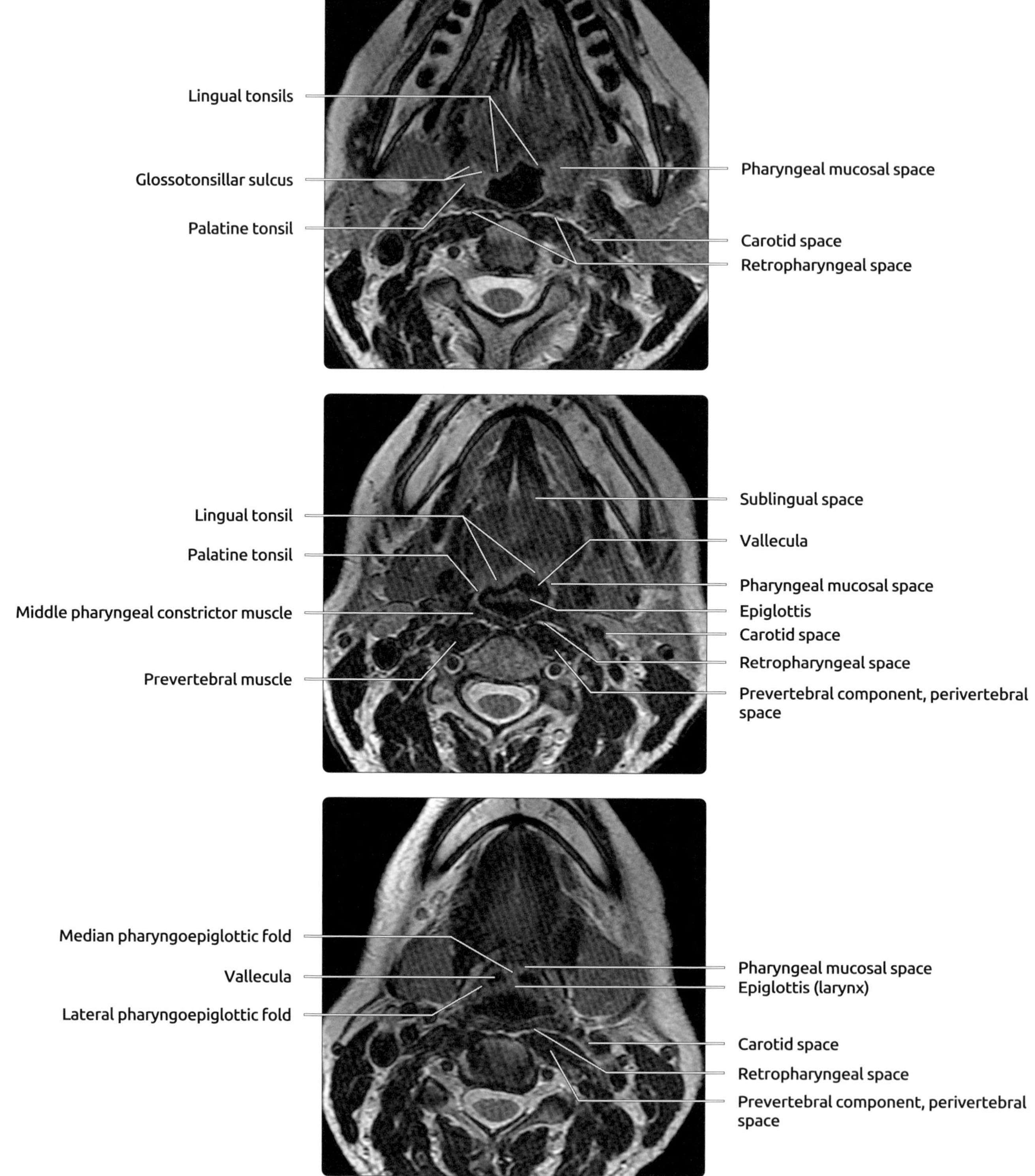

(Top) *In this image, the superior portions of the lingual tonsils are visible at the level of the lower parts of the palatine tonsils. There is a cleft of potential space between the palatine and lingual tonsils, the glossotonsillar sulcus, which is variably visible depending on degree of aeration.* **(Middle)** *Low in the oropharynx, thicker lingual tonsillar tissue can be seen along with an attenuated palatine tonsil. The lingual tonsil is in the oropharynx, not the oral cavity. The vallecula is the space between the lingual tonsil and epiglottis.* **(Bottom)** *At the most inferior aspect of the lingual tonsils, the median pharyngoepiglottic fold is the boundary between the oropharynx and larynx. The lateral pharyngoepiglottic fold is the boundary between oropharynx and hypopharynx.*

GRAPHIC AND CORONAL T1 C+ MR

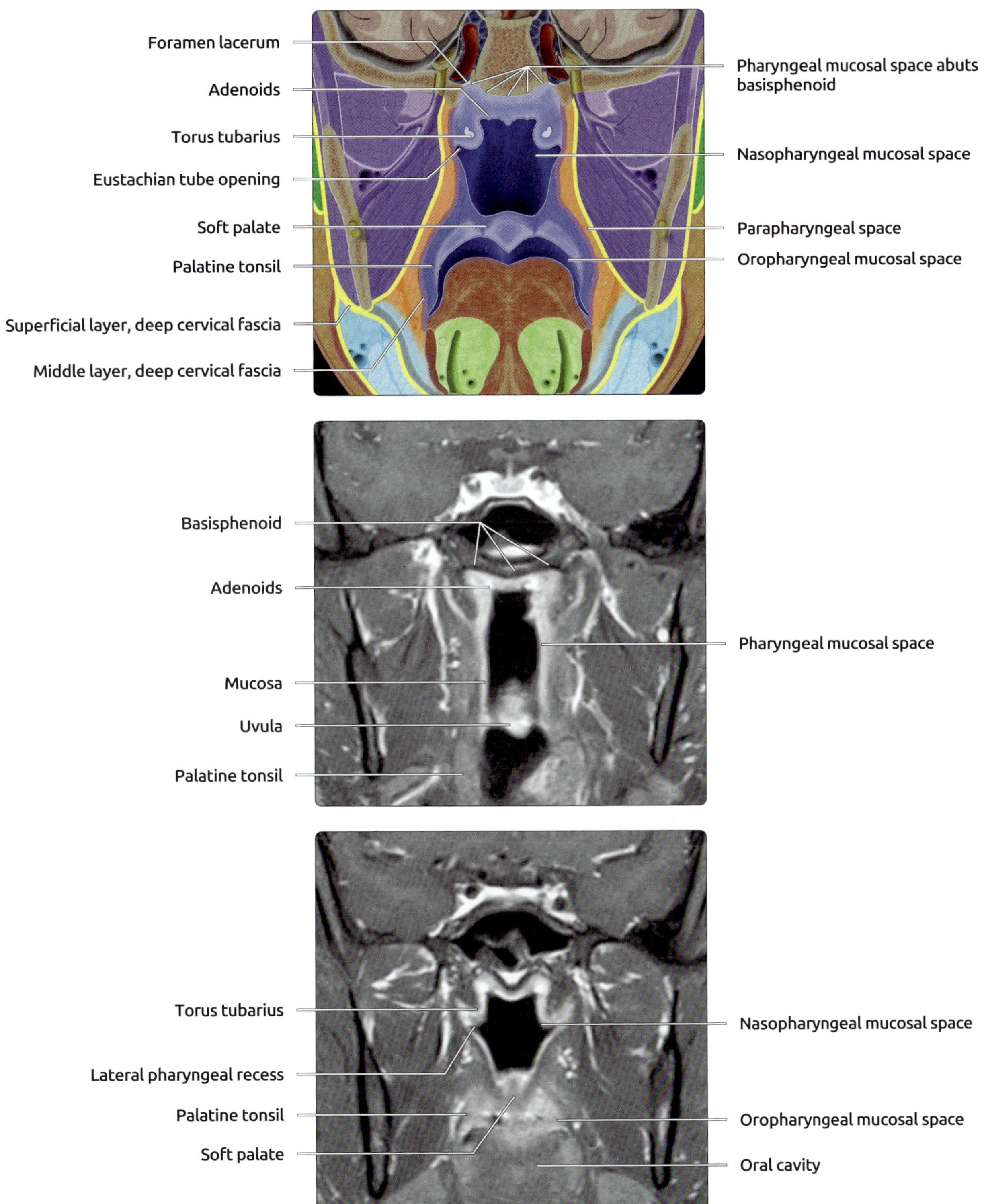

(Top) *Coronal graphic of the nasopharyngeal and oropharyngeal mucosal space is shown. Notice the middle layer of deep cervical fascia defining the lateral margin of the pharyngeal mucosal space. The parapharyngeal spaces are paired fatty spaces lateral to the pharyngeal mucosal space.* **(Middle)** *Coronal T1 C+ FS MR shows the pharyngeal mucosal space surface enhances. Notice that the roof of the nasopharyngeal mucosal space abuts the basisphenoid. Remember that a nasopharyngeal carcinoma that begins in the roof of the nasopharynx will often have invaded the sphenoid sinus at the time of presentation.* **(Bottom)** *Coronal T1 C+ FS MR reveals the enhancing sheet of mucosa with the torus tubarius (cartilaginous eustachian tube) and lateral pharyngeal recess.*

TERMINOLOGY

Abbreviations

- Sublingual space (SLS); floor of mouth (FOM); submandibular space (SMS); submandibular gland (SMG)

Definitions

- SLS: Paired, **non-fascial-lined** spaces of oral cavity below FOM mucosa & superomedial to mylohyoid muscular sling; separated by root of tongue muscles in midline
- FOM: Variable definition
  - Some define FOM as inferior recess of oral cavity, beneath oral tongue, limited to squamous epithelial mucosa, & amenable to clinical visual inspection
  - Some define FOM as region of oral cavity beneath oral tongue, including mucosa & SLS

IMAGING ANATOMY

Overview

- SLS contains sublingual gland (SLG), submandibular duct (SMD)/deep gland, & key neurovascular structures
- Includes hypoglossal nerve (CNXII), lingual nerve (branch of V3), glossopharyngeal nerve (CNIX), lingual artery & vein

Anatomy Relationships

- SLS situated below FOM mucosa & **superomedial to mylohyoid**; lateral to genioglossus/geniohyoid muscles
- Communication between SLSs occurs in midline anteriorly as narrow **isthmus** beneath frenulum
- Lesion in both SLSs across anterior isthmus: "Horizontal horseshoe" parallel to inferior mandibular surface
- SLS communicates with SMS at posterior mylohyoid margin
  - No fascia dividing posterior SLS from adjacent SMS
  - Posterosuperior SMS in turn communicates with inferior parapharyngeal space here
- **Mylohyoid boutonnière:** Variable defects in mylohyoid muscle, allowing SLS lesions to project into anterior SMS **in front of** SMG; most defects < 5 mm, occasionally < 2 cm
  - Bilateral in 2/3, unilateral in 1/3
  - Mostly along lateral margins of mylohyoid muscle, closer to mandible & away from median raphe
  - Defects unusual in thicker, posterior 3rd of mylohyoid
  - Contains fat, blood vessels, & salivary tissue in order of frequency

Internal Contents

- **Hyoglossus muscle** divides posterior aspect of SLS into medial & lateral compartments
- **Lateral compartment contents**: Lingual nerve superolaterally, SMD & sublingual/deep part of submandibular salivary glands in middle, & hypoglossal nerve inferomedially
- SMD & lingual nerve **cross each other** at anterior border of hyoglossus
- **SLG & ducts**: Smallest of major salivary glands, in lateral SLS anteriorly; 2 parts
  - **Anterior lesser SLG**: Mass of 7-5 glands with small ducts of Rivinus joining short main duct to drain onto sublingual fold in FOM
  - **Posterior greater SLG** (not always present)**:** Main duct (Bartholin duct) draining directly onto sublingual papilla or joins SMD
- **SMG deep part & duct**: SMG deep margin extends into posterior opening of SLS
  - Enlarging lesions of SLS, in effect, push this deep margin of SMG out of way as they emerge from SLS into SMS
  - SMD (Wharton) runs anteriorly to open on summit of sublingual papilla in FOM at side of frenulum of tongue
- **Submandibular ganglion**: Fusiform ganglion, lies on hyoglossus muscle just above deep part of SMG
  - Suspended from **lingual nerve** by 2-3 roots; **posterior root** parasympathetic (chorda tympani) to ganglion
  - **Anterior root** has postganglionic parasympathetic fibers reentering lingual nerve to supply SLG; those for SMG reach it through 5-6 direct branches from ganglion
  - **Sympathetic** fibers from **plexus around facial artery** contain postganglionic fibers arising from superior cervical ganglion & pass through submandibular ganglion without relay
  - Sensory fibers from lingual nerve may pass through it
- **Hypoglossal nerve**: Motor to tongue muscles
  - Intrinsic muscles of tongue include inferior lingual, vertical, & transverse muscles
  - Extrinsic muscles of tongue include genioglossus, hyoglossus, styloglossus, & palatoglossus muscles
- **Lingual nerve**: Combined **with chorda tympani** nerve
  - Lingual nerve branch of CNV3 (mandibular division of trigeminal): Sensation to anterior 2/3 of oral tongue
  - Chorda tympani branch of CNVII (facial nerve): Taste to anterior 2/3 of tongue, & parasympathetic secretomotor fibers to SMG & SLG via its preganglionic parasympathetic supply from **pontine superior salivatory nucleus** to **submandibular ganglion**
  - Chorda tympani nerve exits middle ear through petrotympanic fissure into masticator space & joins lingual nerve 2 cm below skull base
- **Medial compartment contents**: Glossopharyngeal nerve above, lingual artery & vein below
- **Glossopharyngeal nerve** (CNIX): Sensation & taste
  - Provides sensation to posterior 1/3 of tongue
  - Carries taste input from posterior 1/3 of tongue
- **Lingual artery & vein**: Supply oral tongue; seen running just lateral to genioglossus muscle

ANATOMY IMAGING ISSUES

Imaging Pitfalls

- Dental amalgam artifact obscures FOM & SLS
- SLG extending through mylohyoid defect mimic SMS lesion

Imaging Issues Related to Malignancy

- Primary tumors of SLG uncommon, but percentage of malignant tumor is high (70-85%)
- Critical to evaluate for deep extension to tongue musculature & bony invasion of mandible in FOM squamous cell carcinoma (SCCa)
- Look for SMG tumor perineural spread in **lingual nerve** between medial pterygoid & mandibular ramus, then in direct contact with mandible medial to 3rd molar tooth, & finally in lateral SLG compartment
- Since neurovascular bundle to tongue travels in SLS, oral cavity SCCa involving posterior SLS challenging to treat

GRAPHIC & AXIAL CECT

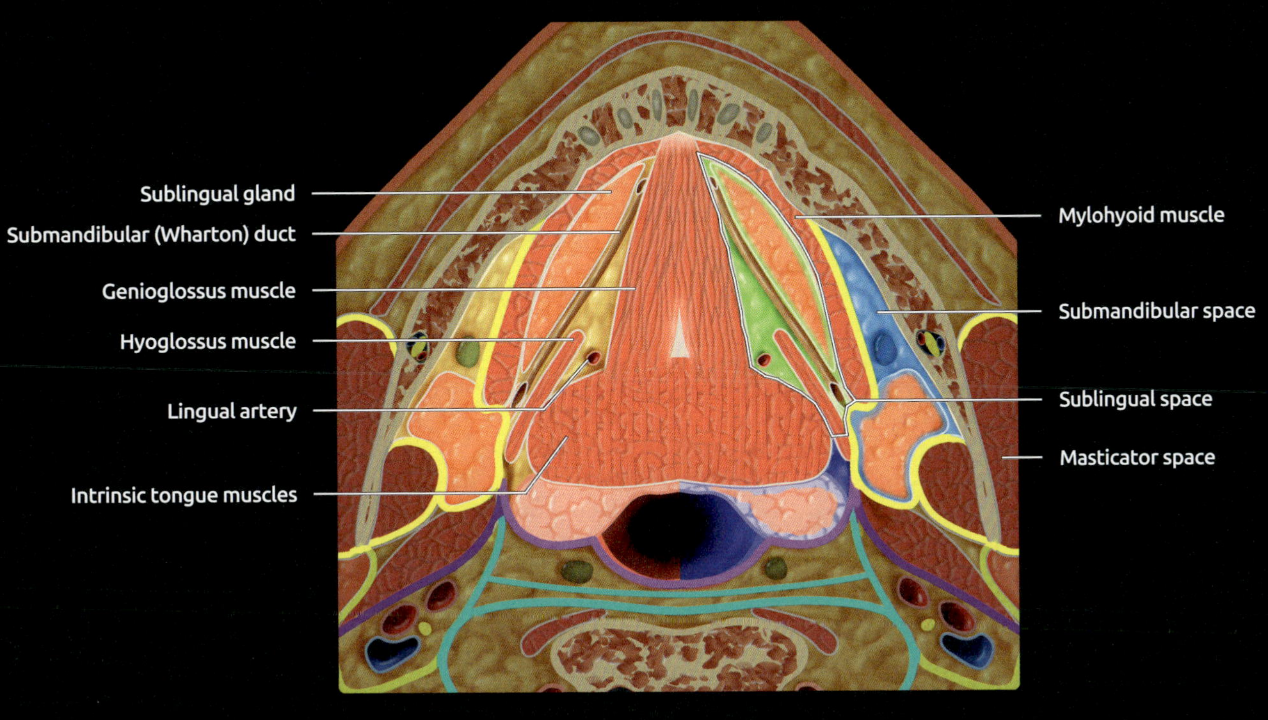

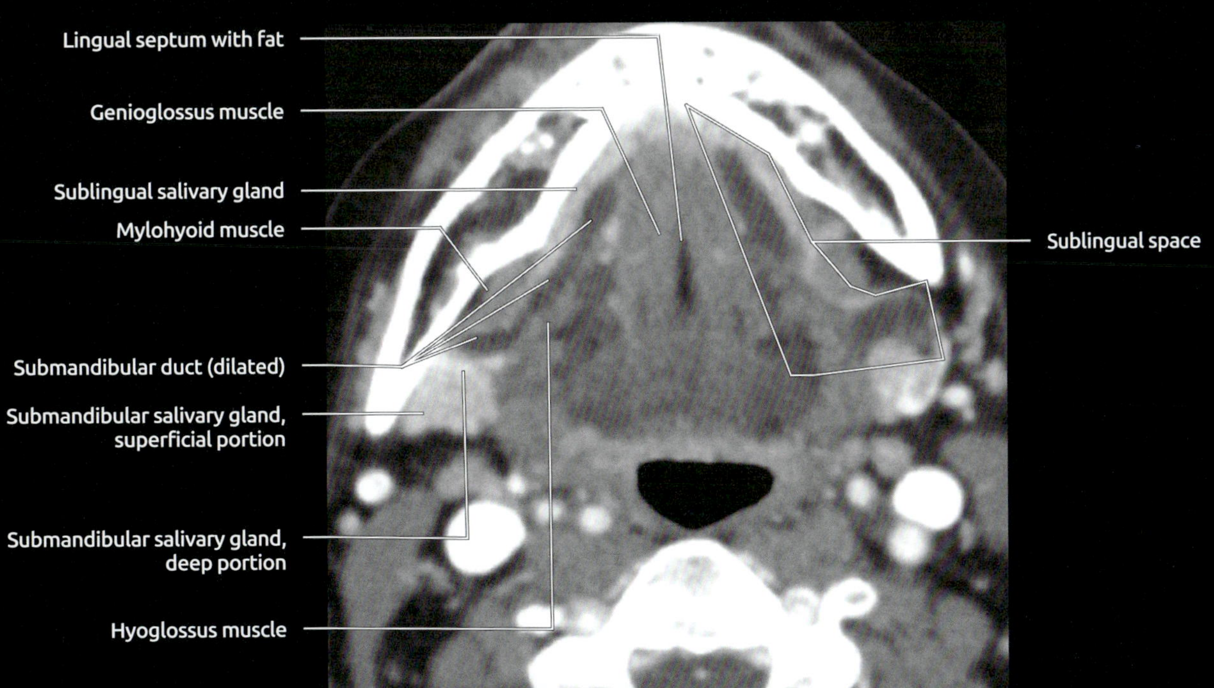

(Top) *Axial graphic through the body of the mandible shows the sublingual space (on the patient's left, shaded in green) situated superomedial to the mylohyoid muscle and lateral to the genioglossus muscle is shown. Notice the absence of fascia surrounding the sublingual space. The yellow line represents the superficial layer of deep cervical fascia.* **(Bottom)** *Axial CECT shows bilateral dilated submandibular (Wharton) ducts in the lateral sublingual space compartments due to midline anterior floor of mouth squamous cell carcinoma (not shown) obstructing their drainage. Sublingual space contents and genioglossus muscle, which is a component of the root of tongue, are marked on the right side. The hyoglossus muscle separates the sublingual space into a lateral and a medial compartment. The deep portion of the submandibular gland, where the Wharton duct originates from it, projects into the posterior margin of the sublingual space. The sublingual space is outlined on the patient's left. The submandibular duct and lingual nerve cross each other at the anterior border of the hyoglossus.*

CORONAL & SAGITTAL GRAPHICS

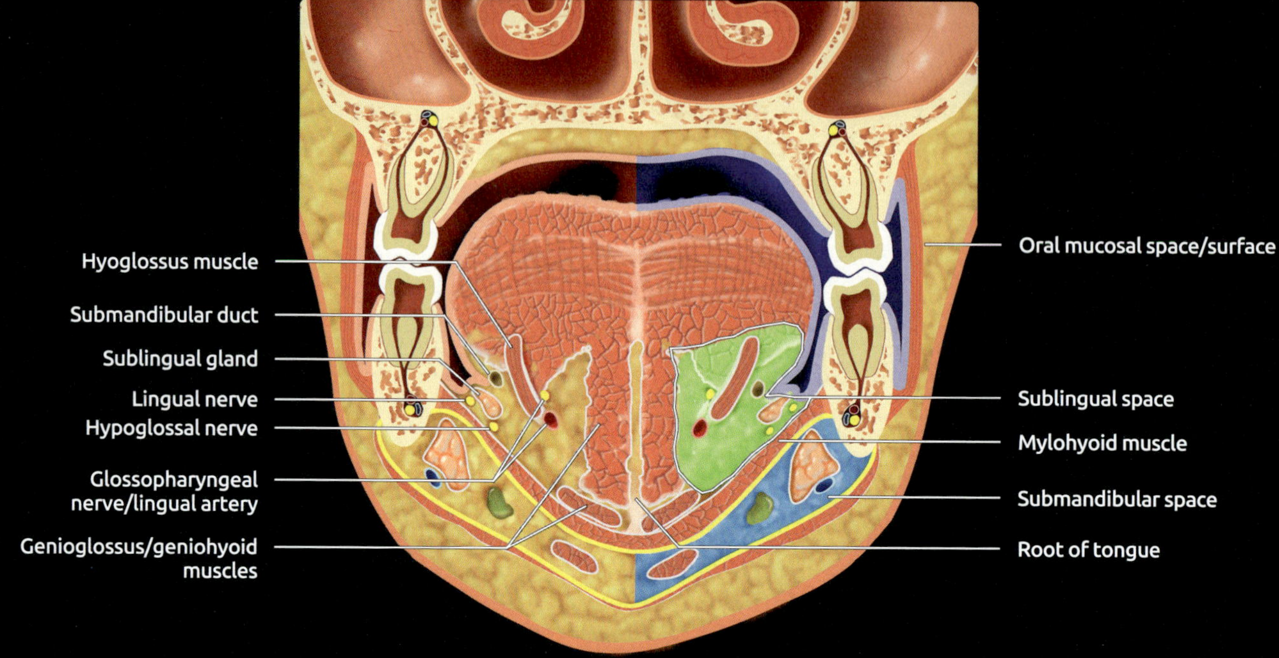

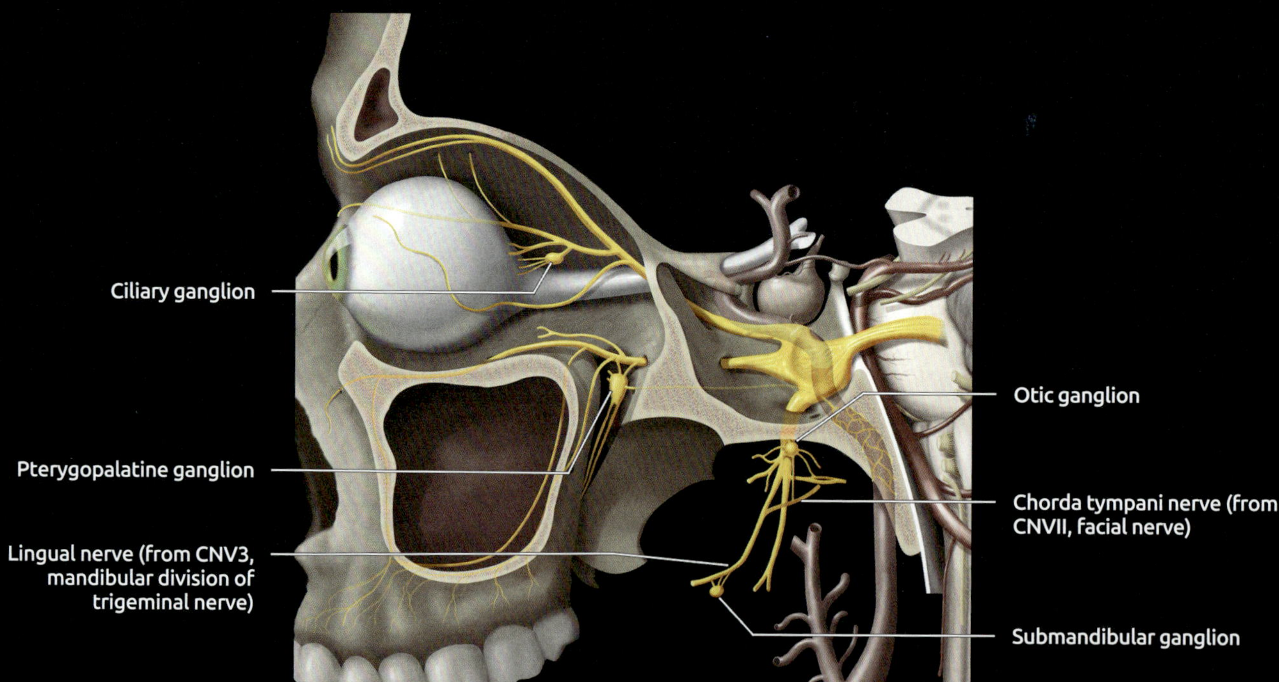

(Top) *In this coronal graphic through the oral cavity, the sublingual space is shaded in green. The sublingual space medial compartment contents include the glossopharyngeal nerve (CNIX) superiorly and the lingual artery and vein inferiorly. Lateral sublingual space compartment contents include the lingual nerve superolaterally; submandibular (Wharton) duct, sublingual salivary gland, deep part of submandibular salivary gland in the middle; and hypoglossal nerve (CNXII) inferomedially. The fascia-lined (yellow line) submandibular space is inferolateral to the mylohyoid muscle.* **(Bottom)** *Sagittal graphic shows 4 parasympathetic ganglia of the head. Submandibular ganglion lies in sublingual space on/lateral to hyoglossus muscle, just above the deep part of submandibular salivary gland. It is topographically connected to trigeminal nerve (CNV3) suspended from the lingual nerve by 2-3 roots, but functionally connected to facial nerve (CNVII branch, chorda tympani). Anterior root has postganglionic parasympathetic fibers reentering lingual nerve. Sympathetic fibers are from plexus around facial artery. Sensory fibers from lingual nerve may pass through the ganglion.*

AXIAL CECT

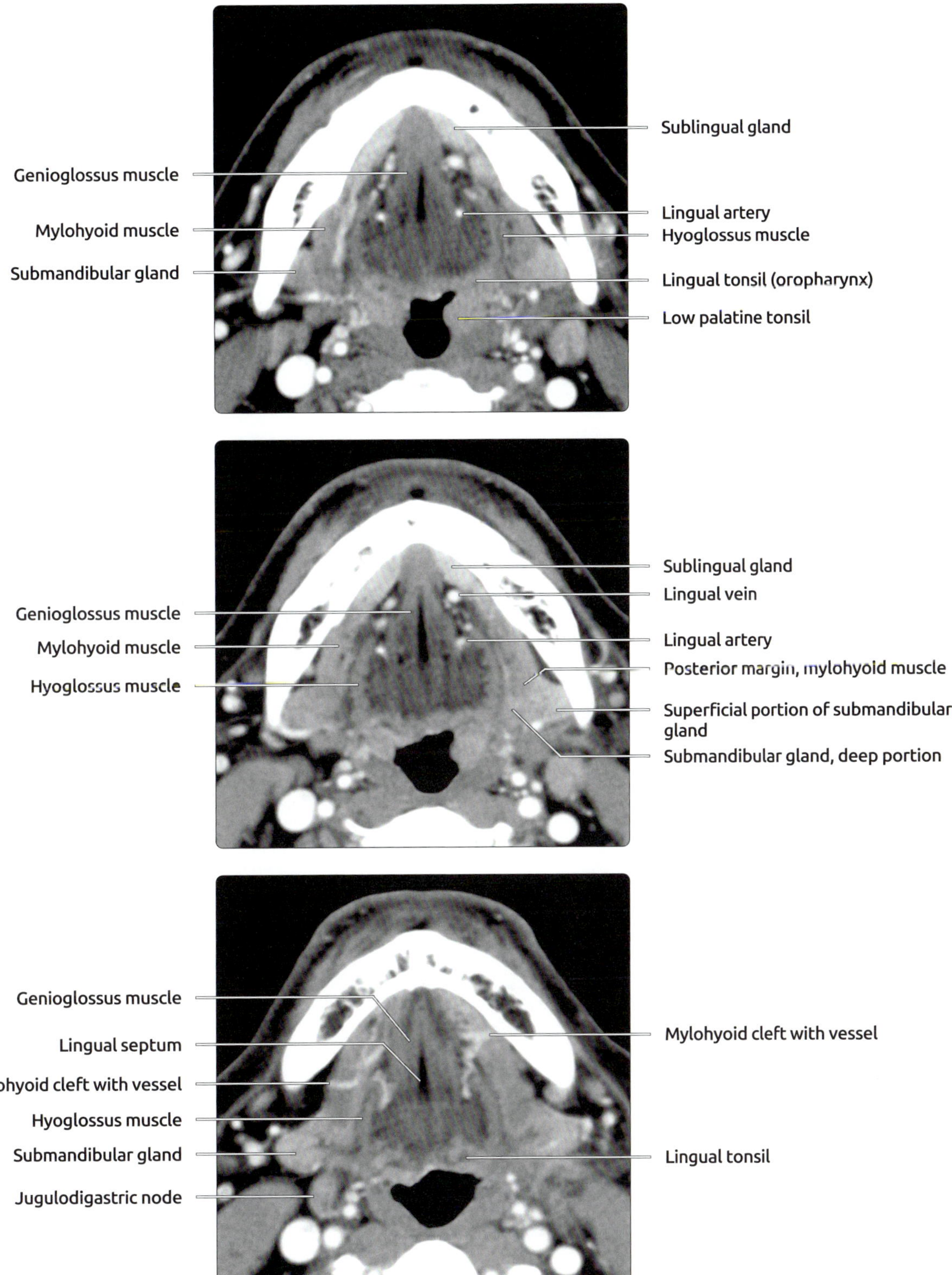

(Top) *The 1st of 3 axial CECT images of the sublingual space within the oral cavity is shown. This most superior image shows that the medial border of the sublingual space is the genioglossus muscle. The hyoglossus muscles are seen projecting into the posterior sublingual spaces. It can sometimes be difficult to separate the mylohyoid muscle from the sublingual gland on CECT.* **(Middle)** *More inferiorly, a larger portion of the mylohyoid muscle can be seen forming the inferolateral border of the sublingual space. Notice the submandibular gland wrapping around the posterior margin of this muscle on the patient's left. The deep portion of the submandibular gland is found in the posterior sublingual space.* **(Bottom)** *Inferiorly, the sublingual spaces become smaller with the hyoglossus muscle filling most of this space. Both mylohyoid muscles demonstrate small clefts with a vessel present bilaterally.*

AXIAL T2 FS MR

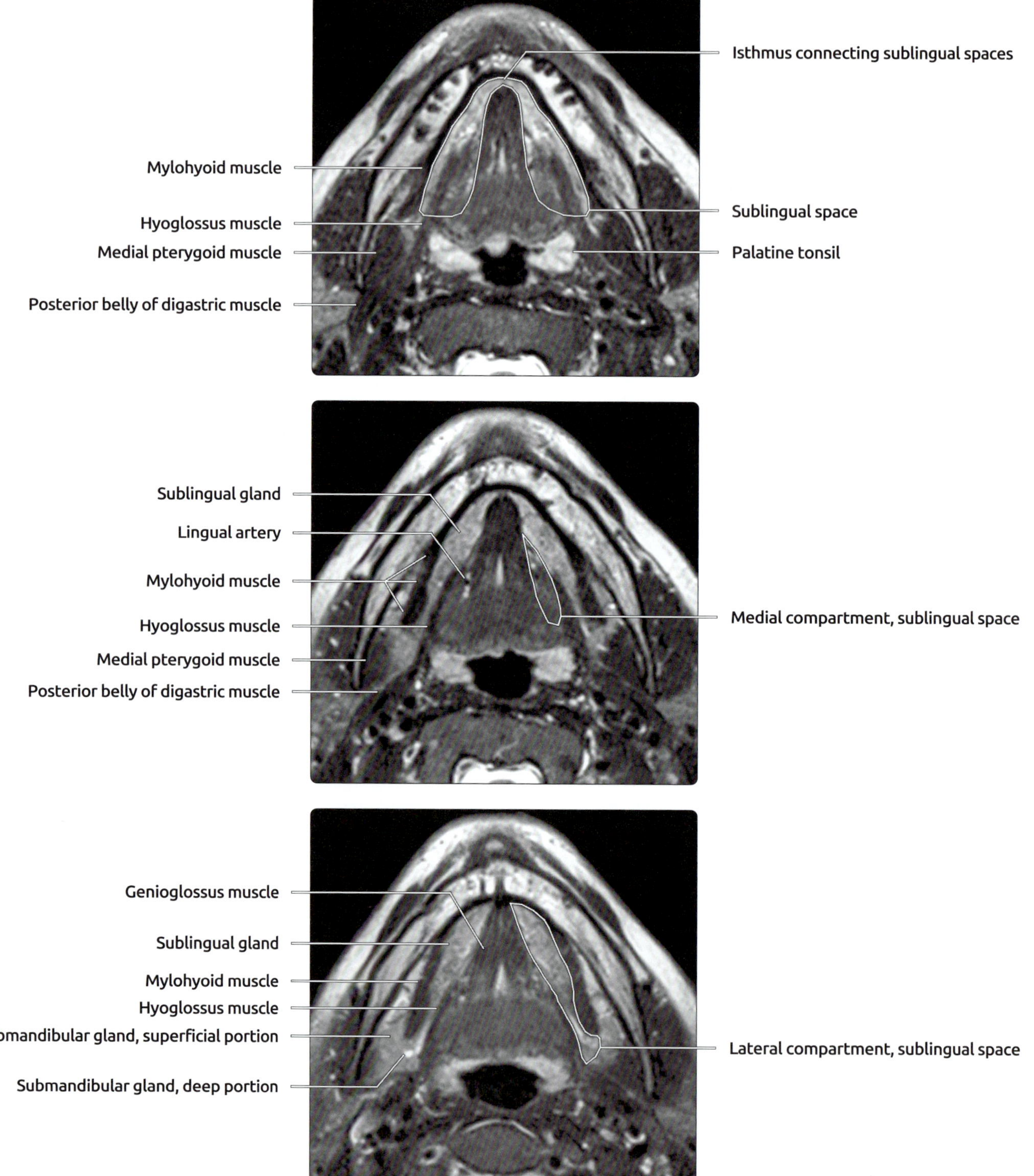

(Top) *The 1st of 3 axial T2 FS MR images presented from superior to inferior through the oral cavity is shown. In this most superior image, the 2 sublingual spaces are outlined to highlight the anterior connecting isthmus that is present under the frenulum of the oral tongue.* **(Middle)** *Slightly inferior, the medial compartment of the sublingual space is outlined on the patient's left. The medial compartment is defined as the sublingual space area medial to the hyoglossus muscle containing the lingual artery and vein as well as the glossopharyngeal nerve (CNIX).* **(Bottom)** *Continuing inferiorly, the submandibular gland deep portion is seen projecting into the posterior margin of the sublingual space. The lateral compartment of the sublingual space is outlined. It is defined as the sublingual space component lateral to hyoglossus muscle. It contains the sublingual gland, lingual nerve, hypoglossal nerve, and submandibular gland duct. The lingual nerve (CNV3 branch) runs anteroinferiorly between the medial pterygoid muscle and mandibular ramus, then in direct contact with the mandible medial to 3rd molar tooth, and finally in the lateral sublingual space compartment.*

CORONAL T1 MR

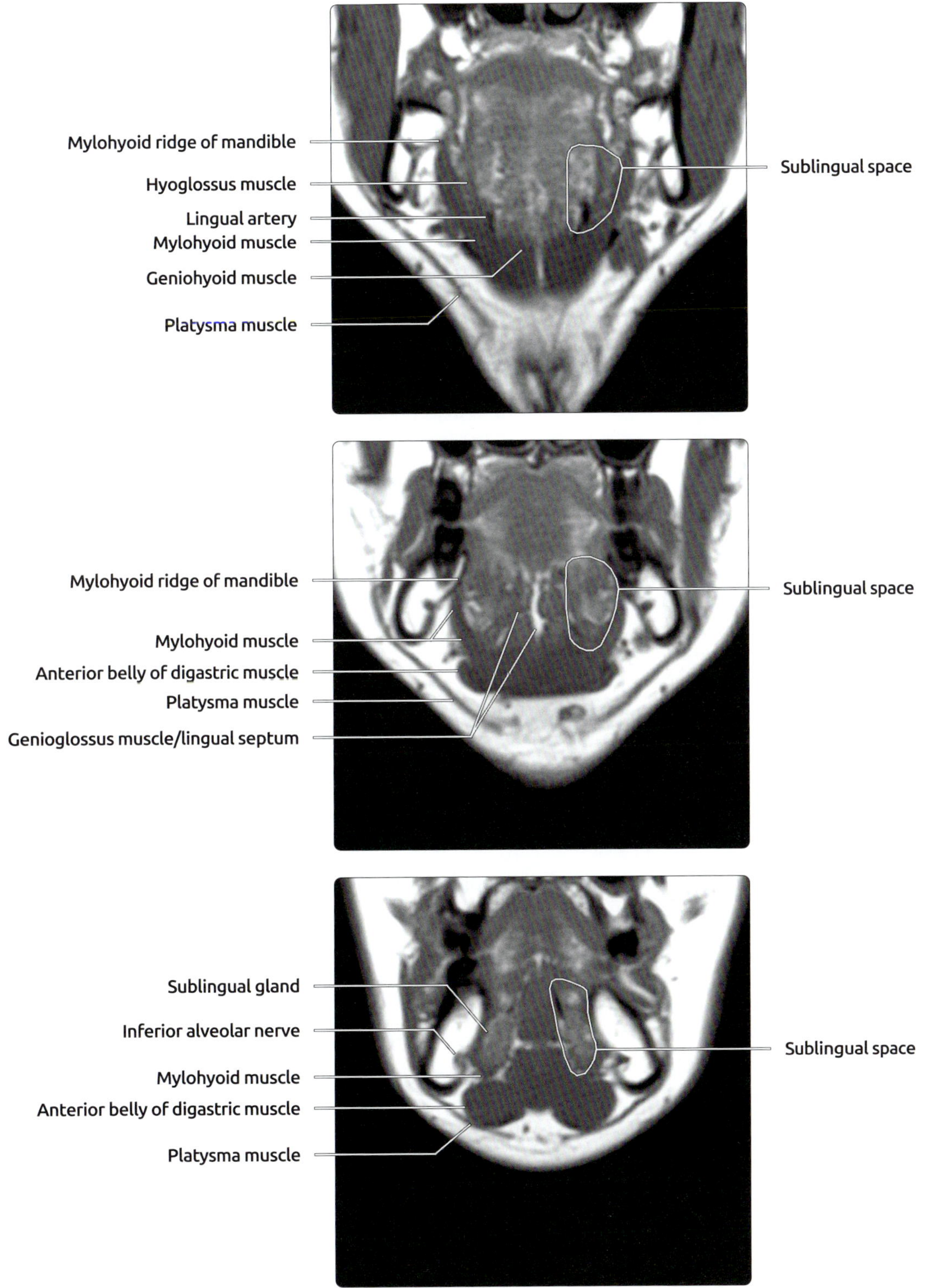

(Top) *The 1st of 3 coronal T1 MR images of a normal oral cavity/sublingual space presented from posterior to anterior is shown. In this most posterior image, the mylohyoid sling is slung from side to side between the mylohyoid ridges of the inner mandibular cortex. The sublingual space is superomedial to the mylohyoid muscle and lateral to the genioglossus and geniohyoid muscles.* **(Middle)** *Anteriorly, in the oral cavity, the true size of sublingual space is visible as delineated on the patient's left. Although it is possible to see the low-signal lingual artery, the remaining normal sublingual space structures are blended into the fibrofatty space itself.* **(Bottom)** *In the very anterior floor of the mouth, the anterior belly of the digastric muscles are the most prominent occupants of the submandibular space. The sublingual gland is mostly found within the anterior sublingual space where it takes up much of the space's volume.*

TERMINOLOGY

Abbreviations

- Submandibular space (SMS)

Definitions

- **Fascial-lined** space inferolateral to mylohyoid muscle containing submandibular salivary gland (SMG), nodes, & anterior belly of digastric muscle

IMAGING ANATOMY

Overview

- SMS is 1 of 4 distinct locations within oral cavity used to develop location-specific differential diagnoses
  - Other 3 locations include oral mucosal space/surface, sublingual space (SLS), & root of tongue

Extent

- Superficial space above hyoid bone deep to platysma & superficial to mylohyoid sling

Anatomy Relationships

- **Inferolateral to mylohyoid muscle**
- Deep to platysma muscle
- Cephalad to hyoid bone
- **Vertical horseshoe-shaped** space between hyoid bone below & mylohyoid sling above
- **Communicates** superiorly with posterior **SLS** & inferior **parapharyngeal space** at posterior margin of mylohyoid
- Continues into infrahyoid neck as **anterior cervical space**

Internal Contents

- **SMG**
  - Superficial layer, deep cervical fascia (SL-DCF) forms SMG capsule
  - **Superficial part:** Larger & in SMS itself
    - Crossed by facial vein & cervical branches of facial nerve (CNVII marginal mandibular branch)
  - **Deep part**: a.k.a. deep "process"
    - Smaller tongue-like extension of gland
    - Projects into posterior aspect of **SLS**
    - Wraps around posterior margin of mylohyoid muscle
    - **Submandibular (Wharton) duct** projects off deep process into **SLS**
  - SMG innervation: Branches from **submandibular ganglion** located **in SLS**
    - Parasympathetic secretomotor supply from chorda tympani (CNVII branch)
      - Via lingual nerve (CNV3)
- **Submental (level IA) & submandibular (level IB) nodes**
  - Lymphatic drainage from anterior facial region, including oral cavity & anterior sinonasal & orbital areas
  - Nodes below mylohyoid muscle, above inferior margin of hyoid bone & anterior to transverse lines drawn along posterior margins of each SMG
  - **Level IA** (**submental** nodes): Found between **medial margins** of anterior bellies of digastric muscles
  - **Level IB** (**submandibular** nodes): Nodes posterior & lateral to medial margin of anterior belly of digastric muscle; around SMG in SMS
- Facial vein & artery pass through SMS
- **Facial vein** in SMS courses **just lateral to SMG** & joins anterior branch of retromandibular vein (coursing along posterior aspect of SMG) to form common facial vein that in turn enters internal jugular vein slightly below this level
- **Caudal loop of CNXII** passes through SMS on its way before looping anteriorly & cephalad into tongue muscles
- **Anterior belly of digastric muscle**
- Tail of parotid gland may "hang down" into posterior SMS

Fascia

- **SMS lined by SL-DCF**
  - Superficial surface of mylohyoid covered by SL-DCF
  - Deep surface of platysma covered by SL-DCF
- **No midline fascia** separating 2 sides of SMS
  - Lesion growth from side to side in SMS unobstructed

ANATOMY IMAGING ISSUES

Questions

- Is mass nodal or SMG in origin?
  - Fatty cleavage plane between mass & SMG identifies lesion as nodal in origin
    - **Facial vein** separates lesion from SMG, then lesion from lymph node
  - "Beaking" of SMG tissue around lesion margin identifies lesion as SMG in origin
- Major diagnoses in SMS differential diagnoses list
  - Congenital: Epidermoid, cystic hygroma
  - Inflammatory: SMG sialoadenitis with ductal calculus; diving ranula; reactive or suppurative adenopathy
  - Benign tumor: Benign mixed tumor of SMG, lipoma
  - Malignant tumor: Salivary gland carcinomas; nodal squamous cell carcinoma & non-Hodgkin lymphoma

Imaging Recommendations

- CECT or T1 C+ fat-saturated MR both effective
- Ultrasound with needle aspiration of lesion also used

Imaging Pitfalls

- Do not mistake obstructed, enlarged SMG for malignant node in setting of anterior floor of mouth primary squamous cell carcinoma
  - Look for **floor of mouth/SLS lesion** when submandibular **(Wharton) duct dilated** & no obstructive salivary stone seen in duct

CLINICAL IMPLICATIONS

Clinical Importance

- Majority of lesions of SMS either from SMG or nodes
  - Sorting lesions into these 2 categories helps work through imaging differential diagnosis
  - SMGs frequently excised during neck dissection due to their proximity to primary lesion & afferent lymph nodes
- Remember, clinicians can see & feel area of SMS
- Incision to perform SMG excision for calculus or tumor must be placed ≥ 4 cm below angle of mandible to preserve marginal mandibular branch of facial nerve, which passes posteroinferior to angle
- **Parotid tail lesions** may appear in posterior SMS clinically
- **Remember: Deep part of SMG, submandibular duct**, & **submandibular ganglion** lie in **SLS** (not SMS)

GRAPHIC AND AXIAL T2 MR

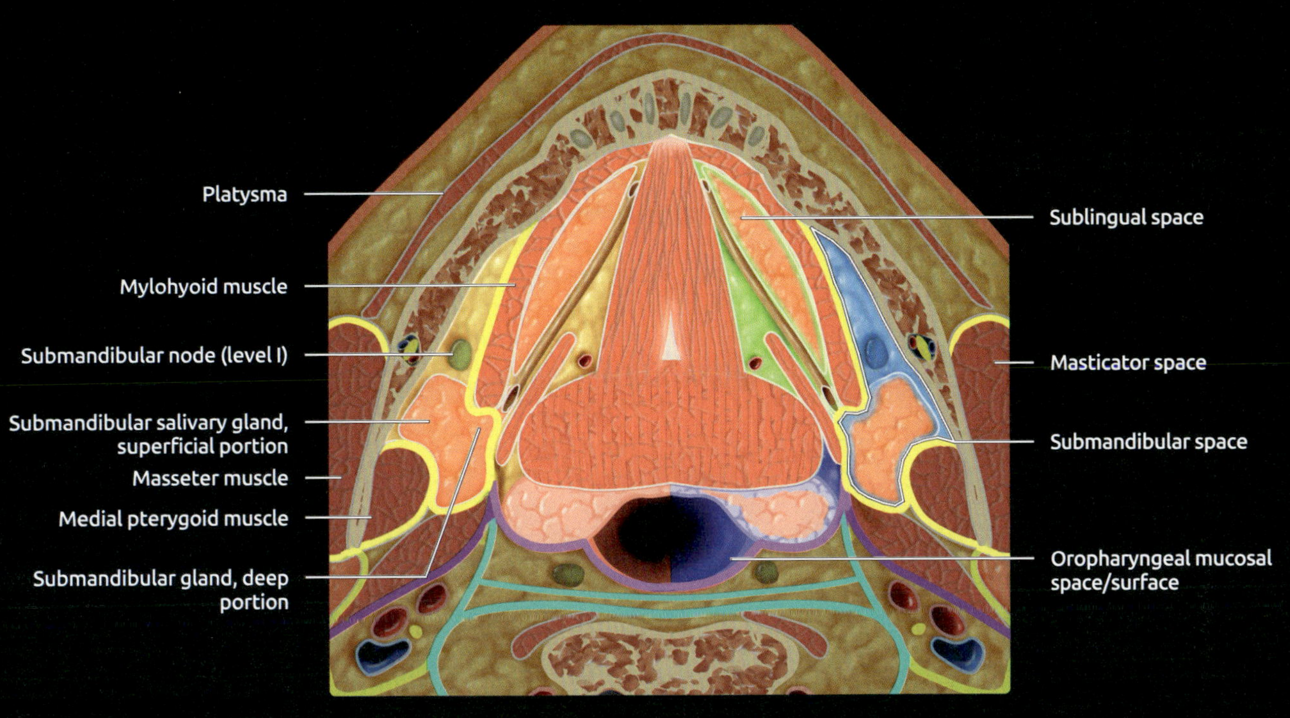

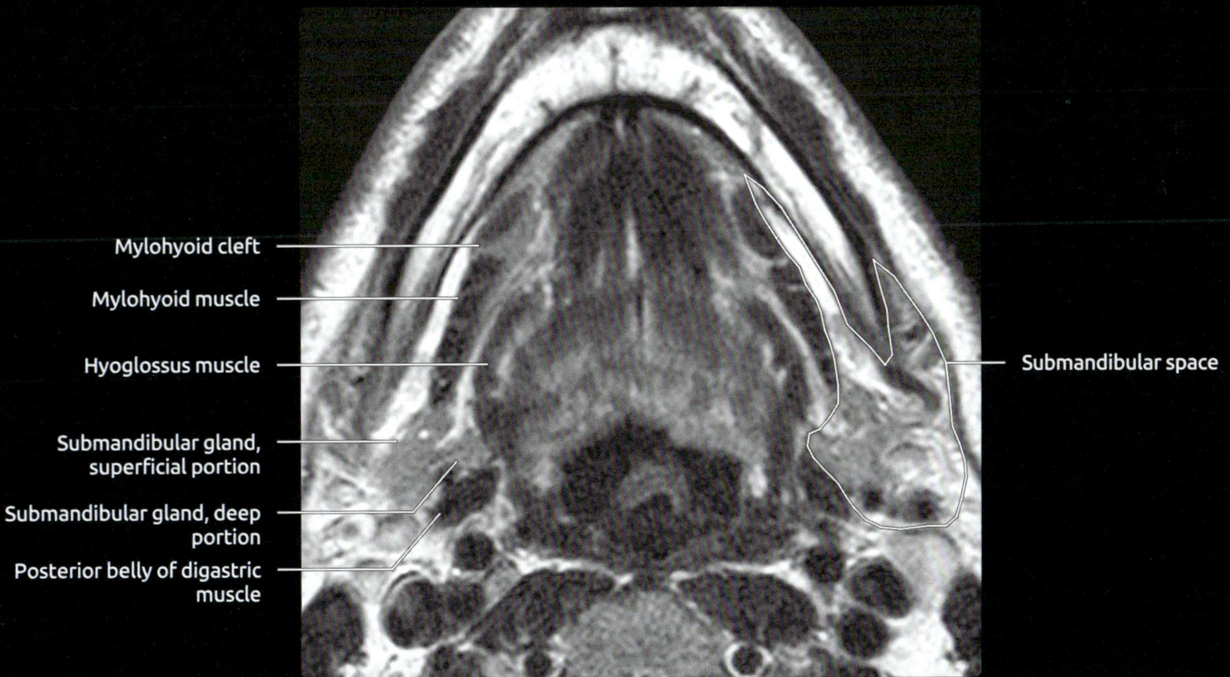

(Top) *Axial graphic shows the oral cavity with emphasis on the submandibular space (SMS) shaded in light blue on the patient's left. The SMS is inferolateral to the mylohyoid muscle. Note the principal occupants of the SMS are the submandibular salivary gland (SMG) and nodes.* **(Bottom)** *Axial T2 MR demonstrates the axial appearance of the SMS outlined on the patient's left. The principal occupants of the SMS are the SMG and nodes. Consequently, the differential diagnosis of lesions of this space includes gland tumors and lymph node diseases.*

GRAPHIC & CORONAL T1 MR

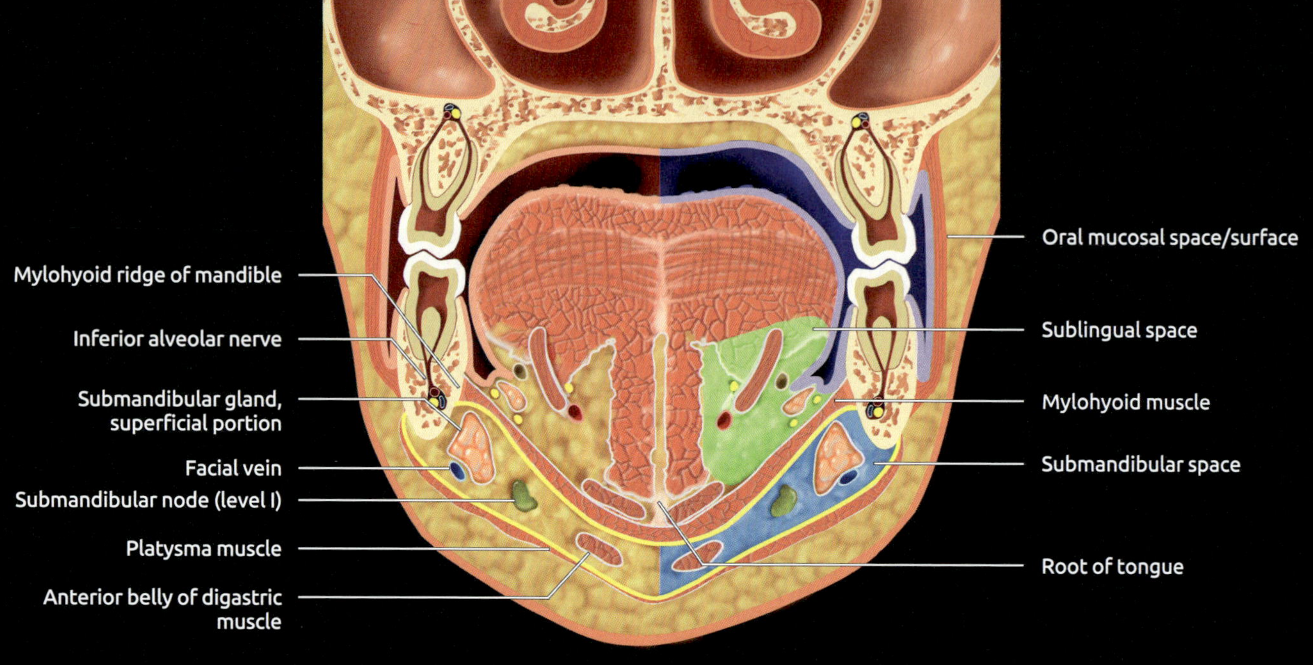

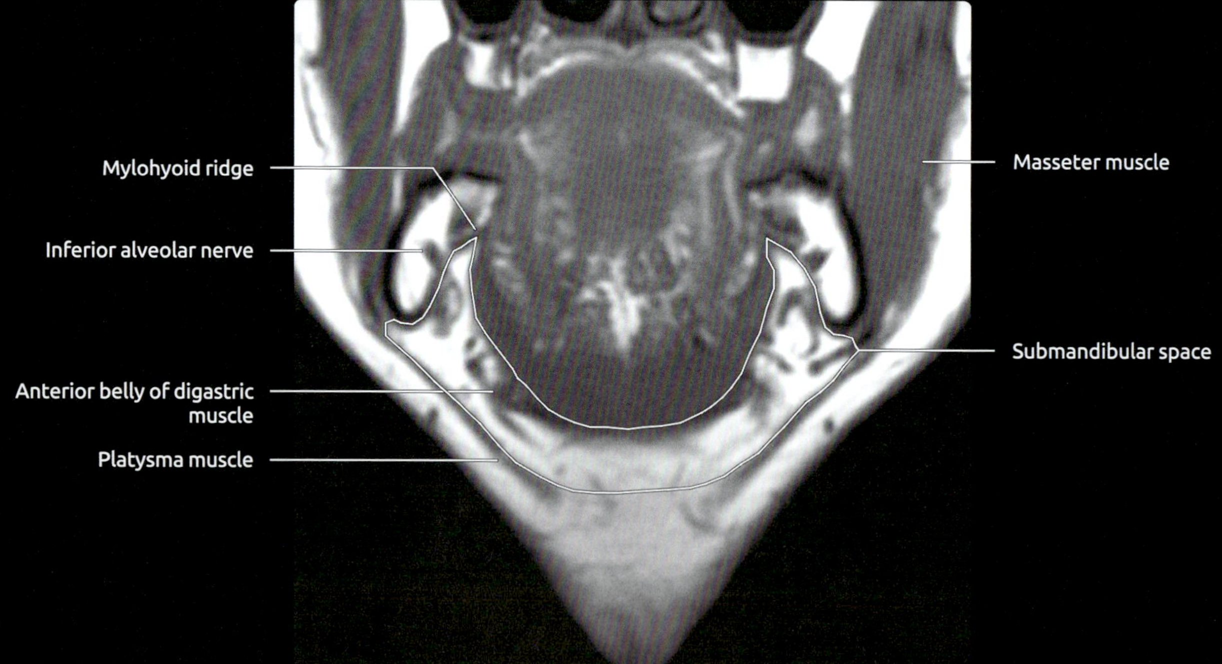

(Top) *In this coronal graphic through the oral cavity, the SMS is shaded in light blue. The superficial layer of deep cervical fascia (yellow line) is seen lining the vertical horseshoe-shaped SMS inferolateral to the mylohyoid muscle. Contents of the SMS are the anterior belly of the digastric muscle, submandibular nodes, SMG, and facial vein. Notice the platysma forms the superficial margin of the SMS.* **(Bottom)** *Coronal T1 MR shows the horseshoe-shaped SMS extending from side to side inferior and inferolateral to the mylohyoid muscle and deep to the platysma muscle. Notice the lack of vertical fascia or septation. Consequently, lesions of the SMS spread readily across the midline.*

AXIAL CECT

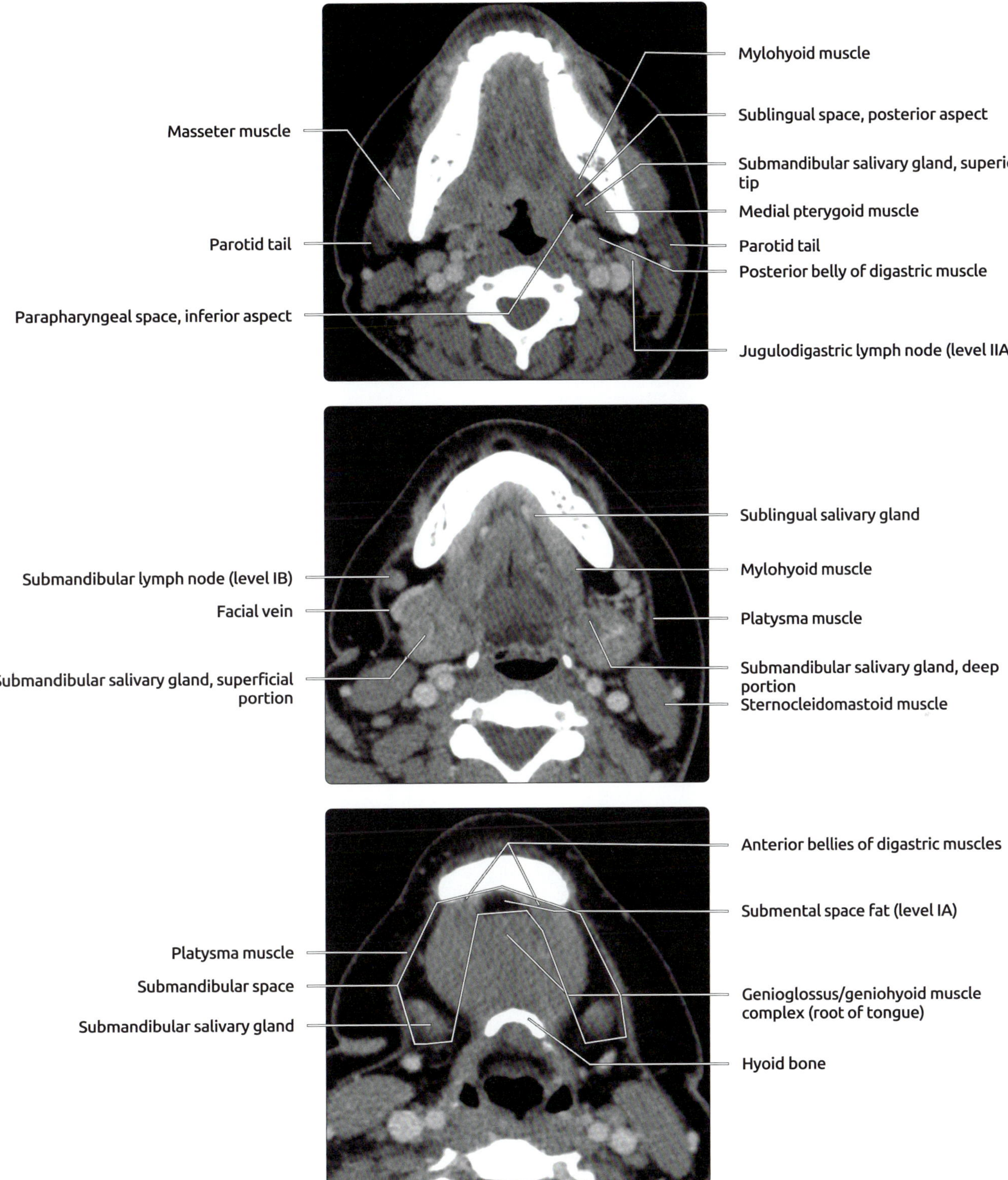

(Top) *First of 3 axial CECT images from superior to inferior is shown. This most superior image reveals the uppermost portion of the SMS. Note the parotid gland tail projecting into the posterior SMS; parotid tail lesions may be palpated clinically in the posterior SMS. The SMS communicates superiorly with the posterior sublingual space and inferior parapharyngeal space at the posterior margin of the mylohyoid muscle.* **(Middle)** *CECT through the mid-SMS shows the bulk of the SMG and the facial vein along its lateral margin, separating the salivary gland from a level IB lymph node. The deep portion of SMG and Wharton duct lies in the sublingual space and not in the SMS.* **(Bottom)** *Low SMS axial CECT highlights the full extent of the horseshoe-shaped SMS. The SMS lies deep to platysma muscle and contains the bilateral anterior bellies of digastric (ABD) muscles filling the anteromedial SMS. The submental space (part of SMS) lies between the medial margins of ABD; level IA submental lymph nodes are situated here. Level IB (submandibular nodes) lie posterior and lateral to the medial margin of ABD; anterior to transverse lines are drawn along the posterior margins of each SMG.*

AXIAL T2 MR

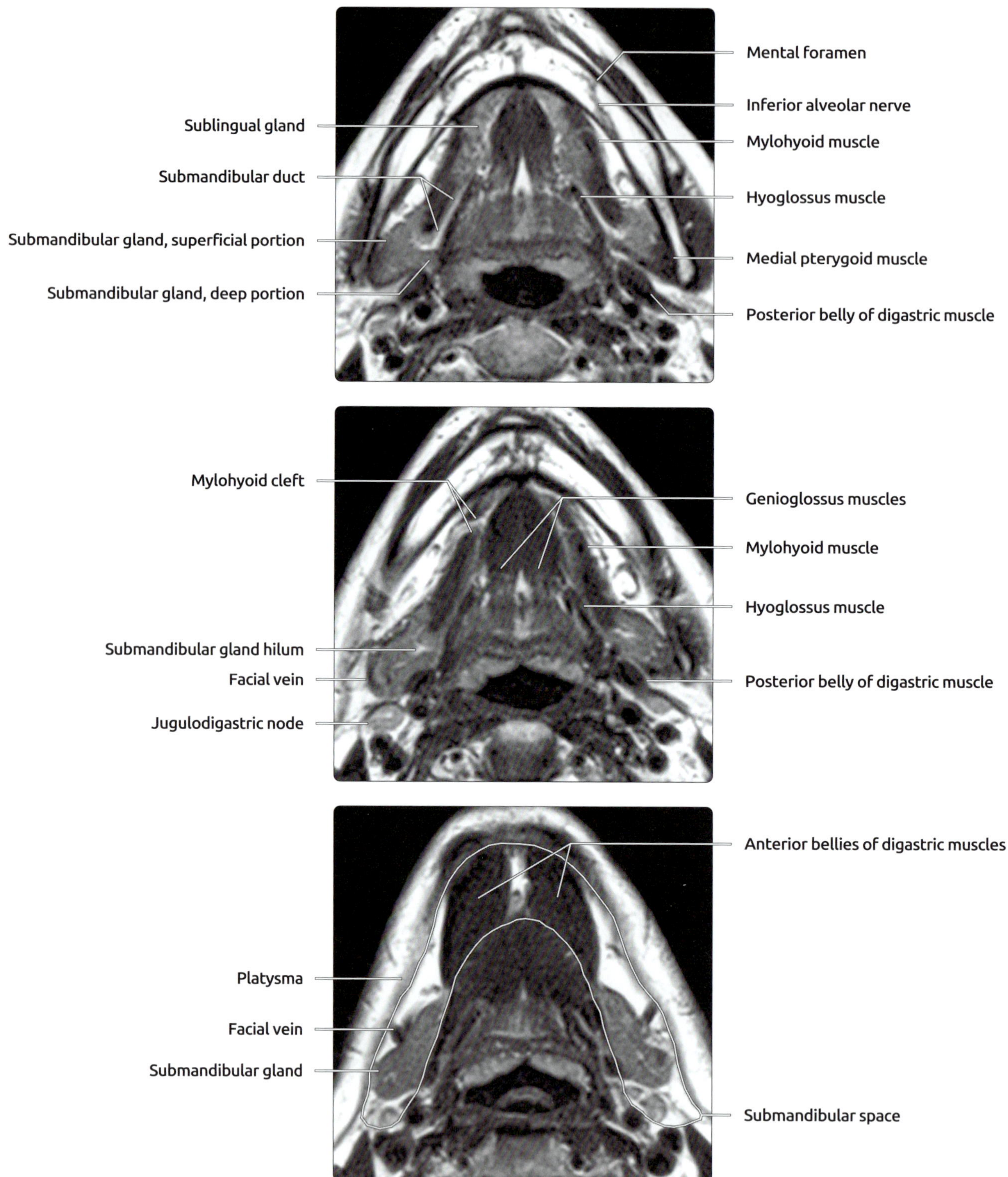

(Top) *First of 3 axial T2 MR images of the oral cavity from superior to inferior is shown. In this most superior image, the upper SMS is evident, filled with fat and the upper SMGs. Notice the high-signal submandibular ducts entering the posterior sublingual spaces bilaterally.* **(Middle)** *Moving inferiorly, more fat is seen in the SMS bilaterally surrounding the SMGs. Both SMGs can be seen wrapping around the posterior margins of the mylohyoid muscles. Remember that the neurovascular pedicle to each side of the tongue enters closely approximated to the hyoglossus muscles.* **(Bottom)** *Low in the SMS, the full extent of both SMSs is visible. Notice that the ABD muscles fill the anteromedial SMS. Remember, there is no midline fascia, so diseases can move across midline from side to side.*

CORONAL T1 MR

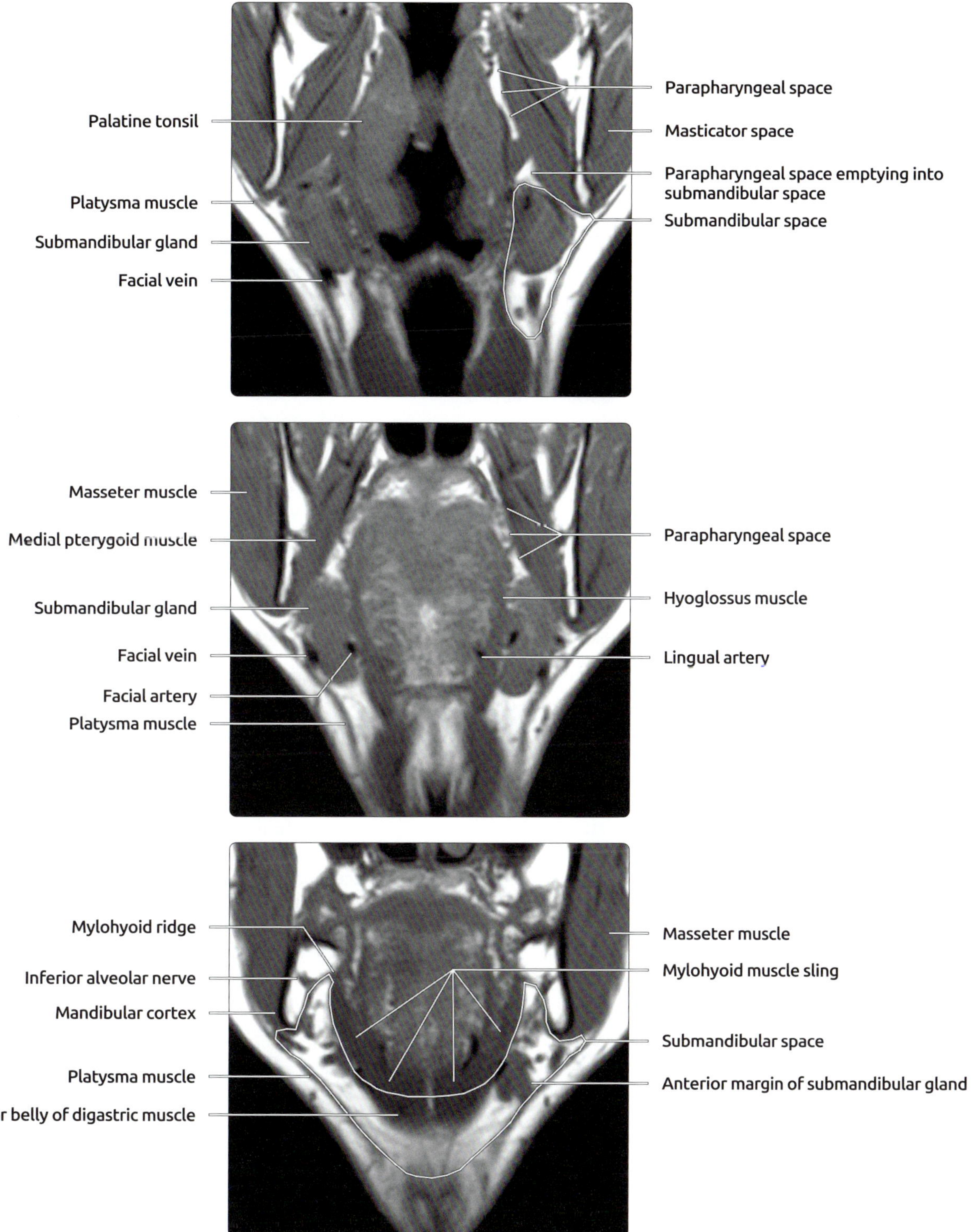

(Top) *First of 3 coronal T1 MR images presented from posterior to anterior is shown. This most posterior image shows the area of the SMS outlined on the patient's left. Notice the parapharyngeal space empties inferiorly into the posterior SMS.* **(Middle)** *More anteriorly, the connection between the parapharyngeal space and the SMS is still visible. The facial vein is visible snaking along the inferolateral margin of the SMG. Remember that if the facial vein is seen between a mass and the gland, it is most likely nodal in origin.* **(Bottom)** *In this image through the midoral cavity, the full extent of the SMS is clearly visible from side to side. The location of the superficial layer of deep cervical fascia is outlined. The mylohyoid sling forms the superomedial border of the SMS. The superficial margin of the SMS is the platysma muscle.*

TERMINOLOGY

Abbreviations

- Buccal space (BS)

Definitions

- Small anatomic space or compartment in deep face situated between buccinator muscle medially, greater and lesser zygomatic muscles laterally, and masticator space posteriorly; contains buccal fat pad, distal parotid duct, facial artery and vein

IMAGING ANATOMY

Overview

- BS received less attention in anatomic and radiologic literature than other spaces in neck
- BS interdigitates between oral cavity, superficial muscular aponeurotic system (SMAS), and masticator space
- Contains adipose tissue with conspicuous **buccal fat pad** that is easily identified with CT and MR
- Buccal fat pad separated from superficial malar fat by zygomaticus muscles and SMAS

Extent

- Medial: Bounded by (but does not include) **buccinator muscle**
  - **BS does not include buccal mucosa** (part of oral cavity mucosal space) or minor salivary glands
  - Separated from buccal mucosa by buccinator muscle and thin layer of submucosal fat
  - Buccinator attachments: Alveolar ridge of maxilla superiorly, alveolar ridge of mandible inferiorly, pterygomandibular raphe posteriorly, and orbicularis oris anteriorly
- Lateral: Several muscles of facial expression in cheek (including greater and lesser zygomatic muscles and risorius muscle) and their associated investing fascia (SMAS)
- Anterior: Orbicularis oris and ventral attachments of zygomatic muscles
- Posterior: Parotid gland laterally and anterior border of lateral pterygoid muscle medially

Internal Contents

- **Buccal fat pad**
  - Represents distinct adipose tissue, composed of fat termed **syssarcosis** (fat that facilitates adjacent muscular motion)
  - Posterior portion of buccal fat pad may represent remnants of succatory fat pad in infants
  - **4 projections** of adipose tissue extend from main buccal fat pad
    - **Posterolateral**: Extends along parotid duct to parotid gland
      - Bounded by superficial layer of deep cervical fascia and facial muscles laterally and parotidomasseteric fascia medially
    - **Posteromedial**: Interposed between mandible laterally and maxilla medially
      - Contiguous with retromaxillary fat
      - Often communicates with masticator space itself
    - **Anterior**: Lies ventral to distal parotid duct and insinuates between buccinator muscle and adjacent muscles of facial expression
    - **Temporal**: Extends superiorly and divides into superficial and deep portion, relative to temporalis muscle
      - Thin superficial portion lies between temporalis muscle and overlying superficial fascia
      - Deep portion passes behind lateral orbital wall and extends to greater wing of sphenoid
- **Distal parotid duct**
  - Passes anteriorly from parotid gland, lateral to masseter muscle, and then turns medially along ventral aspect of masseter muscle
  - Passes through buccal fat pad on its way to its termination in oral cavity at level of maxillary 2nd molar
  - Divides BS into **anterior and posterior divisions**
- **Minor salivary gland tissue**
  - Microscopic submucosal structures found throughout upper aerodigestive tract
  - Occasionally, present in BS; can give rise to minor salivary gland tumors, most common of primary BS tumors
- **Vessels**
  - **Facial vein**: Typically located just anterior to parotid duct on axial images; ultimately drains into external jugular system
  - **Facial artery**: Branch of external carotid artery that extends through BS to nasolabial fold region
  - **Buccal artery**: Branch of internal maxillary artery in masticator space and extends to BS, passing between medial margin of masseter muscle and lateral margin of buccinator muscle; anastomoses with facial artery
- **Nerves**
  - **Buccal branch of facial nerve (CNVII)** innervates buccinator muscles and nearby muscles of facial expression
  - **Buccal branch of mandibular nerve (CNV3)** provides sensory innervation to BS as well as buccal mucosa
- **Accessory parotid tissue**
  - Present in 20%; usually anterior to parotid gland and superficial to masseter muscle
  - Can give rise to common parotid gland pathology, including inflammation and neoplasm
- **Lymph nodes**
  - 1-3 buccal lymph nodes are present along lateral edge of buccinator muscle
  - Buccal nodes ultimately drain into submandibular nodes

ANATOMY IMAGING ISSUES

Imaging Recommendations

- CECT of neck/face: 1st-line imaging tool
- Multiplanar MR, including T1 without fat saturation and T1 C+ with fat saturation in axial and coronal planes

Imaging Approaches

- Location of lesion in relationship to buccinator muscle offers clue regarding etiology, i.e., mucosal vs. minor salivary gland neoplasm (medial/superficial) vs. vascular malformation (deep/lateral)
- Puffed cheek technique to better delineate early buccal mucosal cancer

GRAPHICS

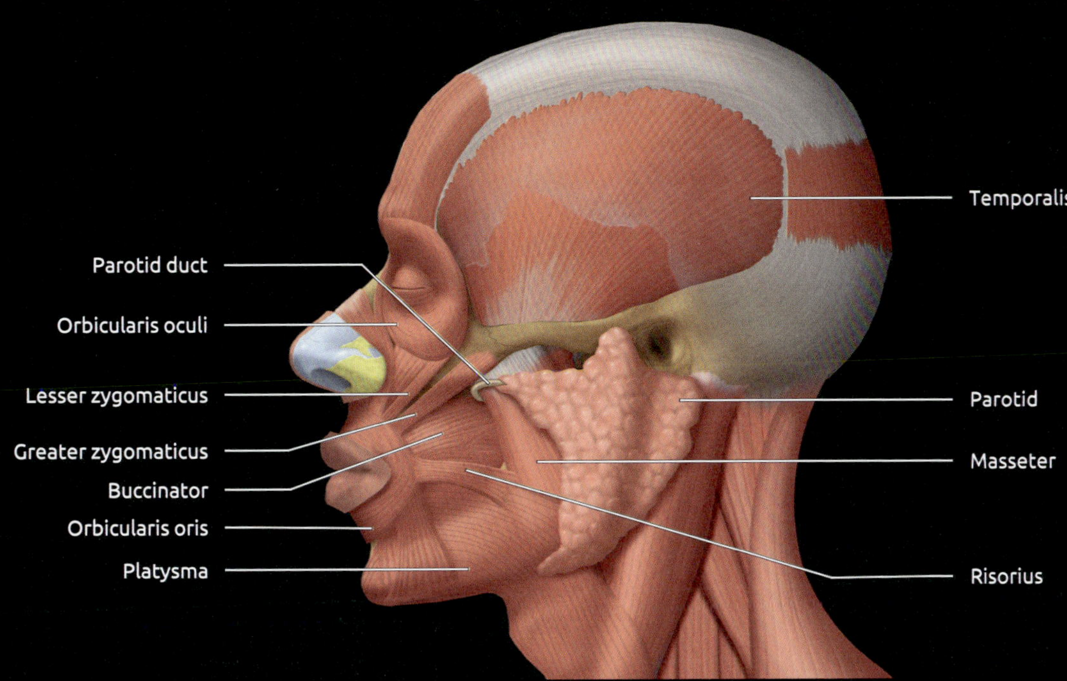

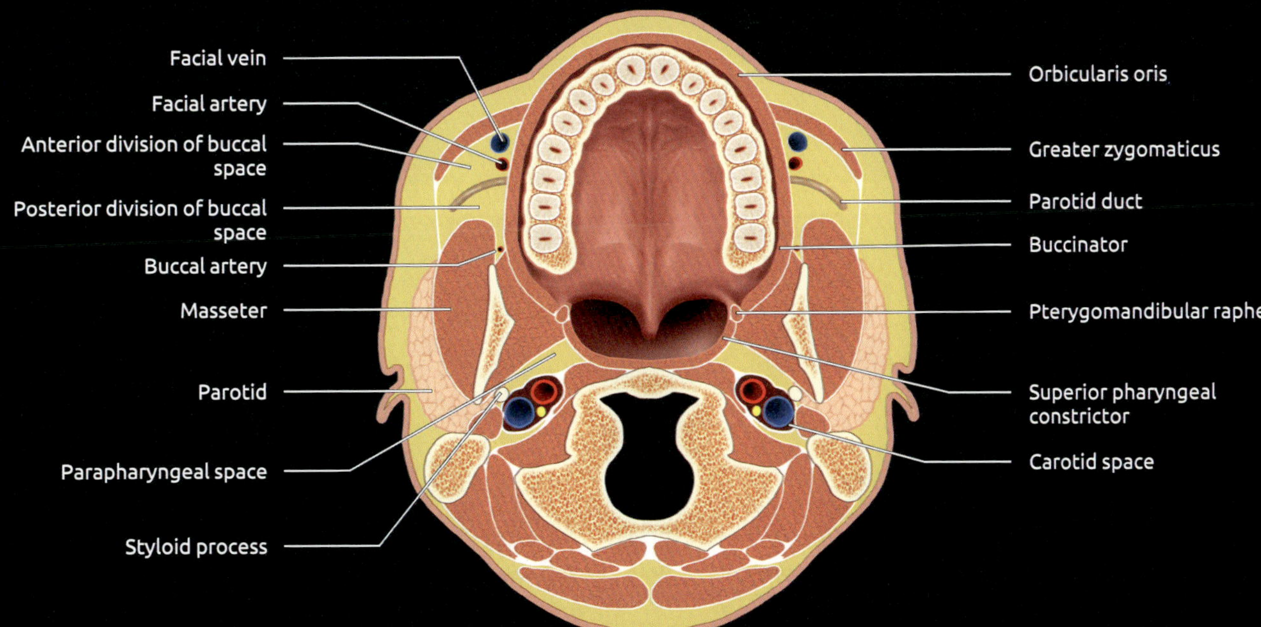

(Top) *Graphic shows extent of buccal space (BS). The medial boundary is formed by buccinator muscle, and the lateral boundary is formed by greater and lesser zygomaticus muscles. Anteriorly, it is limited by the junction of zygomaticus muscles with orbicularis oris and posteriorly by the parotid gland laterally and medially by the masseter muscle.* **(Bottom)** *Graphic shows fat-containing BS. Parotid duct running through the BS divides it into anterior and posterior divisions. The anterior division contains facial vein and facial artery, and the posterior division contains buccal artery. The posterior division is further divided into posteromedial (interposed between mandible and maxilla) and posterolateral (extending along parotid duct). The posteromedial extension is contiguous with retromaxillary fat, which is also an extension of buccal fat.*

BUCCAL SPACE ANATOMY: AXIAL CT

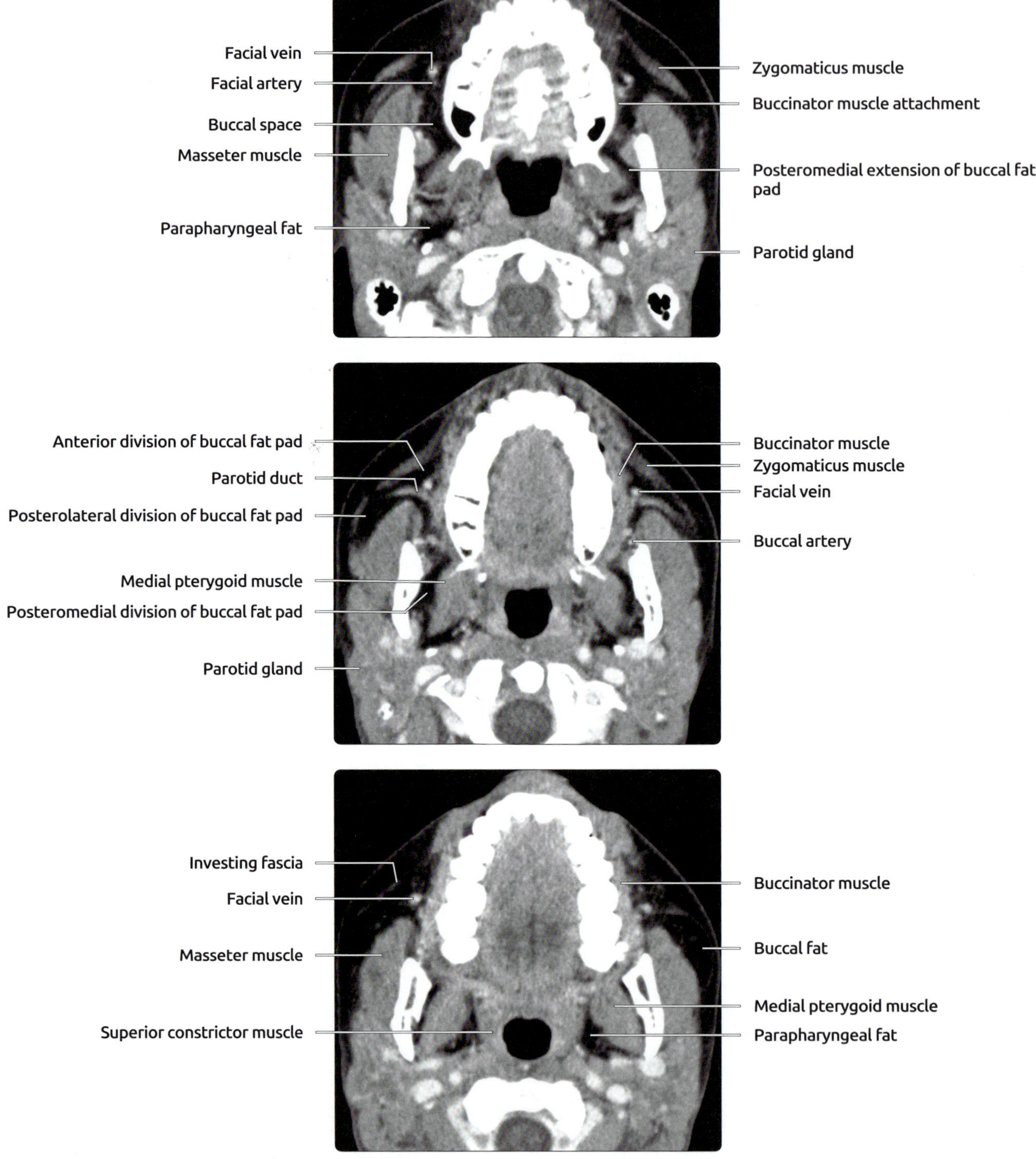

(Top) *Axial CECT shows the upper BS. The medial boundary of this fat-containing BS is formed by the buccinator muscle, which is attached superiorly to the alveolar ridge of the maxilla, and the lateral boundary is formed by zygomaticus muscles. The facial artery and vein are seen in the anterior division of the BS. The posteromedial extension of the BS is contiguous with retroantral buccal fat.* **(Middle)** *Axial CECT shows the mid-BS. The distal parotid duct divides the BS into anterior and posterior divisions. The posterior division is again divided into posteromedial and posterolateral extensions. The buccal artery is seen traversing the posterior division of the BS.* **(Bottom)** *Axial CECT shows the lower BS. A thin investing facia, which is part of superficial muscular aponeurotic system (SMAS), is seen separating buccal fat from subcutaneous fat laterally. The superior pharyngeal constrictor is attached to the buccinator muscle along the pterygomandibular raphe.*

BUCCAL SPACE ANATOMY: AXIAL MR

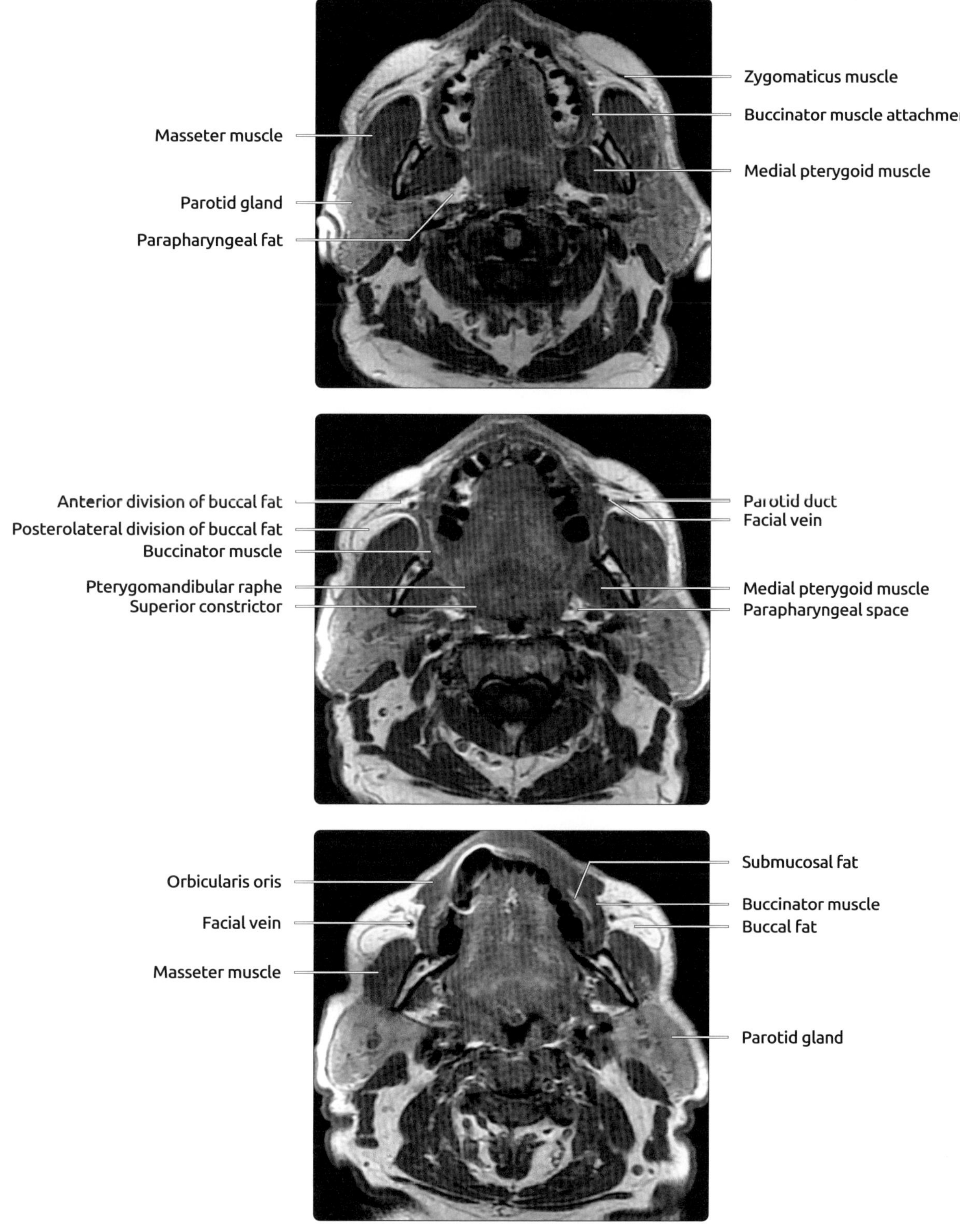

(Top) *Axial T1WI MR shows the upper BS. The lateral boundary of this fat-containing BS is formed by zygomaticus muscles. The buccinator muscle is seen attached to the alveolar ridge of the maxilla superiorly and to the alveolar ridge of the mandible inferiorly (not shown).* **(Middle)** *Axial T1WI MR shows the mid-BS. The distal parotid duct is seen traversing the BS, which divides it into anterior and posterior divisions. The anterior division contains the facial artery and vein. The buccinator muscle is attached posteriorly to the superior constrictor muscles through the pterygomandibular raphe. The posterior border of the BS is defined by the parotid gland laterally and the masticator space medially.* **(Bottom)** *Axial T1WI MR shows the lower BS. The anterior border of this space is formed by the zygomaticus muscle's attachment to the orbicularis oris muscle. The medial boundary formed by the buccinator muscle is separated from the buccal mucosa by the submucosal fat plane.*

BUCCAL SPACE ANATOMY: CORONAL MR

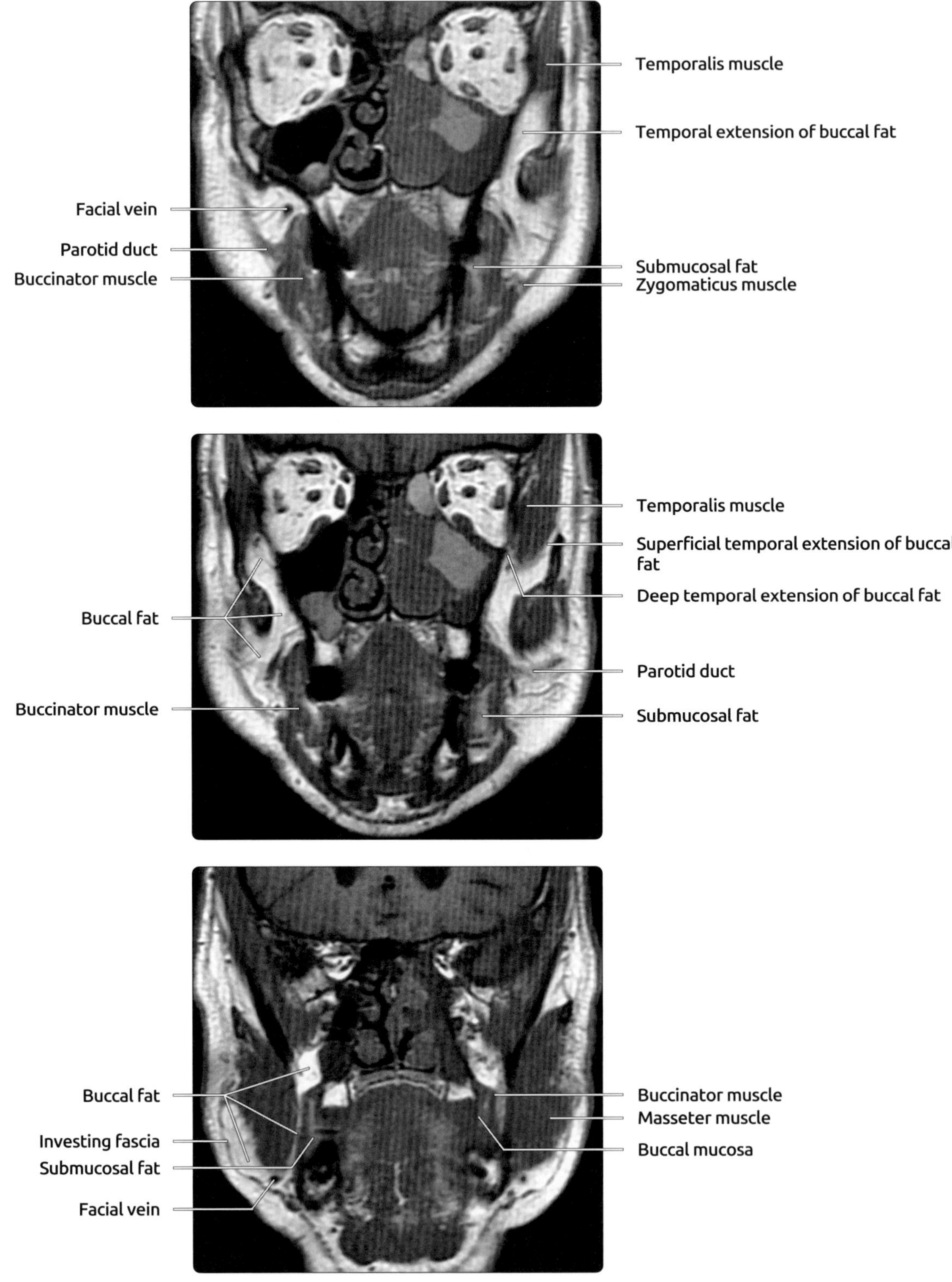

(Top) *Coronal T1WI MR through the anterior BS shows the zygomaticus muscle forming the lateral boundary of the BS on the left, anteriorly attached to the orbicularis oris muscle. On the right, the distal parotid duct is seen piercing the buccinator muscle. The facial vein is seen traversing the BS.* **(Middle)** *Coronal T1WI MR through the mid-BS shows the superior and inferior attachment of the buccinator muscle along the maxillary and mandibular alveolar ridge, respectively. The medial boundary of the BS is formed by the buccinator muscle, which is separated from the buccal mucosa by submucosal fat. The BS shows superior temporal extension both superficial and deep to the temporalis muscle.* **(Bottom)** *Coronal T1WI MR through the posterior BS shows the investing fascia, which is part of the SMAS, separating the BS from subcutaneous fat.*

ANATOMIC-PATHOLOGIC CORRELATION SQUAMOUS CELL CARCINOMA

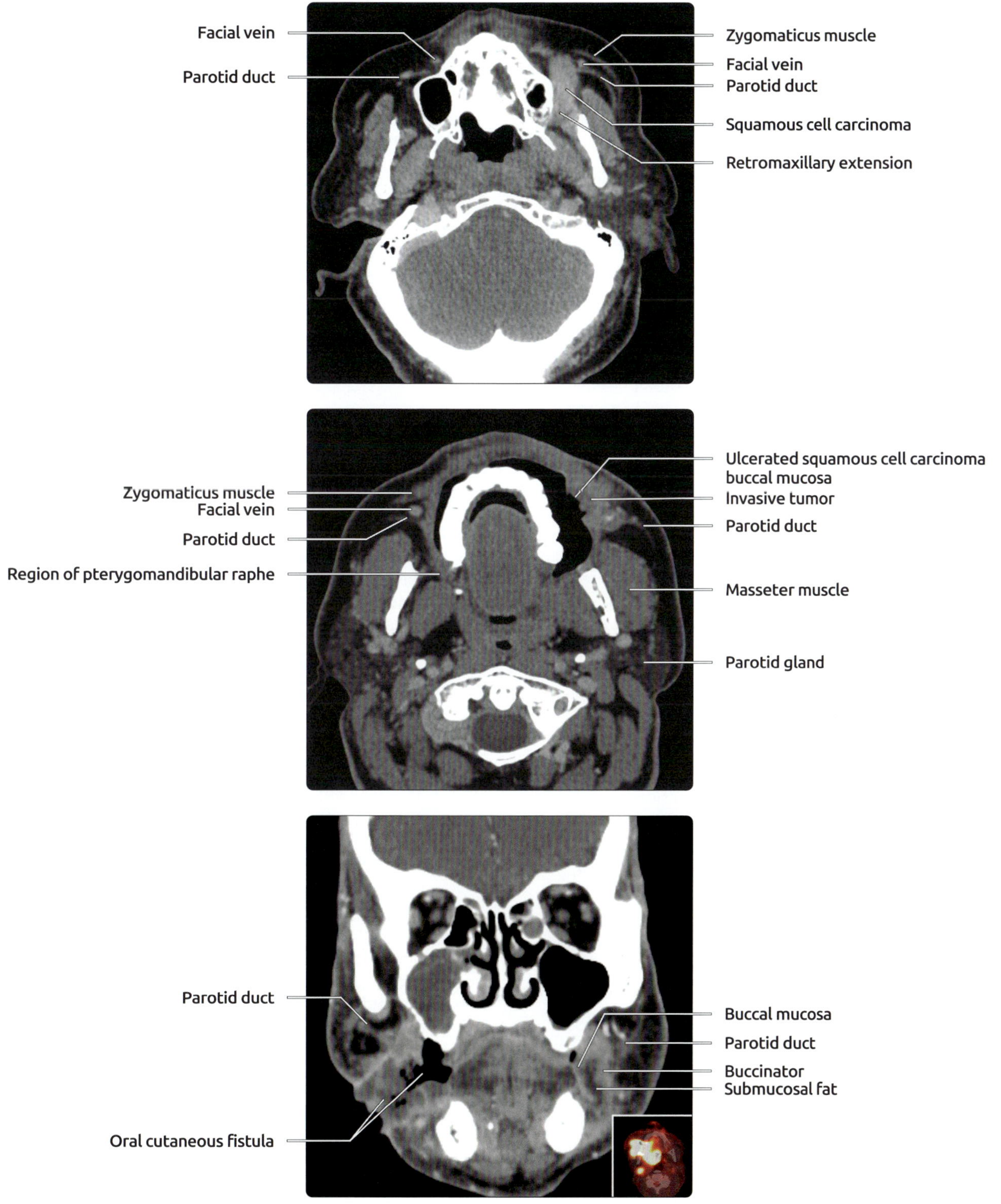

(Top) *Axial CECT through the BS shows a homogeneous mass in the left BS. This is a squamous cell carcinoma that originated on the buccal mucosa and buccal gingival sulcus, then eroded through the mucosa and buccinator space into the BS. The mass causes displacement of the parotid duct but no definite parotid duct enlargement.* **(Middle)** *Axial CECT through the BS was performed using puffed cheek technique, allowing increased air in the lateral oral cavity recesses. There is an ulcerated lesion arising from the buccal mucosa (part of oral cavity mucosa) and invading laterally into the buccinator muscle and BS. There is nodular tissue near the junction of the facial vein and parotid duct. The parotid duct is normal in size despite the potential obstruction.* **(Bottom)** *Coronal CECT was performed after chemoradiation in a patient with a large, unresectable squamous cell carcinoma that extended from the right tonsil to the BS. Pretreatment PET scan is seen in the inset. Posttreatment CECT shows that the tumor has undergone significant necrosis, leaving a large oral cutaneous fistula through the BS.*

TERMINOLOGY

Abbreviations

- Masticator space (MS); lateral pterygoid (LP); medial pterygoid (MP); foramen ovale (FO); internal maxillary artery (Imax)

IMAGING ANATOMY

Overview

- **Suprazygomatic MS**: Contains belly of temporalis muscle
- **Infrazygomatic MS**: MS "proper"; medial to zygomatic arch & lateral to pterygomaxillary fissure; contains masseter, MP, LP, Imax, CNV3, mandible ramus/posterior body

Extent

- Craniocaudal extent of MS more extensive than commonly recognized; reaches parietal bone at top
- Inferior temporal line: Anteroposteriorly arched line crossing middle of parietal bone forming superior limit of muscular origin of temporalis muscle
- Superior temporal line: Just above superior temporal line where temporal fascia covering temporalis muscle attaches

Anatomy Relationships

- Skull base, including **FO** & **foramen spinosum**

Internal Contents

- **Muscles of mastication**
  - **Masseter**: Origin on zygomatic arch
    - Inserts on lateral surface of ramus/angle of mandible
  - **Temporalis**: Origin on suprazygomatic MS parietal bone
    - Inserts on medial surface of coronoid process & anterior surface of mandibular ramus
  - **LP**: Origin on greater wing of sphenoid (superior head) & lateral surface of LP plate (inferior head)
    - Inserts on capsule & articular disc of TMJ (superior head) & neck of mandible (inferior head)
  - **MP**: Origin on medial surface LP plate & pyramidal process of palatine bone
    - Inserts on medial surface of mandibular ramus
- **Mandibular division, trigeminal nerve (V3)**
  - 1st branchial arch's nerve; enters MS through FO
  - Located near skull base medial to LP & lateral to tensor veli palatini (TVP) muscle, within **trigeminal fat pad**
  - **Otic ganglion (OG)**: Below skull base between V3 & TVP
  - Lesser petrosal nerve (branch of tympanic plexus formed by tympanic branch of glossopharyngeal nerve) provides preganglionic parasympathetic supply to OG from medullary inferior salivatory nucleus
    - Lesser petrosal nerve exits middle cranial fossa via FO, or, occasionally, via separate foramen called "canaliculus innominatus"
  - Nonrelaying sympathetic root to OG from plexus on middle meningeal artery (MMA)
  - OG postganglionic secretomotor fibers to parotid join auriculotemporal nerve (V3 branch)
  - **Main trunk of V3** gives off meningeal branch & nerve to MP; latter provides nonrelaying motor root to OG, which supplies TVP & tensor tympani muscles
  - Main trunk soon divides into small **anterior division** & large **posterior division**
  - Anterior division motor branches: Masseteric nerve, 2 deep temporal nerves, & nerve to LP
  - Anterior division sensory branch: Buccal nerve
  - **Auriculotemporal nerve** arises from 2 roots of proximal posterior division, runs backwards encircling MMA & forms single trunk, again runs backwards turning up behind neck of mandible above Imax, & then ascends on temple behind superficial temporal vessels
    - Sensory innervation to external ear, TMJ, parotid, temple, & secretomotor to parotid via OG
  - Posterior division then divides into terminal branches: Inferior alveolar (posterior) & lingual (anterior) nerves
  - **Inferior alveolar nerve** (sensory to mandible & chin) runs downward lateral to MP → enters mandibular foramen (gives off **mylohyoid nerve** just before entering mandible) → runs in mandibular canal → finally emerges at mental foramen as mental nerve
    - Mylohyoid nerve (motor to anterior belly of digastric & mylohyoid muscles) contains all motor fibers of posterior division of V3
  - **Lingual nerve** (V3 sensory to anterior 2/3 of tongue, floor of mouth) begins **1 cm below** skull → runs 1st between TVP & LP → then between LP & MP → then runs anteroinferiorly between MP & mandibular ramus → then in direct contact with mandible medial to 3rd molar tooth → finally in lateral sublingual space compartment
  - **Chorda tympani (CT) nerve** (CNVII branch), distributed through lingual nerve, joins lingual nerve in MS **2 cm below** skull base after exiting petrotympanic fissure
  - CT: Anterior 2/3 of tongue taste; & secretomotor to submandibular/sublingual salivary glands via its preganglionic parasympathetic supply from pontine superior salivatory nucleus to submandibular ganglion
- **Ramus & posterior body of mandible**
- **Imax**: Arises behind neck of mandible as terminal branch of external carotid artery & passes through MS; 3 parts
  - 1st (mandibular) part: Posterior to neck of mandible, inferior to auriculotemporal nerve → then along lower border of LP; 5 branches, most important MMA
  - 2nd (pterygoid) part: Passes anterosuperiorly, superficial to (or deep to or through) inferior head of LP; 4 branches
  - 3rd (pterygopalatine) part: Passes between 2 heads of LP → then through pterygomaxillary fissure → into pterygopalatine fossa; 6 branches, most important sphenopalatine artery (artery of epistaxis)
- **Pterygoid venous plexus**: Along posterior border of LP & parapharyngeal space

Fascia of Masticator Space

- **Superficial layer of deep cervical fascia** (SL-DCF) splits along inferior mandible, creating "sling" enclosing MS
  - **Medial fascial slip** runs along deep surface of pterygoid muscles; inserts at skull base undersurface **medial to FO**
  - **Lateral slip SL-DCF** covers surface of masseter muscle, attaching to zygomatic arch; continues cephalad, covering temporalis muscle to top of suprazygomatic MS
  - **No horizontal fascia** exists deep to zygomatic arch; MS lesions pass freely craniocaudally under zygomatic arch

Potential Subspaces Created by Fibroadipose Tissue

- Masseteric space, pterygoid space, & superficial & deep temporal spaces; more often described in surgical literature

GRAPHICS

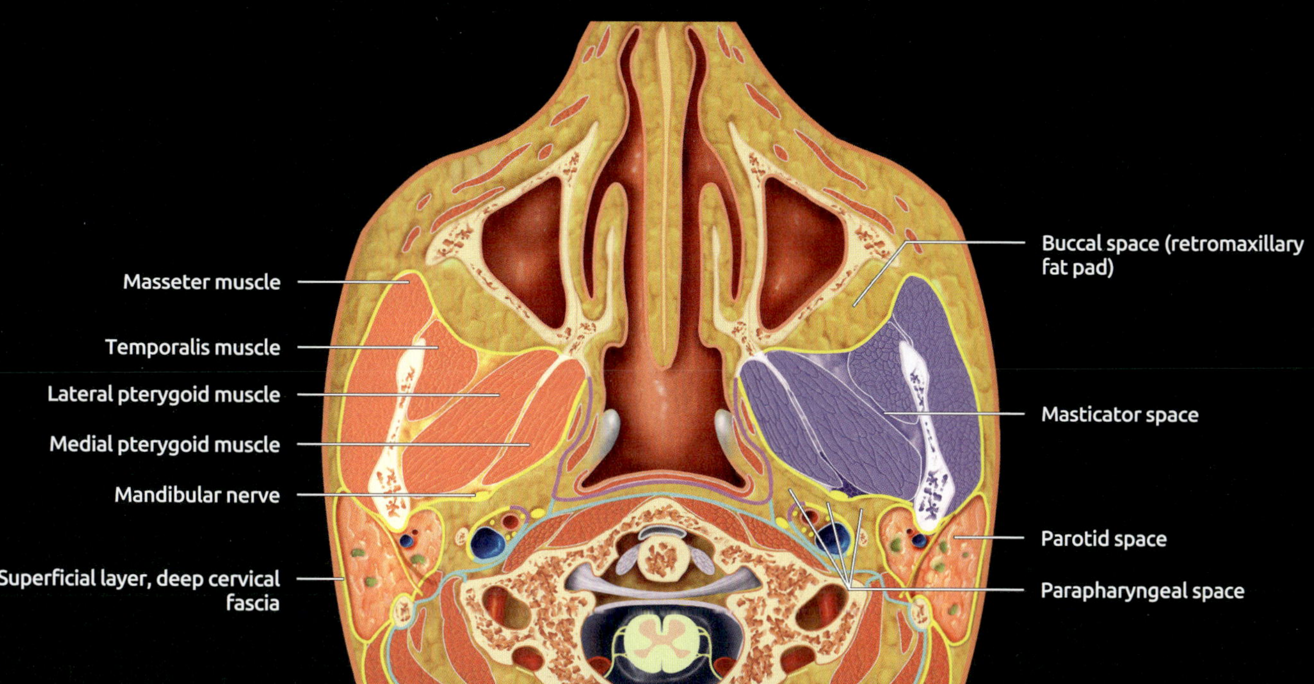

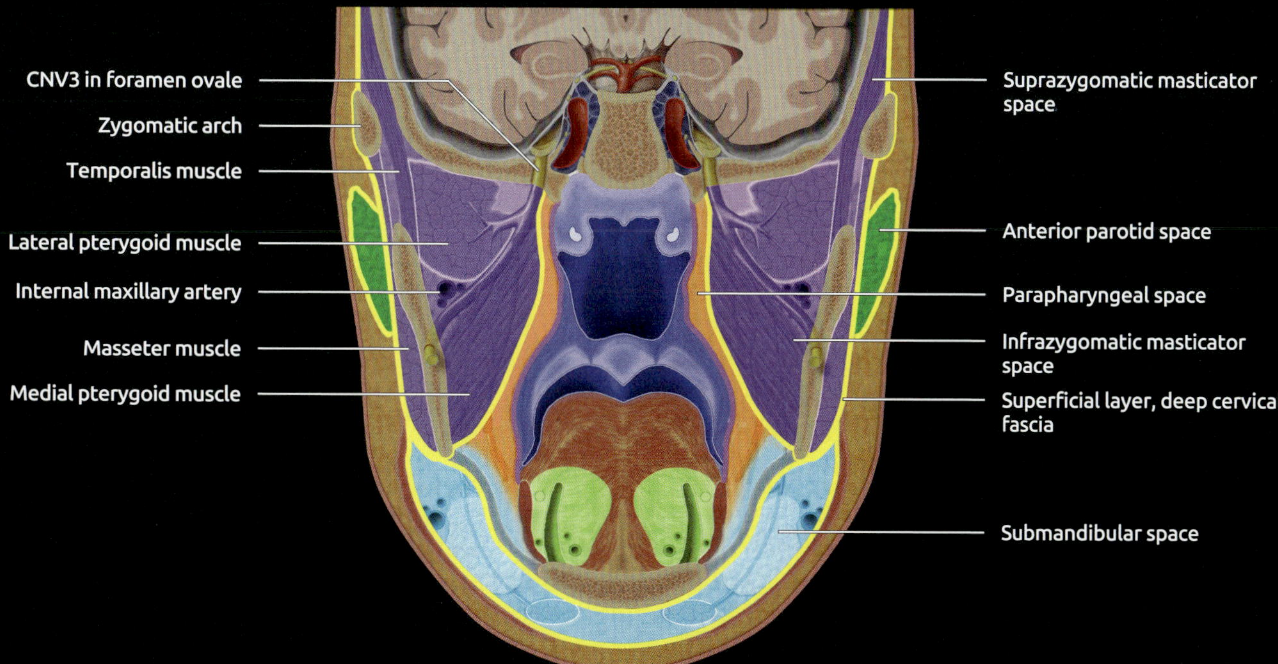

(Top) *Axial graphic shows the masticator space enclosed by superficial layer of deep cervical fascia (yellow line). The muscles of mastication from medial to lateral are the medial & lateral pterygoid, temporalis, & masseter muscles. The buccal space is anterior, while the parapharyngeal & parotid spaces are posterior to the masticator space. Masticator space frequently communicates posteriorly with the buccal space because the parotidomasseteric fascia is sometimes incomplete medially where it joins the buccopharyngeal fascia.* **(Bottom)** *Coronal graphic of the masticator space reveals a suprazygomatic & infrazygomatic component. Notice that the superficial layer of deep cervical fascia attaches to the skull base just medial to the foramen ovale, thereby including the foramen ovale within the confines of masticator space. Foramen spinosum and the occasional canaliculus innominatus (transmitting lesser petrosal nerve), if present, are all contents of the masticator space. There is no "horizontal fascia" beneath the zygomatic arch in order to prevent spread of masticator space disease superiorly into the suprazygomatic masticator space.*

GRAPHICS

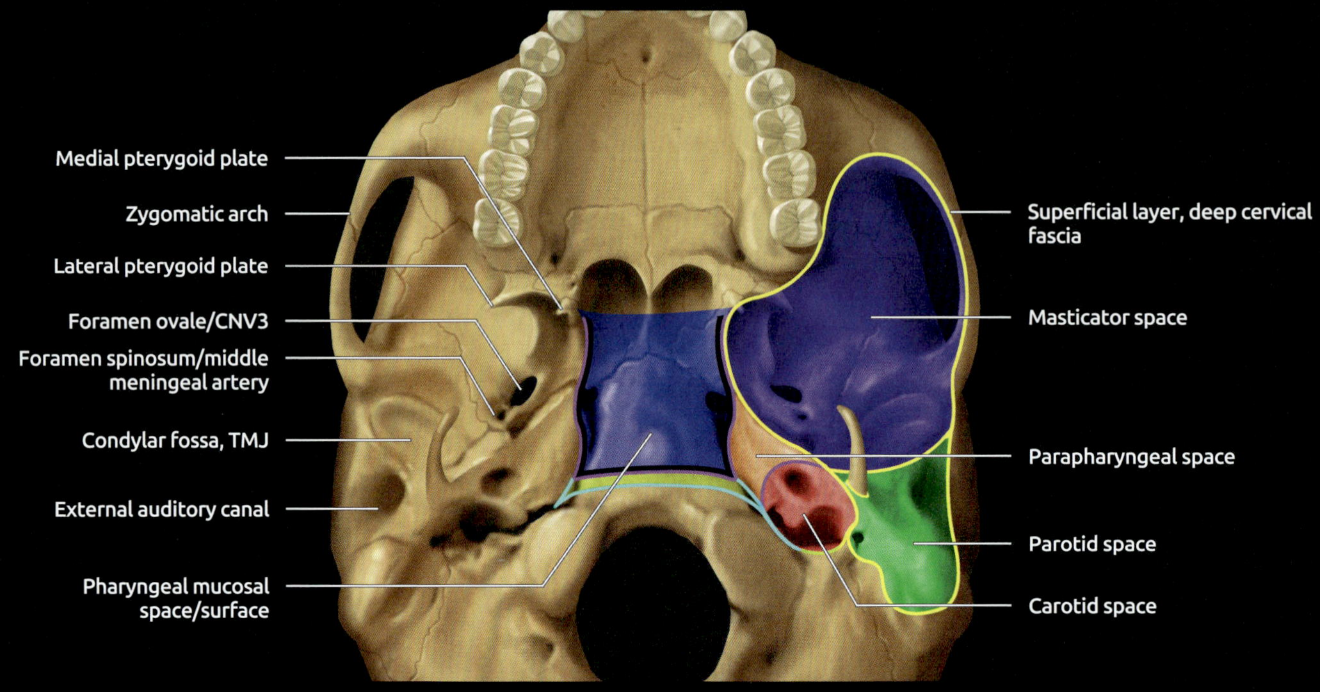

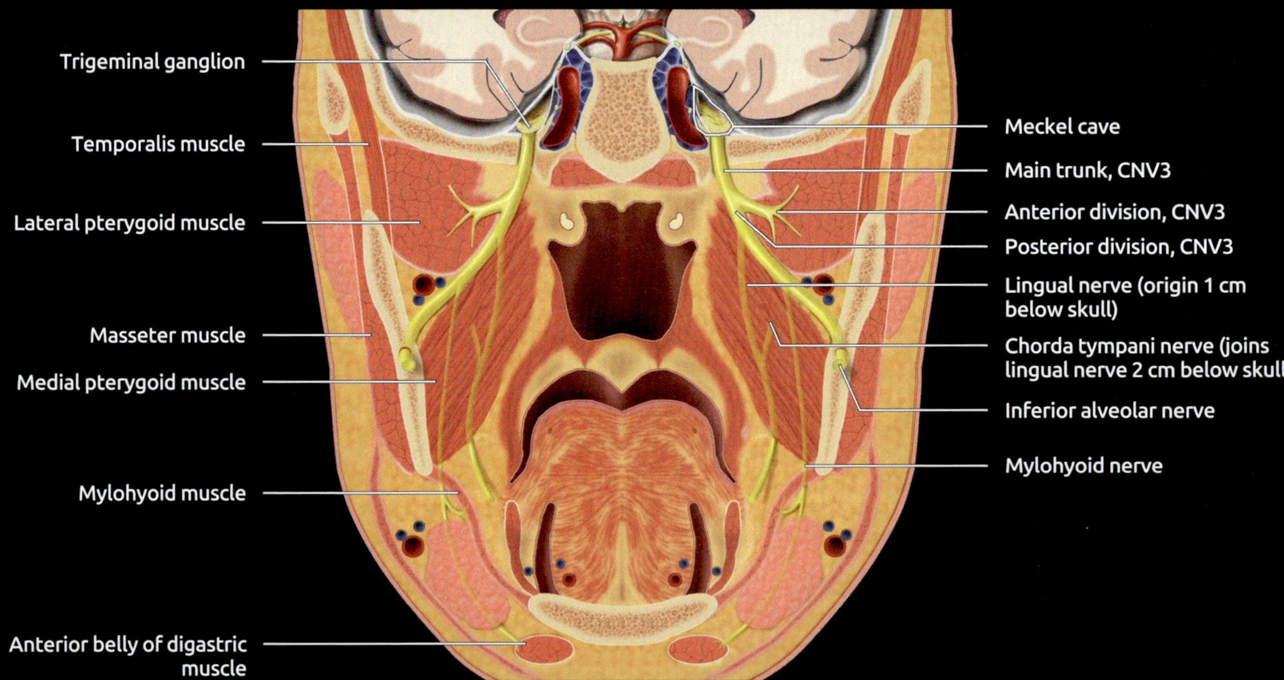

(Top) *Inferior graphic of skull base shows masticator space abutting sphenoid & temporal bones. Masticator space (purple) has a broad abutment with the skull base. CNV3 enters masticator space through foramen ovale while foramen spinosum transmits middle meningeal artery intracranially. Note that the TMJ is within the confines of masticator space.* **(Bottom)** *Coronal graphic of the mandibular division of the trigeminal nerve is shown. CNV3 exits skull base through foramen ovale without entering the cavernous sinus. The motor branches from CNV3 are nerve to medial pterygoid, which also supplies tensor veli palatini & tensor tympani (from main trunk); masseteric nerve, 2 deep temporal nerves to temporalis & nerve to lateral pterygoid (from anterior division); & mylohyoid nerve, which supplies mylohyoid & anterior belly of digastric muscles (branch of inferior alveolar nerve; mylohyoid nerve contains all the motor fibers of posterior division). The main sensory branches are the meningeal branch (from main trunk), buccal nerve (from anterior division), auriculotemporal nerve, & the terminal lingual & inferior alveolar nerves (branches of posterior division).*

GENERIC MASTICATOR SPACE MASS

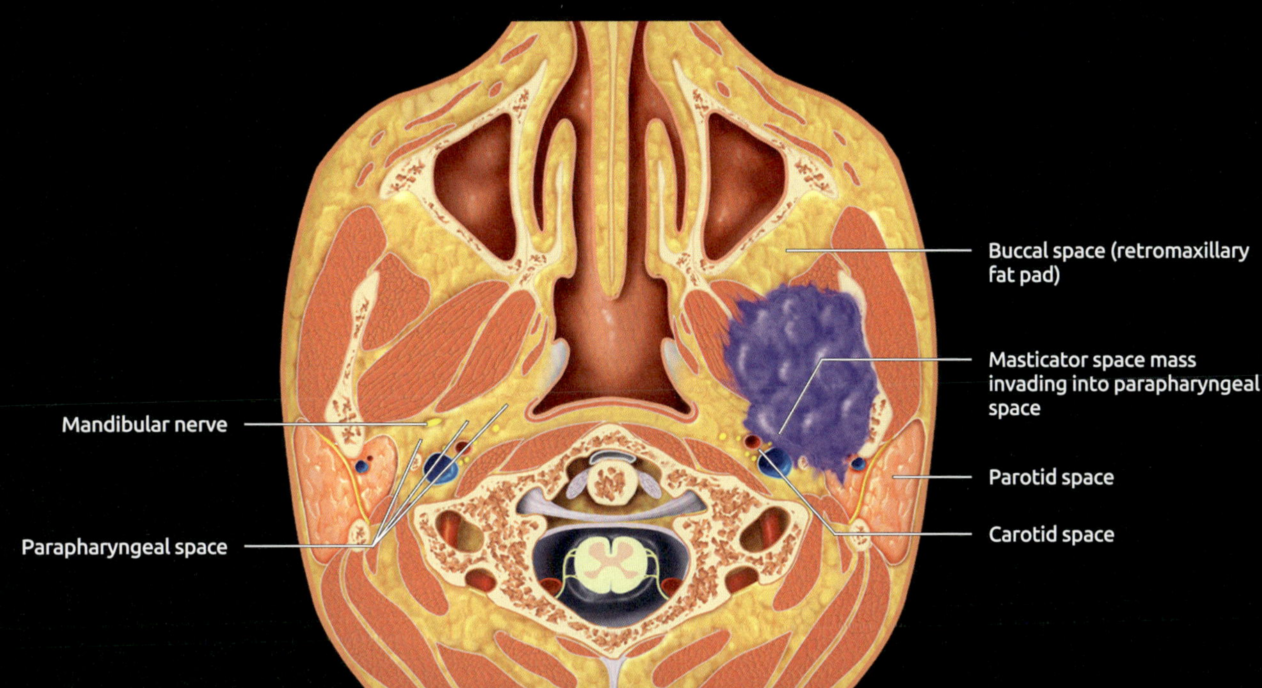

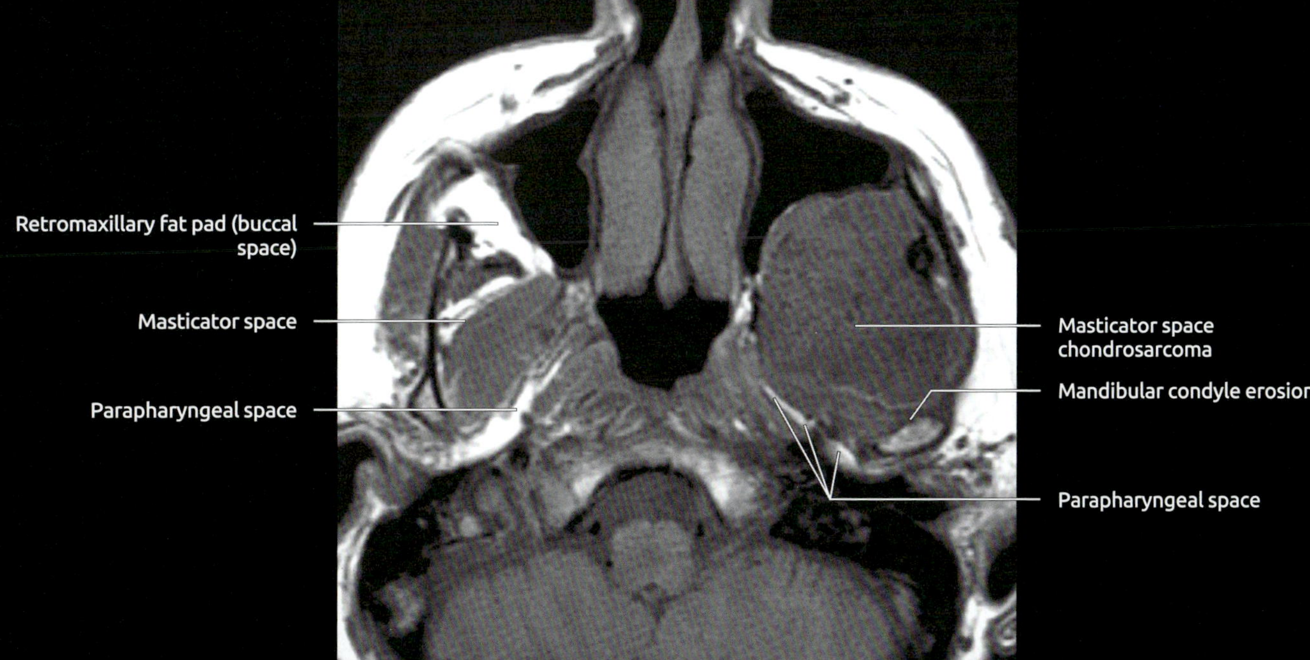

(Top) *Axial graphic at the level of the low nasopharynx demonstrates a generic masticator space mass invading the parapharyngeal space from anterior to posterior. Notice the mandibular nerve is engulfed by the tumor. Masticator space masses invade the masticator muscles & erode the posterior body, ramus, or condylar process of the mandible.* **(Bottom)** *Axial unenhanced T1WI MR through the nasopharynx shows a large mass of the masticator space that displaces the parapharyngeal space from anterior to posterior, invades the muscles of mastication, & erodes the mandibular condyle. The differential diagnosis of primary tumors of the masticator space includes sarcoma & non-Hodgkin lymphoma. In this case, the tumor was a chondrosarcoma. Unenhanced T1WI MR is the best to look for displacement of surrounding T1-hyperintense fat planes & infiltration of masticator space trigeminal fat pad by lesions. Postcontrast fat-suppressed MR is the best for evaluating enhancing tumor, including soft tissue, marrow involvement, & perineural tumor spread. CT best delineates bony lysis/sclerosis of mandible & skull base, but T1, STIR, & postcontrast MR will show early marrow infiltration.*

PERINEURAL CNV3 MALIGNANCY

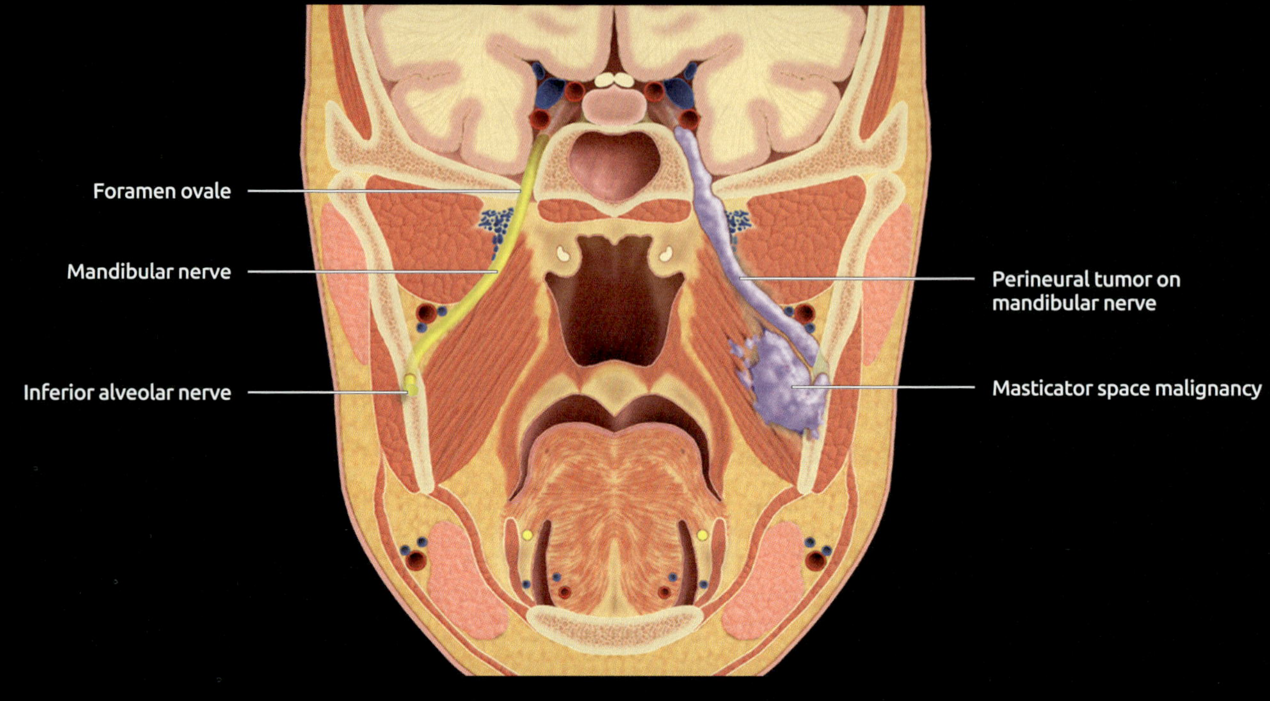

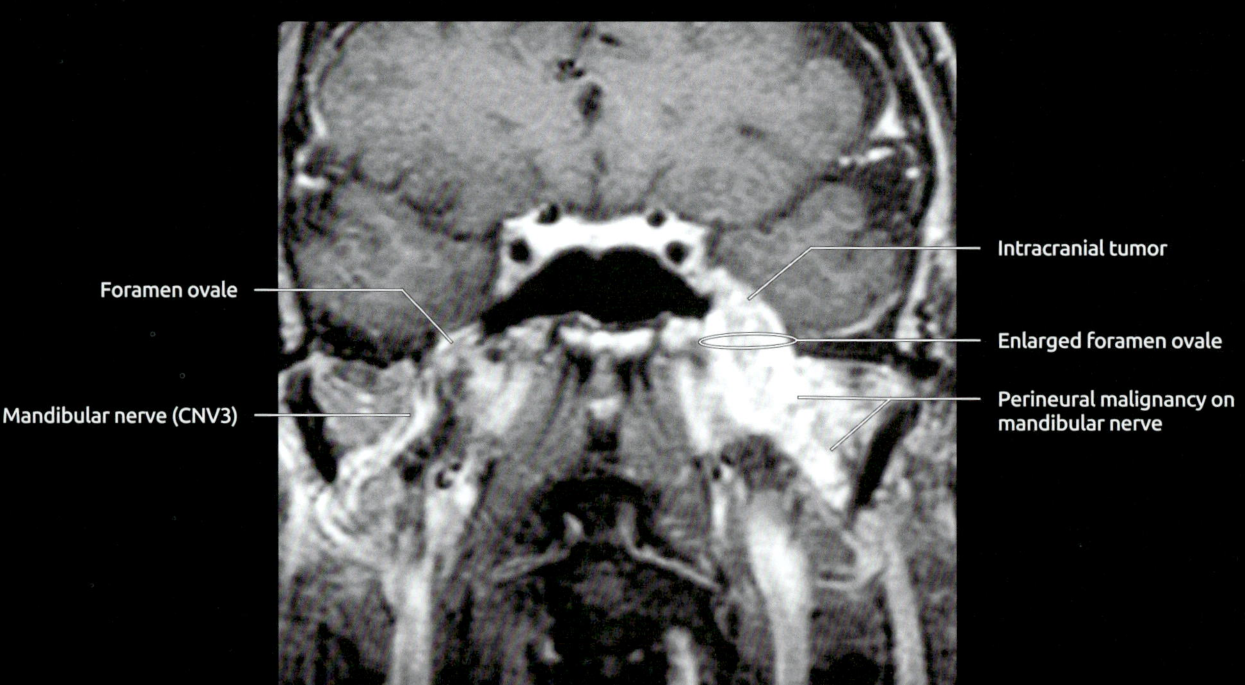

(Top) *Coronal graphic of the suprahyoid neck focused on the masticator space & mandibular nerve is shown. In this drawing, a generic masticator space malignancy is visible invading the lower masticator space, invading the adjacent mandible, & spreading via a perineural route up the mandibular nerve through the foramen ovale into the intracranial compartment. Both primary masticator space malignancy & squamous cell carcinoma of the oral cavity can access the intracranial compartment in this manner.* **(Bottom)** *Coronal T1 C+ FS MR through the foramen ovale shows an enhancing perineural malignant tumor spreading superiorly from the left masticator space along the mandibular nerve. Notice the enlarged left foramen ovale & intracranial tumor. In this case, the tumor came from a primary melanoma on the skin of the chin. If the masticator space lesion affects CNV3, the entire course of the lesion should be imaged from mental foramen anteriorly to trigeminal nerve root entry zone in pons. Epicenter of masticator space lesions lie around muscles of mastication, posterior body & ramus of mandible, & internal maxillary artery & CNV3, which are the primary contents of the space.*

AXIAL CECT

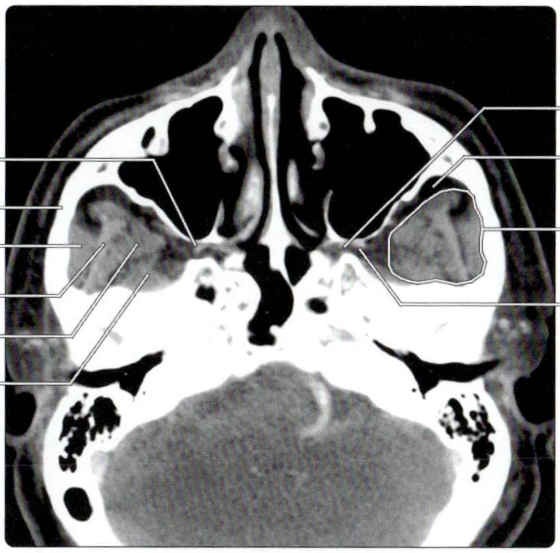

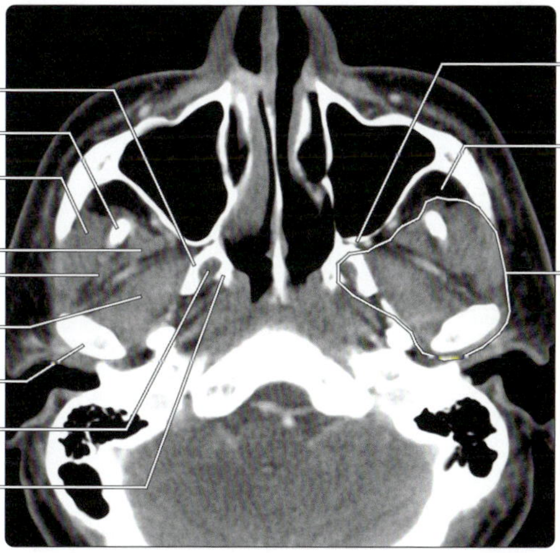

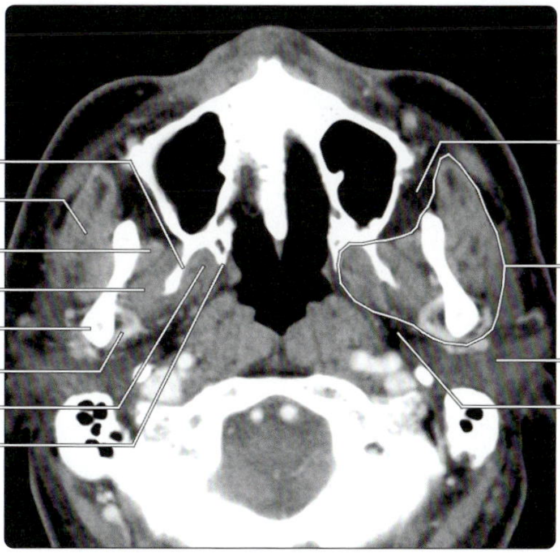

Internal maxillary artery
Zygomatic arch
Masseter muscle
Temporalis tendon
Temporalis muscle
Lateral pterygoid muscle (small superior head)
Pterygopalatine fossa
Buccal space (retromaxillary fat pad)
Masticator space
Pterygomaxillary fissure

Lateral pterygoid plate
Coronoid process of mandible
Masseter muscle
Temporalis muscle
Mandibular notch
Lateral pterygoid muscle (large inferior head)
Mandibular condyle
Medial pterygoid muscle
Medial pterygoid plate
Pterygopalatine fossa
Buccal space (retromaxillary fat pad)
Masticator space

Lateral pterygoid plate
Masseter muscle
Temporalis muscle
Lateral pterygoid muscle
Mandibular ramus
Pterygoid venous plexus
Medial pterygoid muscle
Medial pterygoid plate
Buccal space (retromaxillary fat pad)
Masticator space
Parotid space
Parapharyngeal space

(Top) *First of 6 axial CECT images presented from superior to inferior shows the masticator space medial to the zygomatic arch. Notice the masseter muscle arising from the inferior margin of the zygomatic arch. Also note the superior head of the lateral pterygoid muscle. The 3rd (pterygopalatine) part of the maxillary artery enters the pterygopalatine fossa through the pterygomaxillary fissure, after passing between 2 heads of the lateral pterygoid muscle.* **(Middle)** *At mandibular condyle level, masticator space contains muscles of mastication & parts of mandible. Note inferior head of lateral pterygoid muscle arising from the lateral surface of the lateral pterygoid plate. Medial pterygoid muscle arises from the pterygoid fossa. Supranotch & infranotch masticator space compartments lie above & below an axial plane passing through mandibular notch between coronoid & condyloid processes.* **(Bottom)** *In this image through the low maxillary sinuses, the masticator space is seen between the more anterior buccal space & the more posterior parapharyngeal & parotid spaces. Notice the pterygoid venous plexus as the enhancing area along the posterolateral margin of the masticator space.*

AXIAL CECT

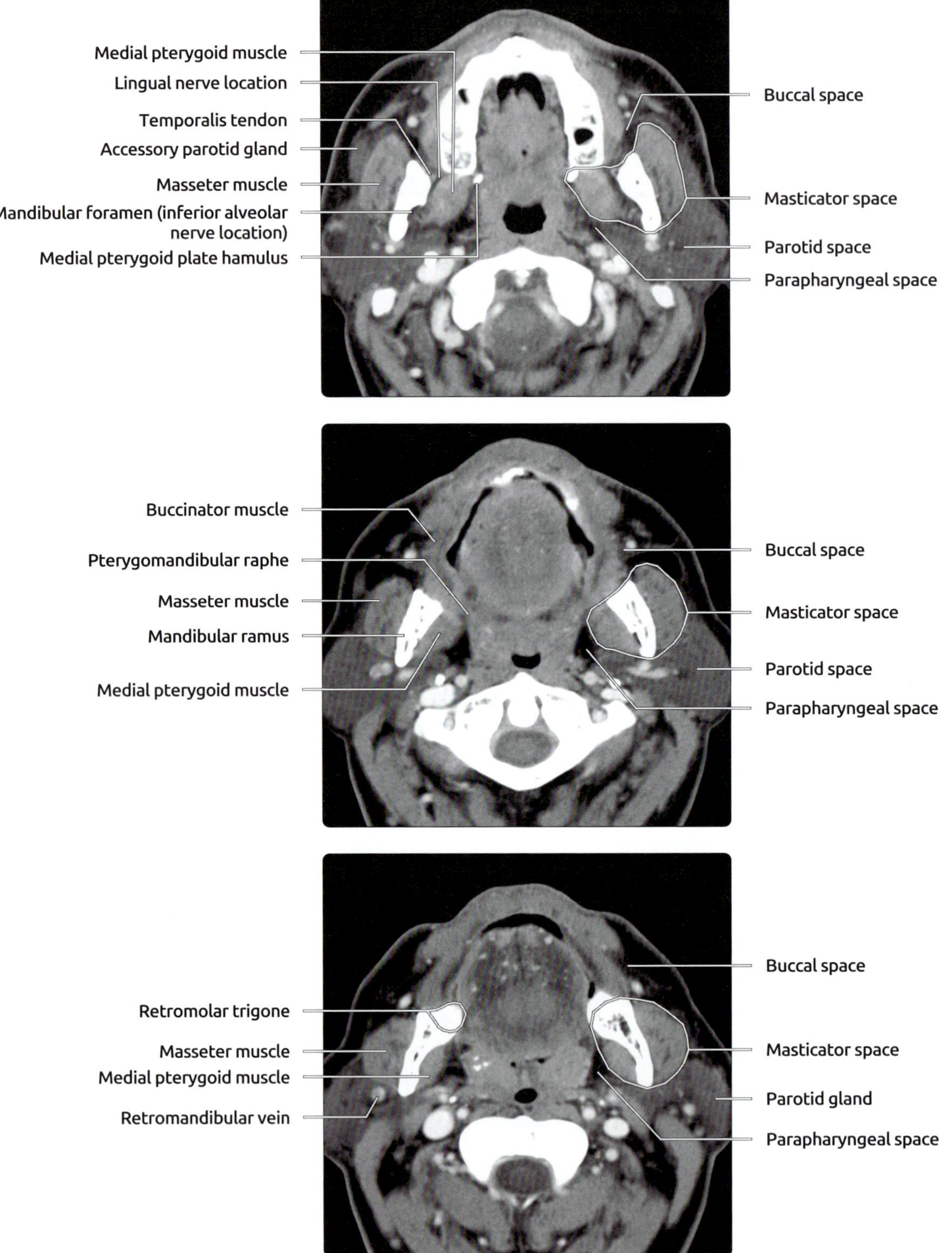

(Top) *In this image through the maxillary ridge, the mandibular foramen is seen where inferior alveolar nerve enters mandible. Lingual nerve is located along the anterior margin of the medial pterygoid muscle at this level. Note the hamulus of the medial pterygoid plate, which acts as a pulley for the tendon of the tensor veli palatini muscle & is the site of superior attachment of the pterygomandibular raphe.* **(Middle)** *In this image, attachment of medial pterygoid is seen along the medial mandibular ramus. Pterygomandibular raphe is the tendinous point of junction between buccinator & superior constrictor muscles.* **(Bottom)** *In this image, the retromolar triangle is seen, which sits on the anterior surface of the masticator space, & squamous cell carcinoma there can directly invade the masticator space with potential of CNV3 perineural tumor spread. Masseteric space (between masseter muscle & ramus of mandible), pterygoid space (between pterygoid muscles & ramus of mandible), & superficial (between temporalis muscle & temporoparietal fascia) & deep (between temporalis fascia & temporal bone) temporal spaces are potential spaces created by fibroadipose tissue in masticator space.*

AXIAL T1 MR

Maxillary sinus
Inferior orbital fissure
Temporalis muscle
Sphenoid bone
Suprazygomatic masticator space

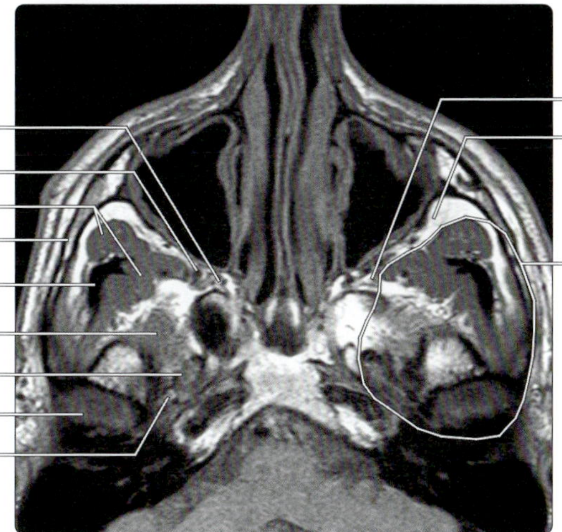

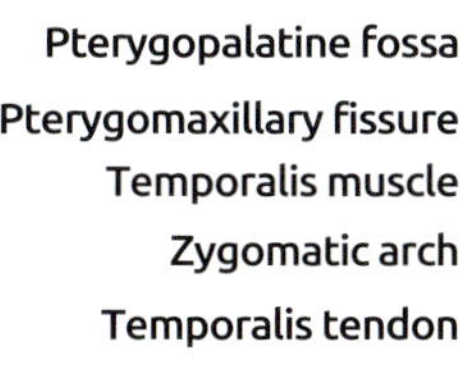

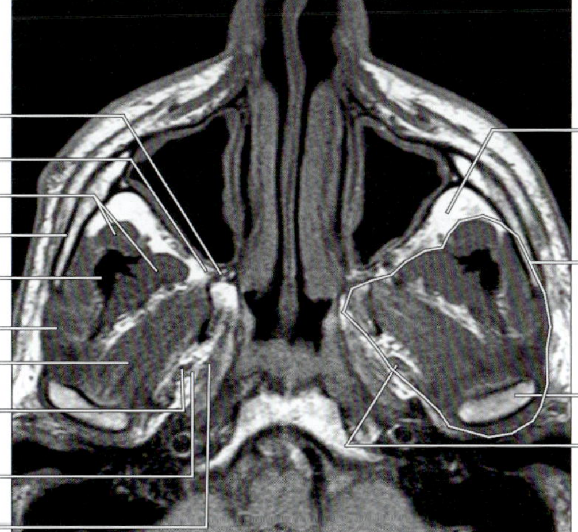

(Top) *First of 6 axial T1 MR images from superior to inferior shows that, above zygomatic arch, the suprazygomatic masticator space is seen. Notice temporalis muscle & fat are only occupants of this portion of masticator space.* **(Middle)** *The mandibular nerve (CNV3) can be visualized within foramen ovale. Middle meningeal artery can be seen posterolateral to foramen ovale within foramen spinosum. Auriculotemporal nerve, which arises by 2 roots of proximal posterior division of CNV3, runs backward, encircling middle meningeal artery, & forms a single trunk. Pterygopalatine fossa opens laterally through pterygomaxillary fissure into masticator space.* **(Bottom)** *Mandibular nerve is visible along posteromedial border of lateral pterygoid muscle. Temporalis muscle & its hypointense tendon fill anterolateral masticator space. Lateral pterygoid muscle inferior head originates from lateral surface of lateral pterygoid plate. Main trunk of mandibular nerve is located near skull base medial to lateral pterygoid & lateral to tensor veli palatini muscle, within T1-hyperintense trigeminal fat pad. Otic ganglion (OG) (not visualized) lies just below skull base between CNV3 & tensor veli palatini.*

AXIAL T1 MR

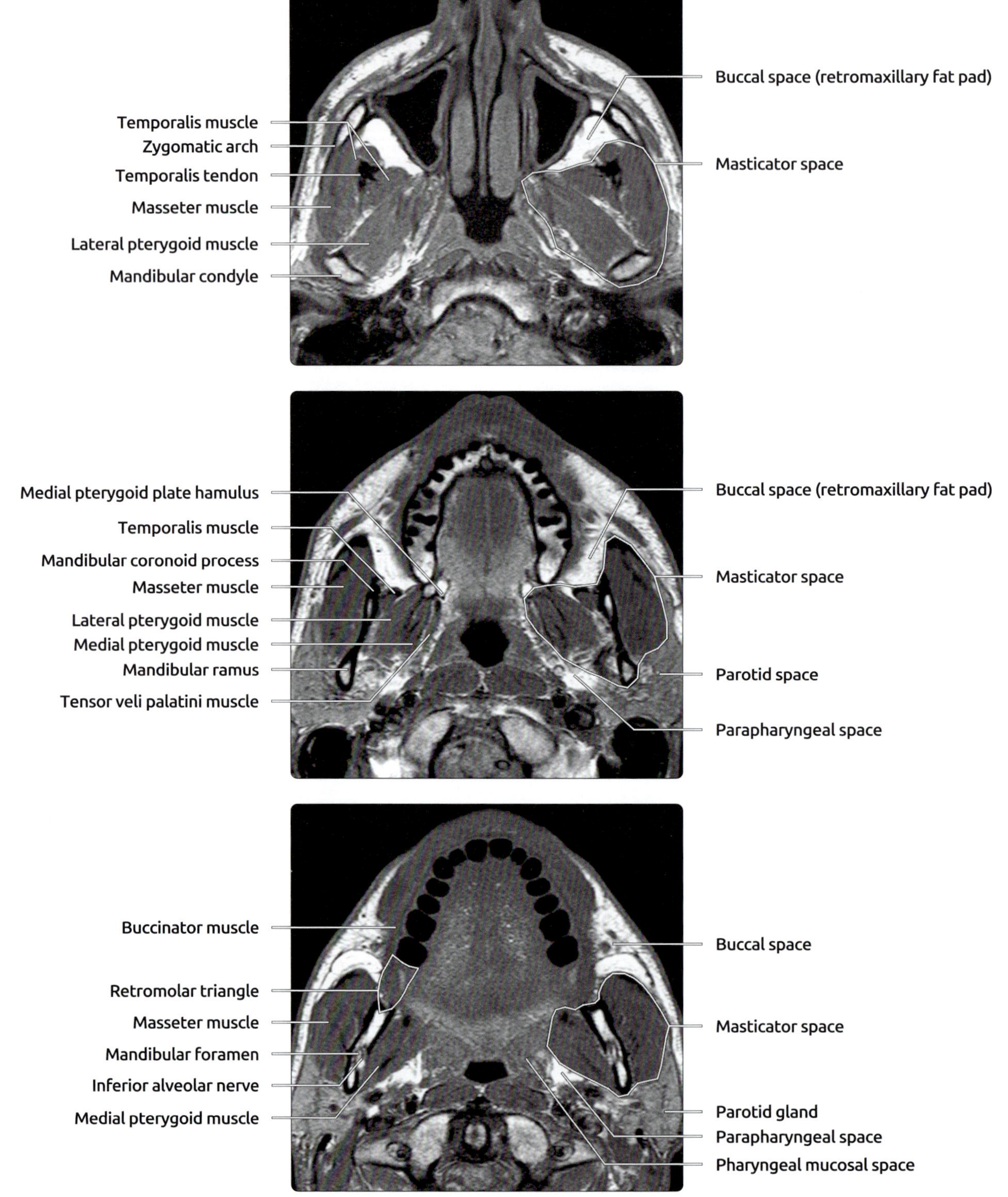

(Top) *In this image, the masseter muscle is seen arising from the inferior surface of the zygomatic arch. The retromaxillary fat pad (superior buccal space) is visible anterior to the masticator space.* **(Middle)** *In this image at the level of the maxillary ridge, the temporalis muscle is seen inserting on the medial surface of the coronoid process of the mandible. The tensor veli palatini muscle approaches the hamulus of the medial pterygoid plate where it will turn medially to the soft palate.* **(Bottom)** *In this image at level of mandibular teeth, inferior alveolar nerve can be seen entering mandibular foramen. Retromolar triangle represents mucosal surface behind 3rd mandibular molar & in front of anterior mandibular ramus. Squamous cell carcinoma of retromolar triangle, when invasive, readily involves masticator space, & may cause CNV3 perineural tumor spread. Supranotch & infranotch masticator space compartments lie above & below axial plane passing through mandibular notch between coronoid & condyloid processes. This compartmentalization is a good division of masticator space in evaluating posterior spread of oral cavity squamous cell cancers.*

CORONAL T1 MR

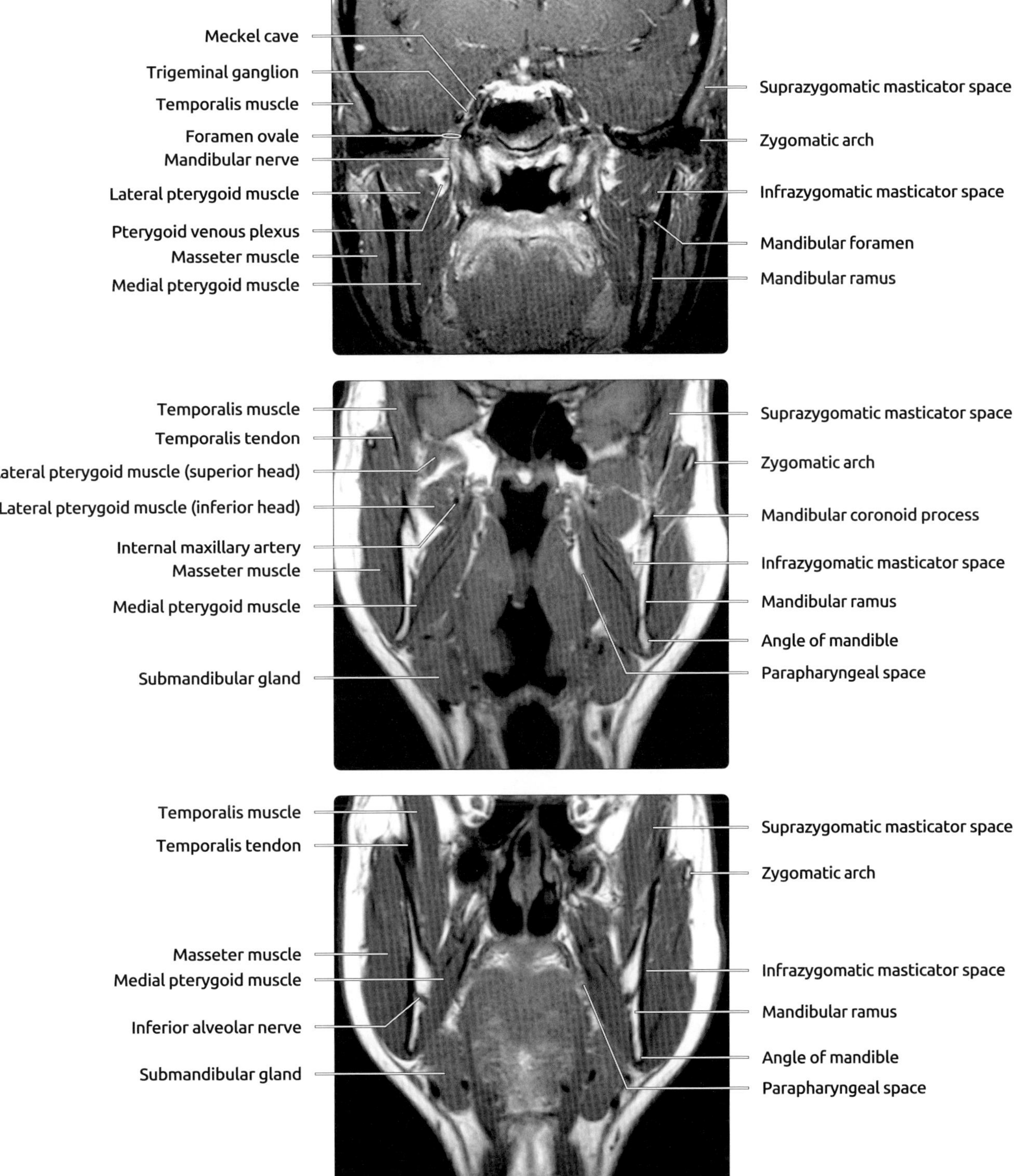

(Top) *Coronal T1 C+ FS MR shows mandibular nerve (main trunk CNV3) descending through foramen ovale. Although not seen on CT/MR, remember that secretomotor supply to parotid gland via auriculotemporal branch of CNV3 functionally comes from parasympathetic fibers of glossopharyngeal nerve (CNIX), relaying in OG; OG is only topographically related to CNV3. Also remember that chorda tympani nerve joining lingual nerve ~ 2 cm below skull base is a facial nerve branch (CNVII), which senses taste from anterior 2/3 of tongue & provides secretomotor supply to submandibular/sublingual salivary glands via its preganglionic parasympathetic supply to submandibular ganglion functionally through CNVII; ganglion is only topographically related to lingual nerve (CNV3) in sublingual space.* **(Middle)** *Coronal unenhanced T1WI MR shows superior & inferior heads of lateral pterygoid muscles. Medial pterygoid muscle arises from pterygoid fossa above & inserts on medial ramus & angle of mandible.* **(Bottom)** *Coronal T1WI MR through posterior nose shows masseter muscle arising from inferior surface of zygomatic arch & inserting on lateral ramus & angle of mandible.*

TERMINOLOGY

Abbreviations

- Parotid space (PS); parotid gland (PG)

Definitions

- **PS**: Paired lateral suprahyoid neck spaces enclosed by superficial layer of deep cervical fascia (SL-DCF)-containing PGs, nodes, & extracranial facial nerve (CNVII) branches

IMAGING ANATOMY

Extent

- PS extends from external auditory canal (EAC) & mastoid tip superiorly to below angle of mandible (parotid tail)
  - Parotid tail extends into posterior submandibular space inferiorly, between sternocleidomastoid & platysma

Anatomy Relationships

- Parapharyngeal space (PPS) directly medial to PS
- Masticator space (MS) anterior to PS
- Buccal space (BS) anterolateral to PS superficially
- Carotid space (CS) posteromedial to PS; **posterior belly of digastric (PBD)** muscle separates upper CS from deep PS

Internal Contents

- **PG**
  - Superficial lobe represents ~ 2/3 of PS
  - Deep lobe projects medially, abuts lateral aspect of PPS
- **Extracranial facial nerve (CNVII)**
  - Exits stylomastoid foramen as single trunk, gives off posterior auricular nerve, & branches to PBD & stylohyoid muscle
  - Ramifies within PS **lateral to** retromandibular vein
  - Ramifying intraparotid facial nerve creates **surgical plane between superficial & deep lobes**
  - Intraparotid facial nerve **not visible** with routine CT or MR except proximally with high-resolution 3T MR
  - Divides into 2 branches, **temporofacial** (divides into temporal & zygomatic branches) & **cervicofacial** (divides into buccal, marginal mandibular, & cervical branches)
  - **Auriculotemporal nerve (CNV3 branch)**: Curves around **neck** of mandible from MS, **just above maxillary artery**
    - Embedded in parotid capsule
    - Crosses through body of PG at right angles to CNVII
    - Usually has direct communications with CNVII here
    - Parotid perineural tumor spread can occur to CNV
    - Parasympathetic secretomotor & sensory supply of PG
  - Facial nerve does not supply parotid
  - Parotid fascia & skin sensory supply from great auricular nerve (C2, C3)
- **External carotid artery (ECA)**
  - Medial, smaller vessel of 2 seen just behind mandibular ramus in PS
- **Retromandibular vein**
  - Lateral, larger vessel of 2 behind mandibular ramus
  - Intraparotid **facial nerve** branches course **just lateral to** retromandibular vein
- **Intraparotid lymph nodes**
  - ~ 20 lymph nodes found in each PG
  - Parotid nodes are 1st-order drainage for EAC, pinna, surrounding deep face & scalp
  - PS undergoes **late encapsulation** in embryogenesis, resulting in intraparotid lymph nodes
- **Parotid duct (Stensen duct)**
  - ~ 5 cm long, emerges from anterior PS, runs along surface of **masseter** muscle in BS
  - Duct then arches through BS to pierce buccinator muscle at level of upper 2nd molar tooth
- **Accessory PGs**
  - Project over surface of masseter muscles, along parotid duct (**facial process** of parotid)
  - Present in ~ 20% of normal anatomic dissections
  - Have their own blood supply & secondary duct emptying into Stensen duct
  - Other small processes are **glenoid process** (superior extension between EAC & TMJ), **pterygoid process** (between medial pterygoid & mandible ramus), & **poststyloid process**

Fascia of Parotid Space

- SL-**DCF** surrounds PS
- Superficial lamina **[parotidomasseteric fascia (PMF)]**: Thick & adherent to PG; parotid swellings very painful due to unyielding nature of fascia
- PMF continues to SL-DCF below, & to temporalis fascia (deep temporal fascia) covering temporalis muscle above
- **Stylomandibular ligament**: Portion of deep lamina
  - Separates parotid **tail** from **submandibular gland**
  - Pierced by **ECA**

ANATOMY IMAGING ISSUES

Imaging Recommendations

- CECT or MR can both readily image PS; T1 C+ fat-saturated axial & coronal MR better for perineural CNVII spread

Imaging Pitfalls

- PG: Soft tissue in children, progressively fatty with age
- Parotid tail mass must be identified as intraparotid or excision may injure facial nerve
- Facial nerve plane in PS can only be estimated

CLINICAL IMPLICATIONS

Clinical Importance

- In cases of tumor, assess relationship of lesion to estimated facial nerve plane & evaluate for perineural spread
- **Facial nerve horizontal** within PS, **blood vessels vertical**
  - Parotid abscess best drained by horizontal incision/small holes (Hilton method) below angle of mandible
- If larger mass lesion of deep lobe, mass displaces PPS from lateral to medial with widening of stylomandibular gap
- **Parotid tumors**: Benign mixed tumor (75%), Warthin tumor (5%), adenoid cystic carcinoma (5%), mucoepidermoid carcinoma (5%), other (10%)
- **Malignancy in salivary gland tumors**: ≈ 20% of parotid, ≈ 50% of submandibular, & ≈ 80% of sublingual tumors
- **Persistent foramen of Huschke (foramen tympanicum)**: Dehiscence in anteroinferior EAC wall; posteromedial to TMJ
  - Anatomic variant normally closing by 5 years age; sometimes persist into adulthood
  - Rarely associated with **salivary discharge into EAC** during mastication/**salivary fistula**

GRAPHICS

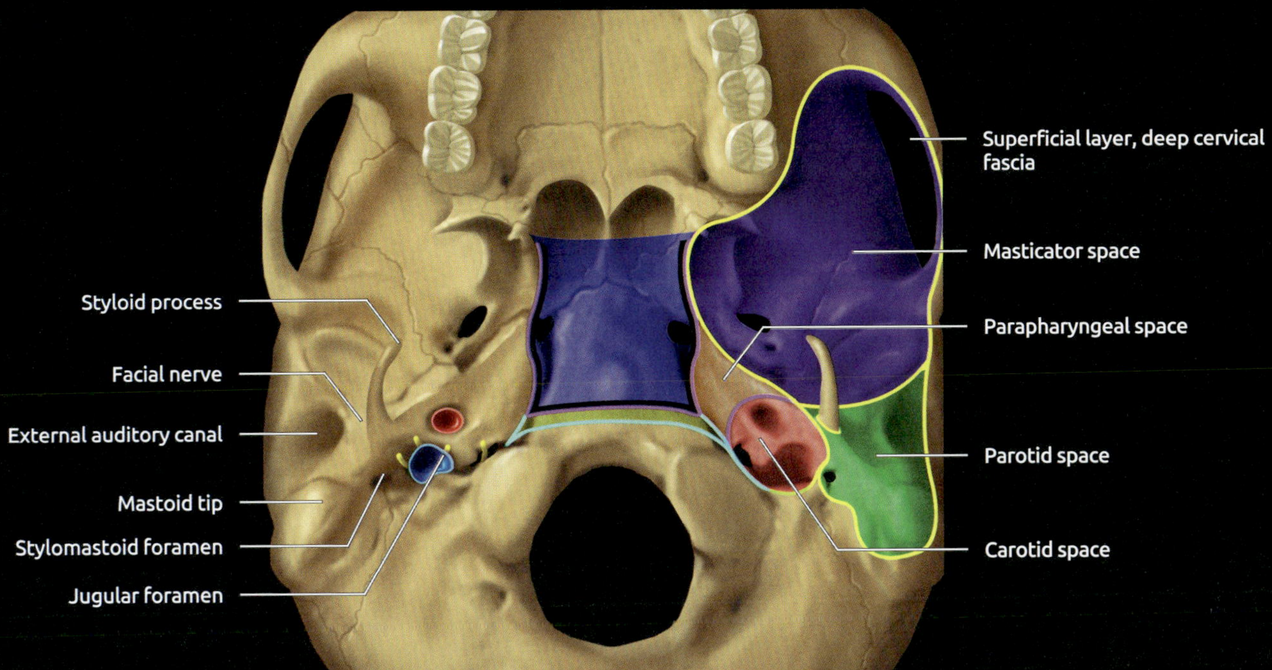

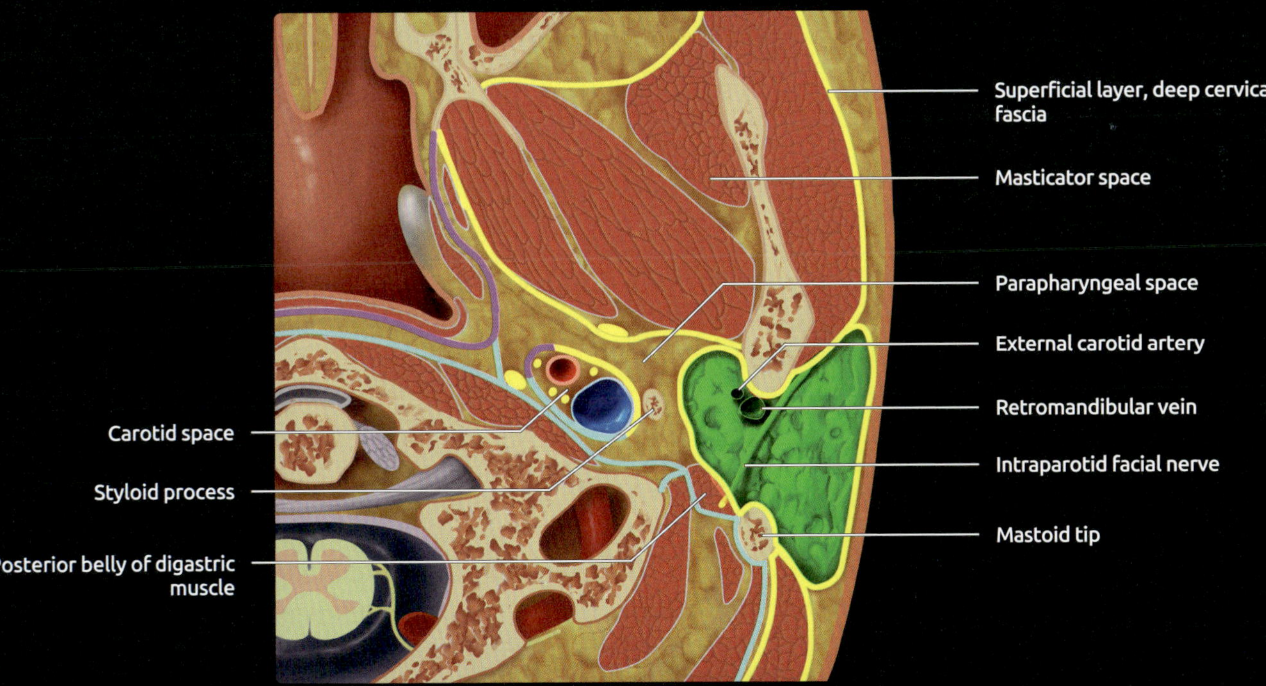

(Top) *Axial graphic of the skull base viewed from below illustrates the interaction between the parotid space and the skull base. CNVII exits through the stylomastoid foramen at the skull base, just posterior to the styloid process and lateral to the jugular foramen. The parotid space is the most lateral space in the nasopharyngeal and oropharyngeal area, extending from the external auditory canal above to the level of the mandibular angle below.* **(Bottom)** *Axial graphic of the parotid space at the level of C1 vertebral body is shown. The parotid space contains the external carotid artery (ECA), retromandibular vein, and facial nerve, from medial to lateral. The intraparotid CNVII creates a surgical plane that divides the gland into superficial and deep lobes. Parotid masses arising in the deep lobe will displace the parapharyngeal space fat medially. The parotid space is enclosed by the superficial layer of the deep cervical fascia. Posterior belly of digastric muscle separates the upper carotid space from deep lobe of parotid gland and can be used to assess the epicenter of tumors in this location.*

GRAPHICS

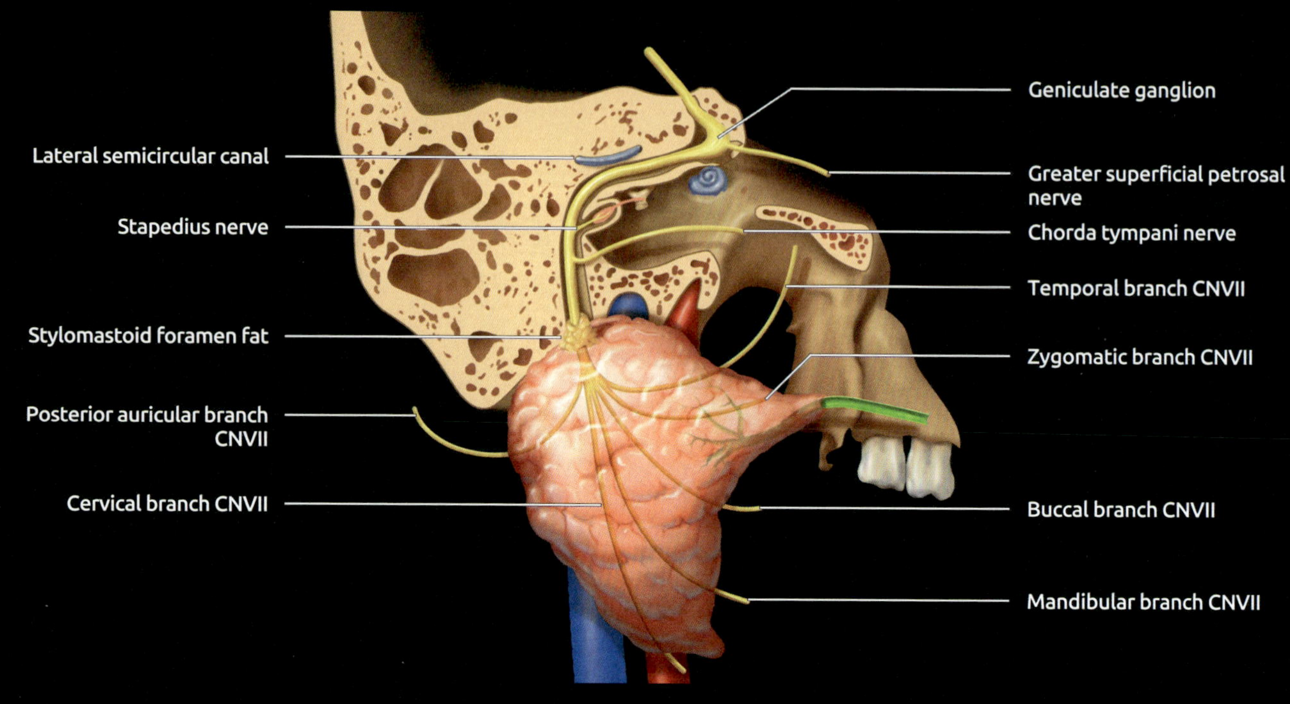

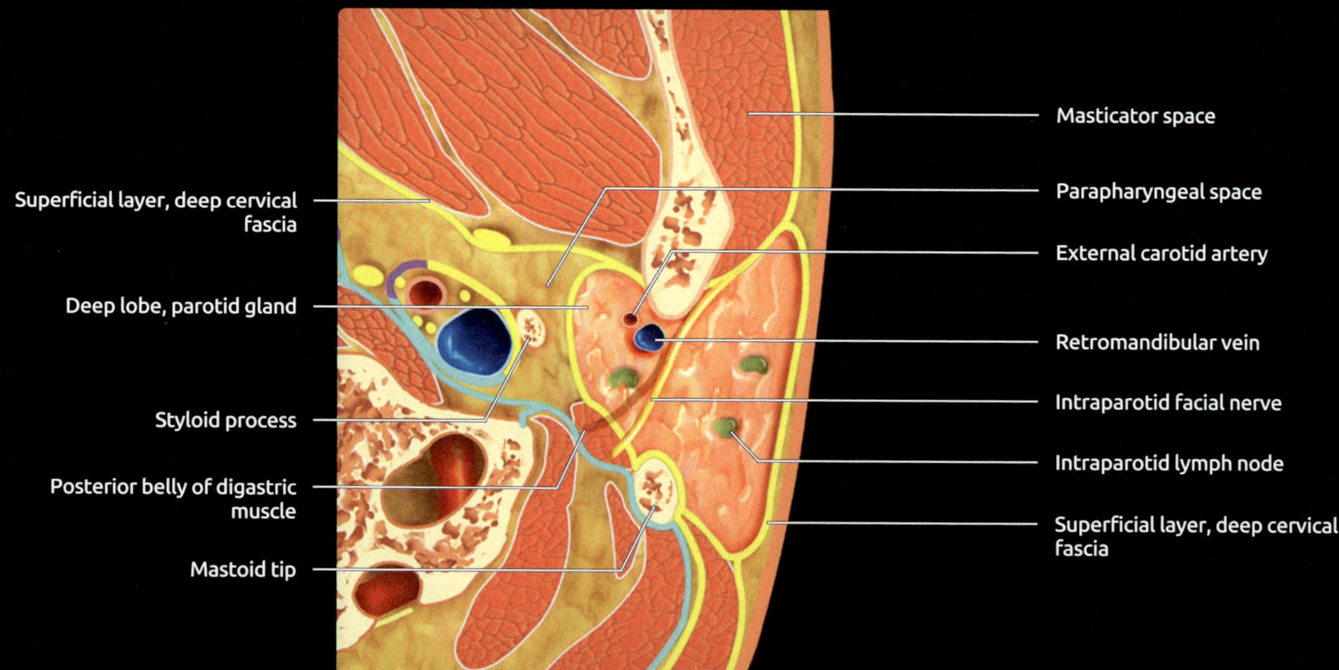

(Top) *Sagittal graphic of the parotid gland and facial nerve is shown. The facial nerve exits the skull base at the stylomastoid foramen, gives off the posterior auricular nerve, and branches to posterior belly of digastric muscle and stylohyoid muscle. Facial nerve then enters the parotid gland where it ramifies into 5 major branches. The plane of the facial nerve branches within the parotid gland is used by the surgeons to define a superficial and deep lobe of the parotid. This is a surgically defined, not a radiologically defined, delineation.* **(Bottom)** *Axial graphic of the parotid space at the level of C1 vertebral body is shown. The intraparotid course of the facial nerve extends from just medial to the mastoid tip to a position just lateral to the retromandibular vein. Late embryologic encapsulation of the parotid gland accounts for intraparotid lymph nodes, which serve as 1st-order drainage for malignancies of the deep face, scalp, and external ear. The normal parotid gland contains ~ 20 nodes.*

GENERIC PAROTID SPACE MASS

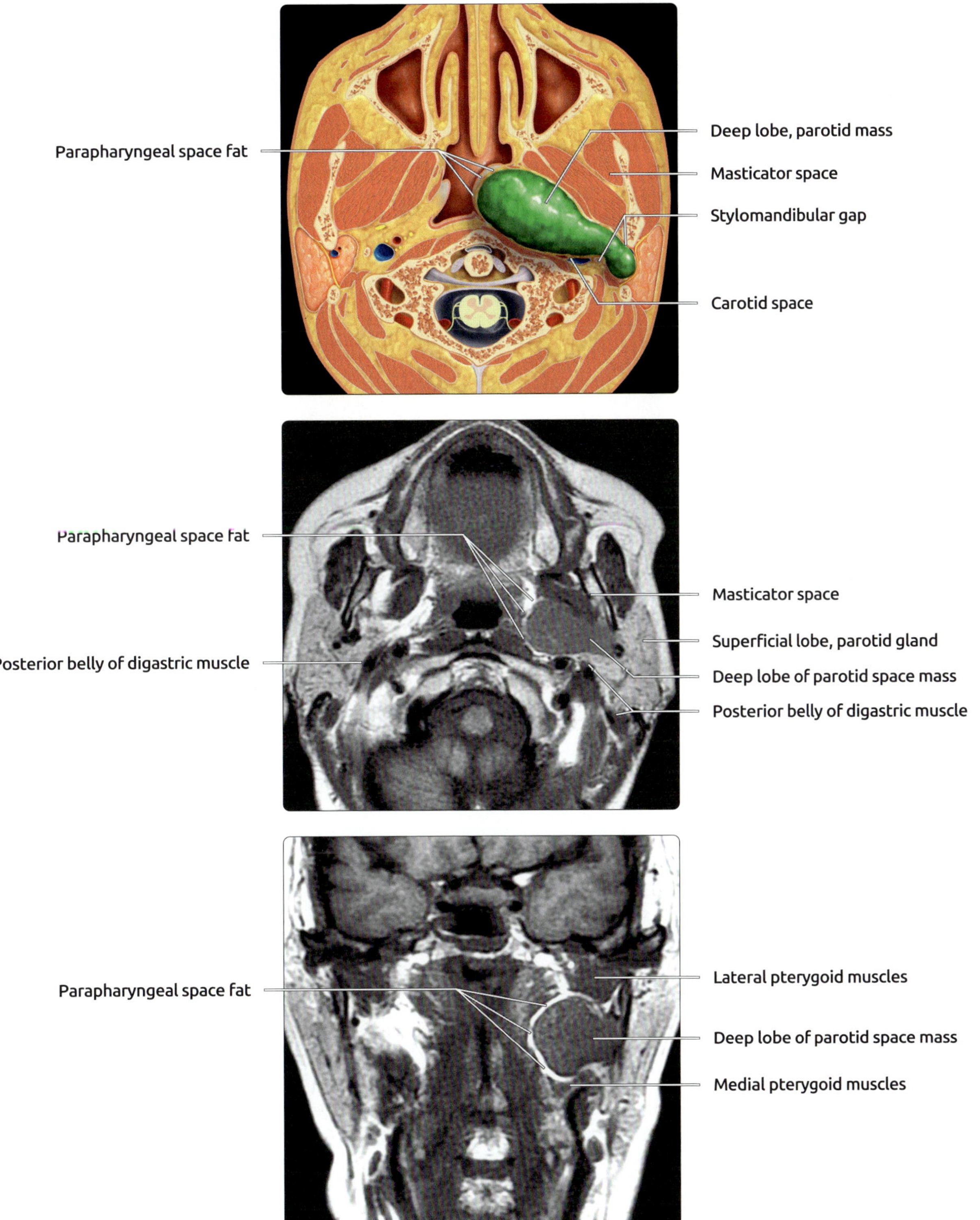

(Top) *Axial graphic of the generic deep lobe of a parotid gland mass demonstrates medial displacement of the parapharyngeal space fat. Also notice the slight enlargement of the stylomandibular gap. Smaller lesions of the superficial lobe of the parotid gland are easily identified as intraparotid. Larger deep lobe lesions may be more difficult to identify as parotid space in origin.* **(Middle)** *Axial T1 MR through the maxillary ridge reveals a pear-shaped mass arising from the deep lobe of the parotid gland. This benign mixed tumor enlarges medially, displacing the parapharyngeal space from lateral to medial. Note the extremely important practical landmark of posterior belly of digastric muscle separating the upper carotid space posteromedial to it from the deep parotid space anterolateral to it.* **(Bottom)** *Coronal T1 MR of a large benign mixed tumor enlarging medially from its origin in the deep lobe of the parotid gland is shown. Note the crescent of parapharyngeal space fat arching medially and still visible despite the large size of this deep lobe tumor.*

PERINEURAL PAROTID SPACE MALIGNANCY

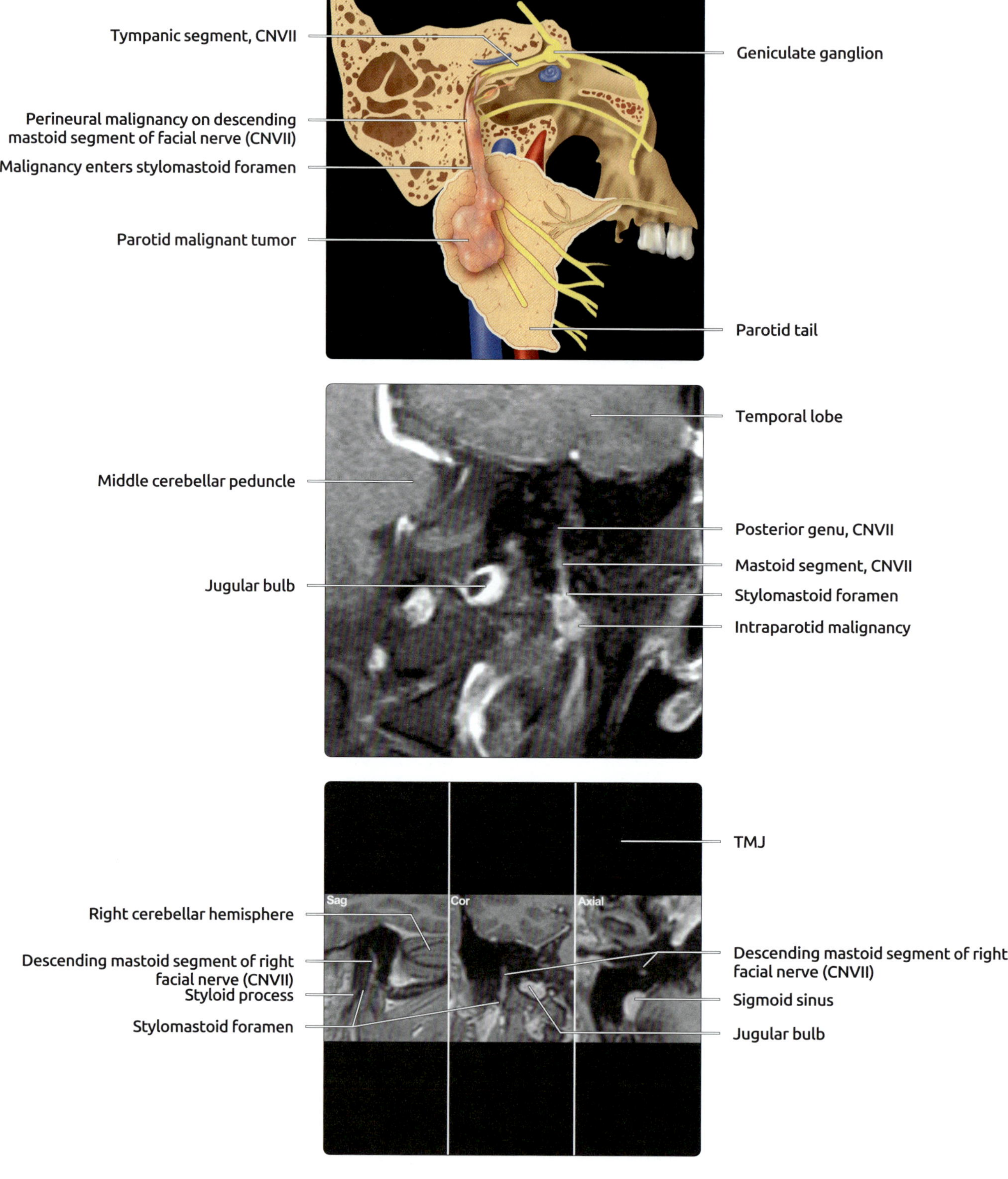

(Top) *Sagittal graphic of a generic parotid malignancy affecting the intraparotid facial nerve is shown. The tumor spreads along CNVII through the stylomastoid foramen to the proximal mastoid segment within the temporal bone. If left untreated, such a perineural malignant tumor will eventually access the intracranial compartment via the internal auditory canal.* **(Middle)** *Coronal T1 C+ FS MR of the left temporal bone shows an enhancing adenoid cystic carcinoma of the parotid gland spreading into the lower flared portion of the stylomastoid foramen. This malignant tumor then spreads in a perineural fashion up the mastoid segment of the facial nerve to the posterior genu.* **(Bottom)** *Multiplanar MPRAGE T1 C+ MR shows normal enhancing right CNVII mastoid segment down to stylomastoid foramen (important anatomy to evaluate in parotid malignancy MR). Frey syndrome (auriculotemporal syndrome) is gustatory sweating due to auriculotemporal nerve injury, which carries parasympathetic fibers to parotid and overlying skin sweat glands. Inappropriate regeneration of parasympathetic nerve fibers may result in sweating in anticipation of eating instead of normal salivatory response.*

AXIAL CECT

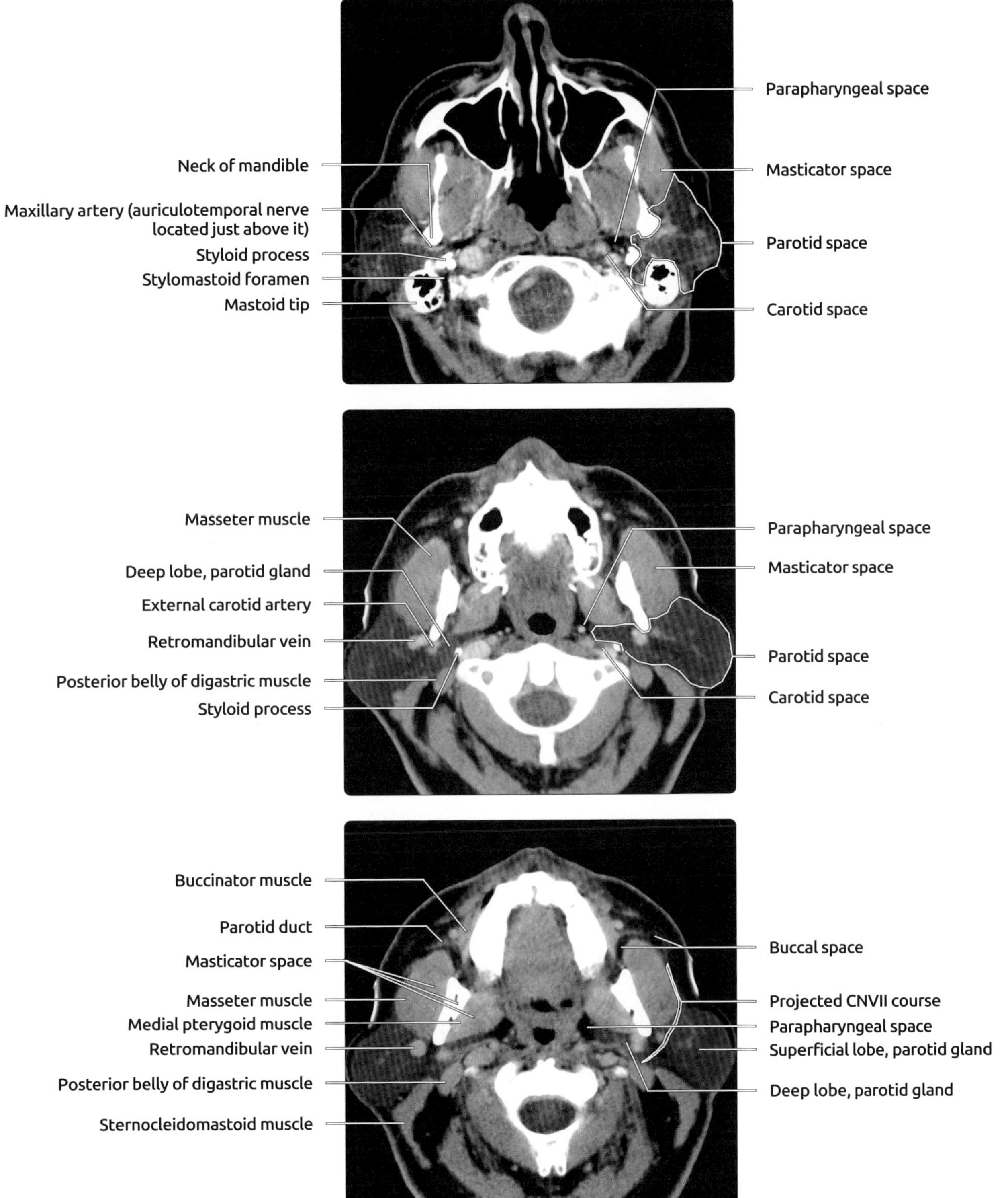

(Top) *First of 6 axial CECT images from superior to inferior shows right stylomastoid foramen with low-attenuation fat. Facial nerve is not seen on CT. If perineural tumor is present, stylomastoid foramen fat will be replaced by tumor. Note maxillary artery, which is 1 of 2 terminal branches of ECA within parotid, leaving the gland at its anteromedial aspect. Auriculotemporal nerve (CNV3 branch) is situated just above maxillary artery at this level posterior to neck of mandible. Auriculotemporal nerve crosses through body of parotid gland at right angles to facial nerve and usually has direct communications with CNVII here with chances for facial to trigeminal perineural tumor spread.* **(Middle)** *Image shows deep lobe of parotid gland projecting through stylomandibular gap to abut parapharyngeal space. Note the medial ECA and more lateral retromandibular vein.* **(Bottom)** *Image shows parotid duct (in buccal space) piecing buccinator muscle just lateral to 2nd maxillary molar tooth. Note the projected course of extracranial CNVII drawn lateral to retromandibular vein and over surface of masseter separating the larger superficial from smaller deep lobe of parotid gland.*

AXIAL CECT

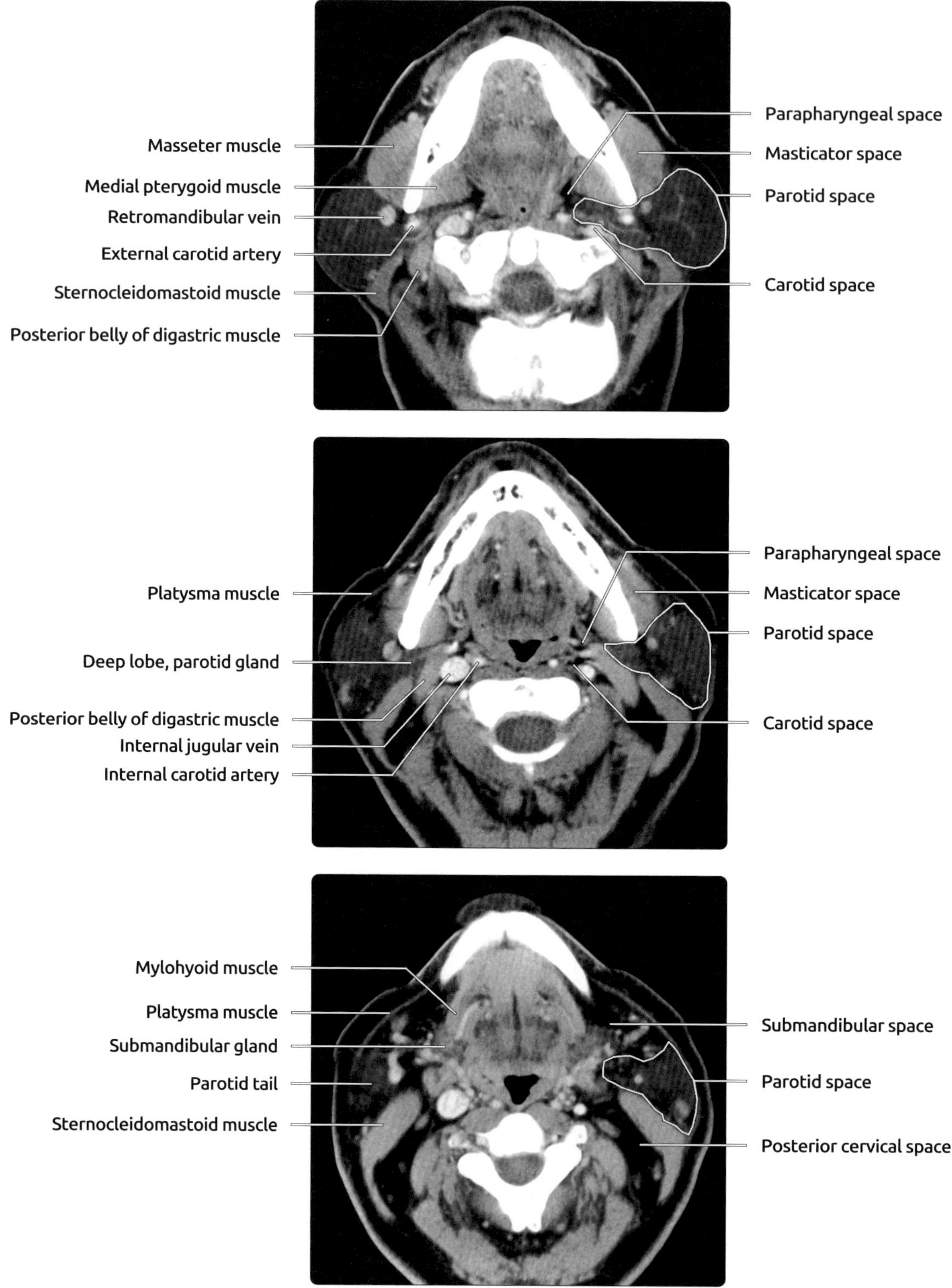

(Top) *In this image at the level of the midoropharynx, the larger laterally placed retromandibular vein can be distinguished from the more medial ECA. Remember that the intraparotid facial nerve cannot be seen on CECT, but its path can be projected along a line just lateral to the retromandibular vein and out over the surface of the masseter muscle.* **(Middle)** *At the level of the mandibular angle, the parotid space is now separated from the carotid space by the posterior belly of the digastric muscle. Note the platysma muscle is now visible over the surface of the parotid gland.* **(Bottom)** *Just below the mandible, the parotid tail is visible projecting into the posterior aspect of the submandibular space. Excisional biopsy of a low-lying mass, unrecognized as being in the parotid tail, may result in facial nerve injury.*

AXIAL T1 MR

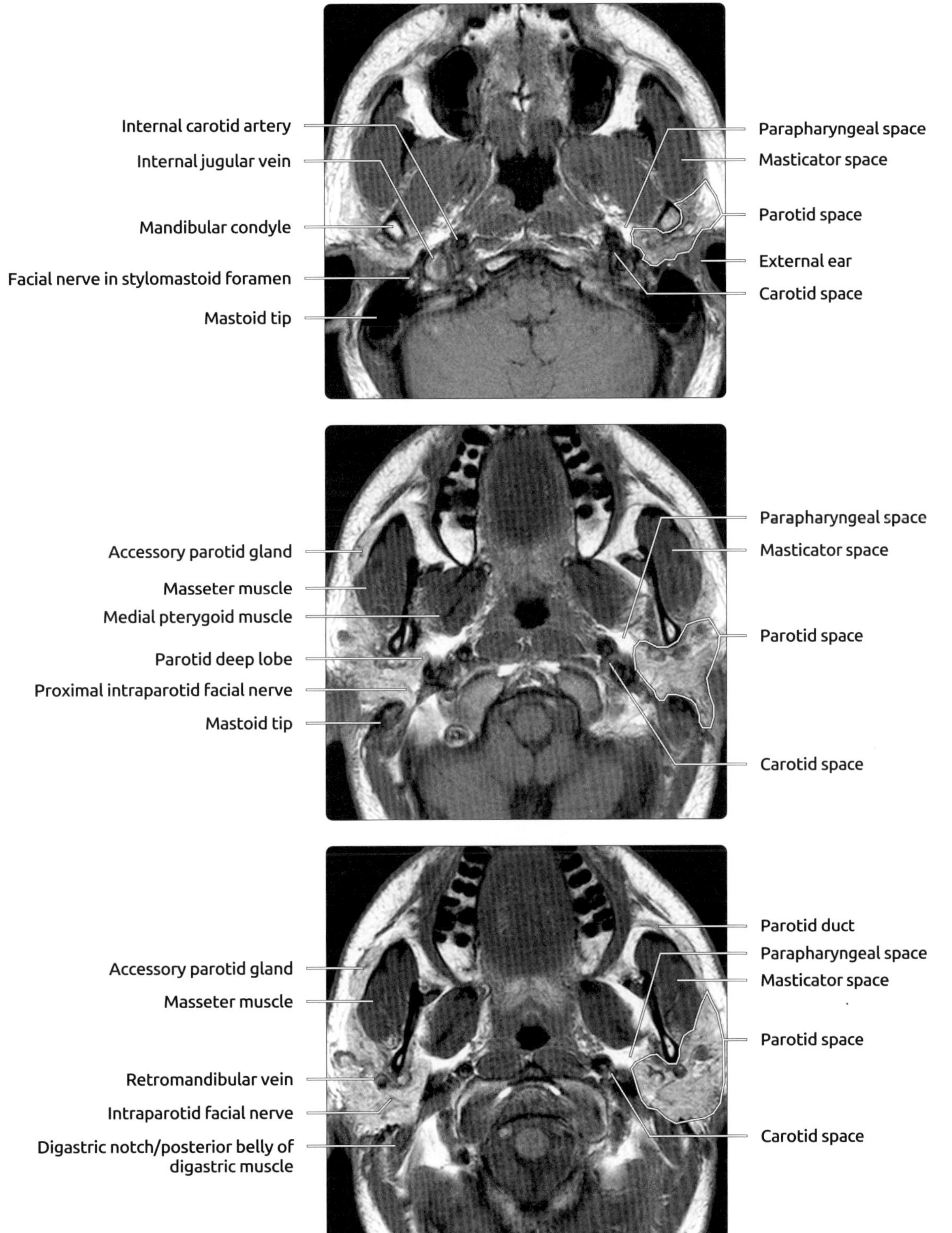

(Top) *First of 6 axial T1 MR images presented superior to inferior shows the right facial nerve exiting the stylomandibular foramen. There is fat in the lower flared aspect of the stylomastoid foramen, so the main trunk of the facial nerve is visible.* **(Middle)** *In this image, the proximal intraparotid facial nerve is seen on the right. Note the accessory parotid gland overlying the right masseter muscle bilaterally.* **(Bottom)** *At the level of the maxillary ridge, a branch of the intraparotid facial nerve is seen projecting anterolaterally around the lateral margin of the retromandibular vein. Usually not visible on routine imaging, the intraparotid facial nerve and its branches follow a predictable course anterolaterally around the lateral margin of the retromandibular vein, and, from there, anteriorly along the lateral surface of the masseter muscle.*

AXIAL T1 MR

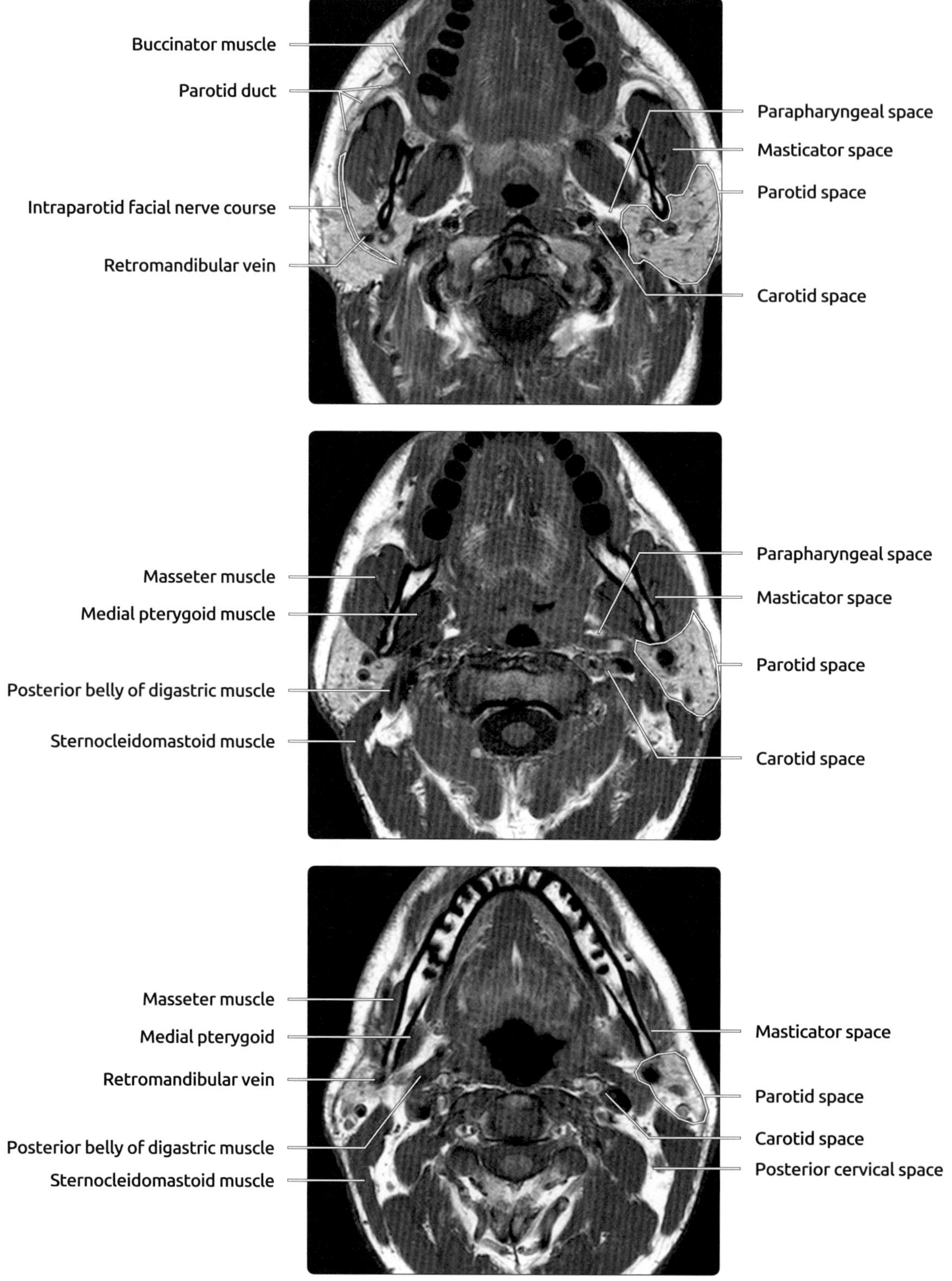

(Top) *At the level of the maxillary teeth, the parotid space is visible posterolateral to the masticator space. Remember that both the masticator and parotid spaces are circumscribed by the superficial layer of the deep cervical fascia. Note the projected intraparotid facial nerve course drawn on the right.* **(Middle)** *In this image, the posterior belly of the digastric muscle is seen on the posteromedial boundary of the parotid space, separating the parotid space from the carotid space. The posterior belly of the digastric muscle is innervated by a branch of the facial nerve.* **(Bottom)** *In this image, the parotid gland is seen at the mandibular angle. The posterior belly of the digastric muscle is seen between the parotid tail and the carotid space on the left. When a parotid space mass is present, the medial displacement of the posterior belly of the digastric muscle helps define its location.*

AXIAL T2 FS MR

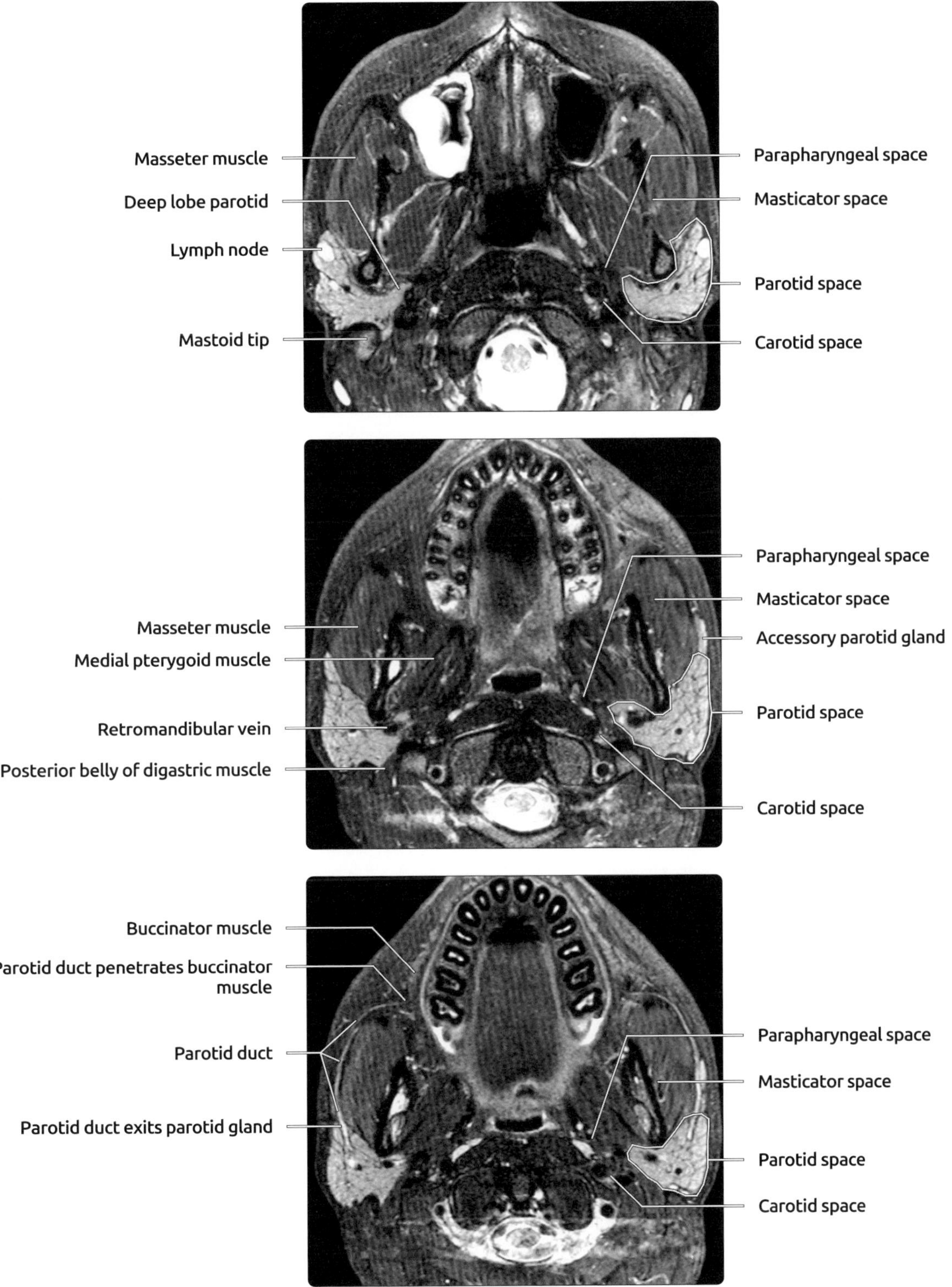

(Top) *First of 3 axial T2 FS MR images presented superior to inferior shows that the adult parotid gland has higher signal than the surrounding muscles of the suprahyoid neck. A few sporadic high-signal intraparotid nodes are present at this level. The parapharyngeal space fat has low signal because of the fat-saturation MR sequence.* **(Middle)** *The parotid space often abuts the accessory parotid gland that may be seen over the surface of the masseter muscle. Both are within the superficial layer of deep cervical fascia.* **(Bottom)** *In this image at the level of the maxillary teeth, the high-signal linear parotid duct is easily visualized extending anteriorly from the parotid gland along the surface of the masseter muscle to penetrate the buccinator muscle.*

TRANSVERSE ULTRASOUND

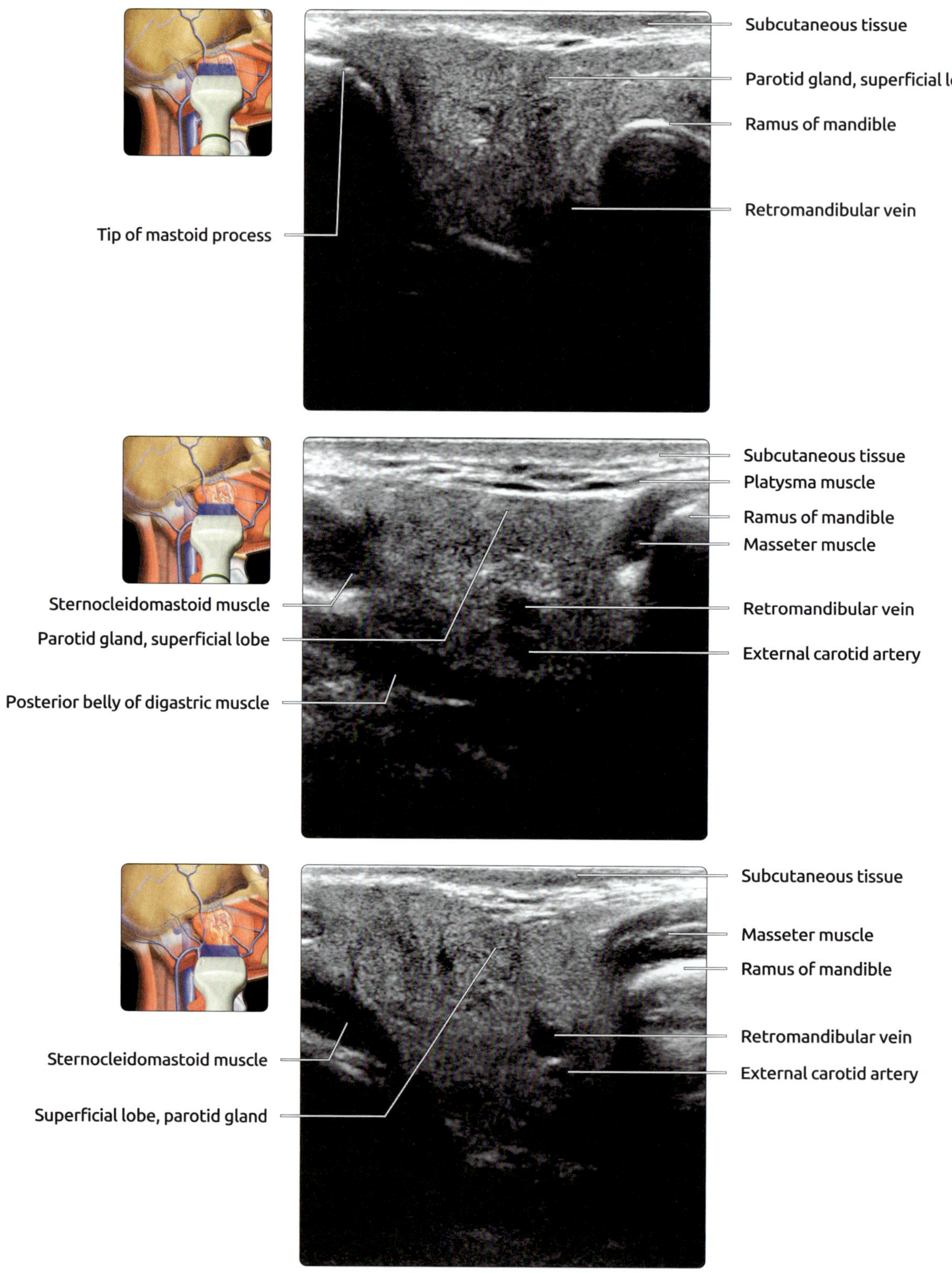

(Top) *Transverse grayscale ultrasound shows the parotid region. Note its relationship to the mastoid process and the mandibular ramus. The glandular parenchyma shows a homogeneous, hyperechoic pattern. The retromandibular vein is visualized as a round, anechoic structure within the parotid gland (partially obscured in this image).* **(Middle)** *Transverse grayscale ultrasound shows the parotid tail region. The sternocleidomastoid muscle and the posterior belly of the digastric muscle are related to the posterior margin of the parotid tail. The retromandibular vein and ECA serve as markers to infer the location of CNVII.* **(Bottom)** *Transverse grayscale ultrasound shows the parotid gland. The retromandibular vein is usually larger and lateral to the ECA within the parotid gland. Note that the deep lobe is obscured by shadowing from the mandibular ramus.*

LONGITUDINAL ULTRASOUND

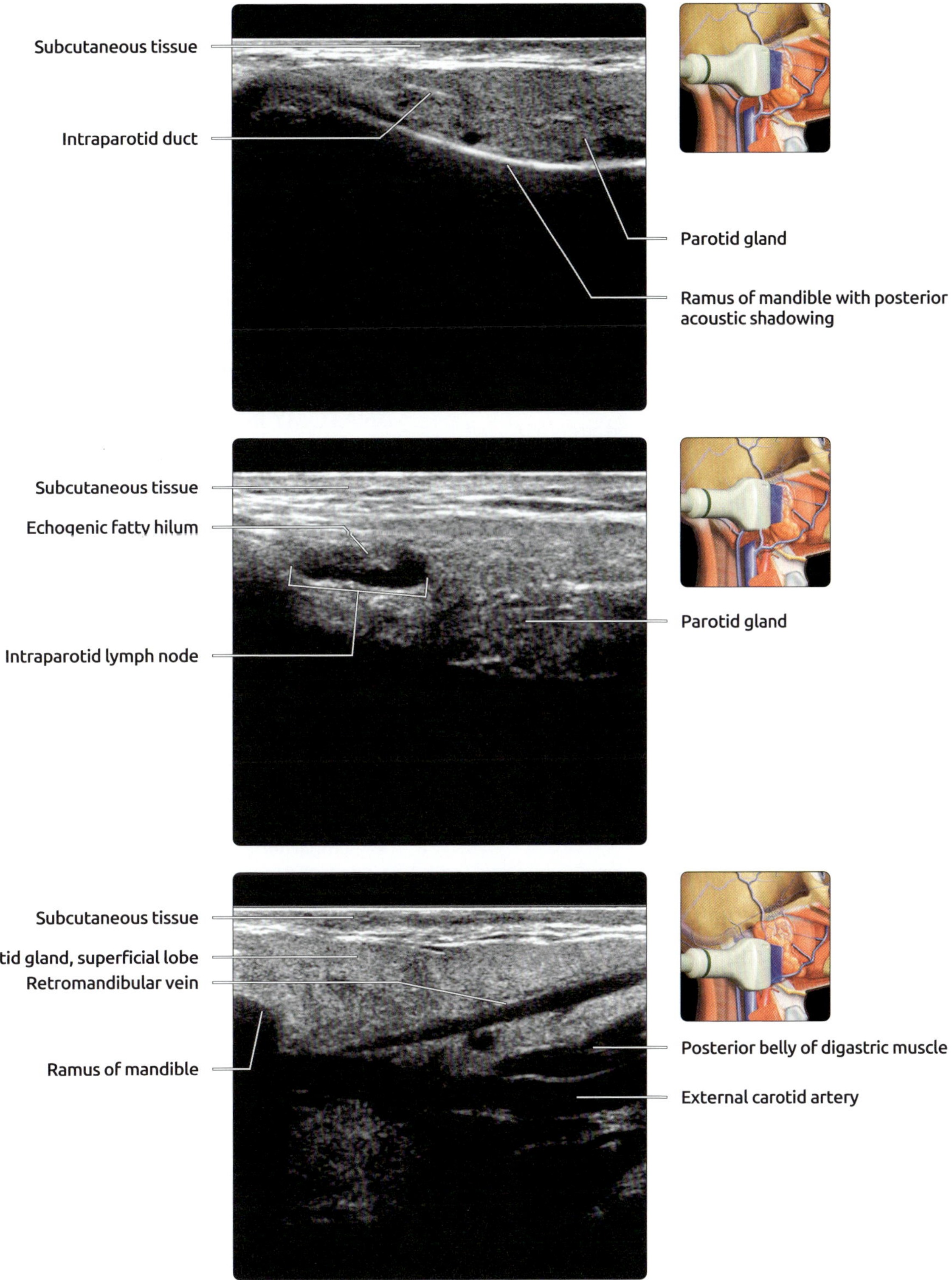

(Top) *This is the 1st image in a series of longitudinal grayscale ultrasound scans of the parotid gland. Intense shadowing from the ramus of the mandible precludes visualization of deeper structures, including the deep lobe of the parotid gland.* **(Middle)** *Second image shows a normal intraparotid lymph node in the superficial lobe of the parotid gland. On high-resolution ultrasound, normal nodes are invariably seen in the parotid tail and in the pretragal parotid gland. The elliptical shape and normal internal architecture with echogenic hilum suggest its benign nature.* **(Bottom)** *Third image at the plane of the retromandibular vein is shown. Such anatomy is best seen in children and young adults where there is not much fat deposition in the gland.*

Carotid Space

TERMINOLOGY

Abbreviations

- Carotid space (CS)
- Suprahyoid neck (SHN); infrahyoid neck (IHN)

Synonyms

- Poststyloid parapharyngeal space (PPS) in SHN
  - Real PPS, a.k.a. prestyloid PPS

Definitions

- Paired, tubular spaces surrounded by carotid sheath that contain carotid arteries, internal jugular veins (IJVs), and **cranial nerves (CNs) IX-XII (SHN) and CNX (IHN)**

IMAGING ANATOMY

Overview

- CS travels from inferior margins of jugular foramen-carotid canal above to aortic arch below
- SHN CS contains CNIX-XII, internal carotid artery (ICA), and IJV
- IHN CS contains CNX only, common carotid artery (CCA), IJV
- IJ nodal chain closely associated with its outer surface

Extent

- CS defined from skull base (carotid canal and jugular foramen) to aortic arch below
- CS can be divided into its major segments
  - Nasopharyngeal, oropharyngeal, cervical, mediastinal

Anatomy Relationships

- **SHN CS adjacent spaces**
  - Retropharyngeal space (RPS) medial; perivertebral space (PVS) posterior; PPS anterior; parotid space (PS) lateral
    - **Posterior belly of digastric (PBD)** muscle separates CS from deep lobe of parotid gland
- **IHN CS adjacent spaces**
  - Visceral space and RPS medial; PVS posterior; anterior cervical space anterior; posterior cervical space lateral

Internal Contents

- **SHN CS**
  - **Vessels: ICA and IJV**
  - **CNIX-XII in nasopharyngeal CS**
  - **Only CNX** in CS from oropharyngeal CS **inferiorly**
  - **CNX** in posterior notch formed by ICA and IJV **within CS**
    - Vagus nerve tumor: **Separates** carotid artery (pushed anteromedially) and IJV (pushed posterolaterally)
  - **Sympathetic trunk** lies **outside CS** posterior to it or between **medial** CS and lateral RPS
    - Plastered to prevertebral fascia
    - Sympathetic trunk tumor: **Displaces both** carotid artery and IJV **together** anteriorly/anterolaterally
    - **Postganglionic** sympathetic fibers pass **around** CCA, ICA, and ECA (within and outside CS) in both SHN and IHN
- **IHN CS**
  - **Vessels**: **CCA and IJV**
  - **Vagus nerve** (within CS between ICA and IJV) and **sympathetic trunk** (outside CS) **posteriorly**
  - **Ansa cervicalis** embedded in anterior wall of CS
  - **Superior root (descendens hypoglossi)**: Descends over **ICA and CCA**; continuation of descending branch of hypoglossal nerve; fibers from **C1** spinal nerve
    - Supplies **superior belly of omohyoid**
  - **Inferior root (descending cervical nerve)**: Descends winding around **IJV**; fibers from **C2**, **C3** spinal nerves
    - Supplies **inferior belly of omohyoid**
    - Joins superior root anteroinferiorly **in front of CCA** to form **ansa cervicalis**
    - Ansa cervicalis supplies **sternohyoid** and **sternothyroid**
  - Internal jugular nodes closely associated (but **not** in CS)

Fascia of CS

- **Carotid sheath** made from components of **all 3 layers of deep cervical fascia (DCF)**
  - SHN CS: Carotid sheath incomplete or less substantial
  - IHN CS: Carotid sheath well-defined, tenacious fascia

ANATOMY IMAGING ISSUES

Questions

- **Lesion in SHN CS**
  - Center of lesion within area of ICA-IJV, posterior to PPS
  - Lesion displaces PPS fat anteriorly; pushes PBD muscle anterolaterally; and nasopharyngeal CS lesion pushes styloid process anterolaterally
  - **Vagus nerve tumor** (schwannoma, neurofibroma, paraganglioma): **Separates** ICA and IJV
    - ICA pushed **anteromedially** and IJV **posterolaterally**
  - **Sympathetic schwannoma**: **Displaces** both ICA and IJV **together** anteriorly or anterolaterally
- **Lesion in IHN CS**
  - May engulf CCA and IJV or push them apart
  - **Vagus nerve tumor**: **Separates** CCA and IJV
  - May **splay ECA** and **ICA** (**carotid body** paraganglioma)
  - **Sympathetic schwannoma**: **Displaces** both CCA and IJV **together** anteriorly or anterolaterally

Imaging Recommendations

- CECT or MR easily identify normal CS anatomy and lesions

Imaging Approaches

- Remember that CS runs from jugular foramen-carotid canal of skull base above to aortic arch below
- If imaging CS because of **left** vagal neuropathy, must reach aortopulmonic window inferiorly

Imaging Pitfalls

- Normal vascular flow phenomenon of IJV may mimic schwannoma or thrombosis

CLINICAL IMPLICATIONS

Clinical Importance

- **CNIX-XII** and **carotid artery** vital structures in CS

Function Dysfunction

- **Injury to nasopharyngeal CS** may result in complex cranial neuropathy involving some combination of **CNIX-XII**
- **Vagus nerve injury**: Vocal cord paralysis
- Look for extranodal extension of internal jugular nodal chain pathology around carotid artery

GRAPHICS

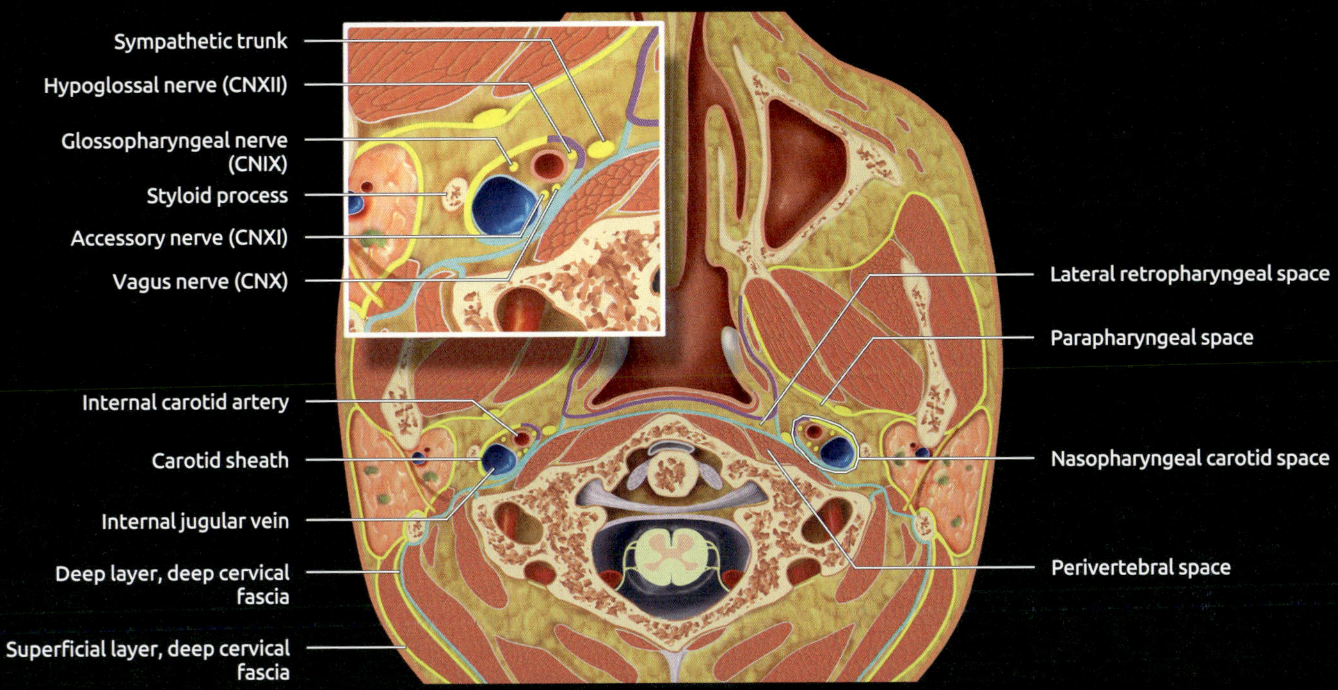

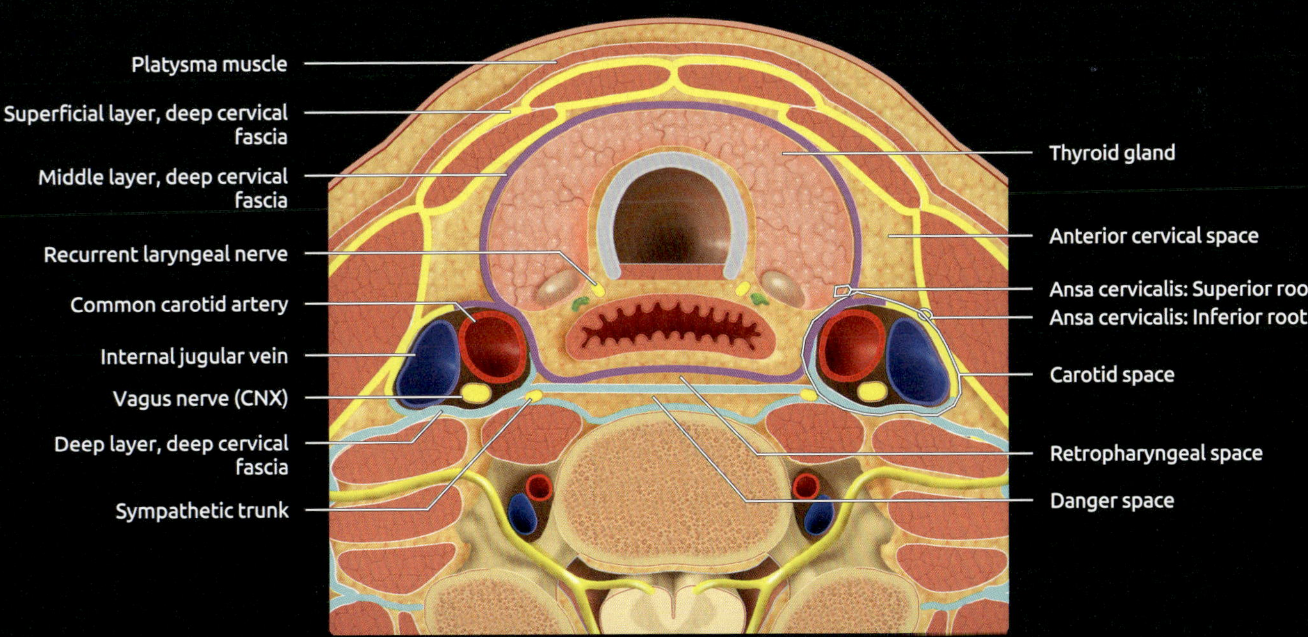

(Top) *Graphic shows the suprahyoid neck (SHN) at the level of C1 vertebral body with insert showing magnified carotid space (CS). SHN CS contains CNIX-XII, internal carotid artery (ICA), and internal jugular vein (IJV). Carotid sheath is made up of components of all 3 layers of deep cervical fascia (tricolor line around CS). In SHN, carotid sheath is less substantial than it is in infrahyoid neck (IHN). Sympathetic trunk runs posteromedial to CS.* **(Bottom)** *In the IHN, the CS is tenacious throughout its length. IHN CS contains the common carotid artery (CCA), IJV, and only the vagus cranial nerve. Note sympathetic trunk lying outside the CS posterior to it, and ansa cervicalis embedded in the anterior wall of the carotid sheath. Postganglionic sympathetic fibers pass around CCA, ICA, and external carotid arteries and branches (within and outside CS) in both SHN and IHN. Postganglionic fibers from superior cervical sympathetic ganglion are distributed in the internal carotid nerve ascending with the ICA into the carotid canal entering the cranial cavity, and also in the lateral, medial, and anterior branches of the ganglion.*

GRAPHICS

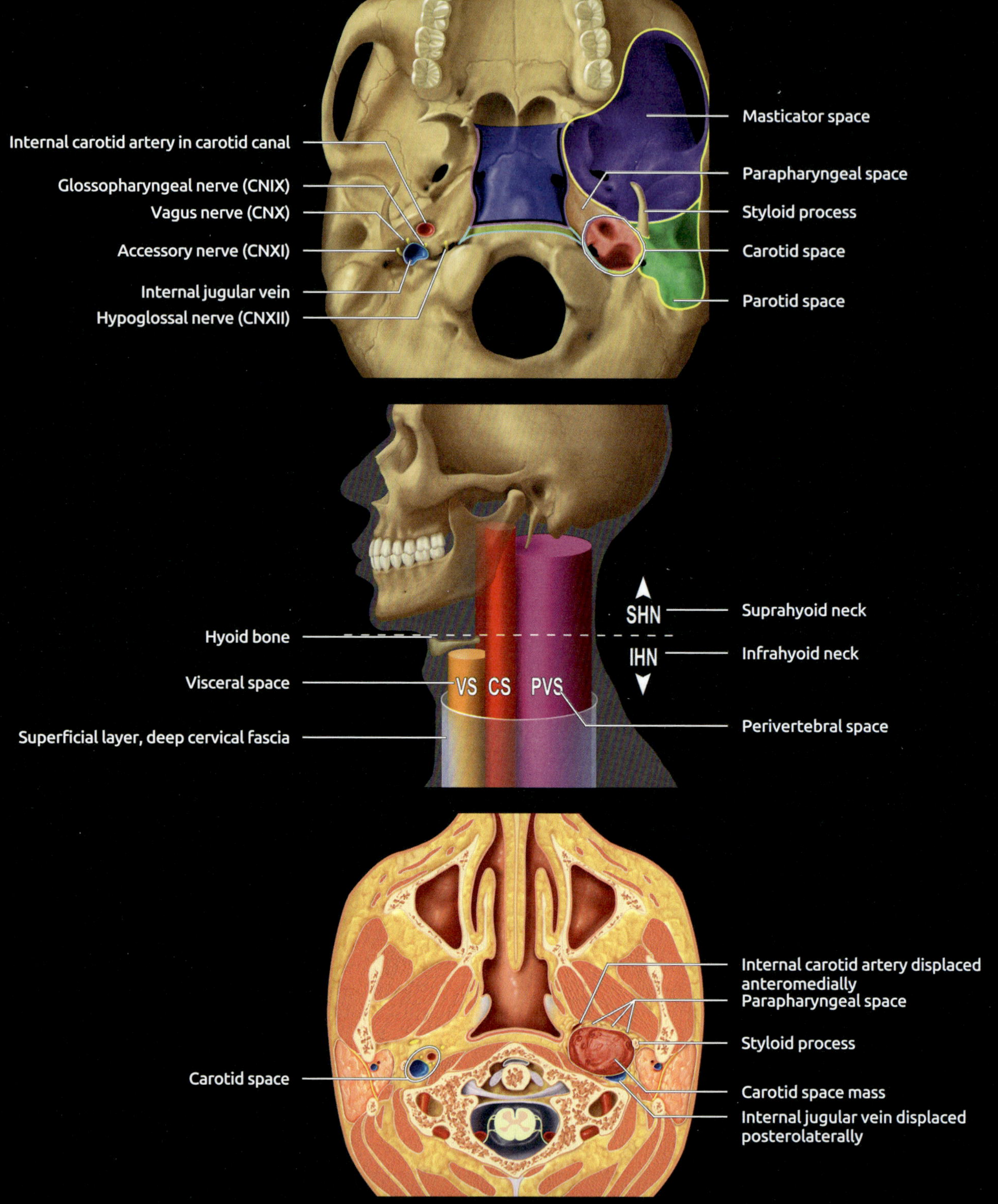

(Top) *Graphic shows the skull base viewed from below, illustrating the interaction between the CS and the skull base. The nasopharyngeal CS is an inferior continuation of the carotid canal, jugular foramen, and hypoglossal canal. The ICA, IJV, and CNIX-XII are found within the CS. The carotid sheath is depicted as a tricolor line because it is formed from all 3 layers of deep cervical fascia.* **(Middle)** *Graphic of the neck shows the CS as a tube running from the skull base to the aortic arch. The CS is divided at the hyoid bone level into suprahyoid and infrahyoid portions. The suprahyoid CS has CNIX-XII within it, and the infrahyoid CS has only a vagus nerve inside.* **(Bottom)** *Graphic shows a generic CS mass. A SHN CS mass displaces the parapharyngeal space fat anteriorly as well as lifts the styloid process anterolaterally. SHN and IHN vagal nerve/sheath tumor separates the carotid artery (pushed anteromedially) and IJV (pushed posterolaterally). In contrast, a sympathetic trunk tumor will displace both carotid artery and IJV together anteriorly/anterolaterally as the sympathetic trunk lies outside the CS posteriorly/posteromedially.*

CECT AND CTA OF CAROTID SPACE VESSELS

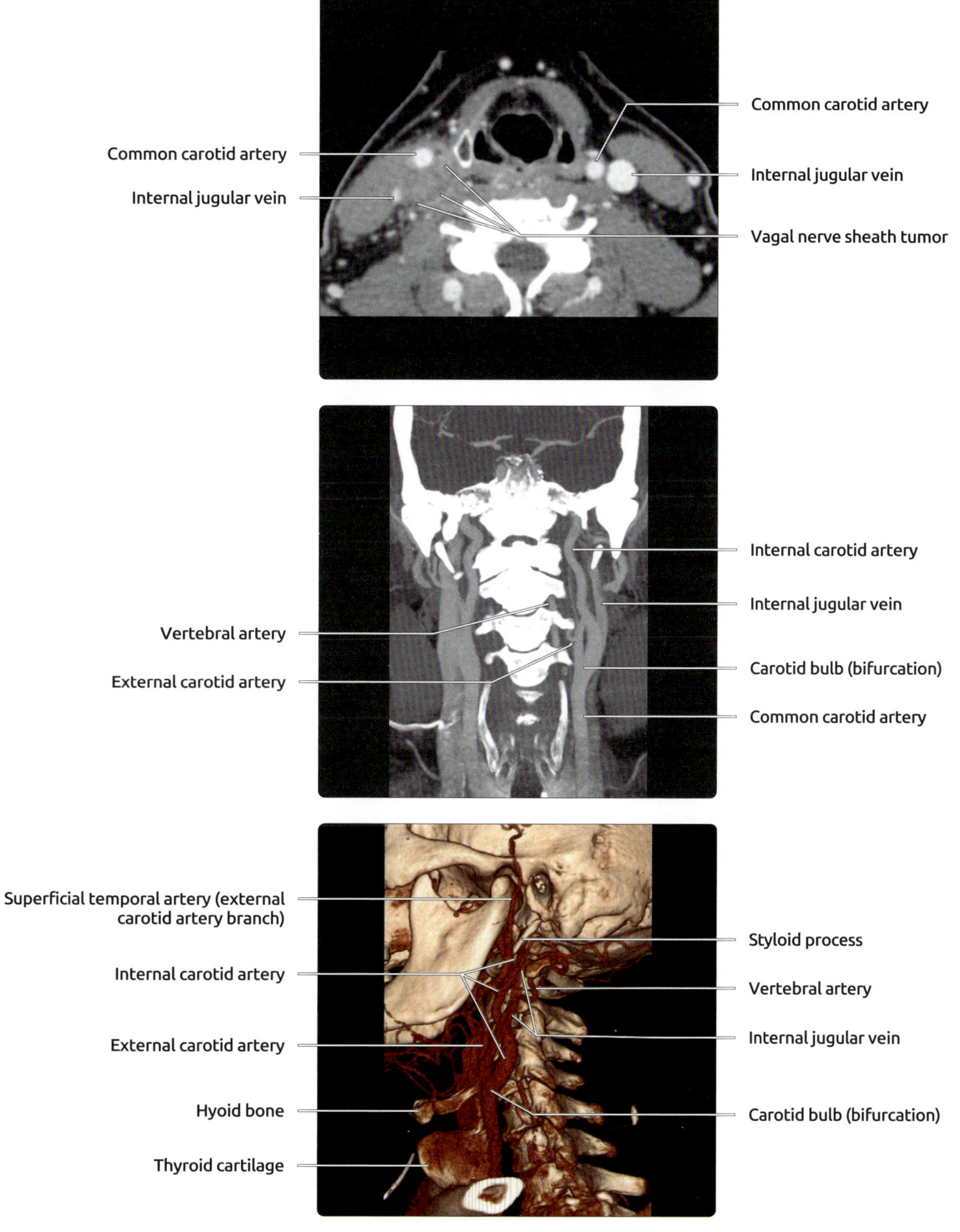

(Top) *Axial CECT of the IHN shows a right vagal nerve sheath tumor splaying the CCA anteromedially and IJV posterolaterally. Note the normal arrangement of the left CCA and IJV.* **(Middle)** *Coronal MIP reconstruction of neck CTA shows the CS vessels, namely, CCA and IJV in IHN and ICA and IJV in SHN. CS nerves, which include CNIX-XII in nasopharyngeal CS and CNX from oropharyngeal CS inferiorly, cannot be visualized on routine CT/MR. ECA and vertebral artery, which are not part of the CS, are also marked.* **(Bottom)** *Lateral view of 3D reconstruction of neck CTA shows the contents of CS. Note that the hyoid bone is approximately at the level of carotid bifurcation with the ICA found in SHN CS and the CCA found in IHN CS. ECA originates from the carotid bulb, exits out of the CS and branches out in the neck, whereas the ICA within the CS has no branches in the neck. IJV runs within the CS in both SHN and IHN. SHN CS is also known as poststyloid parapharyngeal space (PPS) as it lies posterior to the styloid process, just behind the real PPS.*

AXIAL CECT

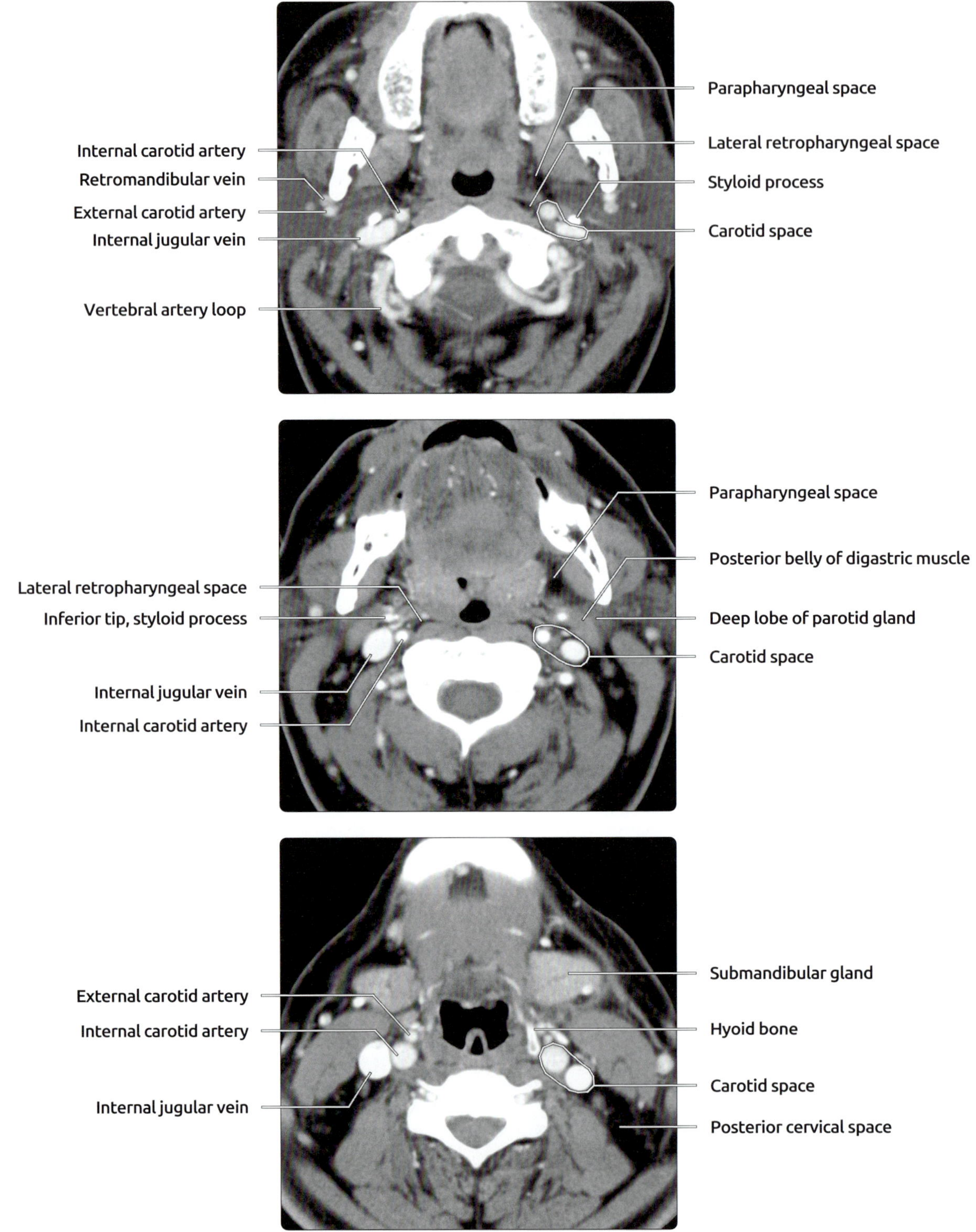

(Top) *First of 6 axial CECT images presented from superior to inferior is shown. In this image at the level of C1 vertebral body, the nasopharyngeal CS contains the ICA, IJV, and CNIX-XII. Notice that the CS is posterior to the styloid process. At the level of the nasopharynx, a CS mass will push from posterior to anterior into the parapharyngeal space and displace the styloid process anterolaterally.* **(Middle)** *In this image at the level of the midoropharynx, the posterior belly of the digastric (PBD) muscle is visible anterolateral to the CS. A CS mass here would push this muscle anterolaterally and the parapharyngeal space anteriorly. CS lies posteromedial to deep lobe of parotid gland in the parotid space and the PBD muscle separates upper CS from deep parotid space. Displacement of PBD muscle can be used to assess the epicenter of tumors in this location. Deep lobe of parotid tumor displaces PBD posteromedially, whereas CS mass here will displace PBD anterolaterally.* **(Bottom)** *At the level of the hyoid bone, the carotid bifurcation can be seen. At this level, only the vagus nerve is left within the CS.*

AXIAL CECT

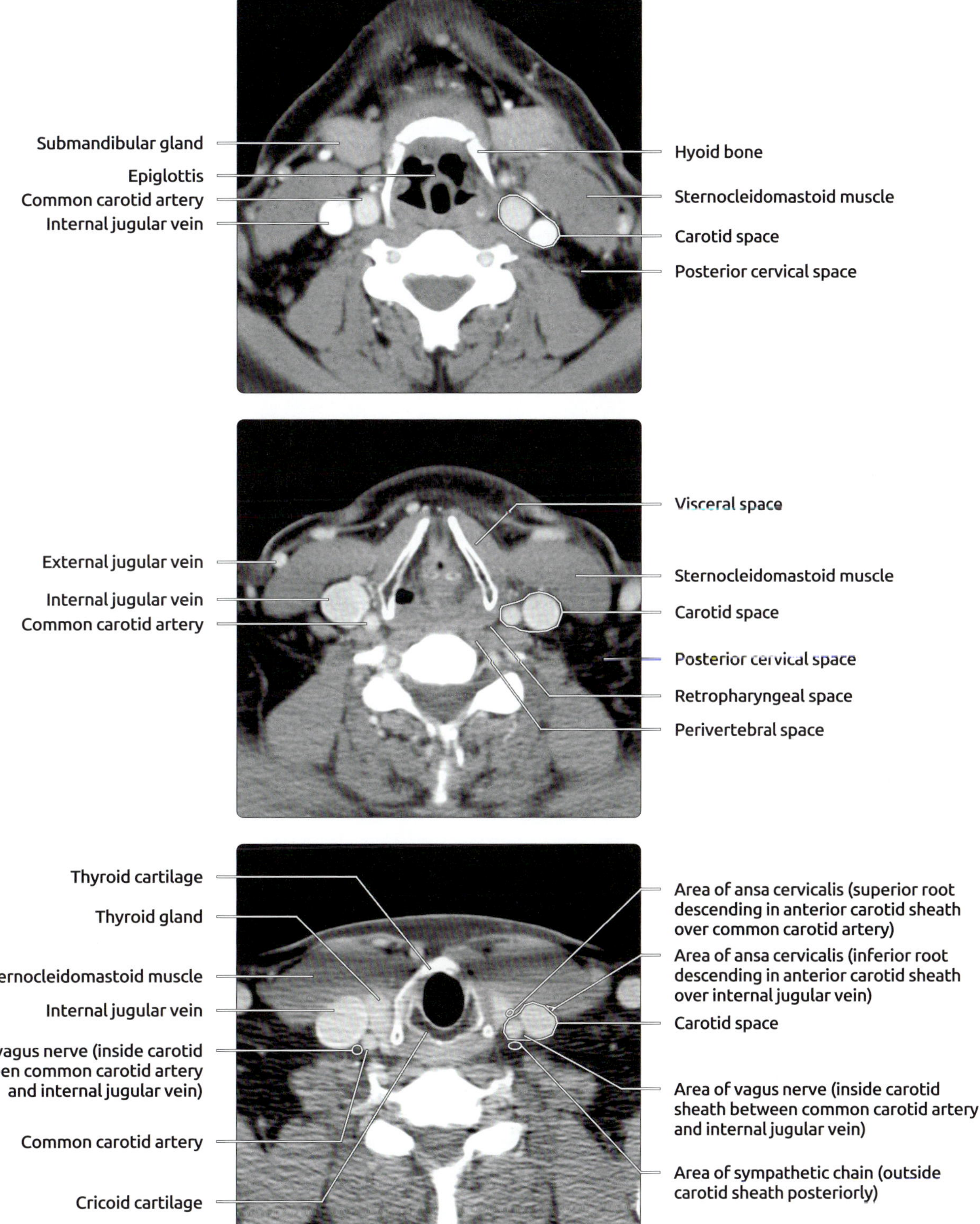

(Top) *At the level of the hyoid bone, the CS has only the CCA, IJV, and vagus nerve within it. Notice that, despite the high-resolution nature of this CT image, it is not possible to see the vagus nerve or the carotid sheath.* **(Middle)** *In this image through the infrahyoid aspect of the CS, the surrounding deep tissue anatomy can be seen. Posterolateral to the CS, the large fat-filled posterior cervical space is visible. Posteromedially, the perivertebral space is found. Medial to the CS are the visceral space and the retropharyngeal space. Anteriorly, the sternocleidomastoid muscle resides.* **(Bottom)** *At the level of the cricoid cartilage, the infrahyoid CS contains the CCA, IJV, and vagus nerve. Despite its large size, the vagal trunk cannot be visualized in its location between the CCA and IJV within the carotid sheath. The sympathetic chain lies outside the carotid sheath posterior to it, and the ansa cervicalis lies embedded in the anterior wall of carotid sheath. These are also not demonstrated (expected locations are marked).*

COMMON CAROTID ARTERY ULTRASOUND

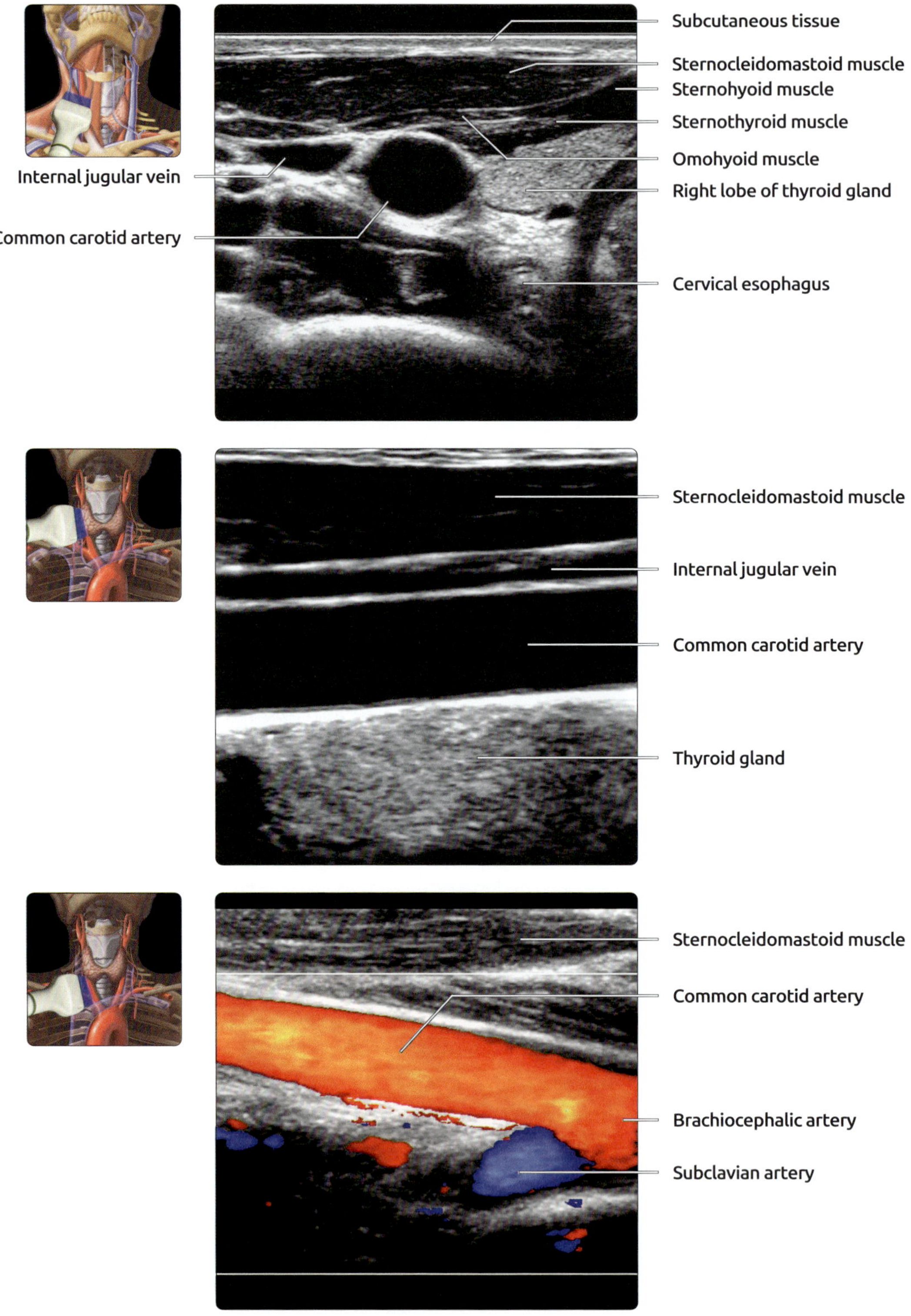

(Top) *Transverse grayscale ultrasound shows the distal CCA at the level of the upper pole of the thyroid gland. Note that the artery wall in a normal individual is smooth with no intimal thickening or atherosclerotic plaque. The lumen is circular in cross section. There is no major named branch of the common carotid proximal to the bifurcation.* **(Middle)** *Longitudinal grayscale ultrasound of the CCA shows the smooth outline of the intimal layer.* **(Bottom)** *Color Doppler ultrasound of the proximal CCA at the root of the neck in the longitudinal plane demonstrates the normal antegrade arterial flow in the cranial direction. Its origin, along with the subclavian artery from the right brachiocephalic artery, is also well demonstrated.*

VAGUS NERVE ULTRASOUND

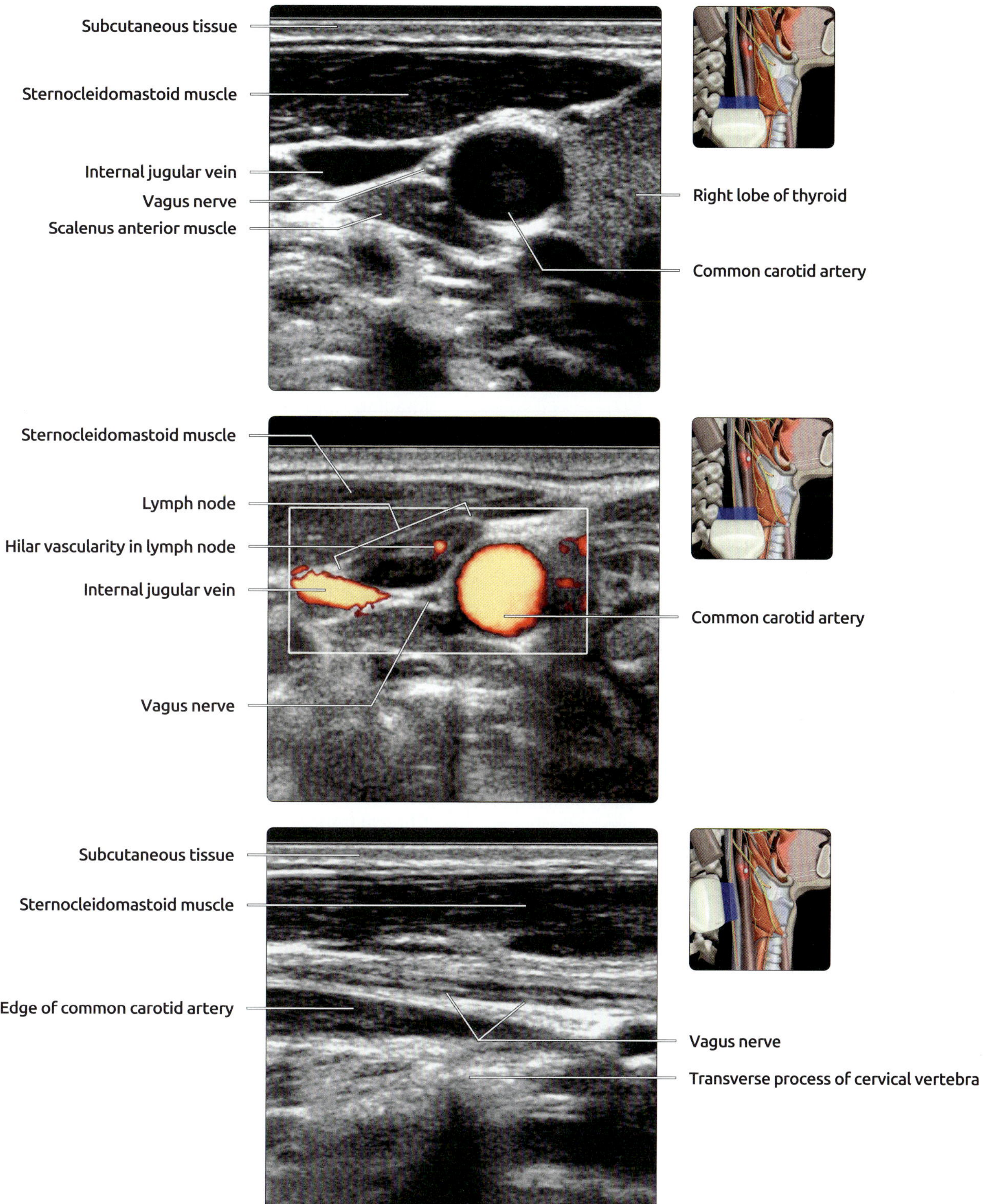

(Top) *Transverse grayscale ultrasound of the lower cervical level at the thyroid gland level shows the vagus nerve as a small, round, hypoechoic structure that exhibits central echogenicity within the carotid sheath and is located between the CCA and the IJV.* **(Middle)** *Power Doppler ultrasound of the midcervical level in the transverse plane demonstrates the avascular nature of the vagus nerve adjacent to the CCA and IJV. Note the presence of hilar vascularity in the adjacent normal deep cervical lymph node.* **(Bottom)** *Longitudinal grayscale ultrasound shows the vagus nerve, which appears as a long, thin, tubular, hypoechoic structure with a central echogenic fibrillary pattern. On ultrasound, the vagus nerve is readily seen from the carotid bifurcation to the lower cervical region.*

Retropharyngeal Space

TERMINOLOGY

Abbreviations

- Retropharyngeal space (RPS); danger space (DS)

Definitions

- RPS: Midline space just posterior to pharynx & cervical esophagus running from skull base to mediastinum
- **Alar fascia** slip of deep layer of deep cervical fascia (DL-DCF) divides RPS into "true" RPS & DS
- **"True" RPS**: Behind posterior wall of pharynx/hypopharynx
  - Anteriorly lined by middle layer of deep cervical fascia (ML-DCF) deep to posterior wall of pharynx/hypopharynx
  - Posteriorly lined by alar fascia (slip of DL-DCF)
- **DS**: Behind "true" RPS (separated by alar fascia) & in front of prevertebral space
  - Anteriorly lined by alar fascia (slip of DL-DCF)
  - Posteriorly lined by prevertebral fascia (layer of DL-DCF)

IMAGING ANATOMY

Extent

- **"True" RPS**: Skull base to T3 vertebral level in mediastinum (variable C6-T6) where alar fascia fuses to ML-DCF
- **DS**: Directly posterior to "true" RPS; continues inferiorly into mediastinum to diaphragm

Anatomy Relationships

- **Suprahyoid neck (SHN) RPS**
  - Pharyngeal mucosal space (PMS) anteriorly
  - DS directly posterior to "true" RPS
- **Infrahyoid neck (IHN) RPS**
  - Hypopharynx & cervical esophagus anteriorly
  - RPS empties via fascial "trap door" inferiorly into DS inferiorly at ~ T3 level (variable C6-T6)
    - Where **alar fascia** fuses to ML-DCF
  - Fascial "trap door" serves as **inferior entry point into DS** for infection from "true" RPS & then into mediastinum
  - Carotid space (CS) lateral to RPS in SHN & IHN
  - Sympathetic trunk lies outside CS posterior to it or between medial CS & lateral RPS
    - Plastered to prevertebral fascia

Internal Contents

- **SHN RPS** (skull base to hyoid bone)
  - Fat is primary occupant of SHN RPS
  - **RPS lymph nodes (RPSLNs): Lateral group**
    - Nodes of **Rouvière:** Skull base/C1 or C1-C2 level
  - **Medial group**: Less often seen; usually at C2-C3 level
  - RPSLNs < 6-8 mm short-axis diameter in adults normal
  - Children may have reactive enlarged RPSLNs
- **IHN RPS** (hyoid bone to T3 vertebral body in mediastinum)
  - **Fat only** in IHN RPS; no RPSLNs in IHN

Fascia of Retropharyngeal Space

- **Anterior wall fascia**: ML-DCF (a.k.a. "buccopharyngeal fascia," especially superiorly)
  - Fascia just behind constrictor muscle of pharynx
- **Alar fascia**: Slip of DL-DCF forming posterior wall of "true" RPS, separating it from DS further behind
- **Posterior wall fascia**: DL-DCF forming posterior wall of DS
  - Anterior to prevertebral muscles of perivertebral space
- **Median raphe** divides RPS into 2 halves
  - Relatively weak fascial slip, more consistent in upper RPS

Recent Concepts on Alar Fascia

- Extension of alar fascia to base of skull controversial
- Classic teaching: Uppermost RPS (nasopharyngeal) "tight" & in RPS abscess, path of least resistance inferiorly
- Recent study: Alar fascia begins at C1 level & loose fibroareolar connective tissue fills transitional space between inferior nuchal line & skull base
  - Transitional level may be alternative **superior entry point into DS** for infection
- Alar fascia comparable in thickness & integrity to buccopharyngeal & prevertebral fasciae
- Lateral fibers of alar fascia large contributor to medial aspect of carotid sheath; may be factor in spread of infection into CS

ANATOMY IMAGING ISSUES

Imaging Approaches

- **CECT best** imaging tool in evaluation of **RPS infection**
- **MR** far more sensitive to detect **RPS tumor/adenopathy**

Imaging Pitfalls

- RPS & DS indistinguishable on CT/MR imaging; consider DS as conduit for RPS disease into mediastinum only
- Lateral RPSLN nodal mass may mimic CS mass
  - Medial to CS; both displace PPS anteriorly
- Not all fluid in RPS is abscess: Nonabscess fluid = no enhancement of wall; minimal mass effect
- **RPS edema**: Internal jugular vein thrombosis, superior vena cava syndrome (transudate), recent chemo-/radiotherapy (lymphedema), pharyngitis, sinusitis, dental infection, angioedema, longus colli tendonitis (cellulitis or transudate)

CLINICAL IMPLICATIONS

Clinical Importance

- **RPSLN** seeded by pharyngitis → RPS abscess
- RPSLNs drain squamous cell carcinoma (SCCa) of nasopharynx & posterior wall of oropharynx & hypopharynx
- Papillary thyroid cancer rarely drains into RPSLN
- Ectopic parathyroid adenoma rarely seen in RPS
- **Benign postradiation hypertrophy of superior cervical sympathetic ganglia** may mimic enlarged lateral RPSLN
  - Majority of enlarged ganglia seen medial to internal carotid artery at C2 & C3 transverse process level
  - Central hypodensity/hypointensity on postcontrast CT/MR: Central black dot sign on axial images & central black line sign on coronal & sagittal images
- **Paucity of fat in RPS in lower neck** makes identification of tissue plane between posterior wall of hypopharynx & prevertebral musculature difficult
- Not detecting intact RPS fat on CT/MR does not imply definite prevertebral space invasion by posterior pharynx/hypopharynx wall SCCa
- Detecting intact retropharyngeal fat stripe provides good negative predictive value for prevertebral tumor invasion
- **RPS lesion**: Anterior to prevertebral muscles; flattens & remains anterior to prevertebral muscles as it enlarges
  - In contrast, perivertebral space mass elevates prevertebral muscles as it enlarges

GRAPHICS

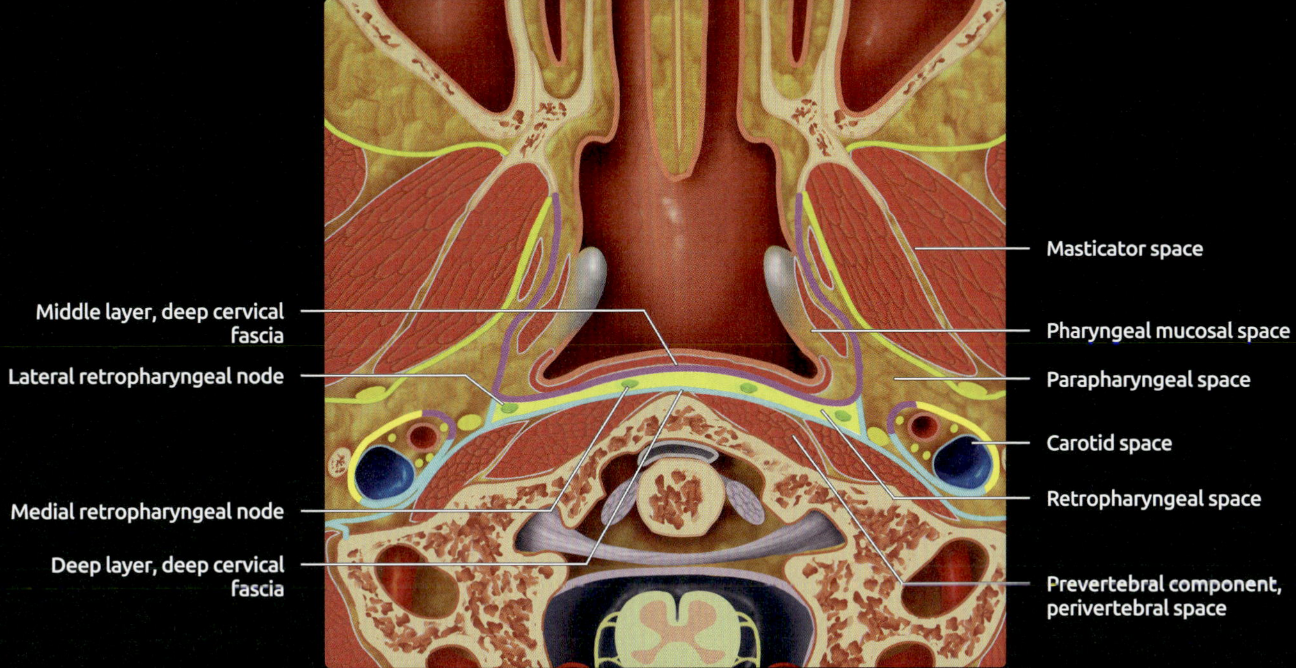

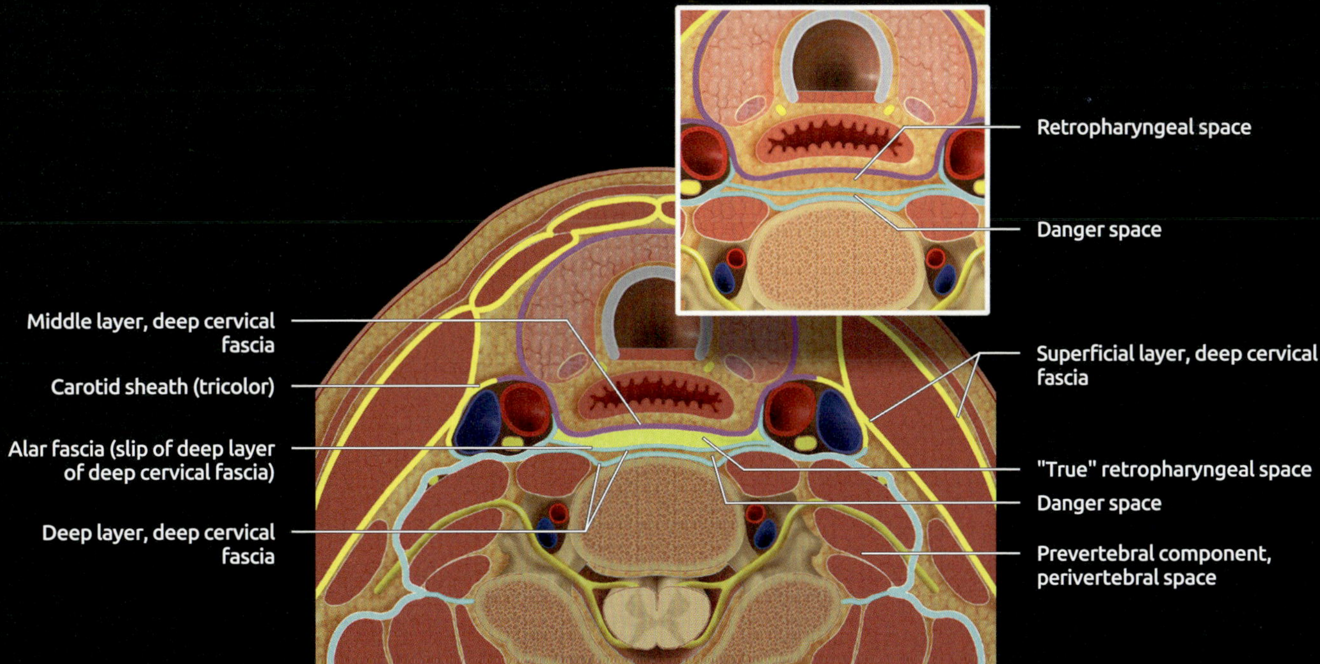

(Top) *Axial graphic shows retropharyngeal space in suprahyoid neck (SHN). In SHN, the retropharyngeal space has medial and lateral retropharyngeal nodes. Notice that the middle layer of deep cervical fascia (called buccopharyngeal fascia here) is the anterior border of the retropharyngeal space, while deep layer of deep cervical fascia is the posterior border. Extension of alar fascia to skull base is controversial, with recent study showing that alar fascia begins at C1 level & loose fibroareolar connective tissue fills transitional space (alternate superior entry point into danger space) between inferior nuchal line & skull base.* **(Bottom)** *Axial graphic depicts the fascia that make up the borders of the retropharyngeal and danger spaces in the infrahyoid neck. Alar fascia is a slip of the deep layer of deep cervical fascia forming the posterior wall of the anteriorly located "true" retropharyngeal space, separating it from the posteriorly located danger space. Posterior wall of danger space is also formed by the deep layer of deep cervical fascia, separating it from the prevertebral space. Notice that there is only fat in the infrahyoid retropharyngeal space. Nodes are only present above the hyoid bone.*

GRAPHICS

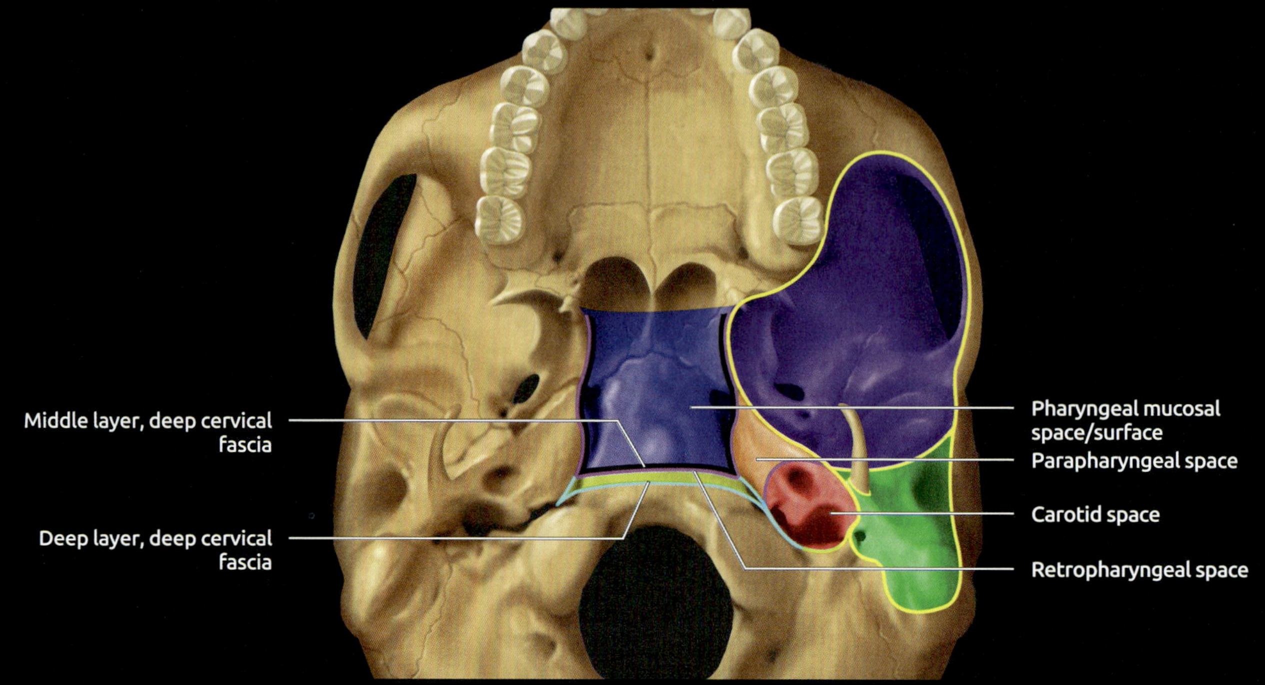

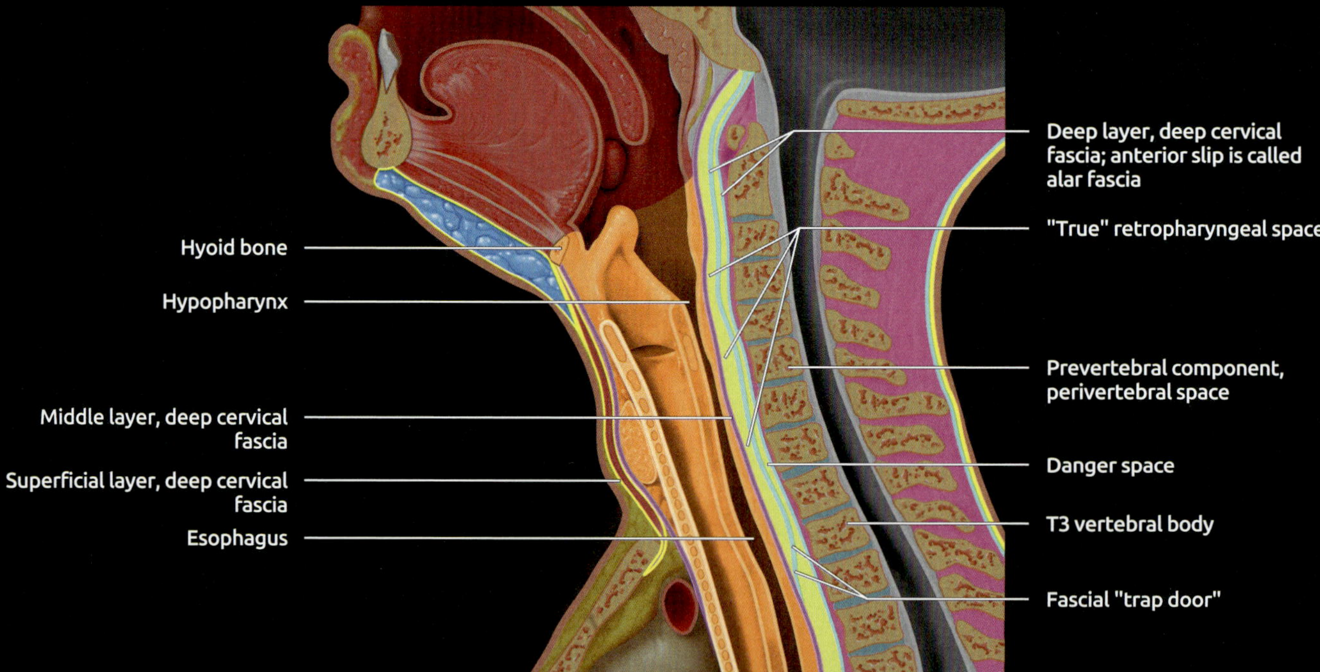

(Top) *Axial graphic of the skull base from below shows the abutment of the retropharyngeal space with the skull base. Notice that the retropharyngeal space abuts the external surface of the basiocciput in an area where there are no foramina.* **(Bottom)** *Sagittal graphic depicts longitudinal spatial relationships of the infrahyoid neck with emphasis on the retropharyngeal and danger spaces. Seen just anterior to the vertebral column, the retropharyngeal and danger spaces run inferiorly from the skull base toward the mediastinum. Notice the fascial "trap door" found at the approximate level of the T3 vertebral body that serves as an inferior conduit from the retropharyngeal to the danger space. Retropharyngeal space infection or tumor may access the mediastinum via this route of spread. Note that the extension of alar fascia to the base of skull is controversial; a recent cadaveric study found that the alar fascia begins at C1 level, and loose fibroareolar connective tissue fills the space between inferior nuchal line and skull base; this transitional level may be an alternative superior entry point into danger space for infection.*

AXIAL SUPRAHYOID NECK RETROPHARYNGEAL SPACE GENERIC MASS

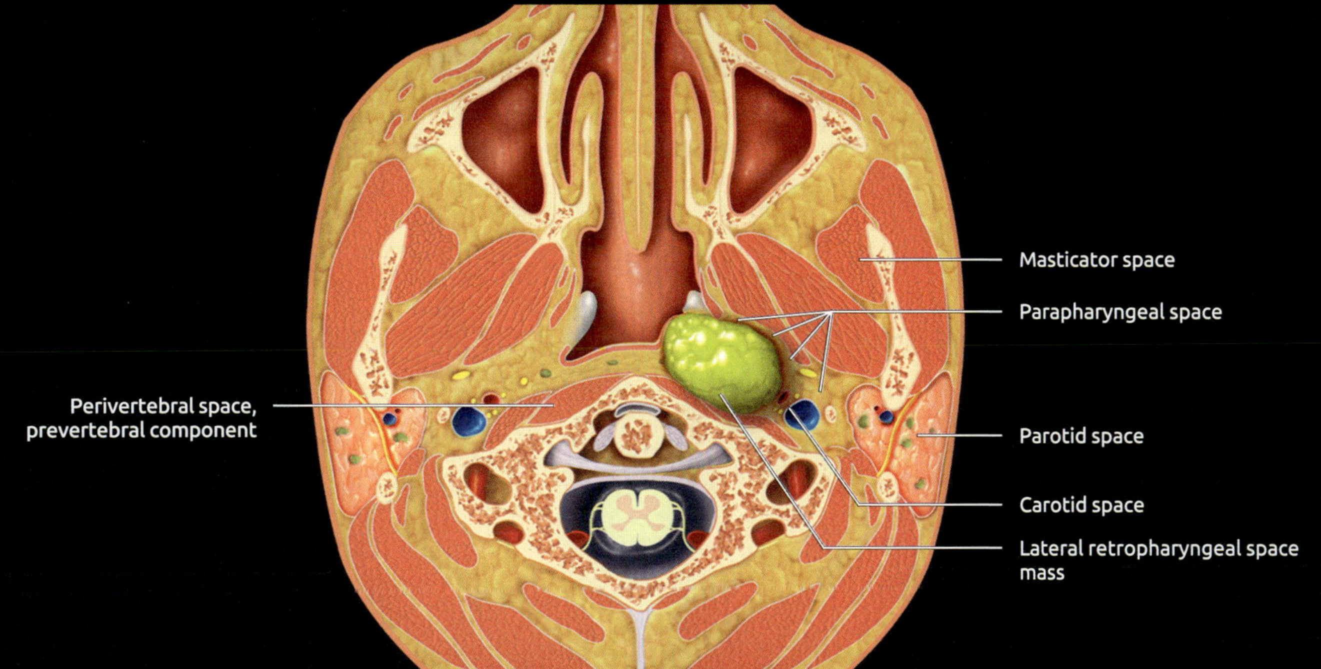

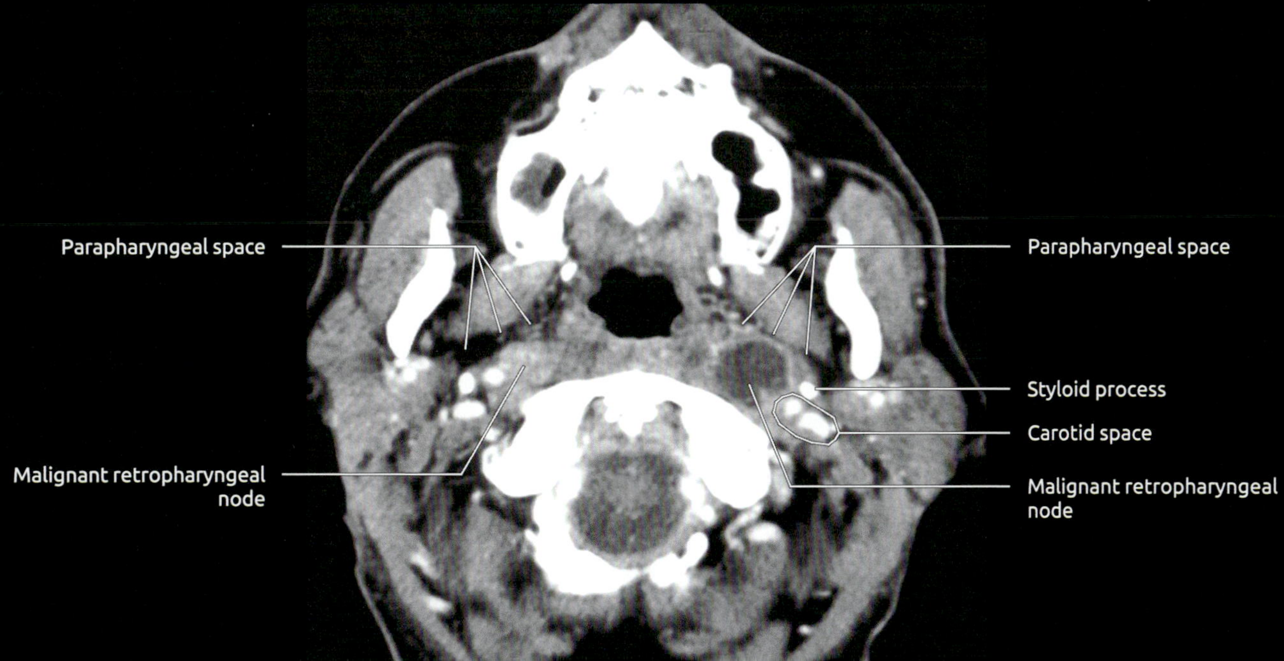

(Top) *Axial graphic depicts generic mass beginning in the lateral retropharyngeal nodal group of the retropharyngeal space. Notice that the lateral retropharyngeal space mass displaces the carotid space posterolaterally and the parapharyngeal space anteriorly. This mass lesion can be mistaken for a carotid space mass if the imager is not cognizant of its more medial location.* **(Bottom)** *Axial CECT at low nasopharynx level reveals bilateral malignant lateral retropharyngeal space lymph nodes (RPSLNs) from a posterior oropharyngeal wall squamous cell carcinoma (not shown). The larger left-sided necrotic node displaces parapharyngeal space anteriorly and carotid space posterolaterally. The smaller right-sided node has not yet caused significant mass effect on either the parapharyngeal or carotid spaces. Benign postradiation hypertrophy of superior cervical sympathetic ganglia may mimic enlarged lateral RPSLNs. Enlarged ganglia are usually seen medial to internal carotid artery at C2 and C3 transverse process level and show central hypodensity/hypointensity on postcontrast CT/MR (central black dot sign on axial images, central black line sign on coronal and sagittal images).*

AXIAL INFRAHYOID NECK RETROPHARYNGEAL SPACE GENERIC MASS

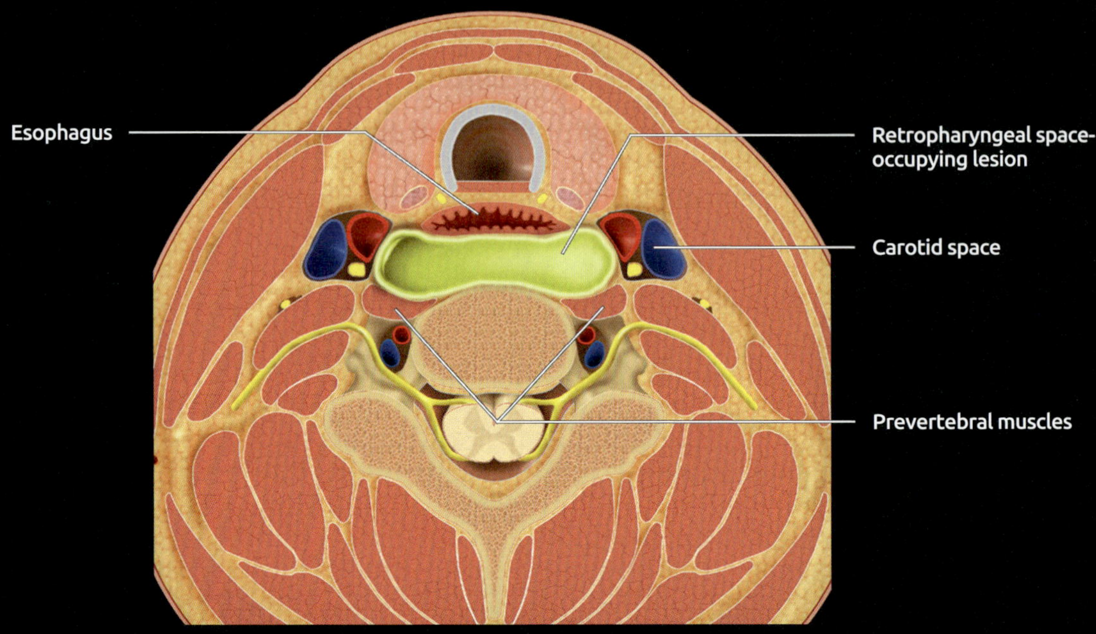

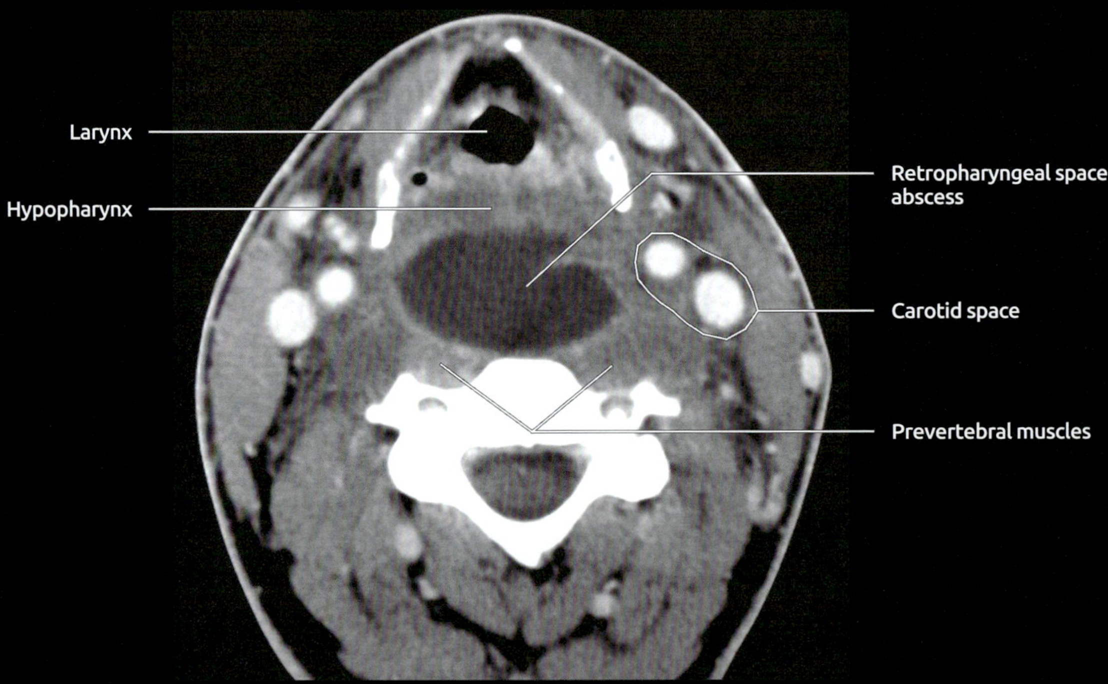

(Top) *Axial graphic of a generic retropharyngeal space lesion in the infrahyoid neck is shown. Note anterior displacement of the visceral space and lateral displacement of the carotid spaces. The prevertebral muscles are flattened, not elevated.* **(Bottom)** *Axial CECT at the level of the infrahyoid neck supraglottic larynx demonstrates an abscess filling the retropharyngeal space. This ovoid-shaped abscess displaces the visceral space (hypopharynx/larynx) anteriorly and the carotid spaces laterally. The prevertebral muscles are posterior to the abscess cavity and flatten them from the anterior aspect. In contrast, the prevertebral space mass elevates the prevertebral muscles as it enlarges.*

AXIAL CECT

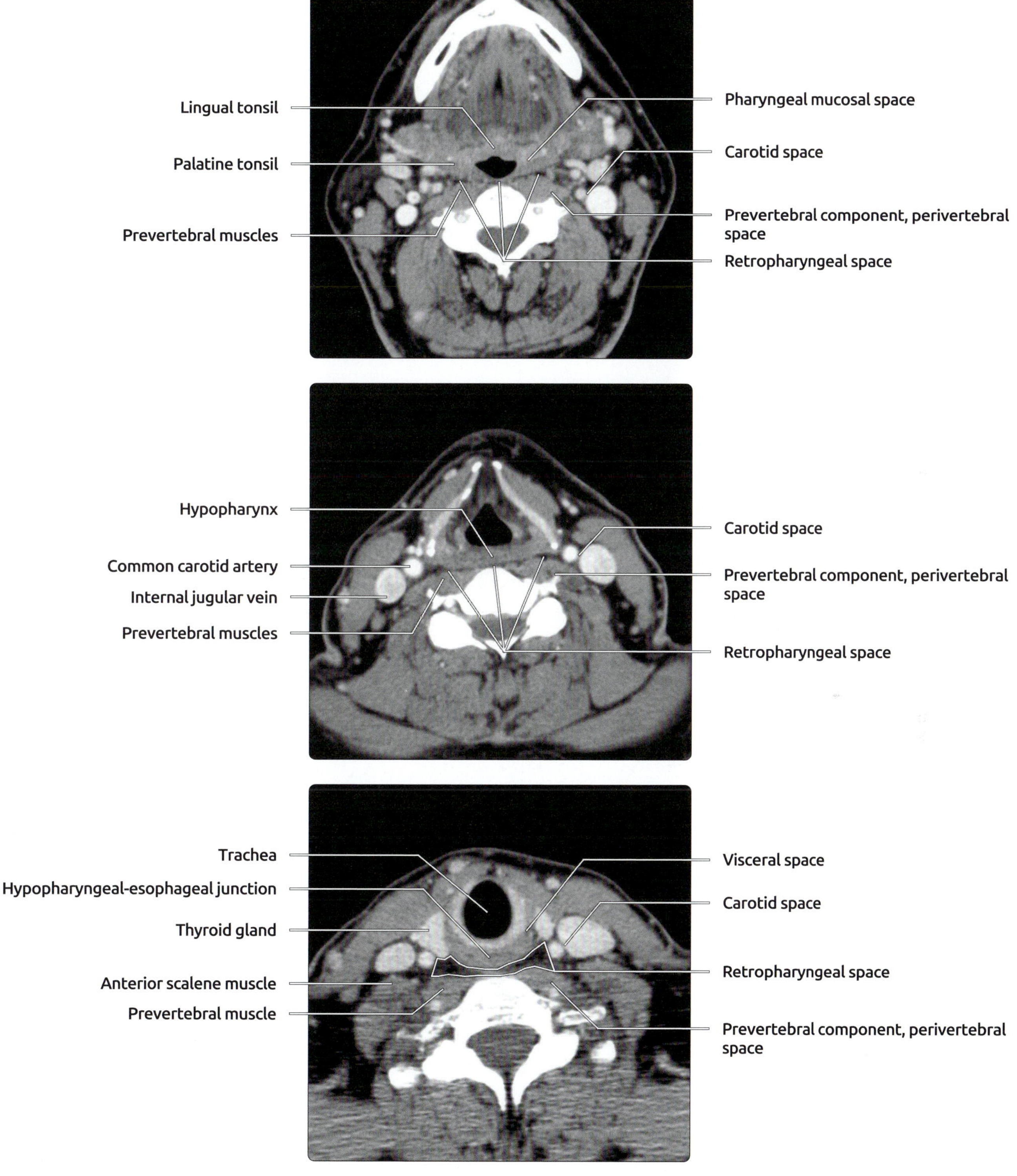

(Top) *First of 3 axial CECT images of the neck is shown. This image at the level of the low oropharynx shows the stripe of fat behind the pharyngeal mucosal space that represents the retropharyngeal space. Posterior to the retropharyngeal space is the prevertebral portion of the perivertebral space; lateral to it are the carotid spaces.* **(Middle)** *In this image at the level of the supraglottis, the stripe of fat behind the larynx and hypopharynx is the retropharyngeal space. The carotid spaces are at the lateral margin of the retropharyngeal space bilaterally.* **(Bottom)** *At the level of the midinfrahyoid neck, the retropharyngeal space is larger and more obvious than in the suprahyoid neck. Anterior is the visceral space with the hypopharyngeal-esophageal junction abutting the retropharyngeal space. The prevertebral component of the perivertebral space is posterior to the retropharyngeal space.*

AXIAL T1 MR

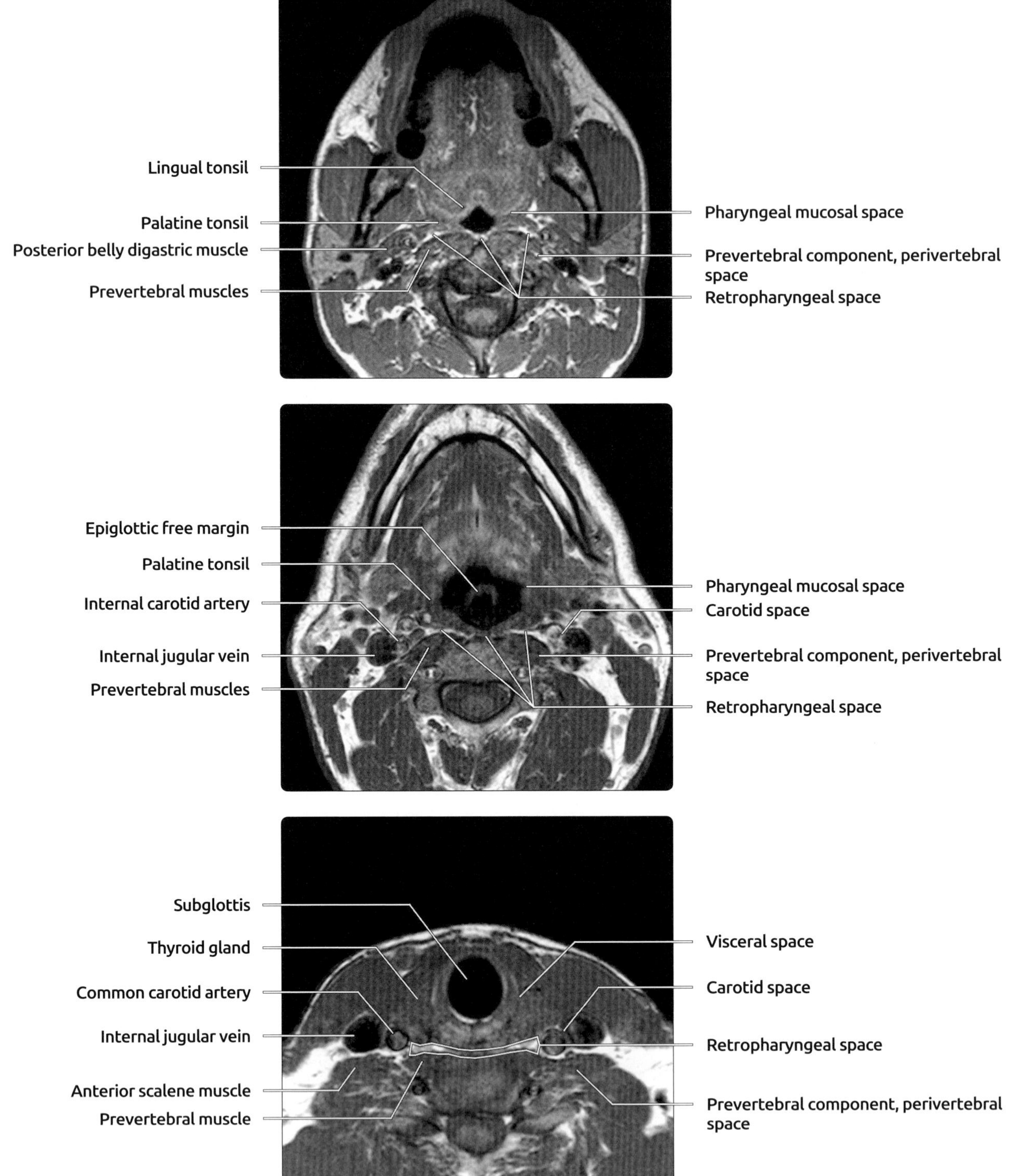

(Top) *First of 3 axial T1 MR images of the extracranial head and neck is shown. This image at the level of the oropharynx shows a thin stripe of high-signal fat behind the pharyngeal mucosal space that represents the retropharyngeal space. Posterior to the retropharyngeal space is the prevertebral portion of the perivertebral space.* **(Middle)** *Image at the low oropharynx level shows the high-signal stripe of fat behind the oropharyngeal mucosal space is the retropharyngeal space. Carotid spaces are at the lateral margin of the retropharyngeal space bilaterally. Prevertebral muscles in the perivertebral space are directly posterior to the retropharyngeal space.* **(Bottom)** *In this image at midinfrahyoid neck, the retropharyngeal space is easily seen between the carotid spaces. The visceral space is the anterior and prevertebral component of the perivertebral space posterior to retropharyngeal space. Not detecting an intact retropharyngeal fat stripe on CT/MR does not imply definite prevertebral space invasion by posterior pharynx/hypopharynx wall tumor as fat paucity can be normal. Detecting an intact fat stripe provides good negative predictive value for prevertebral tumor invasion.*

AXIAL BONE CT AND T2 MR

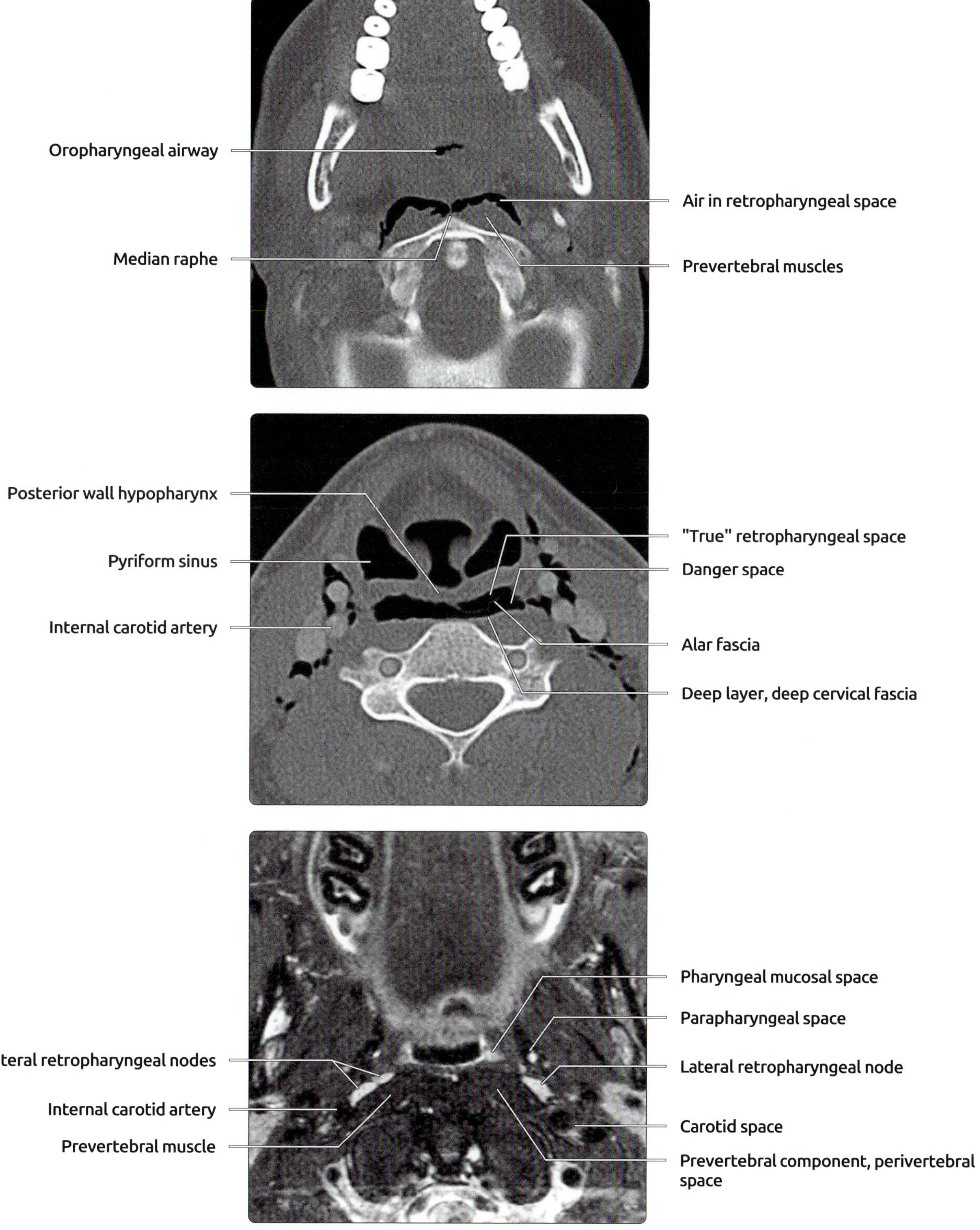

(Top) *Axial bone CT through the midoropharynx in a trauma patient shows air has collected in the retropharyngeal space, allowing the median raphe to be seen. The median raphe functions as an attachment of the constrictor muscles. In addition, it provides an initial barrier to the spread of disease from side to side in the retropharyngeal space.* **(Middle)** *Axial bone CT at the level of the supraglottis in a trauma patient shows air in the "true" retropharyngeal and danger spaces. Air allows identification of the alar fascia that separates these 2 spaces.* **(Bottom)** *Axial fat-saturated T2 MR through the low nasopharynx in a young adolescent reveals normal lateral retropharyngeal space nodes bilaterally. Notice these nodes are positioned just medial to the internal carotid artery and posteromedial to the fat-saturated parapharyngeal space.*

TERMINOLOGY

Abbreviations

- Perivertebral space (PVS)

Definitions

- Perivertebral includes all tissues within cylindrical space surrounding vertebral column and bounded by deep layer of deep cervical fascia (DL-DCF)
- PVS subdivided into anterior **prevertebral** and posterior **paraspinal** components

IMAGING ANATOMY

Extent

- For practical purposes, anterior **prevertebral** component extends from skull base to T4, where ventral DL-DCF attaches to T4
  - Some anatomists contend that prevertebral space extends inferiorly to coccyx
- Posterior **paraspinal** component continues to sacrum

Anatomy Relationships

- **2 major components of PVS**, separated at level of transverse processes (TPs)
  - Prevertebral portion or space
  - Paraspinal portion or space
- **Prevertebral PVS** sits directly behind retropharyngeal and danger space in extracranial head and neck
  - Carotid space lies anterolateral to prevertebral PVS
- **Paraspinal PVS** lies deep to posterior cervical space and posterior to cervical spine TPs

Internal Contents

- **Prevertebral PVS or prevertebral space**
  - Vertebral bodies
  - Prevertebral muscles (longus colli and capitis)
    - Longus capitis: Origin (O): C3-C6 TPs; insertion (I): Basilar occipital bone
    - Longus colli: O: C3-C5 TPs, C5-T3 vertebral bodies; I: Anterior arch C1, C2-C4 vertebral bodies
  - Scalene muscles (anterior, middle, and posterior)
    - O: C3-C6 TPs (anterior), C2-C7 TPs (middle), C5-C7 TPs (posterior)
    - I: Scalene tubercle 1st rib (anterior), upper surface 1st rib (middle), lateral surface 2nd rib (posterior)
  - Brachial plexus (BP) roots
  - Phrenic nerve (C3-C5)
  - Vertebral artery and vein
- **Paraspinal PVS or paraspinal space**
  - Paraspinal muscles (include splenius capitis, splenius cervicis, semispinalis capitis, longissimus capitis, levator scapulae, multifidus, interspinales)
  - Posterior elements, vertebral column
- **BP**, proximal aspect
  - C5-T1 roots leave neural foramina, pass between anterior and middle scalene muscles of prevertebral PVS
  - BP roots pass through sleeves in DL-DCF, into posterior cervical space on their way to axilla

Fascia of PVS

- **DL-DCF completely circumscribes PVS**
  - Anterior portion arches from cervical spine TP across prevertebral muscles to opposite TP
    - Anterior DL-DCF called "**carpet**" by surgeons
    - Pharynx slides on this smooth, carpet-like surface
    - Barrier to disease spread between pharynx and PVS
  - Posterior DL-DCF arches over surface of paraspinal muscles to attach to nuchal ligament of spinous process of vertebral body

ANATOMY IMAGING ISSUES

Questions

- What imaging findings localize lesion to prevertebral PVS?
  - Mass centered in prevertebral muscles or vertebral body
  - Mass lifts or pushes prevertebral muscles anteriorly (retropharyngeal space mass pushes them posteriorly)

Imaging Approaches

- Lateral plain film
  - Assess for prevertebral soft tissue swelling and integrity of cervical vertebral bodies
  - Normal thickness: Adults: < 7 mm at C2, < 22 mm at C6; children: < 14 mm at C6
- CECT (soft tissue, bone algorithm, and sagittal reformation)
  - Most practical imaging evaluation of soft tissue and bones
  - Upper limits of normal thickness on CT: 6 mm at C2, 7 mm at C3, 18 mm at C6/C7
- Cervical MR with contrast and fat saturation best to assess for marrow process and epidural disease

Imaging Pitfalls

- **Hypertrophic levator scapulae muscle** (LSM): Mistaken for enhancing mass or recurrent tumor
  - Secondary to CNXI injury (during neck dissection)
    - Sternocleidomastoid (SCM) and trapezius atrophy
    - LSM hypertrophies to help lift arm
  - Imaging: LSM enlarges and may enhance; SCM and trapezius small, fatty infiltrated
- Limited positive predictive value of MR and CT for PVS invasion from pharyngeal tumor
  - Retropharyngeal fat plane infiltration, ipsilateral muscle concavity, irregular muscle border, muscle T2 hyperintensity and enhancement can also be due to peritumoral edema or posttreatment effects, without actual muscle invasion
  - Preservation of discrete retropharyngeal fat stripe: Reasonably good negative predictor of invasion

CLINICAL IMPLICATIONS

Clinical Importance

- Notable structures: Proximal BP, phrenic nerve, vertebral arteries
- Most PVS lesions originate in vertebral body or disc space (infection or metastatic tumor)
- When prevertebral-PVS disease found on imaging, **always check for epidural space extension**
  - DL-DCF: 1st obstruction to infection or malignancy spread from vertebral body into prevertebral PVS
  - Path of least resistance: Through neural foramen into epidural space

GRAPHICS

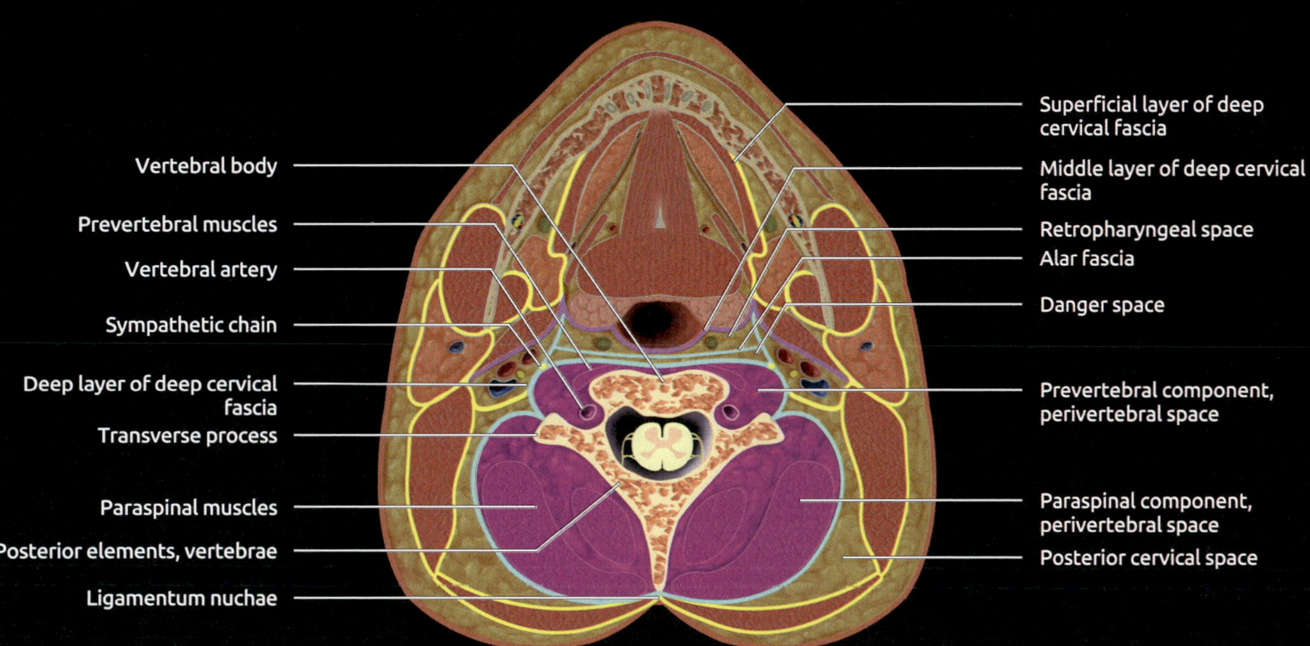

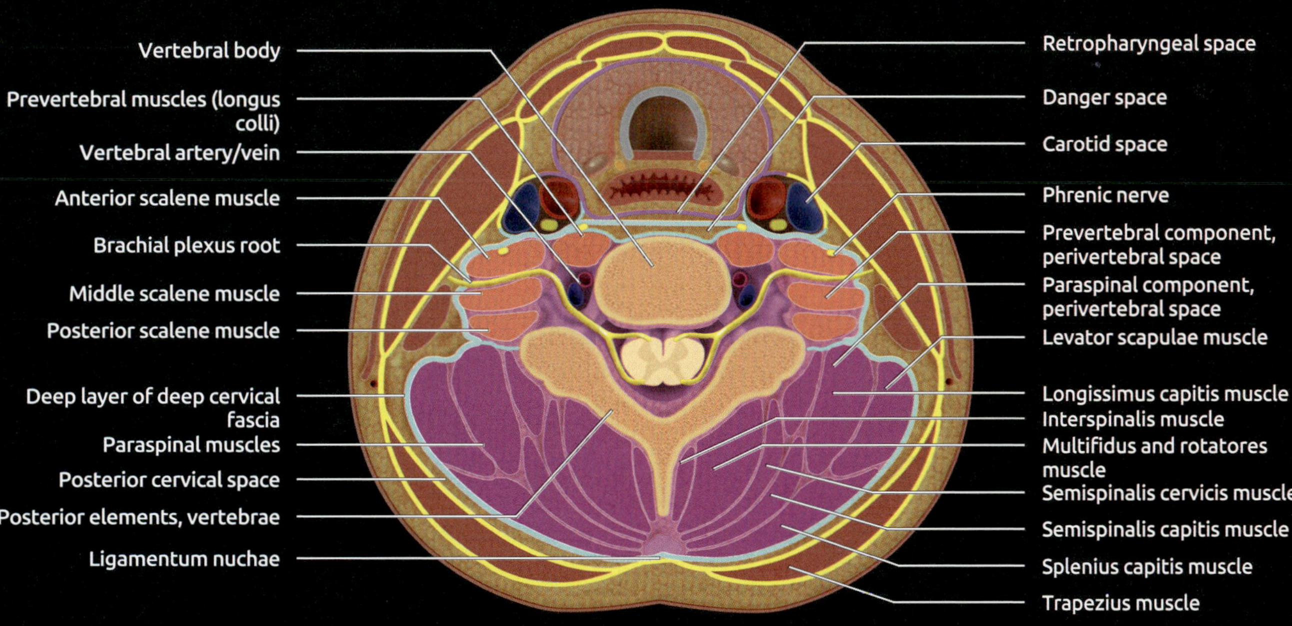

(Top) *Axial graphic through the level of the oropharynx shows prevertebral and paraspinal components of the perivertebral space beneath the deep layer of deep cervical fascia. Notice this fascia curves medially to touch the transverse processes of the vertebra, dividing the perivertebral space into prevertebral and paraspinal components. The danger and retropharyngeal spaces are anterior to the perivertebral space, while the posterior cervical space is lateral and posterior.* **(Bottom)** *Axial graphic through the thyroid bed shows the deep layer of deep cervical fascia curving medially to touch the transverse processes, dividing the perivertebral space into prevertebral and paraspinal components. The prevertebral component contains brachial plexus roots. The paraspinal muscles include rotatores, multifidus, and semispinalis cervicis that form the transversospinalis muscles, producing extension, contralateral rotation and ipsilateral bending. These are also key for cervical spine segmental support with the craniocervical extensors (rectus capitis posterior major and minor and obliquus capitis superior and inferior). Splenius capitis produces extension, ipsilateral bending, and rotation.*

GRAPHICS

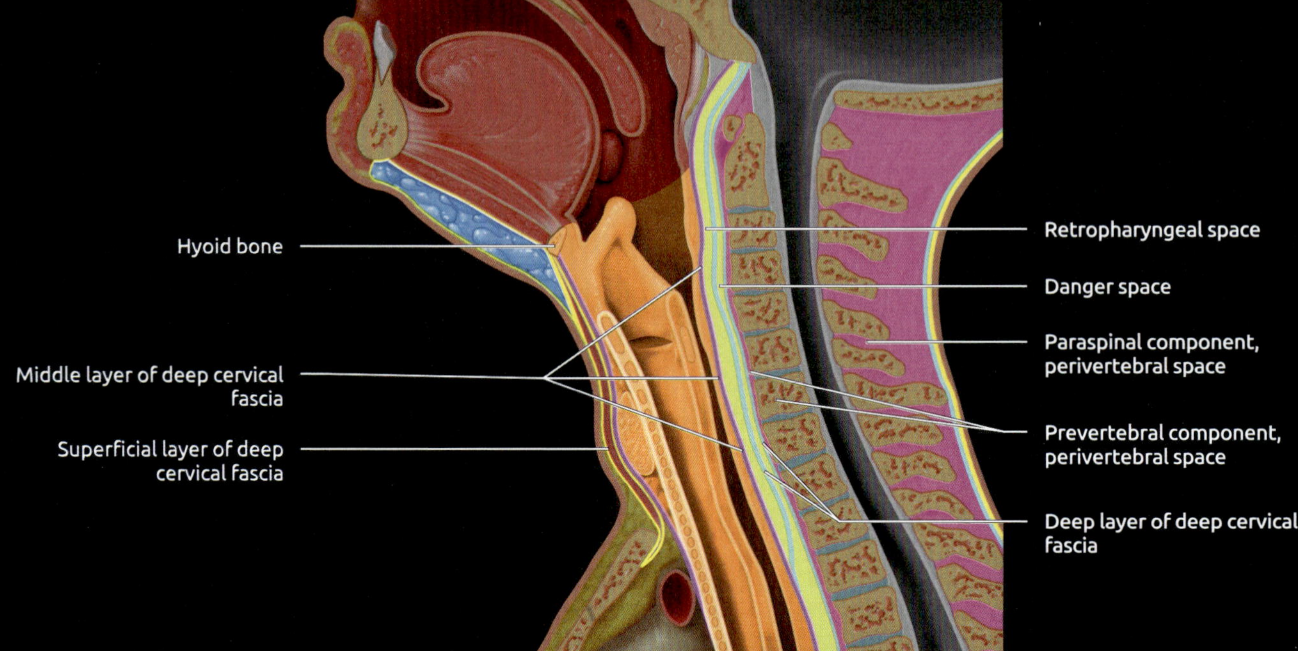

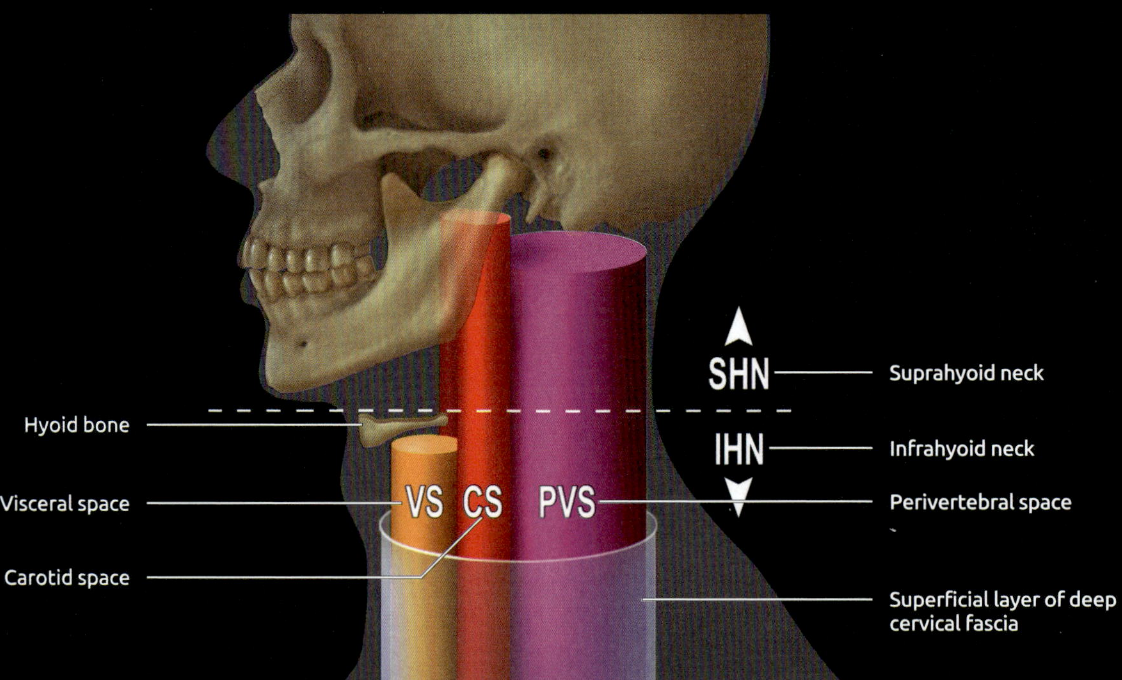

(Top) *Sagittal graphic depicting midline longitudinal spatial relationships of the infrahyoid neck is shown. In the midline, only the vertebral body is seen in the prevertebral component of the perivertebral space. Just anterior to the vertebral column, the retropharyngeal and danger spaces run inferiorly toward the mediastinum. In the midline paraspinal component of the perivertebral space, only the spinous processes are visible.* **(Bottom)** *Lateral graphic of the extracranial head and neck shows the spaces as "tubes" as they traverse the area. The perivertebral space is shown as a tube of tissue that projects from the skull base inferiorly into the thorax. Notice the superficial layer of deep cervical fascia envelops all the spaces of the extracranial head and neck below the hyoid bone.*

GENERIC PERIVERTEBRAL SPACE SUPRAHYOID MASS

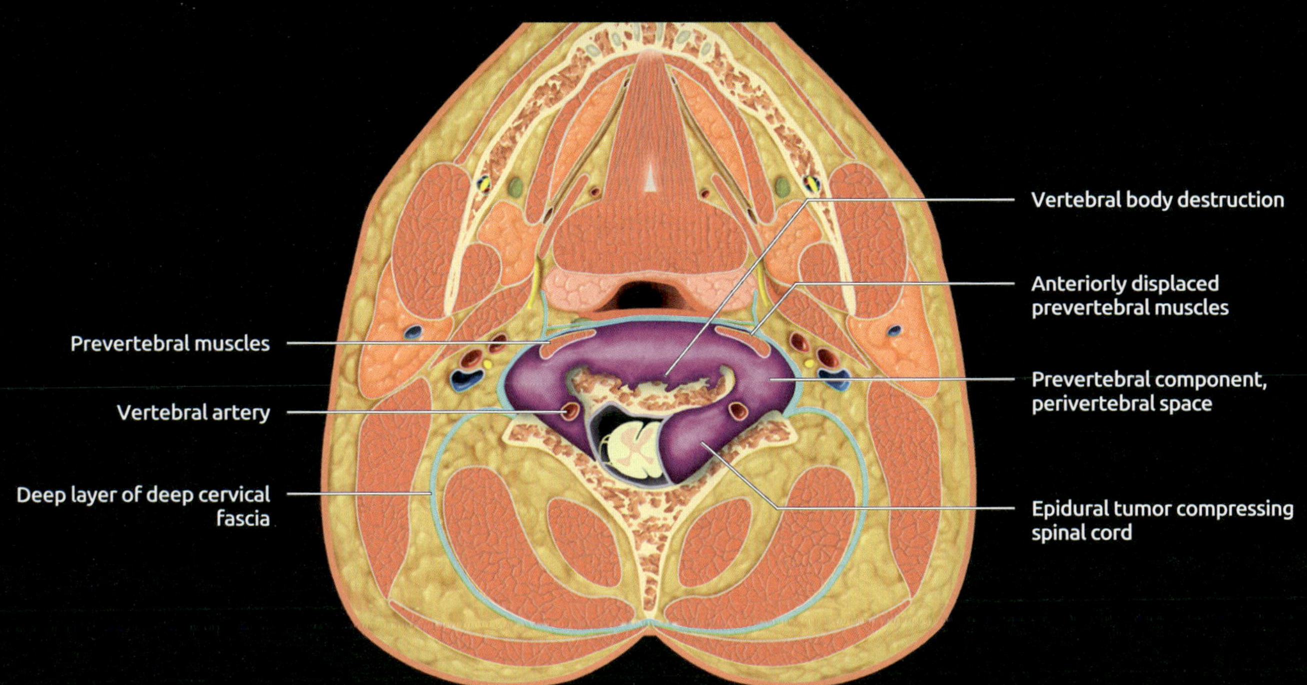

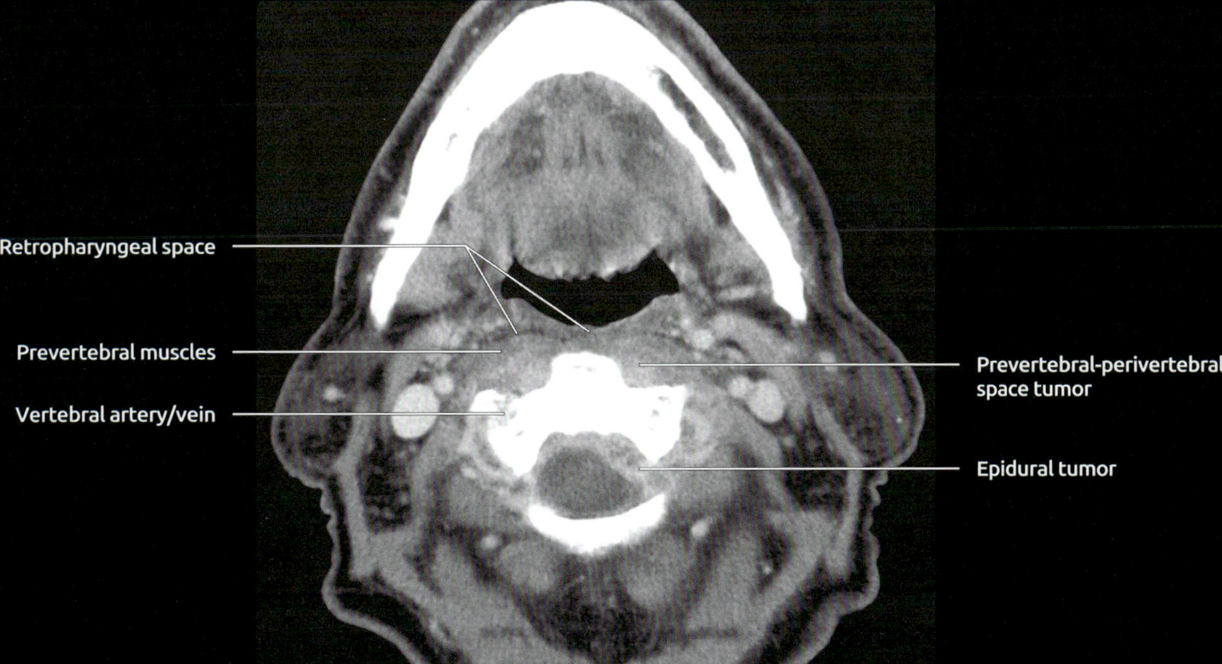

(Top) *Axial graphic through the oropharynx reveals a generic suprahyoid neck perivertebral space mass involving the vertebral body. Notice the vertebral body destruction and the elevation of the prevertebral muscles. The vertebral arteries are engulfed by tumor. In addition, the tumor is confined by the deep layer of deep cervical fascia, forcing it centrally into the epidural space where it is causing spinal cord compression.* **(Bottom)** *Axial CECT demonstrates an enhancing malignant tumor involving the prevertebral component of the perivertebral space. The tumor remains confined to the perivertebral space by the deep layer of deep cervical fascia. Consequently, the tumor spreads centrally into the epidural space where it may cause cord compression.*

GENERIC PERIVERTEBRAL SPACE INFRAHYOID MASS

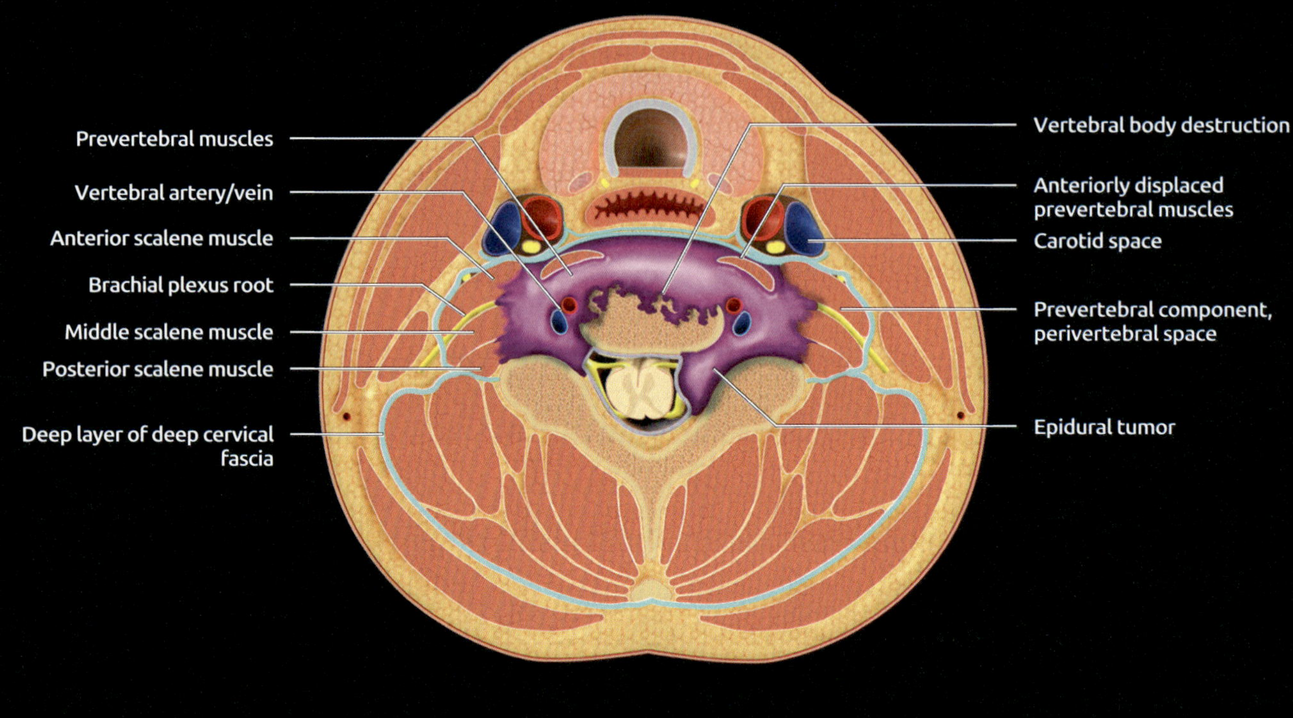

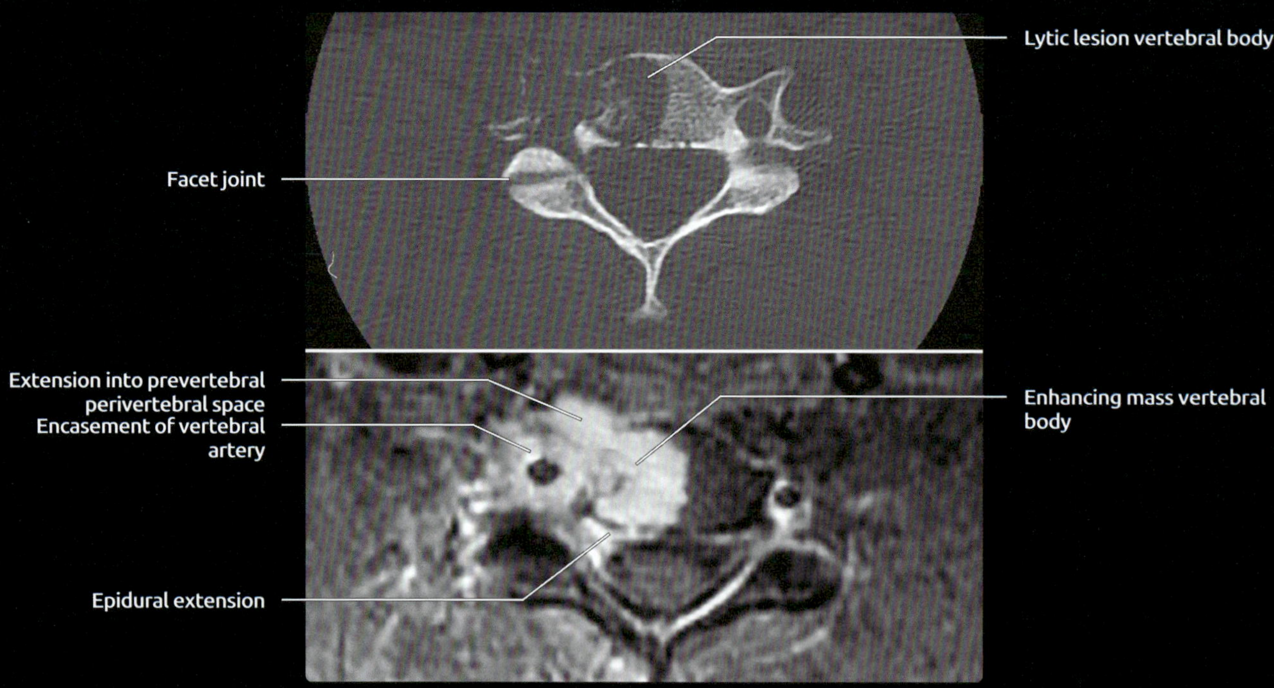

(Top) *Axial graphic through the thyroid bed shows a generic infrahyoid neck perivertebral space mass arising from the vertebral body. Notice the vertebral body destruction and the elevation of the prevertebral muscles. The vertebral artery and vein as well as the brachial plexus roots are engulfed by the tumor. In addition, the tumor is confined by the deep layer of deep cervical fascia, forcing it centrally into the epidural space.* **(Bottom)** *Axial bone CT and axial MR with gadolinium and fat saturation show a tumor arising from the cervical vertebra and extending into the epidural space, neural foramen, and prevertebral component of the perivertebral space. CT best shows the lytic changes of bone; MR best shows the soft tissue components with marrow space involvement.*

AXIAL CECT

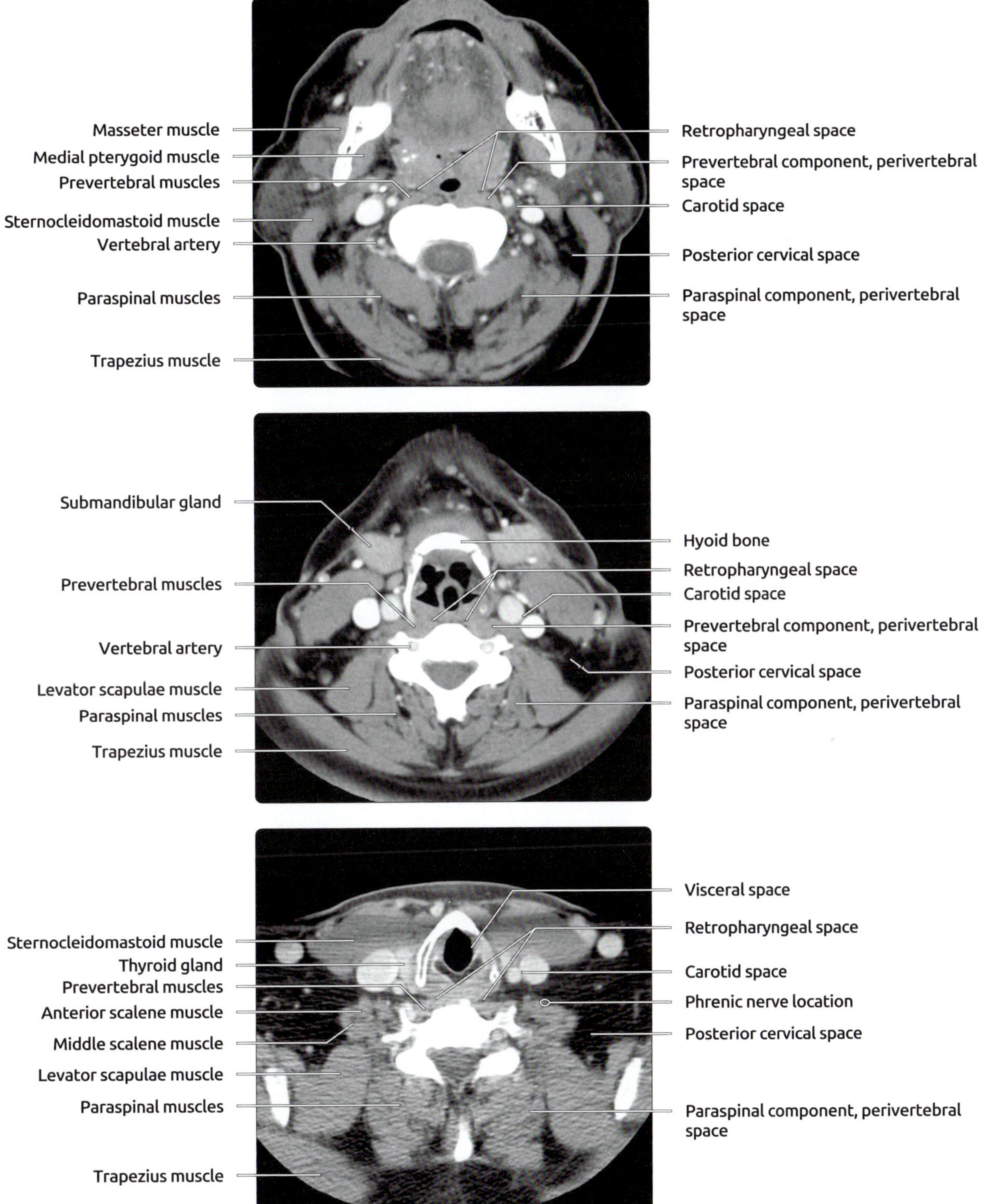

(Top) *First of 6 axial CECT images through the extracranial head and neck show the normal features of the perivertebral space. This image at the level of the C2 vertebral body shows the prevertebral component of the perivertebral space contains the prevertebral muscles, vertebral body, and vertebral artery only. The retropharyngeal space fat stripe is visible anteriorly.* **(Middle)** *In this image at the level of the hyoid bone, the levator scapulae muscles and the paraspinal muscles along with the posterior elements of the vertebral body are the principal occupants of the paraspinal component of the perivertebral space.* **(Bottom)** *At the level of the cricoid cartilage, the scalene muscles are visible. The phrenic nerve location is marked on the left, although it is not visible on imaging.*

AXIAL CECT

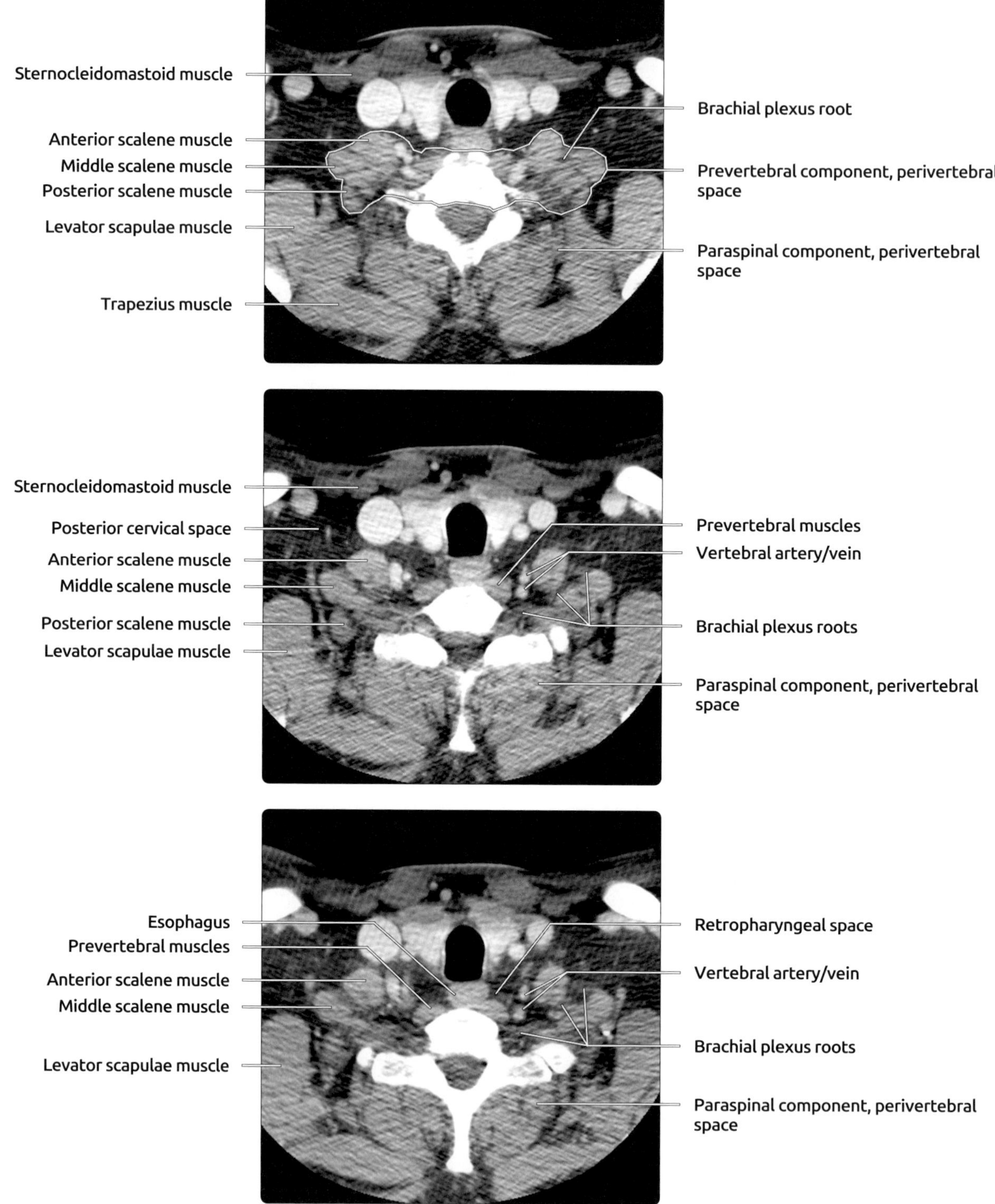

(Top) *At the level of the upper thyroid bed, the scalene muscles are seen in the prevertebral component of the perivertebral space. The anterior band of the deep layer of deep cervical fascia is referred to as the "carpet."* **(Middle)** *In this image at the level of the midthyroid bed, the low-density ovoid brachial plexus roots can be seen emerging from the cervical neural foramina to pass anterolaterally between the anterior and middle scalene muscles in the prevertebral component of the perivertebral space.* **(Bottom)** *At the level of the low thyroid bed, the low-density brachial plexus roots are visible passing anterolaterally between the anterior and middle scalene muscles in the prevertebral component of the perivertebral space. These roots continue through openings in the deep layer of deep cervical fascia into the posterior cervical space on their way to the axillary apex.*

AXIAL T2 FS AND CORONAL STIR MR

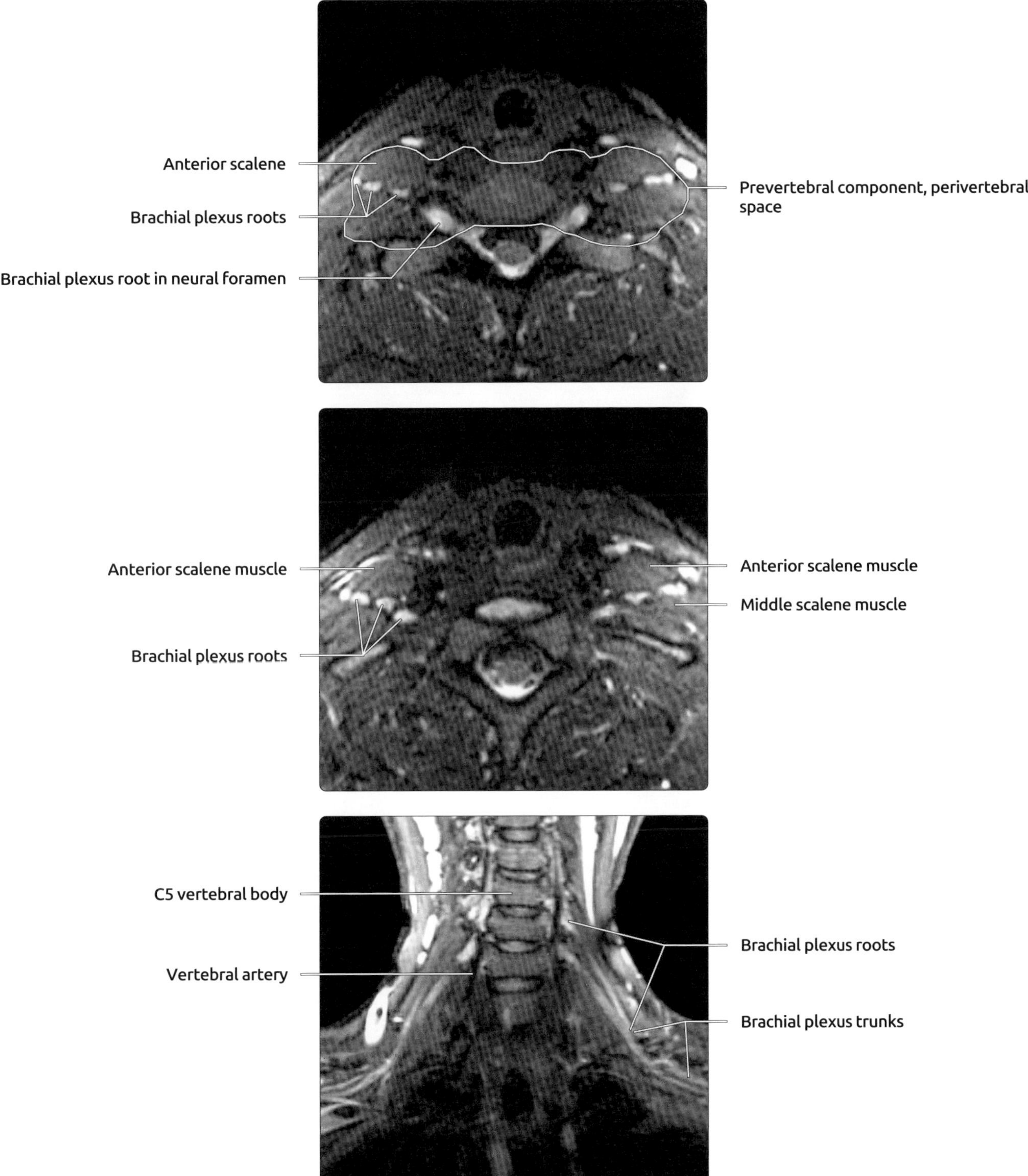

(Top) *Axial T2 FS MR at the level of the thyroid gland shows the normal high-signal brachial plexus roots between the anterior and middle scalene muscles. Notice a single root passes through the neural foramen bilaterally. The brachial plexus arises from the ventral rami of C5 through T1.* **(Middle)** *In this axial T2 FS MR, the anterior and middle scalene muscles can be seen on the anterior and posterior sides of the high-signal brachial plexus roots. Distally, the 5 roots become 3 trunks (upper, middle, and lower) as they emerge from their interscalene muscle location.* **(Bottom)** *Coronal STIR MR through the lower cervical vertebral bodies shows both the 5 brachial plexus roots and the 3 trunks in the same plane. The brachial plexus transitions from roots to trunks to divisions to cords to end in branches.*

MULTICOMPARTMENT ABSCESSES

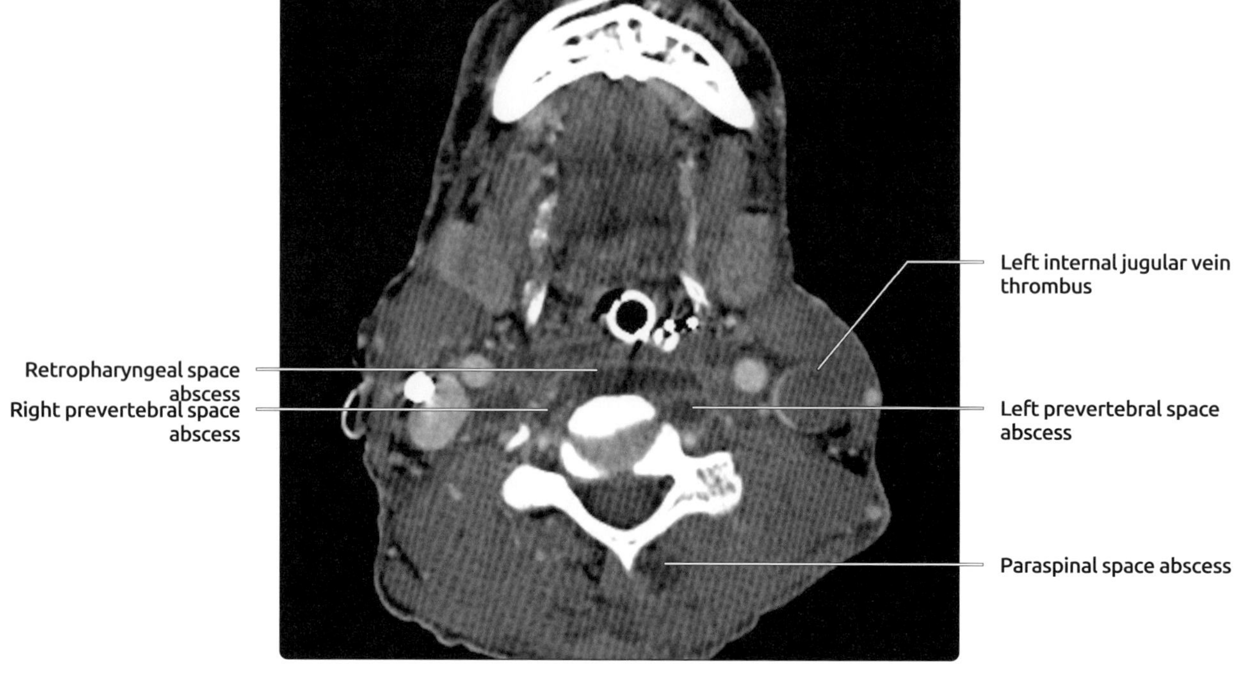

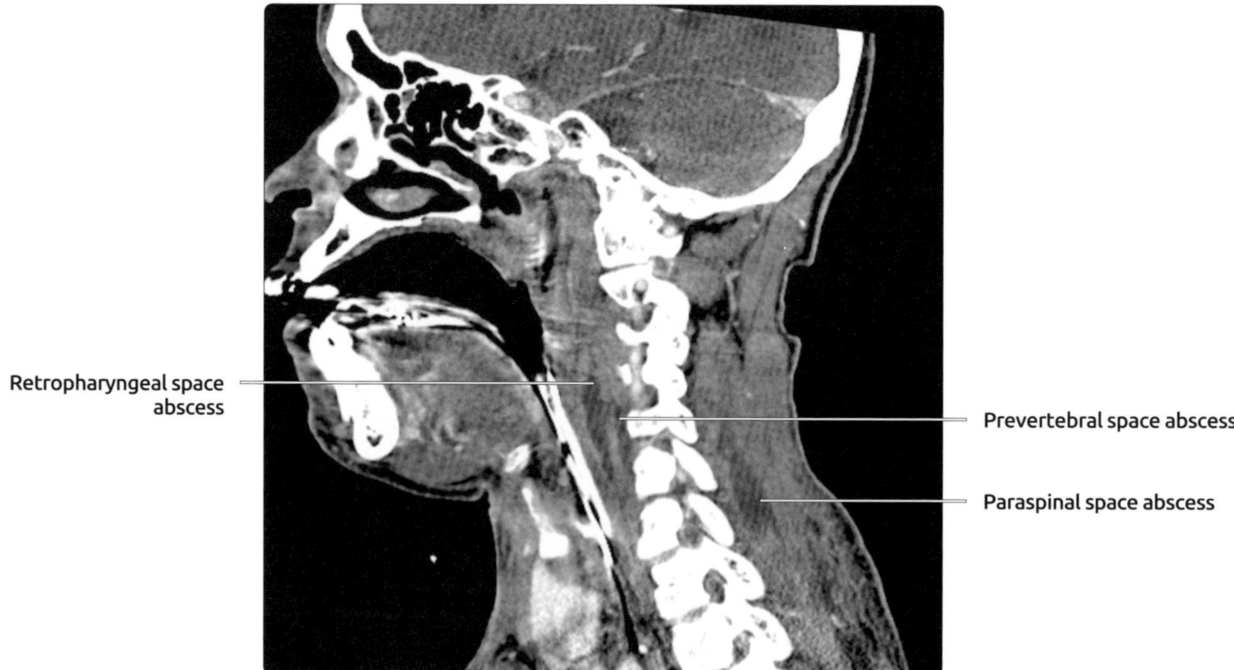

(Top) *Axial CECT through the neck demonstrates multicompartment rim-enhancing collections, consistent with abscesses. These include bilateral prevertebral muscles abscesses, a retropharyngeal space abscess, and a left paraspinal space abscess posteriorly. There is lateral extension of the abscesses on the right adjacent to the carotid space. Incidental note is also made of near-occlusive left internal jugular vein thrombosis.* **(Bottom)** *Left parasagittal CECT demonstrates the multiple rim-enhancing fluid collections in the neck, consistent with abscesses (retropharyngeal, prevertebral, and paraspinal). The source of infection was cervical spondylodiscitis (not shown).*

GRAPHICS

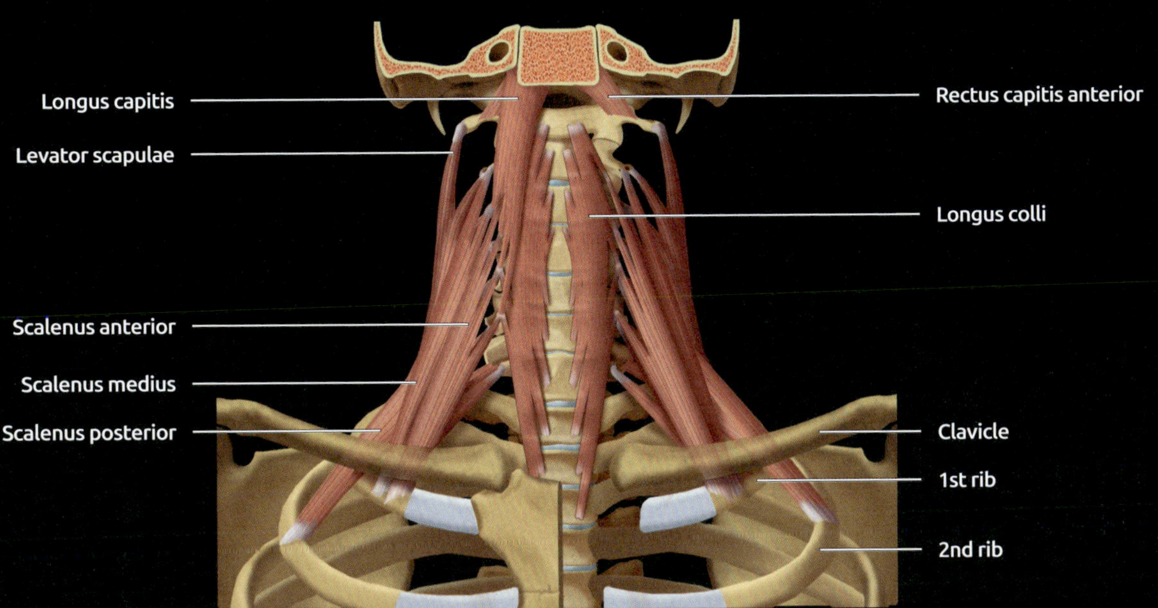

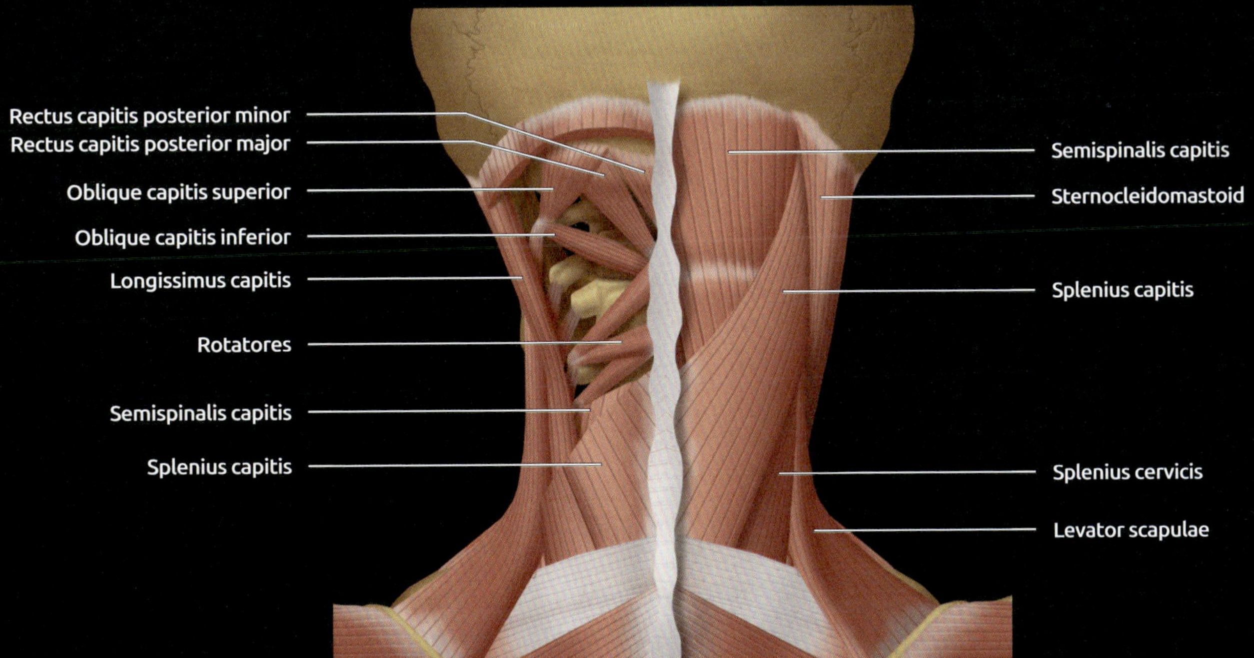

(Top) *Anterior view of neck muscles mainly shows the insertions and origins of the longus colli and longus capitis muscles and portions of the scalene anterior, middle, and posterior muscles.* **(Bottom)** *Graphic shows posterior muscles of the neck, including the sternocleidomastoid, splenius capitis, semispinalis capitis, levator scapulae, splenius cervicis, and suboccipital muscles.*

Posterior Cervical Space

TERMINOLOGY

Abbreviations

- Posterior cervical space (PCS)

Definitions

- Posterolateral fat-containing space in neck with complex fascial boundaries; extends from posterior mastoid tip to clavicle
- Encompasses major portion of posterior triangle

IMAGING ANATOMY

Overview

- Posterolateral fat-filled space just deep and posterior to sternocleidomastoid (SCM) muscle
- Lymphadenopathy: Infection, inflammation, and tumor constitute vast majority of lesions in PCS

Extent

- PCS extends from narrow superior component near mastoid tip to broader base at level of clavicle

Anatomy Relationships

- Anterolateral: SCM
- Anteromedial: Carotid space
- Deep to PCS: Perivertebral space
  - Anterior PCS: Superficial to **prevertebral component of perivertebral space**
  - Posterior PCS: Superficial to **paraspinal component of perivertebral space**

Internal Contents

- Fat is major content
- Spinal accessory nerve (CNXI)
- Lymph nodes
  - Level II, III, and IV: Anterior PCS
  - Level V: Posterior PCS
- Preaxillary brachial plexus
  - Segment of brachial plexus from scalene triangle passes through PCS
- Dorsal scapular nerve
  - Arises from ventral ramus of CNV
  - Motor innervation to rhomboid and levator scapulae muscles

Fascia of Posterior Cervical Space

- Complex fascial boundaries surround PCS
  - Superficial: Superficial layer of deep cervical fascia
  - Deep: Deep layer of deep cervical fascia
  - Anteromedial: Carotid sheath (all 3 layers, deep cervical fascia)

Surgical Triangles

- **Posterior triangle**
  - Region of neck posterolateral to SCM and anteromedial to trapezius muscle
  - Subdivided by inferior belly of omohyoid muscle into **occipital and subclavian triangles**
- **Occipital triangle**
  - Boundaries: Anteromedial-SCM muscle; posterolateral-trapezius muscle; inferior-inferior belly of omohyoid muscle
  - Contents: Fat, accessory nerve (CNXI), dorsal scapular nerves, and SAN chain
  - Includes majority of PCS
- **Subclavian triangle**
  - Boundaries: Superior-inferior belly of omohyoid muscle; anteromedial-SCM muscle; posterolateral-trapezius muscle
  - Contents: 3rd portion of subclavian artery, cervical brachial plexus
  - Subclavian triangle is lower, smaller portion of posterior triangle

ANATOMY IMAGING ISSUES

Questions

- What are criteria for defining cervical neck mass lesion as primary to PCS?
  - Lesion must be **centered within fat of PCS**
  - Lesion displaces carotid space anteromedially
  - Lesion elevates SCM muscle
  - Lesion flattens deeper perivertebral space structures
- How can you tell internal jugular node from spinal accessory node (SAN)?
  - Lower PCS
    - Jugular chain nodes abut carotid space
    - SANs (level VB) are separated from carotid space by fat and are lateral to oblique line drawn from posterior edge of SCM to posterior edge of anterior scalene muscle
  - Upper PCS
    - Internal jugular and SAN chain converge cephalad toward jugulodigastric group
    - Nodes that abut anterior, lateral, or posterior carotid space: Consider internal jugular nodes
    - Nodes posterior to coronal line along posterior margin of SCM: Consider SAN (level VA)

CLINICAL IMPLICATIONS

Clinical Importance

- Common: Malignant lymphadenopathy from primary head & neck malignancy or lymphoma; inflammatory lymphadenopathy
- Less common: Nerve sheath tumors, lipoma, congenital lymphatic malformation, 3rd branchial cleft cyst
- Pseudomasses: Cervical ribs, prominent transverse processes, and levator scapulae muscle hypertrophy

Function Dysfunction

- Spinal accessory cranial neuropathy results when CNXI injured
  - Most commonly injured during neck dissection for malignant squamous cell carcinoma nodes
  - Dysfunction: Sternomastoid and trapezius muscle paresis; difficulty lifting arm
    - Acute denervation: Muscles may swell and enhance
    - Chronic denervation: Muscles atrophy and fatty infiltrate
    - Levator scapulae muscle hypertrophies

GRAPHICS

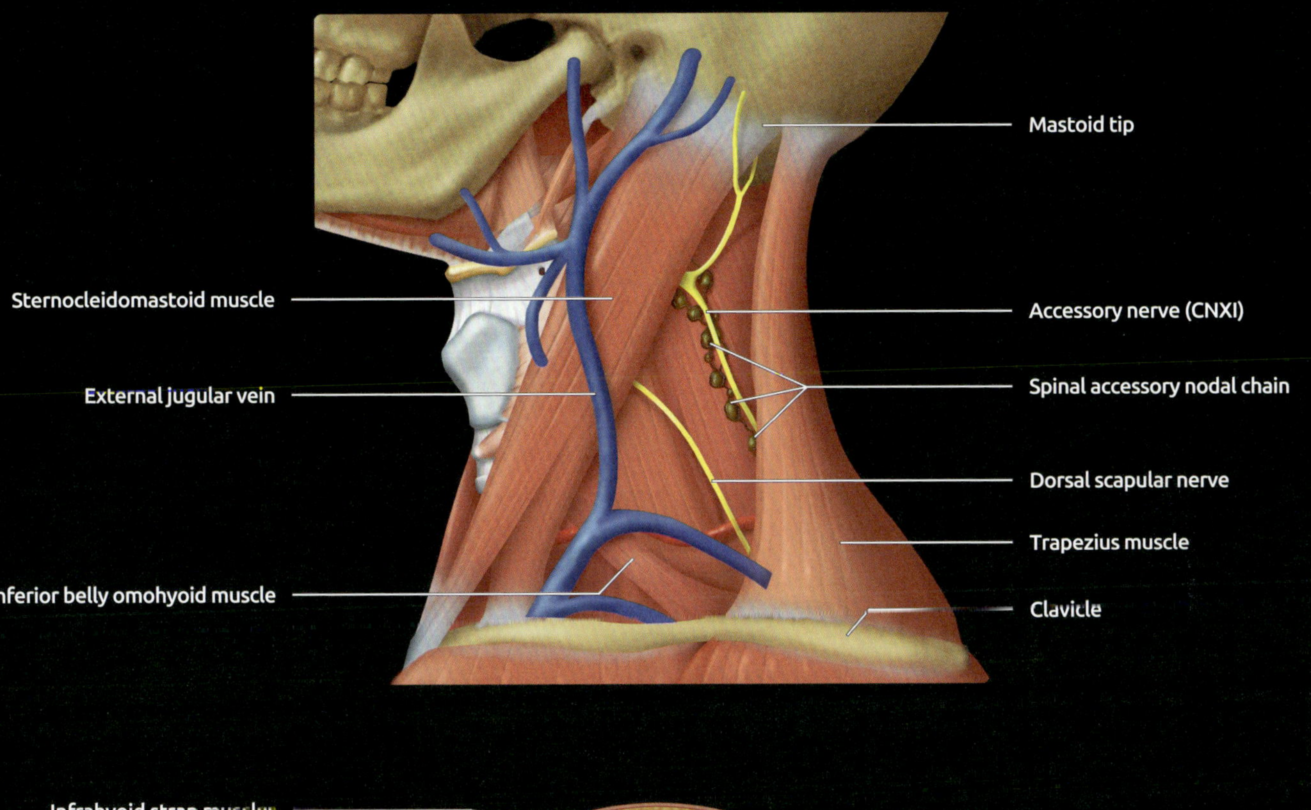

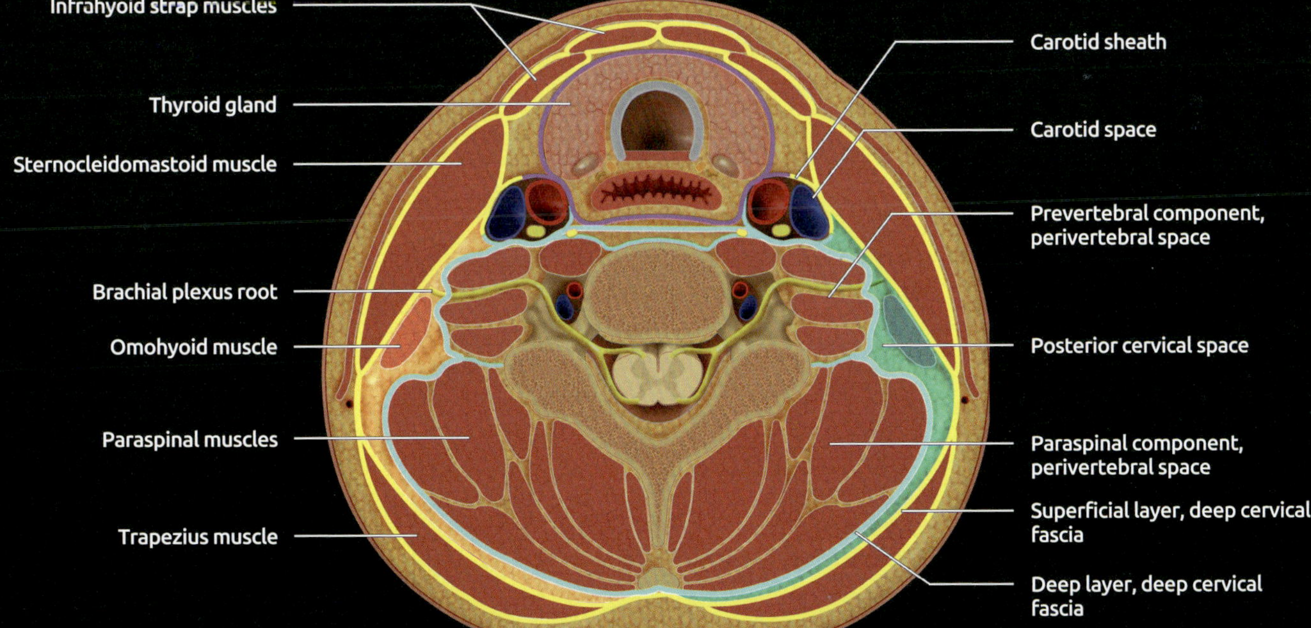

(Top) *Lateral graphic of extracranial head and neck shows the posterior cervical space (PCS) as a "tilting tent" with its superior margin at the level of the mastoid tip and its inferior border at the clavicle. It has 2 main nerves in its floor, the spinal accessory nerve (CNXI) and the dorsal scapular nerve. The spinal accessory nodal chain is its key occupant with regards to the kind of lesions found in the PCS.* **(Bottom)** *Axial graphic through the thyroid bed of the infrahyoid neck depicts the PCS with its complex fascial borders. The superficial layer of the deep cervical fascia (SL-DCF) (yellow outline covering the sternocleidomastoid and trapezius muscles) is its superficial border, while the deep layer of the deep cervical fascia (blue outline) is its deep border. Note the tricolored carotid sheath is its anteromedial border. The brachial plexus roots travel through the PCS on their way to the axillary apex. Coverage of strap muscles by SL-DCF (yellow outline) is controversial in the literature, with many considering it to be covered by the middle layer of deep cervical fascia (ML-DCF) (pink outline covering the visceral space/thyroid gland as well).*

POSTERIOR CERVICAL SPACE NODAL STATIONS/DISEASES

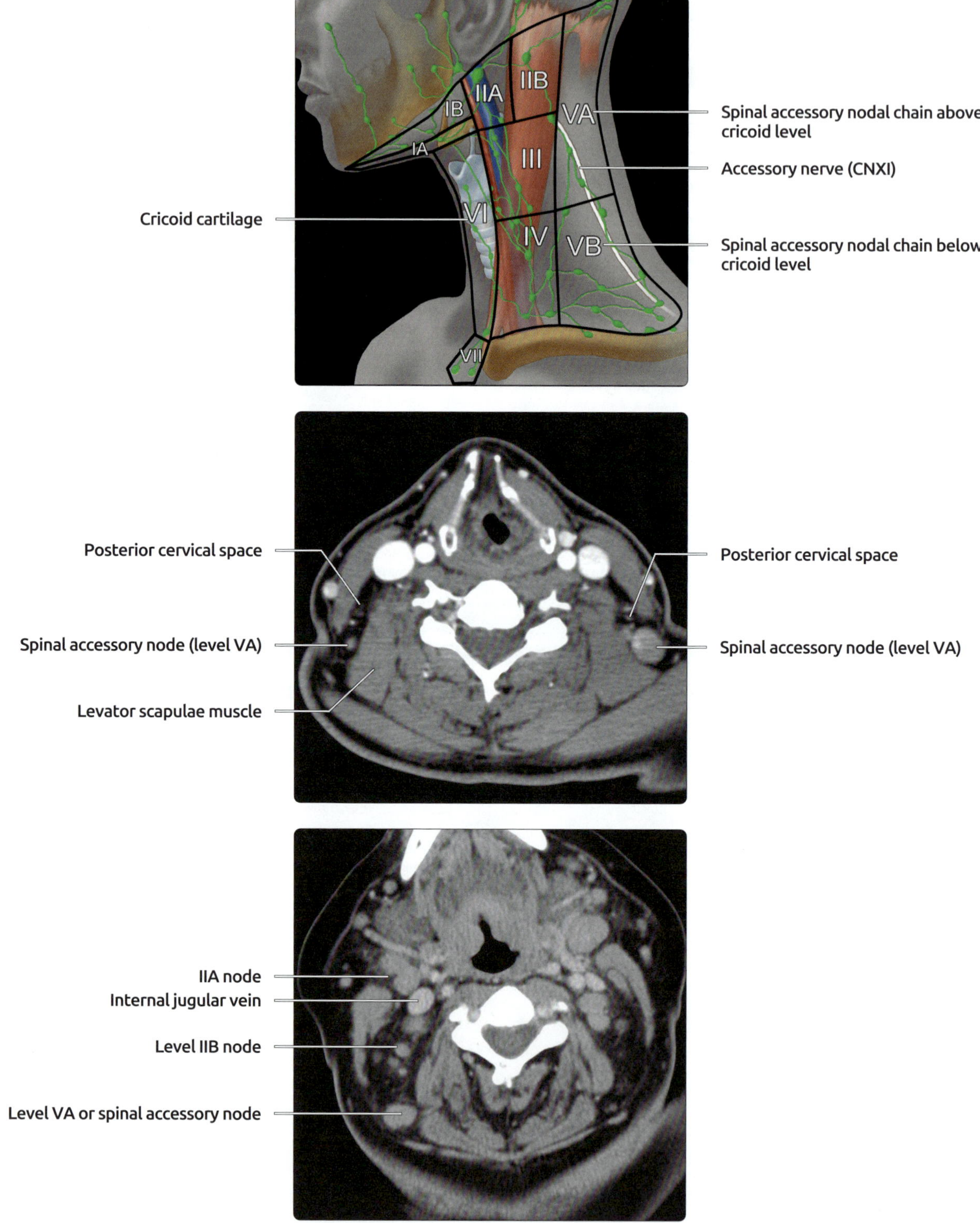

(Top) *Oblique graphic of the extracranial head and neck depicts the principal nodal chains and their assigned levels. The spinal accessory chain (level V) is divided at the axial level of the cricoid cartilage into the upper level VA and lower level VB groups. Levels II, III, and IV nodes are in the internal jugular chain.* **(Middle)** *Axial CECT of the cervical neck at the level of the supraglottis shows bilateral level VA nodes in the PCS of the neck. These are considered VA because they are in the PCS above the cricoid cartilage.* **(Bottom)** *Axial CECT demonstrates an enlarged spinal accessory nerve chain lymph node level VA in the PCS. The lymph nodes anterior to the carotid sheath or in contact with the carotid sheath are level IIA nodes, and lymph nodes posterior to the carotid sheath are level IIB nodes.*

AXIAL CECT

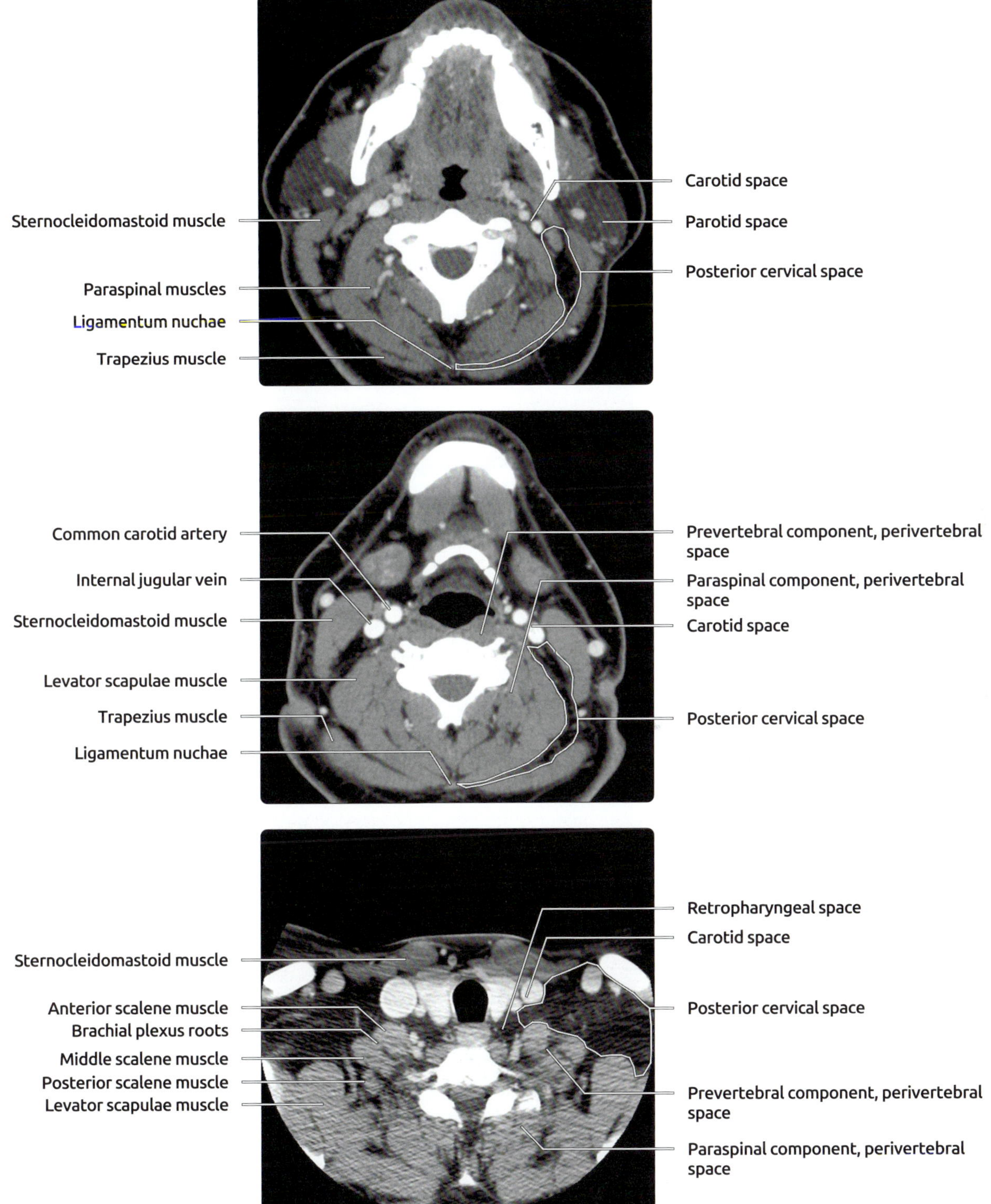

(Top) *First of 3 axial CECT images at the level of the midoropharynx shows the fat-filled PCS. Notice the posteromedial extension of the PCS between the paraspinal muscles and the trapezius where it reaches as far as the ligamentum nuchae.* **(Middle)** *At the level of the hyoid bone, the anteromedial border of the PCS abuts the carotid space. Deep to the PCS is the paraspinal component of the perivertebral space. The lateralmost muscle in the paraspinal muscle group is the levator scapulae muscle.* **(Bottom)** *At the level of the clavicle, the PCS is seen enlarging in the inferolateral direction to meet the axillary apex. Notice the brachial plexus roots must traverse the posterior cervical space as they emerge from between the anterior and middle scalene muscles.*

TRANSVERSE ULTRASOUND

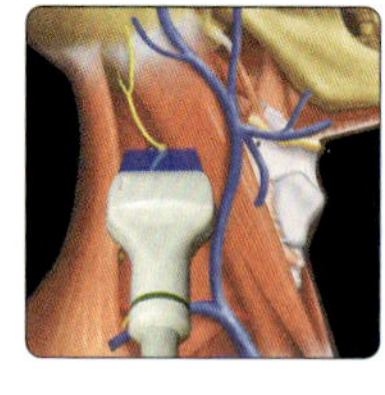

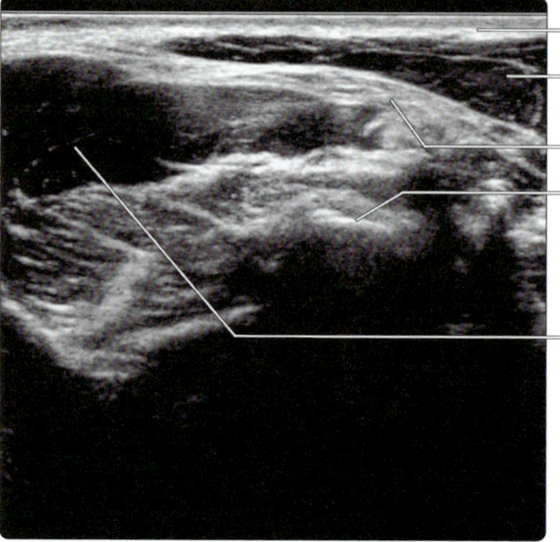

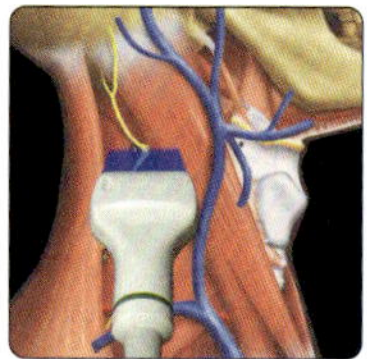

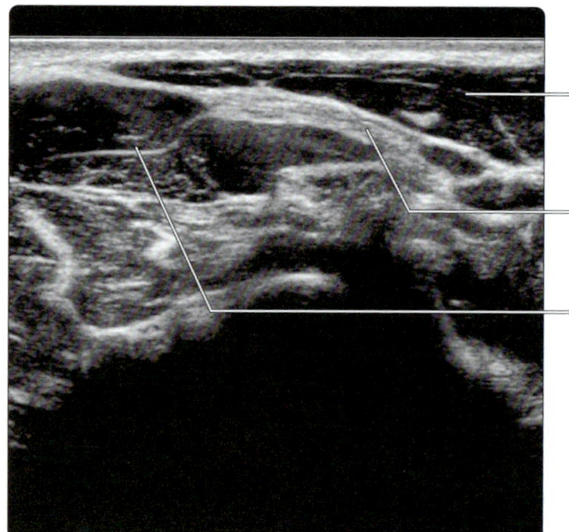

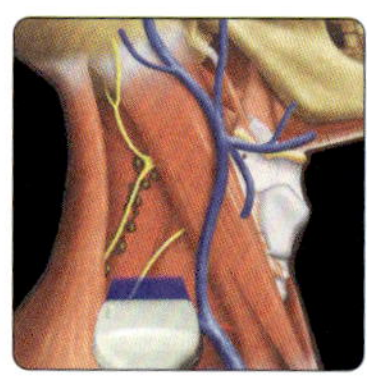

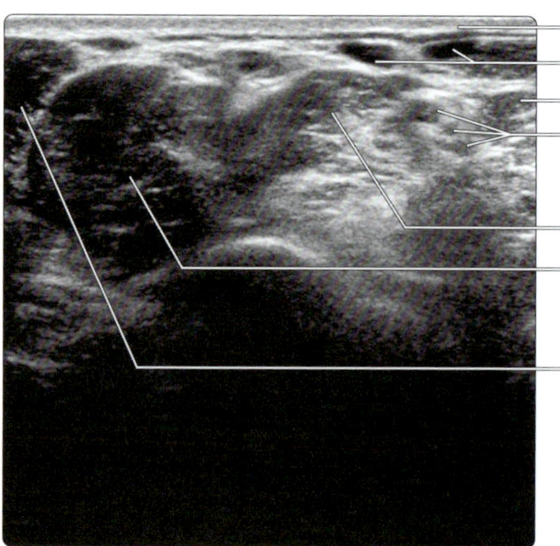

(Top) *First of 3 transverse grayscale ultrasound images shows the posterior triangle. The sternocleidomastoid muscle marks the anterior border of the posterior triangle. Muscles form the floor of the posterior triangle. Note the accessory nerve and nodes lie in the intermuscular fat plane.* **(Middle)** *Transverse grayscale ultrasound shows the intermuscular fat plane, which is best screened in this plane. Once pathology is detected, further examination, particularly Doppler, is best done longitudinally.* **(Bottom)** *Lower level of the posterior triangle is shown. The trapezius muscle marks the posterior margin of the posterior triangle. The main bulk of the levator scapulae muscle forms the muscular floor.*

LONGITUDINAL AND TRANSVERSE ULTRASOUND

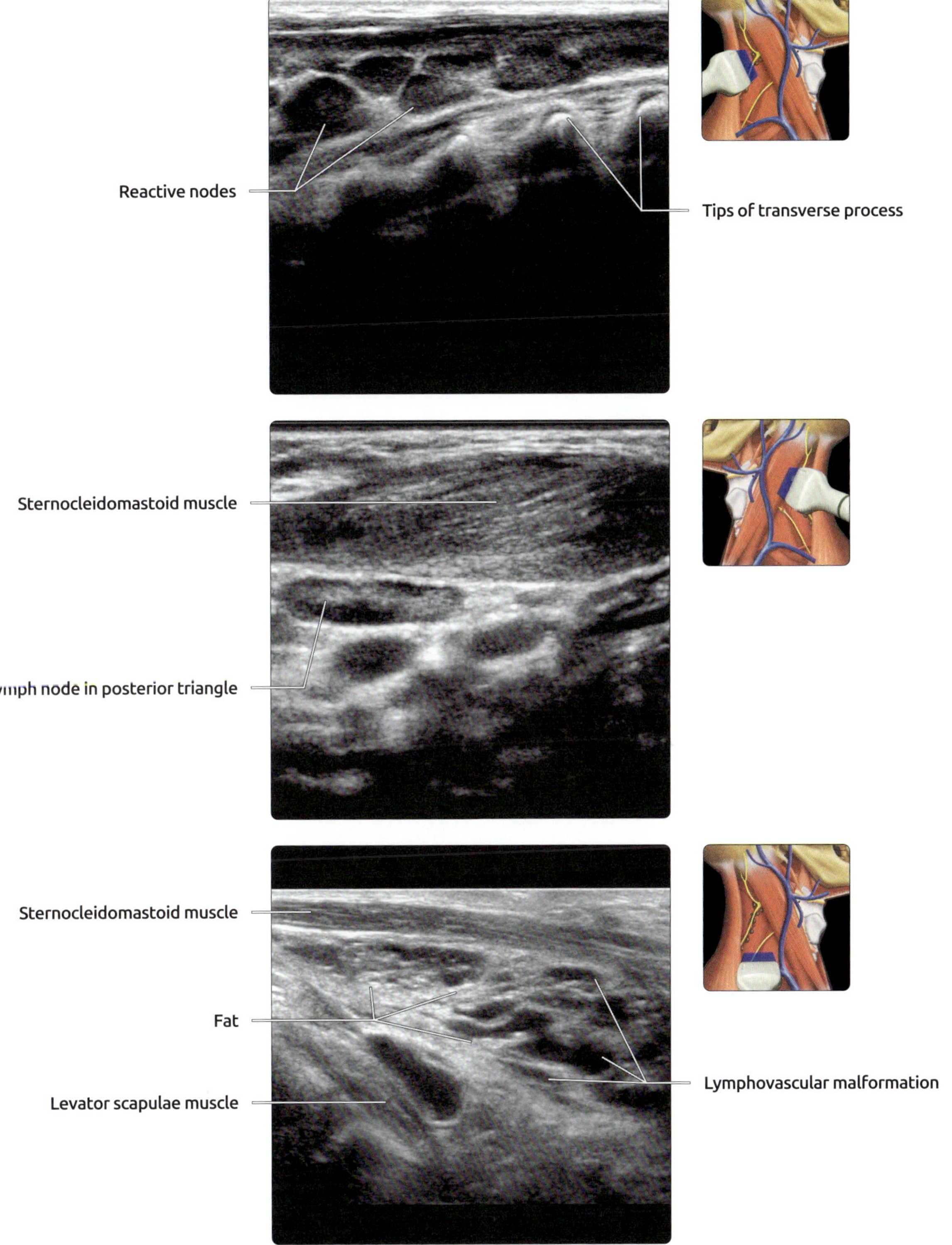

(Top) *Longitudinal grayscale ultrasound of the posterior triangle shows a chain of reactive accessory nodes. Note their location in the intermuscular fat plane. Do not mistake the tips of the transverse processes with calcified nodes.* **(Middle)** *Longitudinal grayscale ultrasound shows hypertrophy of the sternocleidomastoid muscle (pseudotumor) in an infant with torticollis. Note the internal muscular striations are preserved, helping to identify this as a muscle and not a mass.* **(Bottom)** *Oblique transverse grayscale ultrasound of a child who underwent 2 treatments of ultrasound-guided sclerotherapy for a large, multiloculated lymphovascular malformation is shown. Note that small cystic locules persist; however, much of the lymphatic malformation has been replaced by fatty tissue. Ultrasound safely guides intralesional injection and readily monitors posttreatment change in size and appearance.*

GENERIC MASS IN POSTERIOR CERVICAL SPACE

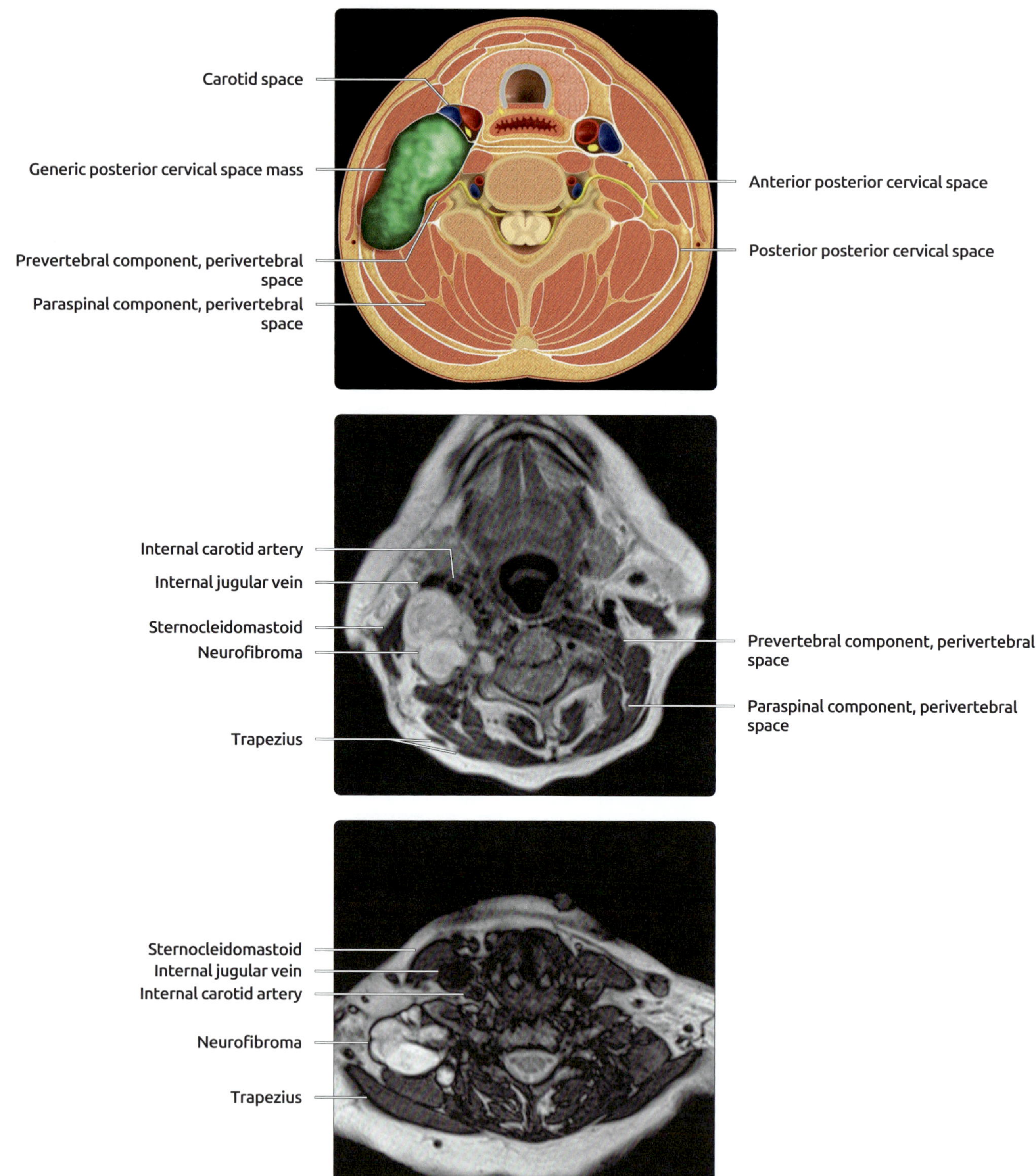

(Top) *Axial graphic in the infrahyoid neck shows a generic mass in the posterior cervical space on the left. Notice the lesion is centered within fat of the PCS. A PCS mass typically displaces the carotid space anteromedially, elevates the sternocleidomastoid muscle, and flattens the deeper perivertebral space structures. Anterior PCS is superficial to the prevertebral component of perivertebral space, and posterior PCS is superficial to the paraspinal component of perivertebral space.* **(Middle)** *Axial T2-weighted MR at the suprahyoid level-superior portion of a neurofibroma is seen filling the anterior PCS.* **(Bottom)** *Axial T2-weighted opposed-phase MR at the infrahyoid level shows the inferior portion of the neurofibroma in posterior PCS.*

CORONAL & SAGITTAL T1 MR

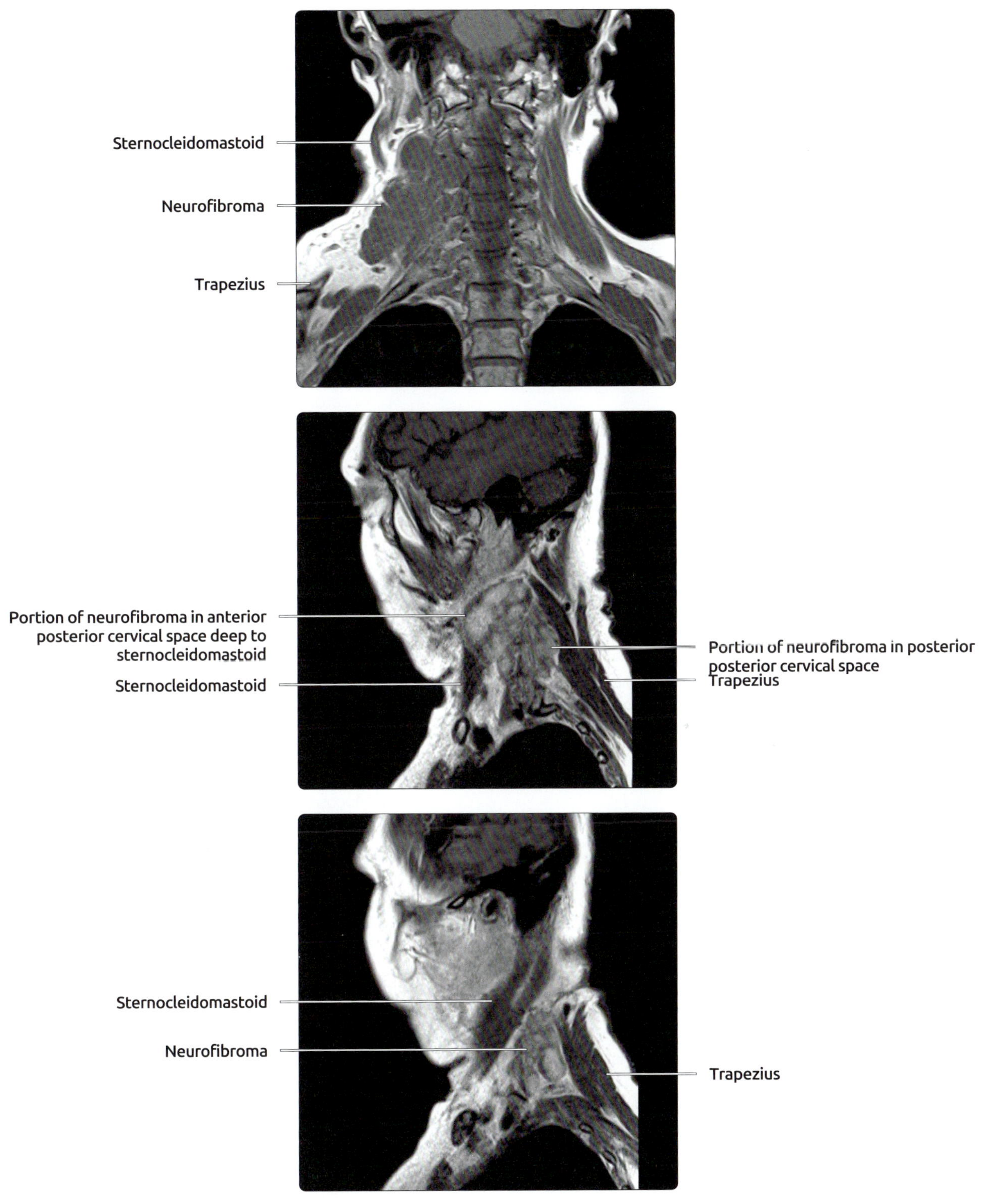

(Top) *Coronal T1-weighted MR shows plexiform neurofibroma in the PCS. The superior portion of the lesion is in the anterior PCS, deep to the sternocleidomastoid. The inferior portion of the lesion is in the posterior PCS. This is due to the oblique direction of the sternocleidomastoid extending from the mastoid tip, anteriorly to the sternum and clavicle.* **(Middle)** *Sagittal T1-weighted postcontrast MR shows a plexiform neurofibroma in the PCS. The anterosuperior portion of the lesion is deep to the sternocleidomastoid in the anterior PCS. The posterior and inferior portion of the lesion is in the posterior PCS.* **(Bottom)** *Sagittal T1-weighted postcontrast MR shows a plexiform neurofibroma in the posterior PCS.*

TERMINOLOGY

Abbreviations

- Visceral space (VS)

Definitions

- Cylindrical space in midline infrahyoid neck (IHN) enclosed by middle layer of deep cervical fascia (ML-DCF)

IMAGING ANATOMY

Overview

- Cylindrical space containing central contents of IHN; extends from hyoid bone to upper mediastinum
- Largest space of IHN with multiple important anatomic subunits
- **Critical contents**: Larynx, trachea, hypopharynx (HP), esophagus, thyroid and parathyroid glands, and recurrent laryngeal nerves (RLNs)

Anatomy Relationships

- Anterior: Strap muscles
- Lateral: Paired anterior cervical spaces
- Posterolateral: Paired carotid spaces (CSs)
- Posterior: Retropharyngeal space (RPS)

Internal Contents

- **Larynx**
  - Hollow, mucosal-lined, muscular, and cartilaginous organ
  - Functions: Breathing, phonation, and prevents aspiration
  - **Supraglottis**: Top of epiglottis to laryngeal ventricle, includes false vocal cords
  - **Glottis**: True vocal cords (TVCs), anterior and posterior commissures, and central air space within
  - **Subglottis**: From undersurface of TVC to inferior cricoid
- **Cervical trachea**
  - Superior portion of trachea extending from larynx to thoracic inlet
  - Trachea: Semirigid tube extending from larynx to main bronchi (carina) comprised of cartilage, smooth muscle, connective tissue, and mucosal lining
    - 15-20 incomplete rings of hyaline cartilages surrounding anterior 2/3
    - Flat, cartilage-deficient posterior portion: Fibromuscular tissue
  - Smooth muscle fibers in posterior membrane (trachealis muscle) attach to free ends of tracheal cartilages and can alter cross-sectional area of airway
  - Mucosa: Pseudostratified ciliated columnar epithelium interspersed with goblet cells, both lying on basal lamina
  - Variable measurement: Both AP and transverse dimensions ~ 10-25 mm
  - Anterior: Strap muscles and fat plane superiorly, thyroid isthmus inferiorly
  - Lateral: Thyroid gland
  - Posterior: Esophagus, separated by thin layer of fat
  - Functions: Airway protection, humidification and warming of inspired air, and mucociliary clearance
- **HP**
  - Inferior continuation of oropharynx
  - Begins at level of pharyngoepiglottic folds, at approximately horizontal level of hyoid bone, and merges with esophagus below at esophageal verge
  - Complex mucosal and muscular tube consisting of 5 principal layers
    - **Mucosa**: Stratified squamous epithelium that lines lumen
    - **Submucosa**: Loose stroma that can contain fat and can be identified on cross-sectional imaging as thin fat plane
    - Fibrous layer that represents limited inferior continuation of **pharyngobasilar fascia** (pharyngeal aponeurosis)
    - **Muscular layer** consisting of middle and inferior constrictors
    - Outer fascial layer originating from buccopharyngeal fascia
  - Consists of 3 major regions
    - **Pyriform sinuses (PSs)**
      - Anterolateral recesses of HP
      - Each PS has shape of inverted pyramid with base of pyramid positioned superiorly at level of pharyngoepiglottic fold and inferior tip (PS apex) positioned at level of TVC
      - Majority of hypopharyngeal squamous cell carcinomas (2/3) originate in PS
    - **Posterior wall**
      - Inferior continuation of posterior oropharyngeal wall from approximate level of hyoid bone to inferior tip of cricoid cartilage
      - Muscular layer formed by middle and inferior constrictor muscles
      - Posterior wall separated from **perivertebral space** by **RPS**
    - **Postcricoid region**
      - Anterior wall of lower HP
      - Mucosa of postcricoid region faces posteriorly: Normally directly apposed to mucosa of posterior wall during routine cross-sectional imaging
      - Air-filled HP lumen between postcricoid HP anteriorly and lower posterior wall of HP posteriorly only rarely visualized on CT/MR
      - Anterior-posterior dimension of postcricoid soft tissue should be < 1 cm normally
- **Cervical esophagus**
  - HP merges with esophagus below at esophageal verge
  - Esophageal verge is best defined by cricopharyngeus muscle that encircles junction, but this muscle cannot be identified easily on cross-sectional imaging
  - Cricopharyngeus muscle is located at approximate level of inferior margin of cricoid cartilage
  - Descends posterior to trachea and thyroid, lying in front of lower cervical vertebrae
  - Positioned slightly to left in lower cervical neck and upper mediastinum
  - Nonkeratinized stratified squamous epithelium
  - Thin layer of fat separates posterior wall of trachea from esophagus
  - Thin fat planes are generally present on lateral margins of cervical esophagus
  - Variable diameter depending on degree of distension

- Esophageal wall is generally < 5 mm thick
- **RLNs**
  - Recurrent, courses opposite to "parent" nerve
  - Arise from vagus nerves, innervate all intrinsic muscles of larynx except cricothyroid muscle
  - Left: Recurs under aortic arch and ascends in tracheoesophageal (TE) groove
  - Right: Recurs under subclavian artery and ascends to side of trachea behind common carotid artery to TE groove
  - Enter larynx deep to lower border of inferior constrictor muscle
  - Left RLN is longer than right
  - Injury or insult to RLN (or proximal vagus nerve) can lead to ipsilateral vocal cord paralysis
  - Right RLN close to bifurcation of right inferior thyroid artery and is more prone for injury during thyroid surgery
  - Extralaryngeal branching of RLN, which is relatively common variation, predisposes to injury during surgery
  - Non-RLN (NRLN) exits vagus nerve and enters larynx with short and straight course in neck
    - Clues: Aberrant right subclavian artery: NRLN on right; situs inversus with aberrant left subclavian artery: NRLN on left
    - Rare: Both recurrent and nonrecurrent branch on same side without associated vascular anomaly
- **Thyroid gland**
  - Shield-shaped endocrine organ in lower neck that produces thyroid hormones (T3 and T4) that are involved in many functions, including metabolism (cardiac rate and output) and protein synthesis (growth); also produces calcitonin
  - Lies anterior and lateral to trachea in VS of IHN at C5-T1 level
  - 2 lobes connected by isthmus
  - High levels of iodine normal, hyperdense in CT
  - Lower than normal density = hypothyroid state
  - High iodine content and vascularity protect against infection
- **Parathyroid glands**
  - Small glands in VS of neck, intimately associated with posterior margin of thyroid gland, which produce parathormone, hormone that regulates calcium concentration in serum and interstitial fluids
  - 4 glands, 2 pairs behind upper and lower poles of thyroid gland
  - Superior 2 glands consistent in location
  - Inferior 2 glands less reliable in location
    - May be normally found in cervicothoracic junction or superior mediastinum
- **VS lymph nodes**
  - Considered **level VI nodal group**
  - Paratracheal lymph node group
    - **1st-order drainage for thyroid malignancy**
    - Serves as primary conduit for nodal spread into superior mediastinum
  - Prelaryngeal nodal group
  - Pretracheal nodal group

Fascia

- **ML-DCF** completely encloses VS
- ML-DCF also referred to as "visceral fascia"

ANATOMY IMAGING ISSUES

Imaging Approaches

- Imaging approach is determined by clinical symptoms and anatomic subunit under investigation
- **Thyroid**
  - **Ultrasound** ± needle aspiration biopsy is **1st-line approach** to lesions of thyroid gland
  - Differentiated thyroid carcinoma = total thyroidectomy and I-131 diagnostic scan 6 weeks after surgery
  - If suspected nodes from clinical examination, I-131 study, or significant residual uptake remaining in thyroid bed, therapeutic I-131 dose is administered
  - MR: Preferred imaging tool to stage superior mediastinum as it prevents iodine load-delaying iodine-based nuclear medicine therapy
  - Suspected VS malignancy: Image to carina to include level VI (paratracheal, prelaryngeal, and pretracheal) nodes and superior mediastinal nodes (level VII)
- **Parathyroid**
  - Ultrasound is best 1st-line approach
  - Tc-99m sestamibi useful for localizing parathyroid adenoma (PTA)
  - CT, CTA, and MR useful in challenging cases, especially ectopic PTA cases
  - Searching for PTA includes upper mediastinal search
  - Symptoms associated with hypercalcemia produced by excessive parathyroid hormone
- **HP and cervical esophagus**
  - CECT is best overall modality for evaluating soft tissue masses of HP and cervical esophagus
  - MR is useful in problem solving, especially evaluation of local invasion
  - Barium swallow can evaluate for motility disorder, obstruction, aspiration
  - Symptoms include dysphagia, intolerance to solid foods
- **Larynx and cervical trachea**
  - CECT is best overall approach for evaluating lesion of larynx and proximal trachea
  - Symptoms include cough, stridor, aspiration, hoarseness
  - RLN: Distal vagal neuropathy with isolated vocal cord paralysis; hoarseness

Imaging Pitfalls

- Patulous esophagus may project from behind left tracheal margin, mimicking PTA
- Ending VS cross-sectional imaging at cervicothoracic junction is significant imaging mistake
  - **Multiple VS lesions require imaging to carina**
    - When staging VS tumor, especially differentiated thyroid carcinoma, must evaluate upper mediastinal nodes (level VII)
    - Vocal cord paralysis requires continuing to carina if on **left**
- Small lymph nodes in VS can be mistaken for PTAs on cross-sectional imaging; hypervascularity on arterial-phase CTA can help distinguish PTA, but sestamibi scan is more specific for identifying PTAs
- Exophytic thyroid nodules can mimic PTA; noncontrast CT density, hypervascularity on arterial phase, and washout on venous phase can help

GRAPHICS

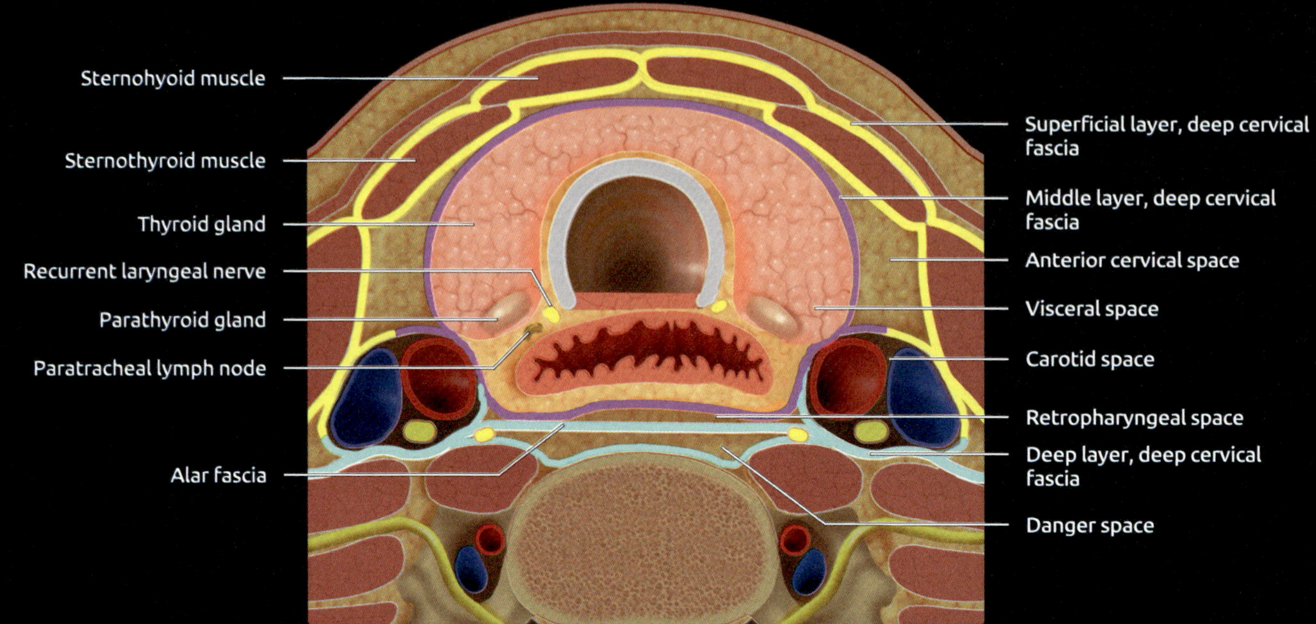

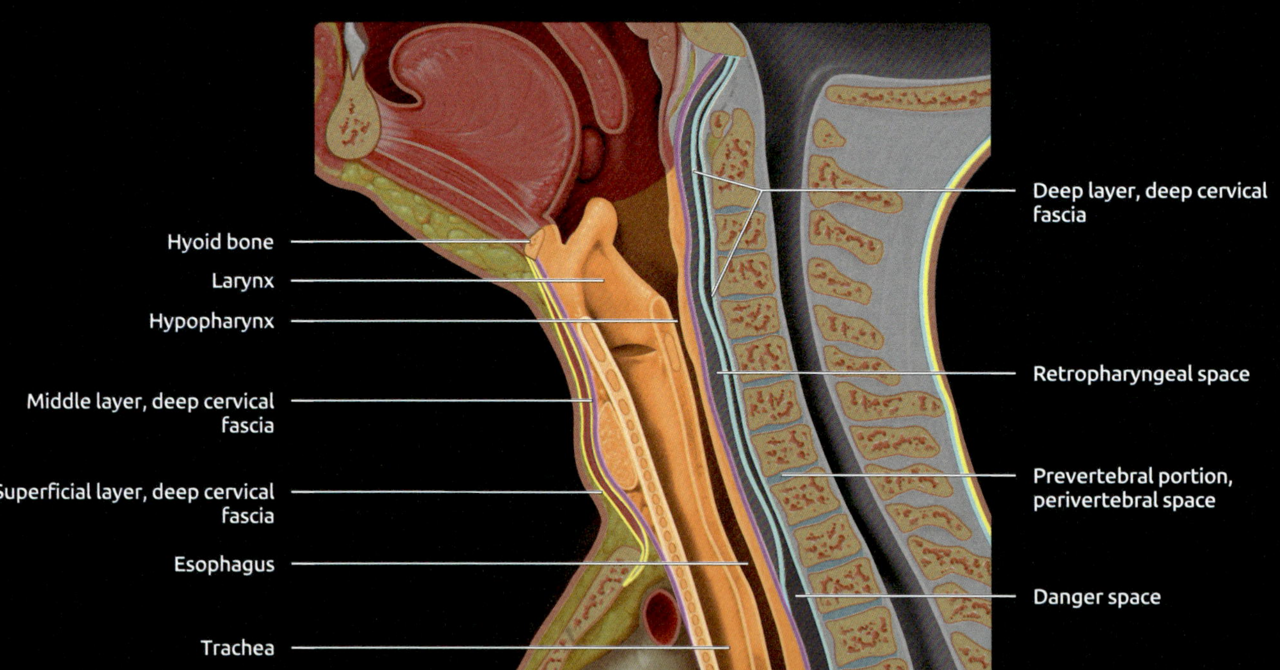

(Top) *Axial graphic shows the visceral space defined by the middle layer of the deep cervical fascia [(ML-DCF) pink]. The ML-DCF, a.k.a. visceral fascia, runs along the deep surface of the strap muscles, merges anteriorly with the superficial layer of deep cervical fascia [(SL-DCF) yellow], and splits to encapsulate the thyroid gland. The ML-DCF also forms the anterior margin of the retropharyngeal space and contributes to the carotid sheath. The recurrent laryngeal nerve lies in the tracheoesophageal groove; injury there results in vocal cord paralysis and hoarseness. Coverage of the strap muscles by the SL-DCF (yellow outline) is controversial in literature with many considering it to be covered by the ML-DCF (pink outline), which covers the visceral space/thyroid gland also.* **(Bottom)** *Sagittal graphic shows the longitudinal relationships of the infrahyoid neck. Note that the visceral space (orange) is the only space unique to the infrahyoid neck, extending from the hyoid bone to the superior mediastinum. The visceral space is the cylindrical space in the anterior midline neck surrounded by the ML-DCF (pink).*

AXIAL CECT

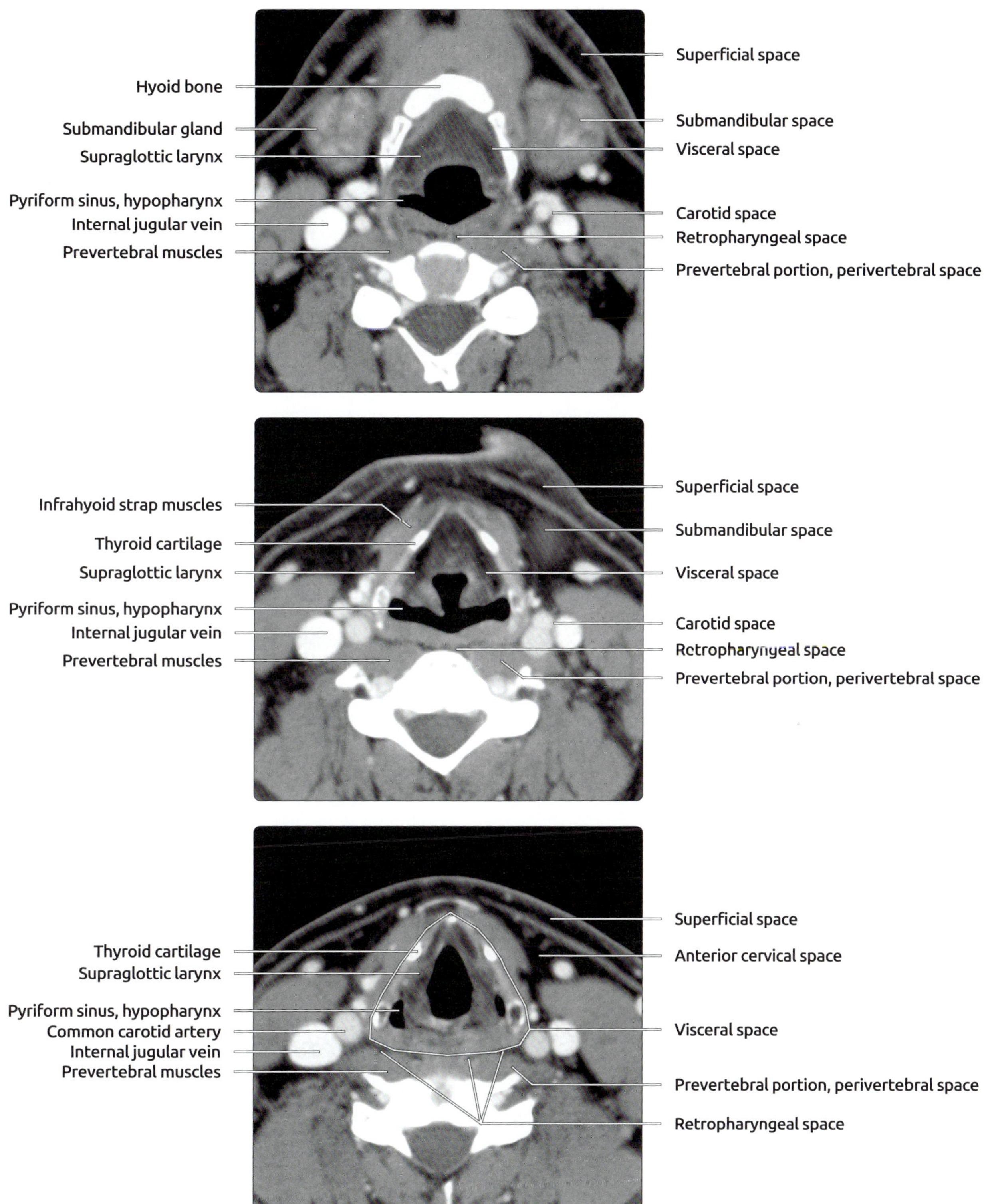

(Top) *First of 6 axial CECT images of the visceral space presented from superior to inferior shows the hyoid bone, which represents the superior extent of the visceral space. This cylindrical space in the midline infrahyoid neck is enclosed by the ML-DCF and extends to the superior mediastinum. The submandibular space is continuous with the anterior cervical space.* **(Middle)** *This image shows the visceral space contains the larynx and hypopharynx at this level. It is bordered posteriorly by the retropharyngeal space and posterolaterally by carotid spaces.* **(Bottom)** *This image shows the visceral space is completely enclosed by the ML-DCF, represented by outline drawn. The paired anterior cervical spaces are lateral to the visceral space and are continuous with submandibular spaces superiorly. The retropharyngeal space is seen as a stripe of fat between the posterior hypopharynx and prevertebral muscles.*

AXIAL CECT

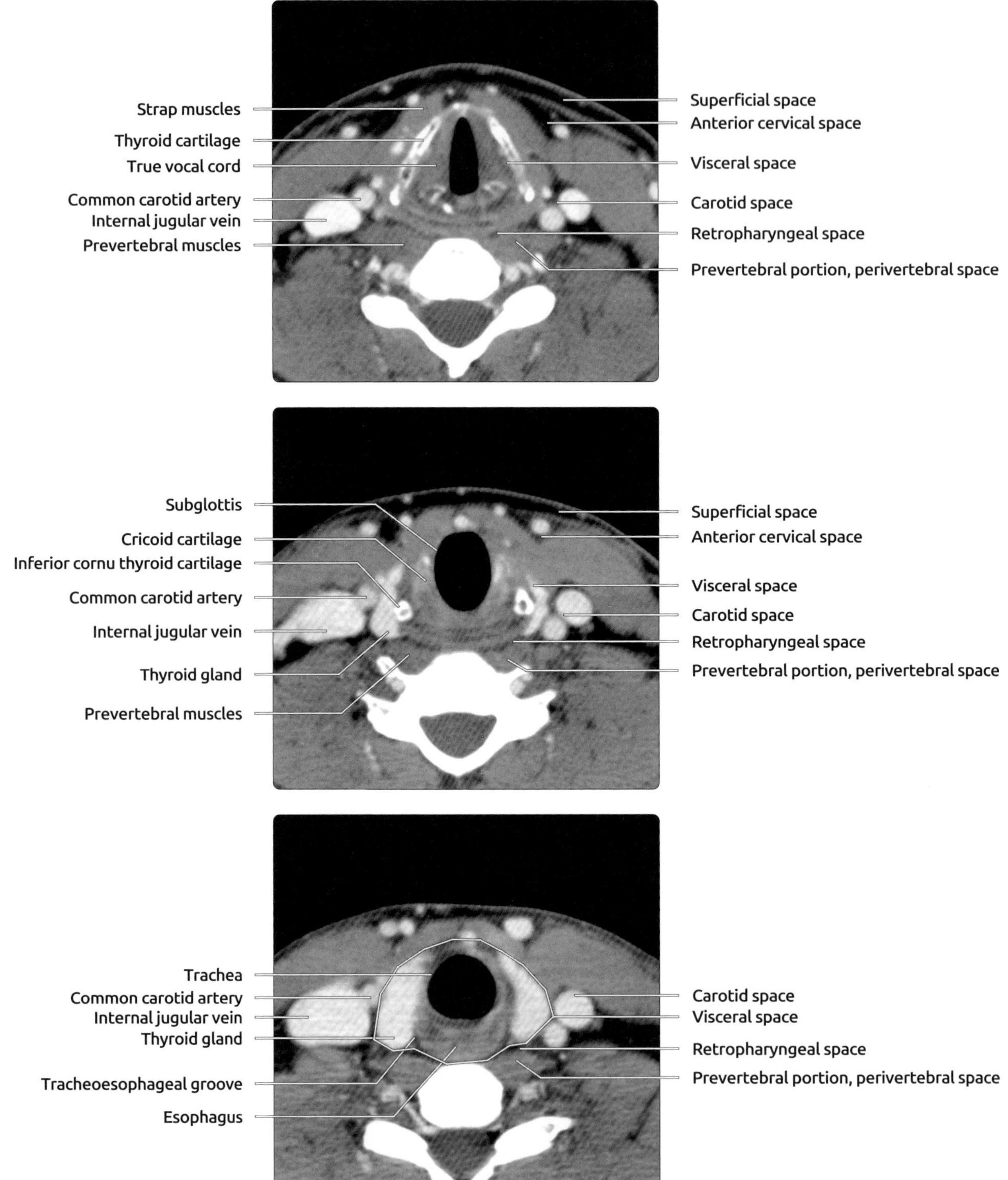

(Top) *Image at the level of the glottis shows the visceral space in the anterior midline surrounded by the anterior cervical space, carotid space, and retropharyngeal space.* **(Middle)** *Image at the subglottic larynx level shows the upper thyroid lobes.* **(Bottom)** *Image at the thyroid gland level shows the inferior visceral space, which includes the esophagus and trachea. The recurrent laryngeal nerve is located in the tracheoesophageal groove but cannot be seen on conventional imaging. Injury of this nerve results in vocal cord paralysis, and imaging should extend to the carina in patients with left-sided injury. Thyroid disease is one of the most common lesions of the visceral space and is often best evaluated by ultrasound. If differentiated thyroid disease is present, nuclear medicine I-131 study is the next best study. CECT may delay therapy in patients planned for iodine-based nuclear medicine therapy.*

THYROID MASS GRAPHIC AND CORONAL CECT

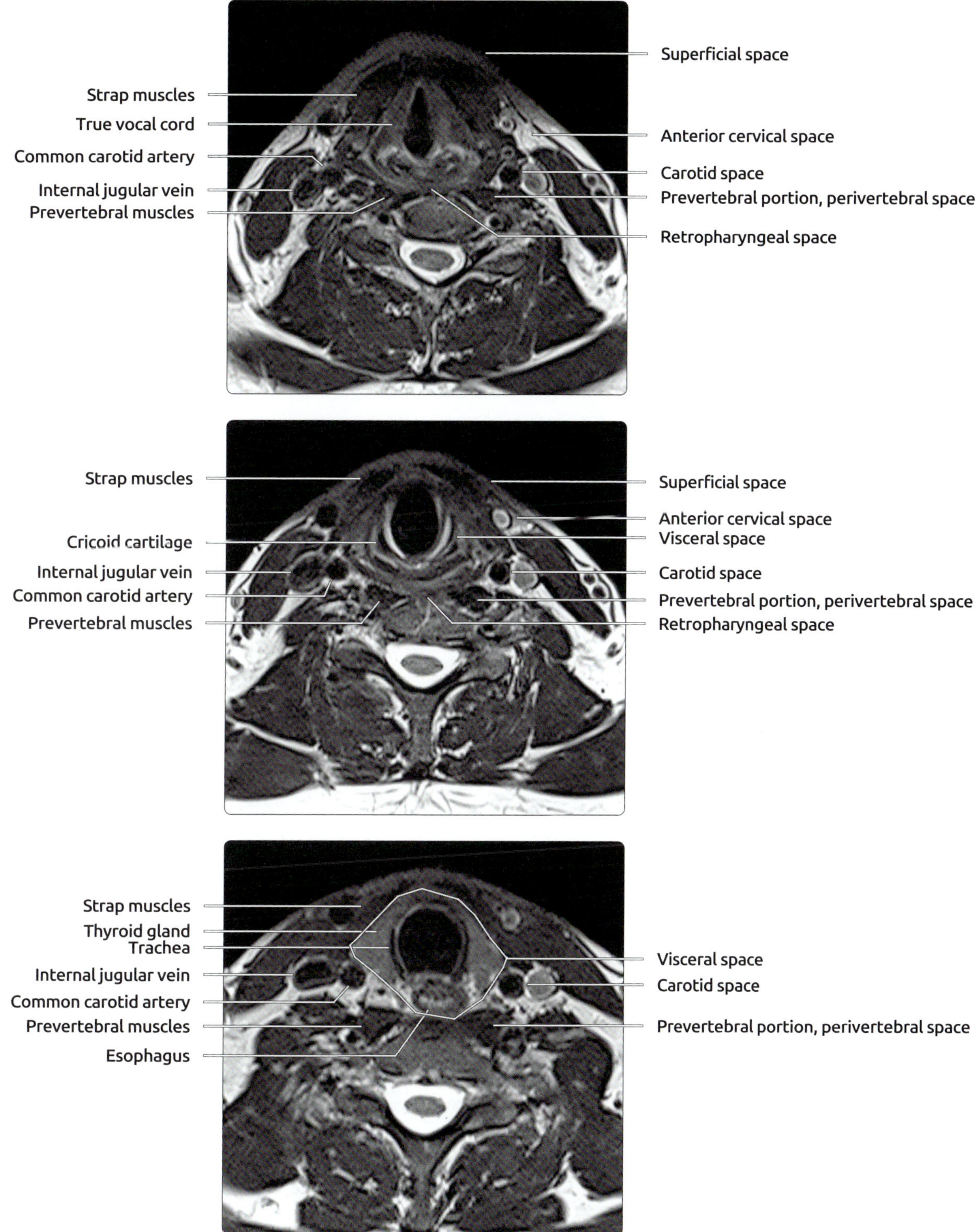

(Top) *Axial T2 MR at the level of the glottis shows the visceral space in the anterior midline surrounded by strap muscles, the anterior cervical space, carotid space, and retropharyngeal space.* **(Middle)** *Axial T2 MR is shown at the level of the subglottic larynx.* **(Bottom)** *Axial T2 MR at the thyroid gland level shows the inferior visceral space, which includes the esophagus and trachea.*

GENERIC VISCERAL SPACE MASS GRAPHIC AND SAGITTAL ANATOMY

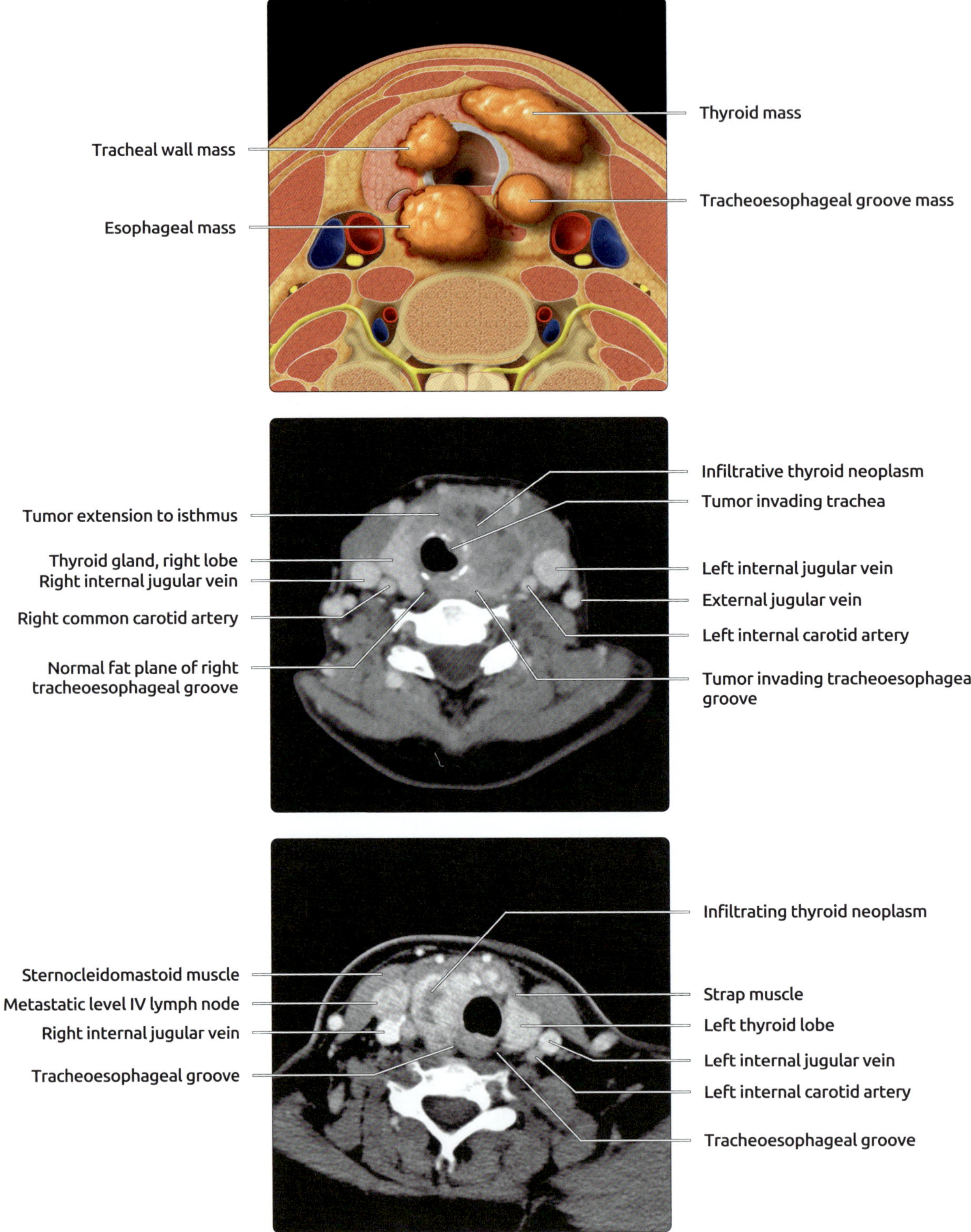

(Top) *Axial graphic shows 4 distinct generic visceral space mass locations. A thyroid mass is defined by a mass at least partially surrounded by thyroid tissue. A mass involving the tracheoesophageal groove typically results in recurrent laryngeal nerve injury. A tracheal wall mass is centered in the tracheal wall and displaces the thyroid gland laterally and esophagus posteriorly. An esophageal mass is typically midline and displaces the trachea and thyroid anteriorly.* **(Middle)** *Axial CECT through the thyroid gland demonstrates a large, infiltrative anaplastic thyroid carcinoma involving the left lobe and isthmus of the thyroid gland. Tumor extends beyond the medial capsular margin of the thyroid through the tracheal wall. Tumor obliterates the normal fat plane of the left tracheoesophageal groove.* **(Bottom)** *Axial CECT through the level of the thyroid gland in a patient with right vocal cord paralysis and hoarseness shows a heterogeneously enhancing right thyroid lobe tumor with extracapsular extension to the right tracheoesophageal groove. There is a level IV lymph nodal metastasis.*

VISCERAL SPACE: RADIOLOGIC CORRELATION

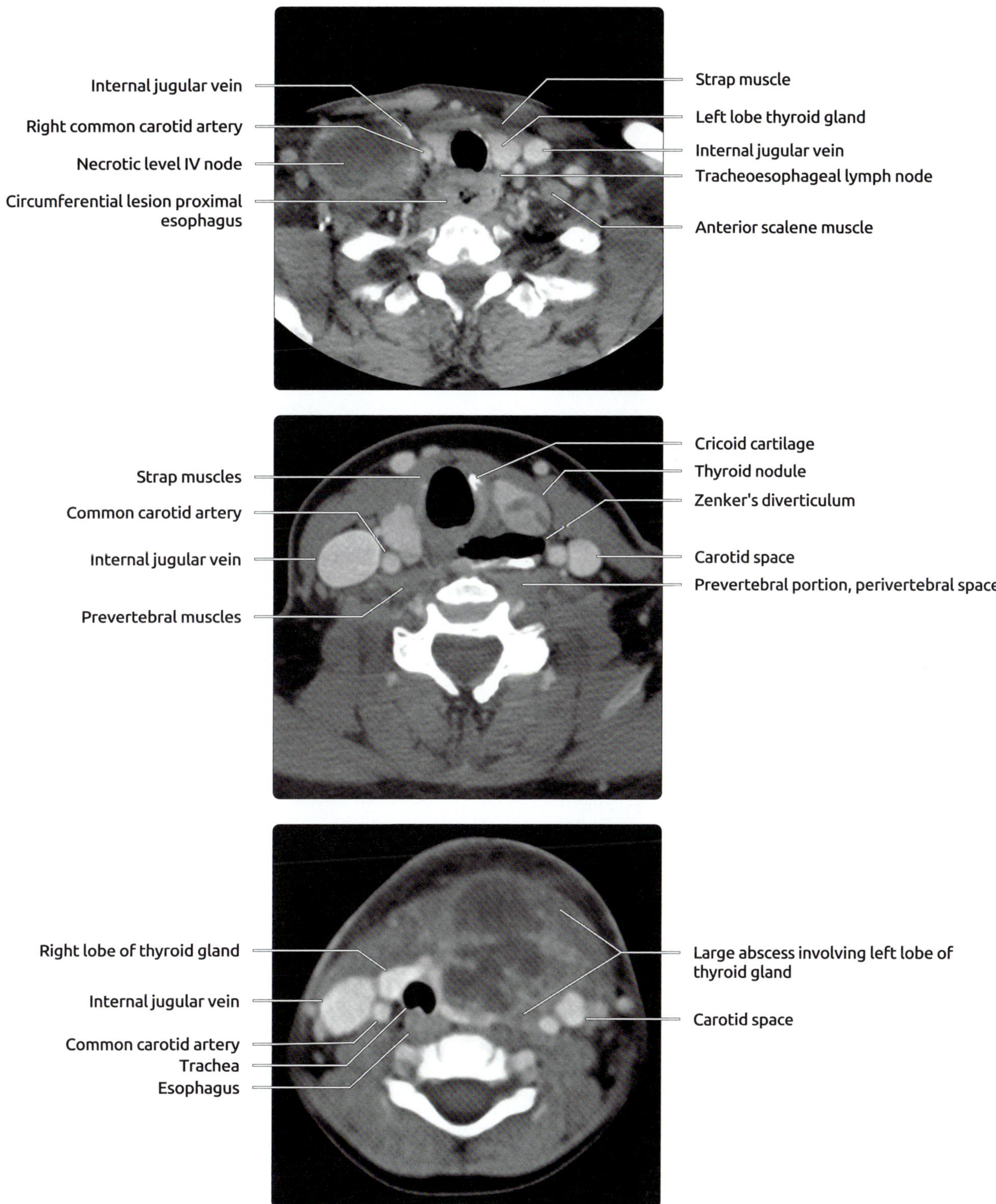

(Top) *Axial CECT through the level of the thyroid gland shows a large, circumferential lesion involving the cervical esophagus, consistent with squamous cell carcinoma. There is a large necrotic level IV lymph node (that demonstrates peripheral enhancement and central low density) on the patient's right. Air density in the central lumen of the esophagus is present.* **(Middle)** *Axial CECT shows Zenker diverticulum containing air and layering density from oral contrast to the left side of the esophagus and posterior to the thyroid gland. The lesion displaces the carotid space laterally and the thyroid lobe with an incidental nodule anteriorly.* **(Bottom)** *Axial CECT shows suppurative thyroiditis with a large abscess due to infection of 4th branchial cleft cyst in an infant. The lesion involves the left lobe of thyroid, which is a diagnostic clue. The lesion displaces the carotid space laterally and the strap muscles anteriorly. Infection of the thyroid gland is rare due to its high iodine content and vascularity.*

TERMINOLOGY

Abbreviations

- True vocal cord (TVC); false vocal cord (FVC)
- Hypopharynx (HP); aryepiglottic fold (AEF)

IMAGING ANATOMY

Extent

- Located in ventral aspect of neck, suspended from hyoid bone, and extending superiorly to inferiorly between ~ C3 and C6 vertebrae
- Continuous below with trachea, opens above into pharynx

Internal Contents

- **Laryngeal cartilages**
  - Thyroid, cricoid, and base of arytenoid (hyaline cartilage) ossify after 25 years age
  - Epiglottis, corniculate, cuneiform, and processes of arytenoid (elastic cartilage) do not ossify usually
    - May rarely see calcifications, especially in epiglottis
  - **Thyroid cartilage**: Largest cartilage; "shields" larynx
    - 2 lateral laminae meet anteriorly at acute angle; thyroid notch just superior to this angle
    - Superior cornua elongated and narrow, attach to lateral thyrohyoid ligament
    - Inferior cornua short and thick, articulating medially with sides of cricoid cartilage
    - Thyrohyoid membrane extends from superior margin of thyroid cartilage to hyoid bone
      - **Median thyrohyoid ligament**: Focal midline thickening of membrane
      - **Lateral thyrohyoid ligament**: Thickened lateral margins of membrane
      - **Triticeous cartilage**: Calcified cartilage occasionally seen centrally within lateral thyrohyoid ligament
      - Small aperture in lateral thyrohyoid membrane allows passage of superior laryngeal artery and internal branch of superior laryngeal nerve
  - **Cricoid cartilage**: Only complete ring in endolarynx
    - Broad posterior "lamina" and narrow anterior "arch"
    - Lower border of cricoid cartilage forms junction between larynx above and trachea below
  - **Arytenoid cartilage**: Paired pyramidal cartilages that sit atop posterior cricoid cartilage
    - Vocal and muscular processes at level of TVC
    - **Vocal processes**: Anterior projections of arytenoids where posterior margins of TVC attach
  - **Corniculate cartilage**: Rests on top of superior process of arytenoid cartilage within AEF
  - **Cuneiform cartilage**: Within AEF just ventral to corniculate cartilage
- **Supraglottis of endolarynx**
  - Supraglottis extends from top of epiglottis to laryngeal ventricle below
  - Contains epiglottis, AEFs, FVCs, preepiglottic space, paraglottic space, upper 1/2 of laryngeal ventricles, and upper arytenoid cartilages
  - **Laryngeal aperture**: Superior opening of larynx formed by epiglottis, AEFs, and interarytenoid space
  - **Laryngeal vestibule**: Supraglottic larynx airway from laryngeal aperture superiorly to TVCs inferiorly
  - **Epiglottis**: Leaf-shaped cartilage; larynx lid with free margin (suprahyoid) and fixed portion (infrahyoid)
    - **Petiole**: "Stem" of leaf, which attaches epiglottis to thyroid lamina via thyroepiglottic ligament
    - **Hyoepiglottic ligament**: Attaches epiglottis to hyoid
    - **Glossoepiglottic fold**: Median mucous membrane covering superior aspect of hyoepiglottic ligament
    - Median glossoepiglottic fold connects upper free margin of epiglottis to tongue and divides space between them into 2 sacs called valleculae
  - **Preepiglottic space**: Fat-filled space between hyoid bone anteriorly and epiglottis posteriorly
    - Devoid of lymph nodes
  - **AEFs**: Projects from cephalad tip of arytenoid cartilage to inferolateral margin of epiglottis bilaterally
    - Represents superolateral margin of supraglottis, dividing it from pyriform sinus (HP)
  - **FVCs (a.k.a. vestibular folds)**: Medially bulging mucosal surfaces of larynx mildly narrowing lower vestibule
    - Mucosa covers supportive vestibular ligament (= inferior margin of quadrangular membrane)
    - **Paraglottic space**: Fat-filled space deep to FVCs
    - **Rima vestibuli**: Airway opening between FVCs
  - **Quadrangular membrane**: Membrane extending from lateral margin of epiglottis anteriorly to apex and fovea triangularis of ipsilateral arytenoid cartilage
    - Free upper/lower (AE/vestibular ligaments) borders
    - Upper border slopes posteriorly to form **AE ligament**, which forms central component of **AEF**
    - **Free lower border** forms **vestibular ligament**, within **vestibular fold (FVC)**
    - Posterior border passes through fascial plane of esophageal suspensory ligament, aiding in formation of **median corniculopharyngeal ligament**
  - **Paraglottic space**: Paired fat-containing spaces lateral/deep to FVC (mainly) and TVCs
    - Superiorly, paraglottic space merges with preepiglottic space
    - **Quadrangular membrane** superiorly and **conus elasticus** inferiorly lie along medial aspect of paraglottic space
    - Easily seen by abundant fat at FVC level
    - At level of true cords, fat lateral to thyroarytenoid muscles (TAMs) very thin and can be imperceptible
    - Authors disagree as to whether thyroarytenoid/vocalis muscles are within paraglottic space or medial to it
  - Respiratory pseudostratified columnar epithelium with abundant mucous glands and lymphatics
  - Main blood supply: Superior laryngeal artery
  - Main sensory afferent to supraglottic laryngeal mucosa: Internal branch of superior laryngeal nerve
  - **Laryngeal ventricles**: Lateral outpouchings situated between false vocal folds above and true vocal folds (cords) below
    - Upper 1/2 in supraglottis, lower 1/2 in glottic larynx
  - **Laryngeal saccule (appendix)**: Small outpouching that functions to lubricate ipsilateral cord (that lack glands) along anterior roof of each laryngeal ventricle
    - Dilatation of saccule → **laryngocele** formation
    - Saccule curves slightly backwards and ascends forwards from anterior end of laryngeal ventricle

        - Within paraglottic space fat, between vestibular fold and thyroid cartilage
    - **Thyroepiglottic muscle** separates saccule from thyroid cartilage laterally, compresses saccule
        - To express secretions onto vocal folds
    - Saccule has more density of mucous glands in submucosa of whole larynx
- **Glottis of endolarynx**
    - ~ 1-cm thick region from axial level of midlaryngeal ventricle to lower margin of TVC
    - Consists of **TVCs (a.k.a. true vocal folds)**, anterior and posterior commissures, and central air space
    - **TVC complex microanatomy**: **5 layers**
        - **(1) Mucosal nonkeratinized squamous epithelium**: Most superficial layer, attached to underlying superficial lamina propria by basement membrane
            - Can give rise to squamous cell carcinoma of TVC
        - **(2) Superficial lamina propria (Reinke space)**: Hypocellular, mainly loose, fine collagen (reticular fibers) and elastic fibers
            - Structure essential for normal voice function
            - **Reinke edema** in smokers (a.k.a. polypoid corditis): Swelling of entire layer of superficial lamina propria
            - Only loosely attached to underlying vocal ligament
        - **(3) Middle layer of lamina propria**: Predominantly elastic fibers oriented parallel to vocalis muscle
        - **(4) Deep layer of lamina propria**: Predominantly collagen fibers oriented parallel to vocalis muscle
            - **Vocal ligament**: Thin linear tissue band formed by combination of **middle and deep layers** of lamina propria: provides strength and elasticity to TVCs
            - Vocal ligaments course anteriorly from vocal process of arytenoid cartilage to thyroid cartilage
            - Vocal ligament **merges inferiorly with conus elasticus**
        - **(5) Muscles of TVC**: **Thyroarytenoid and vocalis**
            - **Vocalis muscle:** Medial belly of TAM; muscle fibers arranged longitudinally parallel to vocal ligament
        - **Rima glottidis**: Airway opening in between TVCs
    - **Anterior commissure**
        - Midline, anterior meeting point of TVC, ≤ **1 mm** thick
        - **Broyle ligament (BL)**: Dense connective tissue at insertion of vocal ligaments to thyroid cartilage
            - Above glottic plane, BL resists tumor invasion from glottic carcinoma
            - Just caudal to glottic plane, BL is replaced by thin layer of connective tissue and is more vulnerable to tumor invasion
            - At point of attachment of BL to thyroid cartilage, cartilage is devoid of perichondrium, making region more vulnerable to tumor invasion
    - **Posterior commissure**
        - Fixed midline posterior wall of glottis, ≤ **1 mm** thick
- **Subglottis of endolarynx**
    - Extends from undersurface of TVC to inferior cricoid
    - Mucosal surface closely applied to cricoid cartilage
    - **Conus elasticus**: Fibroelastic supporting membrane extends from medial margin of TVC above to cricoid below; forms median cricothyroid ligament anteriorly
        - Lateral aspects of conus elasticus thinner than anterior median cricothyroid ligament
        - **Median cricothyroid ligament**: Attaches inferiorly to upper margin of midline cricoid arch
            - Superiorly to lower thyroid cartilage margin, extending upwards up to TAM attachment on inner surface of thyroid angle
        - **Lateral aspects of conus elasticus**: Attach inferiorly to upper margin of of cricoid arch and lamina
            - Superiorly to just below inner midpoint of thyroid cartilage anteriorly, and to tip/upper surface of vocal process and fovea oblonga of arytenoid cartilage
        - Thick, horizontal, **free upper border of conus elasticus** between anterior thyroid cartilage and posterior arytenoid cartilage attachments **merge with vocal ligament**
- **Laryngeal muscles**
    - **Extrinsic muscles**: Function to raise and lower larynx
        - Digastric, mylohyoid, geniohyoid, stylohyoid, sternothyroid, sternohyoid, thyrohyoid, omohyoid
    - **Intrinsic muscles**: Aryepiglottic, oblique arytenoid, thyroepiglottic, thyroarytenoid, posterior cricoarytenoid, lateral cricoarytenoid, transverse arytenoid, and cricothyroid
        - **Thyroepiglottic muscle**: From upper border of thyroid lamina to side of epiglottis, compresses mucous glands in saccule to lubricate larynx
        - **TAM**: From anterior inner thyroid cartilage to arytenoid cartilage, paralleling vocal ligament
            - Makes up bulk of tissue of TVCs
            - Medial component referred to as vocalis muscle
        - **Posterior cricoarytenoid muscle:** From posterior cricoid cartilage to muscular process of arytenoid
            - **Abduction** of TVCs, seen **active in F18-FDG PET**
- **Innervation of larynx**
    - Vagus nerve (CNX) provides sensory and motor innervation to larynx
    - **Superior laryngeal nerve** arises from inferior ganglion of vagus nerve and descends toward larynx
        - **Internal branch**: Perforates thyrohyoid membrane posteriorly, enters larynx, and supplies sensory innervation to laryngeal mucosa
        - **External branch**: Remains external to larynx, supplies **motor** innervation **to cricothyroid** muscle
    - **Recurrent laryngeal nerve (RLN)**: Branch of vagus nerve that initially descends, then ascends lower neck in tracheoesophageal groove, returning to larynx
        - Left RLN loops around aorta inferiorly
        - Right RLN loops around right subclavian artery
        - RLN innervates **all intrinsic muscles** of larynx **except cricothyroid** muscle
- **Embryology**
    - Supraglottic larynx from primitive buccopharyngeal anlage and has rich lymphatics
    - Glottic and subglottic larynx from tracheobronchial buds and has few lymphatics
    - Clinical implication: **Supraglottic** squamous cell carcinoma has much higher incidence of **nodal metastases** at presentation than glottic and subglottic

GRAPHICS

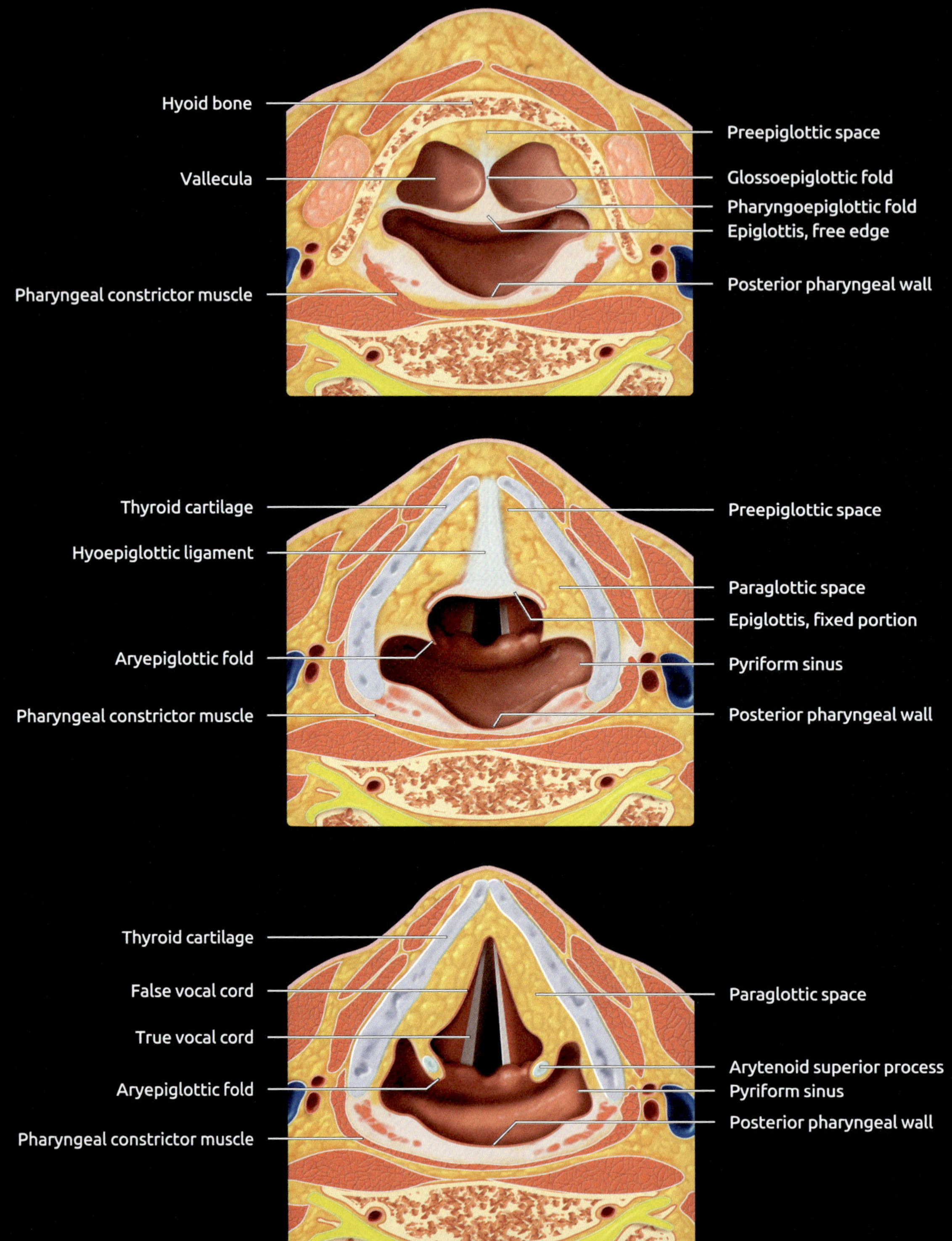

(Top) *First of 6 axial graphics of the larynx and hypopharynx from superior to inferior shows the roof of the hypopharynx at the hyoid bone level and high supraglottic structures. The supraglottis consists of the epiglottis, aryepiglottic fold, false vocal cord, and the fat-filled preepiglottic fat and paraglottic spaces. The free edge of the epiglottis is attached to the hyoid bone via the hyoepiglottic ligament, which is covered by a glossoepiglottic fold, a ridge of mucous membrane.* **(Middle)** *Graphic at the midsupraglottic level shows the hyoepiglottic ligament dividing the lower preepiglottic space. No fascia separates the preepiglottic space from the paraglottic space. These 2 endolaryngeal spaces are submucosal locations where tumors hide from clinical detection. The aryepiglottic fold (marginal supraglottis) represents the junction between the larynx and hypopharynx.* **(Bottom)** *Graphic at the low supraglottic level shows false vocal cords formed by mucosal surfaces of the laryngeal vestibule. The paraglottic space is beneath false vocal cords, a common location for submucosal tumor spread.*

GRAPHICS

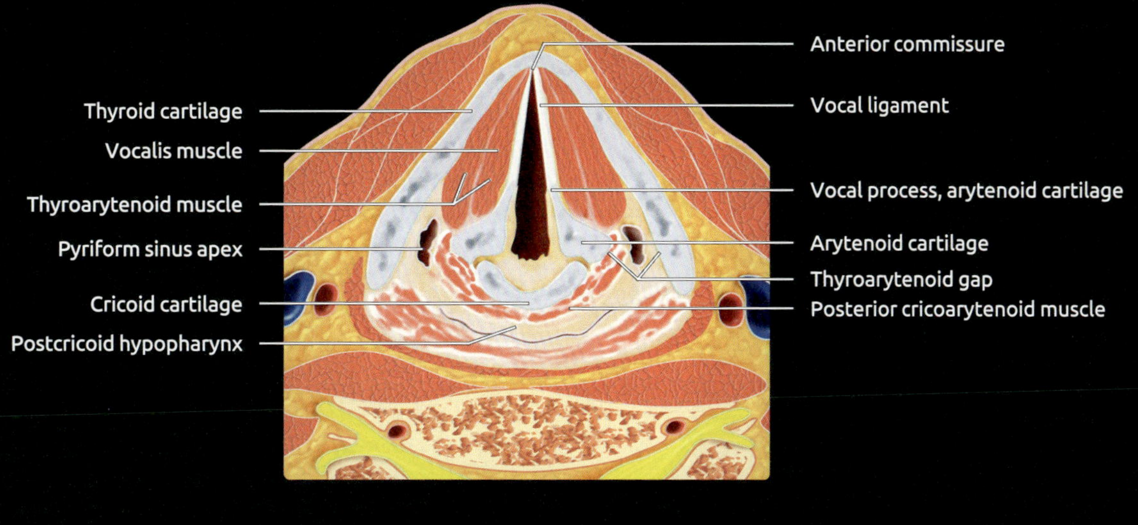

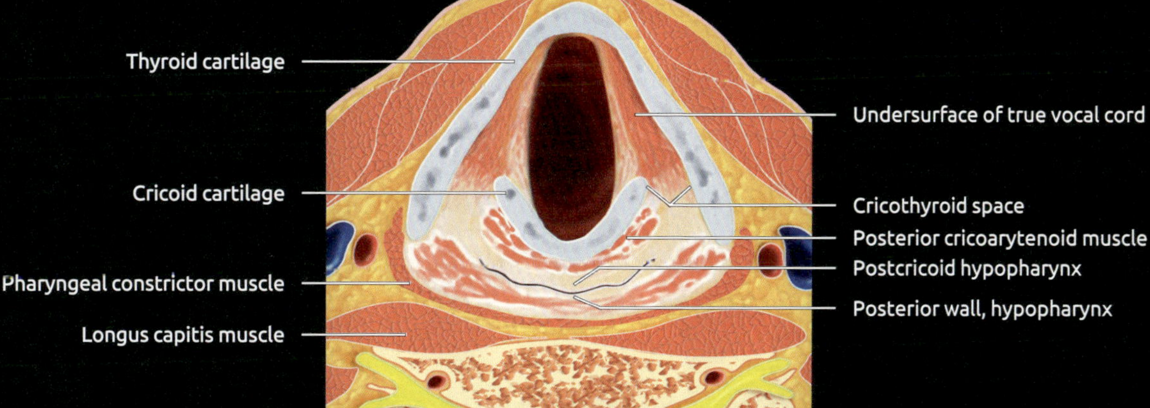

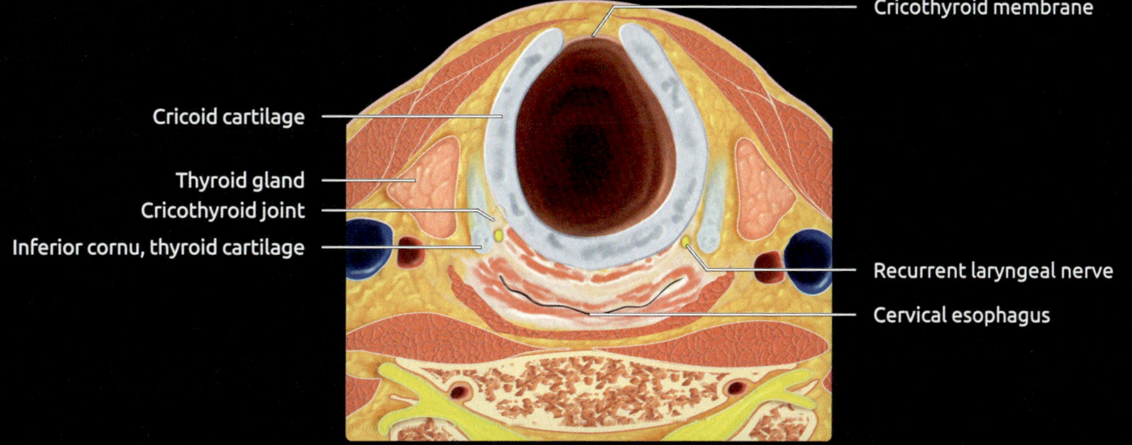

(Top) *Graphic at the glottic true vocal cord level shows the thyroarytenoid muscle, which makes up the bulk of the true vocal cord. Medial fibers of the thyroarytenoid muscle are known as vocalis muscle. Glottic larynx consists of a 1-cm thick region from the axial level of the midlaryngeal ventricle to the lower margin of the true vocal cord. Thyroarytenoid gap is where tumors may spread between larynx and hypopharynx.* **(Middle)** *Graphic at the level of the undersurface of true vocal cord shows posterior lamina of cricoid cartilage. Postcricoid hypopharynx represents the anterior wall of the lower hypopharynx and extends from cricoarytenoid joints to the lower edge of cricoid cartilage at the cricopharyngeus muscle. The posterior wall of the hypopharynx represents inferior continuation of the posterior oropharyngeal wall and extends to the cervical esophagus.* **(Bottom)** *Graphic of the subglottic larynx (below lower margin of true vocal cord at cricoid level) shows the cricothyroid joint close to the recurrent laryngeal nerve, located in the tracheoesophageal groove. The life-saving emergency laryngotomy procedure is done by inserting a needle through the cricothyroid membrane.*

GRAPHICS

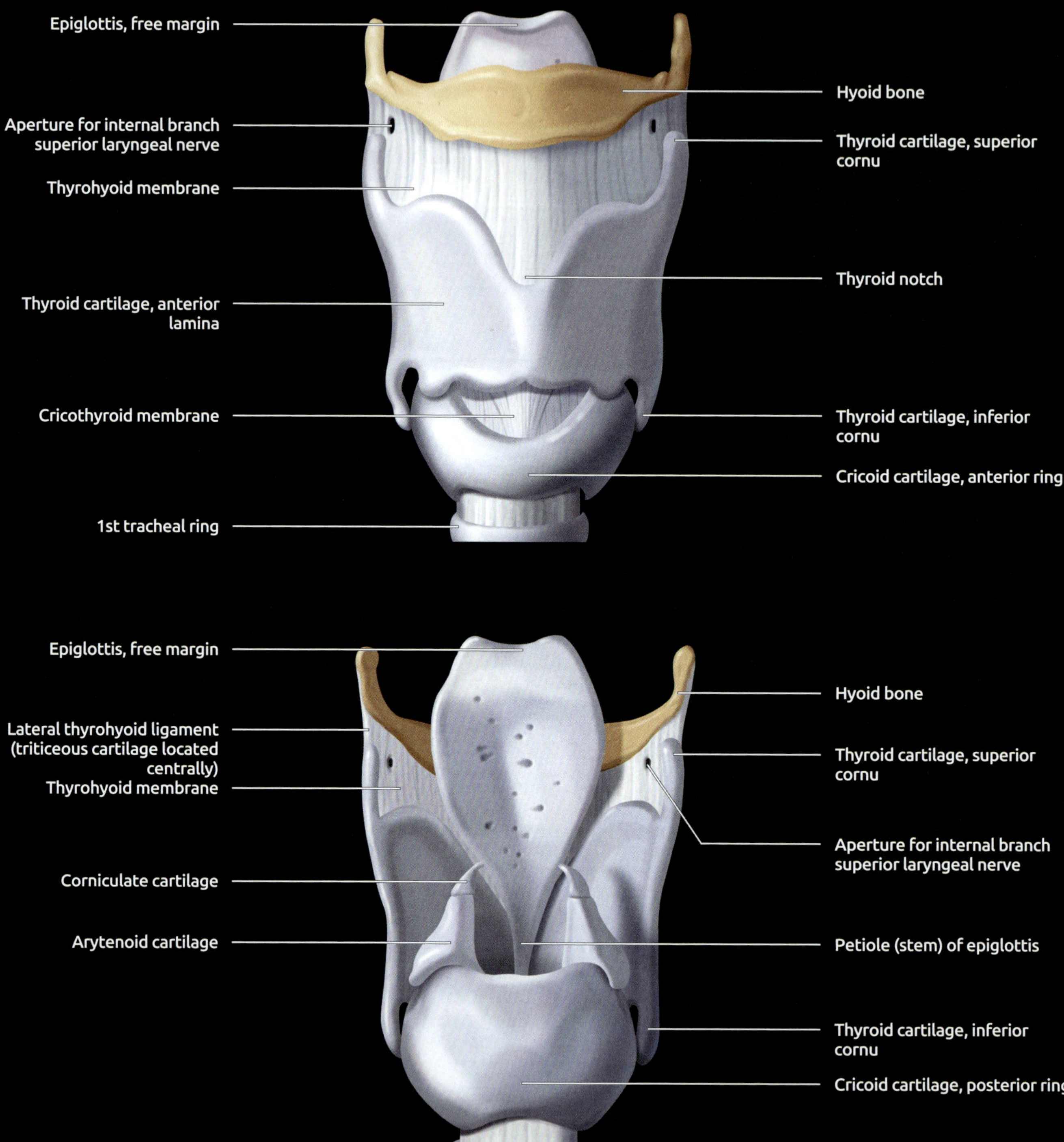

(Top) *Anterior view of the laryngeal cartilages is shown. Note 2 large anterior laminae of the thyroid cartilage that "shield" the larynx. The thyrohyoid membrane contains an aperture through which the internal branch of superior laryngeal nerve and associated vessels course. An internal laryngeal nerve then passes beneath mucosa of the pyriform sinus; removal of foreign bodies from the sinus may damage this nerve, leading to supraglottic anesthesia and impaired protective cough reflex. Mixed (external) laryngoceles herniate through the thyrohyoid membrane to extend into the submandibular space.* **(Bottom)** *Posterior view shows arytenoid cartilage sitting on top of the posterior cricoid cartilage. The true vocal cord attaches to the vocal process of arytenoid cartilage and forms the glottis. The epiglottis is a leaf-shaped cartilage, which forms the lid of the larynx and contains fixed and free margins. Cricoid cartilage is the only complete ring in the endolarynx and provides structural integrity. Calcified triticeous cartilage could be mistaken for a foreign body in radiographs.*

GRAPHICS

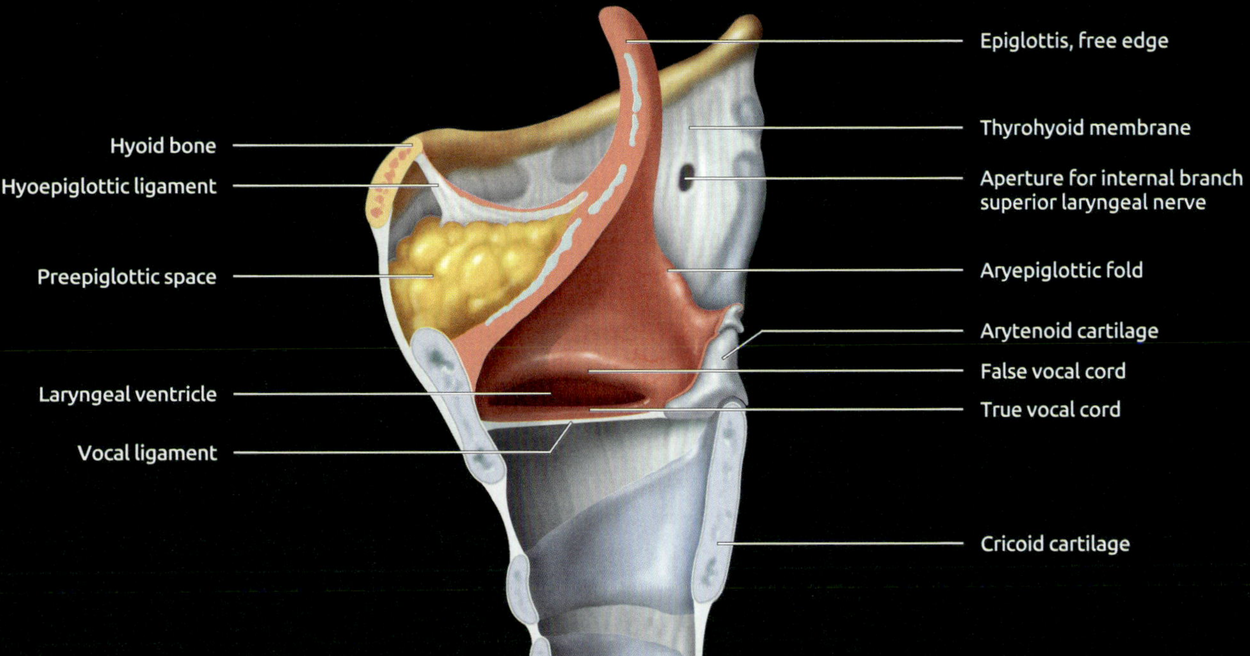

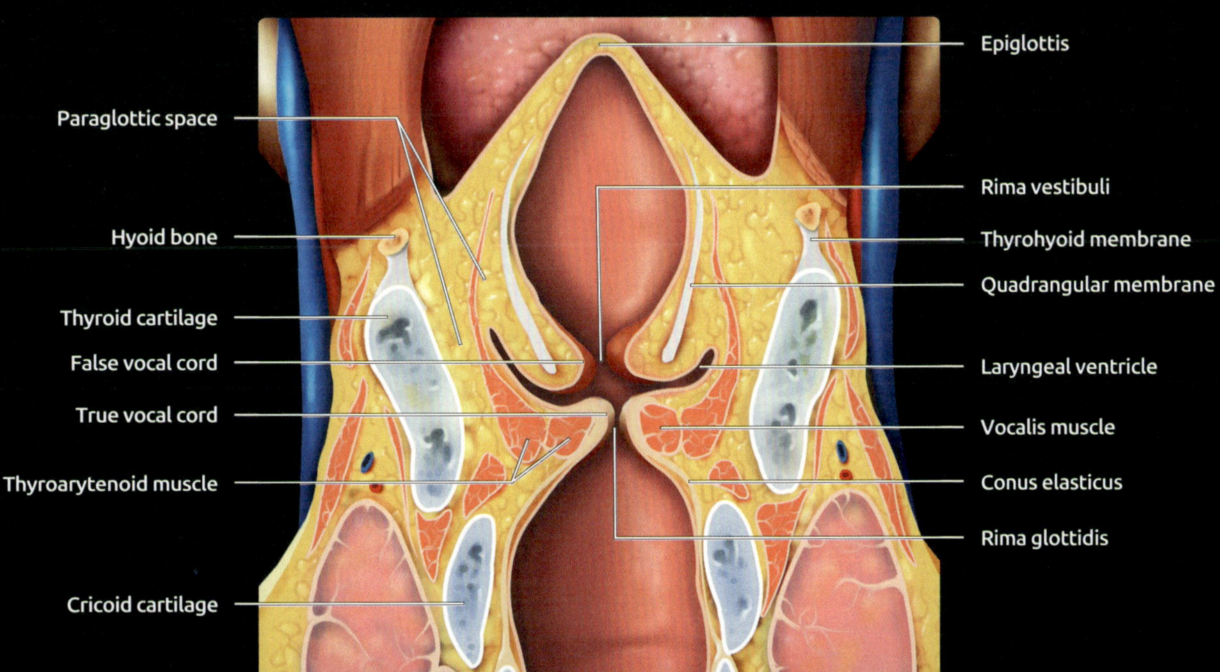

(Top) *Sagittal graphic of midline larynx shows laryngeal ventricle, the air-space that separates false vocal cords above with true vocal cords below. Aryepiglottic folds project from the tip of arytenoid cartilage to inferolateral margin of epiglottis and separate supraglottic larynx anteromedially from pyriform sinus (hypopharynx) posterolaterally.* **(Bottom)** *Coronal posterior view shows false and true vocal cords separated by laryngeal ventricle. Fibroelastic structures of the larynx, not seen on conventional CT/MR, lie inside cartilaginous framework along medial aspect of paraglottic space, underneath laryngeal mucosa. The upper part, called quadrangular membrane (QM), extend from lateral margin of epiglottis anteriorly to ipsilateral arytenoid cartilage. Free upper border of QM forms aryepiglottic ligament (central component of aryepiglottic fold); free lower border forms vestibular ligament (within false vocal cord vestibular fold). The lower part, called conus elasticus (CE), extends from medial margin of true vocal cord above to cricoid cartilage below. CE forms median cricothyroid ligament anteriorly, and its free upper border merges with vocal ligament (within true vocal cord).*

GRAPHIC AND REFORMATTED CT

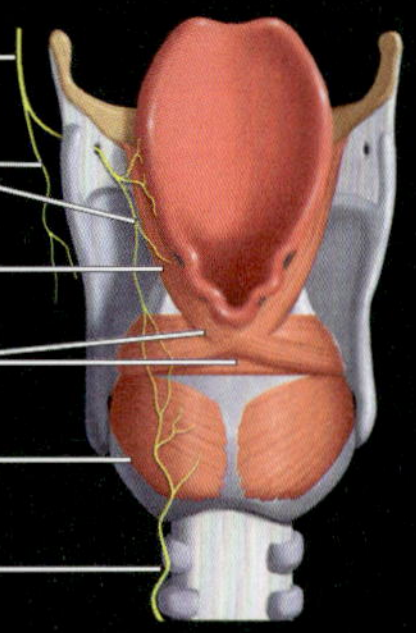

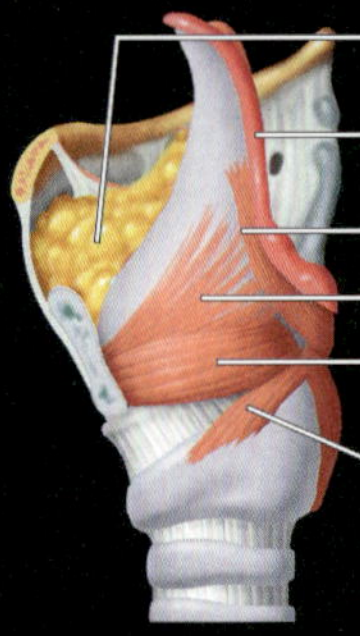

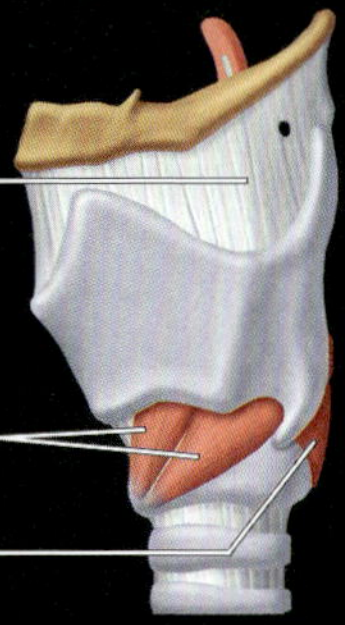

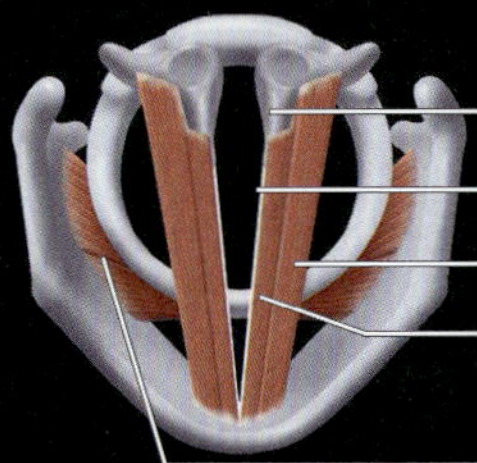

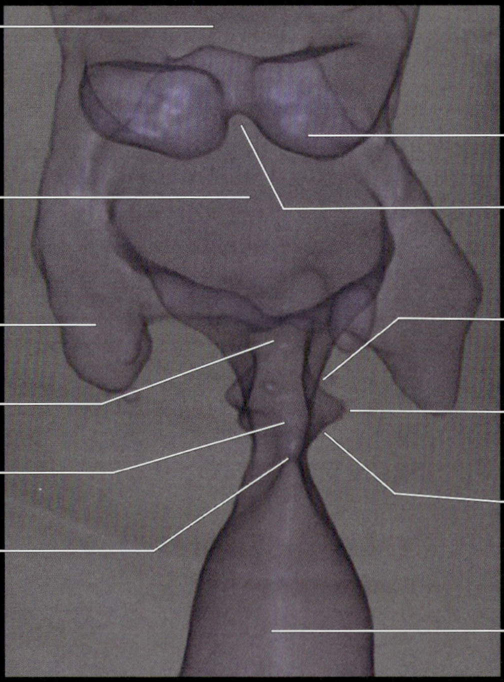

(Top) *Multiple graphics demonstrate internal laryngeal muscles. The posterior cricoarytenoid muscle is the only muscle directly functioning to abduct (separate) the vocal cords. The recurrent laryngeal nerves innervate all of the internal laryngeal muscles except the cricothyroid muscle (external branch of the superior laryngeal nerve). The thyroarytenoid muscle makes up much of the bulk of the vocal fold and includes the medial component, the vocalis muscle.* **(Bottom)** *3D reformatted CT shows the airway of the larynx and hypopharynx. Supraglottic airway (laryngeal vestibule) is located at and above the level of false vocal cord indentation on the airway and upper 1/2 of laryngeal ventricle. Glottic airway is a 1-cm region from the midlaryngeal ventricle level to lower margin of true vocal cord indentation. Subglottic larynx airway lies at cricoid cartilage level, below the lower margin of true vocal cord indentation. Pyriform sinus represents the anterolateral recess of the hypopharynx and is the most common location for hypopharyngeal tumors. The pyriform sinus apex (inferior tip) lies at the level of the true vocal cord, which allows pyriform sinus tumors access to true vocal cords.*

AXIAL CECT CORDS ABDUCTED (APART)

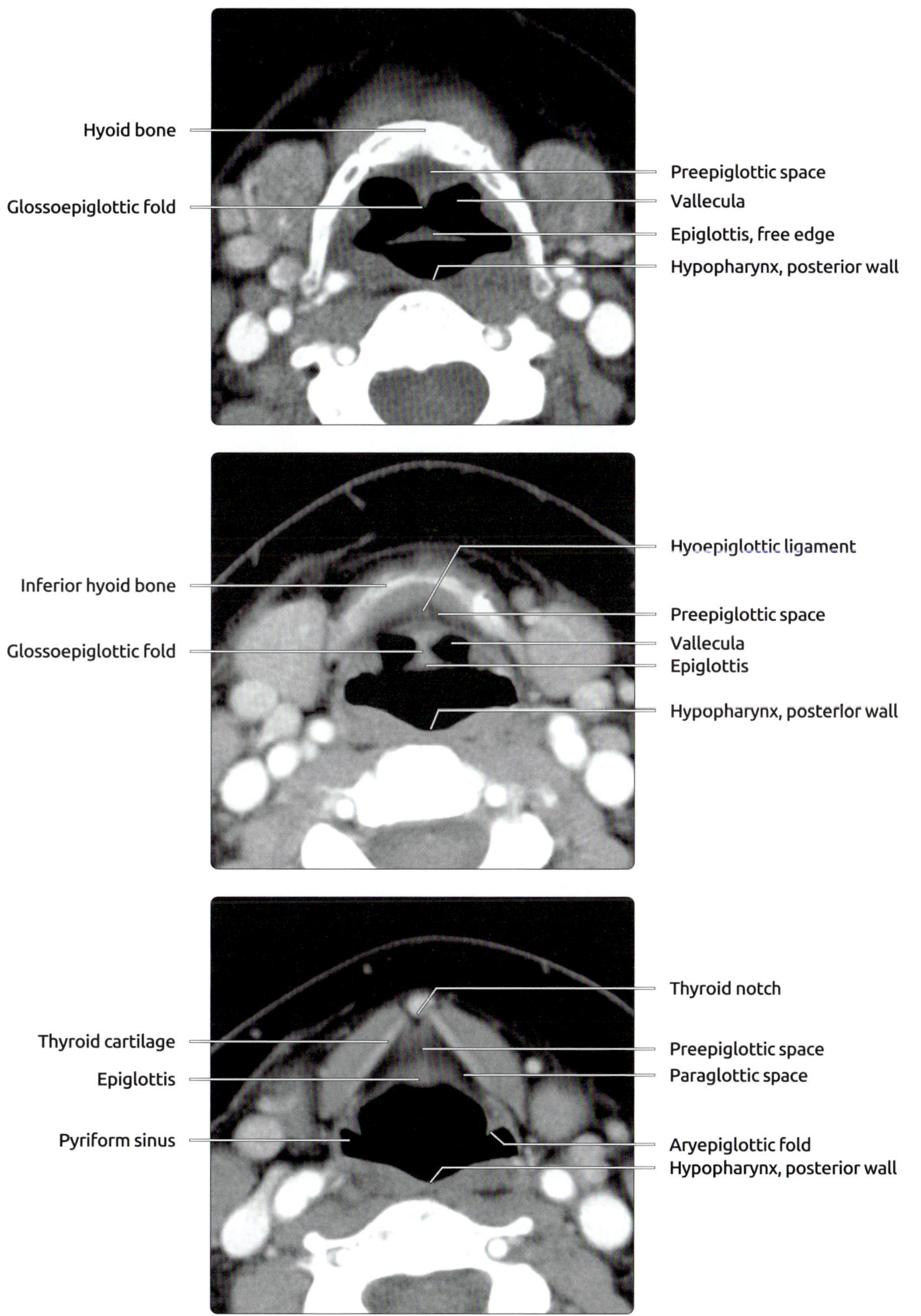

(Top) *First of 9 axial CECT images from superior to inferior of the larynx and hypopharynx is shown of a patient in quiet respiration. The hyoid bone represents the level of the roof of the larynx and hypopharynx. The glossoepiglottic and pharyngoepiglottic folds represent transition from the oropharynx above to the larynx and hypopharynx below.* **(Middle)** *Image of the high supraglottic level of the larynx shows a C-shaped preepiglottic space, a common location for tumors to hide. If supraglottic tumor extends to the preepiglottic space, it becomes a T3 tumor.* **(Bottom)** *Image of the high supraglottic level shows that the preepiglottic and paraglottic spaces are continuous with no intervening fascia. This allows tumors to spread submucosally in these locations. The aryepiglottic fold, part of the larynx, represents transition between the larynx and the hypopharynx. The posterolateral wall of the aryepiglottic fold is the anteromedial margin of the pyriform sinus.*

AXIAL CECT CORDS ABDUCTED (APART)

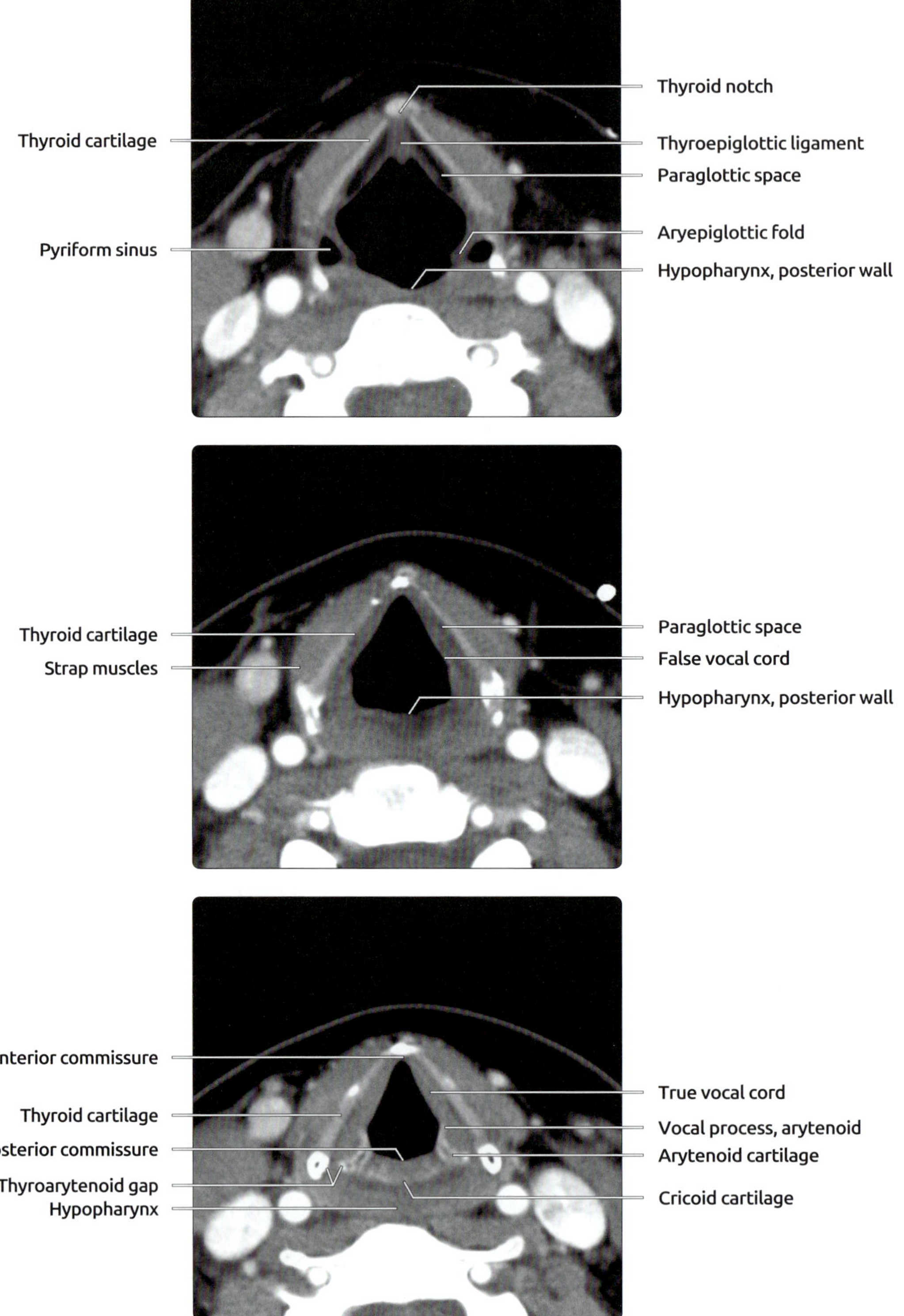

(Top) *Image at the midsupraglottic level shows the thyroepiglottic ligament dividing the preepiglottic space. Aryepiglottic folds are at the margin of the pyriform sinus and larynx; a tumor primary to the aryepiglottic fold is considered a "marginal supraglottic" tumor.* **(Middle)** *Image of the low supraglottic level shows the false vocal cord level. The paraglottic space represents the deep fatty space beneath the false vocal cords. Tumors that cross the laryngeal ventricle from supraglottic false vocal cords to involve glottic true vocal cords, or involve glottic true vocal cords and extend to the subglottis (> 10 mm below the free margin of true vocal cord), or both, are called transglottic tumors.* **(Bottom)** *Image at the glottic level shows true vocal cords in abduction in quiet respiration. The true vocal cord level is identified on CT when arytenoid and cricoid cartilages are seen and muscle fills the inferior paraglottic space. Anterior and posterior commissures of true vocal cords should be < 1 mm in normal patients. The postcricoid hypopharynx is typically collapsed.*

AXIAL CECT CORDS ABDUCTED (APART)

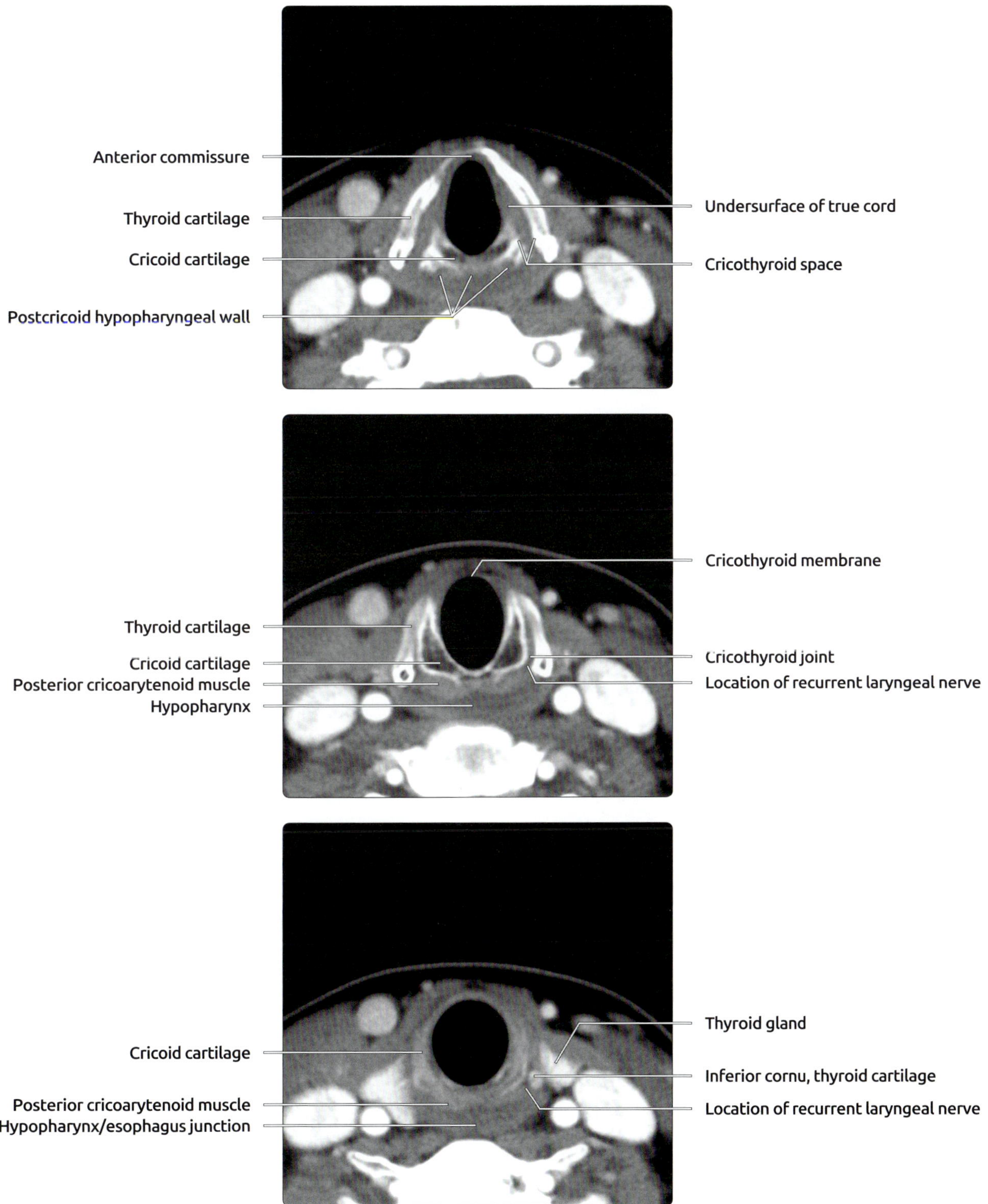

(Top) *In this image through the undersurface of the true cord level, the cricothyroid space is seen. Lack of arytenoid cartilage identifies the undersurface of the true cord level.* **(Middle)** *Image more inferior shows the subglottic level with the cricoid ring nearly complete. Cricoid is the only complete cartilage ring in the larynx and provides structural integrity. Dislocations of the cricothyroid joint may result in vocal cord paralysis secondary to recurrent laryngeal nerve injury. There may be associated atrophy of the posterior cricoarytenoid muscle on the involved side of vocal cord paralysis. Posterior cricoarytenoid is the only abductor of the vocal cord and could be seen to be slightly hypermetabolic physiologically in F-18 FDG PET/CT scans.* **(Bottom)** *At the level of the inferior cricoid cartilage, the inferior margin of the larynx and hypopharynx are transitioning to the trachea and cervical esophagus. Mucosa along the subglottis should be no more than 1 mm in normal patients. Thickened mucosa raises concern for tumor.*

AXIAL CECT CORDS ADDUCTED (TOGETHER)

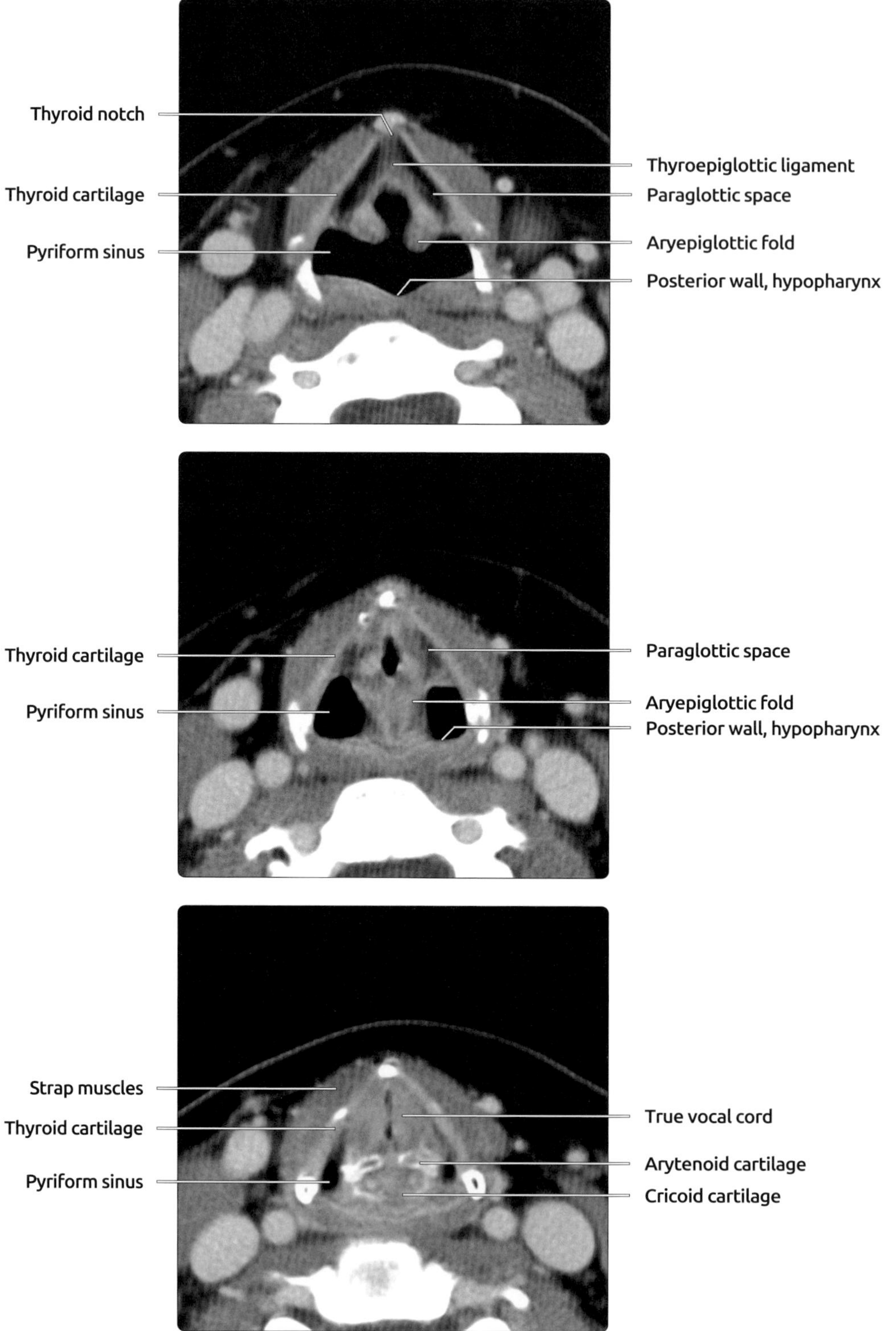

(Top) *First of 3 axial CECT images from superior to inferior in a patient with breath holding shows adduction of false and true vocal cords as well as aryepiglottic folds.* **(Middle)** *Image at the low supraglottic level shows the level of false vocal cords in adduction. Note the mucosa of the aryepiglottic folds contacts the posterior hypopharyngeal wall.* **(Bottom)** *Image at the glottic level shows adduction of the true vocal cords. With breath holding, true vocal cords oppose in the midline. A cord that remains paramedian is either paralyzed or mechanically fixed. Vocal cord paralysis typically results in paramedian true vocal cords with associated abnormal location of arytenoid cartilage, which is fixed in an anteromedial position. With breath holding, the paralyzed cord remains fixed, while the opposite normal cord crosses the midline in attempt to close the glottis. There may be ipsilateral dilation of laryngeal ventricle (sail sign) and an associated patulous pyriform sinus.*

CORONAL NECT

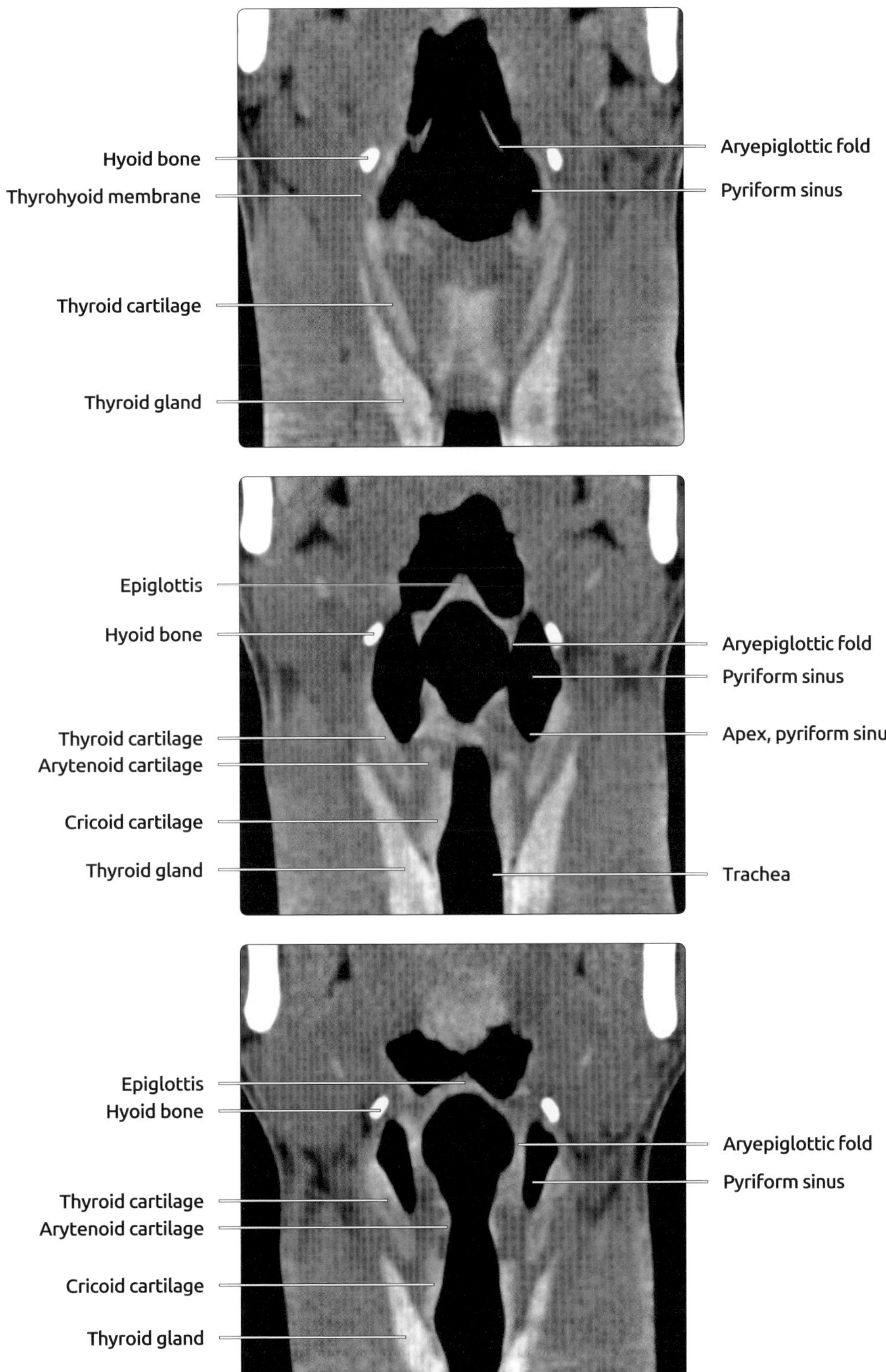

(Top) *First of 6 NECT coronal reformation images of the larynx and hypopharynx presented from posterior to anterior shows the hyoid bone, which represents the level of the roof of the larynx and hypopharynx. CT is particularly good for evaluation of patients with diseases of the larynx and hypopharynx, as these patients often have difficulty with secretions, coughing, and swallowing, making a short exam time vital.* **(Middle)** *Image more anterior shows laryngeal cartilages. These cartilages are variably ossified in adults, which makes pathologic conditions, such as cartilage invasion, difficult to diagnose with certainty. Apex of the pyriform sinus extends inferiorly to the level of true vocal cord.* **(Bottom)** *In this image, aryepiglottic folds are well seen as they extend from the lateral epiglottis to arytenoid cartilage. The pyriform sinus is the most common location for tumors of the hypopharynx.*

CORONAL NECT

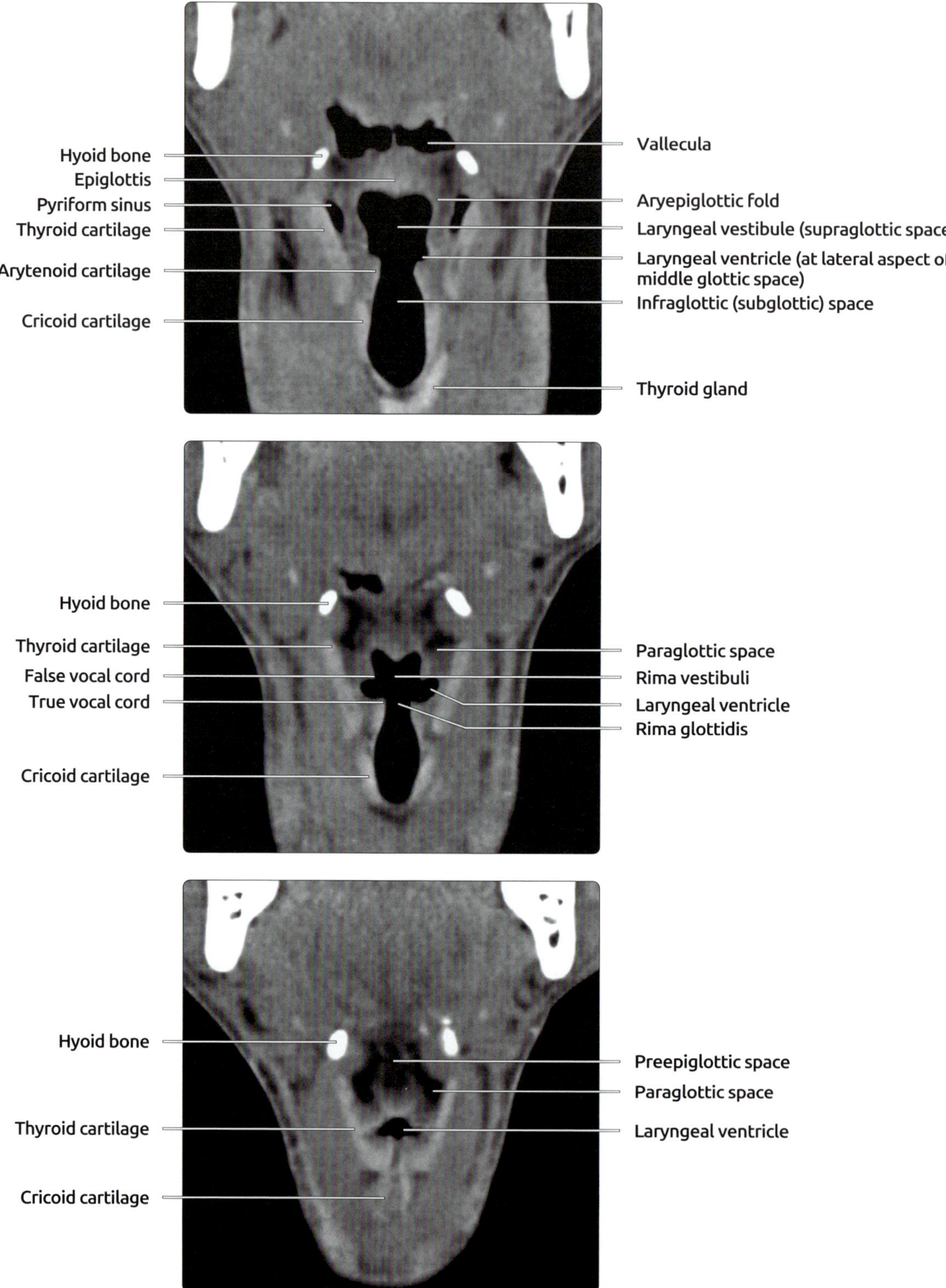

(Top) *This image shows the fixed portion of the epiglottis in the midline. The aryepiglottic fold, which represents the junction between the larynx anteriorly and hypopharynx posteriorly, is noted. The supraglottic, middle glottic, and subglottic spaces are also demarcated.* **(Middle)** *In this image, the laryngeal ventricle is visible as an air space between false vocal cords above and true vocal cords below. When a tumor crosses the laryngeal ventricle to involve true and false cords, it is transglottic, which has important treatment implications. Coronal imaging is particularly useful for evaluation of transglottic disease. The rima vestibuli is the opening between false vocal cords. The rima glottidis is the opening between true vocal cords and is the narrowest part of the laryngeal cavity.* **(Bottom)** *This image reveals preepiglottic fat to be continuous with paraglottic fat. These are the most important spaces of the endolarynx, as they allow submucosal spread of tumors, which is undetectable by clinical exam.*

SAGITTAL NECT

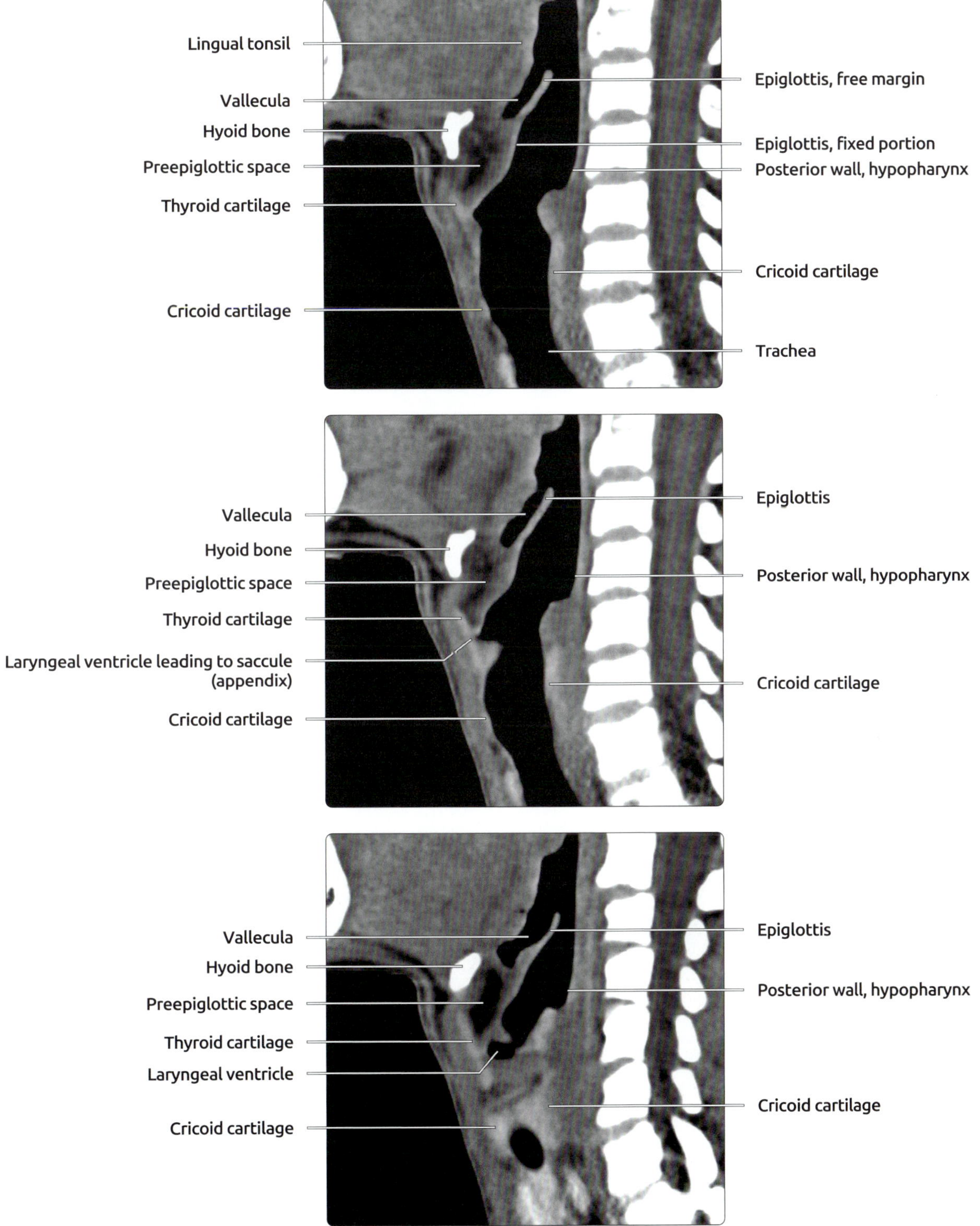

(Top) *First of 3 sagittal NECT images from medial to lateral shows the midline larynx/hypopharynx. Preepiglottic fat is seen posterior and inferior to the hyoid bone. Posterior hypopharyngeal wall pathology is well seen on sagittal images and also helps define the craniocaudal extent of lesions.* **(Middle)** *A more lateral image shows the laryngeal ventricle, the lateral air space of the middle glottic cavity separating false vocal cords above from true cords below. The laryngeal ventricle can have an anterosuperior tubular extension between the vestibular fold and thyroid cartilage, called the laryngeal saccule or ventricular appendix. They have mucous glands to lubricate vocal folds that are termed "oil can of larynx." Laryngoceles are dilated air or fluid-filled laryngeal saccules.* **(Bottom)** *More lateral image shows laryngeal cartilages, variably ossified in adults, making pathology difficult to evaluate, particularly cartilage invasion from tumors and traumatic injury. Cricoid cartilage, the only complete ring in the larynx, has a signet ring shape with the larger signet portion projecting posteriorly.*

AXIAL T1 MR

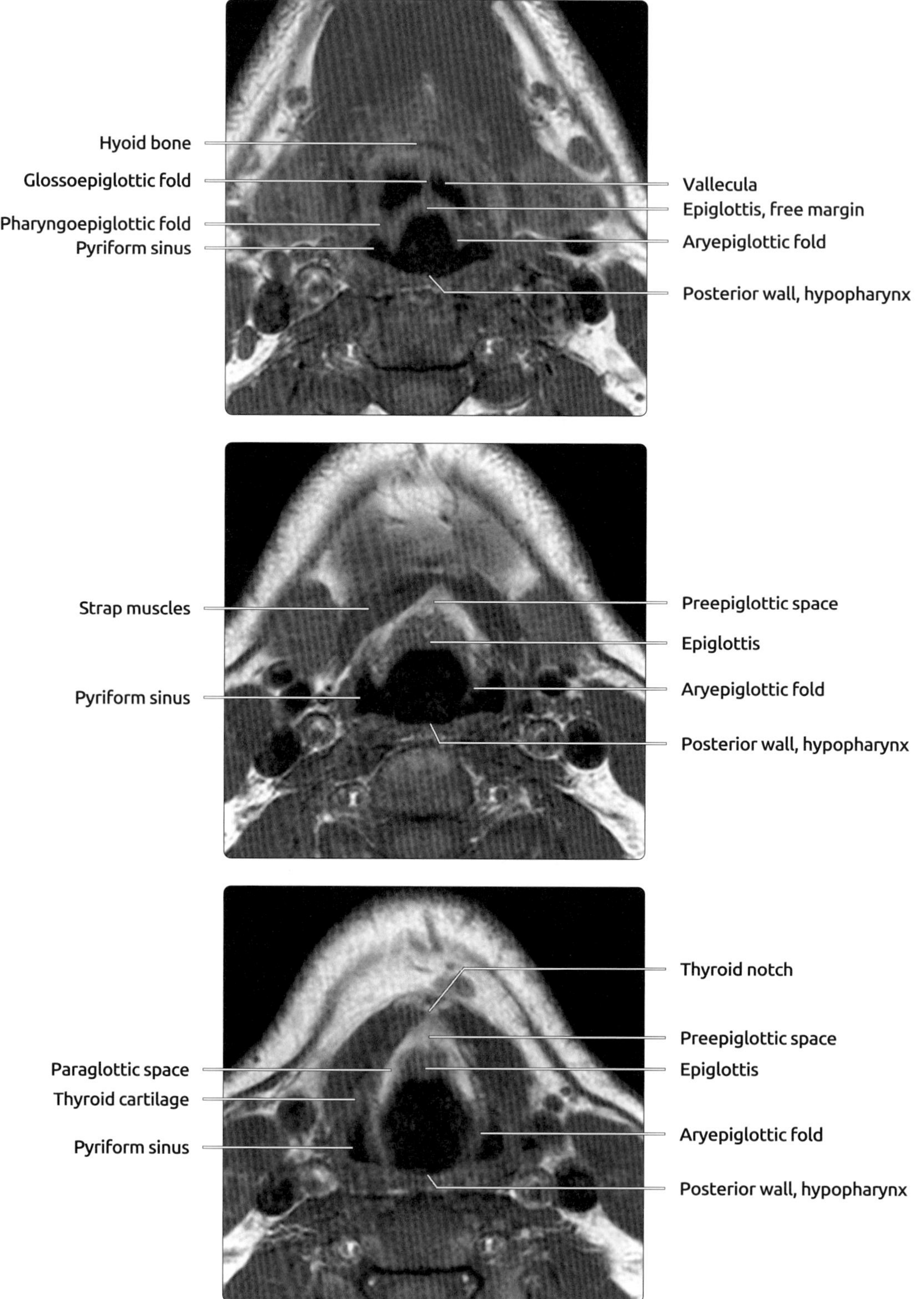

(Top) *First of 6 axial T1 MR images from superior to inferior of the larynx and hypopharynx with the patient in quiet respiration shows the roof of the larynx, which is defined by the epiglottis, glossoepiglottic, and pharyngoepiglottic folds. MR is typically reserved for answering specific questions, such as cartilage invasion, rather than as a 1st imaging study of a patient with larynx or hypopharynx disease.* **(Middle)** *Image at the level of the high supraglottis shows a C-shaped, fat-filled preepiglottic space and fixed portion of the epiglottis. Cartilage is variably ossified, which makes it somewhat difficult to visualize on T1 MR images.* **(Bottom)** *Image at the midsupraglottic level shows fat of the preepiglottic space continuous with fat of the paraglottic space. Lack of fascia between these 2 submucosal spaces allows tumor to travel from one to the other and hide from clinical detection.*

AXIAL T1 MR

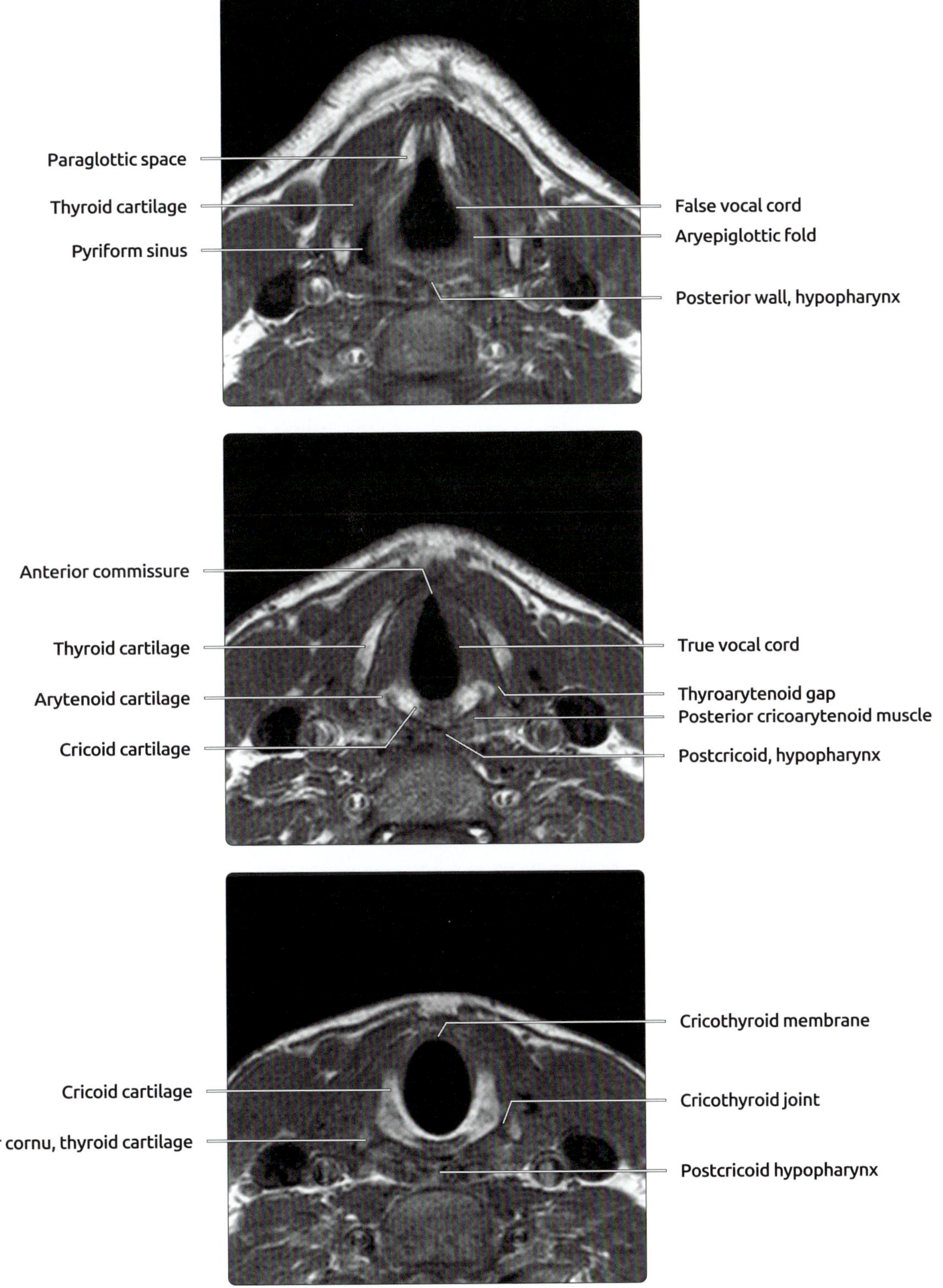

(Top) *Image at the level of the low supraglottis demonstrates false vocal cords and aryepiglottic folds. The paraglottic space beneath false vocal cords is primarily fat-filled. Aryepiglottic folds often contact the posterior wall of the hypopharynx in normal patients.* **(Middle)** *Image at the glottic level shows muscle in the paraglottic space beneath the true vocal cords. Both cricoid and arytenoid cartilage are seen at the true vocal cord level. The thyroarytenoid muscle makes up the bulk of true vocal cords. The posterior cricoarytenoid muscle is often atrophied in patients with vocal cord paralysis.* **(Bottom)** *Image at the subglottic level shows large, broad, posterior cricoid cartilage. The cricothyroid joint is where the recurrent laryngeal nerve is located. Dislocation of this joint is associated with recurrent laryngeal nerve injury. The postcricoid hypopharynx extends from the cricoarytenoid joints to the lower cricoid cartilage.*

SAGITTAL T1 MR

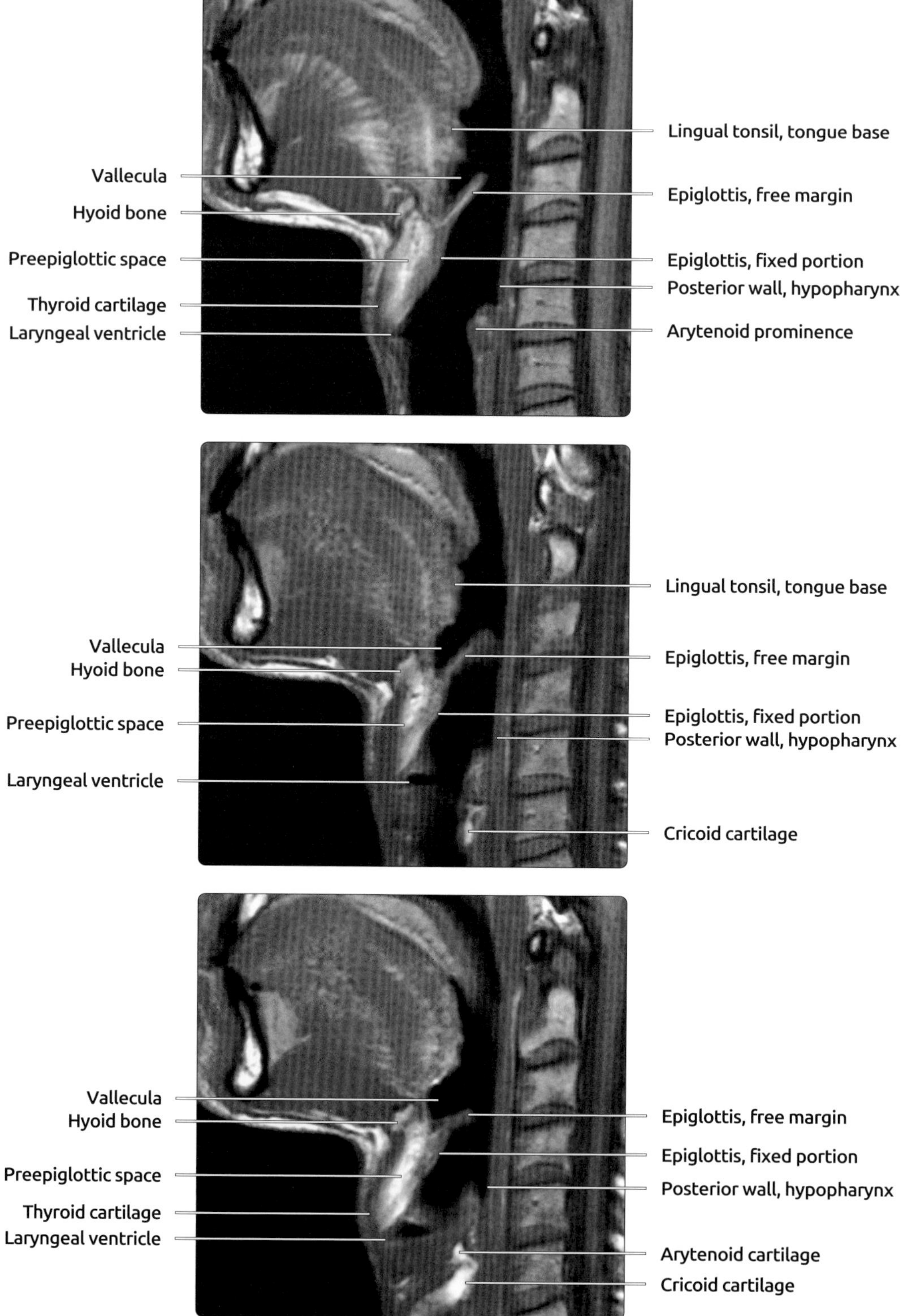

(Top) *First of 3 sagittal T1 MR images from medial to lateral of the larynx and hypopharynx shows midline structures. The preepiglottic space is T1 hyperintense as it is primarily fat-filled. The free margin (suprahyoid) and fixed portion (infrahyoid) of the epiglottis is well visualized, making sagittal imaging useful for evaluation of epiglottic lesions.* **(Middle)** *Image just lateral to the midline shows the laryngeal ventricle, which is important as it is the air space that separates false vocal cords above from true vocal cords below. Knowing if a tumor crosses the laryngeal ventricle is vital for surgical planning.* **(Bottom)** *Paramedial image through the cricoarytenoid joint shows arytenoid cartilage sitting on top of posterior cricoid cartilage. Traumatic dislocation of arytenoid cartilage may mimic vocal cord paralysis clinically and on imaging. Posterior arytenoid dislocation may occur during withdrawal of the endotracheal tube with an incompletely deflated cuff, whereas the mechanism of anterior dislocation is the arytenoid tip being caught on the distal opening of the tube lumen during intubation.*

CLINICAL CORRELATES

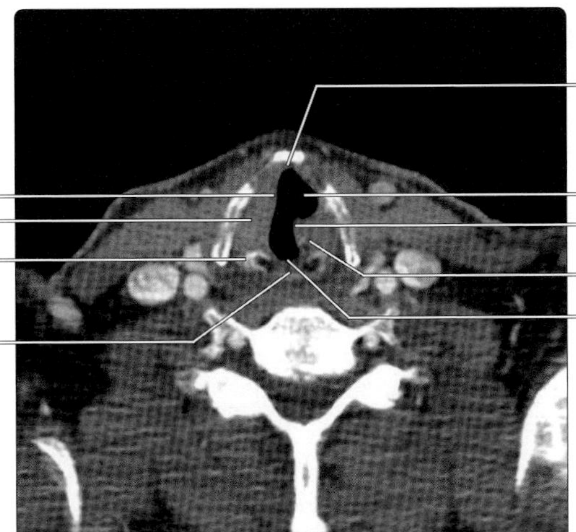

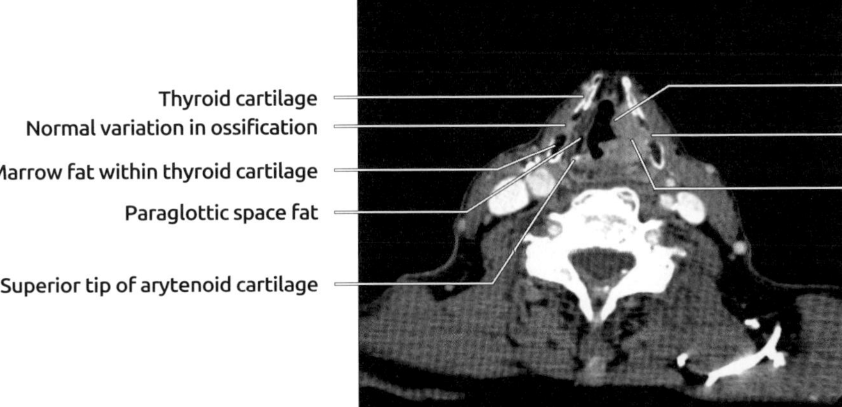

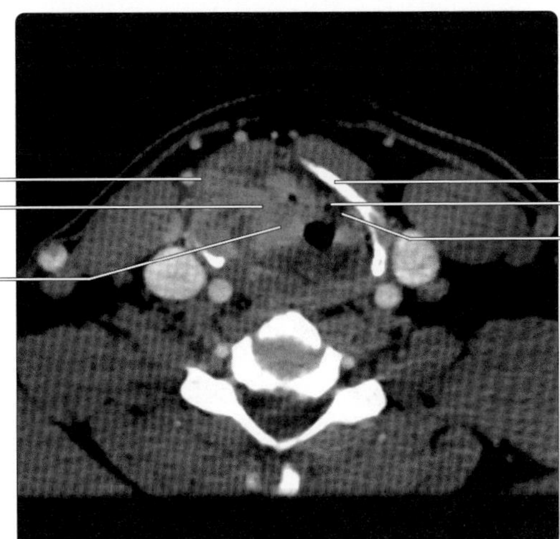

(Top) *Axial CT through the vocal cords in a case of left vocal cord paralysis shows that left arytenoid cartilage is rotated medially and slightly inferior to normal. The laryngeal ventricle on the left is also widened slightly and comes into view anteriorly. The right vocal cord is in normal position during quiet respiration and its soft tissue is primarily of thyroarytenoid muscle (including the vocalis muscle). Note very little, if any, paraglottic space fat at the true cord level. Superior cricoid cartilage supports the posterior midline wall of the glottis, which is called the posterior commissure.* **(Middle)** *Axial CECT through the false cord shows an invasive neoplasm on the left. Enhancing tumor encroaches upon the airway medially and extends into left paraglottic space fat. Note the superior tip of arytenoid cartilage and fat in the right paraglottic space. Tumor involved the false and true cords (not shown), making it a "transglottic" tumor.* **(Bottom)** *Large, invasive supraglottic carcinoma on the right extends from mucosa medially, through paraglottic fat, destroys thyroid cartilage lamina, and extends into extralaryngeal soft tissues.*

TRANSVERSE ULTRASOUND

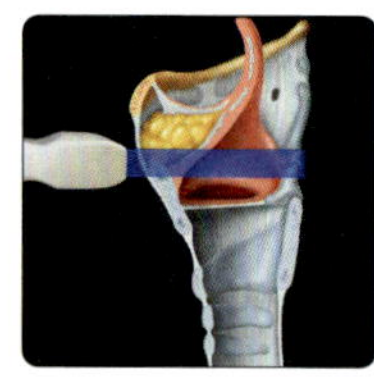

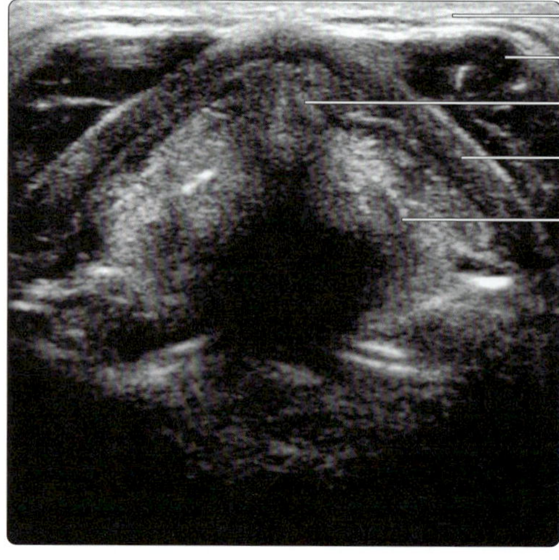

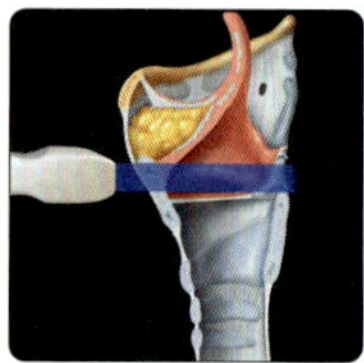

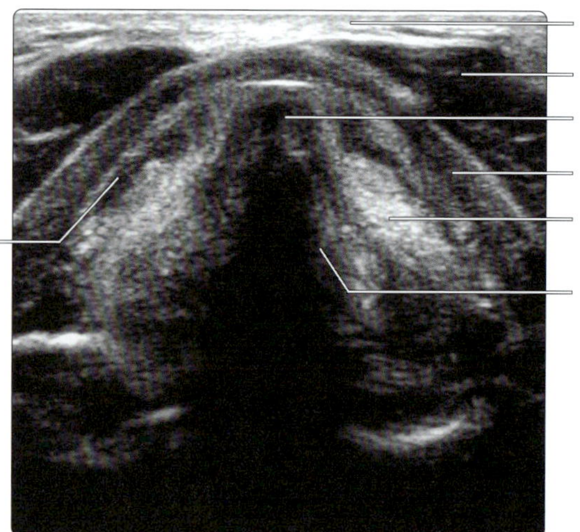

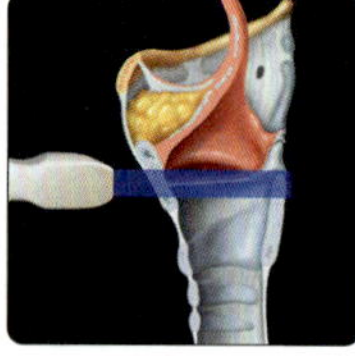

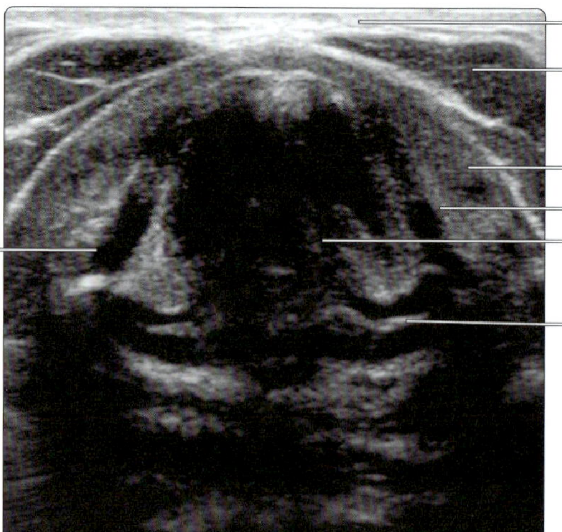

(Top) *Axial grayscale ultrasound of the larynx at the supraglottic larynx level shows that the thyroid laminae are the largest cartilaginous structures of the larynx and appear as thin, hypoechoic bands that join at the midline anteriorly. The hyperechoic, fat-filled paraglottic and preepiglottic spaces are important surgical landmarks for the staging of laryngeal carcinoma.* **(Middle)** *Transverse grayscale ultrasound of the larynx at the level of the false vocal cords shows abundant fat in the paraglottic spaces. The echo-poor intrinsic muscles of the larynx are embedded within the echogenic paraglottic fat.* **(Bottom)** *Transverse grayscale ultrasound of the larynx at the level of the true vocal cords shows that the arytenoid cartilage appears as echogenic foci posteriorly with attachments to the true vocal cords, which have distinct echo-poor appearances.*

LONGITUDINAL ULTRASOUND

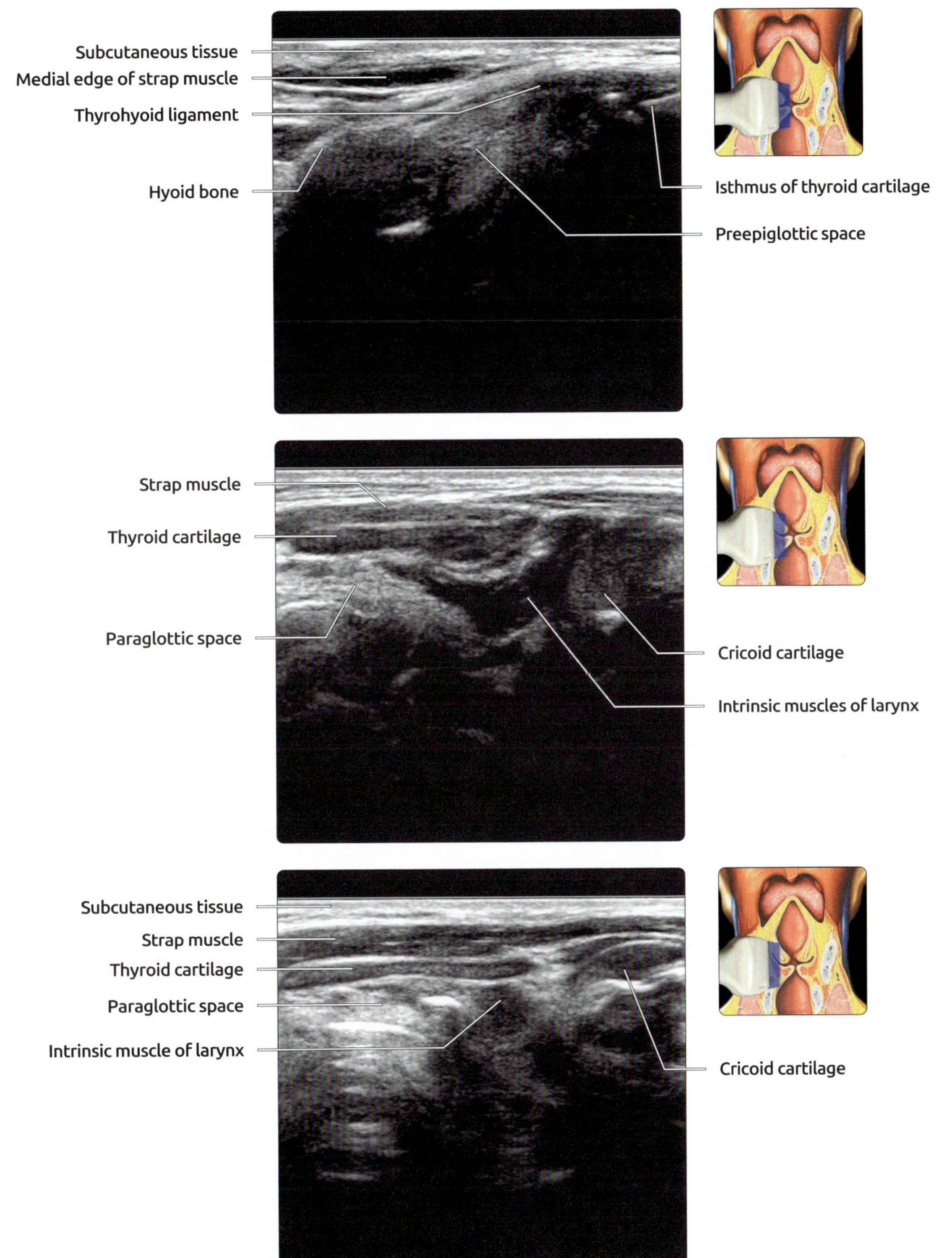

(Top) *Midline sagittal longitudinal grayscale ultrasound of the supraglottic larynx shows the fat-filled, echogenic, preepiglottic space underneath the thyrohyoid membrane. Tumor spread at this location is readily assessed by ultrasound.* **(Middle)** *Parasagittal longitudinal grayscale ultrasound of the larynx shows sonolucent thyroid and cricoid cartilages with no laryngeal calcification/ossification in a young adult. The paraglottic space is fat-filled and appears echogenic. The intrinsic muscles of the larynx are embedded within the paraglottic space and are hypoechoic on ultrasound.* **(Bottom)** *Parasagittal longitudinal grayscale ultrasound shows the larynx further lateral. Gas within the laryngeal lumen appears highly echogenic, casting posterior acoustic shadowing.*

Hypopharynx

TERMINOLOGY

Abbreviations

- Hypopharynx (HP)

Definitions

- **HP** consists of 3 regions starting with letter **P**
  - **P**osterior wall of HP
  - **P**yriform sinuses (PSs) (paired anterolateral recesses)
  - **P**ostcricoid region (anterior wall of lower HP)
- Caudal continuation of pharyngeal mucosal space, between oropharynx & esophagus

IMAGING ANATOMY

Extent

- HP (laryngopharynx): Extends from level of glossoepiglottic & pharyngoepiglottic folds superiorly (inferior margin of vallecula lying at hyoid bone level) to inferior cricoid cartilage (cricopharyngeus muscle)
- Caudal continuation of pharyngeal mucosal space, between oropharynx & esophagus
- Anterior wall formed by inlet of larynx (above) & posterior surfaces of cricoid & arytenoid cartilages (below)

Anatomy Relationships

- HP inferior continuation of oropharynx
- HP begins at level of pharyngoepiglottic folds at approximate horizontal level of hyoid bone
- HP merges with esophagus below at esophageal verge
- Esophageal verge best defined by cricopharyngeus muscle that encircles junction, but this muscle cannot be identified easily on cross-sectional imaging
- Cricopharyngeus muscle located at approximate level of inferior margin of cricoid cartilage
- Relative to cervical vertebrae, HP extends from approximate C3 level to C6 level
- HP posterior to larynx, medial to carotid spaces bilaterally, & ventral to retropharyngeal space

Internal Contents

- **Posterior wall**: Inferior continuation of posterior wall of oropharynx formed by superior constrictor of pharynx
  - Inferior continuation of posterior oropharyngeal wall, from hyoid bone level to inferior tip of cricoid cartilage
  - Posterior wall of HP separated from **prevertebral space** by **retropharyngeal space**
- HP posterior wall by middle & inferior constrictors
- Posterior wall supported mainly by 4th & 5th cervical vertebrae & partly by 3rd & 6th vertebrae
- **PS**: Bilateral anterolateral recesses of HP
- PS: Inverted pyramid shape with **superior base (3rd branchial arch)** at pharyngoepiglottic fold level & **inferior** tip **(PS apex, 4th branchial arch)** at true vocal cord level
- Bounded laterally by inner surface of thyrohyoid membrane (above) & thyroid cartilage (below)
- Anteromedial margin of PS formed by posterolateral wall of aryepiglottic (AE) (a.k.a. marginal supraglottis)
- AE folds project from cephalad tip of arytenoid cartilages to inferolateral margin of epiglottis
- AE folds represent superolateral margins of supraglottis, dividing it from PS (HP)
- During swallowing, nasopharynx & laryngeal vestibule are sealed, & food is usually deviated laterally away from larynx into piriform sinuses by epiglottis & AE folds
- Posterior boundary formed by posterior wall of HP
- 2/3 HP squamous cell carcinomas (SCCas) originate in PS
- **Postcricoid region**: Lower HP anterior wall (< 1 cm AP thickness)
- Extends from cricoarytenoid joints to lower edge of cricoid
- Anteriorly, lower border of cricoid cartilage forms junction between larynx above & trachea below
- **Mucosa** of postcricoid region **faces posteriorly** & is normally directly apposed to mucosa of posterior wall on cross-sectional imaging
- **Layers**: Pharynx consists of 5 layers from inner luminal to outer deep aspect, present in HP also
- Mucosa, submucosa, pharyngobasilar fascia (pharyngeal aponeurosis) forming median raphe posteriorly, muscular coat of inner longitudinal (stylopharyngeus, palatopharyngeus, & salpingopharyngeus) & outer circular (superior, middle, & inferior constrictors) layers & buccopharyngeal fascia covering outer surface of muscles
  - **Mucosa**: Stratified squamous epithelium lining lumen
  - **Submucosa**: Loose stroma that can contain fat & can be identified on cross-sectional imaging as thin fat plane
- **Pharyngobasilar fascia** hardly extends below superior constrictor & so not essential layer in HP
- **Buccopharyngeal fascia** also best developed in upper pharynx & extends anteriorly across pterygomandibular raphe to cover buccinator muscle
- Pharyngeal plexuses of veins & nerves lies between muscular coat (mainly middle constrictor) & buccopharyngeal fascia
- **Muscles**: Constrictors of pharynx attached to bones or cartilages in relation to larynx anteriorly & expand posteriorly, ending in midline tendinous raphe
- Inferior constrictor arising anteriorly from thyroid & cricoid cartilages & middle constrictor from hyoid bone forms part of HP; superior constrictor part of oro-/nasopharynx above arises from mandible & sphenoid
- Lower constrictors overlap constrictor muscles above them like **flower pots placed inside one another**
- Stylopharyngeus muscle & glossopharyngeal nerve pass through **gap between superior & middle constrictors**
- Internal laryngeal nerve & superior laryngeal vessels pierce thyrohyoid membrane in **gap between middle & inferior constrictors** & run through PS to reach larynx
- Inferior constrictor muscle: 2 parts: Thyropharyngeus with oblique fibers & cricopharyngeus with transverse fibers continuous with circular fibers of esophagus
  - **Killian dehiscence**: Potential gap between these 2 parts
- Recurrent laryngeal nerve & inferior laryngeal vessels pass through **gap between inferior constrictor & esophagus**
- **Nerve supply**: Pharyngeal plexus (CNIX-X branches & sympathetic fibers of superior cervical ganglion)
- Motor fibers in plexus from pharyngeal branch of vagus carry cranial accessory nerve fibers & supply all pharyngeal & soft palate muscles except stylopharyngeus (by CNIX) & tensor veli palatini (by CNV)
- Sensory fibers in plexus are from glossopharyngeal nerve & supply all 3 parts of pharynx
- **Blood supply**: HP by branches of external carotid artery (ascending pharyngeal) & subclavian (inferior thyroid)

- Venous plexus at posterolateral aspect of pharynx receives blood from pharynx, soft palate, & prevertebral region & drains to internal jugular vein

ANATOMY IMAGING ISSUES

Imaging Recommendations

- CECT best overall modality for evaluating HP pathology
- MR for problem solving, especially evaluation of laryngeal cartilage & prevertebral soft tissue invasion by HP tumor
- PET/CT useful especially in occult PS primary tumor

Imaging Sweet Spots

- Removal of foreign bodies from piriform sinus may damage internal laryngeal nerve beneath its mucosa, leading to supraglottic laryngeal anesthesia
- Pharyngeal (Zenker) diverticulum: Outpouching of Killian dehiscence due to neuromuscular incoordination between thyropharyngeus & cricopharyngeus parts of inferior constrictor
- If sphincteric cricopharyngeus (supplied by recurrent laryngeal nerve) fails to relax when propulsive thyropharyngeus (supplied by pharyngeal plexus) contracts, then food bolus gets pushed backwards & tends to form Zenker diverticulum through Killian dehiscence
- Killian dehiscence called "gateway of tears" as perforation can occur at this site during esophagoscopy
- Do not confuse Zenker diverticulum with upper esophageal Killian-Jamieson diverticulum (KJD)
  - KJD just below cricopharyngeus muscle, anteriorly & laterally through Killian-Jamieson space
  - Left sided or, occasionally, bilateral
  - Smaller (< 1.5 cm), less frequent, & less symptomatic than Zenker diverticulum
  - KJD & Zenker diverticulum both mucosal outpouchings through muscular defect (pseudodiverticula)
- Barium esophagram best imaging tool
  - Confirms diagnosis & shows diverticular neck
  - Evaluates associated reflux & hiatal hernia
- **Referred otalgia**
  - Referred otalgia (ear pain) in patients with pathology outside temporal bone due to complex neural pathway interconnections in temporal bone & neck
  - Sensory nerves from superior laryngeal nerve & pharyngeal plexus can ultimately communicate with Arnold nerve (sensory to ear) at level of jugular foramen
  - HP carcinoma can be source of referred otalgia
  - When no source of otalgia is found in temporal bone, further clinical & radiologic evaluation with CECT or PET/CT recommended to exclude another source of referred pain in head & neck, including HP
- **PS tumor evaluation**
  - Small tumor in PS can be occult & represent clinical & radiologic blind spot; could be primary etiology in some cases of metastatic SCCa of unknown primary
  - Tumors of PS can extend in multiple directions given anatomic location
    - Anterior: Larynx
    - Lateral: Thyrohyoid membrane, thyroid cartilage
    - Posterior: Prevertebral invasion
    - Inferior: Postcricoid subsite of HP & to esophagus
    - Superior: Oropharynx extension common
  - Majority HP SCCa (2/3) originate in PS
- **Posterior wall tumor evaluation**
  - SCCa in posterior wall of HP can invade prevertebral soft tissues & prevent complete surgical resection
  - Accuracy for CT & MR in predicting prevertebral invasion & fixation limited
  - **Intact retropharyngeal fat plane on CT/MR (MR best)** between HP posterior wall tumor & prevertebral space **good negative predictor for tumor invasion**
- **Postcricoid tumor evaluation**
  - With conventional cross-sectional imaging, HP typically nondistended, & postcricoid mucosa normally directly apposed to mucosa of posterior wall
  - Distinguishing postcricoid soft tissue components can be difficult on CT or MR but is possible with optimal mucosal enhancement & presence of visible intramural fat planes
  - **Normal AP** dimension of **postcricoid soft tissue < 1 cm**
  - Consider neoplasia if postcricoid soft tissue > 1 cm AP
  - Soft tissue posterior to cricoid cartilage region
    - Posterior cricoarytenoid muscles
    - Fatty submucosa of postcricoid HP
    - Conglomerate of mucosa of postcricoid HP, collapsed lower HP lumen, & mucosa of posterior wall of HP
    - Fatty submucosa of posterior wall of HP
    - Inferior constrictor (cricopharyngeus) muscle in posterior wall of HP
    - Retropharyngeal fat stripe
    - Prevertebral fascia & longus coli muscles

Imaging Pitfalls

- Paucity of fat in retropharyngeal space in lower neck makes identification of tissue plane between posterior wall of HP & prevertebral musculature difficult
- Not detecting intact retropharyngeal fat on CT/MR does not imply definite prevertebral space invasion
- Detecting intact retropharyngeal fat stripe provides good negative predictive value for prevertebral tumor invasion

EMBRYOLOGY

Embryologic Events

- Pharynx develops from most cranial aspect of foregut, buccopharyngeal anlage
- Endodermal pouches formed in relation to lateral wall of foregut here, most lose contact with pharyngeal wall
- Floor of foregut gives rise to midline tracheobronchial diverticulum from which entire respiratory system develops
- Site of midline diverticulum becomes inlet of larynx
- Pharynx subdivides into nasopharynx, oropharynx, & HP with establishment of palate & mouth
- Pharyngeal wall muscles develop from 3rd & subsequent pharyngeal arches
- **3rd branchial arch** tract anomalies arise superiorly from **base of PS**, whereas **4th branchial arch** tract anomalies arise inferiorly from **PS apex**; 90% of both left sided
- Both tract anomalies pass through throat **near cricothyroid joint** with external sinus/fistula skin orifice situated along anterior border of sternocleidomastoid muscle
- 4th branchial pouch anomaly presents as recurrent left lobe of thyroid abscess; look for tract connecting to PS apex

GRAPHICS

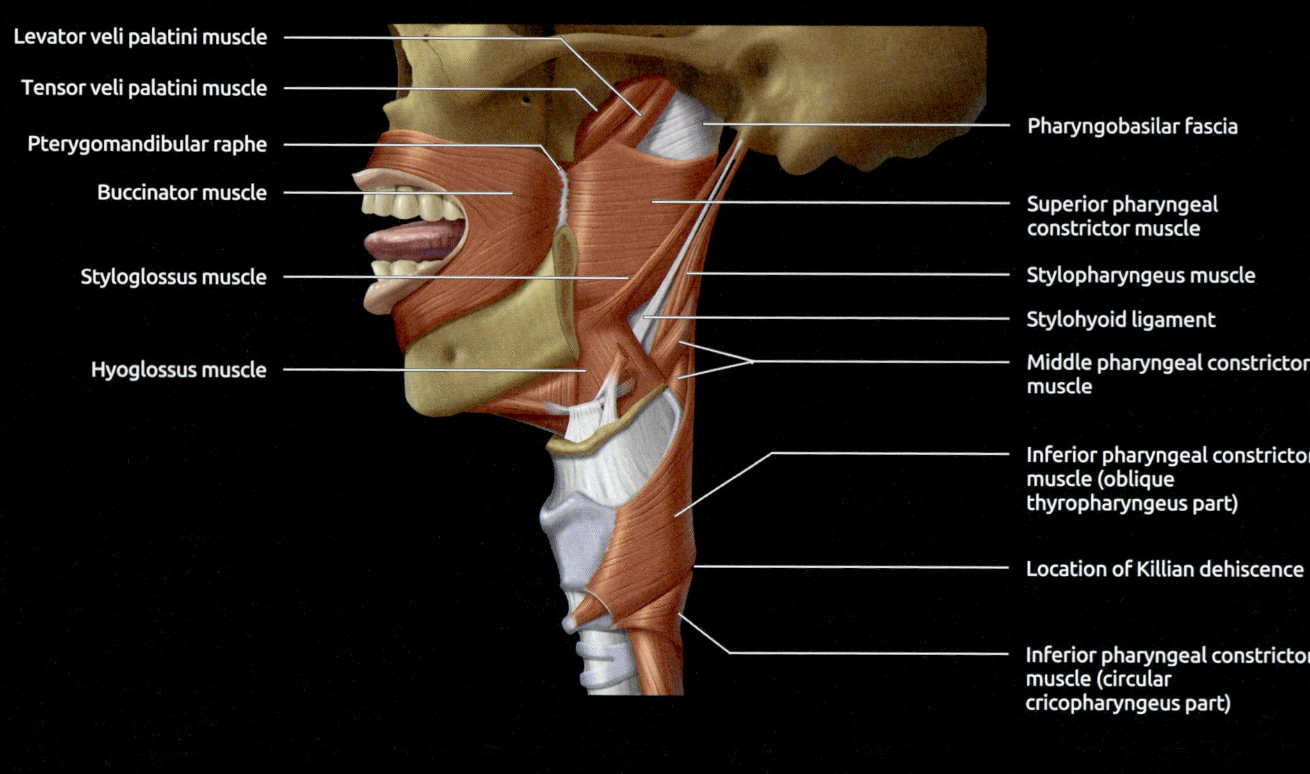

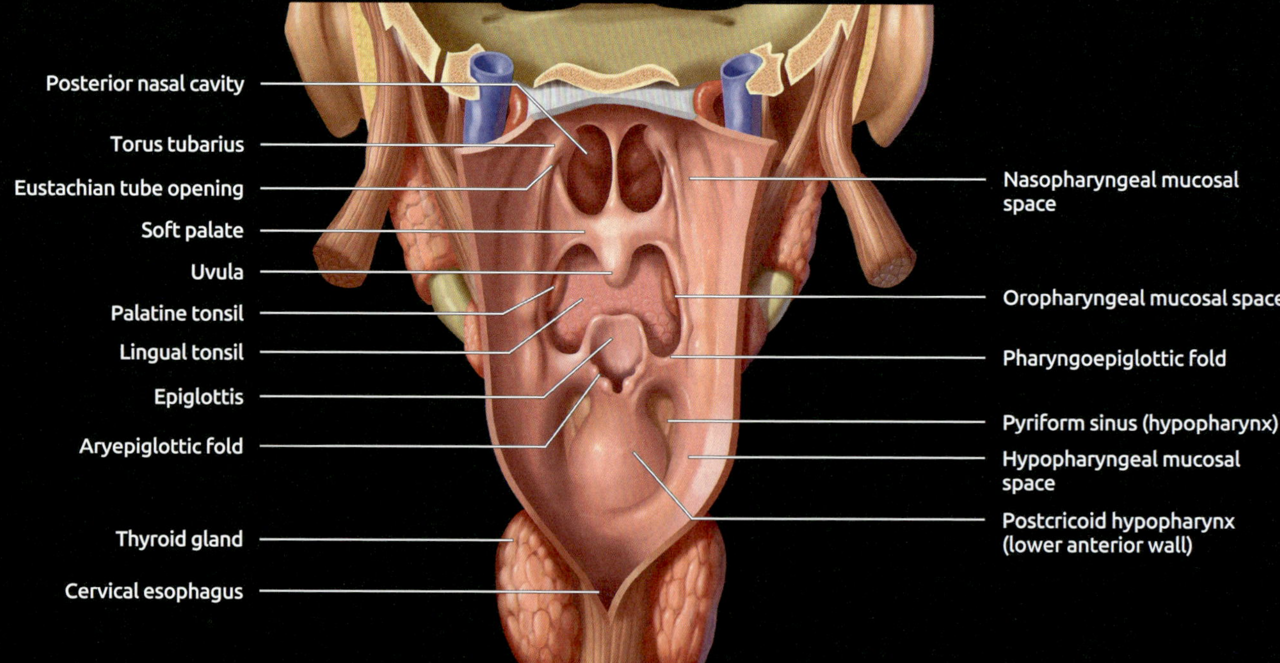

(Top) *Lateral graphic shows the major muscles of the pharyngeal mucosal space (PMS). Note that the superior (naso-/oropharynx), middle, & inferior pharyngeal constrictor (hypopharynx) muscles are in the posterior wall of the PMS from the nasopharynx through the oropharynx to the hypopharynx. Note also that the inferior constrictor muscle has 2 parts: Thyropharyngeus with oblique fibers & cricopharyngeus with transverse fibers continuous with circular fibers of the esophagus; between these is a potential gap called Killian dehiscence (KD). Pharyngobasilar fascia (at nasopharyngeal level) attaches the superior pharyngeal constrictor to the skull base. The distal end of the levator veli palatini muscle is on the airway side of the middle layer of deep cervical fascia, making it a part of PMS.* **(Bottom)** *Graphic of the PMS/surface seen from behind shows this space can be divided into nasopharyngeal, oropharyngeal, & hypopharyngeal areas. The lymphatic ring of the PMS contains nasopharyngeal adenoids, oropharyngeal palatine, & lingual tonsils. The anterior wall of the hypopharynx is formed by the laryngeal inlet above & posterior surfaces of the cricoid & arytenoid cartilages below.*

GRAPHICS

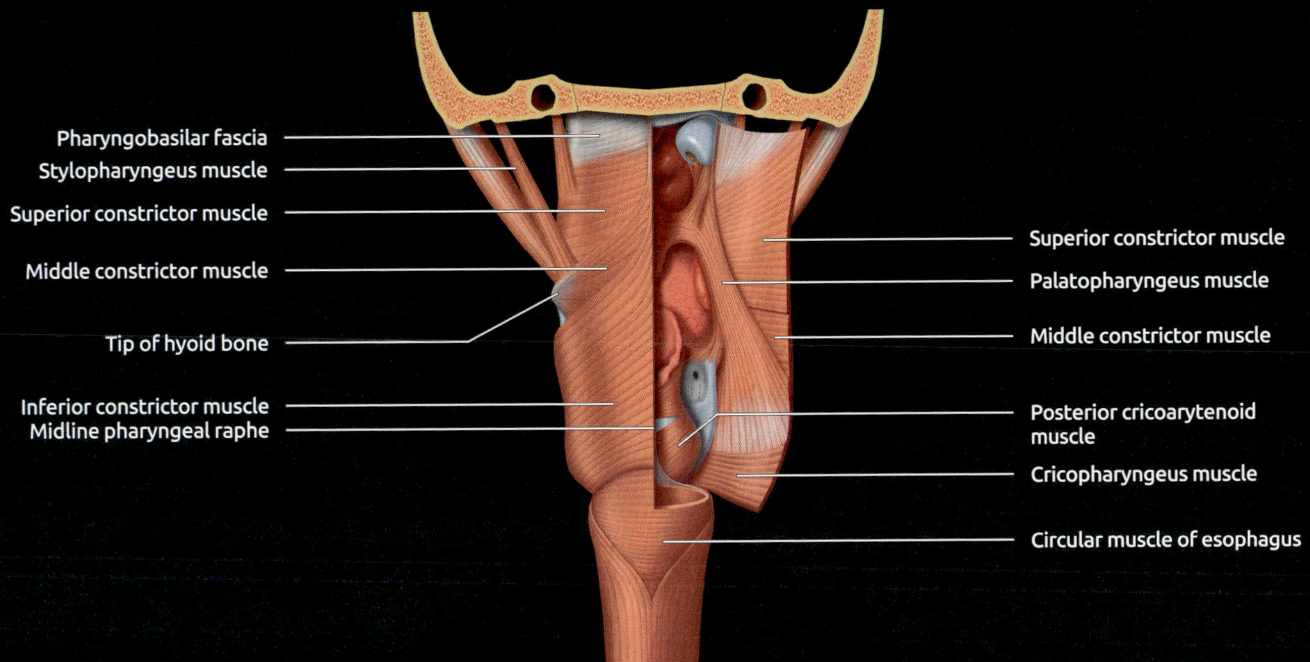

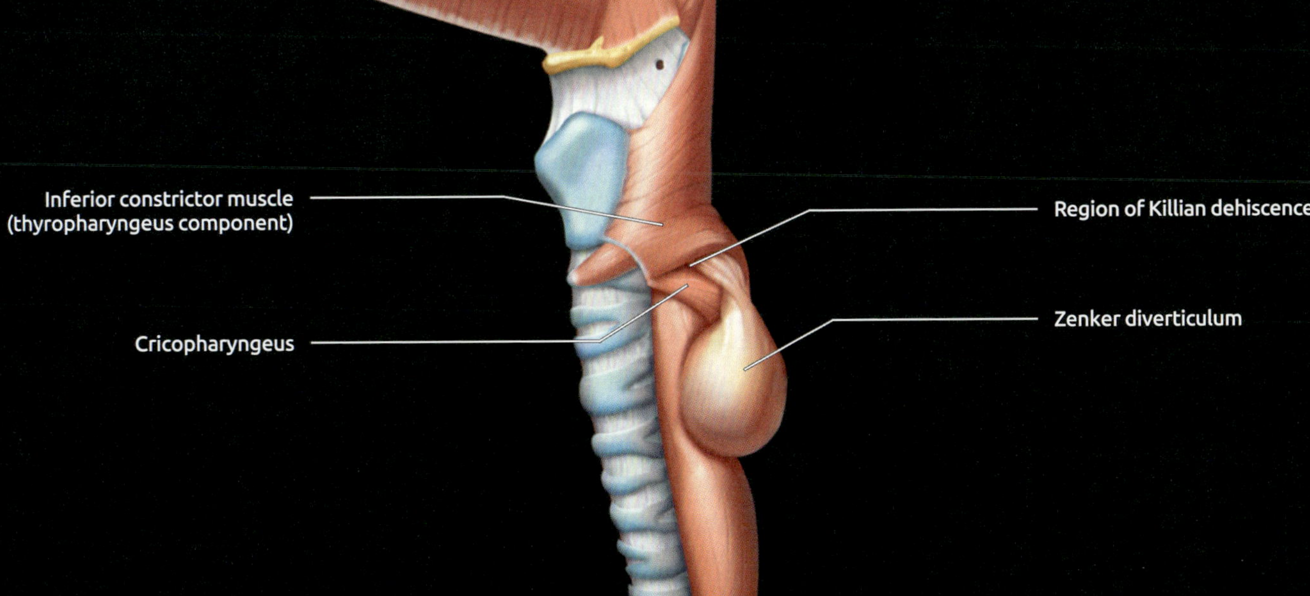

(Top) *Posterior view of the pharynx shows lower constrictors overlapping constrictor muscles above them like flower pots placed one inside the other. Pharyngeal constrictors attach to bones or cartilages in relation to the larynx anteriorly & expand posteriorly, ending in a midline tendinous raphe. Pharyngobasilar fascia is the thickened fibrous attachment at the skull base. The stylopharyngeus muscle & glossopharyngeal nerve pass through the gap between superior & middle constrictors. Internal laryngeal nerve & superior laryngeal vessels pierce thyrohyoid membrane in the gap between middle & inferior constrictors & run through the pyriform sinus to reach the larynx. Inferior constrictor muscle: 2 parts; oblique thyropharyngeus & transverse cricopharyngeus. KD is a potential gap between these 2 parts. The recurrent laryngeal nerve & inferior laryngeal vessels pass through the gap between the inferior constrictor & esophagus.* **(Bottom)** *Graphic shows hypopharyngeal Zenker diverticulum (ZD) with herniation at KD between thyropharyngeal & cricopharyngeal fibers of inferior constrictor muscle. Do not confuse ZD with upper esophageal Killian-Jamieson diverticulum.*

GRAPHICS

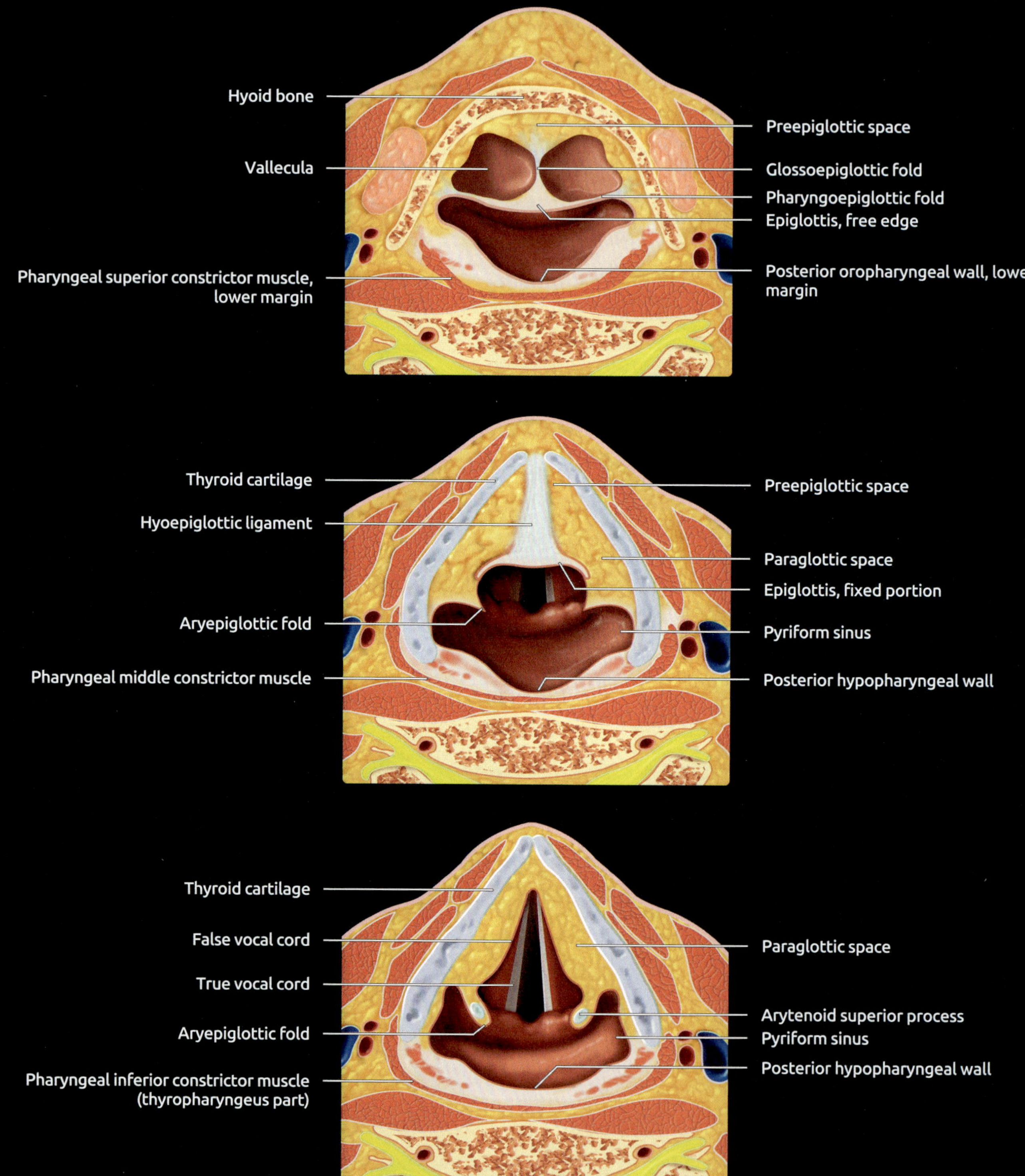

(Top) *First of 6 axial graphics of the larynx & hypopharynx from superior to inferior shows the roof of hypopharynx/lower margin of the oropharynx junction at the hyoid bone level & high supraglottic structures. The free edge of the epiglottis is attached to the hyoid bone via the hyoepiglottic ligament, which is covered by the glossoepiglottic fold, a ridge of mucous membrane. The hypopharynx extends from the level of the glossoepiglottic & pharyngoepiglottic folds superiorly (inferior margin of vallecula, which is at hyoid bone level) to cricoid cartilage (cricopharyngeus muscle) inferiorly.* **(Middle)** *Graphic at midsupraglottic level shows hyoepiglottic ligament dividing lower preepiglottic space. No fascia separates preepiglottic space from paraglottic space. These 2 endolaryngeal spaces are submucosal locations where tumors hide from clinical detection. Aryepiglottic fold represents the junction between the larynx & hypopharynx. Middle constrictor muscle is now seen deep to upper posterior hypopharyngeal wall.* **(Bottom)** *Graphic at low supraglottic level shows false vocal cords. Inferior constrictor muscle (upper thyropharyngeus part) is seen in the deep midposterior hypopharyngeal wall.*

GRAPHICS

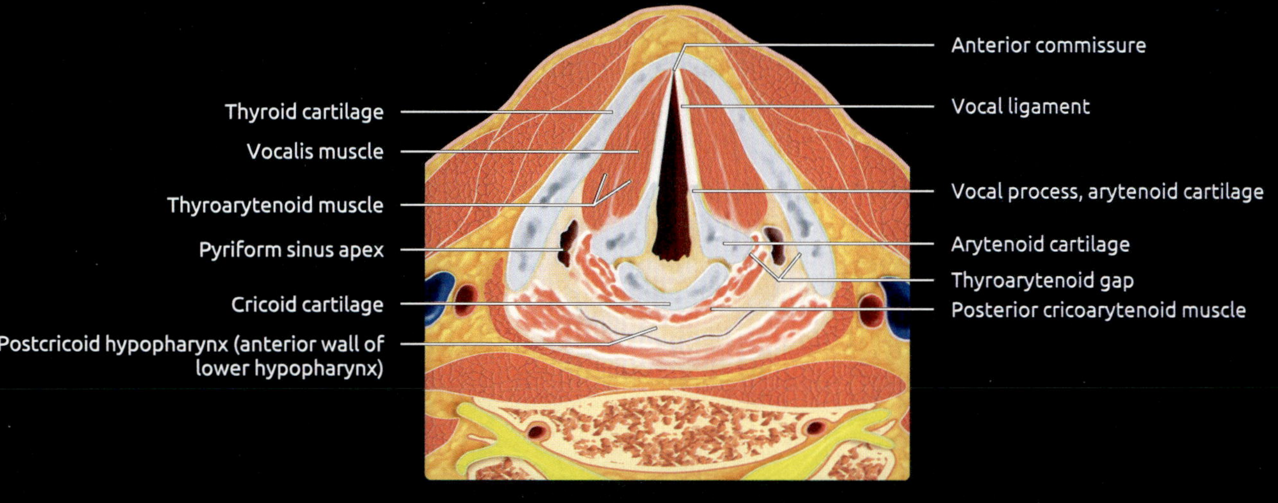

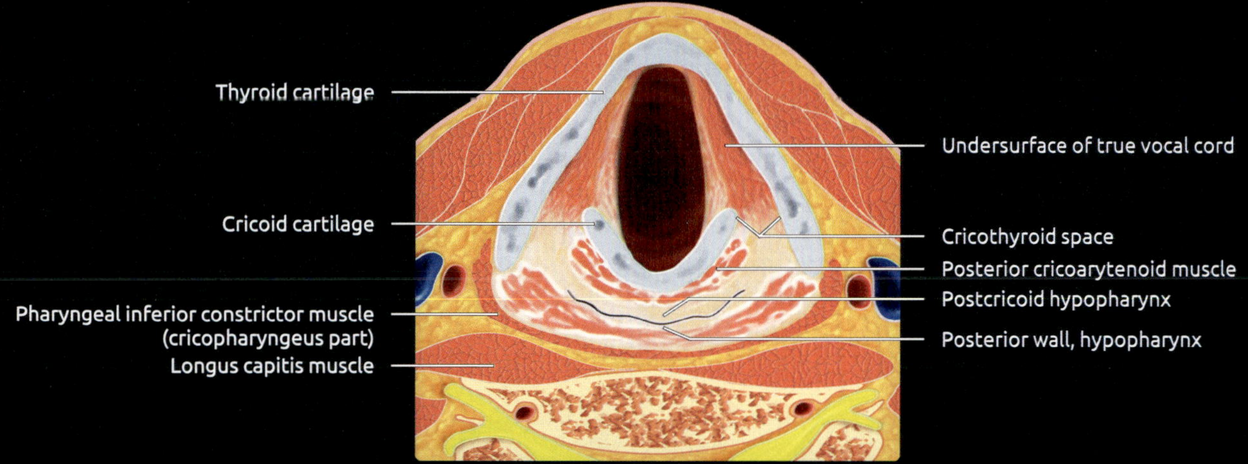

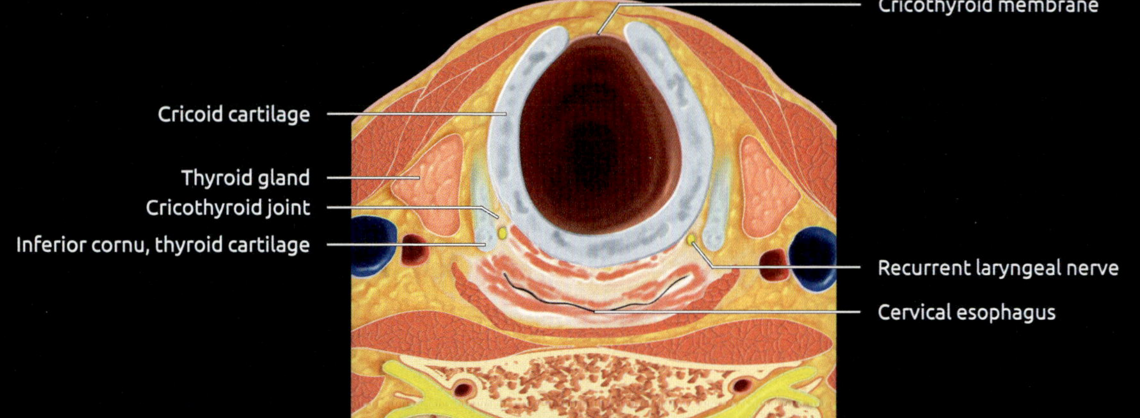

(Top) *Graphic at the glottic, true vocal cord level shows thyroarytenoid muscle; this makes up bulk of true vocal cord. Medial fibers of thyroarytenoid muscle are known as the vocalis muscle. Pyriform sinus apex (hypopharynx) is seen at glottic level. Thyroarytenoid gap is location where tumors may spread between larynx & hypopharynx. Postcricoid region is anterior wall of lower hypopharynx.* **(Middle)** *Graphic at undersurface level of true vocal cord shows posterior lamina of cricoid cartilage. Postcricoid hypopharynx represents anterior wall of lower hypopharynx & extends from cricoarytenoid joints to lower edge of cricoid cartilage at cricopharyngeus muscle. Posterior wall of lower hypopharynx at this level is formed by inferior circular cricopharyngeus part of inferior constrictor muscle. Unlike other pharyngeal constrictors, fibers in this lower part of inferior constrictor muscle bypass pharyngeal raphe & inserts itself into circular fibers of esophagus to serve as a superior esophageal sphincter.* **(Bottom)** *Subglottic level graphic shows upper cervical esophagus. Note cricothyroid joint immediately adjacent to recurrent laryngeal nerve, located in tracheoesophageal groove.*

AXIAL CECT

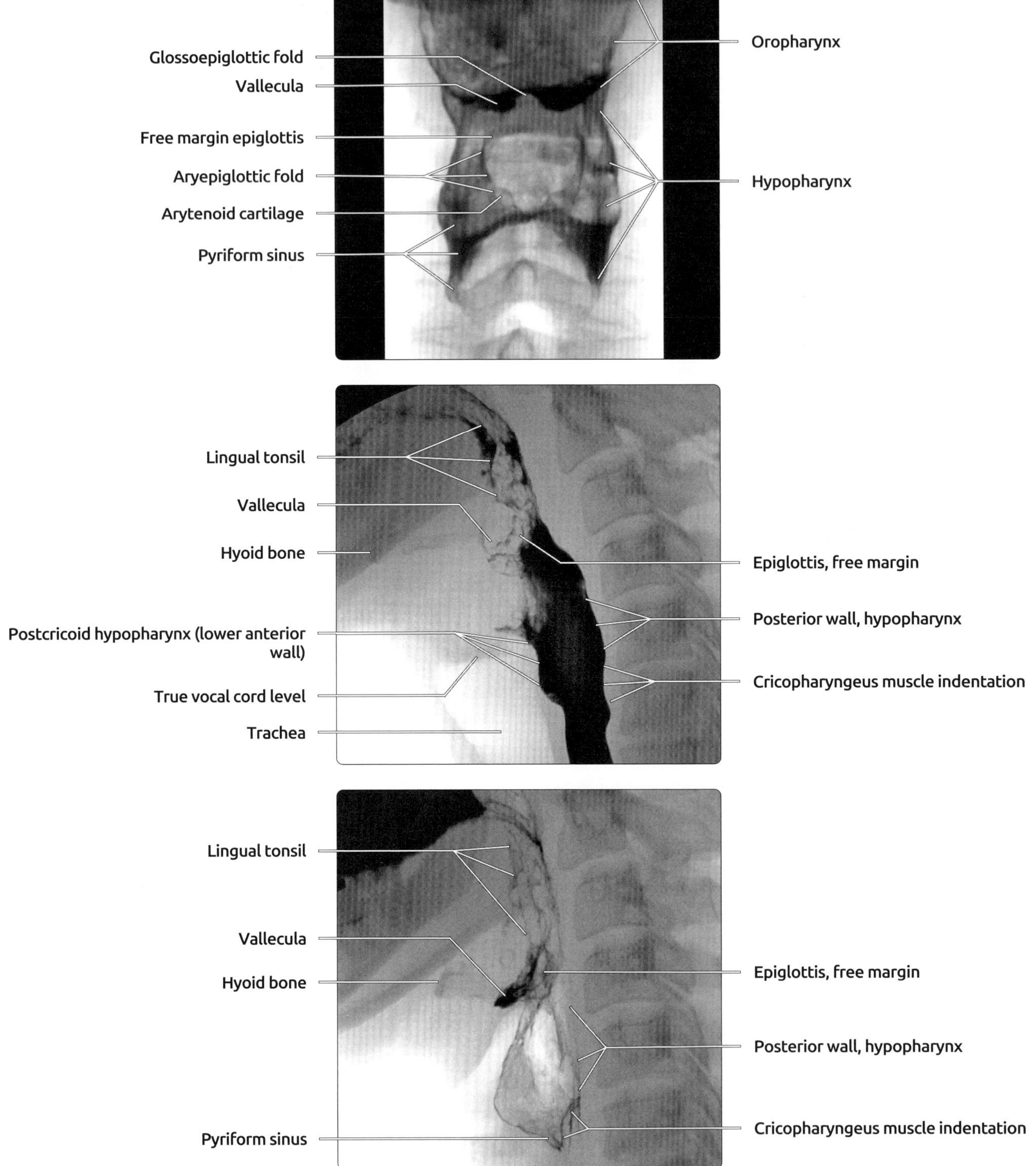

(Top) *AP barium swallow focused on the low oropharyngeal & hypopharyngeal mucosal space surfaces shows that the hypopharynx extends from the level of the vallecula & glossoepiglottic fold superiorly to the inferior margin of the pyriform sinus. The inferior margin of vallecula marks the transition from oropharynx to hypopharynx. Pyriform sinuses are bilateral anterolateral recesses of the hypopharynx & have an inverted pyramid shape with the superior base at the pharyngoepiglottic fold level & inferior tip/apex at true vocal cord level.* **(Middle)** *In this lateral view of a barium swallow, the irregular surface of the lingual tonsil is recognized along the posterior margin of the tongue. The postcricoid area (lower anterior hypopharynx wall) & the posterior wall of the hypopharynx make up 2 of the 3 major subsites within the hypopharynx. The 3rd subsite is the pyriform sinus.* **(Bottom)** *Lateral barium swallow shows cricopharyngeus muscle indentation in the lower hypopharynx. The inferior constrictor muscle has 2 parts: Oblique thyropharyngeus & transverse cricopharyngeus (continuous with circular fibers of the esophagus) with KD in between.*

AXIAL CECT

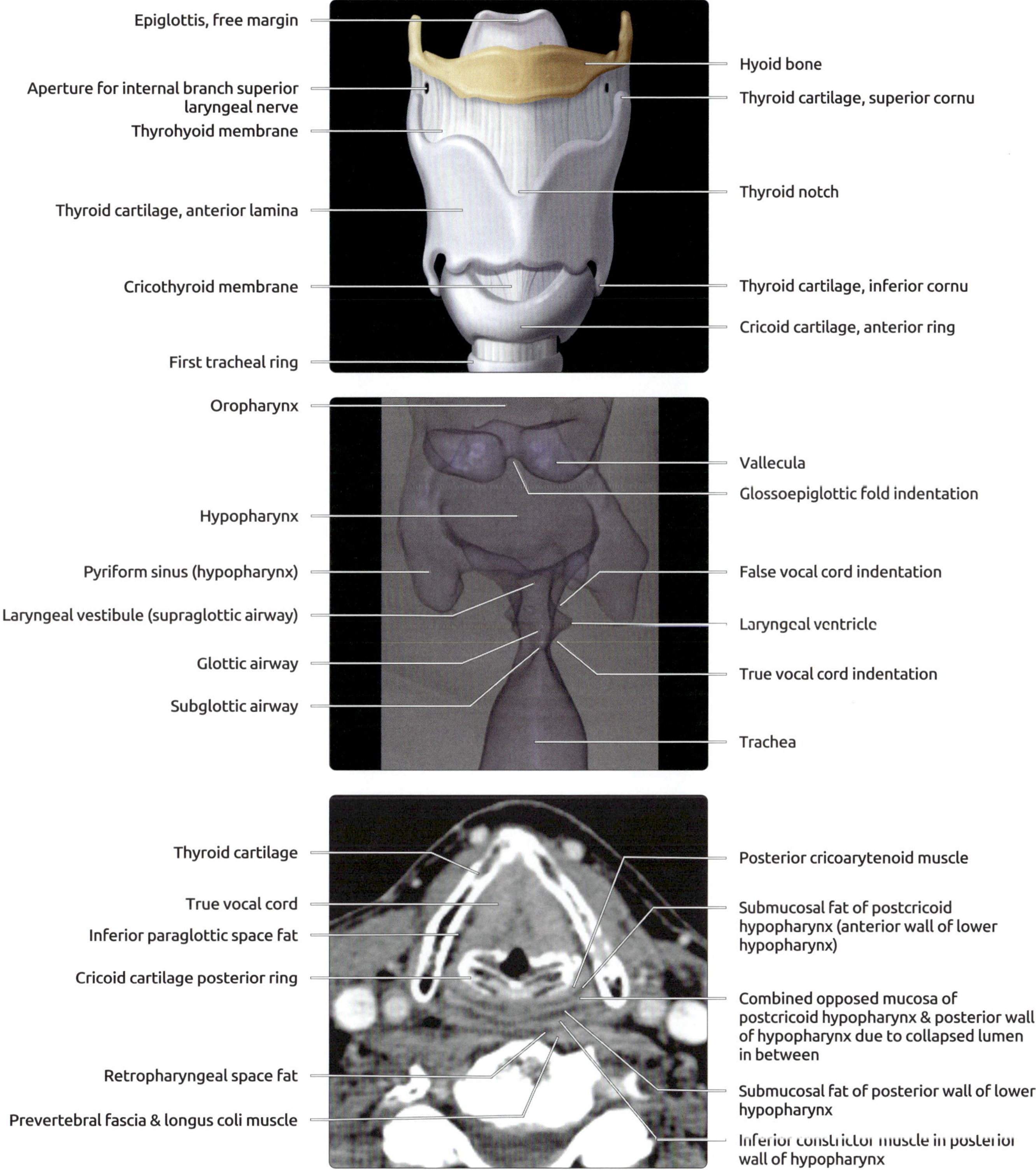

(Top) *Anterior view of laryngeal cartilage provides the structural framework for soft tissues of the larynx to drape over. Two large anterior laminae of thyroid cartilage "shield" the larynx. Note the aperture in thyrohyoid membrane for the internal laryngeal nerve & superior laryngeal vessels. They pierce the membrane in the gap between the middle & inferior constrictor muscles & run through the pyriform sinus to reach the larynx. Removal of foreign bodies from pyriform sinus may damage the internal laryngeal nerve beneath its mucosa, leading to supraglottic laryngeal anesthesia.* **(Middle)** *3D reformatted CT shows the larynx & hypopharynx airway. Pyriform sinuses are the paired anterolateral recess of the hypopharynx & the most common site of squamous cell carcinoma in the hypopharynx. The pyriform sinus apex (inferior tip) lies at the level of true vocal cord, which allows pyriform sinus tumors access to true vocal cords.* **(Bottom)** *Axial CECT through a normal hypopharynx/larynx at cricoid cartilage level shows the laminated appearance of multiple tissue layers posterior to cricoid cartilage & anterior to vertebra. Normal AP thickness of postcricoid soft tissue is < 1 cm.*

AXIAL CECT

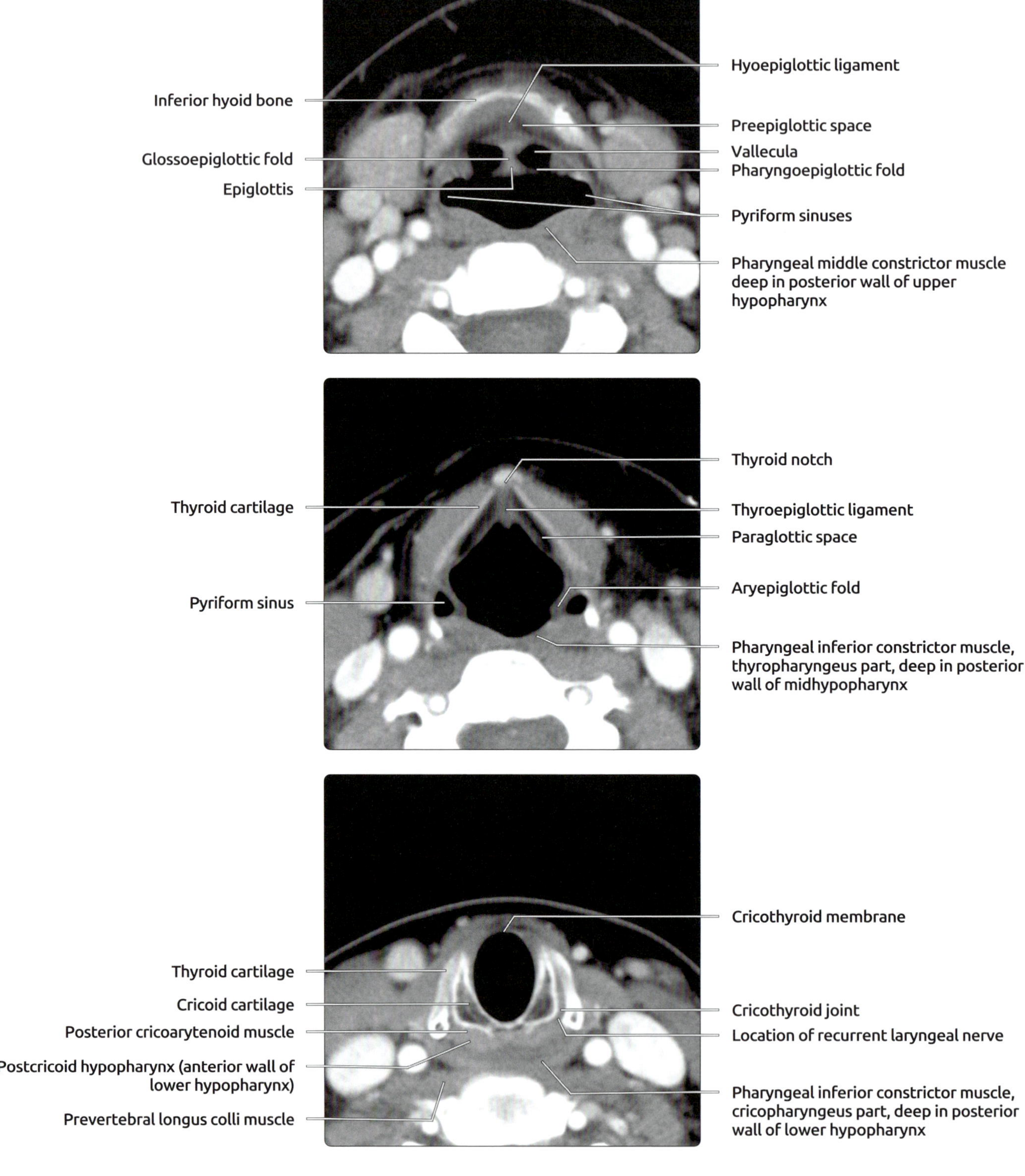

(Top) *First of axial 4 CT images from top to bottom shows the hypopharynx, which extends from the level of the glossoepiglottic & pharyngoepiglottic folds superiorly (inferior margin of vallecula lying at hyoid bone level) to inferior cricoid cartilage (cricopharyngeus muscle) where the esophagus begins. This image at the high supraglottic level of the larynx shows the upper hypopharynx, including its upper posterior wall & pyriform sinuses. Note the lowermost aspect of vallecula, glossoepiglottic, & pharyngoepiglottic folds, the undersurface of which form the roof of the hypopharynx. The C-shaped preepiglottic space, a common location for tumors to hide, is also seen.* **(Middle)** *CT at the midsupraglottic level shows the thyroepiglottic ligament dividing the preepiglottic space. Aryepiglottic folds at the margin of the pyriform sinus & larynx & a tumor primary to the fold is considered a "marginal supraglottic" tumor.* **(Bottom)** *CT more inferiorly at the subglottic level with the cricoid ring nearly complete is shown. The postcricoid hypopharynx is the anterior wall of the lower hypopharynx, whereas its posterior wall here is formed by the cricopharyngeus part of the inferior constrictor muscle.*

AXIAL CECT

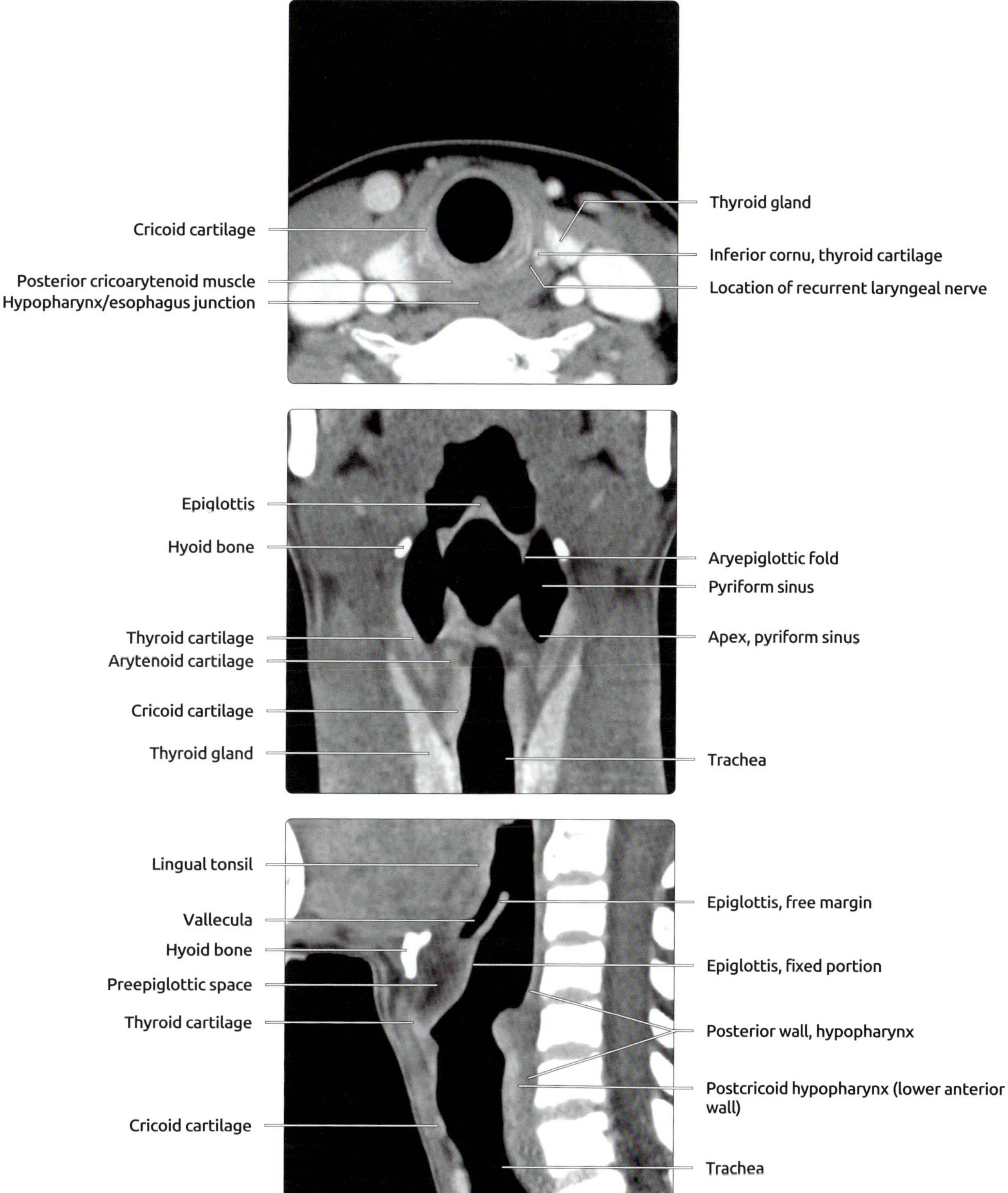

(Top) *At the level of the inferior cricoid cartilage, the inferior margin of the larynx & hypopharynx are transitioning to the trachea & cervical esophagus. Mucosa along the subglottis should be no > 1 mm in normal patients. If there is thickened mucosa, it raises concern for tumor.* **(Middle)** *Coronal reformatted CT shows the laryngeal cartilages & pyriform sinus. Note that the pyriform sinuses on both sides are inverted pyramid-shaped with a superior base (3rd branchial arch derivative) at the pharyngoepiglottic fold level & an inferior tip (apex, 4th branchial arch derivative) at true vocal cord level. Both 3rd & 4th tract anomalies pass through the throat near the cricothyroid joint with external sinus/fistula skin orifice situated along the anterior border of the sternocleidomastoid muscle. Pyriform sinus is bound laterally by the inner surface of thyrohyoid membrane above & thyroid cartilage below.* **(Bottom)** *Midsagittal reformatted CT shows midline larynx & hypopharynx. Preepiglottic fat is seen at midline, posterior & inferior to hyoid bone. Diseases of posterior hypopharyngeal wall are well seen on sagittal imaging. Sagittal imaging also helps define cranial to caudal extent of lesions.*

TERMINOLOGY

Abbreviations

- Parathyroid gland (PTG)

THYROID

Imaging Anatomy

- **Overview**
  - Batwing-shaped thyroid gland
    - 2 prominent lateral lobes
    - Connected by smaller median isthmus
- **Anatomy relationships**
  - Thyroid gland lies anterior & lateral to trachea in **visceral space** of infrahyoid neck at C5-T1 level
  - Posteromedially: Tracheoesophageal (TE) groove
    - TE groove contains paratracheal lymph nodes (LNs), recurrent laryngeal nerve (RLN), & PTGs
  - Posterolaterally: Carotid spaces
  - Anteriorly: Infrahyoid strap muscles
  - Anterolaterally: Sternocleidomastoid muscles
  - Superior PTGs: Posterior to & close to thyroid, usually within thyroid false capsule or in TE groove
  - Inferior PTGs: More anteriorly & can be more distant
- **Internal contents**
  - **Thyroid gland** (average: 25 grams weight)
  - **Right & left lobes** ~ 5.0 x 2.5 x 2.5 cm each, larger in females, commonly asymmetric
    - Each lobe: Apex, base & lateral, medial & posterior surfaces; anterior & posterior borders
    - Apex limited superiorly by **sternothyroid** strap muscle attaching to oblique line of thyroid cartilage medially
  - Lateral lobes joined by midline **isthmus** at 2nd-4th tracheal ring level
  - **Pyramidal lobe** present in ~ 40% of cases; ascends in midline from isthmus or, rarely, from 1 of lobes
    - **Levator glandulae thyroidea**: Fibromuscular band from hyoid body to isthmus or pyramidal lobe
  - **Zuckerkandl tubercle**: Protuberance from posterior aspect of gland to TE groove
    - Surgeons use as landmark for superior PTG & recurrent laryngeal nerve
    - Seen in 70% patients; R > L, may be bilateral
- **Arterial supply of thyroid gland**
  - **Superior thyroid arteries (STA)**
    - STA: 1st anterior branch of external carotid artery
    - Proximal course closely associated with external (superior) laryngeal nerve
    - Anterior branch descends on anterior border of thyroid lobe, sending branch deep into gland
      - Then curves along upper border of isthmus & anastomoses with contralateral anterior branch
    - Posterior branch descends on posterior border of thyroid lobe & anastomoses with ascending branch of inferior thyroid artery, supplying PTG
    - Anastomosis good guide to PTG, usually lie near it
  - **Inferior thyroid arteries (ITA)**
    - From thyrocervical trunk, branch of subclavian artery
    - Ascends vertically, then curves medially to enter TE groove in plane posterior to carotid space
    - Most of its branches penetrate posterior aspect of thyroid lobe
    - 1 ascending branch anastomose with STA
    - Terminal part near thyroid closely associated with recurrent laryngeal nerve, proximally away from nerve
    - **ITA** ligated **away** from gland during thyroidectomy to protect recurrent laryngeal nerve
    - **STA** ligated **close to** gland to protect external laryngeal nerve
  - **Thyroidea ima artery** occasionally present (3%)
    - Single vessel originating from aortic arch or innominate artery
    - Enters thyroid gland at inferior border of isthmus
- **Venous drainage from thyroid**
  - 3 pairs from venous plexus on thyroid surface
  - Superior & middle thyroid veins → internal jugular vein
  - Inferior thyroid veins → left brachiocephalic vein
- **Lymphatic drainage**
  - Extensive & multidirectional drainage to LN
  - Superomedial lymphatic trunk → prelaryngeal (delphian) LN (level VI)
  - Inferomedial trunk → pre-/paratracheal LN (level VI)
    - Paratracheal nodes drain along RLN into mediastinum
  - Superolateral trunk → upper jugular chain LN (levels II-V)
  - Inferolateral trunk → supraclavicular/jugulosubclavian LN
  - Additional pathways: Retrograde from jugular chain lymphatics & direct posterosuperior lymphatic trunk pathway from upper pole of thyroid gland to lateral retropharyngeal LN (RPLN)
  - Papillary thyroid cancer with metastatic cervical lymphadenopathy or prior neck dissection might alter lymphatic drainage direction to retrograde pathway, resulting in unusual RPLN metastasis
- **Fascia**
  - **Middle layer of deep cervical fascia** surrounds visceral space & ensheathes thyroid & PTG
  - Thyroid gland **inner true capsule** formed by peripheral condensed connective tissue of gland
    - Dense capillary plexus deep to true capsule: Thyroid removed along with true capsule at thyroidectomy
  - **Outer false capsule** from pretracheal (middle) layer of deep cervical fascia; thick medially & forms **suspensory ligament of Berry** connecting thyroid lobe to cricoid cartilage

Embryology: Thyroid

- **Embryologic events**
  - 1st endocrine gland to develop (24th gestational day)
  - Originates from 1st & 2nd pharyngeal pouches (medial anlage) as proliferation of endodermal cells at **foramen cecum** (median surface of developing pharyngeal floor)
  - Bilobed thyroid gland descends anterior to pharyngeal gut along **thyroglossal duct (TGD)**
    - Tubular TGD later solidifies & ultimately obliterated (gestational weeks 7-10)
  - Inferior descent carries thyroid gland anterior to hyoid bone & laryngeal cartilages to pretracheal location
  - RLN derived from 6th pharyngeal arch: Anchored to 4th arch-derived subclavian artery on right & aortic arch on left when 5th arch & distal portions of 6th arch regress, leaving behind RLN

- RLN normally descend into thorax with these arterial structures, hence, typical recurrent course
- RLN normal descent can be altered with formation of **nonrecurrent** laryngeal nerve course
  - On right side with aberrant right subclavian artery
  - On left side with right-sided aortic arch & aberrant left subclavian artery
- 4th branchial (pharyngeal) pouch contains dorsal & ventral wings
  - Ventral wings develop into ultimobranchial body & parafollicular C cells of thyroid
  - Dorsal wings develop into superior PTGs

- **Practical implications**
  - **TGD cyst**: From failure of involution of part of TGD
    - Anywhere along TGD course from foramen cecum at tongue base to just anterior to thyroid lobes
    - 50% at hyoid bone level, in midline
    - 20-25% in suprahyoid neck, often in midline
    - 25% in infrahyoid neck, in midline or paramedian **within strap muscles**
    - 65% have thyroid tissue in wall microscopically
    - < 2% of TGD cysts harbor carcinoma
  - **Thyroid ectopia**
    - Most common location: Deep to foramen cecum in tongue base = **lingual thyroid (> 90%)**
    - **Submandibular & lateral neck** region thyroid ectopia: Defective lateral thyroid component that cannot migrate & fuse with median thyroid anlage
    - **Mediastinum** & **subdiaphragmatic** locations: Over descent of TGD remnants
    - Ectopic thyroid tissues in **distant** locations: Aberrant migration or heterotopic differentiation of uncommitted endodermal cells
    - Ectopic thyroid tissue in **genital tract**: Parthenogenetic development of germ cells into thyroid tissue after failure of these cells to migrate to genital crest in early embryological development
  - **4th branchial pouch anomaly**: May present as **recurrent left thyroiditis**
    - Look for **sinus tract to pyriform sinus (PS) apex**, which also develop from 4th branchial pouch
  - **Non-RLN**: ↑ risk of up to 13% nerve injury at thyroidectomy

Imaging Approaches

- US best 1st-line approach; CT & MR can evaluate thyroid lesion, its relationship to other structures & adenopathy
- If thyroid neoplasia is suspected, iodinated contrast should not be given; will delay therapeutic iodine I-131 treatment

PARATHYROID

Imaging Anatomy

- **Anatomy relationships**
  - **Superior** PTG lie **posterior** to RLN
  - **Inferior** PTG lie **anterior** to RLN
- **Internal contents**
  - ~ 6 mm length, 3-4 mm transverse, & 1-2 mm in anteroposterior diameter; 40-50 mg weight
  - Parathyroid adenoma mean weight 1 g
  - **Normal number = 4**, 2 superior & 2 inferior
    - > 4 PTGs in 3-5%; < 4 PTGs in 3%
  - **Superior PTG locations: Posterior to** & close to **thyroid**, usually within thyroid false capsule or in **TE groove**
    - 70-75% found on posterior border of middle 1/3 of thyroid gland
    - 20-25% found behind upper or lower 1/3 of thyroid
    - 7% located below inferior thyroid (dropped superior PTG in TE groove)
    - Retropharyngeal or retroesophageal (< 2-3% ectopic)
    - Within scalene fat pad (< 1%)
    - PS: 4th branchial pouch gives rise to PS apex
  - **Inferior PTG locations**: Anteriorly **(anterolateral to trachea, posterior to strap muscles)**; can be distant
    - 50% located lateral to lower thyroid pole
    - 15% within 1 cm of inferior thyroid poles
    - 25% ectopic along thyrothymic ligament into superior/lower anterior mediastinum
    - Within carotid sheath (< 1%), intrathyroidal (< 1%)
    - Undescended PTG near angle of mandible (near submandibular salivary gland), carotid bifurcation
    - PS: 3rd branchial pouch gives rise to base of PS
    - Embedded in vagus & hypoglossal nerves (3rd branchial pouch contacts ectodermal structures from which vagus & hypoglossal nerves arise)
    - Rarely, intrathyroidal superior/inferior PTG
- **Arterial supply**: ITA & anastomosis between STA & ITA

Embryology

- **Superior PTG** develop from 4th branchial pouch along with primordial **thyroid gland &** migrate caudally along **TGD**
- **Inferior PTG** develop from 3rd branchial pouch along with anlage of **thymus**
  - Migrate caudally along thymopharyngeal duct
  - May descend into anterior mediastinum

Imaging Approaches

- Primary hyperparathyroidism: Majority single adenoma (80%), then multigland disease, such as PTG hyperplasia (10%) or multiple adenomas (10%); rarely, PTG carcinoma (1%)
- Imaging to localize PTG lesions: Anatomic study for patients suitable for surgery, such as minimally invasive parathyroidectomy or uni-/bilateral neck exploration
- Imaging does not make hyperparathyroidism diagnosis [serum calcium, parathyroid hormone (PTH), & urine calcium make diagnosis]
- US best 1st examination for localizing most PTA
- Tc-99m sestamibi concentrates in PTG lesions & useful for locating ectopic PTA
- 4D CT detects smaller lesions better than sestamibi scan
  - 3 phases of scan acquisition to compare density of lesion with that of thyroid: Precontrast, arterial at 25-30 s, 7 delayed (venous) at 80-90 s
  - 4th dimension of 4D CT: Time (multiple data points)
- Dynamic contrast-enhanced (DCE) parathyroid MR
  - Pros: No radiation; can be repeated many times
  - Cons: No native bright thyroid signal for comparison
- **Predictors of multigland disease on 4D CT**
  - Smaller PTG lesion size on 4D CT (< 7 mm, 85% specific)
  - Either multiple PTG lesions or no PTG lesion on 4D CT
  - Lower Wisconsin index score (product of serum calcium in mg/dl & PTH levels in picogram/ml)

GRAPHICS

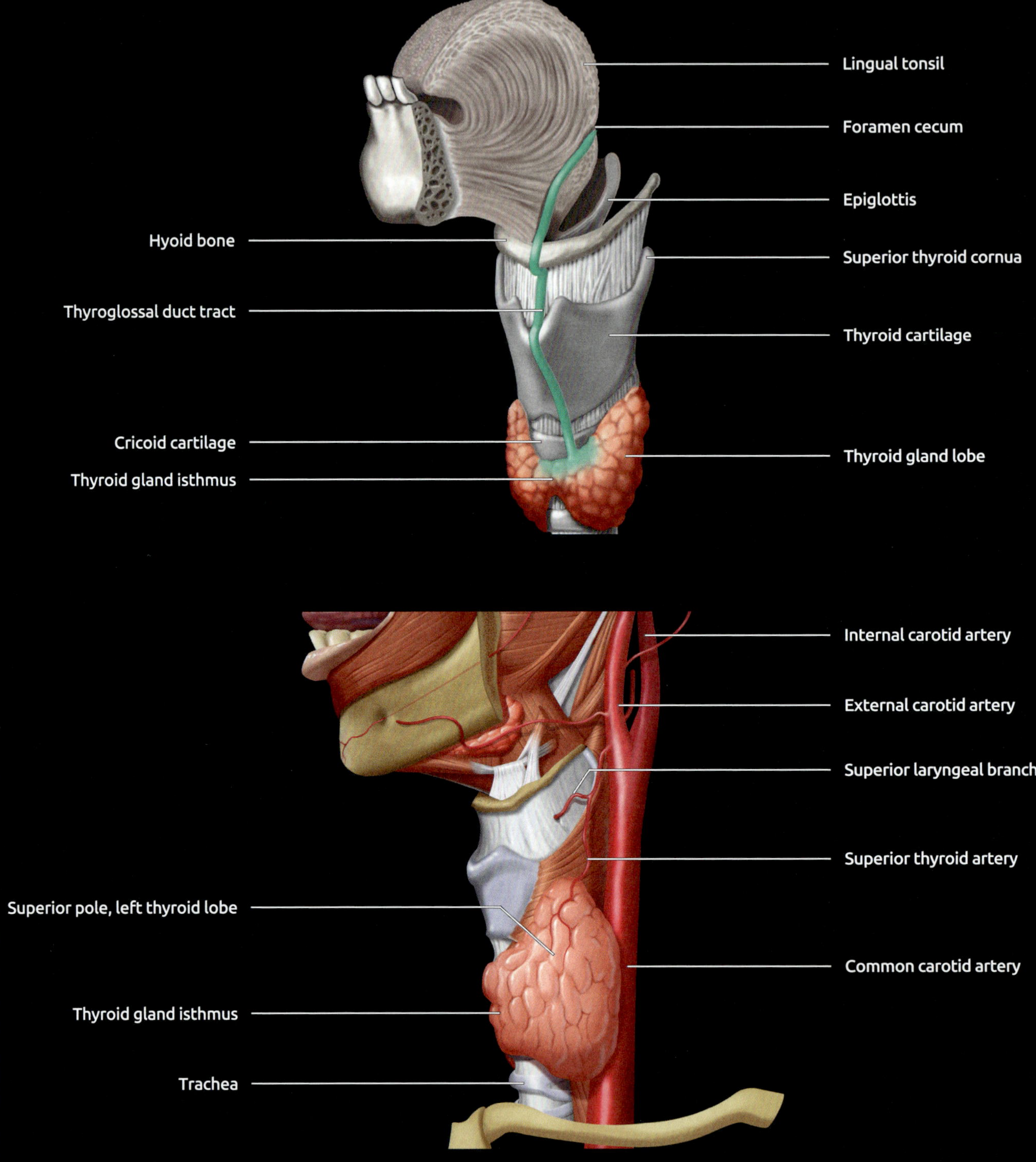

(Top) *Sagittal oblique graphic displays thyroglossal duct tract as it traverses the cervical neck from its origin at the foramen cecum to its termination in the anterior & lateral visceral space of the infrahyoid neck. The thyroid is the 1st endocrine gland to develop. At ~ 24-days gestation, it develops from a median endodermal thyroid diverticulum, the medial anlage, arising from the paramedian aspect of the 1st & 2nd branchial pouches (foramen cecum of tongue area). The lower end of diverticulum enlarges to form the gland, & the rest remains narrow (called thyroglossal duct). It descends through the tongue base, floor of mouth, around & in front of the hyoid bone, & through an area of infrahyoid strap muscles to a final position in thyroid bed of visceral space. Thyroglossal duct begins to involute by 7-10 weeks of gestation; its lower end often persists as pyramidal lobe. Lateral thyroid lobes may form from 4th & 6th branchial pouches (lateral anlagen). The fetal thyroid becomes functional during the 3rd month of gestation.* **(Bottom)** *Oblique graphic of the neck shows superior thyroid artery as 1st branch of external carotid artery. Its proximal course is closely associated with superior laryngeal nerve.*

GRAPHICS

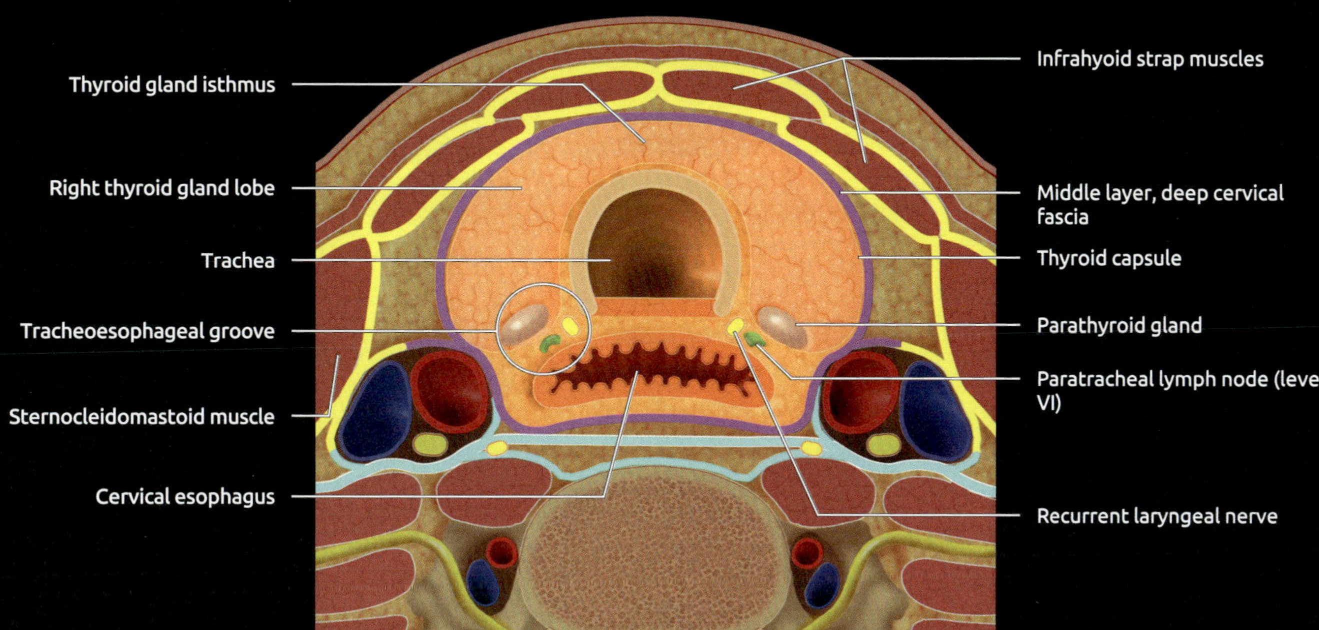

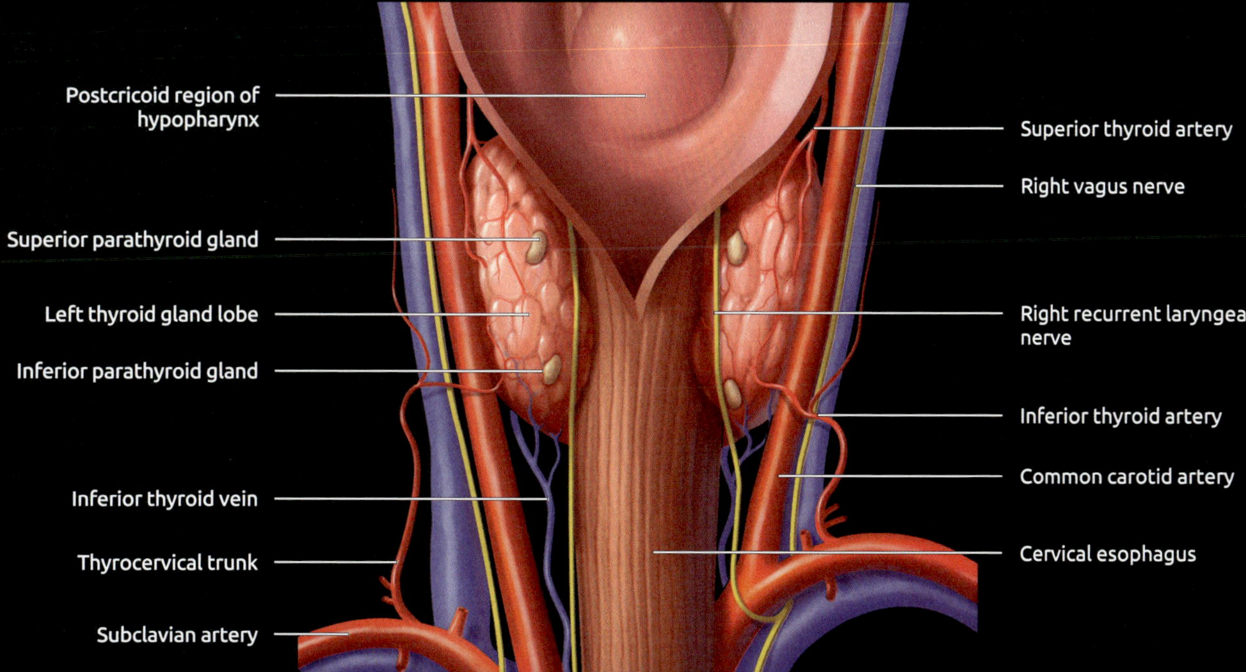

(Top) *Axial graphic at the thyroid level depicts the thyroid lobes and isthmus in the anterior visceral space wrapping around the trachea. Note that the coverage of strap muscles by the superficial layer of deep cervical fascia (SL-DCF, yellow outline) is controversial in literature with many considering it to be covered by the middle layer of deep cervical fascia (ML-DCF, pink outline), which covers the visceral space/thyroid gland also. SL-DCF surrounds sternomastoid muscles. Notice that there are 3 key structures found in the area of the tracheoesophageal groove: The recurrent laryngeal nerve, paratracheal lymph node chain, & parathyroid gland (PTG). The PTGs may be inside or outside of the thyroid capsule. Thyroid gland inner true capsule is formed by peripheral condensed connective tissue of gland, whereas the outer false capsule is formed by ML-DCF.* **(Bottom)** *Coronal graphic shows the thyroid and PTGs from behind. It depicts the typical anatomic relationships of the paired superior & inferior PTGs closely applied to the posterior lobes of the thyroid gland. Note the arterial supply to the superior & inferior thyroid lobes & the superior & inferior thyroid arteries, respectively.*

AXIAL CECT

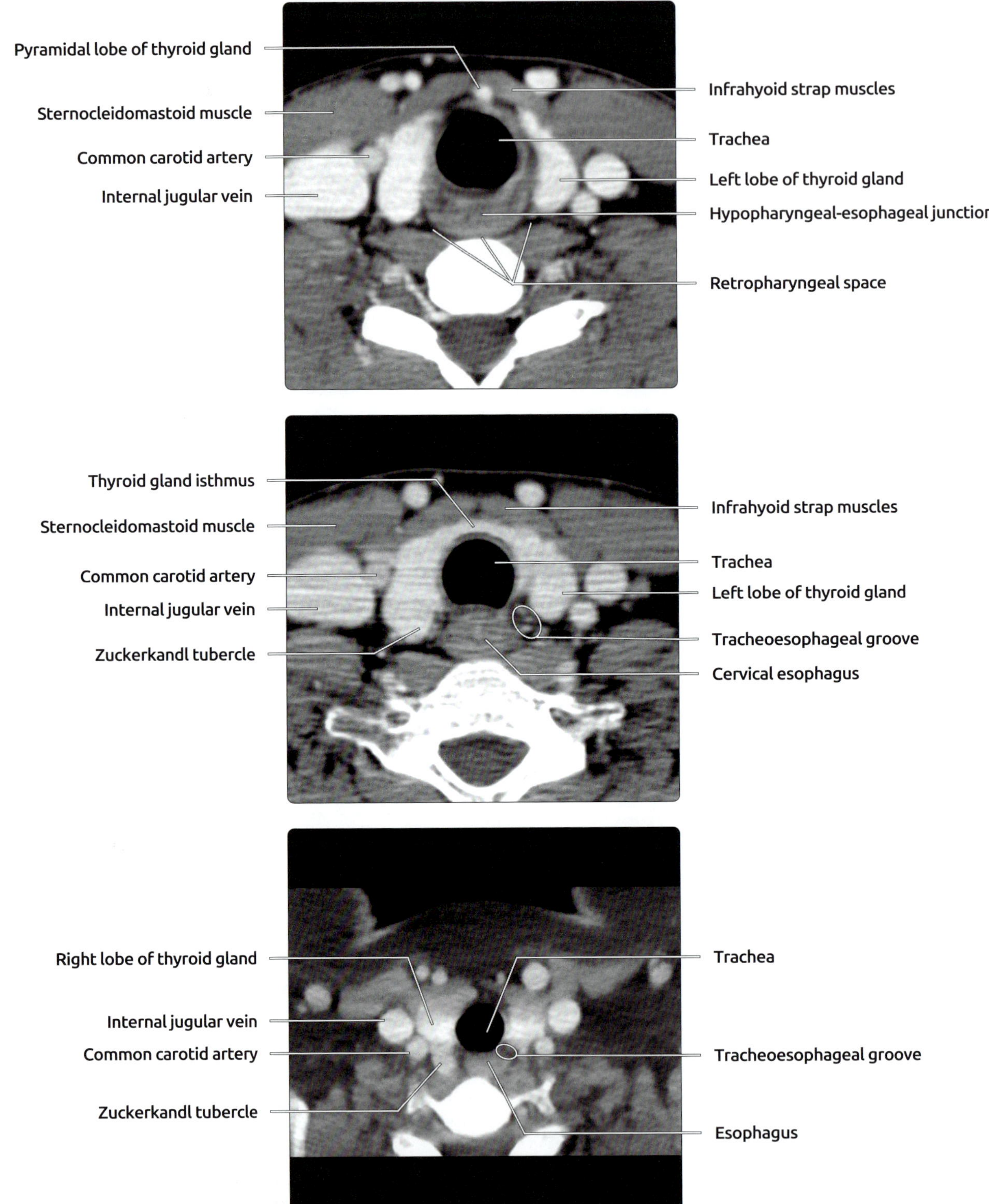

(Top) *First of 2 axial CECT images presented from superior to inferior shows a small, superiorly projecting pyramidal lobe in the anterior midline just beneath the infrahyoid strap muscles. Notice the retropharyngeal space fat stripe extends posterior to the thyroid lobes & esophagus.* **(Middle)** *In this image, the thyroid lobes are found along the lateral margin of the trachea. A more prominent right posterior thyroid protuberance is described as the Zuckerkandl tubercle, which is a landmark for surgeons for the location of the recurrent laryngeal nerve & superior PTG. Nodularity in this gland portion can mimic a tracheoesophageal groove node or enlarged PTG.* **(Bottom)** *Axial CECT in another patient shows a prominent Zuckerkandl tubercle on the right side, which shows an enhancement pattern the same as that of the rest of the thyroid gland. This should not be mistaken for a differentially enhancing parathyroid adenoma. The tracheoesophageal groove has been circled on the left. Remember that the recurrent laryngeal nerve, paratracheal nodes, and PTGs can all be normally found in this location. None of these structures are typically visible on routine enhanced CT images.*

CORONAL CECT

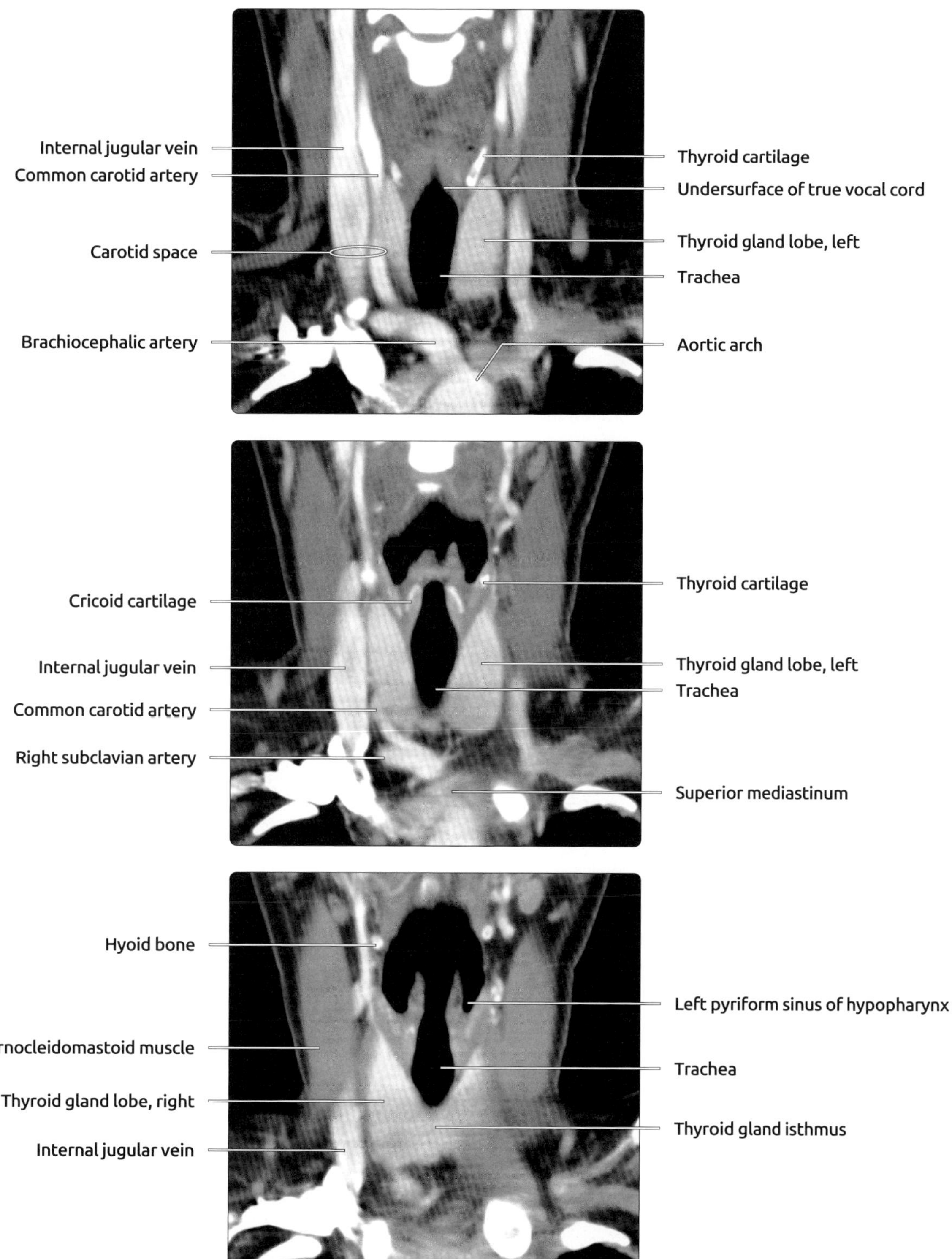

(Top) *First of 3 coronal CECT reformations presented from posterior to anterior demonstrates the 2 lobes of the thyroid gland with the trachea on their medial borders. Lateral to each of the thyroid lobes are the carotid spaces containing the vagus nerve, common carotid artery, & internal jugular vein.* **(Middle)** *In this image, the chevron-shaped lobes of the thyroid gland are particularly well seen. Notice the intimate relationship between the superomedial thyroid gland & the larynx. Remember that thyroid gland malignancy 1st-order nodes are the paratracheal nodes. The paratracheal nodes drain inferiorly into the superior mediastinum. Consequently, it is important for the radiologist to image to the aortic arch in cases of thyroid gland malignancy.* **(Bottom)** *The isthmus of the thyroid gland is visible just anterior to the trachea in this image. Malignancy evaluation of the thyroid & adjacent structures like the larynx & hypopharynx should include careful scrutiny of the images both in soft tissue [window width/level of ~ 300 Hounsfield units (HU)/100 HU] & cartilage windows (width/level of ~ 1700 HU/600 HU).*

TRANSVERSE ULTRASOUND

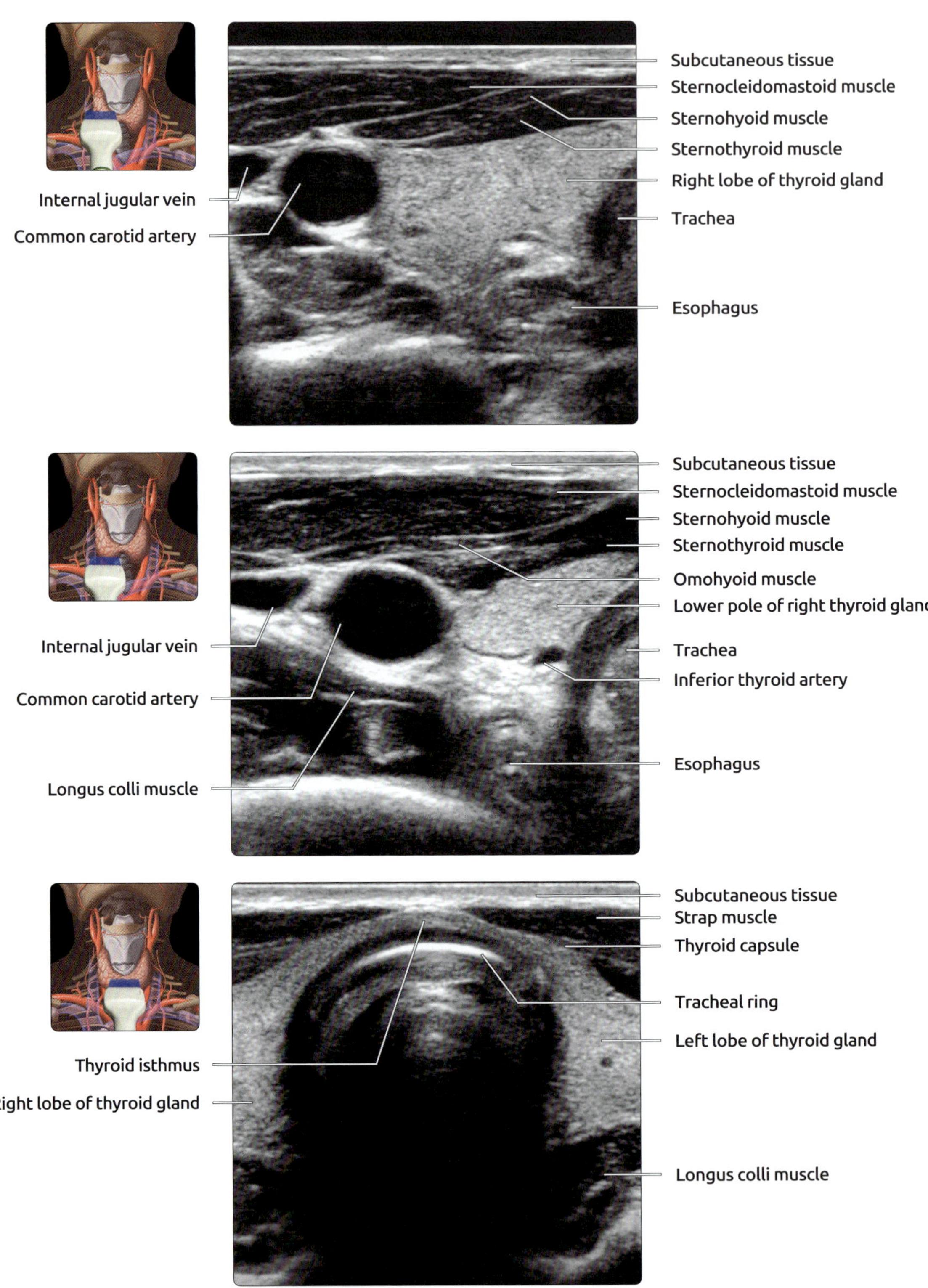

(Top) *Transverse grayscale ultrasound of the right lobe of the thyroid gland shows the homogeneous, hyperechoic echo pattern of the glandular parenchyma. Note its close anatomic relationship with the major vessels of the carotid sheath (internal jugular vein & common carotid artery) laterally, the trachea medially, & the cervical esophagus posteromedially.* **(Middle)** *Transverse grayscale ultrasound shows the level of the inferior pole of the thyroid gland. The inferior thyroid artery is a consistent finding related to & supplying the inferior pole.* **(Bottom)** *Midline transverse grayscale ultrasound shows the thyroid isthmus connecting the 2 lobes. The isthmus lies on the anterior surface of the trachea. In view of the intimate anatomic relationship between the thyroid gland & the trachea, a local tumor invasion into the trachea from malignant thyroid carcinoma can occur, rendering surgical excision more extensive than total thyroidectomy.*

LONGITUDINAL ULTRASOUND

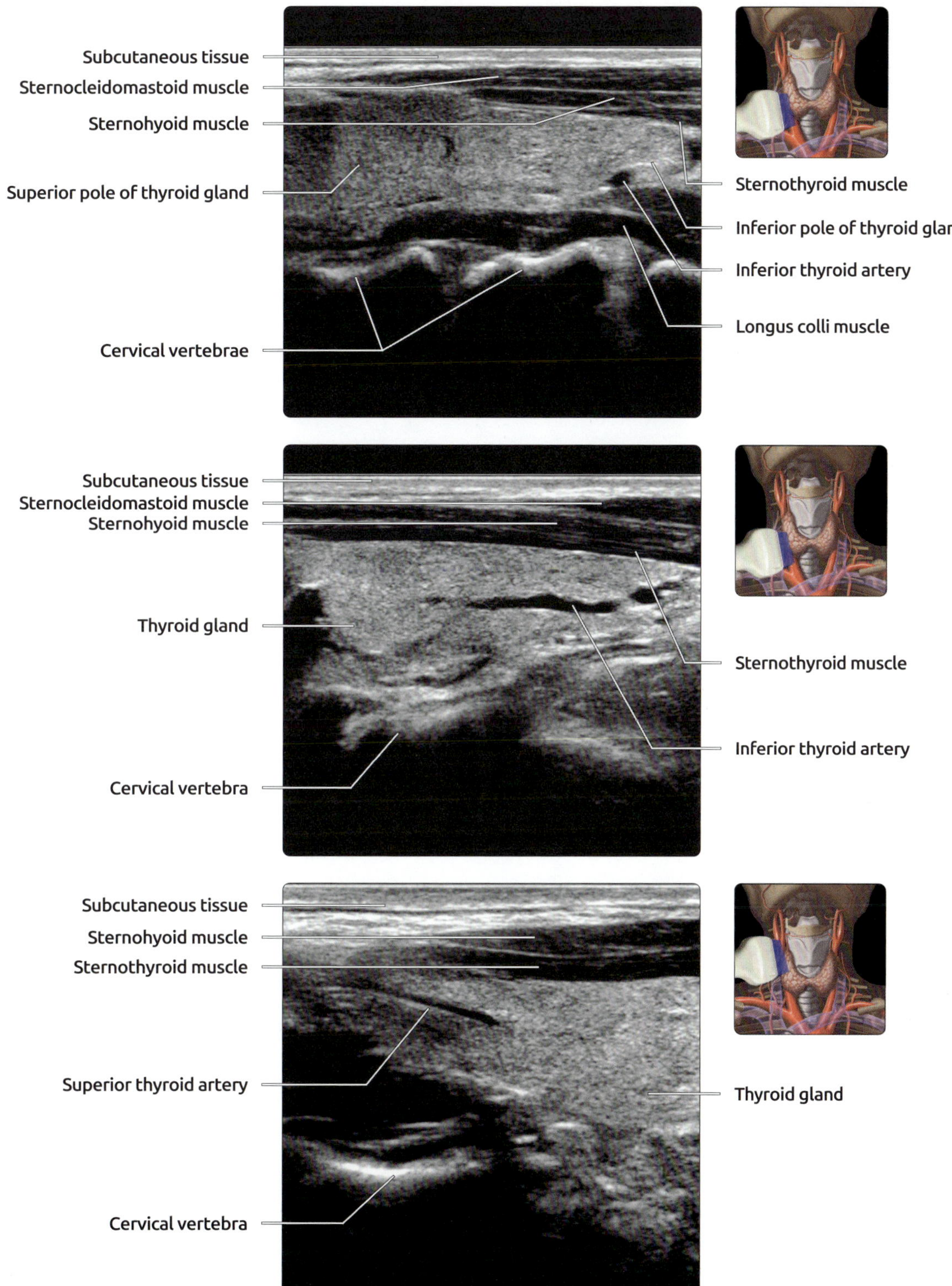

(Top) *Parasagittal longitudinal grayscale ultrasound shows the thyroid gland. The homogeneous, hyperechoic echo pattern of the glandular parenchyma is better assessed on longitudinal scans. Part of the tortuous course of the inferior thyroid artery is seen in relation to the lower pole.* **(Middle)** *Parasagittal longitudinal grayscale ultrasound shows the inferior thyroid artery coursing superiorly from the inferior pole within the glandular parenchyma.* **(Bottom)** *Parasagittal longitudinal grayscale ultrasound shows the superior thyroid artery, the 1st anterior branch of the external carotid artery, running inferiorly within & supplying the upper pole of the thyroid gland. Longitudinal scans best evaluate the glandular parenchyma & vascularity.*

GRAPHICS OF THYROID LESION

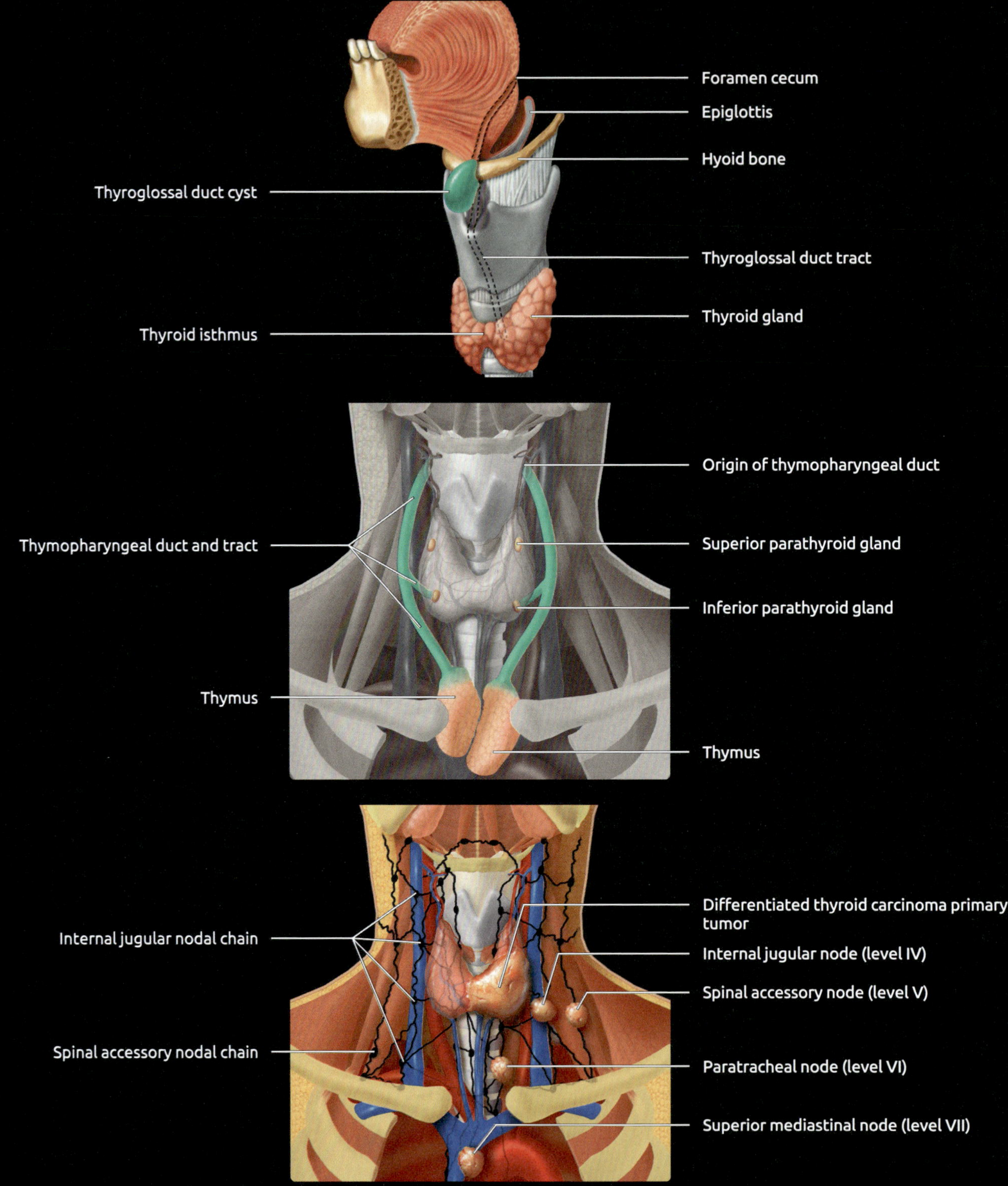

(Top) *Sagittal oblique graphic shows a thyroglossal duct cyst (TDC) at hyoid bone level. TDCs (failure of involution of duct) or thyroid tissue remnants may be found anywhere along its tract from foramen cecum at tongue base to just anterior to thyroid lobes. Most TDCs are located near the hyoid bone with 50% at hyoid bone & 20-25% in suprahyoid neck, often in midline; remaining 25% are located in the infrahyoid neck, in midline, or within strap muscles in a paramidline location. Most common thyroid ectopia is in the lingual thyroid.* **(Middle)** *AP graphic of the cervical neck shows the course of inferomedial migration of thymic primordia & inferior PTGs along paired thymopharyngeal duct tracts. Note that the tracts extend from lateral hypopharyngeal area to anterior mediastinum. Variable descent of inferior PTGs may result in ectopic locations along thymopharyngeal ducts.* **(Bottom)** *Coronal graphic of infrahyoid neck & superior mediastinum shows left thyroid lobe & isthmus differentiated thyroid carcinoma primary. Notice that in addition to nodal metastases in internal jugular & spinal accessory chains, there are also nodal metastases in paratracheal & superior mediastinal nodal groups.*

GENERIC TRACHEOESOPHAGEAL GROOVE MASS

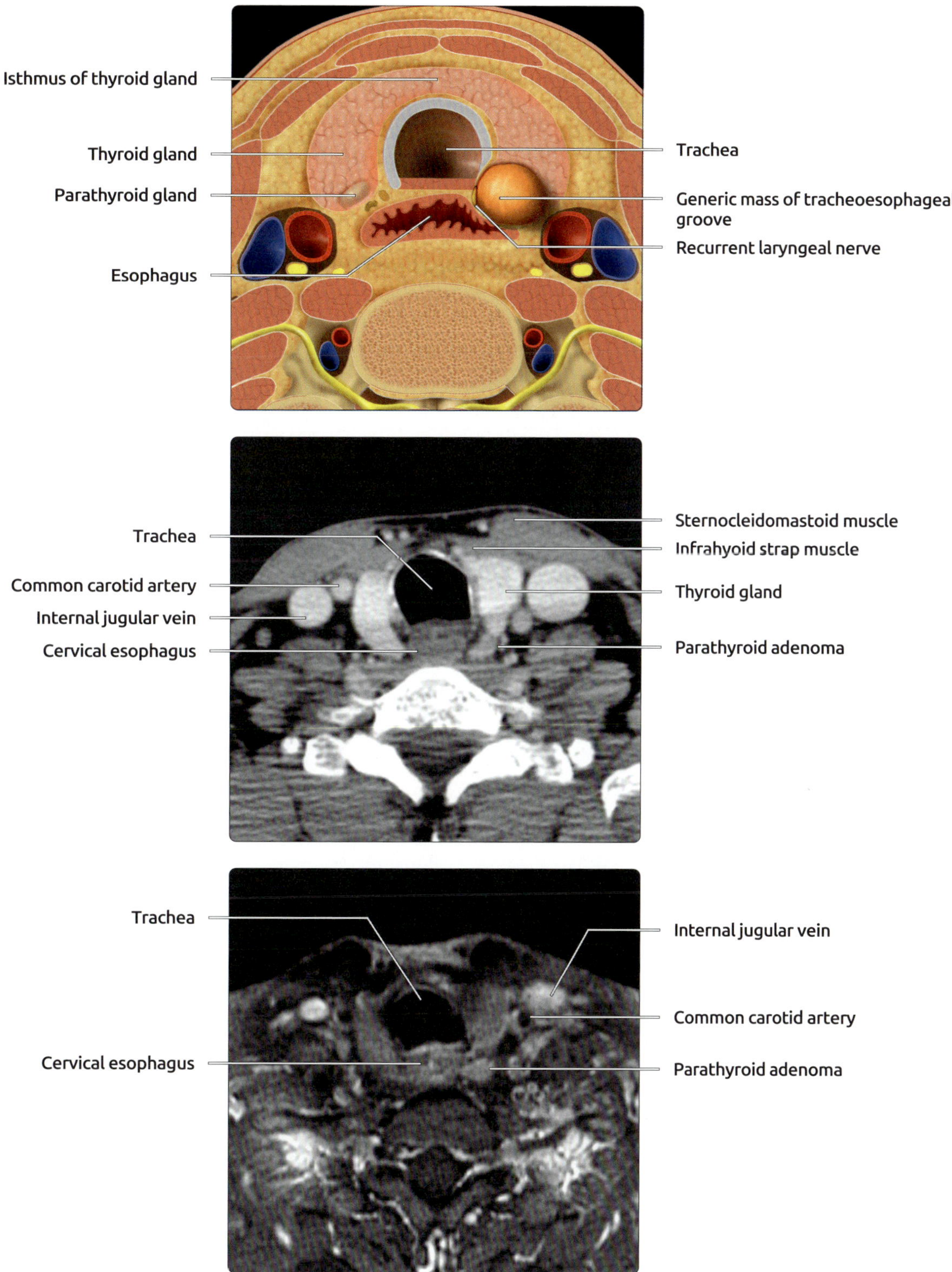

(Top) *Axial graphic shows a well-circumscribed generic mass in the left tracheoesophageal groove, causing mass effect on the recurrent laryngeal nerve, esophagus, trachea, & left thyroid lobe. Parathyroid adenoma (PTA), recurrent laryngeal nerve schwannoma, & nodal disease in the paratracheal nodal chain all could cause such an appearance.* **(Middle)** *Axial CECT at the level of the thyroid gland shows an enhancing PTA in the left tracheoesophageal groove, posterior to the left thyroid lobe. In a patient with hypercalcemia & elevated parathormone, this location & appearance is diagnostic.* **(Bottom)** *Axial T1 contrast-enhanced fat-saturated MR at the level of the thyroid bed demonstrates an enhancing PTA posterior to the left lobe of the thyroid in the left tracheoesophageal groove.*

GRAPHICS OF PARATHYROID AND GLAND EMBRYOLOGY & 3D CTA

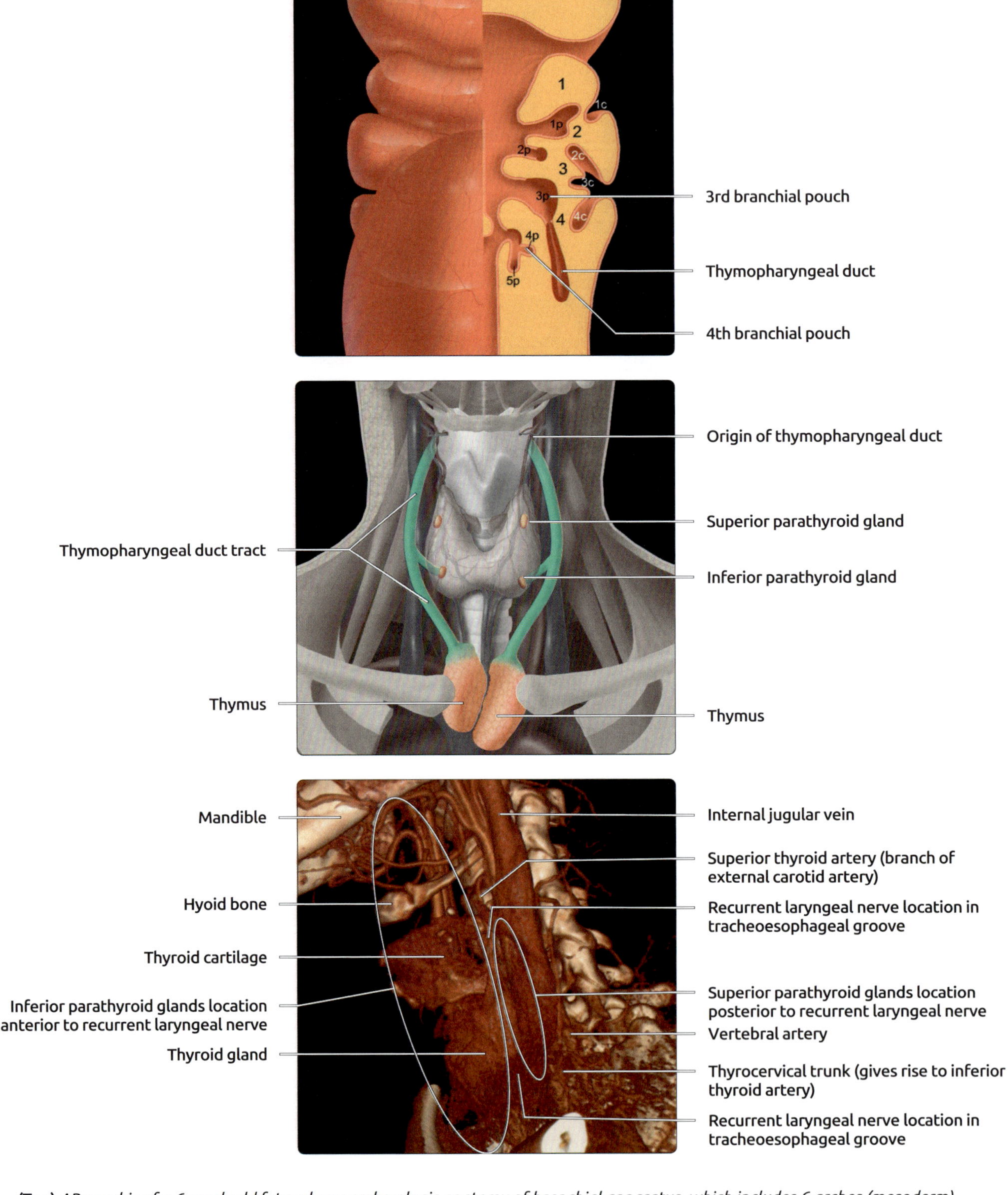

(Top) *AP graphic of a 6-week-old fetus shows embryologic anatomy of branchial apparatus, which includes 6 arches (mesoderm) interfaced by 4 clefts (ectoderm) & pouches (endoderm) on each side at the end of the 4th week of embryonic life. 5th arch is rudimentary & does not contribute to formation of any adult structure. Superior PTGs develop from 4th branchial pouches along with primordial thyroid. Superior PTGs & thyroid gland migrate caudally along thyroglossal duct. Less than 2% of superior PTGs are ectopic. Inferior PTGs develop from 3rd branchial pouches along with anlage of thymus. Inferior PTGs & primordial thymus migrate caudally along thymopharyngeal duct & may descend into anterior mediastinum. Up to 35% of inferior PTGs can be in ectopic locations.* **(Middle)** *AP graphic of the neck shows the course of inferomedial migration of thymic primordia & inferior PTGs along paired thymopharyngeal duct tracts from the lateral hypopharyngeal area to the anterior mediastinum.* **(Bottom)** *Left lateral oblique CTA reformat shows the expected locations of superior & inferior PTGs, posterior to & anterior to the recurrent laryngeal nerve in the tracheoesophageal groove.*

ECTOPIC PARATHYROID ADENOMA

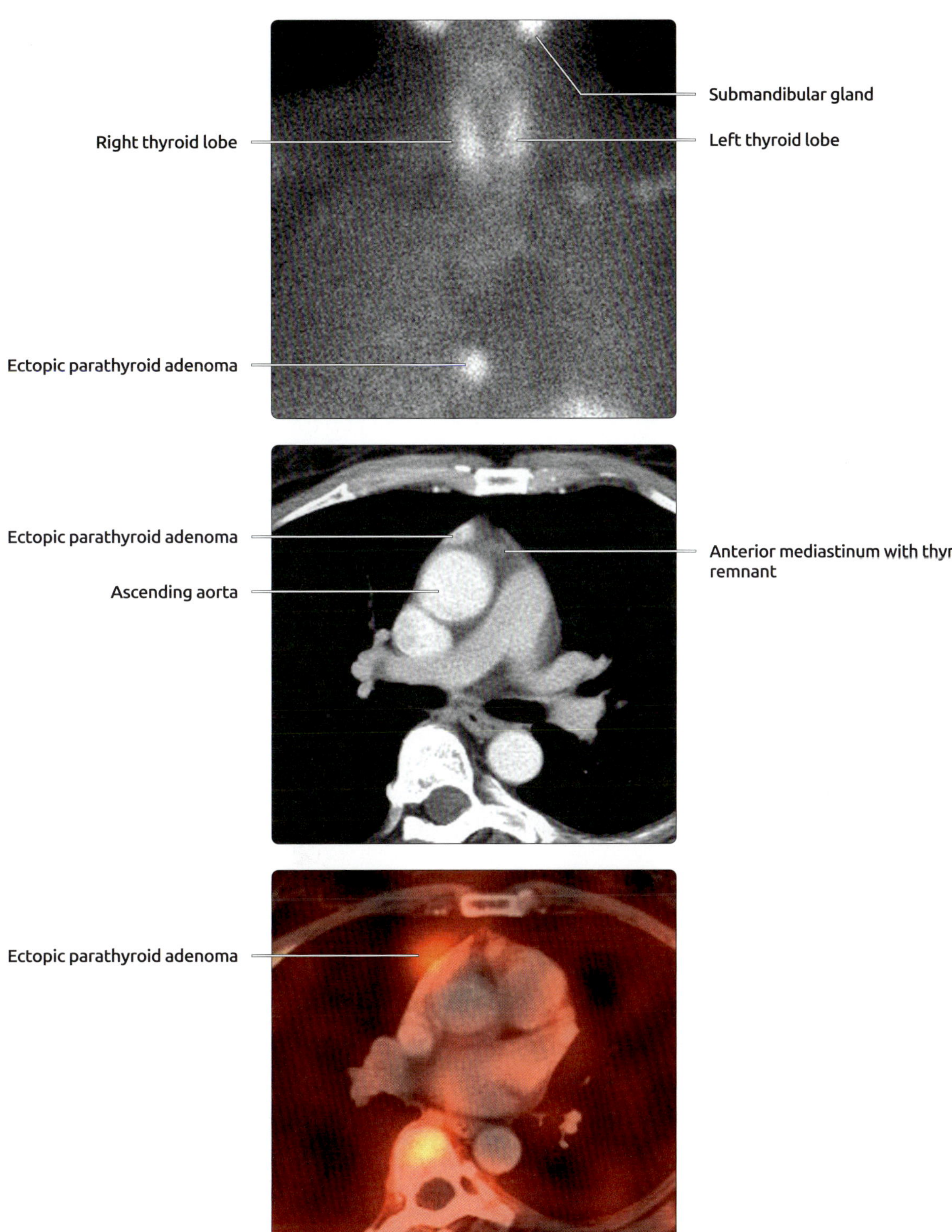

(Top) *Hypercalcemic patient with elevated parathormone underwent a Tc-99m sestamibi nuclear medicine scan. In this 120-minute delayed scan, an area of persistent concentration of isotope is visible in the mediastinum. In this clinical setting, an ectopic PTA can be diagnosed. Persistent activity is also visualized in the thyroid & submandibular salivary glands. CECT is ordered for presurgical localization.* **(Middle)** *Axial CECT at the level of the main pulmonary artery demonstrates an enhancing PTA in the anterior mediastinum, anterior to the ascending aorta.* **(Bottom)** *Axial fusion image of a CECT & Tc-99m sestamibi nuclear medicine scan at the level of the left atrium shows ectopic radiotracer activity in an anterior mediastinal PTA.*

CLINICAL CORRELATES: PARATHYROID ADENOMA

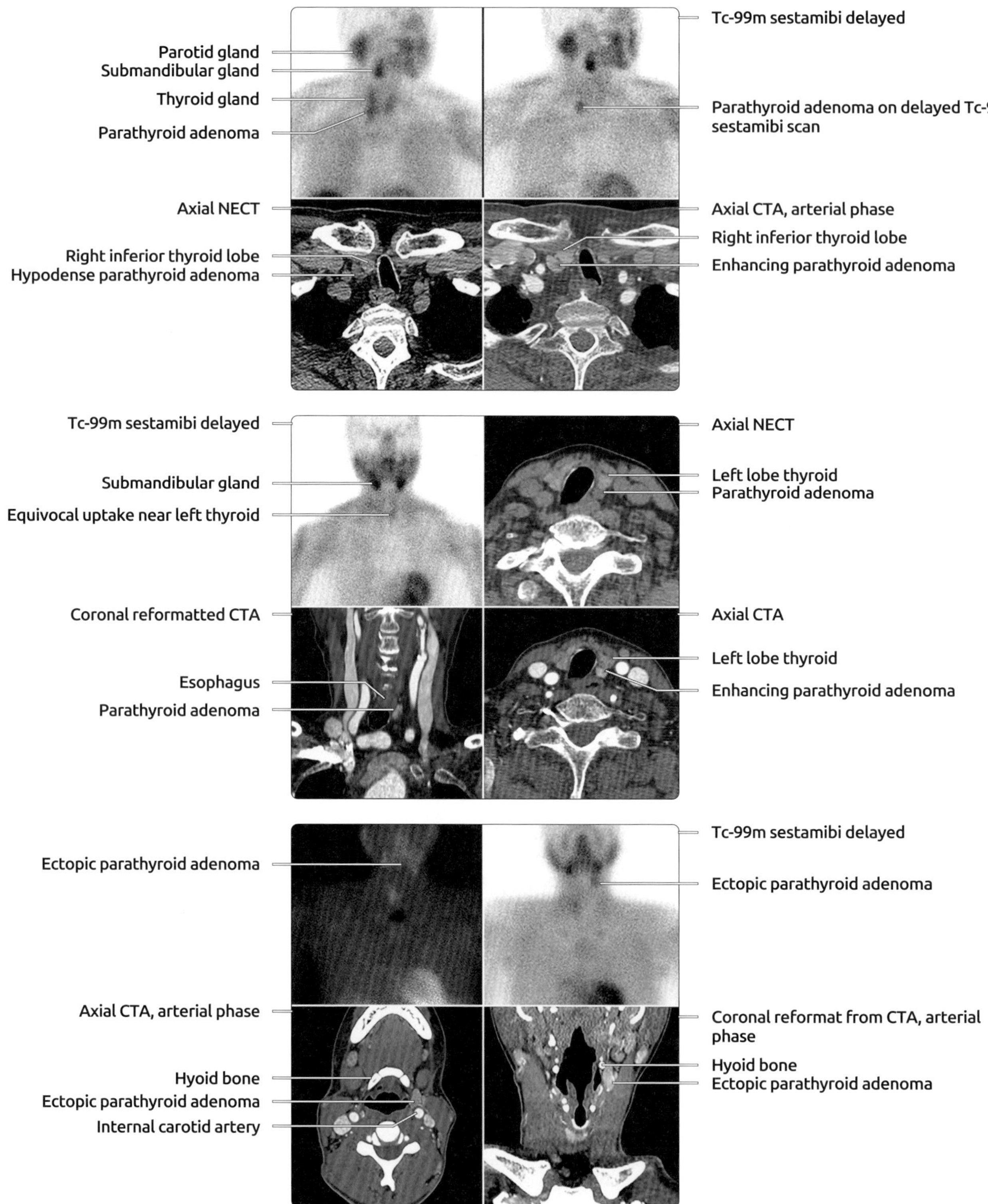

(Top) *Hyperparathyroidism & PTA are shown. Early & delayed Tc-99m sestamibi scans demonstrate uptake in PTA just adjacent to the inferior margin right lobe thyroid gland. Thyroid uptake disappears on delayed images, allowing greater conspicuity of PTA. NECT through this region demonstrates slightly hyperdense thyroid tissue medially & hypodense PTA posterolaterally. During the early arterial phase, PTA enhances & is now isodense to the thyroid gland.* **(Middle)** *Hyperparathyroidism & PTA are shown. Sestamibi scan is equivocal in demonstrating left PTA. NECT demonstrates small soft tissue nodule in the left tracheoesophageal groove. CTA, arterial phase, demonstrates brisk enhancement of nodule, helping localize the PTA.* **(Bottom)** *Hyperparathyroidism & PTA are shown. Patient underwent exploration for PTA, but no PTA was found. Sestamibi revealed a small focus of abnormal uptake in the left suprahyoid neck, just below the submandibular gland; CTA shows enhancing PTA just anterior to the internal carotid artery & just below the submandibular gland.*

PARATHYROID ULTRASOUND

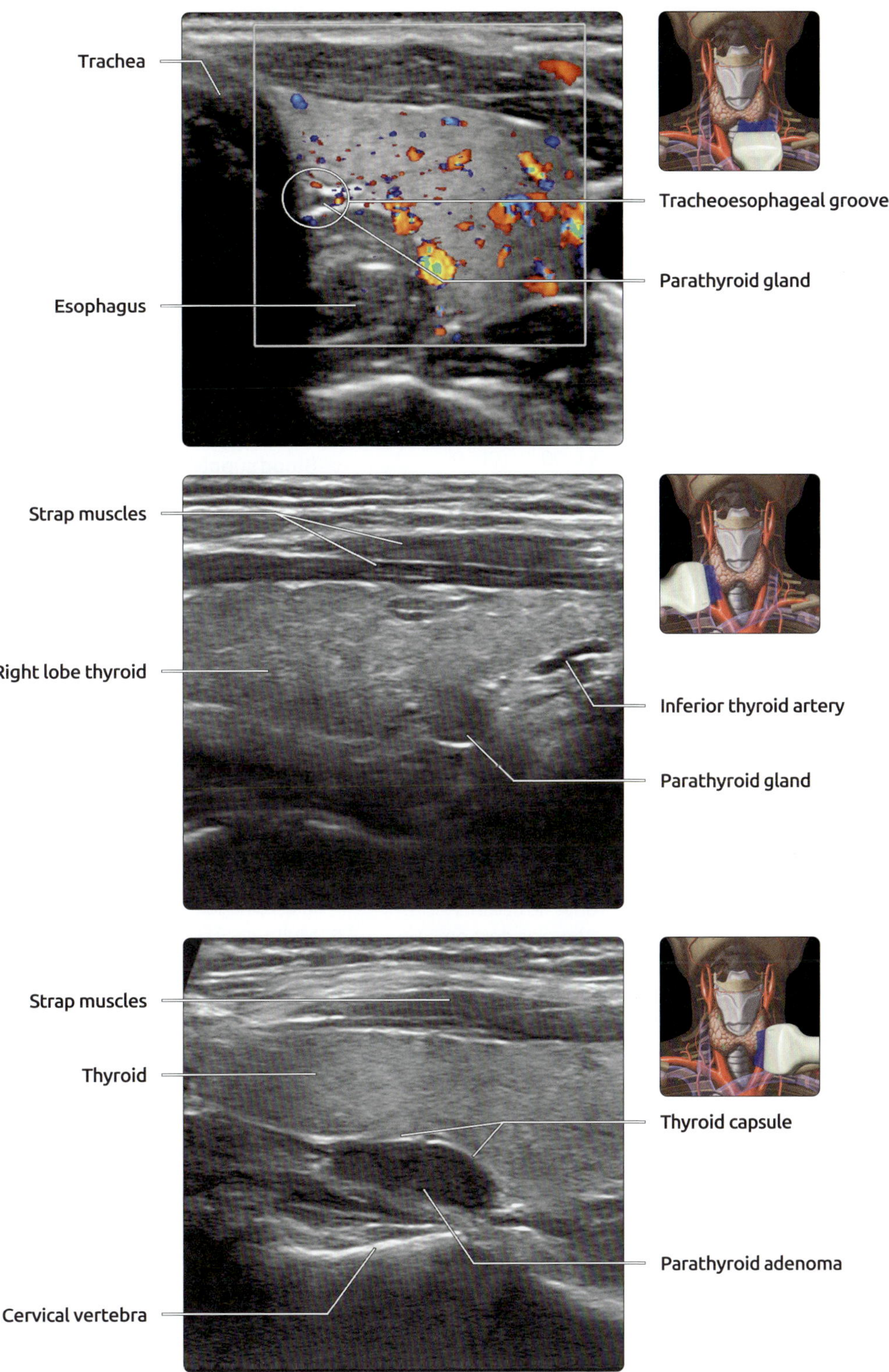

(Top) *Transverse color Doppler ultrasound of the midportion of the left thyroid lobe shows the tracheoesophageal groove. The normal PTG is located in this area & is small, round to elliptical, & hypoechoic, but is often difficult to identify with certainty.* **(Middle)** *Longitudinal scan of the right thyroid shows a larger, hypoechoic nodule in the expected location of the PTG, posterior middle 1/3 of the thyroid gland. This is the typical location of the superior PTGs. Careful analysis during a real-time scan should be done to prove they are outside the thyroid capsule & not a thyroid nodule. A PTG may also sometimes be confused with a small lymph node, but a normal lymph node should have an echogenic hilum.* **(Bottom)** *Longitudinal ultrasound of the left lobe of the thyroid in a patient with hypercalcemia shows a well-defined, ovoid, hypoechoic mass. Note the distinct thyroid capsule, confirming this is posterior to the thyroid & therefore likely a PTG rather than a thyroid nodule.*

TERMINOLOGY

Definitions

- Cervical trachea: Superior portion of trachea extending from larynx to thoracic inlet
- Cervical esophagus: Superior portion of esophagus extending from pharynx to thoracic inlet

IMAGING ANATOMY

Overview

- Trachea
  - 10- to 13-cm semirigid tube extending in midline from inferior larynx at ~ 6th cervical vertebral body to carina at upper margin of 5th thoracic vertebral body
- Esophagus
  - Muscular tube connecting hypopharynx to stomach, extending ~ C6 to T11 vertebral levels in adults, ~ 25 cm in adults and 8-10 cm at birth
  - Descends behind trachea and thyroid, lying in front of lower cervical vertebrae
    - Inclines slightly to left in lower neck and upper mediastinum, returning to midline at T5 vertebral level

Anatomy Relationships

- **Cervical trachea**
  - Anterior: Infrahyoid strap muscles; isthmus of thyroid gland (2nd-4th tracheal cartilages)
  - Lateral: Lobes of thyroid gland
    - Tracheoesophageal groove structures: Recurrent laryngeal nerve, paratracheal nodes, parathyroid glands
  - Posterior: Cervical esophagus
- **Cervical esophagus**
  - Anterior: Cervical trachea
  - Anterolateral: Tracheoesophageal groove structures
  - Lateral: Carotid spaces on both sides, thoracic duct on left side at C6 level
  - Posterior: Retropharyngeal/danger spaces

Internal Contents

- **Cervical trachea**
  - **Cartilage anatomy**
    - Trachea has 15-20 "incomplete ring" of cartilage forming anterior 2/3
    - Flat, cartilage-deficient posterior portion of fibromuscular tissue
    - D-shaped with flat side posterior on cross section
    - Smooth muscle fibers in posterior membrane (trachealis muscle) provide alteration in tracheal cross-sectional area
  - **Cervical tracheal mucosa**
    - Continuous sheet from larynx above
    - Layer of pseudostratified ciliated columnar epithelium interspersed with goblet cells with both lying on basal lamina
    - Minor salivary glands sporadically distributed in tracheal mucosa
    - Trachea has 3 layers: Mucosa, cartilage, and adventitia
  - **Blood supply**: Inferior thyroid arteries and veins
  - **Lymphatic drainage**: Level VI, pretracheal and paratracheal nodes
- **Cervical esophagus**
  - Begins at lower border of cricoid cartilage as continuation of hypopharynx
    - Cricopharyngeus muscle arises from either side of cricoid cartilage and creates muscular sling that encircles proximal esophagus, helping to form upper esophageal sphincter complex
    - Innervated by pharyngeal plexus
    - Unlike inferior pharyngeal constrictor, cricopharyngeus does not insert upon median raphe
    - Narrowest portion is at beginning, at level of cricopharyngeal sphincter
  - **Cervical esophageal mucosa**
    - Nonkeratinized stratified squamous epithelium
  - **Musculature**: Outer longitudinal and inner circular muscle layers
    - Circular muscle layer: Peristalsis
  - **Blood supply and drainage**: Inferior thyroid arteries and veins
  - **Lymphatic drainage**: Level IV, level VI, and paratracheal nodes

Fascia

- Middle layer, deep cervical fascia surrounds visceral space with trachea and esophagus inside

ANATOMY IMAGING ISSUES

Imaging Approaches

- **Cervical trachea**
  - **Multislice CT** with sagittal and coronal reformations is exam of choice for trachea
- **Cervical esophagus**
  - **Air-contrast barium swallow** is primary diagnostic tool in esophageal evaluation
  - Multislice CECT for esophageal tumor staging

CLINICAL IMPLICATIONS

Clinical Importance

- Cervical tracheal lesions present with shortness of breath and stridor
  - May be treated for asthma prior to diagnosis
- Cervical esophageal lesions present with dysphagia
  - Aspiration pneumonia may occur prior to diagnosis

EMBRYOLOGY

Embryologic Events

- During 4th gestational week, respiratory primordium begins with formation of laryngotracheal groove that extends lengthwise in floor of gut just caudal to pharyngeal pouches
- Groove then deepens into laryngotracheal diverticulum whose ventral ectoderm become larynx and trachea
- Lateral furrows develop on either side of laryngotracheal diverticulum, then deepen to form laryngotracheal tube
- Tracheoesophageal septum then develops caudally to cranially, separating respiratory system from esophagus
- Esophageal atresia and tracheoesophageal fistula usually occur together

BARIUM SWALLOW

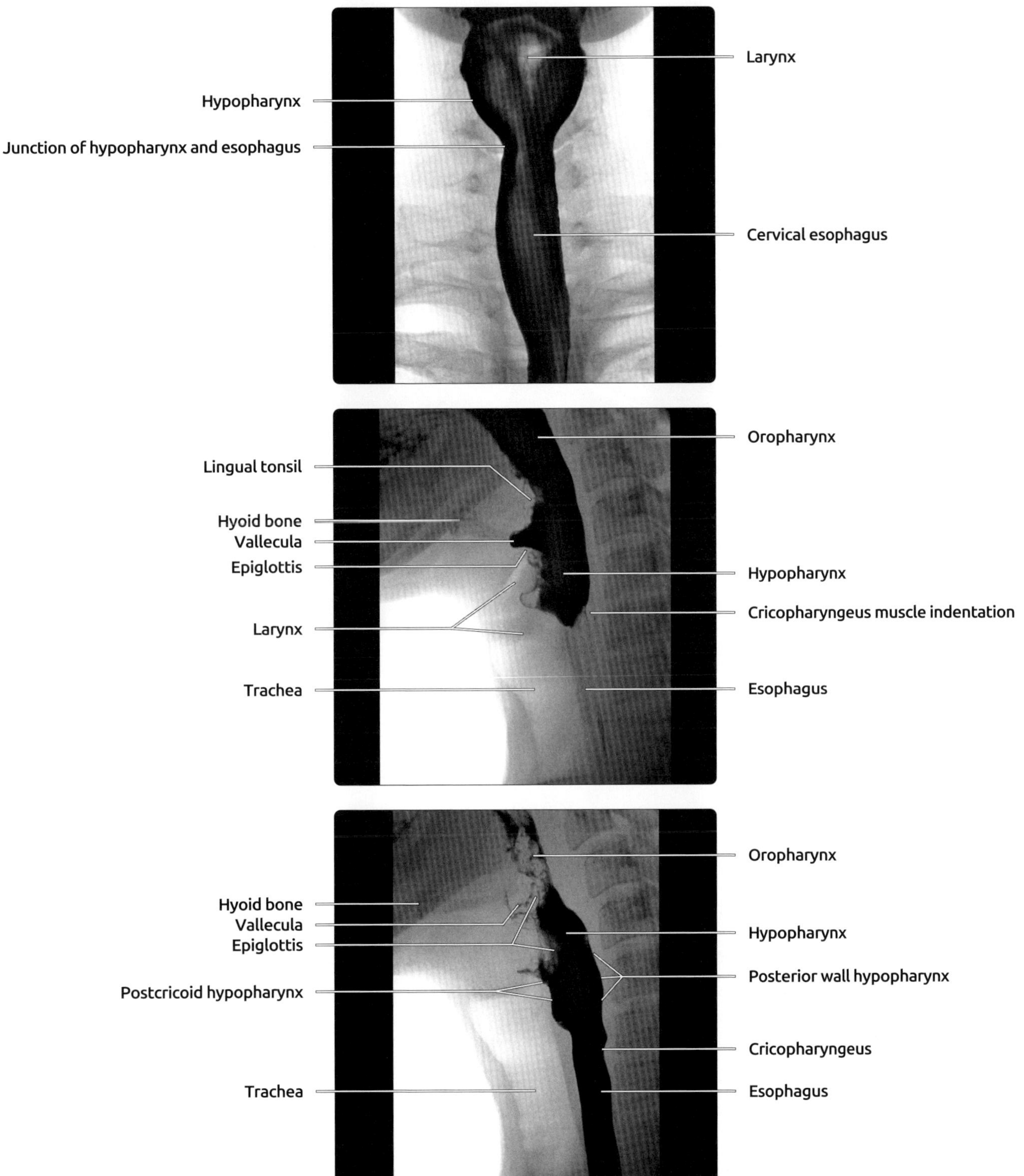

(Top) *Frontal view of a normal barium swallow shows barium deflected around the larynx that appears as a filling defect. Inferior cricoid cartilage delineates the inferior larynx and hypopharynx on CT studies as well as the junction of the hypopharynx with the cervical esophagus.* **(Middle)** *Lateral view of a barium swallow of the upper pharynx shows the junction of the oropharynx and hypopharynx at the hyoid bone. The lingual tonsil (base of tongue) causes a lobulated impression upon the anterior oropharynx. Epiglottis closes during swallowing to protect the larynx from aspiration. Valleculae are recesses between the tongue and epiglottis.* **(Bottom)** *Lateral view of a barium swallow shows the hypopharynx and cervical esophagus posterior to the larynx and trachea. The hypopharynx extends from the hyoid bone to the cricopharyngeus muscle. The cricopharyngeus muscle demarcates the hypopharynx from the cervical esophagus on barium studies and is typically located at the C5/C6 level.*

GRAPHICS: MUSCLES AND SPACES

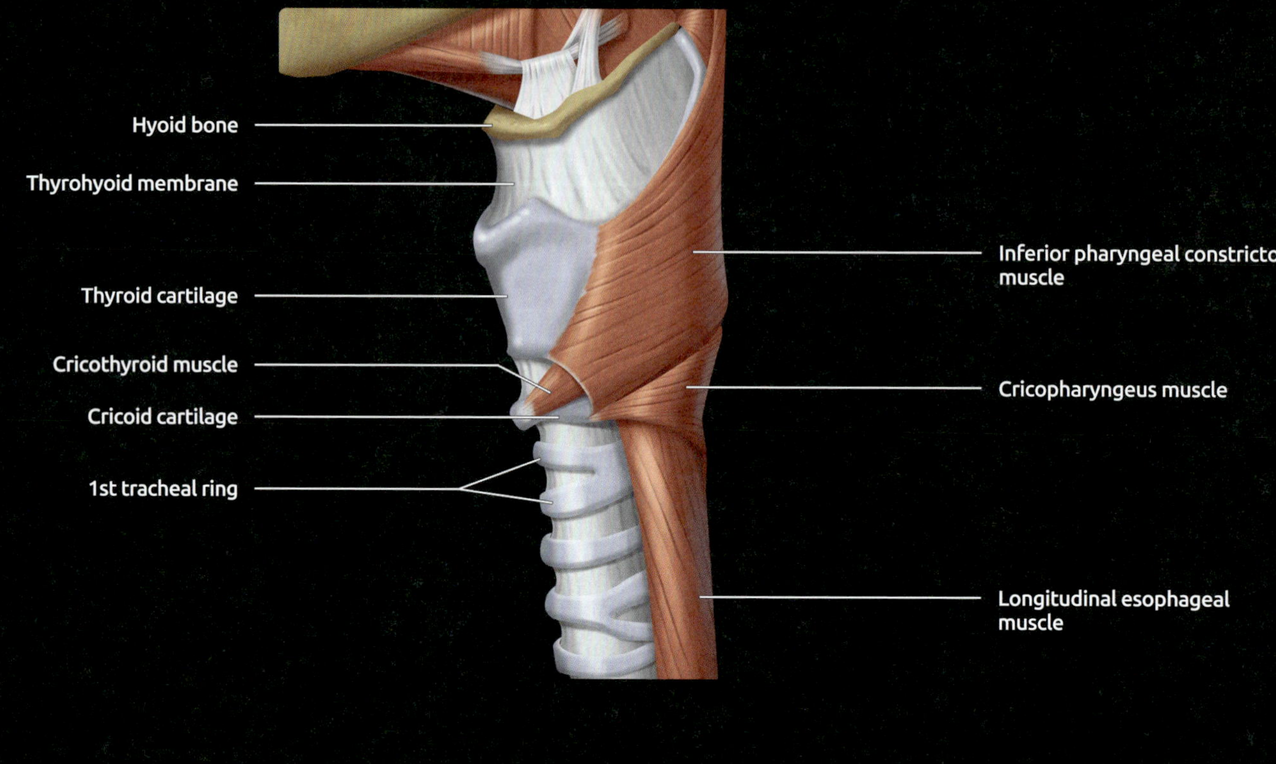

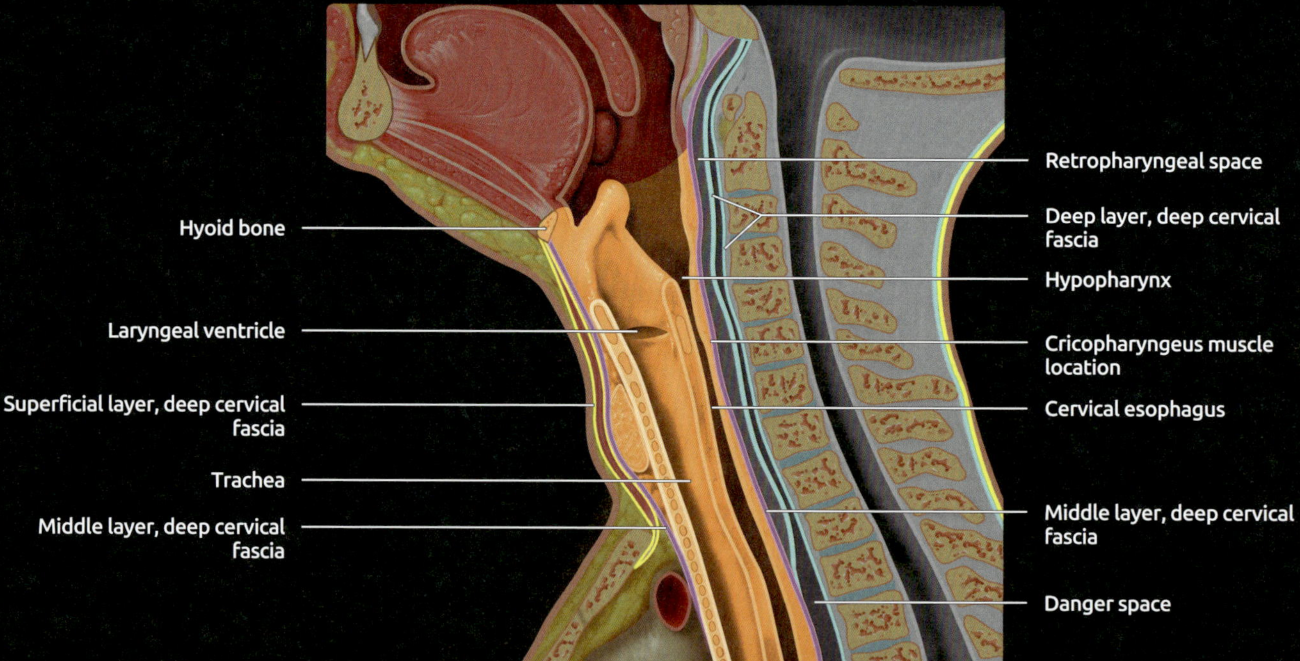

(Top) *Lateral graphic shows the junction of the larynx and hypopharynx with the trachea and esophagus. The cricopharyngeus muscle, which separates the hypopharynx from the cervical esophagus, is part of the inferior constrictor muscle. The esophagus is composed of outer longitudinal muscles and an inner circular muscle layer (not shown). The 1st tracheal ring is the broadest of all tracheal cartilages and is often merged to cricoid cartilage or the 2nd tracheal ring. Mucosal portions of the posterior trachea are separated from the esophagus by a thin layer of connective tissue, often called the "party wall," as it separates the trachea anteriorly from the esophagus posteriorly.* **(Bottom)** *Sagittal graphic shows the longitudinal relationships of the infrahyoid neck. Note the middle layer of deep cervical fascia (ML-DCF) (pink outline) encircles the trachea and esophagus as part of the visceral space. The trachea and esophagus are an inferior continuation of the airway and pharynx. Coverage of strap muscles by the superficial layer of deep cervical fascia (SL-DCF) (yellow outline) is controversial in the literature with many considering it to be covered by the ML-DCF.*

GRAPHICS

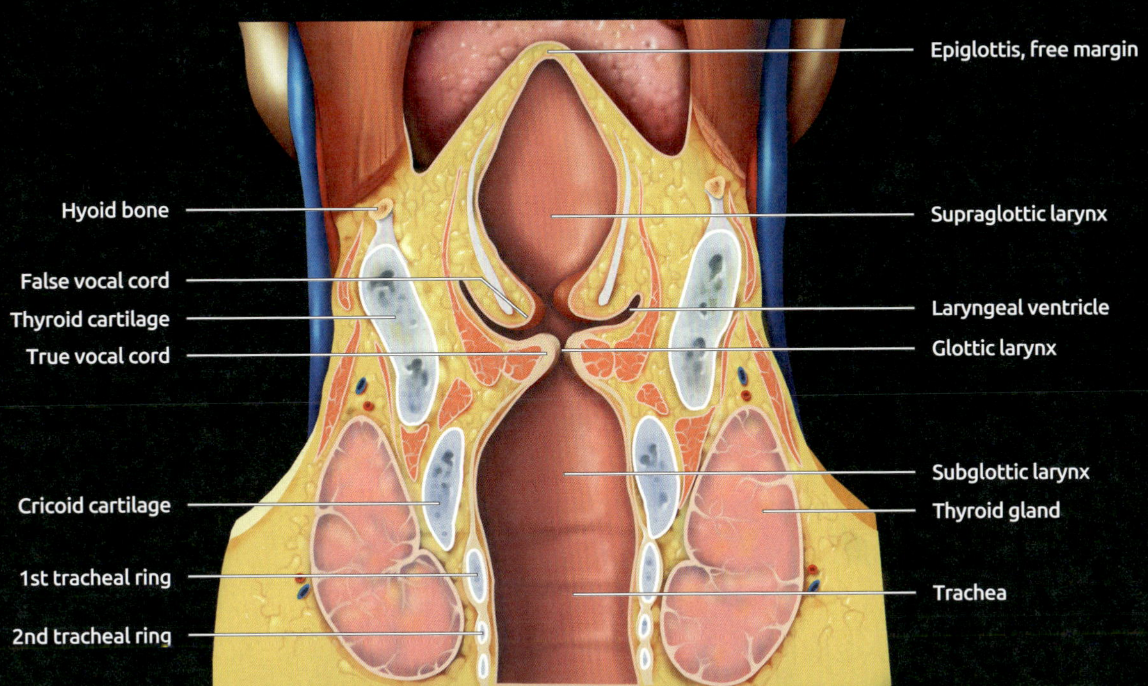

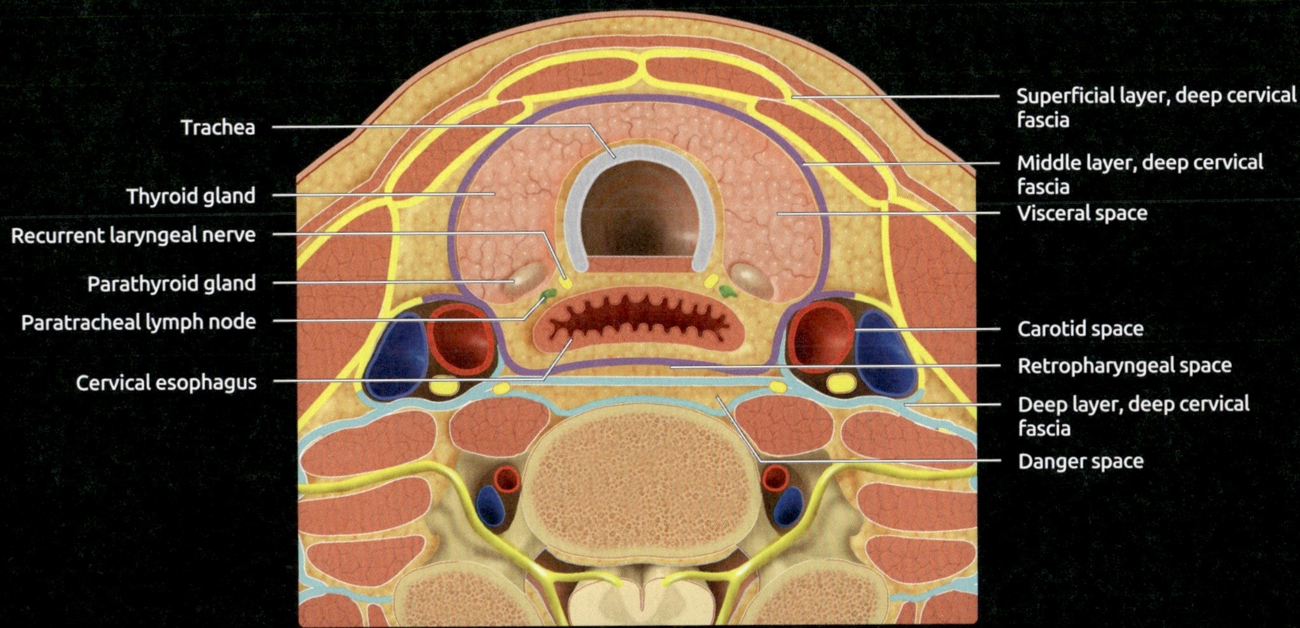

(Top) *Coronal graphic shows the larynx and trachea. The supraglottic larynx includes the epiglottis, aryepiglottic folds, false vocal cords, and preepiglottic and paraglottic spaces. The glottic larynx includes true vocal cords. The subglottic larynx is separated from the trachea at the inferior cricoid cartilage. The 1st tracheal ring is located 1.5-2 cm below the true vocal cords and is broadest of all the cartilage rings. The 2nd, 3rd, and 4th tracheal rings are surrounded by the thyroid gland, anteriorly and laterally. Coronal and sagittal reformatted images are particularly helpful in evaluation of tracheal stenosis and other disorders.* **(Bottom)** *Axial graphic shows layers of deep cervical fascia in the infrahyoid neck. Note the ML-DCF as it surrounds the visceral space. Important components of the tracheoesophageal groove include the recurrent laryngeal nerve, paratracheal nodes, and parathyroid glands. Coverage of strap muscles by SL-DCF is controversial in the literature with many considering it to be covered by the ML-DCF, which covers the visceral space/thyroid gland as well.*

AXIAL CECT

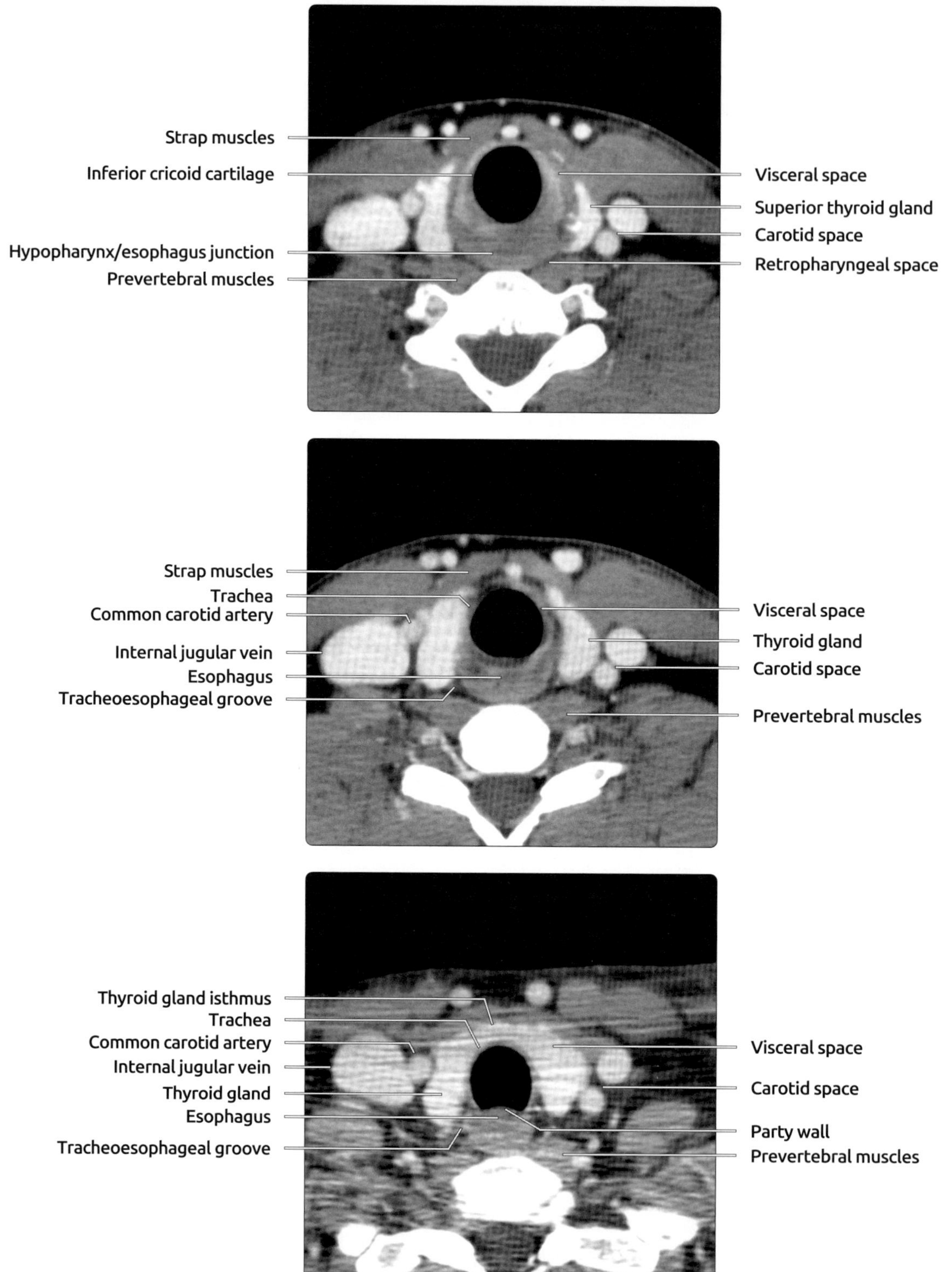

(Top) *The junction of the hypopharynx and larynx is defined by the cricopharyngeus muscle on barium swallow studies. This muscle is an inferior portion of the inferior pharyngeal constrictor muscle and is typically present at C5/C6.* **(Middle)** *Image more inferior shows the cervical trachea and esophagus. The upper 2nd through 4th tracheal rings are surrounded by the thyroid gland.* **(Bottom)** *This image shows the "party wall," the thin layer of connective tissue that separates the mucosal portions of the posterior trachea from the anterior esophagus. Tracheoesophageal groove structures include the recurrent laryngeal nerve, paratracheal lymph nodes, and parathyroid glands.*

AXIAL CECT

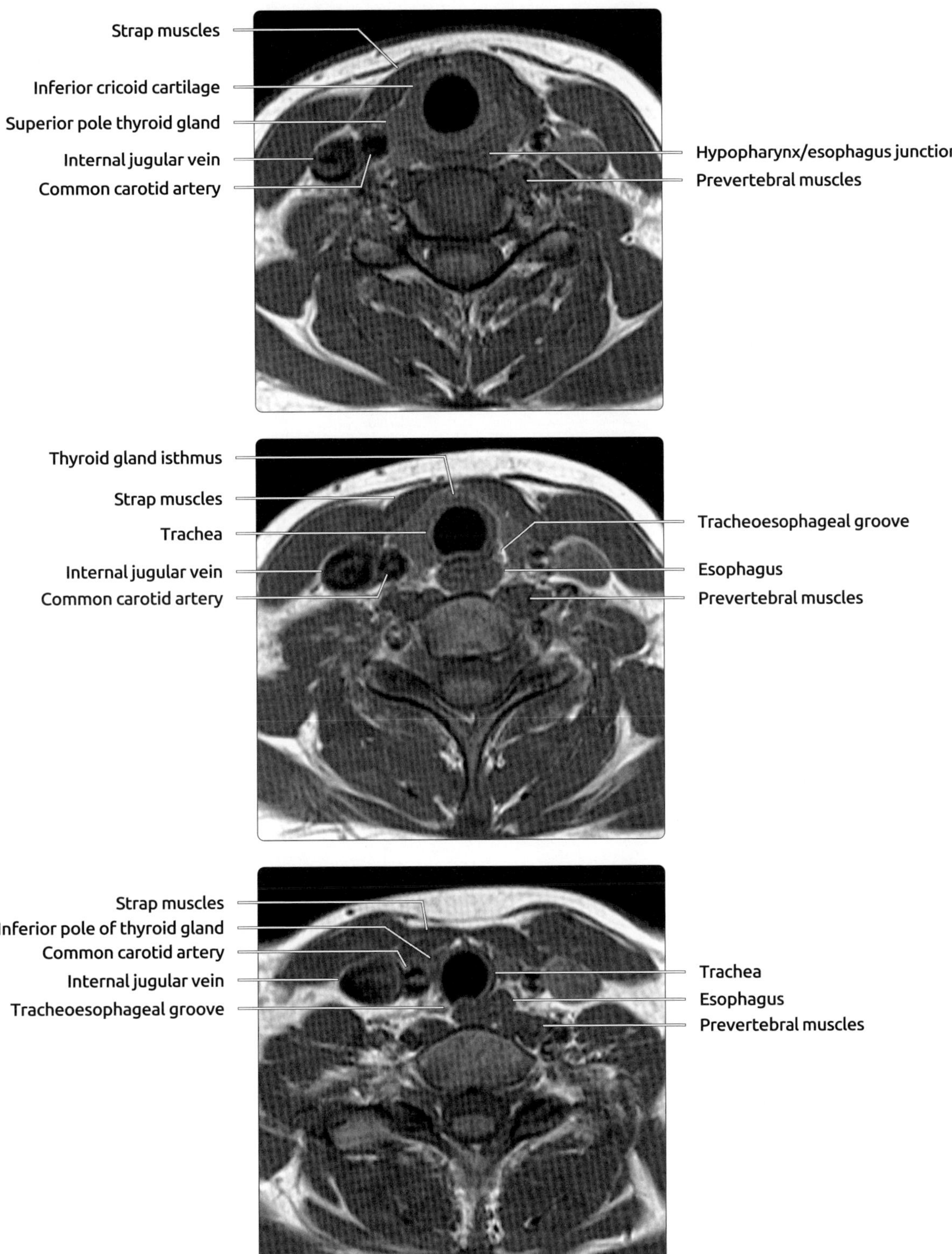

(Top) *Axial T1 MR shows the junction of the hypopharynx and esophagus.* **(Middle)** *Image more inferior shows the cervical trachea and esophagus. The upper 2nd through 4th tracheal rings are surrounded by the thyroid gland.* **(Bottom)** *Image at the inferior portion of cervical trachea and esophagus at the C7 level shows the esophagus posterior and slightly to the left of the trachea.*

GENERIC TRACHEAL MASS GRAPHIC AND CECT

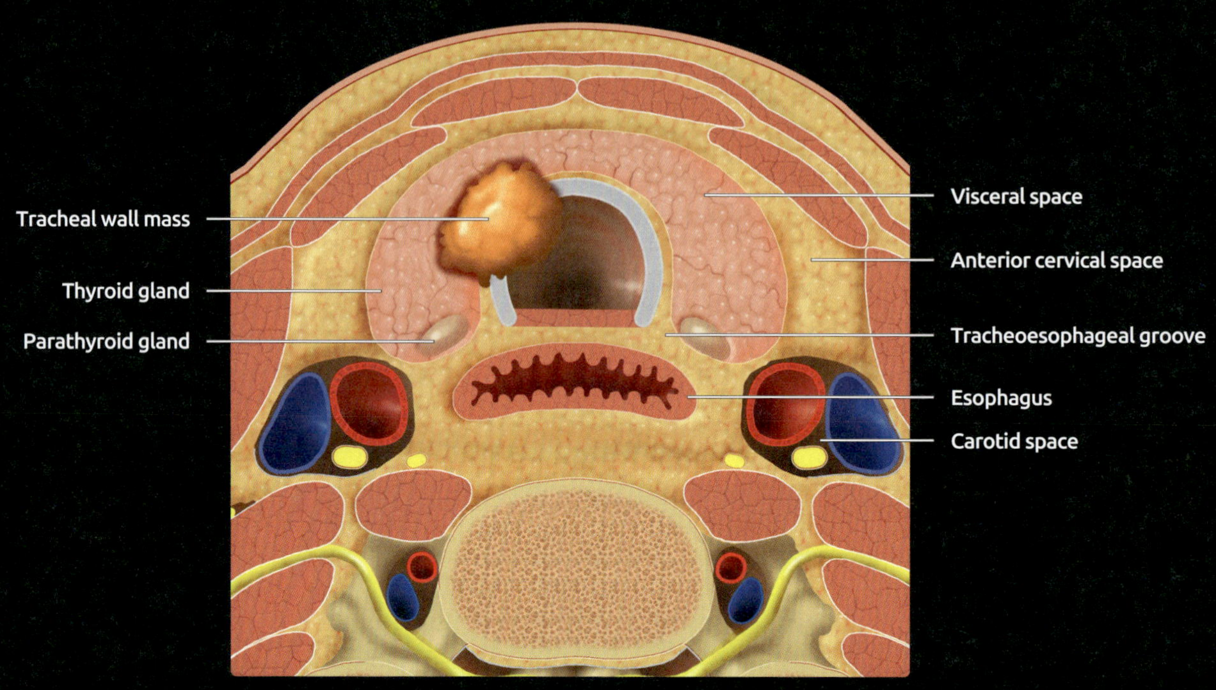

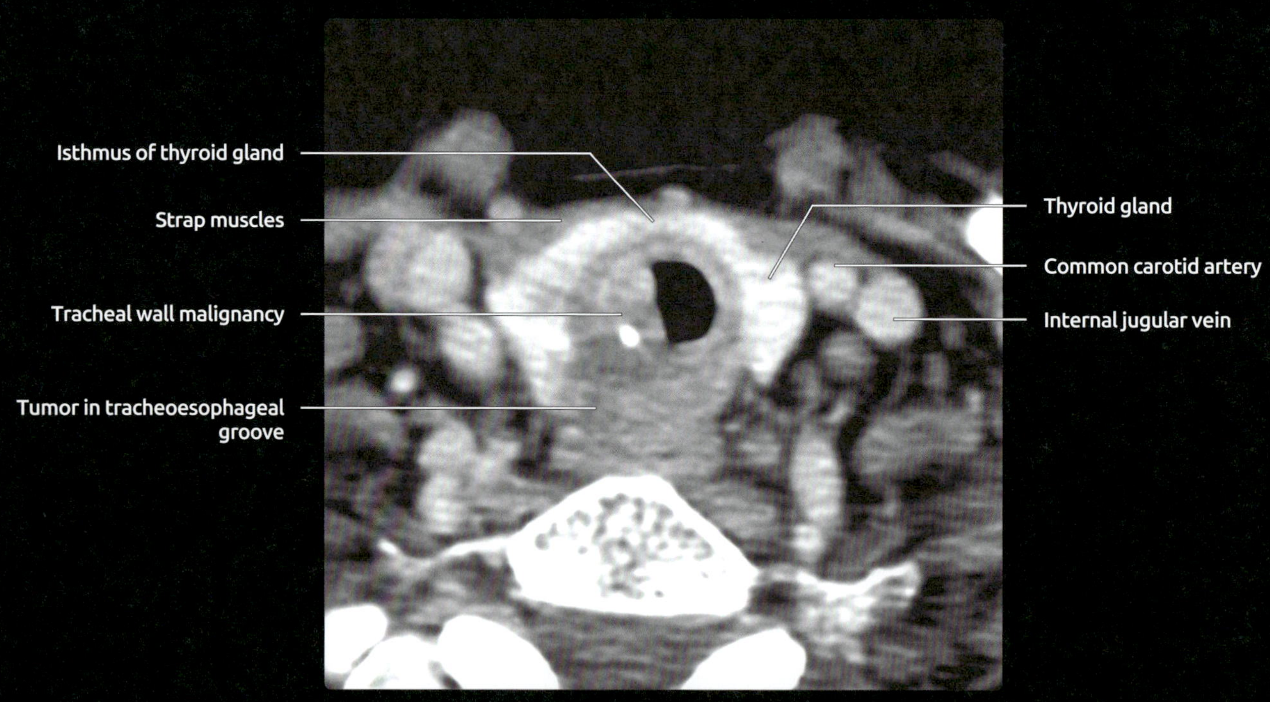

(Top) *Axial graphic shows a generic tracheal wall mass. A mass within the tracheal wall typically displaces the thyroid gland laterally and the esophagus posteriorly. Primary tumors of the trachea are rare, representing 2% of upper airway tumors. The most common primary malignant tumors include squamous cell carcinoma (SCCa) and adenoid cystic carcinoma. SCCa usually arises in the lower trachea and carina. Adenoid cystic carcinomas are usually located on the posterolateral tracheal wall.* **(Bottom)** *Axial CECT demonstrates a right tracheal wall adenoid cystic carcinoma that has spread posteriorly to involve the right tracheoesophageal groove and the anterior wall of the cervical esophagus. Such lesions can be relatively asymptomatic until stridor supervenes.*

GENERIC ESOPHAGEAL MASS GRAPHIC AND CECT

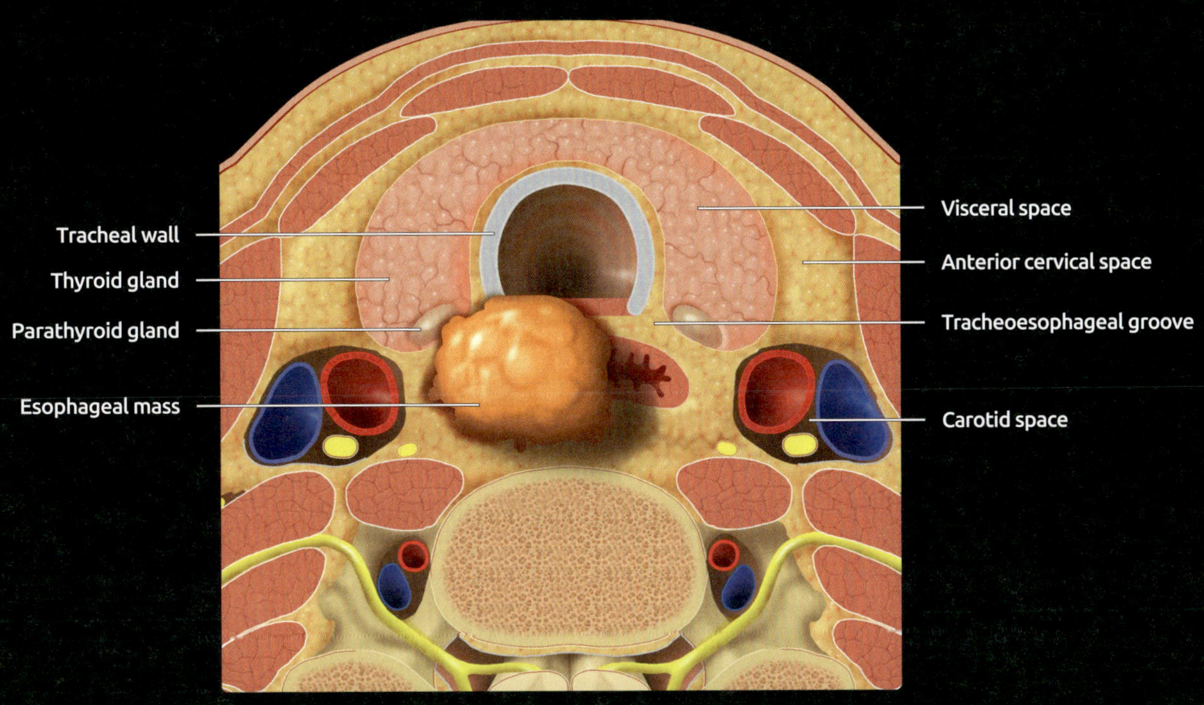

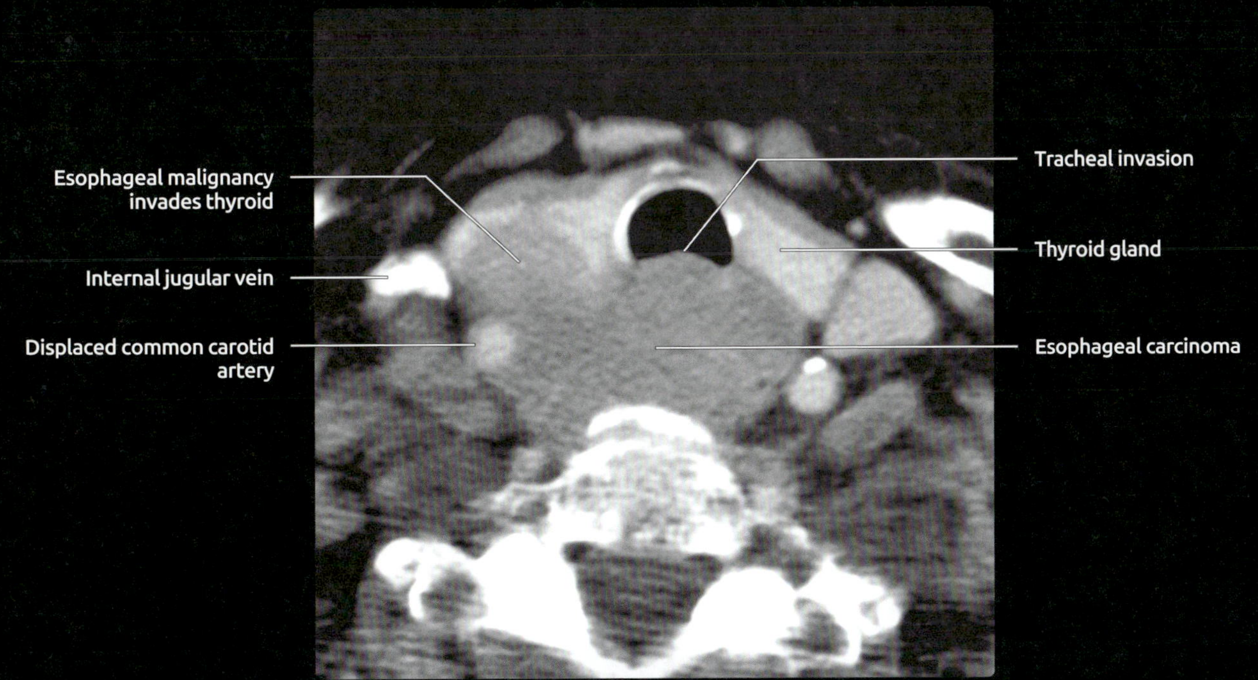

(Top) *Axial graphic of a generic esophageal mass, which is typically midline and displaces the trachea and thyroid gland anteriorly, is shown. 90% of esophageal carcinomas are SCCa, while the remainder are adenocarcinomas related to Barrett esophagus. CT is particularly useful to define the extent of disease and associated metastases, typically to periesophageal, paratracheal, supraclavicular, and mediastinal lymph nodes and the liver. Leiomyoma is the most common benign tumor of the esophagus and is usually incidentally discovered.* **(Bottom)** *Axial CECT through the lower thyroid bed in the cervical neck reveals a large retrotracheal invasive mass (esophageal carcinoma) that has lifted the trachea and left thyroid lobe anteriorly. The right common carotid artery is displaced laterally. The tumor has invaded the right thyroid lobe and the posterior trachea.*

TRANSVERSE ULTRASOUND

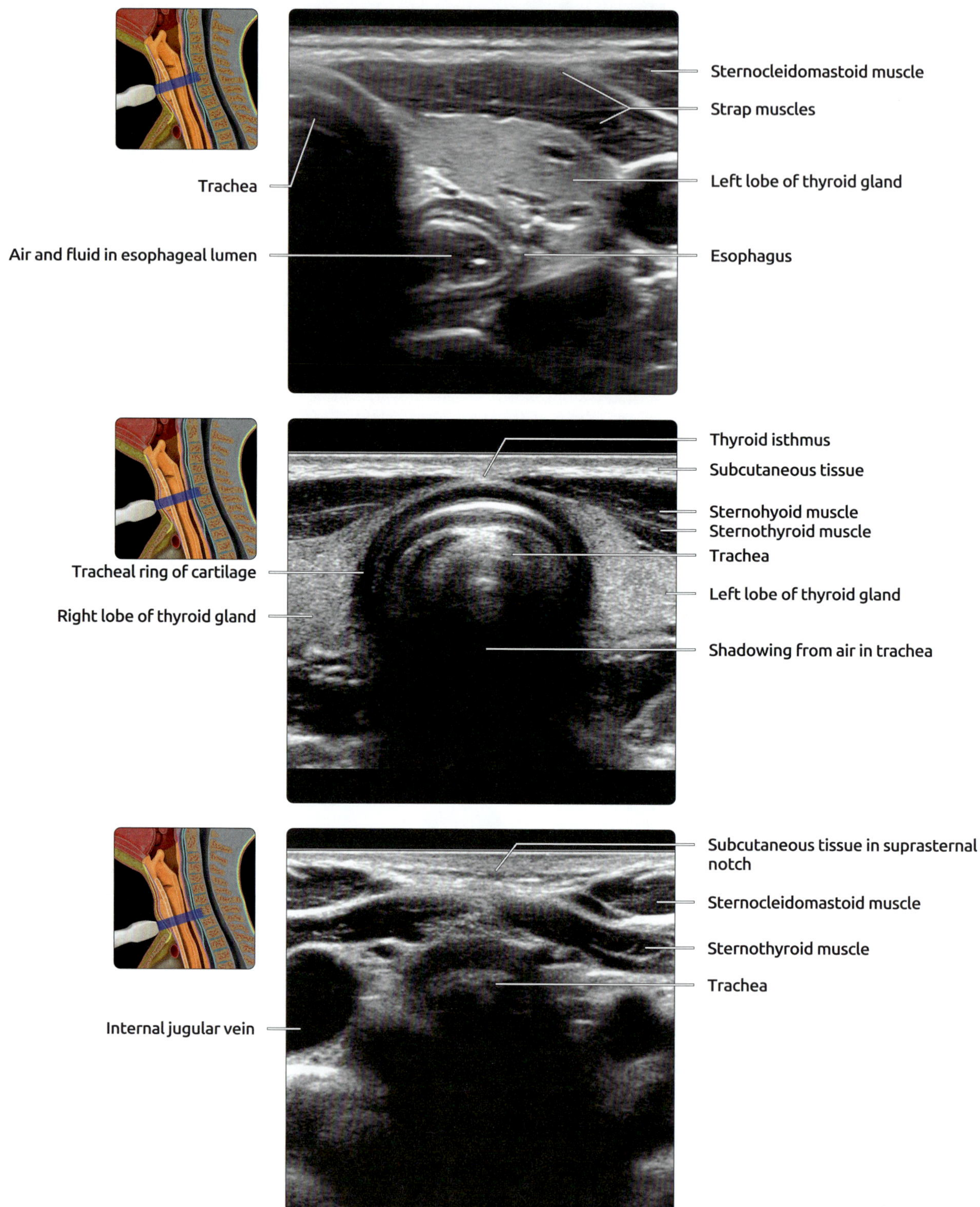

(Top) *Transverse grayscale ultrasound of the left lower cervical level shows the location of the cervical esophagus posterior to the left lobe of the thyroid gland and posterolateral to the trachea. It is easily recognized by the alternating hypo-/hyperechoic rings (gut signature). If there is any question, have the patient swallow. The recurrent laryngeal nerve is located in the tracheoesophageal groove. The nerve is not visualized on ultrasound.* **(Middle)** *Transverse grayscale ultrasound of the midline anterior neck at the level of thyroid gland shows the trachea as a midline structure underneath the isthmus of the thyroid gland and related laterally to the thyroid lobes. Note the hypoechoic tracheal ring composed of hyaline cartilage that is incomplete posteriorly.* **(Bottom)** *Transverse grayscale ultrasound of the suprasternal region shows the lower cervical trachea underneath the insertion sites of the strap muscles.*

LONGITUDINAL ULTRASOUND AND CT

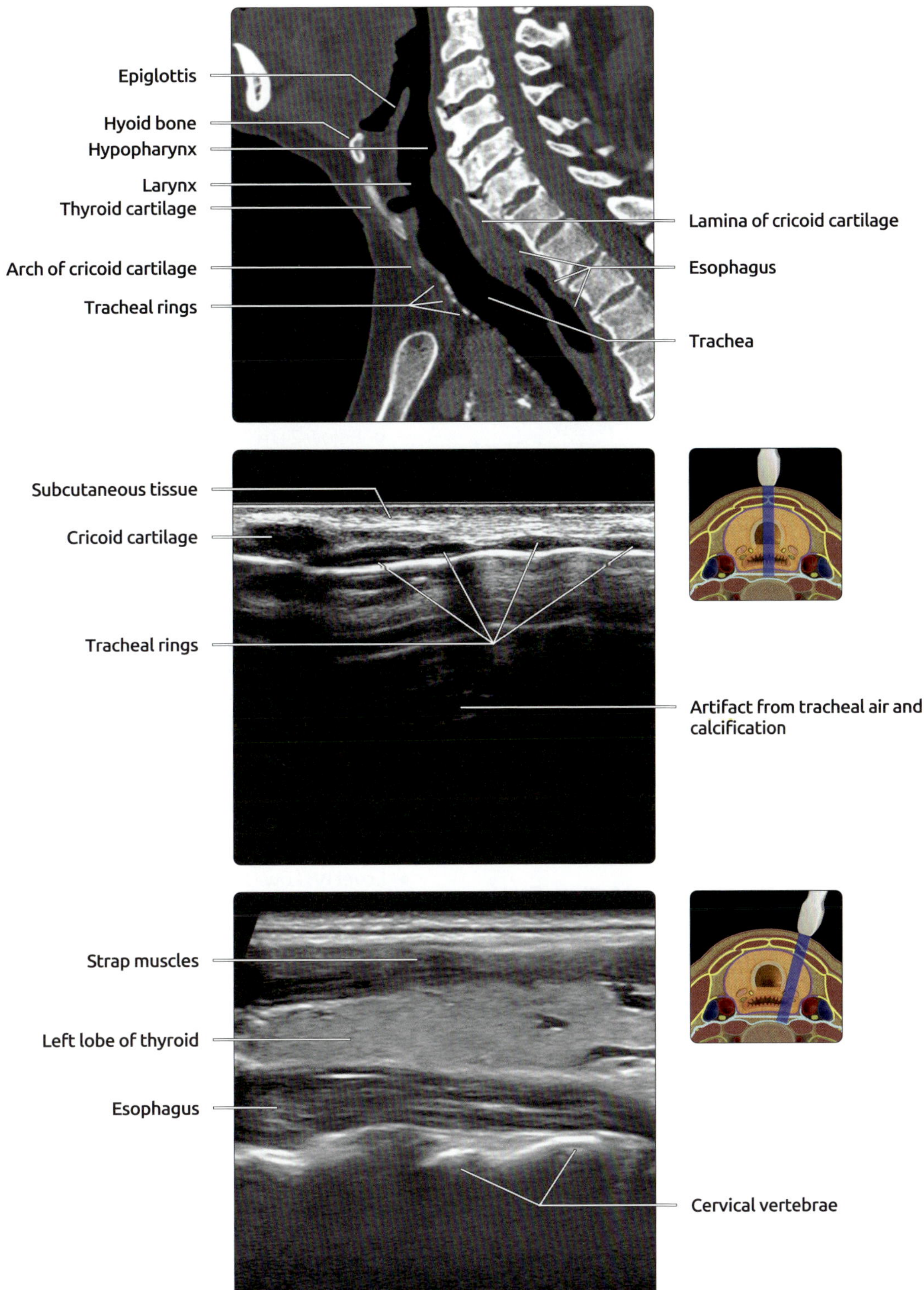

(Top) *Sagittal CT reformation of the midline neck shows calcified tracheal rings anteriorly. These rings form an arch around the trachea and are incomplete posteriorly. The posterior wall is composed of a thick fibromuscular membrane and is immediately anterior to the esophagus.* **(Middle)** *Longitudinal grayscale ultrasound of the midline anterior neck shows the presence of hypoechoic tracheal rings along the cervical portion of the trachea. Note the hypoechoic, noncalcified, cricoid cartilage above the tracheal rings.* **(Bottom)** *Longitudinal grayscale ultrasound of the lower left neck at the thyroid gland level shows the cervical esophagus posterior to the left lobe of the thyroid gland. It is a long tubular structure with alternating echogenic/hypoechoic layers representing the mucosal, submucosal, muscular, and serosal layers.*

TERMINOLOGY

Abbreviations

- Lymph nodes (LNs); internal jugular chain (IJC); internal jugular vein (IJV); sternocleidomastoid muscle (SCM); internal carotid artery (ICA); common carotid artery (CCA); spinal accessory chain (SAC); retropharyngeal space (RPS)

IMAGING ANATOMY

Overview

- **Lymphatic system** in neck: Extensive lymphatic capillary & vessel network, up to 300 individual LNs, & Waldeyer ring [palatine, nasopharyngeal (adenoid), & lingual tonsils]
- LN: Bean-shaped gland that receives 1 or more **afferent** lymphatic vessels piercing LN outer capsule & bringing lymph from tissues (or from upstream LN) to **subcapsular sinus**
- Hilum: Focal concavity along margin of LN, contains small arterioles, venules, & **efferent** lymphatic vessels
- Supporting architecture of LN includes **peripheral capsule** of thin, fibrous connective tissue, internal fibrous trabeculae that penetrate gland from capsule, & fine network of reticular cells
- LN contains variety of immune cells specifically organized into functional regions to maximize cellular exposure to antigens & provoke immune response
  - **Cortex:** Responsible for humoral immunity; located in periphery of LN, contains **lymphoid follicles** composed mostly of B-cell lymphocytes
  - **Paracortex:** Main site of cellular immunity; T cells reside here & proliferate when stimulated
  - **Medulla:** Main antibody production site; contains lymphocytes, plasmacytoid lymphocytes, & plasma cells
- Cervical LNs drain into **thoracic duct on left** & **right lymphatic duct on right;** both open into their respective angle of internal jugular & subclavian veins

Cervical Lymph Node Nomenclature & Classifications

- Earliest classifications (Rouvière, Trotter, & Poirier & Charpy) largely based on palpable landmarks of neck
- Shah suggested level-based nomenclature system in 1981
- Since 1981, several level-based systems developed to standardize head & neck cancer staging & surgical approaches based on predictable patterns of tumor spread
- 1997: American Joint Committee on Cancer classification
- 1998: American Academy of Otolaryngology-Head & Neck Surgery classification
- 1999: Imaging-based classification based on cross-sectional CT or MR images (Som, Curtin, & Mancuso)

Image-Based Lymph Node Classification Method

- **Axial CT plane**: Head in comfortable neutral position with **hard palate perpendicular** to table top & shoulders down as far as possible
  - CT gantry aligned along **inferior orbitomeatal plane**
- Relies on identification of anatomic landmarks, easily determined on cross-sectional CT or MR images
- Requires drawing **lines** along margins of specific anatomic structures **in axial plane** to determine LN level boundaries
- Lines defining boundaries of LN levels must be **drawn separately for each side** of neck
- **LN** lying **in both adjacent levels** on either side of line **assigned to** level with **most cross-sectional area** of node
- **Level I: Submental & submandibular nodes**
  - LN below mylohyoid muscle, above inferior margin of hyoid bone, & anterior to transverse lines drawn along posterior margins of **each** submandibular gland (SMG)
  - Level IA (submental nodes): LN between **medial margins** of anterior bellies of digastric (ABD) muscles
  - Level IB (submandibular nodes): LN posterior & lateral to medial margin of ABD muscle, around SMG in submandibular space
- **Level II: Upper IJC nodes (suprahyoid)** from skull base at lower jugular fossa to **lower margin** of hyoid bone body
  - Anterior to **transverse line** along posterior border of SCM, & posterior to transverse line along posterior edge of SMG on either side
  - **LN within 2 cm of skull base**: Lateral, anterior, or posterior to carotid sheath: Level II node
    - **Medial to ICA here**: Retropharyngeal LN **(RPLN)**
  - Below 2 cm of skull base, level II node can lie medial, lateral, anterior, or posterior to IJV
  - Level IIA: Level II node anterior, medial, lateral, anterior, or posterior to IJV; if **posterior** to IJV, node **inseparable from IJV**
  - Level IIB: Level II node posterior to IJV with **fat plane visible** between node & IJV
    - Lies above & behind spinal accessory nerve (CNXI)
- **Level III: Mid-IJC nodes** from lower margin of hyoid bone to **lower margin** of cricoid cartilage arch
  - Anterior to **transverse line** along SCM posterior border
  - **Lateral** to **medial margin** of CCA/carotid bulb
  - Note: Level VI nodes **medial to** medial margin of CCA/carotid bulb
  - **Remember**: Hyoid bone lies at level of carotid bulb; hence, LNs in relation to ICA (above hyoid) lie in level II
- Anterior boundary of levels III & IV: Sternohyoid muscle
- **Level IV: Low IJC nodes (infracricoid)** from **lower margin** of cricoid arch to clavicle
  - Anterior & medial to **oblique line** along posterior border of SCM/posterolateral border of anterior scalene muscle
  - **Lateral** to **medial margin** of CCA
  - Note: Level VI nodes **medial to** medial margin of CCA
- **Level V: Nodes of posterior cervical space (SAC)**
  - Anterior to transverse line along **anterior border** of trapezius muscle
  - Level VA: Upper SAC nodes from skull base to lower margin of cricoid cartilage arch; posterior to **transverse line** along posterior border of SCM
  - Level VB: Lower SAC (transverse cervical) nodes from lower margin of cricoid cartilage arch to clavicle; posterior to **oblique line** along posterior border of SCM & posterolateral border of anterior scalene muscle
- **Level VI: Visceral nodes** found from **lower margin** of hyoid bone above to **top** of manubrium below; includes prelaryngeal, pretracheal, & paratracheal subgroups
  - Medial to **medial margin** of CCA/bulb
- **Level VII: Superior mediastinal nodes** found between carotid arteries from top of manubrium above to innominate vein below; medial to medial margin of CCA
- **Supraclavicular nodes**: LN lateral to medial margin of CCA if **any portion of clavicle seen on that side** in axial image

- If level of axial image is cranial & does not show any portion of clavicle on that side, then lower lateral neck node classified as either level IV (anteriorly) or VB (posteriorly)
- **Axillary nodes**: Nodes below clavicle level & **lateral to ribs**
- **Parotid nodal group**: Intraglandular or extraglandular
  - Both intraglandular & extraglandular nodes within fascia circumscribing parotid space
  - Drains into upper IJC nodes (level II)
- **RPLN**: 2 subgroups
  - RPLN **within 2 cm of skull base** & **medial to ICA**
  - Lateral RPLN: Anterolateral to prevertebral muscles, medial to ICA
    - Nodes of Rouvière: Skull base/C1 or C1-C2 level
  - Medial RPLN: Less often seen, usually at C2-C3 level
- **Facial nodal groups**
  - Mandibular nodes: Along external mandibular surface
  - Buccinator nodes: In buccal space
  - Infraorbital nodes: In nasolabial fold
  - Malar nodes: On malar eminence
  - Retrozygomatic nodes: Deep to zygomatic arch

ANATOMY IMAGING ISSUES

Imaging Approaches

- **Squamous cell carcinoma (SCCa) nodal staging**: CECT or T1 C+ MR; scan extent: Skull base to clavicles
- PET/CT utility in head & neck SCCa nodal work-up: Small active malignant node identification & treatment planning
- **Thyroid or cervical esophageal cancer**
  - Scan extent: Skull base to **carina to include superior mediastinum**
  - MR preferred for thyroid cancer as iodinated contrast for CECT may interfere with decision for I-131 radioiodine thyroid ablation treatment
- **High-resolution ultrasound**: Micrometastasis in small LN **subcapsular** sinus where metastatic tumor cells grow first
  - Also differentiate LN (hilar vessels) from other tumors
  - Parathyroid adenoma may have polar vessel

CLINICAL IMPLICATIONS

Clinical Importance

- Recognizing enlarged or pathologic-appearing nodes in infectious, inflammatory, & neoplastic processes
- Differentiation between **benign vs. malignant nodes**
  - Most normal LNs in neck not visualized by routine imaging
  - Normal nodes oval & smoothly marginated
  - Metastatic nodes critical for cancer staging & treatment
  - **Normal short-axis** diameter size criteria in older adults in axial plane: < 10 mm, except
    - Occasionally slightly larger level II jugulodigastric & level I submandibular nodes, especially in children & young adults
    - Lateral RPLN: < 6 mm, normally slightly larger in children & young adults
    - Medial RPLN: Any visible LN in adult (normally seen in ~ 20% children)
  - Nodes smaller than cutoff size criteria may be malignant, especially if in drainage areas of primary tumor; evaluate for abnormal morphology & micrometastasis
  - Normal **long-axis** diameter size criteria < 12-15 mm for levels II & III, but jugulodigastric node commonly above 15 mm in younger adults
  - Morphology: Oval nodes with central fatty hila normally
    - Metastatic nodes: May be round, replace normal fatty hila, & show necrosis, cystic change, calcification, or hyperenhancement
  - **Micrometastasis**: In **subcapsular sinus** where metastatic tumor cells deposited by **afferent** lymphatics grow first
    - **High-resolution ultrasound** of LN peripheral region
- IJC final common pathway for all lymphatics of upper aerodigestive tract & neck, emptying into thoracic duct on left & right lymphatic duct on right (both opening into angle of IJV & subclavian vein on their respective sides)
  - Neck SCCa do not normally drain into mediastinum
  - Neck imaging to stage SCCa: Skull base to clavicles
- Distal thoracic duct or right lymphatic duct could be mistaken for supraclavicular lymphadenopathy
  - Also for neurogenic tumor, such as schwannoma, due to their location near carotid sheath
  - For congenital cystic mass, such as branchial anomaly or lymphatic malformation in younger patients
  - For pseudoaneurysm on NECT
- **RPLN**
  - Reactive-appearing RPS nodes commonly seen in younger patients on brain MR exam
  - Important when identified on imaging in SCCa setting as often clinically silent
  - RPLN drain SCCa nasopharynx & posterior wall of oropharynx & hypopharynx
  - Papillary thyroid cancer (PTC) rarely drain into RPLN
  - PTC with metastatic cervical LNs or prior neck dissection might alter lymphatic drainage direction to retrograde pathway, resulting in unusual RPLN metastasis
  - Benign postradiation hypertrophy of **superior cervical sympathetic ganglia** may mimic enlarged lateral RPLN
- **Parotid nodal group**
  - Receives lymph drainage from external auditory canal, eustachian tube, skin of lateral forehead & temporal region, posterior cheek, gums, & buccal mucous membrane (especially due to skin SCCa & melanoma)
  - Parotidectomy & nodal dissection of neck necessary if malignancy of superficial ear area presents as cervical neck malignant adenopathy
- **Notable named nodes**
  - **Signal (Virchow) node**: Lowest node in IJC; if no primary tumor in neck, consider chest or abdomen primary with metastasis carried via thoracic duct; left > right
  - **Rouvière node**: Highest node in retropharyngeal group; lies within 2 cm of skull base; site of spread for nasopharyngeal carcinoma, esthesioneuroblastoma
  - **Jugulodigastric node**: Lies within IJC just above hyoid bone; larger than surrounding nodes
    - First **(sentinel) node** to receive lymphatic drainage from face, mouth, pharynx, & tonsils
    - Near IJV crossing by posterior belly of digastric muscle
  - **Delphian (prelaryngeal/precricoid) node**: Not normally identified on imaging; pathologically enlarged in cases of advanced thyroid cancer & head & neck SCCa
  - **Juguloomohyoid node (level III)**: "LN of tongue," near intermediate tendon of omohyoid muscle

GRAPHIC LYMPH NODE ANATOMY AND HISTOLOGY

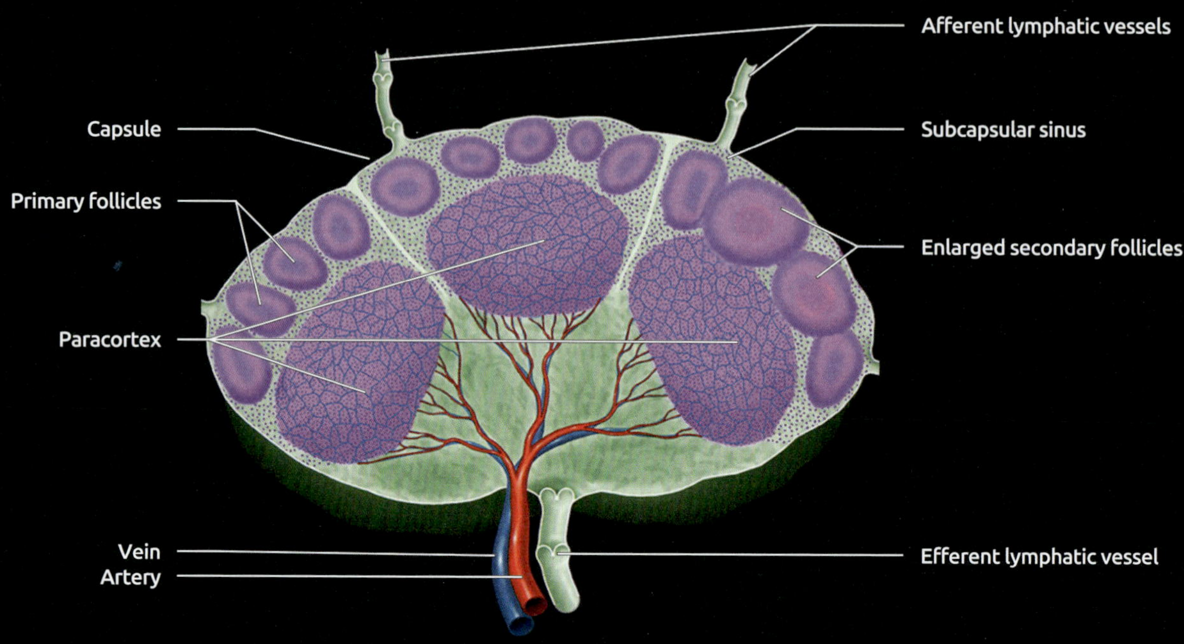

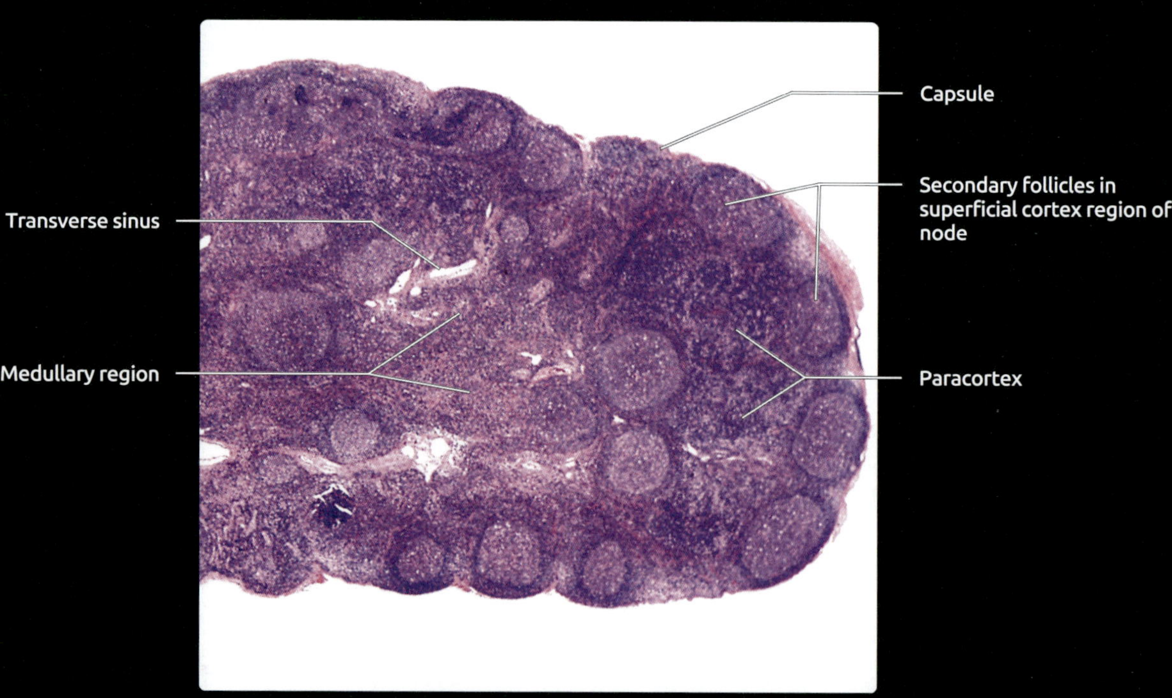

(Top) *Several afferent lymphatic vessels enter the broad convex capsular side of the lymph node (LN). Lymph flows through a series of sinuses from the periphery toward the hilum. Micrometastasis occurs in the subcapsular sinus, where metastatic tumor cells deposited by the afferent lymphatics piercing LN cortex first start to grow. High-resolution ultrasound may detect these under the cortex in normal-sized LNs. Peripherally, the lymphatic tissue is organized into the superficial cortex that contains the primary follicles. When the primary follicles are stimulated, secondary follicles with germinal centers are formed. The follicles preferentially contain B cells. The paracortex contain the so-called deep cortical units where T cells congregate and proliferate when stimulated. Plasma cell precursors produced by B-cell proliferation migrate to the medulla where they ultimately secrete antibodies.* **(Bottom)** *Histologic slide of a reactive LN demonstrates the principle regions of the node from the superficial cortex that contains the follicles (B cells), the paracortex that contains the deep cortical units (T cells), and the medullary region where B cells mature and produce antibodies.*

GRAPHICS

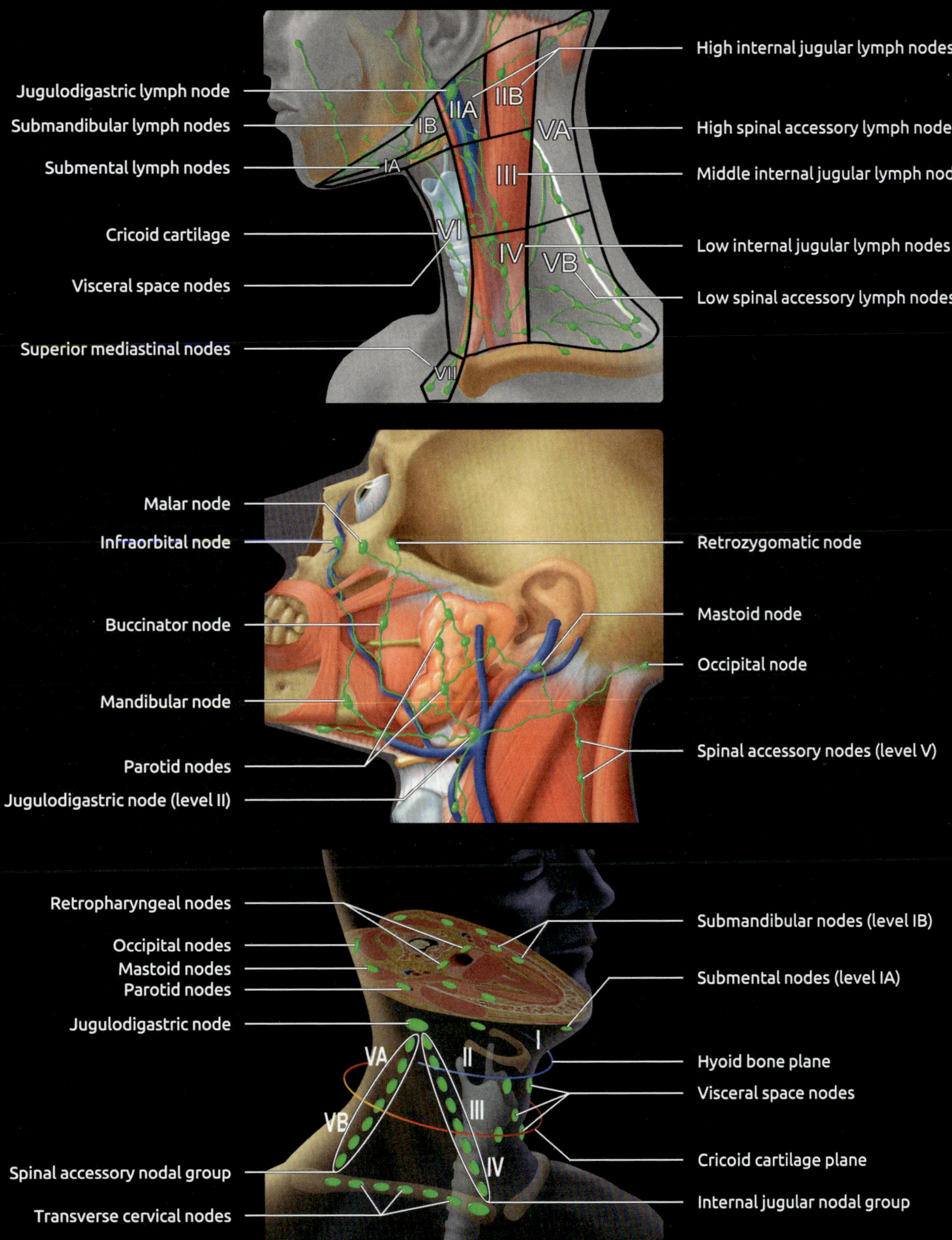

(Top) *Lateral oblique graphic of the neck shows anatomic locations of major nodal groups of the neck. Division of the internal jugular nodal chain into high, middle, and low regions is defined by the level of the lower borders of the hyoid bone and cricoid cartilage. Similarly, the spinal accessory nodal chain is divided into high and low regions by lower cricoid cartilage level.* **(Middle)** *Lateral view of facial nodes and parotid nodes is shown. None of these nodes bear level numbers and must be described by their anatomic location. The jugulodigastric node (level II) and spinal accessory nodes (level V) are also marked.* **(Bottom)** *Lateral oblique graphic of the cervical nodes depicts an axial slice through the suprahyoid neck. Note retropharyngeal nodes behind the pharynx, which are often clinically occult. Lower margins of the hyoid bone (blue arc) and cricoid cartilage (orange circle) planes are highlighted as they serve to subdivide the internal jugular and spinal accessory nodal group levels. Neck LNs empty into the thoracic duct on the left and right lymphatic duct on the right, both opening into an angle of the internal jugular and subclavian veins on their respective sides.*

IMAGING CLASSIFICATION: AXIAL CT

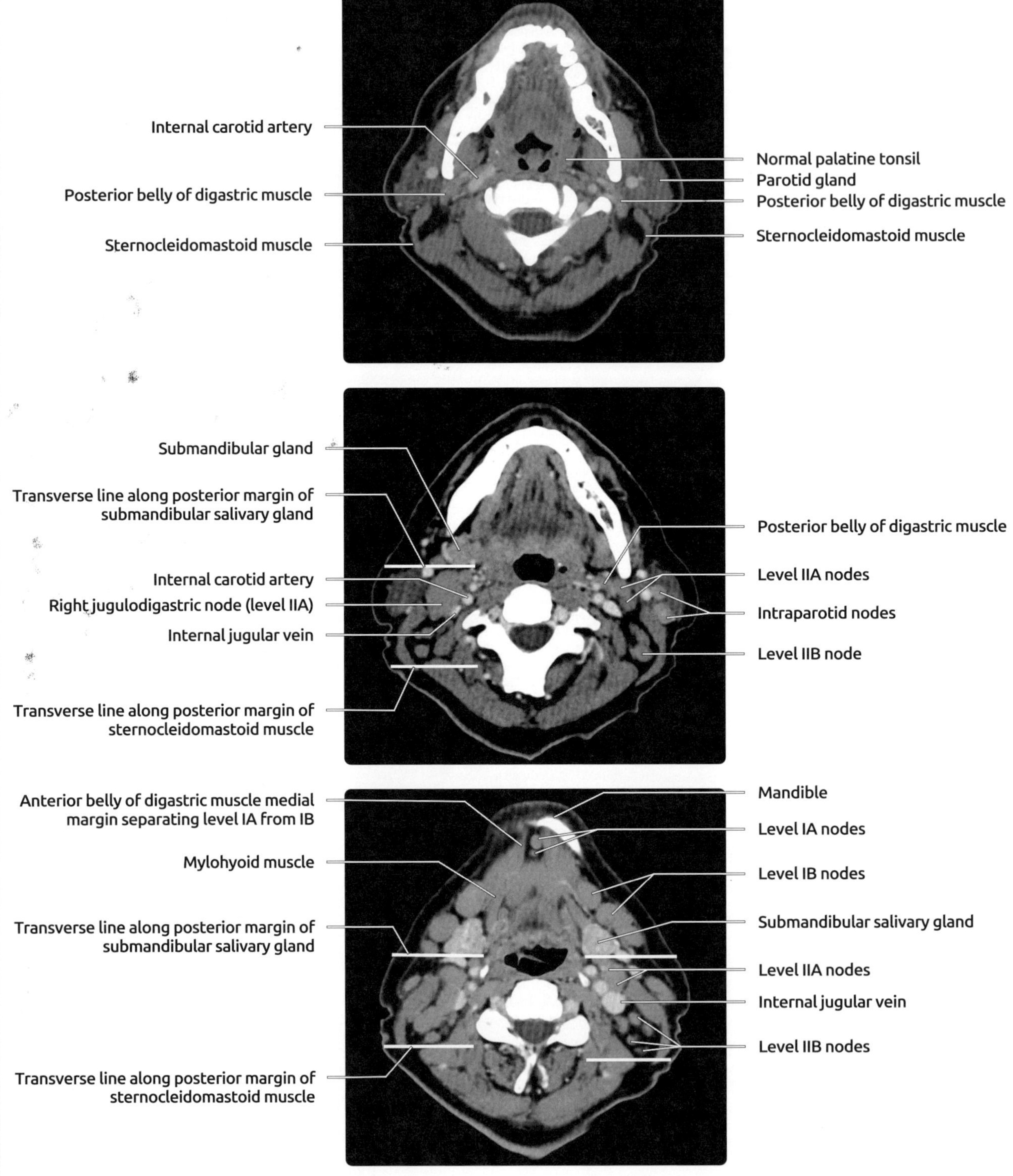

(Top) *Axial CECT from skull base to clavicle in a patient with newly diagnosed leukemia demonstrates diffuse bilateral adenopathy. The posterior belly of digastric (PBD) muscle arises from the mastoid tip and passes between the deep lobe of the parotid gland and carotid space and helps to determine neck space of origin of mass lesions here. Jugulodigastric node lies immediately below PBD, often the largest LN in normal neck and can be larger than 10 mm in short axis and 15 mm in long-axis diameter.* **(Middle)** *In this section, multiple enlarged nodes are present, including a significantly enlarged right level II jugulodigastric node. Transverse lines are drawn along the posterior margin of the submandibular salivary gland (to demarcate level IB from level IIA nodes) and along the posterior margin of sternocleidomastoid muscle (SCM) (to distinguish level II from level VA nodes).* **(Bottom)** *Axial CECT shows the submandibular region above the hyoid bone. Transverse lines are drawn along the posterior margins of submandibular salivary glands and SCMs. In a normal subject, a small number of these nodes would be identifiable on CT. All lines should be drawn separately for each side of neck.*

IMAGING CLASSIFICATION: AXIAL CT

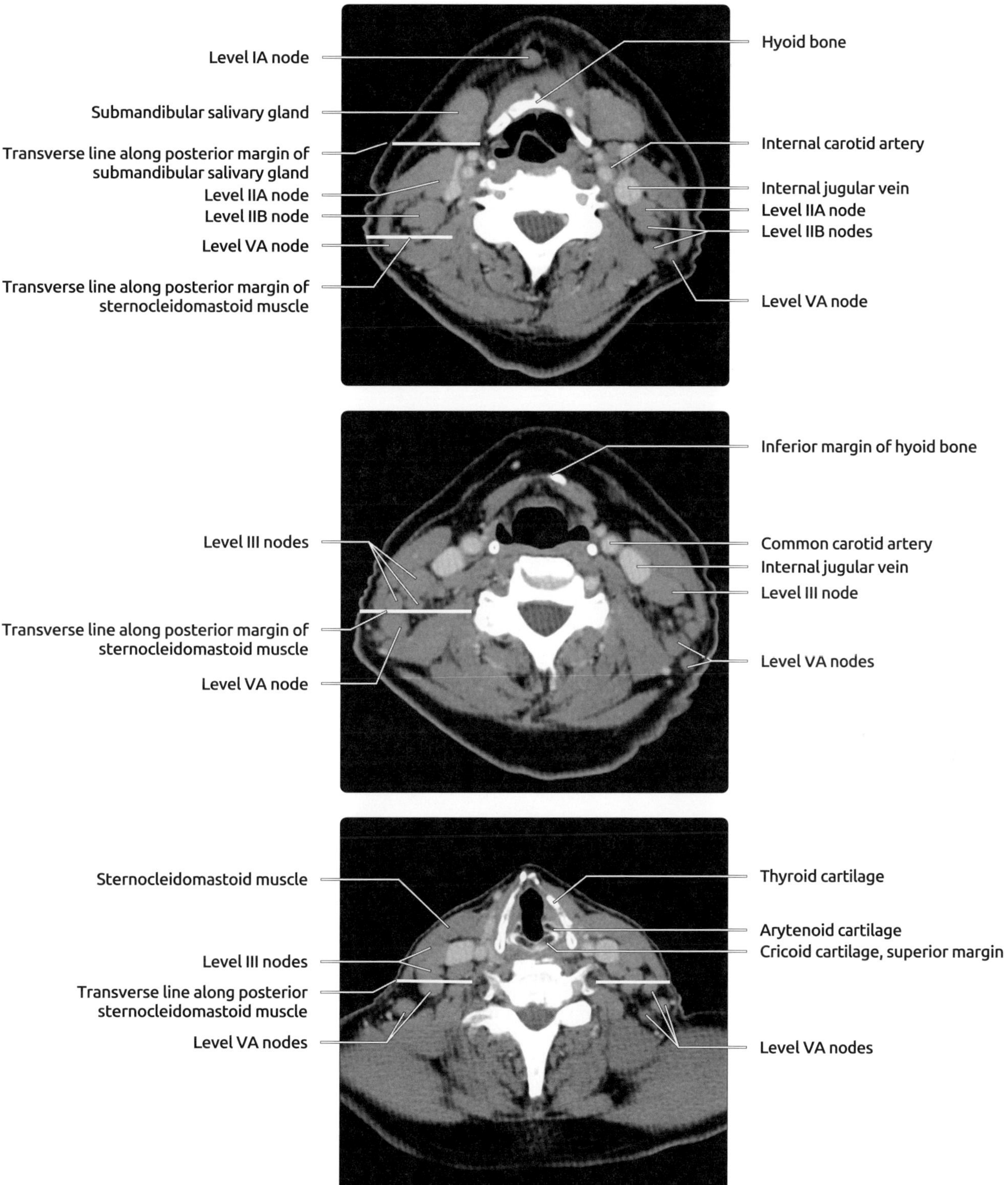

(Top) *Axial CECT from the level of the hyoid bone shows the midbody of the hyoid bone anteriorly. Transverse lines drawn on the patient's right again separate level I from level II and level II from level VA. Level IIB nodes lie posterior to the internal jugular vein (IJV) with the fat plane visible between the node and IJV. Note that one of the nodes posterior to left IJV contacts the vein without an interposed fat plane and is denoted as level IIA node even though posterior.* **(Middle)** *Axial CECT just below the level of the hyoid bone is shown. The inferior margin of the hyoid bone is an important landmark, marking the transition from level II IJV nodes above to level III IJV nodes below. Level III extends from the inferior margin of the hyoid bone to the inferior margin of the cricoid cartilage. A transverse line is drawn on the patient's right, along the posterior margin of the SCM, separating the level II nodes from more posterior level VA nodes.* **(Bottom)** *Axial CECT below the hyoid and above the inferior margin of cricoid cartilage is shown. A transverse line is drawn bilaterally along the posterior margins of SCMs. This separates the level III nodal group from level VA.*

IMAGING CLASSIFICATION: AXIAL CT

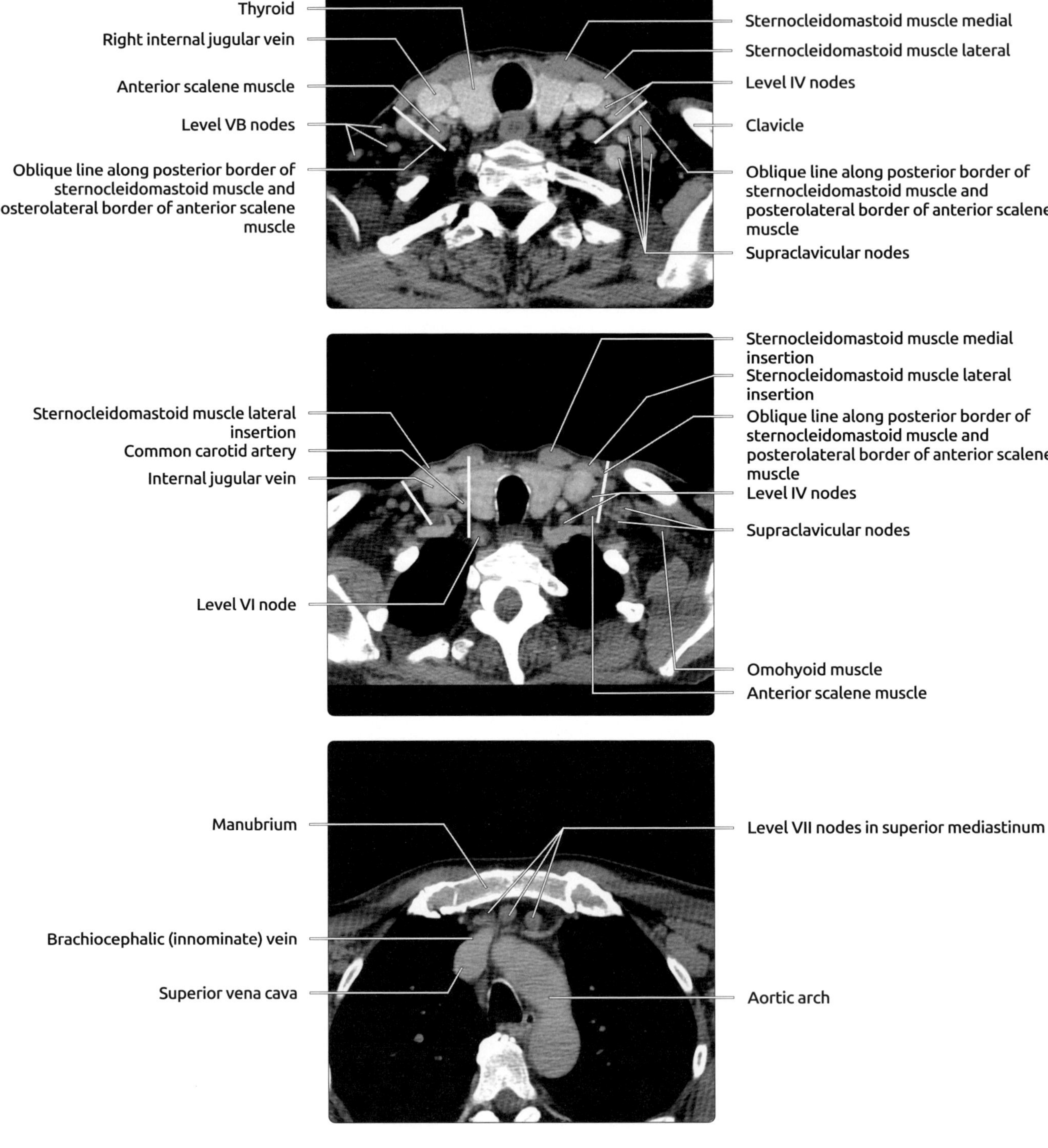

(Top) *Axial CECT just below the inferior margin of the cricoid cartilage is shown. The inferior margin of the cricoid is important because it separates level III internal jugular chain (IJC) nodes above from level IV IJC nodes below and also marks the inferior extent of level VA. Notice on the patient's right, the clavicle is not in view, and the nodes posterior to the oblique line is designated as level VB. On the patient's left, the clavicle is in view, and, by convention, the nodes posterior to the oblique line is designated as supraclavicular nodes.* **(Middle)** *Axial CECT at the thyroid level is shown. Oblique lines separate the level IV nodes from more lateral supraclavicular nodes bilaterally as clavicles are visualized in the image on both sides. An AP line is drawn in the sagittal plane along the medial margin of the right common carotid artery (CCA) to separate level IV nodes lateral to it from the more medially located level VI nodes. A single level VI node is identified in the right tracheoesophageal groove.* **(Bottom)** *Axial CECT below the upper margin of the manubrium shows the top of the manubrium marks the separation between level VI nodes above and level VII superior mediastinal nodes below.*

3D CTA & CECT AXIAL, SAGITTAL

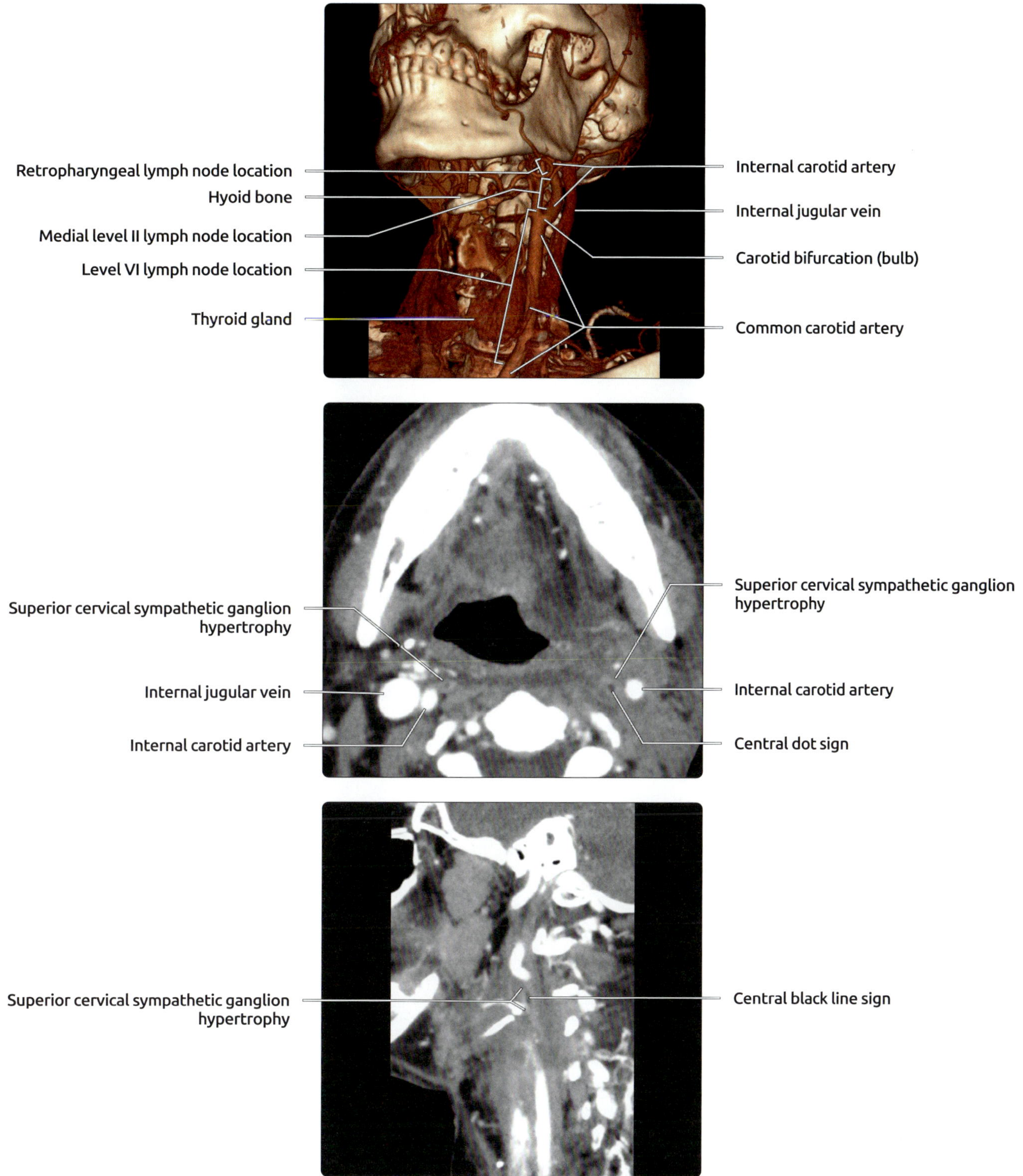

(Top) *3D reformat of a neck CTA shows the hyoid bone lies at the level of the carotid bulb; this makes the medial LNs in the suprahyoid neck medial to the carotid sheath lie medial to the internal carotid artery (ICA), where it is classified as level II superiorly up to 2 cm below the skull base. A level II node can lie medial, lateral, anterior, or posterior to IJV. But, if a node lies more superiorly within 2 cm of the skull base and medial to ICA, it is classified as a retropharyngeal node. Infrahyoid nodes medial to the medial margin of the carotid sheath will be medial to the CCA/carotid bulb (not ICA) and classified as level VI, inferiorly down to the top of manubrium sterni.* **(Middle)** *Axial CECT shows bilateral benign postradiation hypertrophy of superior cervical sympathetic ganglia (SCG), mimicking enlarged lateral retropharyngeal LNs (RPLNs). Most hypertrophic SCG lie medial to the ICA at the C2 and C3 transverse process levels with central hypodensity/hypointensity on CECT/MR (central black dot sign on axial images), which become oblong on coronal and sagittal images (central black line sign).* **(Bottom)** *Sagittal CECT shows the central black line sign in the hypertrophic SCG.*

AXIAL T1 & T2 MR

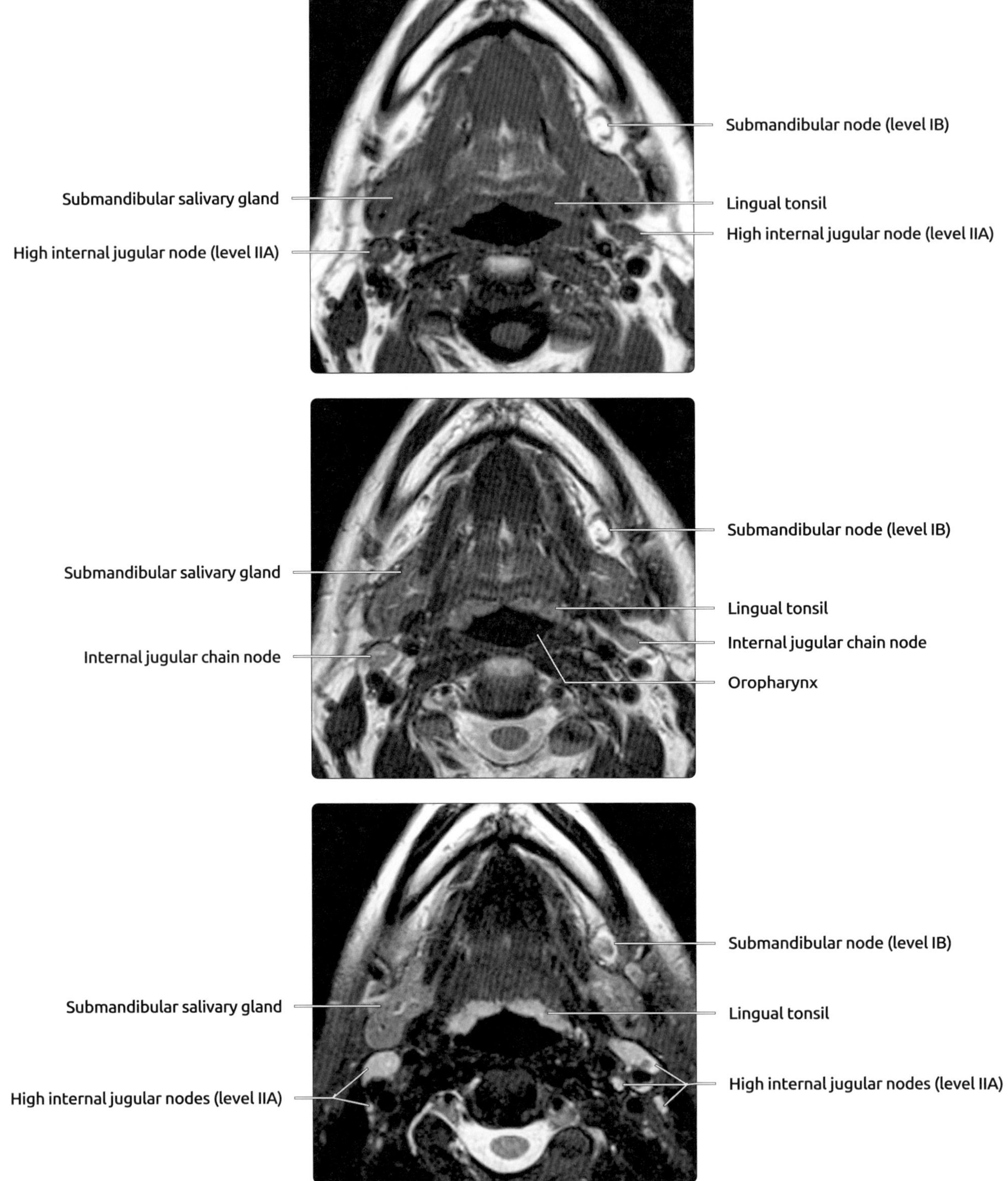

(Top) *Axial T1 MR through the low oropharynx shows the characteristic low T1 signal of LNs. A prominent submandibular node with a fatty hilum is seen on the left. Level IIA internal jugular nodes are observed bilaterally.* **(Middle)** *Axial T2 MR at the level of the low oropharynx shows high internal jugular nodes as intermediate signal intensity.* **(Bottom)** *Axial T2 MR with fat saturation creates increased conspicuity of LNs. The smaller high internal jugular nodes surrounding the carotid space are easily identified on this fat-saturated T2 MR. STIR MR sequences create the same level of nodal conspicuity. Lingual tonsil tissue is also made more conspicuous with the fat-saturation T2 sequence.*

RETROPHARYNGEAL NODES

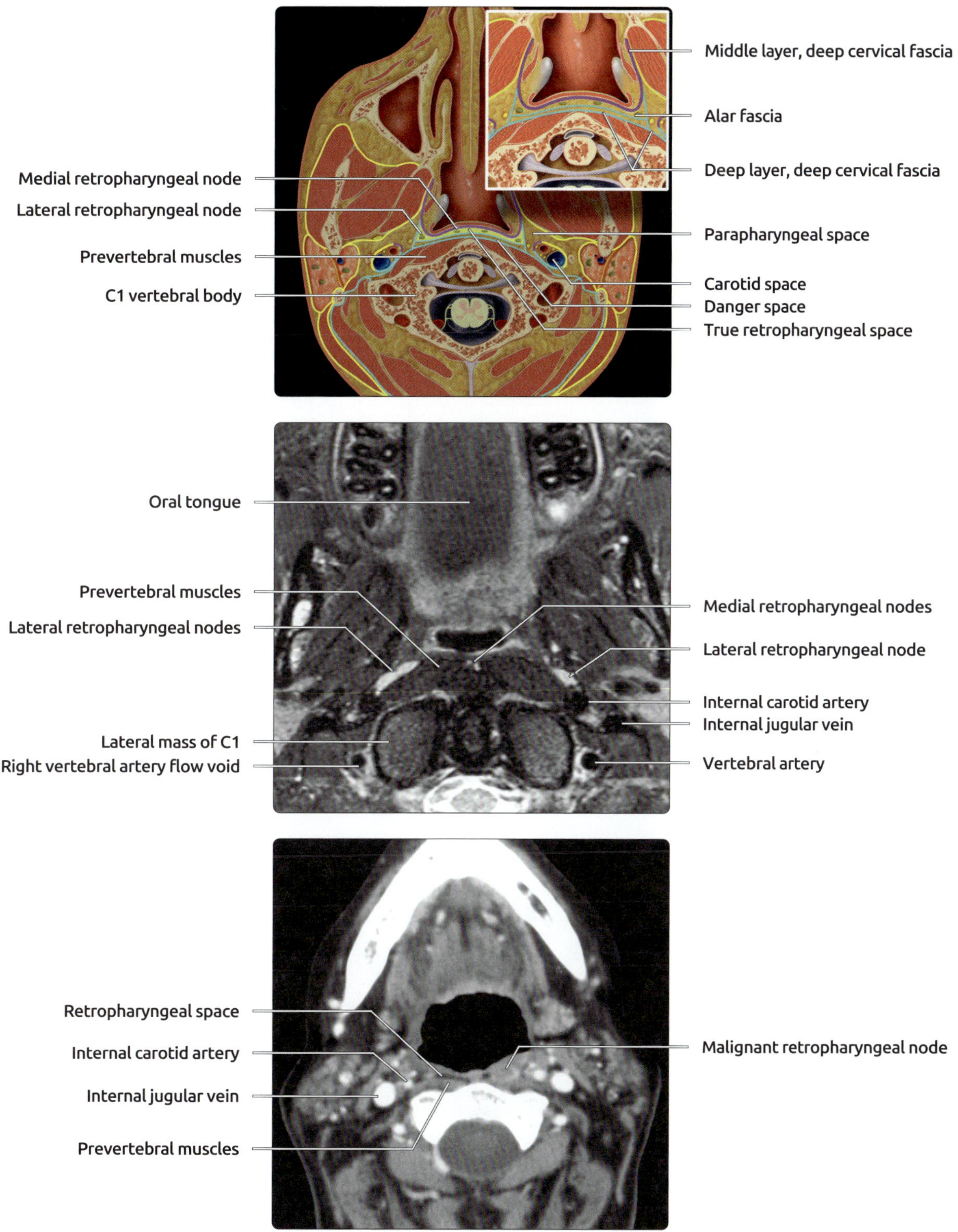

(Top) *Axial graphic at the base of the skull demonstrates medial retropharyngeal nodes in the paramedian retropharyngeal space; the lateral retropharyngeal nodes are lateral to the prevertebral muscles and medial to the ICA. If a node lies within 2 cm of the skull base and medial to ICA, it is classified as retropharyngeal node, whereas if a node within 2 cm of skull base lies lateral, anterior, or posterior to the carotid sheath, it is a level II node. Note that below 2 cm of the skull base and above the lower margin of the hyoid bone, a level II node can lie medial, lateral, anterior, or posterior to the IJV. Infrahyoid nodes medial to the medial margin of the CCA/carotid bulb lie in level VI.* **(Middle)** *Axial T2 MR with fat saturation shows the location of both medial and lateral RPLNs. Note the lateral group is located on the anterolateral surface of prevertebral muscles, just medial to the carotid space.* **(Bottom)** *Axial CECT at the level of the low oropharynx shows a small medial retropharyngeal node in a patient with posterior wall hypopharynx squamous cell carcinoma (not shown). Central low density suggests a malignant node despite the small size.*

NORMAL AND REACTIVE NODES: GRAYSCALE ULTRASOUND

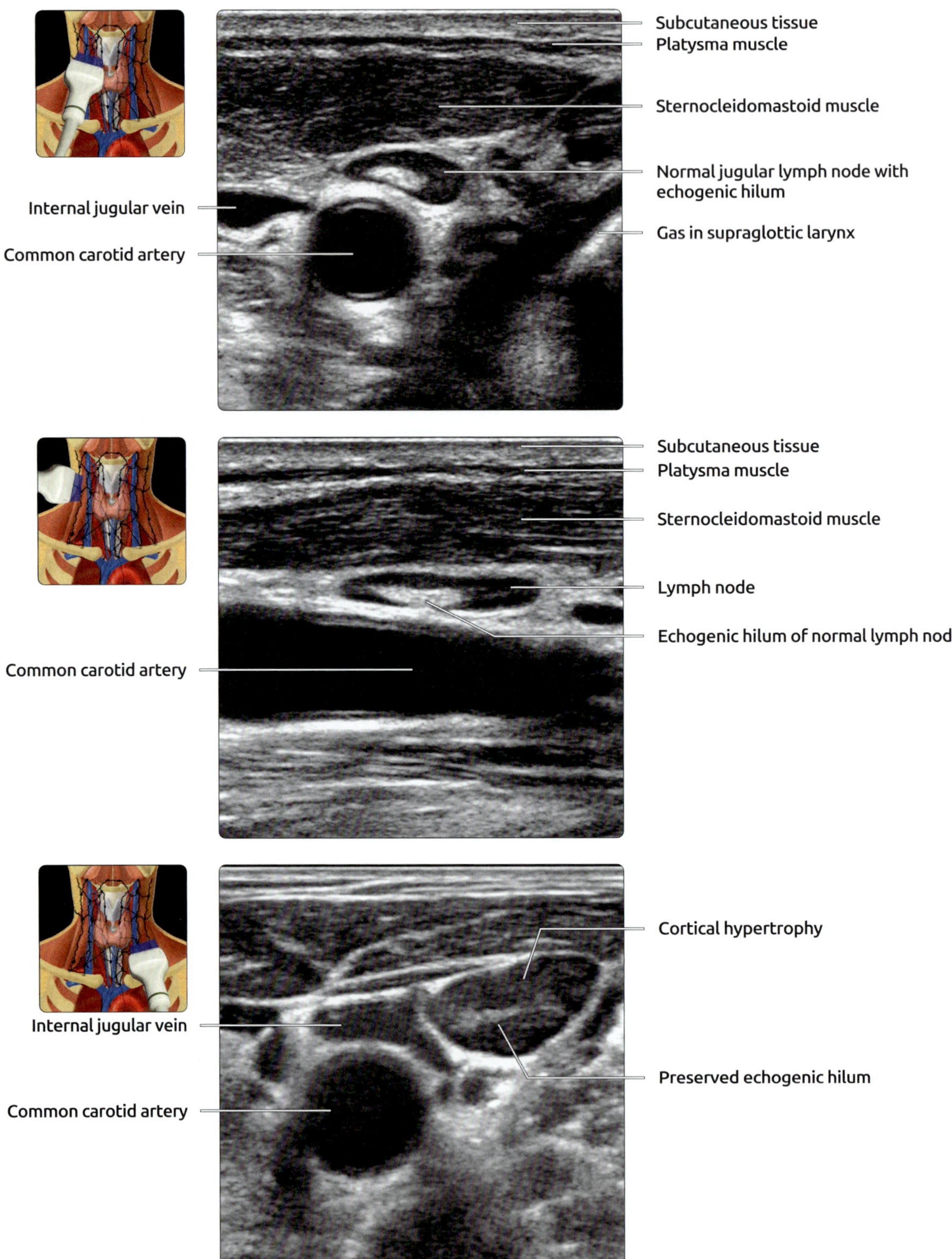

(Top) *Transverse grayscale ultrasound of the midcervical level shows the normal appearance of a cervical LN (i.e., ovoid shape with echogenic hilum). It is commonly found anterior to the carotid artery/internal jugular vein.* **(Middle)** *Longitudinal grayscale ultrasound of the midcervical level shows a normal elliptical hypoechoic LN with echogenic hilum anterior to the CCA. Micrometastasis initially occurs in the subcapsular sinus where metastatic tumor cells deposited by the afferent lymphatics piercing the LN outer cortex first start to grow. High-resolution ultrasound may detect these micrometastatic deposits just underneath the outer cortex in normal-sized LNs.* **(Bottom)** *Transverse grayscale ultrasound shows a hypoechoic node with cortical hypertrophy and preserved echogenic hilum along the deep cervical/jugular chain. This is the classic appearance of a reactive node. Note its relation to the IJV and CCA. This is a common site of reactive nodes, which are often bilateral and symmetric.*

NORMAL AND REACTIVE NODES: POWER DOPPLER ULTRASOUND

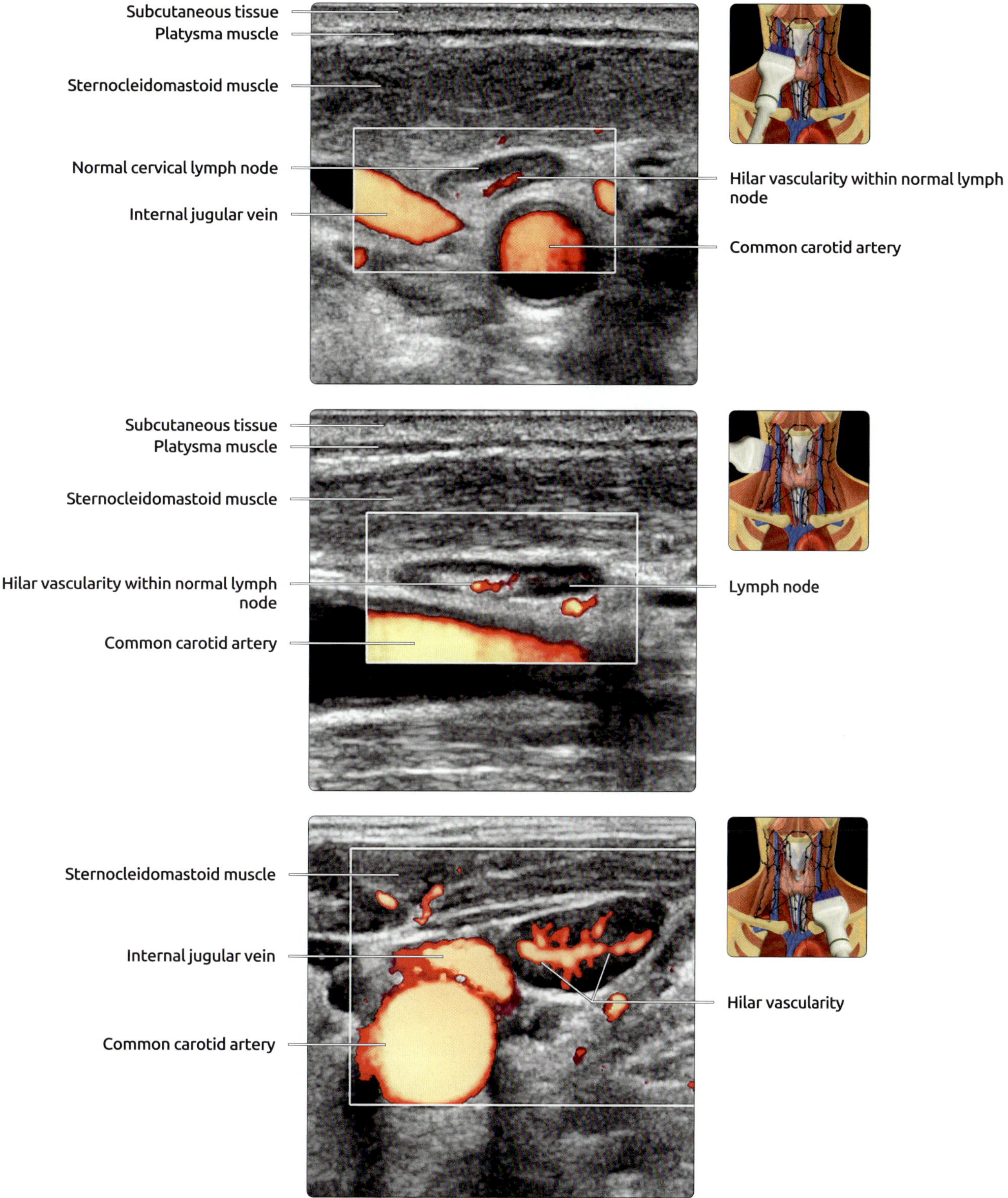

(Top) *Transverse power Doppler ultrasound shows the presence of hilar vascularity within the echogenic hilum of a normal cervical LN.* **(Middle)** *Longitudinal power Doppler ultrasound shows hilar vascularity within the echogenic hilum of a normal cervical LN. The presence of echogenic hilum and hilar vascularity are good signs of cervical LN benignity.* **(Bottom)** *Power Doppler ultrasound of a reactive node clearly defines radiating hilar vascularity and its relation to the IJV and CCA.*

PATHOLOGY: GRAYSCALE ULTRASOUND

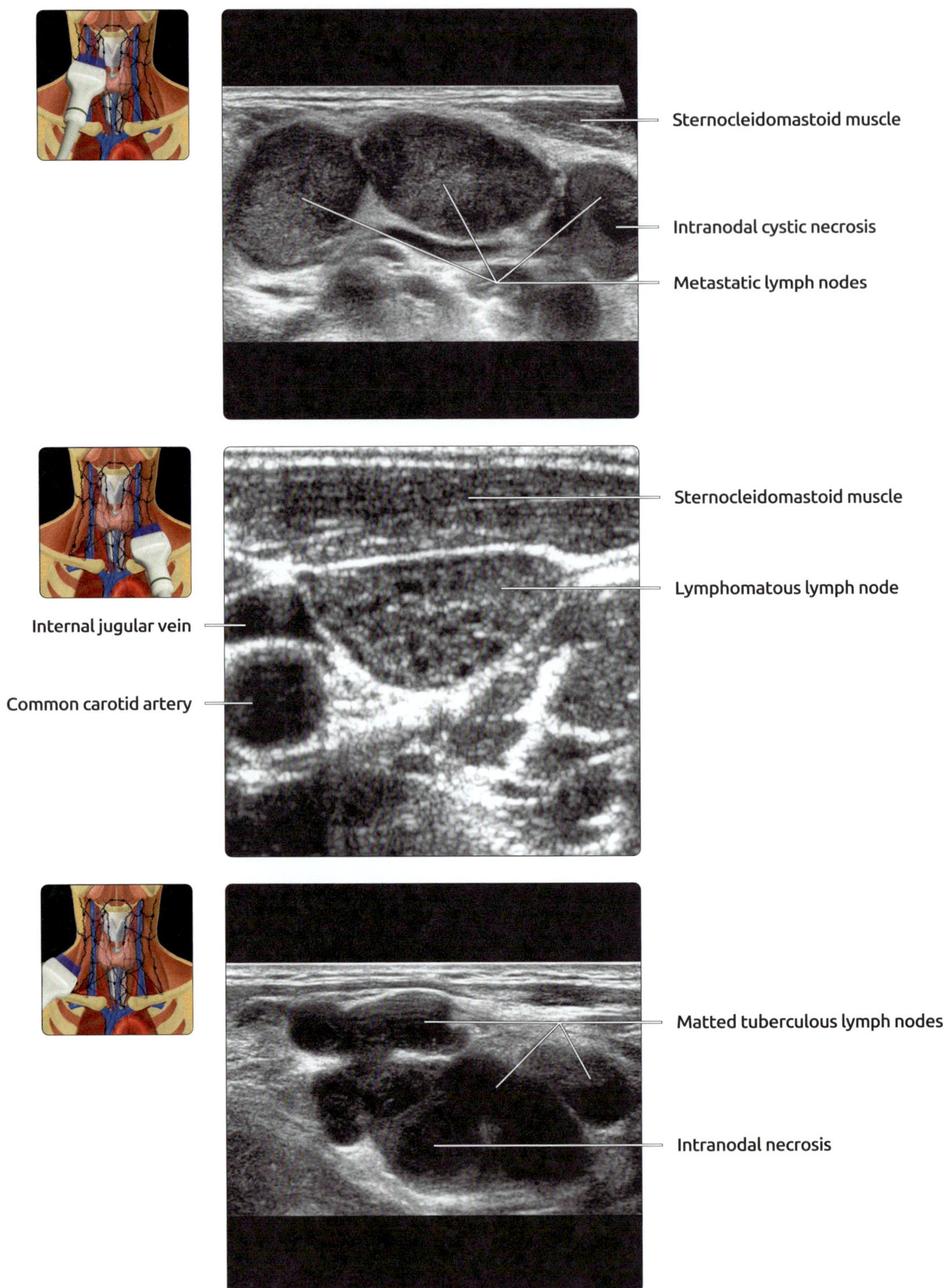

(Top) *Axial grayscale ultrasound of the upper neck shows multiple enlarged, round, predominantly solid, hypoechoic LNs. The patient has a known history of head and neck cancer. Presence of intranodal cystic necrosis in a patient with known primary malignancy is indicative of the metastatic nature of LNs.* **(Middle)** *Transverse grayscale ultrasound of a lymphomatous LN in a midjugular chain demonstrates the typical reticulated echo pattern without central necrosis.* **(Bottom)** *Transverse grayscale ultrasound shows multiple matted, enlarged, heterogeneous, hypoechoic LNs in the posterior triangle of a patient with tuberculosis. Some of them demonstrate intranodal necrosis. A mild degree of edema is noted in the adjacent soft tissue. Features are compatible with tuberculous lymphadenitis.*

PATHOLOGY: POWER DOPPLER ULTRASOUND

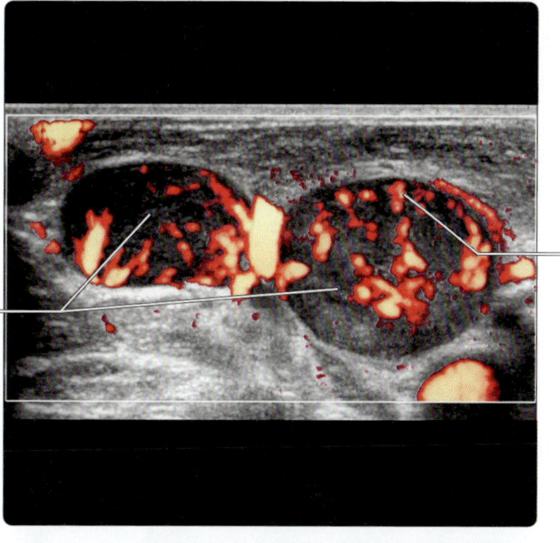

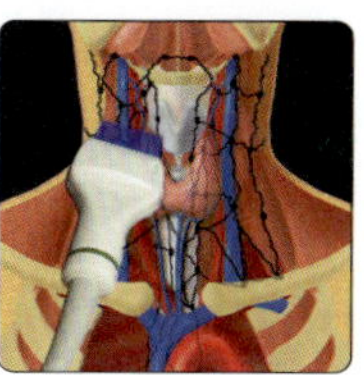

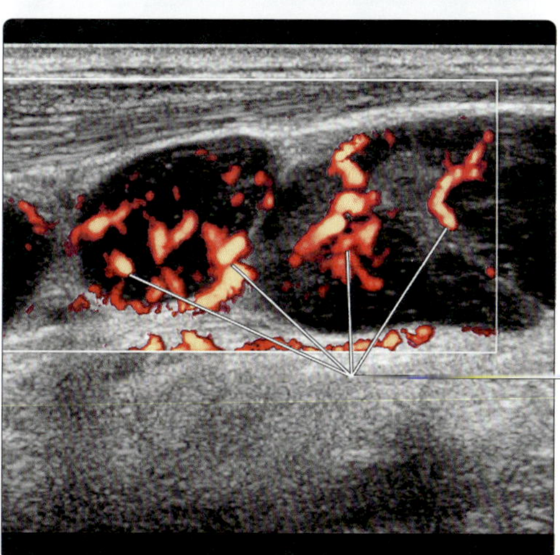

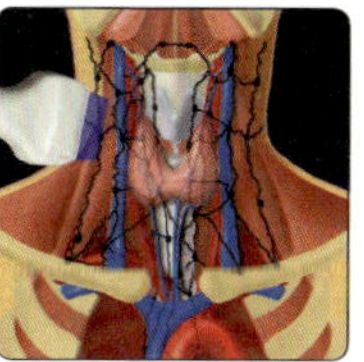

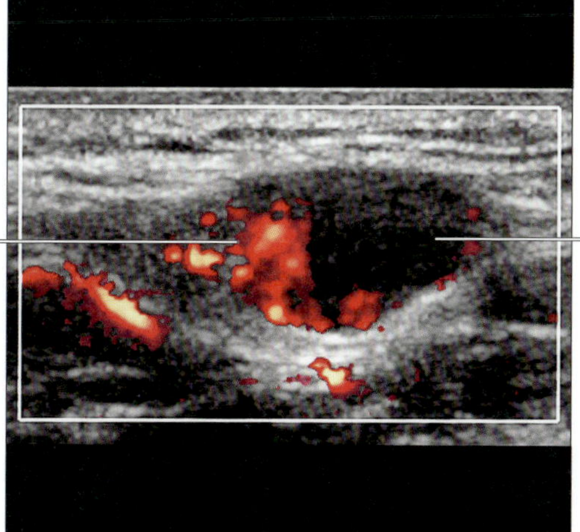

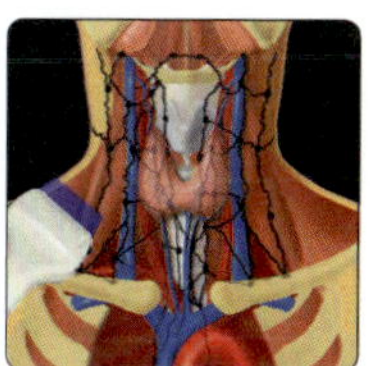

(Top) *Transverse power Doppler ultrasound shows multiple subcapsular/peripheral intranodal vessels in multiple round, hypoechoic, solid LNs at the upper cervical level. Pathology confirmed metastatic squamous cell carcinoma.* **(Middle)** *Longitudinal power Doppler ultrasound of multiple lymphomatous LNs shows chaotic peripheral and central intranodal vessels. Note that hilar vascularity is more prominent than peripheral vascularity.* **(Bottom)** *Transverse power Doppler ultrasound shows a tuberculous LN in the posterior triangle that is predominantly hypovascular with displaced hilar vascularity. The hypovascular portion corresponds to intranodal caseating necrosis.*

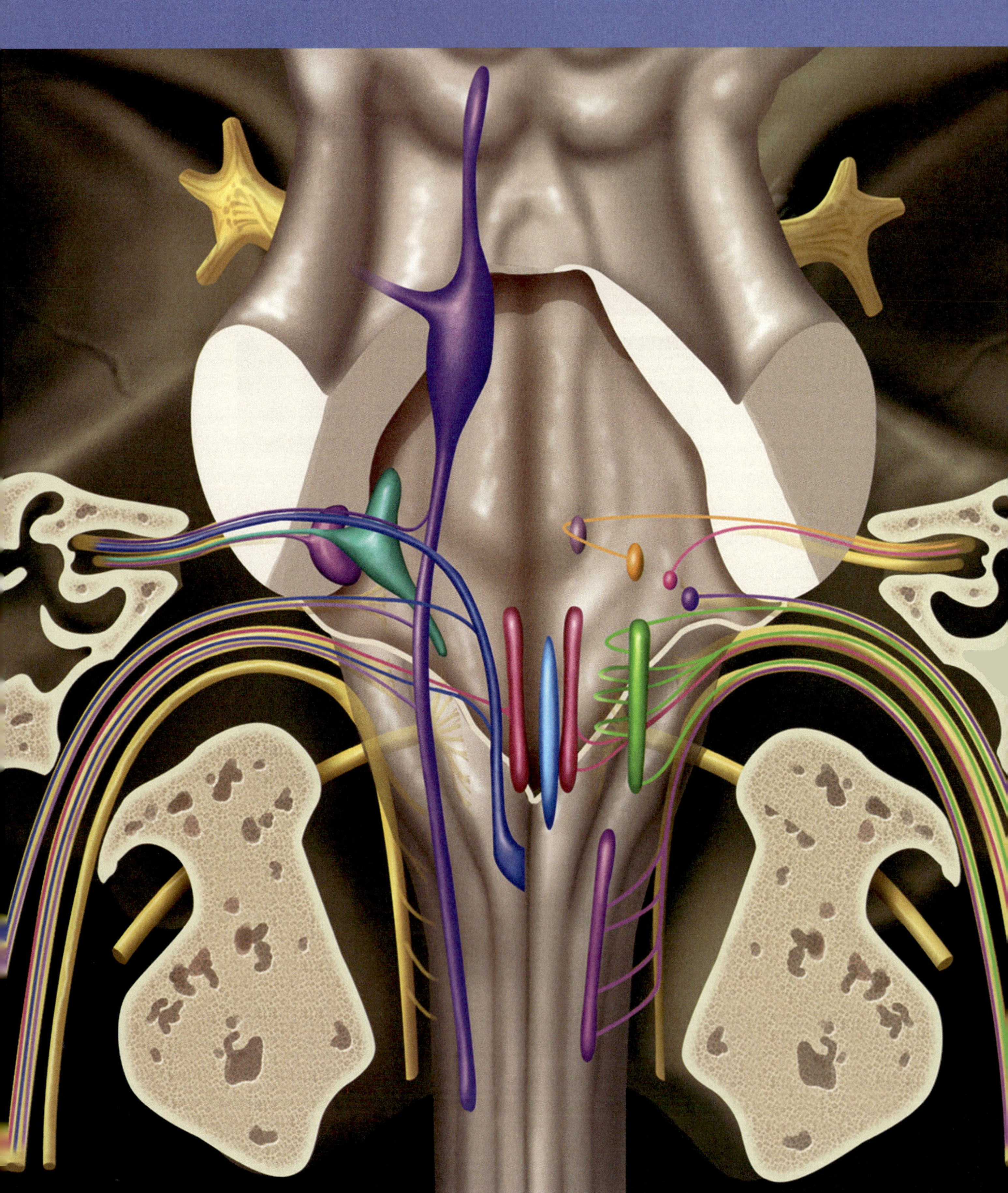

SECTION 8

Cranial Nerves

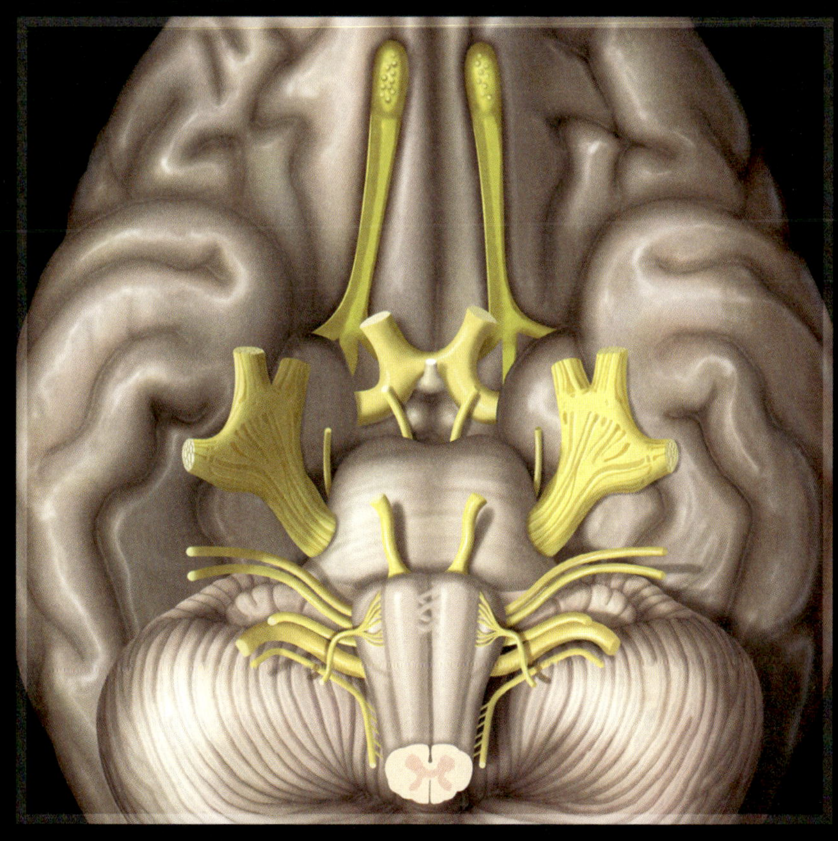

TERMINOLOGY

Synonyms

- Olfactory nerve: CNI
- Optic nerve: CNII
- Oculomotor nerve: CNIII
- Trochlear nerve: CNIV
- Trigeminal nerve: CNV
- Abducens nerve: CNVI
- Facial nerve: CNVII
- Vestibulocochlear nerve: CNVIII
- Glossopharyngeal nerve: CNIX
- Vagus nerve: CNX
- Accessory nerve: CNXI
- Hypoglossal nerve: CNXII

IMAGING ANATOMY

Overview

- Cranial nerve groupings based on area of brainstem origin
  - Diencephalon: CNII
  - Mesencephalon (midbrain): CNIII and CNIV
  - Pons: CNV, CNVI, CNVII, and CNVIII
  - Medulla: CNIX, CNX, CNXI, and CNXII

ANATOMY IMAGING ISSUES

Imaging Recommendations

- Best imaging modality for any simple or complex cranial neuropathy: **MR**
  - Single exception to this directive is distal vagal neuropathy where imaging down to aortopulmonic window on left is necessary
    - CECT better here, as less affected by breathing, swallowing, and coughing movements
- If lesion located in bony area, such as skull base, sinuses, or mandible, bone CT highly recommended to provide complementary bone anatomy and lesion-related information
  - Contrast enhancement of CT not necessary if full T1, T2, and T1 C+ MR available

Imaging Approaches

- Remember: Cranial nerves do **not** stop at skull base
- Radiologist must image entire extent of affected cranial nerve
  - **CNI, CNII, CNIII, CNIV, and CNVI**: Include focused **orbital sequences**
  - **CNV**: Include entire **face to inferior mandible if V3** affected
  - **CNVII**: Include **cerebellopontine angle (CPA), temporal bone, and parotid space**
  - **CNVIII**: Include **CPA-internal auditory canal (IAC) and inner ear**
  - **CNIX-XII**: Include **basal cistern, skull base, nasopharyngeal carotid space**
    - **CNX**: To fully evaluate for recurrent laryngeal nerve lesion, follow carotid space to just below aortopulmonic window on left and subclavian artery on right
    - **CNXII**: Remember to reach hyoid bone to include distal loop as it rises into sublingual space

Imaging Pitfalls

- Radiologist forgets to image extracranial structures associated with cranial nerve affected

CLINICAL IMPLICATIONS

Clinical Importance

- Cranial nerves and their functions
  - Olfactory nerve (CNI)
    - Sense of **smell**
  - Optic nerve (CNII)
    - Sense of **vision**
  - Oculomotor nerve (CNIII)
    - **Motor** to all **extraocular muscles** except lateral rectus and superior oblique
    - **Parasympathetic** supply to ciliary and pupillary constrictor muscles
  - Trochlear nerve (CNIV)
    - **Motor** to **superior oblique** muscle
  - Trigeminal nerve (CNV)
    - **Motor** (V3) to **muscles of mastication**, anterior belly digastric, mylohyoid, tensor tympani and palatini
    - **Sensory** innervation to surface of **forehead and nose** (V1), **cheek** (V2), and **jaw** (V3)
    - **Sensory** innervation to surfaces of nose, sinuses, meninges, and external surface of tympanic membrane (auriculotemporal nerve)
  - Abducens nerve (CNVI)
    - **Motor** to **lateral rectus** muscle
  - Facial nerve (CNVII)
    - **Motor** to **muscles of facial expression**
    - **Motor** to **stapedius muscle**
    - **Parasympathetic** to lacrimal, submandibular, and sublingual glands
    - Anterior 2/3 tongue **taste** (chorda tympanic nerve)
    - General sensation for periauricular skin, external surface of tympanic membrane
  - Vestibulocochlear nerve (CNVIII)
    - Senses of **hearing and balance**
  - Glossopharyngeal nerve (CNIX)
    - **Motor** to **stylopharyngeus** muscle
    - **Parasympathetic** to parotid gland
    - Visceral sensory innervation to carotid body
    - Posterior 1/3 tongue **taste**
    - General sensation to posterior 1/3 of tongue and internal surface of tympanic membrane
  - Vagus nerve (CNX)
    - **Motor** to **pharynx-larynx**
    - Parasympathetic to pharynx, larynx, thoracic and abdominal viscera
    - Visceral sensation from pharynx, larynx, and viscera
    - General sensation from small area around external ear
  - Accessory nerve (CNXI)
    - **Motor** to **sternocleidomastoid and trapezius** muscles
  - Hypoglossal nerve (CNXII)
    - **Motor** to intrinsic and extrinsic **tongue muscles** except palatoglossus

GRAPHICS, GLOBAL CRANIAL NERVES

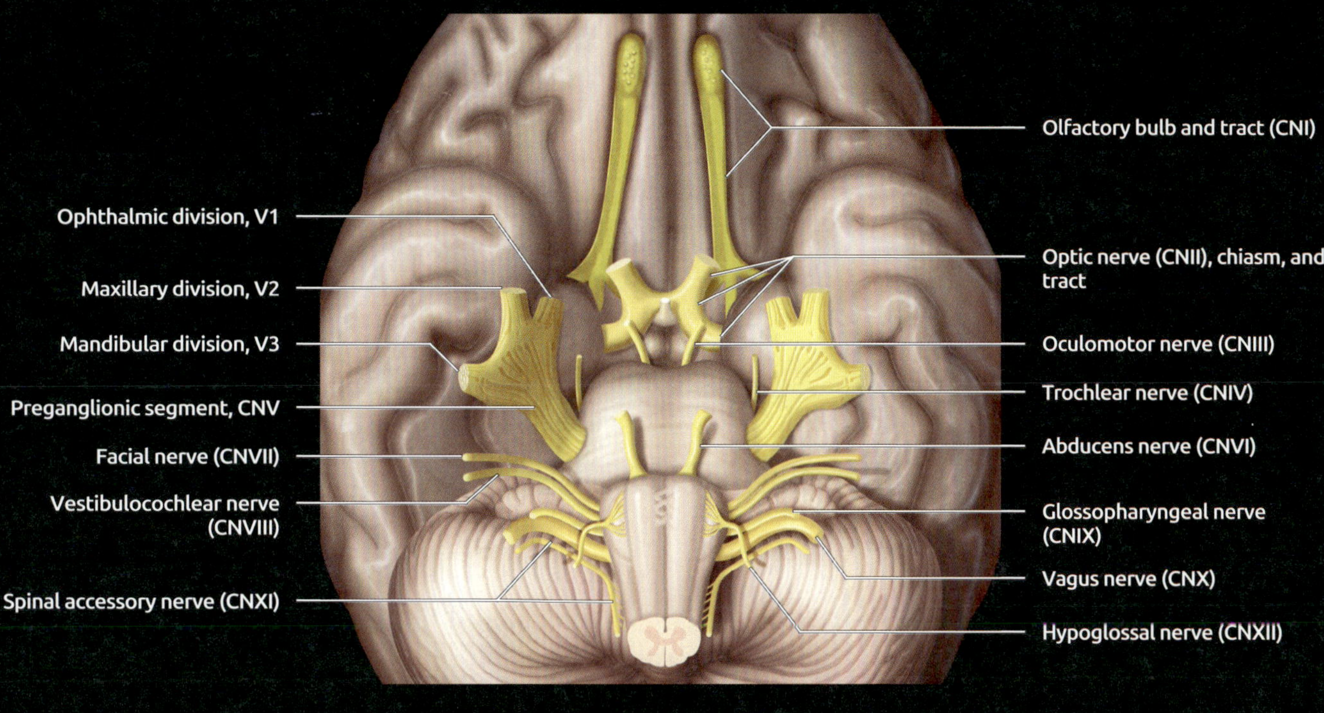

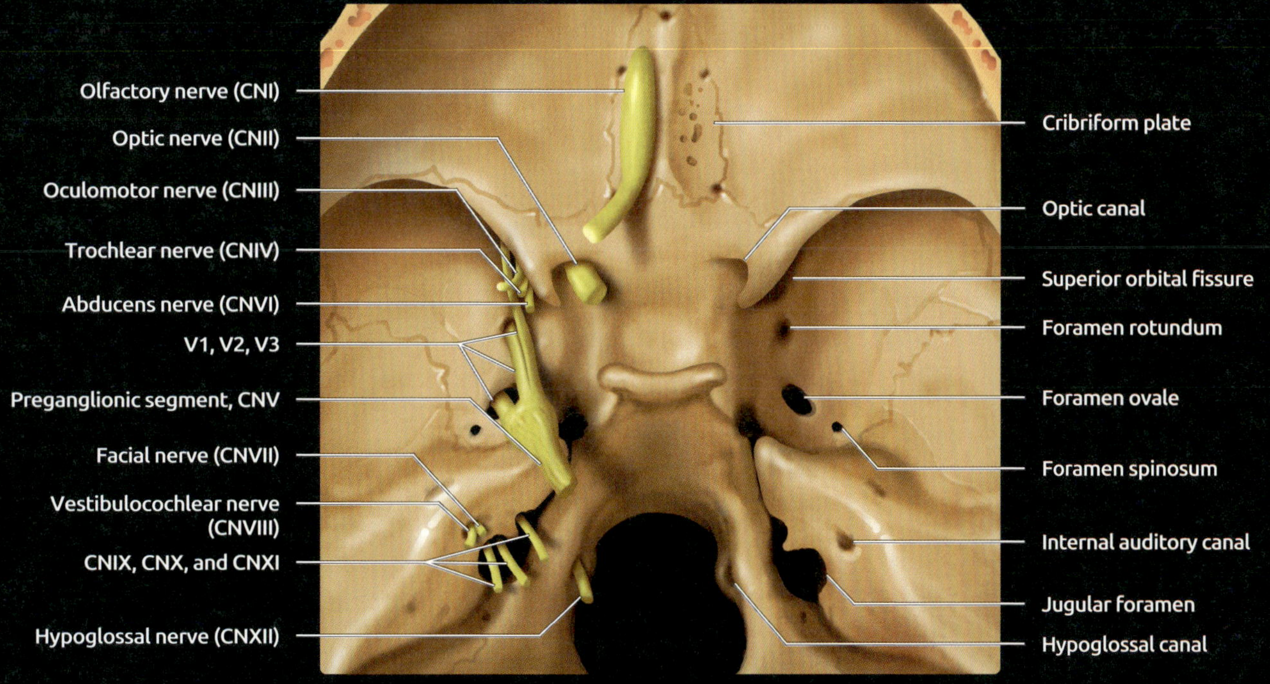

(Top) *Graphic shows all cranial nerves, viewing the brainstem from below. Remember that CNIII-IV are associated with the midbrain (mesencephalon), while CNV-VIII are affiliated with the pons. CNIX-XII emerge from various aspects of the medulla.* **(Bottom)** *In this graphic of the skull base, viewed from above, the foramina are illustrated on the right, and the associated cranial nerves are illustrated on the left. The terminal branches of CNI exit the skull base through many openings in the cribriform plate of the ethmoid bone. CNII exits via the optic canal, while CNIII, CNIV, CNVI, and CNV1 all go through the superior orbital fissure. V2 traverses foramen rotundum, and V3 is seen exiting the foramen ovale. CNVII and CNVIII are seen in the internal auditory canal with CNIX-XI found in the jugular foramen. Finally, CNXII uses its own hypoglossal canal to leave the basal cistern.*

GRAPHICS, UPPER CRANIAL NERVES

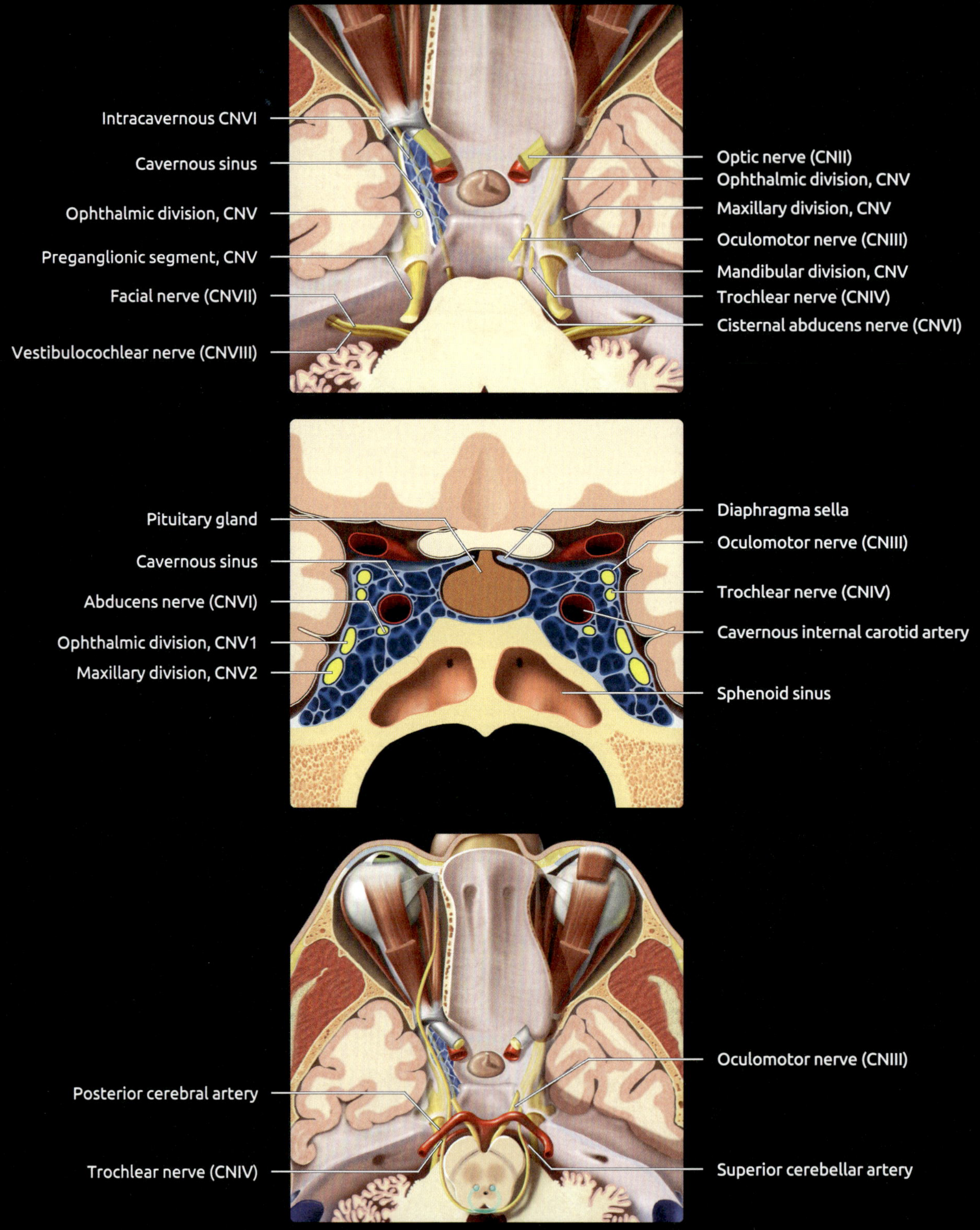

(Top) *Axial graphic shows the prepontine cistern and cavernous sinus (CS) areas viewed from above. The preganglionic segment of CNV can be seen in the lateral prepontine cistern, entering the Meckel cave through the porus trigeminus.* **(Middle)** *Coronal posterior graphic of CS is shown. Abducens nerve (CNVI) is the only cranial nerve with a purely intracavernous course. Thick inner endosteal layer of CS lateral wall envelops CNIII, CNIV, CNV1, and CNV2. CNIII and CNIV enter the roof of CS. CNIII travels a short distance in a tubular CSF-containing cistern before becoming incorporated into the lateral wall of CS. CNIV becomes immediately embedded in the lateral wall. CNV1 also lies in lateral wall. CNV2 lies at inferior margin of CS lateral wall or just outside CS envelope. CNV3 is invested by contiguous dura but not considered component of CS wall. Sympathetic nerves travel along the intracavernous internal carotid artery (ICA) as well.* **(Bottom)** *Axial graphic shows that CNIII passes in between the posterior cerebral artery (PCA) and superior cerebellar artery (SCA) near the arterial origins. CNIV also passes between PCA and SCA but more laterally in the perimesencephalic cistern.*

GRAPHICS, LOWER CRANIAL NERVES

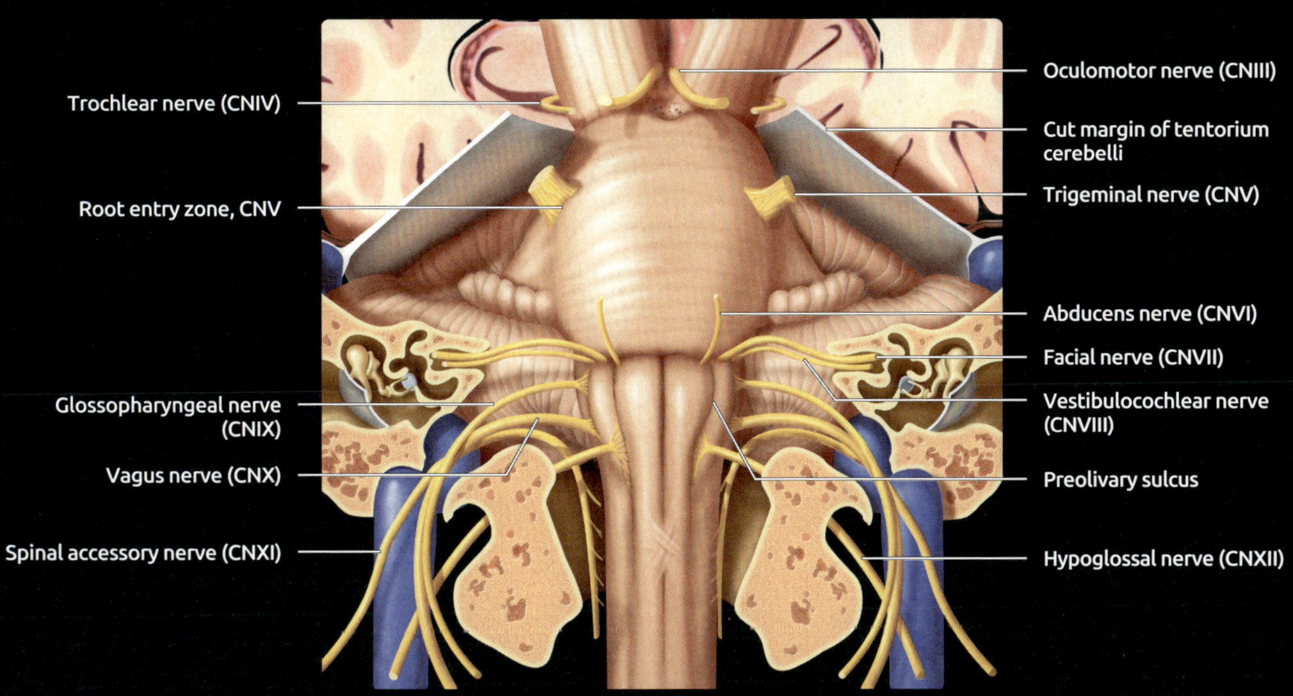

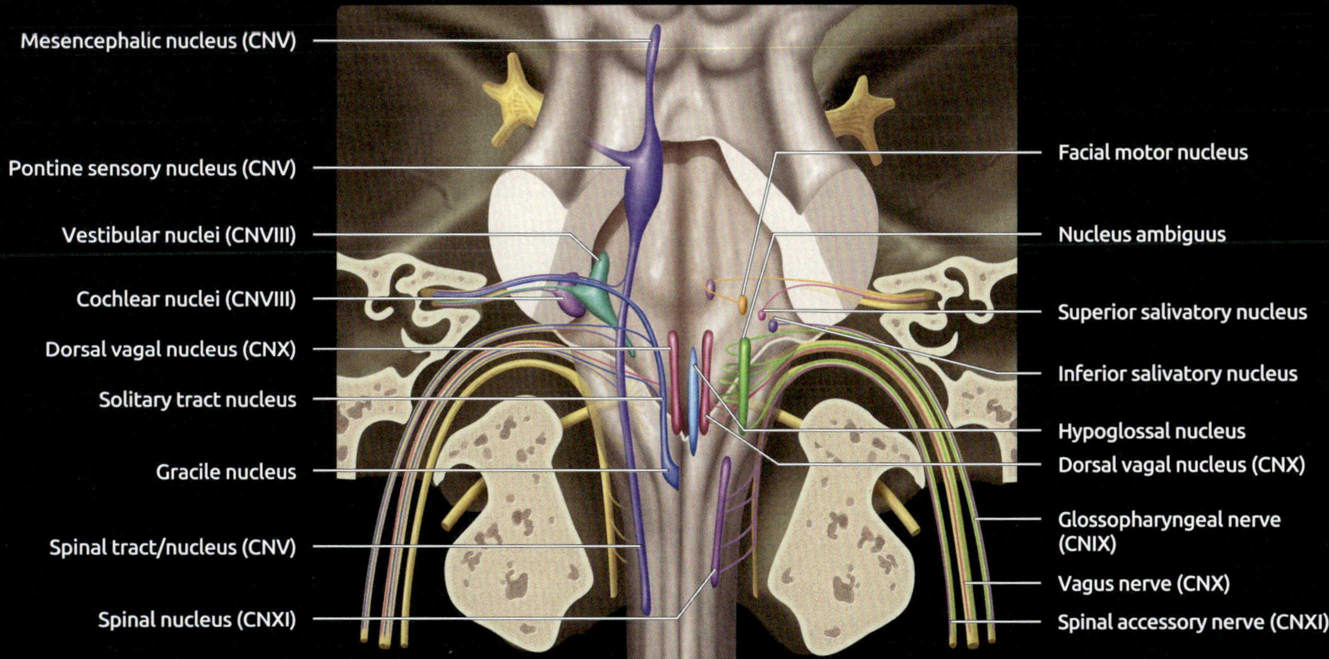

(Top) *Graphic shows frontal view of brainstem and exiting cranial nerves. CNIII is seen exiting the midbrain into the interpeduncular cistern. CNIV wraps around lateral midbrain in tentorial margin. CNVI exits at pontomedullary junction. CNVII and CNVIII exit brainstem at cerebellopontine angle. Inferiorly, CNIX-XI leave the lateral medulla in the postolivary sulcus. CNXII exits via the preolivary sulcus.* **(Bottom)** *Graphic shows brainstem from behind, emphasizing lower cranial nerve nuclei. On the right are efferent fibers, and on the left are afferent fibers connecting to brainstem nuclei. Note nucleus ambiguus providing voluntary motor fibers to CNIX and CNX. Pontine superior salivatory nucleus provides parasympathetic supply functionally through facial nerve/chorda tympani to submandibular ganglion (topographically hanging down from lingual nerve) and through facial nerve/vidian nerve to pterygopalatine ganglion (topographically hanging down from maxillary nerve). Inferior salivatory nucleus provides secretomotor fibers to the parotid via CNIX. Dorsal motor nucleus provides involuntary motor and sensory fibers to CNX. Solitary tract receives taste from CNVII and CNIX.*

AXIAL BONE CT

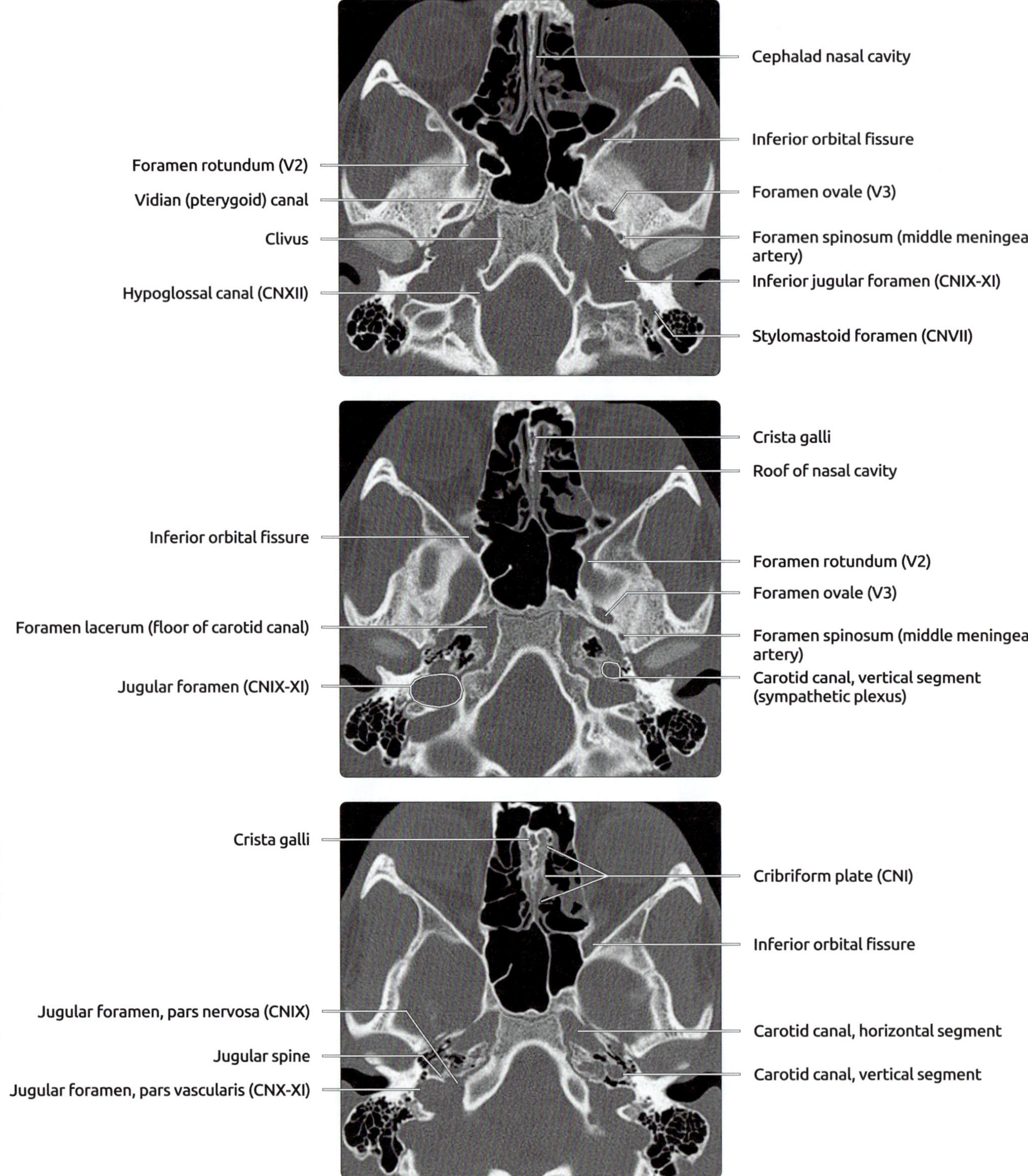

(Top) *First of 6 sequential axial bone CT images through the skull base, presented from inferior to superior, shows foramina of sphenoid bone, including foramen rotundum (CNV2) and foramen ovale (CNV3). More posteriorly oblique, the hypoglossal canal is visible bilaterally in the occipital bone.* **(Middle)** *At the level of the inferior jugular foramen, the entry to the vertical segment of the carotid canal is also seen just anterior to the jugular foramen. Notice the ovoid shape of the jugular foramen at this level. The floor of the anteromedial aspect of the horizontal segment of the petrous ICA is called the foramen lacerum.* **(Bottom)** *At the level of the cribriform plate, the jugular foramen is now divided by the jugular spine into the more anterior pars nervosa (CNIX, Jacobsen nerve, and the inferior petrosal sinus) and more posterolateral pars vascularis (CNX, CNXI, Arnold nerve, and jugular bulb).*

AXIAL BONE CT

Crista galli
Subfrontal cistern (olfactory bulb here)
Superior orbital fissure (CNIII, CNIV, CNVI, and CNV1)
Internal carotid artery, lacerum segment
Carotid canal, horizontal segment
Jugular foramen, pars nervosa (CNIX)
Jugular spine
Jugular foramen, pars vascularis (CNX-XI)
Facial nerve canal, mastoid segment (CNVII)
Jugular tubercle

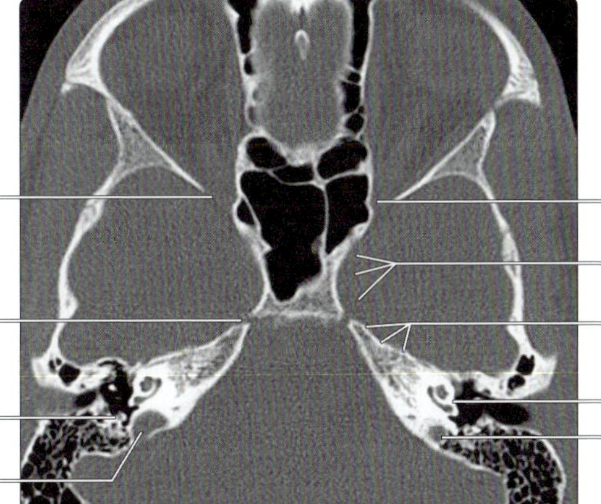

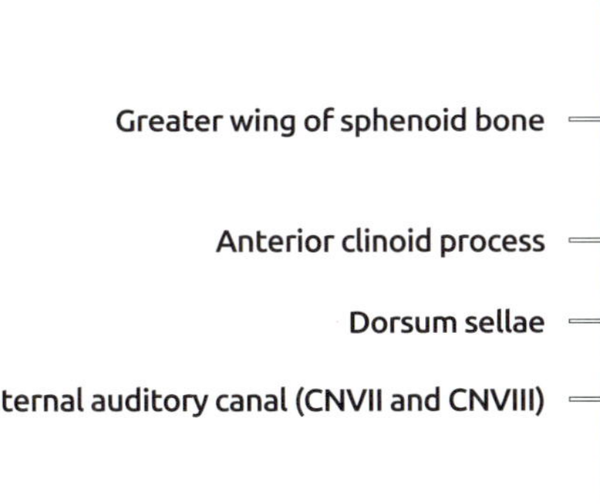

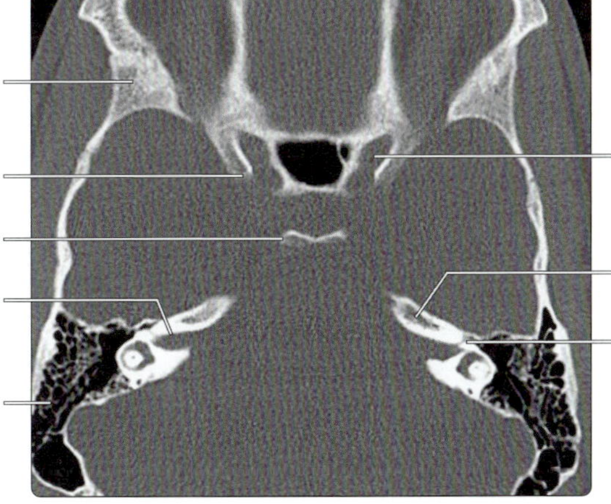

(Top) *At the level of the midhorizontal portion of the petrous ICA, the superior orbital fissure is seen. Remember that CNIII, CNIV, and CNVI as well as the ophthalmic division of CNV and the superior ophthalmic vein all enter the orbit through this structure.* **(Middle)** *At the level of the cochlea and upper petrous apex, the petrooccipital fissure is seen. This is approximately the location of CNVI after it pierces the dura to leave the prepontine cistern on its way to the CS. On bone CT, the area of the CS can only be approximated. Notice also the inferior margin of the porus trigeminus.* **(Bottom)** *The internal auditory canal is visible on this most cephalad CT. The facial (CNVII) and vestibulocochlear (CNVIII) nerves pass through the internal auditory canal. The optic nerve (CNII) enters orbit via the optic canal, which lies medial to the anterior clinoid process.*

AXIAL T2 MR

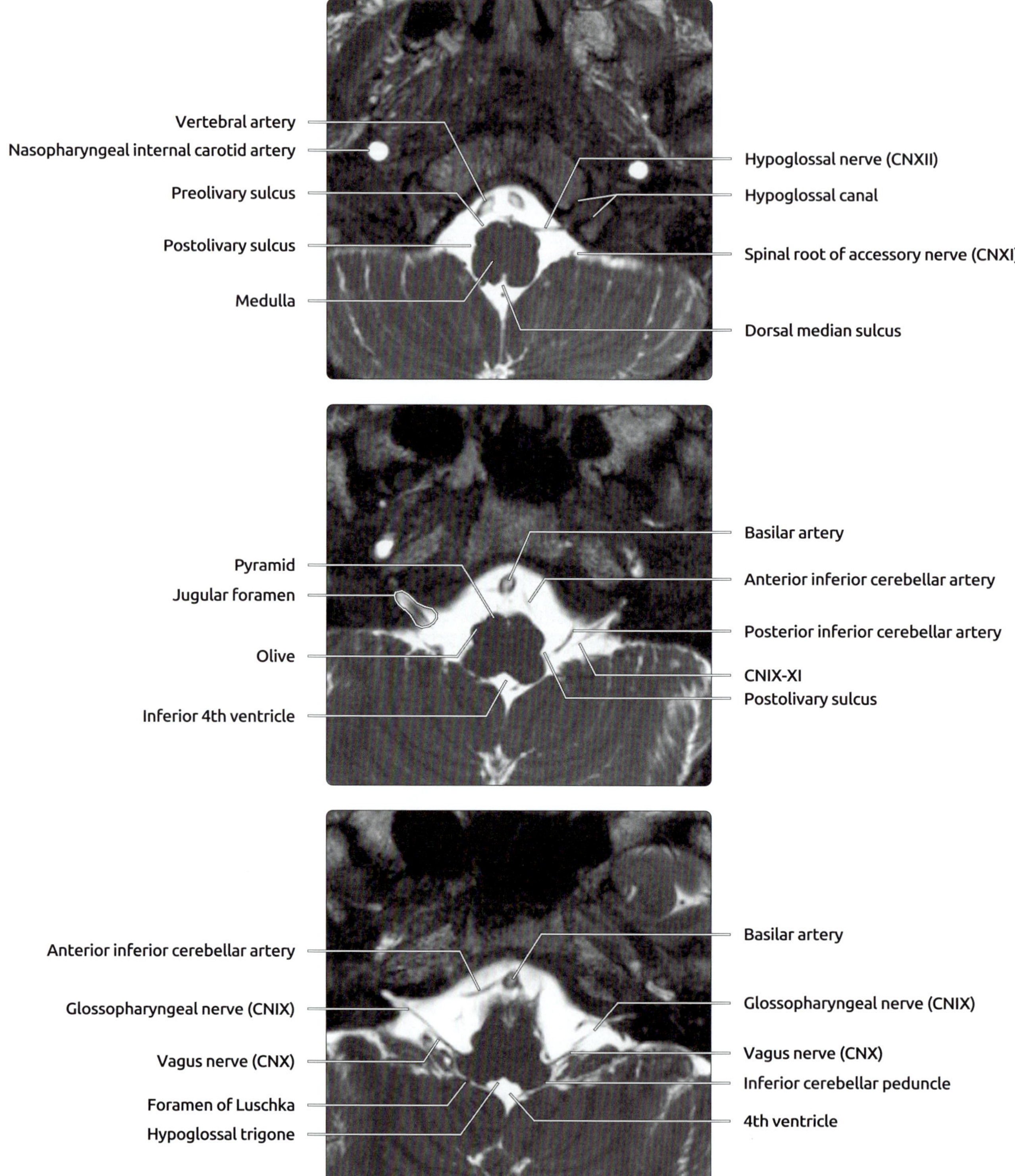

(Top) *First of 12 axial T2 MR images presented from inferior to superior shows the left hypoglossal nerve leaving the preolivary sulcus of the medulla. Spinal root of accessory nerve (CNXI) ascends through the foramen magnum, lateral to the brainstem, to unite with the cranial roots of the accessory nerve before exiting via the jugular foramen.* **(Middle)** *Glossopharyngeal (CNIX), vagus (CNX), and cranial (bulbar) roots of spinal accessory (CNXI) nerves emerge from lateral brainstem posterior to the olive in the postolivary sulcus and exit the skull base via jugular foramen. Do not confuse the posterior or anterior inferior cerebellar arteries for cranial nerves.* **(Bottom)** *Nucleus of hypoglossal nerve (CNXII) forms a characteristic bulge on the floor of the 4th ventricle called the hypoglossal trigone. It is often difficult to separate CNIX from CNX in the basal cistern.*

AXIAL T2 MR

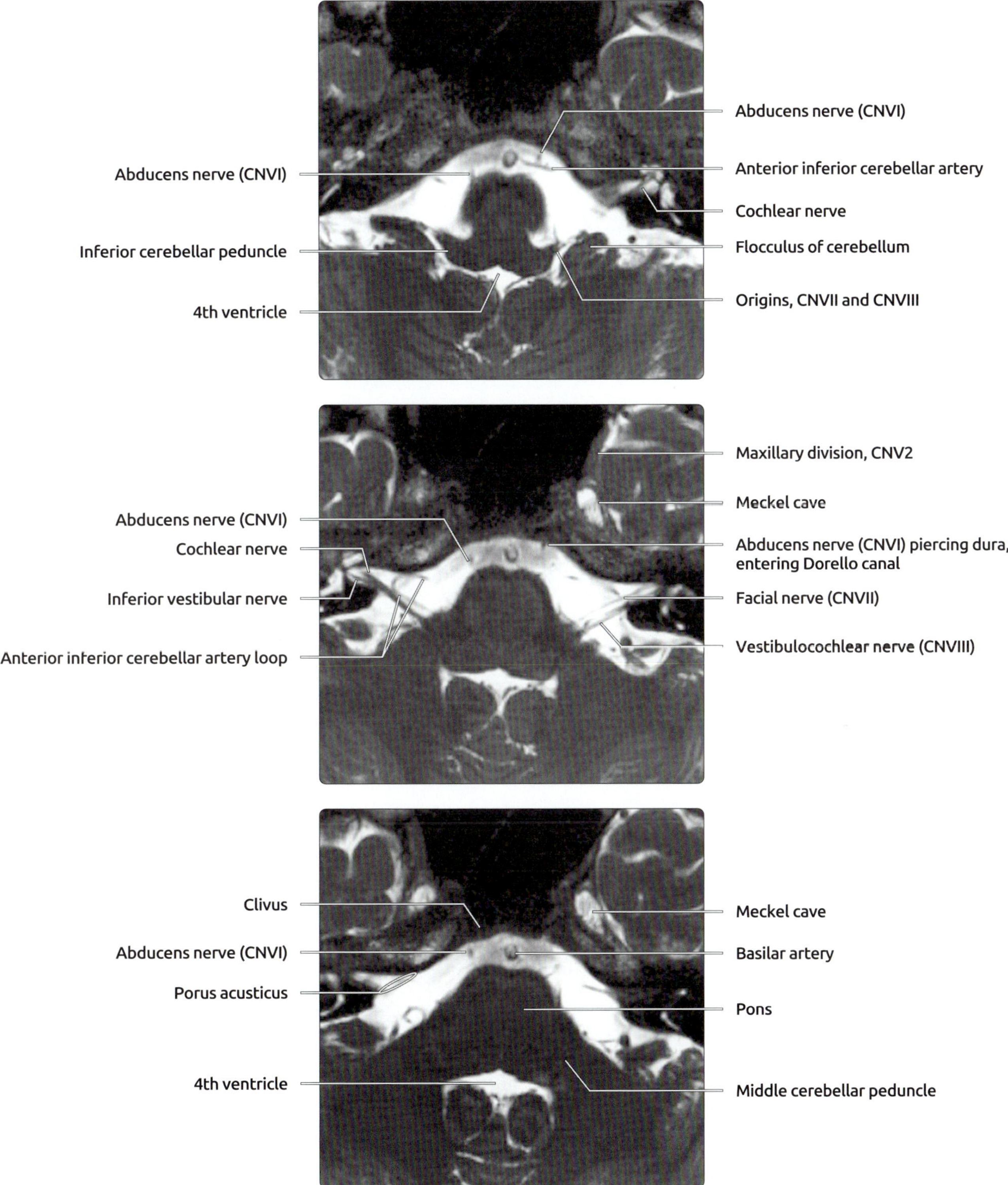

(Top) *Abducens (CNVI) nerves exit the brainstem anteriorly at the pontomedullary junction just above pyramid, ascending from there through the prepontine cistern toward the clivus. Cochlear nerve nuclei are found on the lateral surface of the inferior cerebellar peduncle (restiform body).* **(Middle)** *CNVII and CNVIII exit the brainstem laterally at the pontomedullary junction to enter the cerebellopontine angle cistern. CNVII lies anterior to CNVIII in the cerebellopontine angle cistern. Notice CNVI piercing dura on the patient's left to enter the Dorello canal, an interdural channel passing along the dorsal surface of the clivus within the basilar venous plexus toward the CS.* **(Bottom)** *Meckel cave is formed by a dural reflection, lined with arachnoid and containing CSF. The gasserian ganglion (trigeminal ganglion) is semilunar in shape and lies anteroinferiorly in the Meckel cave.*

AXIAL T2 MR

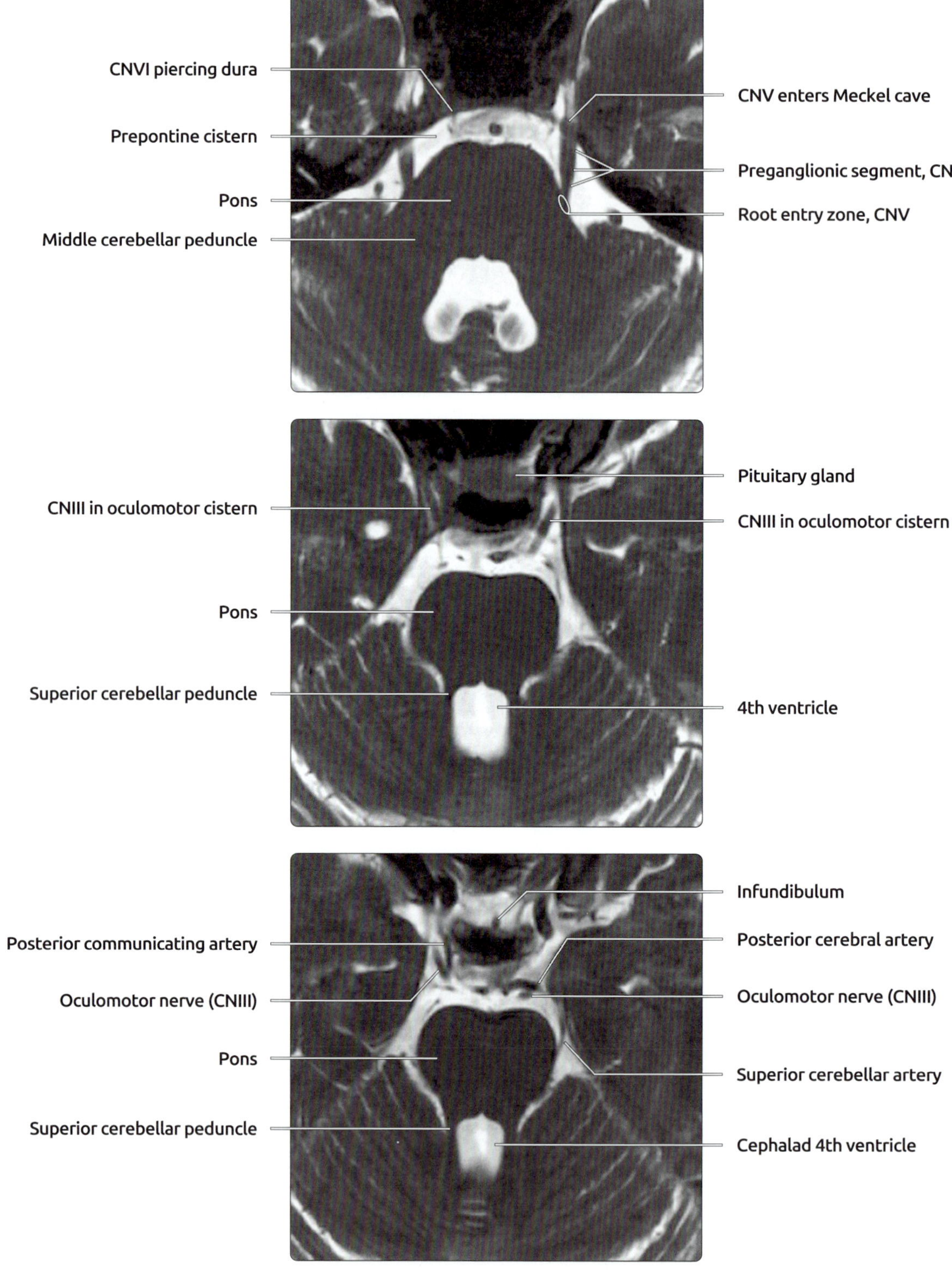

(Top) *CNV exits the lateral pons at a point referred to as the root entry zone. Preganglionic segment courses anteriorly through the prepontine cistern and passes over the petrous apex to enter the Meckel cave via the porus trigeminus (entrance to Meckel cave).* **(Middle)** *In this image, the oculomotor nerve (CNIII) can be seen surrounded by high-signal CSF as it enters the roof of the CS. This area is referred to as the oculomotor cistern. CNIII travels anterolaterally, becoming incorporated into the lateral wall of the CS near the anterior clinoid process.* **(Bottom)** *At the level of the upper pons, important vascular relationships of CNIII passing between the PCA and SCA are visible. Notice CNIII coursing anteriorly within the suprasellar cistern adjacent to the posterior communicating artery. An aneurysm of the posterior communicating artery will result in compression of CNIII. More laterally in the perimesencephalic cistern, CNIV (trochlear nerve) also passes between PCA and SCA.*

AXIAL T2 MR

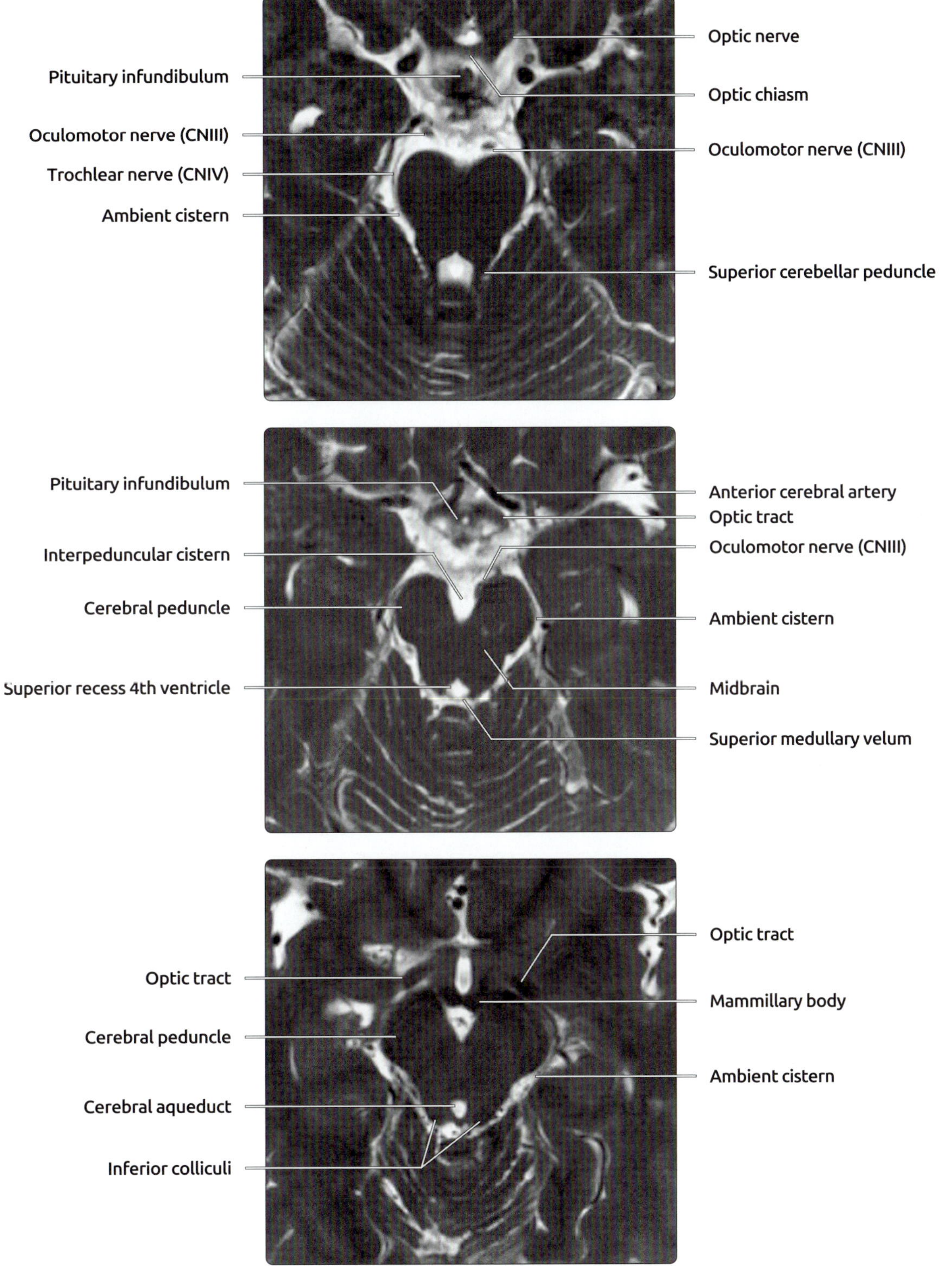

(Top) *Anteriorly, note the optic nerves (CNII) form the optic chiasm in the suprasellar cistern. Fibers originating from the nasal halves of the retina cross within the optic chiasm. CNIII courses anteriorly within the suprasellar cistern toward the CS.* **(Middle)** *CNIII is seen on the patient's left, exiting the brainstem along the medial aspect of the cerebral peduncle, where it enters the interpeduncular cistern. The trochlear nerve (CNIV) decussates in the superior medullary velum, then exits along the dorsal surface of the midbrain below the inferior colliculus to enter the quadrigeminal plate cistern. From there, CNIV courses around the brainstem below the tentorium cerebelli in the ambient cistern passing between the PCA and SCA.* **(Bottom)** *Optic tracts connect the lateral geniculate body to the optic chiasm. Only a portion of the optic tracts are visible here.*

CORONAL T2 MR

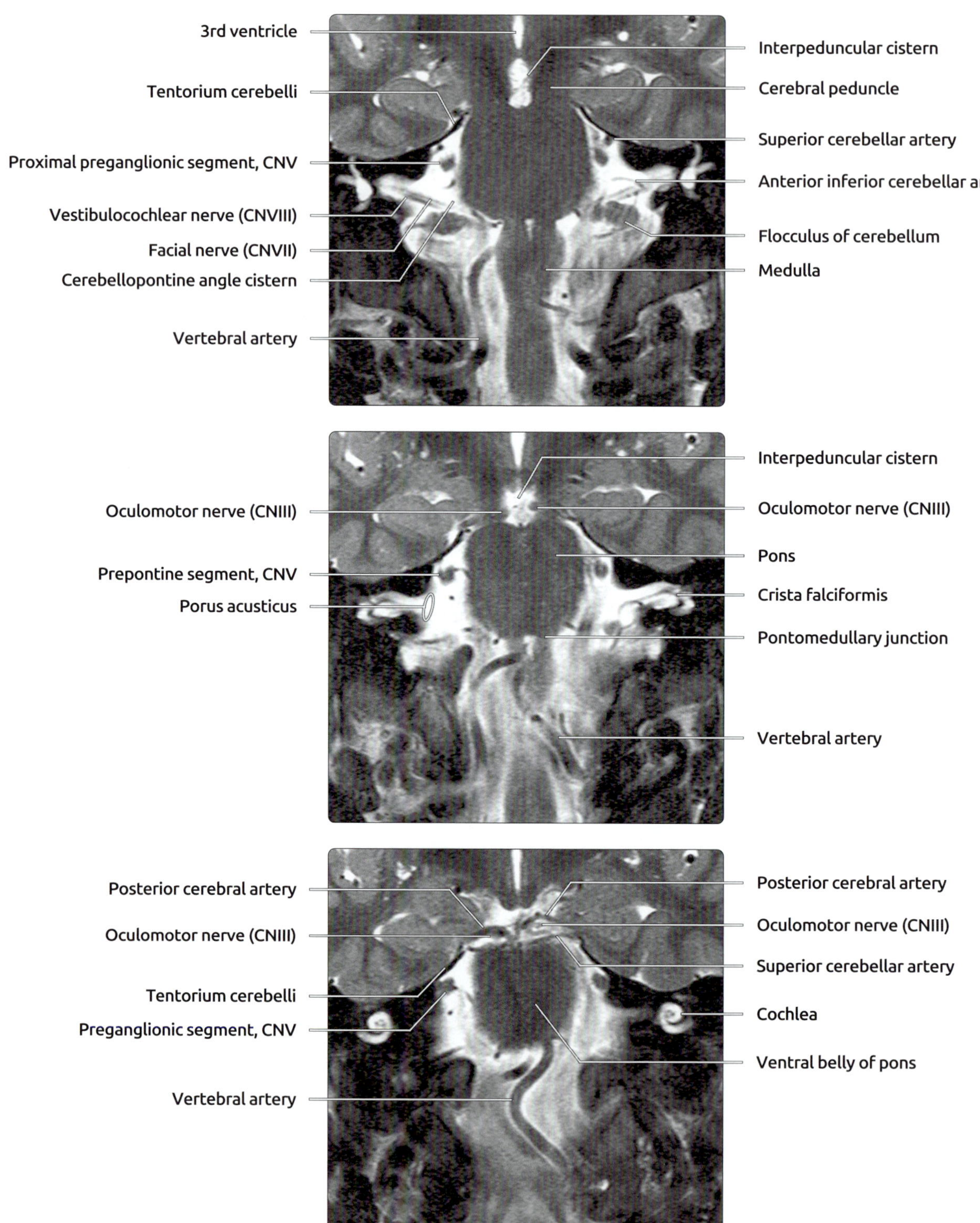

(Top) *First of 6 coronal T2 MR images of the brainstem, cisterns, and cranial nerves presented from posterior to anterior is shown. Preganglionic segment of the trigeminal nerve is seen arising from the lateral pons. Also seen are the facial and vestibulocochlear nerves traversing the cerebellopontine angle cistern into the internal auditory canal.* **(Middle)** *Oculomotor nerves are seen emerging from the medial aspect of the cerebral peduncle into the interpeduncular cistern. Basal cistern cranial nerves are not visible. The abrupt transition between the pons and the medulla is termed the pontomedullary junction.* **(Bottom)** *In this image, notice the oculomotor nerves passing between the PCA above and the SCA below. The distal preganglionic segment of CNV is poised to enter the porus trigeminus on its way into the Meckel cave.*

CORONAL T2 MR

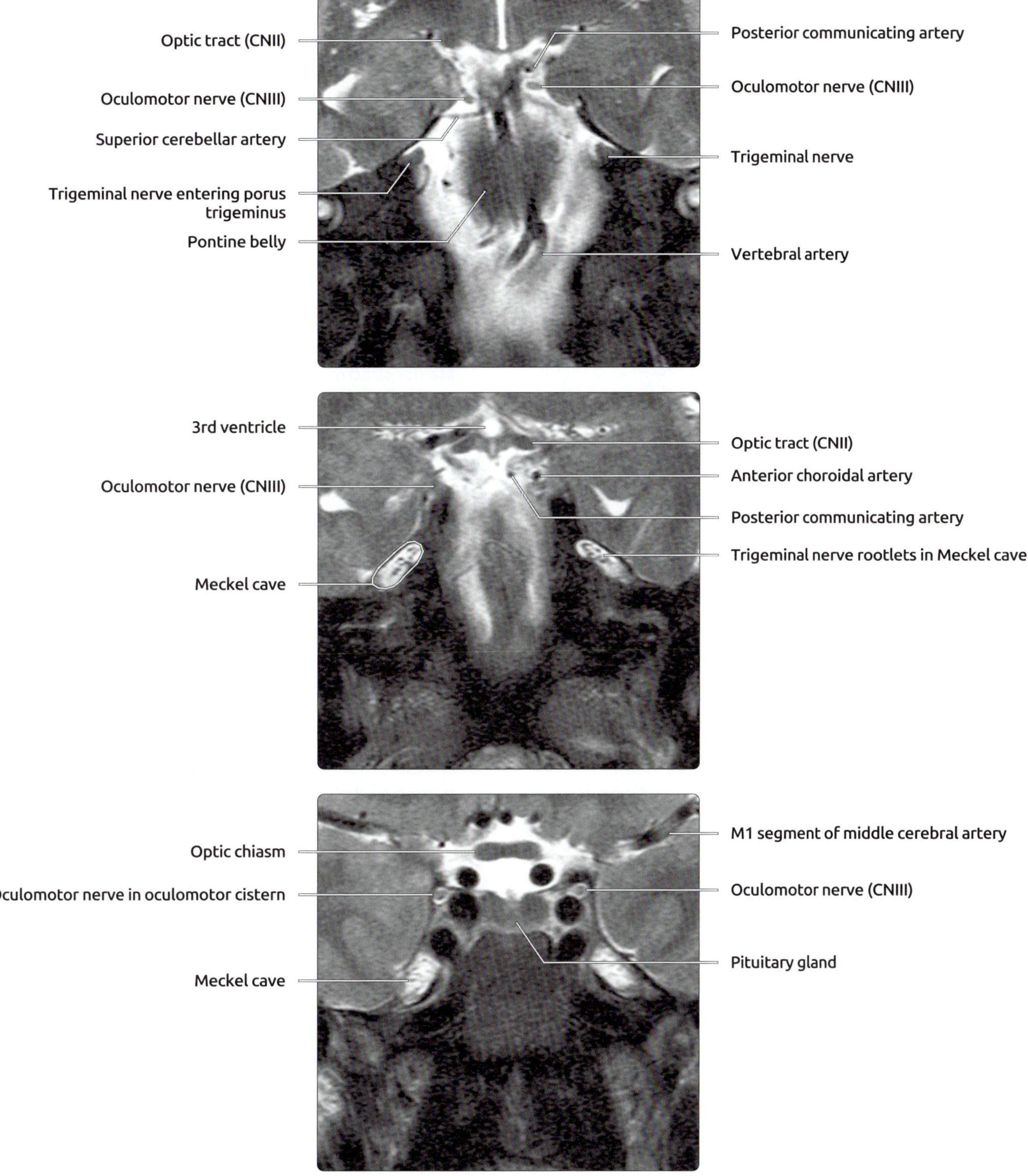

(Top) *This image shows the oculomotor nerve between the posterior communicating artery above and the SCA below. The trigeminal nerve is visible entering the porus trigeminus of the Meckel cave.* **(Middle)** *Here, the optic tracts are seen converging toward the optic chiasm. Note a large left anterior choroidal artery coursing posterolaterally within the suprasellar cistern. Preganglionic fibers of the trigeminal nerve are seen within the Meckel cave. The Meckel cave is formed by a reflection of dura, which is lined with arachnoid, contains CSF, and communicates freely with prepontine cistern.* **(Bottom)** *In this most anterior coronal T2 image, the pituitary is seen below the optic chiasm. Notice the oculomotor nerve is entering the CS in the oculomotor cistern. The high-signal ring around CNIII is CSF.*

TERMINOLOGY

Abbreviations

- Olfactory nerve (CNI)

Synonyms

- 1st cranial nerve

Definitions

- Visceral afferent cranial nerve for sense of smell

IMAGING ANATOMY

Overview

- Olfactory nerve segments
  - Receptor neurons in olfactory epithelium in nasal vault
  - Transethmoidal segment through cribriform plate
  - Intracranial olfactory bulb, tract, and cortex

Nasal Epithelium

- Pseudostratified columnar epithelium (~ 2 cm^2), classically described in roof of each nasal cavity, adjacent septum, and lateral nasal cavity wall, including superior turbinates
  - More extensive distribution up to middle turbinate, posterior and middle septum in recent studies
- Contains **bipolar olfactory receptor cells**
  - Their peripheral processes/dendrites are sensory receptors for smell, each neuron expressing single type of odorant receptors out of ~ 400-500 types
- Olfactory glands (of Bowman) secrete mucous, which solubilizes inhaled scents (odorant molecules)

Transethmoidal Segment

- Hundreds of central processes/axons of receptor cells are bundled into unmyelinated fascicles (fila olfactoria) interleaved with specialized glial cells called olfactory ensheathing cells
  - **Fila olfactoria: True olfactory nerves**
  - ~ 20 fila traverse **cribriform plate** on each side of nasal cavity to synapse with olfactory bulb neurons

Intracranial Olfactory Bulb and Tract

- Olfactory bulb and tracts: Extensions of brain, not nerves, but historically referred to as 1st cranial nerve
- **Olfactory bulb** (mean volume 125 ±17 mm^3) closely apposed to cribriform plate at ventral surface of medial frontal lobe
  - Histologically, bulb contains 6 concentric cell layers
  - Axons within fila from receptor cells expressing same type of odorant receptor converge to spherical "glomerulus" in glomerular layer of bulb where they synapse with processes of secondary neurons (mitral and tufted cells) in deeper layers of bulb
    - Short axon and granule cells modulate secondary neurons
  - Axons of mitral and tufted cells coalesce to form lateral olfactory tract
- **Olfactory tract** (mean length 28-30 mm) trifurcates to medial, intermediate, lateral striae at **anterior perforated substance**, where intermediate striae terminate
  - This trifurcation creates **olfactory trigone**
  - Anterior olfactory nucleus formed by some neurons along olfactory tract
  - Olfactory tubercle: Immediately behind division of olfactory stria, fused with anterior perforated substance

Intracranial, Central Pathways

- Complex connections, incompletely elucidated in humans
- **Olfactory cortex**
  - Cortical areas that receive input from olfactory bulb
  - Composed of anatomically distinct areas: Piriform cortex, olfactory tubercle, anterior olfactory nucleus, anterior cortical nucleus of amygdala and periamygdaloid cortex, and anterior parts of entorhinal cortex
- **Lateral olfactory striae**
  - Formed by majority of fibers of olfactory tracts
  - Course over limen of insula to piriform (previously called prepiriform) cortex anterior to uncus and then to medial surface of amygdala
  - Projections from piriform cortex go to orbitofrontal cortex, thalamus (medial dorsal thalamic nucleus), hypothalamus, amygdala, and hippocampal formation
- **Medial olfactory striae**
  - Majority terminate in parolfactory area of Broca (medial surface in front of subcallosal gyrus), some in subcallosal gyrus and anterior perforated substance
  - Few fibers go contralaterally in anterior commissure
- **Medial forebrain bundle**
  - Formed by fibers from basal olfactory region, periamygdaloid area, and septal nuclei
  - Some fibers terminate in hypothalamic nuclei
  - Most fibers go to autonomic areas in brainstem (reticular formation, salivatory nuclei, dorsal vagus nucleus)
  - In human imaging studies, olfactory tubercle seen between uncus and medial forebrain bundle

ANATOMY IMAGING ISSUES

Imaging Recommendations

- Olfactory dysfunction imaging depends on clinical context
  - Sinus CT with coronal reconstructions typically done in post-URI anosmia, head trauma, or sinus surgery
  - Brain and sinonasal MR used with suspected neurodegenerative disease (Alzheimer, Parkinson), neurologic symptoms, olfactory hallucinations, hypogonadism, or anosmia, especially post COVID-19

Imaging Pitfalls

- Coronal sinus CT includes nasal vault and cribriform plate but insensitive to intracranial pathology
- Remember to include medial temporal lobes in assessment

CLINICAL IMPLICATIONS

Clinical Importance

- CNI dysfunction produces **unilateral anosmia**
- **Esthesioneuroblastoma** arises from olfactory epithelium
- Olfactory ensheathing cells can give rise to schwannomas
- Head trauma may cause anosmia: Cribriform plate fracture or shear forces; anterior temporal lobe injury
- Seizures involving olfactory network produce "uncinate fits" with olfactory hallucinations, variable oroglossal automatisms, and impaired awareness
- Olfactory bulb volumes decreased in head trauma, chronic rhinosinusitis, Alzheimer disease, multiple sclerosis, and schizophrenia

GRAPHICS

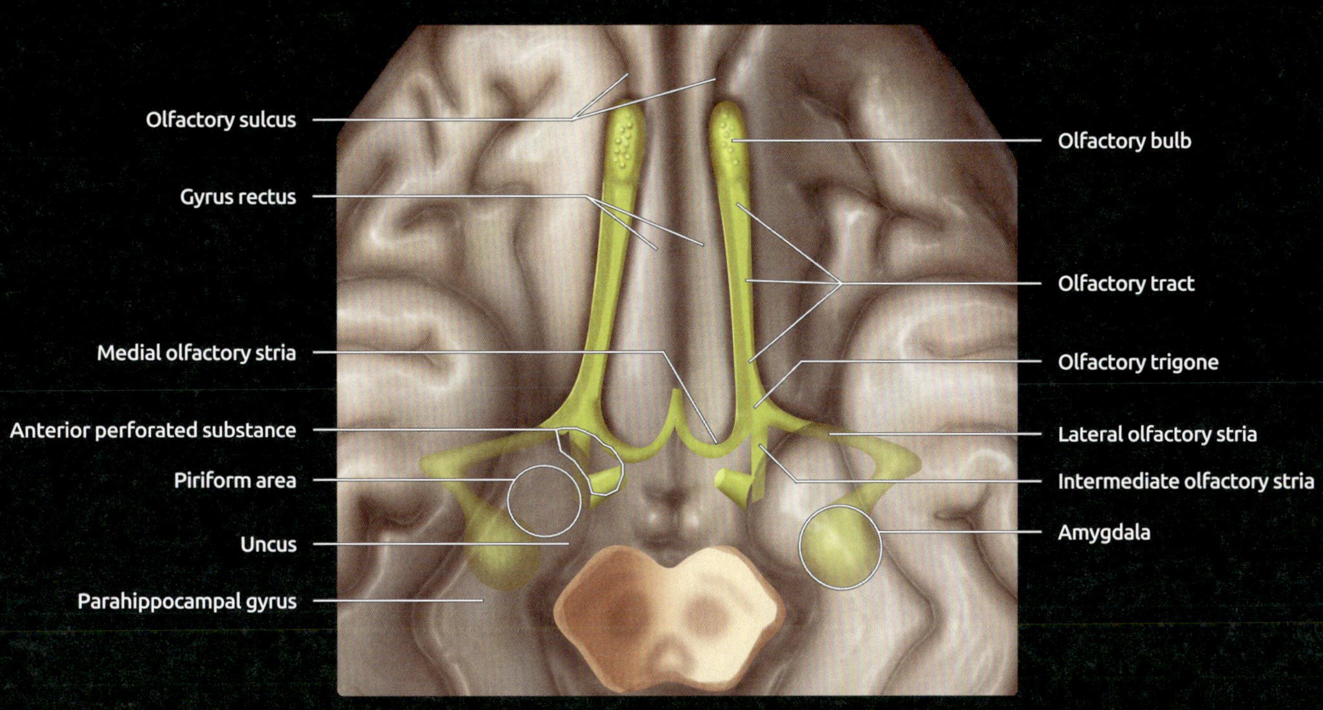

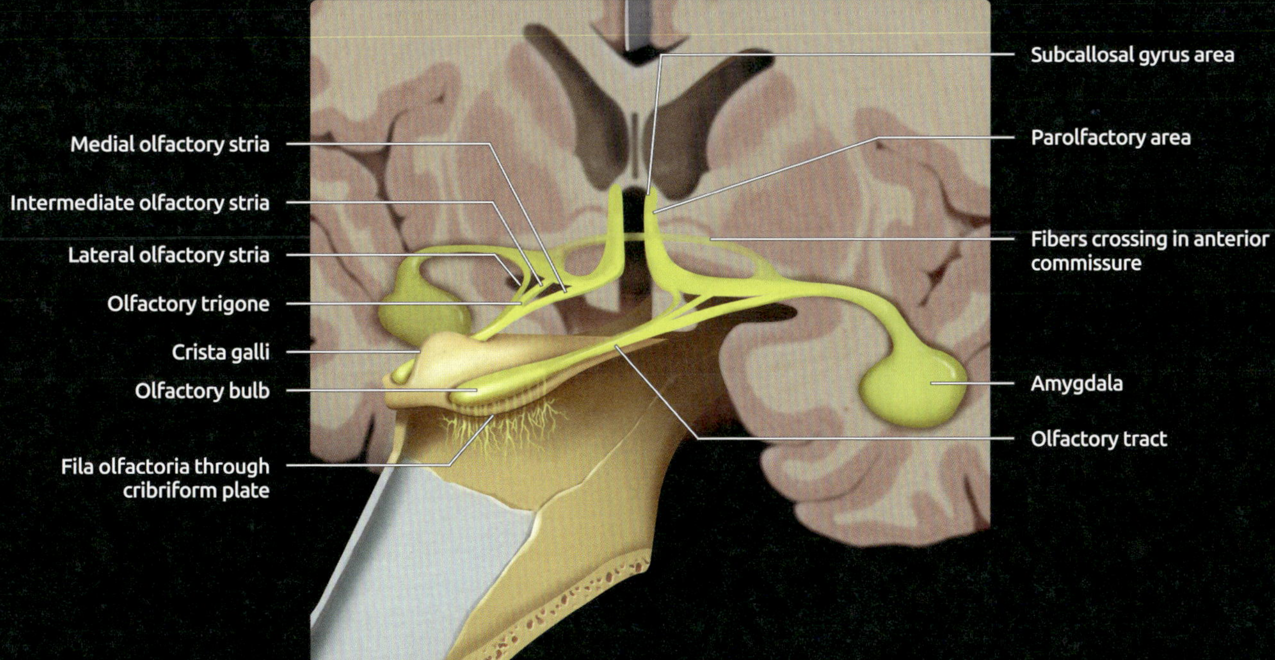

(Top) *Graphic of olfactory system viewed from below shows olfactory tracts coursing from olfactory bulbs to the olfactory trigone. In the olfactory trigone, fibers split up into lateral, intermediate, and medial striae. The majority of fibers course through the lateral stria to the piriform area and amygdala. Some fibers in the medial stria course through the anterior commissure to connect to the opposite tract. The majority of intermediate stria fibers terminate in the anterior perforated substance.* **(Bottom)** *Graphic of the olfactory system seen from an anterolateral oblique perspective shows central processes from bipolar olfactory cells in the olfactory epithelium crossing the cribriform plate, bundled as fila olfactoria (~ 20 per side) and connecting with secondary neurons in the olfactory bulbs. The olfactory trigone is visible dividing into lateral, intermediate, and medial striae.*

CORONAL NECT

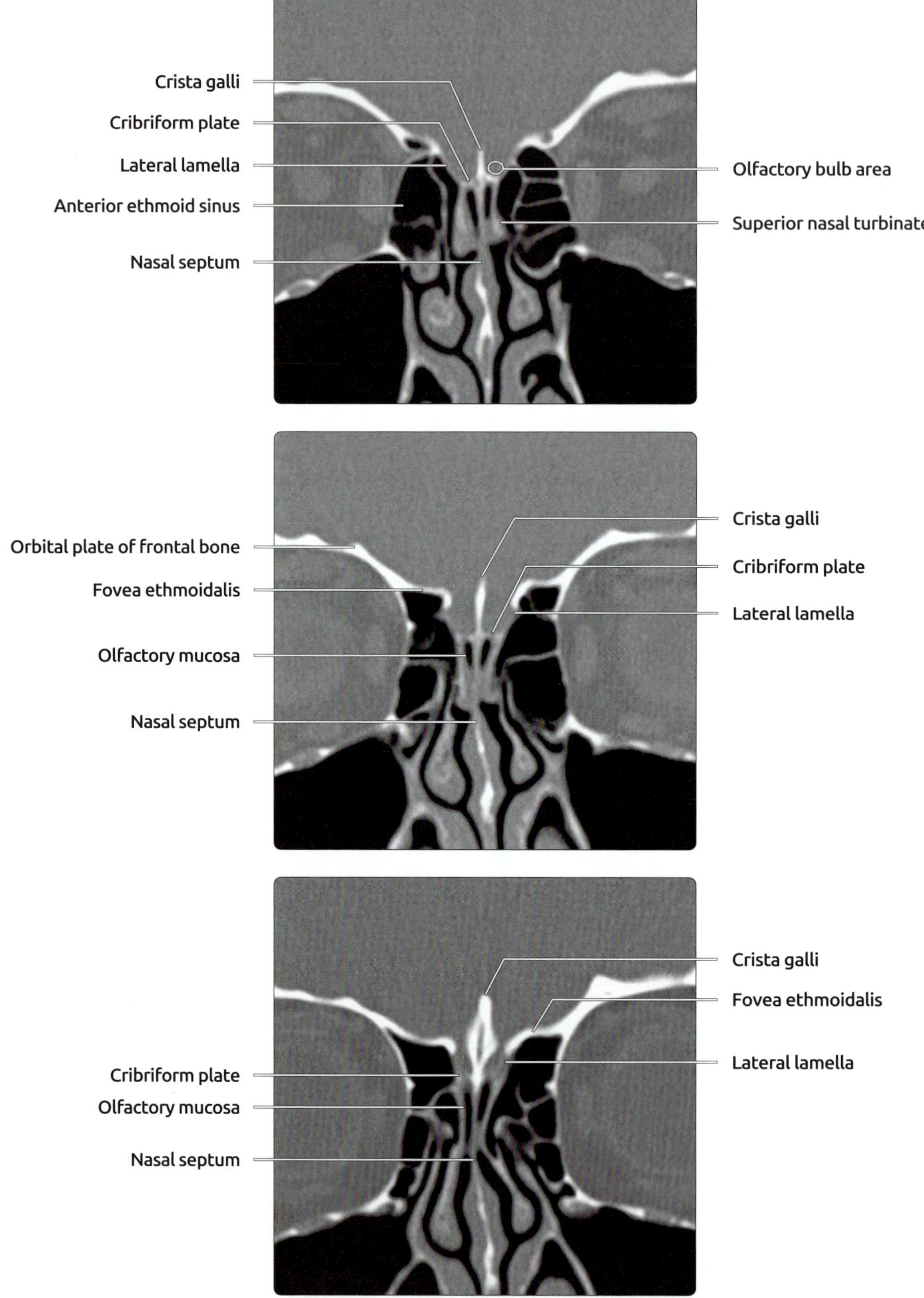

(Top) *First of 3 coronal bone CT images through the anterior cranial fossa are presented from posterior to anterior. The olfactory epithelium is found on the roof of the nasal cavity, extending inferolaterally on the superior turbinate and inferomedially on the nasal septum. The olfactory nerves pass through perforations in the cribriform plate. The olfactory bulbs sit just above the cribriform plates.* **(Middle)** *In this CT, the ethmoid bone forms the medial floor of the anterior cranial fossa and consists of the cribriform plate and crista galli. The fenestrated cribriform plate is depressed relative to the orbital plate of the frontal bone. The fovea ethmoidalis is the most medial portion of the orbital plate of the frontal bone and separates the ethmoid labyrinth from the anterior cranial fossa.* **(Bottom)** *On this CT the anterior cribriform plate is seen at the base of the larger anterior crista galli.*

CORONAL T2 MR

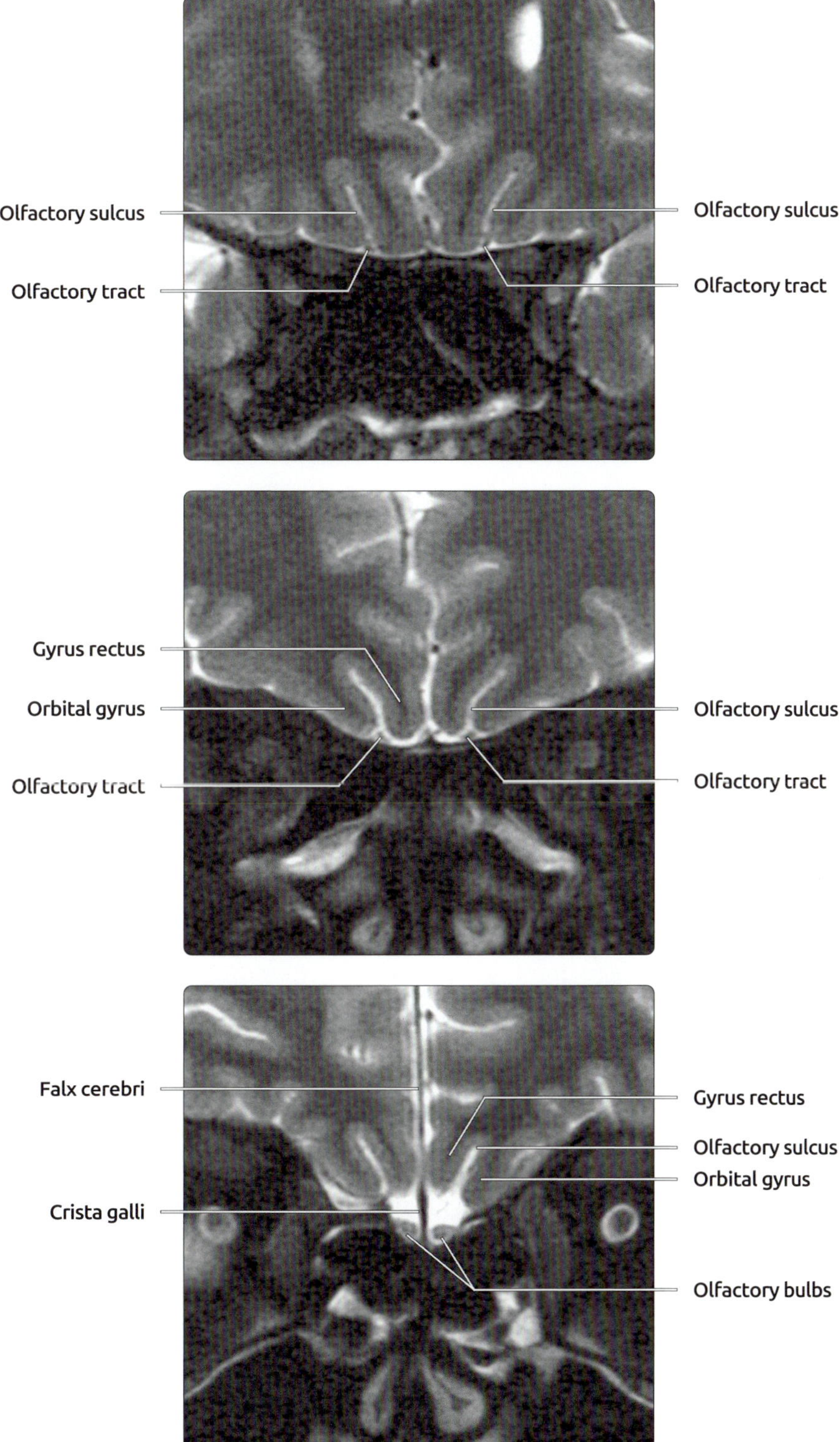

(Top) *First of 3 sequential coronal T2 MR images presented from posterior to anterior shows the triangular olfactory tracts, which are composed of centrally projecting axons, embedded within the olfactory sulcus.* **(Middle)** *The olfactory sulcus is easily identified separating the gyrus rectus medially from the orbital gyrus laterally. Again note the olfactory tracts at the base of the olfactory sulcus.* **(Bottom)** *In this image through the anterior cribriform plate, note the olfactory bulbs. The olfactory bulbs are rostral enlargement of the olfactory tracts, which lie on either side of the midline on the intracranial surface of the cribriform plate. The olfactory nerves arise from the olfactory epithelium located in the roof nasal cavity and pass through the fenestrated cribriform plate to end in the olfactory bulbs.*

CORONAL T2

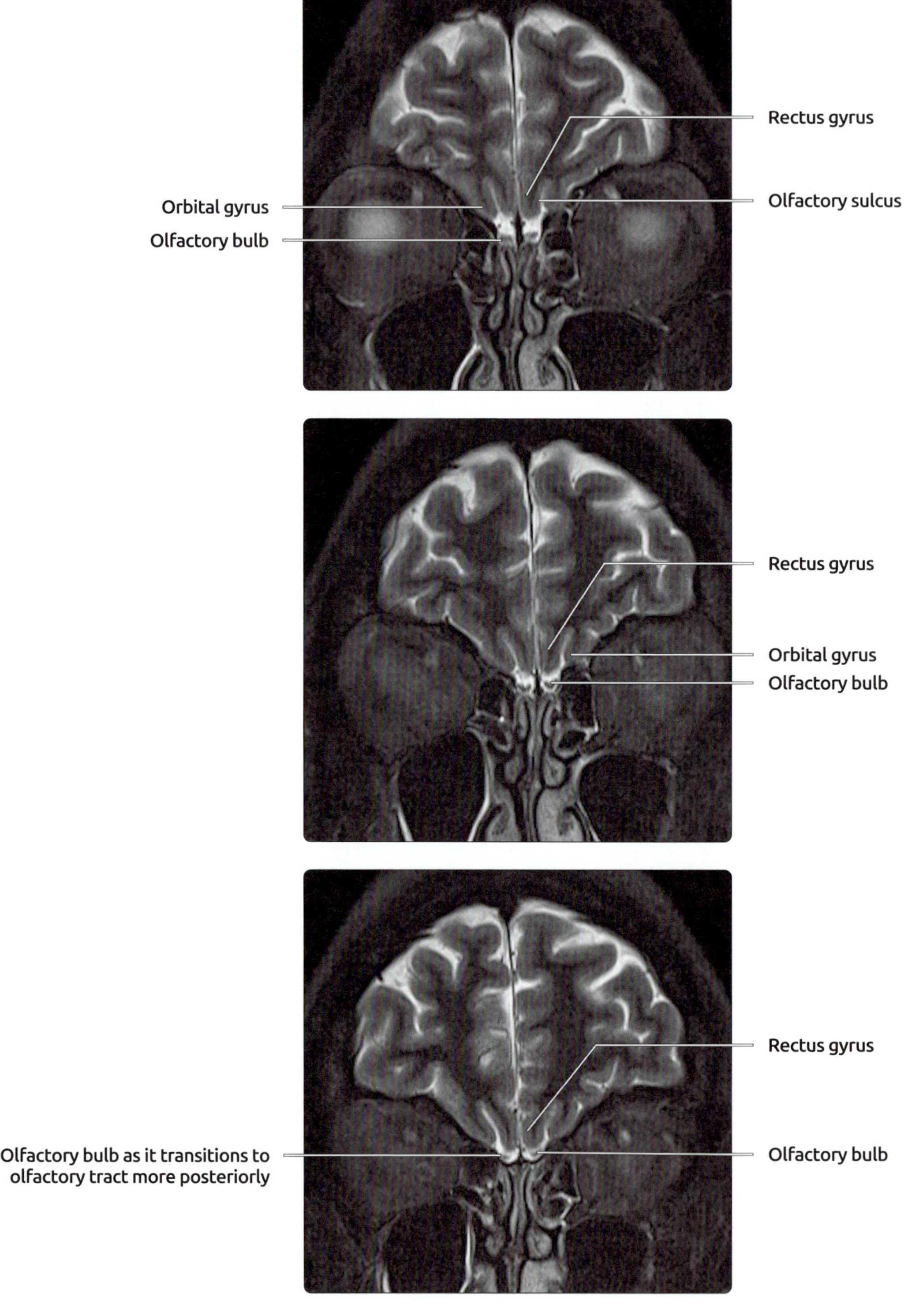

(Top) *Images from anterior to posterior demonstrate the configuration of the olfactory bulb as it transitions posteriorly to the olfactory tract.* **(Middle)** *The olfactory bulb may demonstrate an oval or inverted J-shaped morphology.* **(Bottom)** *The olfactory bulb's signal can be compared with the gyrus rectus to evaluate for any abnormal intensity.*

FLOWCHART: OLFACTORY NERVE PATHWAY

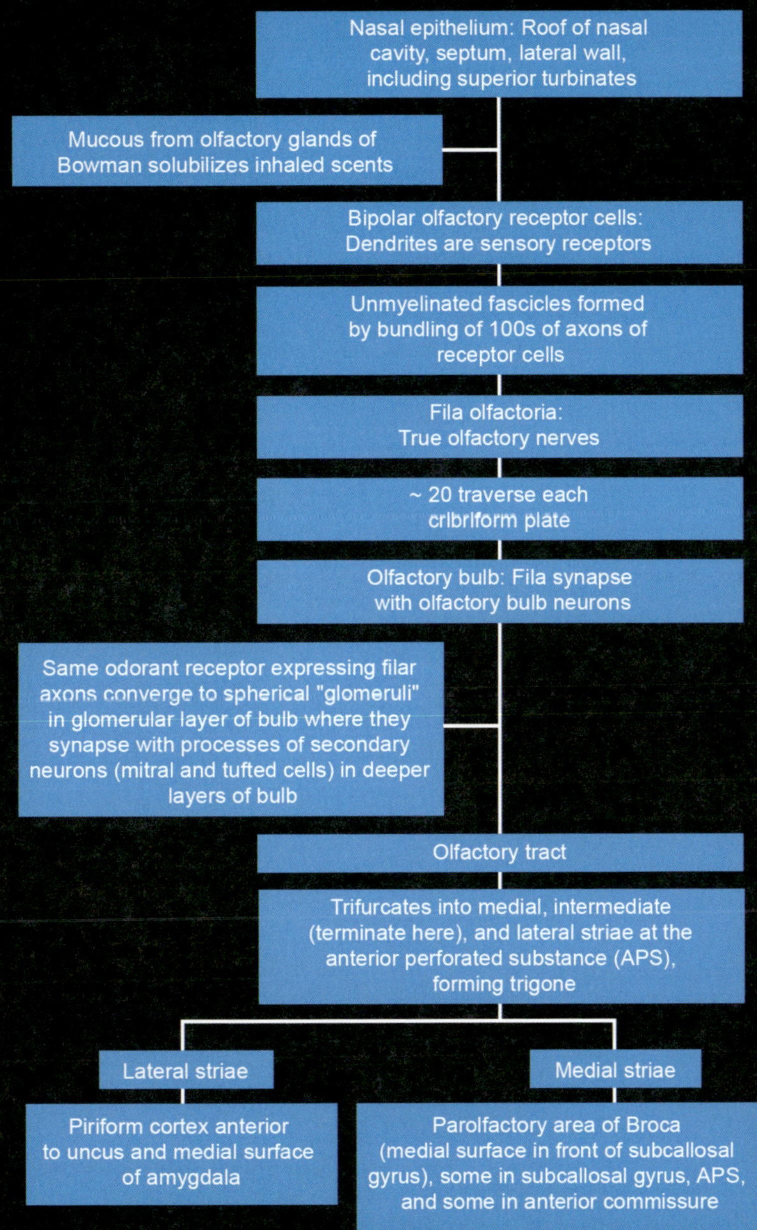

This flowchart summarizes sequential structures in the olfactory nerve pathway beginning at the nasal epithelium to the initial areas of the cortex. Please refer to the text for further details regarding the cortex connections.

TERMINOLOGY

Abbreviations

- Cranial nerve II (CNII)

Synonyms

- 2nd cranial nerve

Definitions

- CNII: Nerve of sight
- Visual pathway consists of optic nerve, optic chiasm, and retrochiasmal structures

IMAGING ANATOMY

Overview

- Optic nerve **not** true cranial nerve but rather **extension of brain**
  - Represents collection of retinal ganglion cell axons
  - Myelinated by **oligodendrocytes** not by Schwann cells as with true cranial nerves
  - Enclosed by meninges
  - Throughout its course to visual cortex, nerve fibers are arranged in **retinotopic order**
- Optic nerve has 4 segments
  - Intraocular, intraorbital, intracanalicular, and intracranial
- Partial decussation of CNII fibers within optic chiasm
  - Axons from medial portion of each retina cross to join those from lateral portion of opposite retina
- Retrochiasmal structures: Optic tract, lateral geniculate body, optic radiation, and visual cortex

Optic Pathway

- **Optic nerve**: **Intraocular segment**
  - 1 mm in length
  - Region of sclera termed **lamina cribrosa** where ganglion cell axons exit globe
- **Optic nerve**: **Intraorbital segment**
  - 20-30 mm in length
  - Extends posteromedially & superiorly from back of globe to orbital apex within intraconal space of orbit
  - Tortuous course allowing for movements of eye
  - Covered by same 3 meningeal layers as brain
    - Outer dura, middle arachnoid, and inner pia
    - Subarachnoid space (SAS) between arachnoid and pia contains CSF; continuous with SAS of suprasellar cistern
    - Fluctuations in intracranial pressure transmitted via SAS of optic nerve-sheath complex
  - Central retinal artery
    - 1st branch of ophthalmic artery
    - Enters optic nerve halfway along intraorbital segment
- **Optic nerve**: **Intracanalicular segment**
  - ~ 10-mm segment within bony optic canal
  - Ophthalmic artery lies inferolateral to CNII
  - Dura of CNII fuses with orbit periosteum (periorbita)
  - Weakest point of anterior orbital pathway as it is fixed to bony canal
- **Optic nerve**: **Intracranial segment**
  - ~ 10 mm in length from optic canal to chiasm
  - Surrounded by optic sheath and dorsal surface covered by falciform ligament
  - Ophthalmic artery runs inferolateral to nerve
- **Optic chiasm**
  - Horizontally oriented; X-shaped structure within suprasellar cistern
  - Forms part of floor of 3rd ventricle between optic recess anteriorly and infundibular recess posteriorly
  - Positioned over diaphragma sellae (normofixed) or tuberculum sellae (prefixed) or dorsum sellae (postfixed)
  - Anteriorly, chiasm divides into optic nerves
  - Axons representing temporal visual fields decussate in chiasm
  - Posteriorly, chiasm divides into optic tracts
  - Medial fibers of optic tracts cross in chiasm to connect lateral geniculate bodies of both sides (commissure of Gudden)
- **Optic tracts**
  - Posterior extension of optic chiasm
  - Fibers pass posterolaterally, curving around cerebral peduncle, and divide into medial and lateral bands
    - Lateral band (majority of fibers) ends in **lateral geniculate body** of thalamus
    - Medial band goes by medial geniculate body to pretectal nuclei deep to superior colliculi
- **Optic radiation and visual cortex**
  - Axons from lateral geniculate body form **optic radiations** (geniculocalcarine tracts)
  - Fan out from lateral geniculate body and run as broad fiber tract to calcarine fissure
    - Initially pass laterally behind posterior limb internal capsule and basal ganglia
    - Extend posteriorly around lateral ventricle passing through posterior temporal and parietal lobes
    - Terminate in calcarine cortex (primary visual cortex) on medial surface of occipital lobes

ANATOMY IMAGING ISSUES

Imaging Recommendations

- CT best for skull base and optic canal bony anatomy
- MR for CNII, optic chiasm, and retrochiasmal structures
  - Axial and coronal thin-section T2, T1, and T1 C+ images

Imaging Pitfalls

- Orbital CT may see subtle calcified optic sheath meningioma when MR may not

CLINICAL IMPLICATIONS

Clinical Importance

- Lesion location
  - Optic nerve pathology: **Monocular visual loss**
  - Central optic chiasm pathology: **Bitemporal heteronymous hemianopsia**
  - Peripheral optic chiasm pathology: **Ipsilateral nasal hemianopsia**
  - Retrochiasmal pathology: **Homonymous hemianopsia**
- Increased intracranial pressure transmitted along SAS of optic nerve-sheath complex presenting as papilledema
  - Imaging demonstrates flattening of posterior sclera, tortuosity and elongation of intraorbital optic nerves, and dilatation of perioptic SAS

GRAPHICS

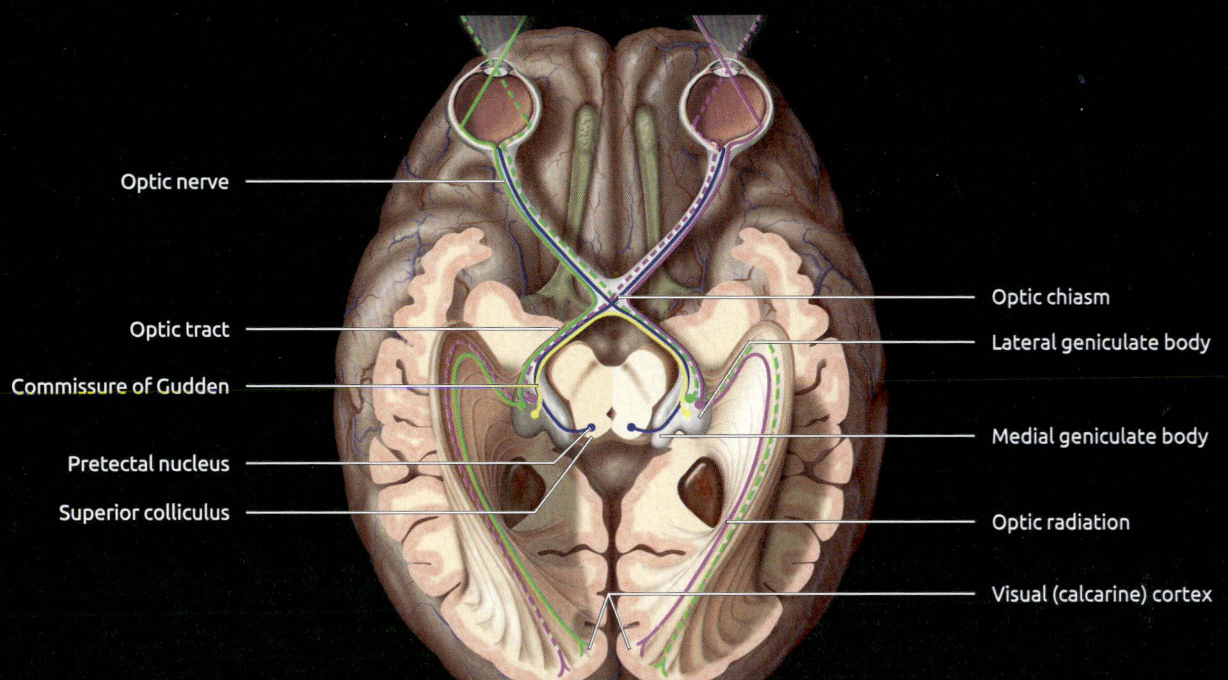

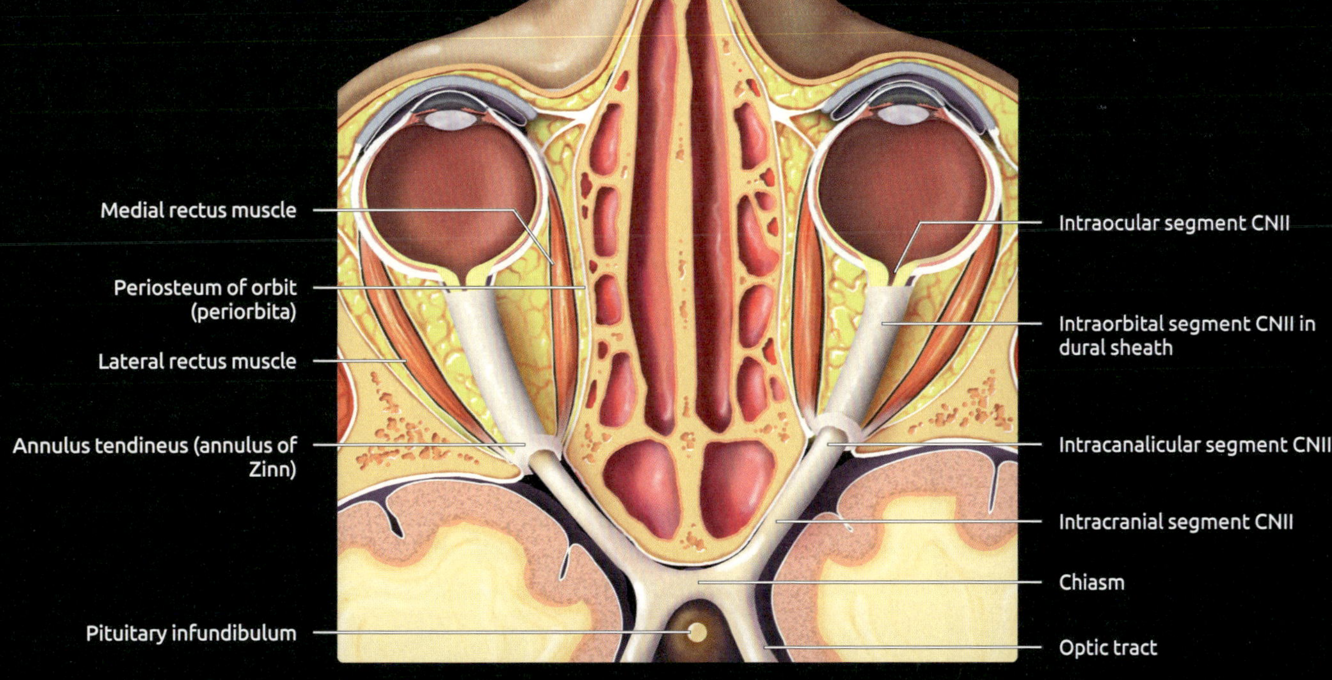

(Top) *Axial graphic through the visual pathway shows medial retinal fibers crossing in the optic chiasm so that fibers from the left 1/2 of both retinas course in the left optic tract, and fibers in the right 1/2 of both retinas course in the right optic tract (purple and green, respectively). The majority of retinal nerve fibers terminate in the lateral geniculate bodies, where synaptic neuronal cell bodies give rise to optic radiations, which extend to the visual cortices. A few retinal nerve fibers (blue) involved in optic reflexes bypass the lateral geniculate bodies and terminate in the pretectal nuclei. Medial fibers of optic tracts cross in chiasm to connect lateral geniculate bodies of both sides (yellow).* **(Bottom)** *Axial graphic of the orbit shows the 4 segments of the optic nerve (intraocular, intraorbital, intracanalicular, and intracranial). At the annulus of Zinn, the dural sheath of the intraorbital segment becomes contiguous with periorbita.*

GRAPHICS

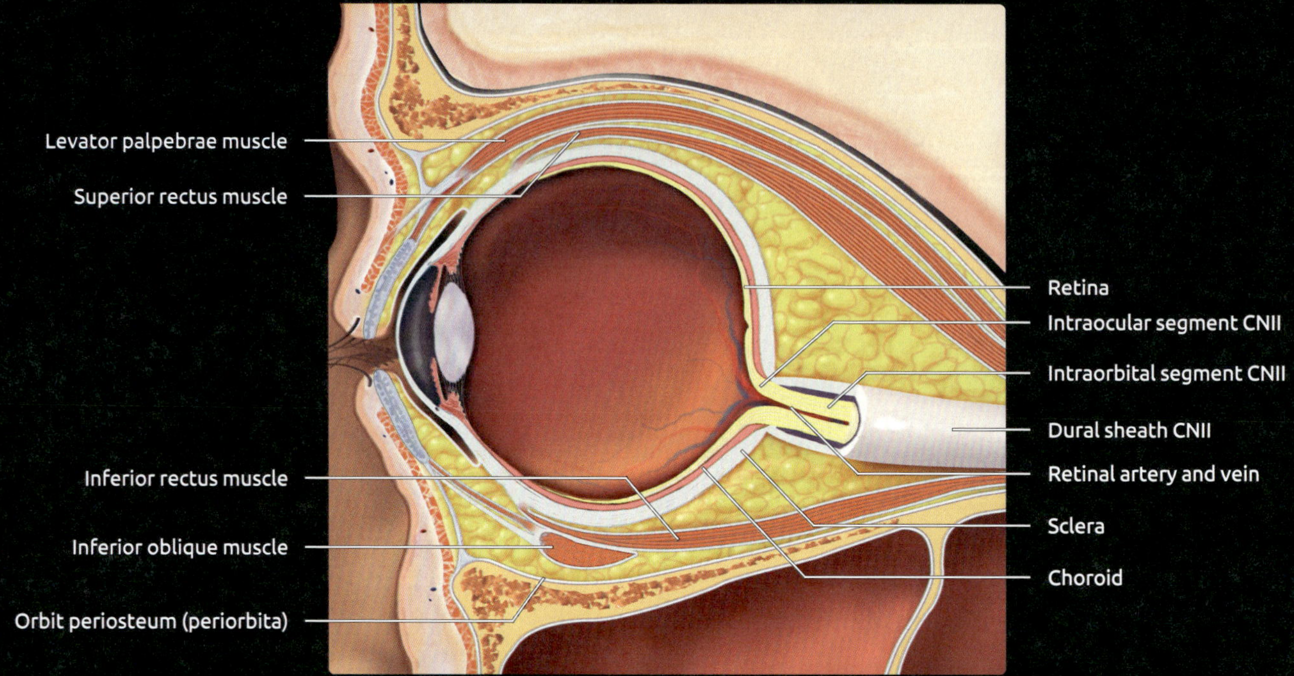

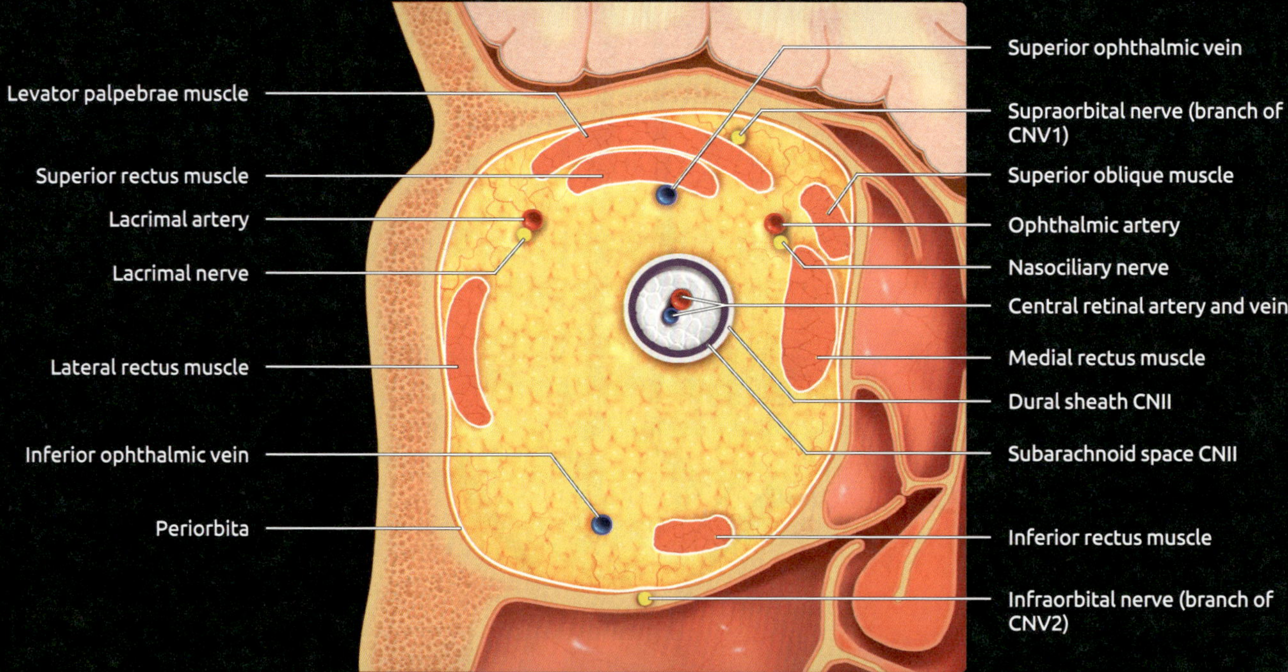

(Top) *Sagittal graphic through the orbit shows continuity of the dural sheath of the intraorbital segment of CNII with the sclera. At the annulus of Zinn, the dural sheath is continuous with the periorbita (not seen in this graphic). The central retinal artery and vein enter the midintraorbital segment of CNII to supply the retina.* **(Bottom)** *Coronal graphic through the distal optic nerve shows encasement of the optic nerve by the arachnoid and dura. The subarachnoid space of CNII is continuous with the cerebral subarachnoid space. The central retinal artery and vein pierce the dura of the distal intraorbital segment and continue to the retina in the center of CNII.*

AXIAL T2 FS MR

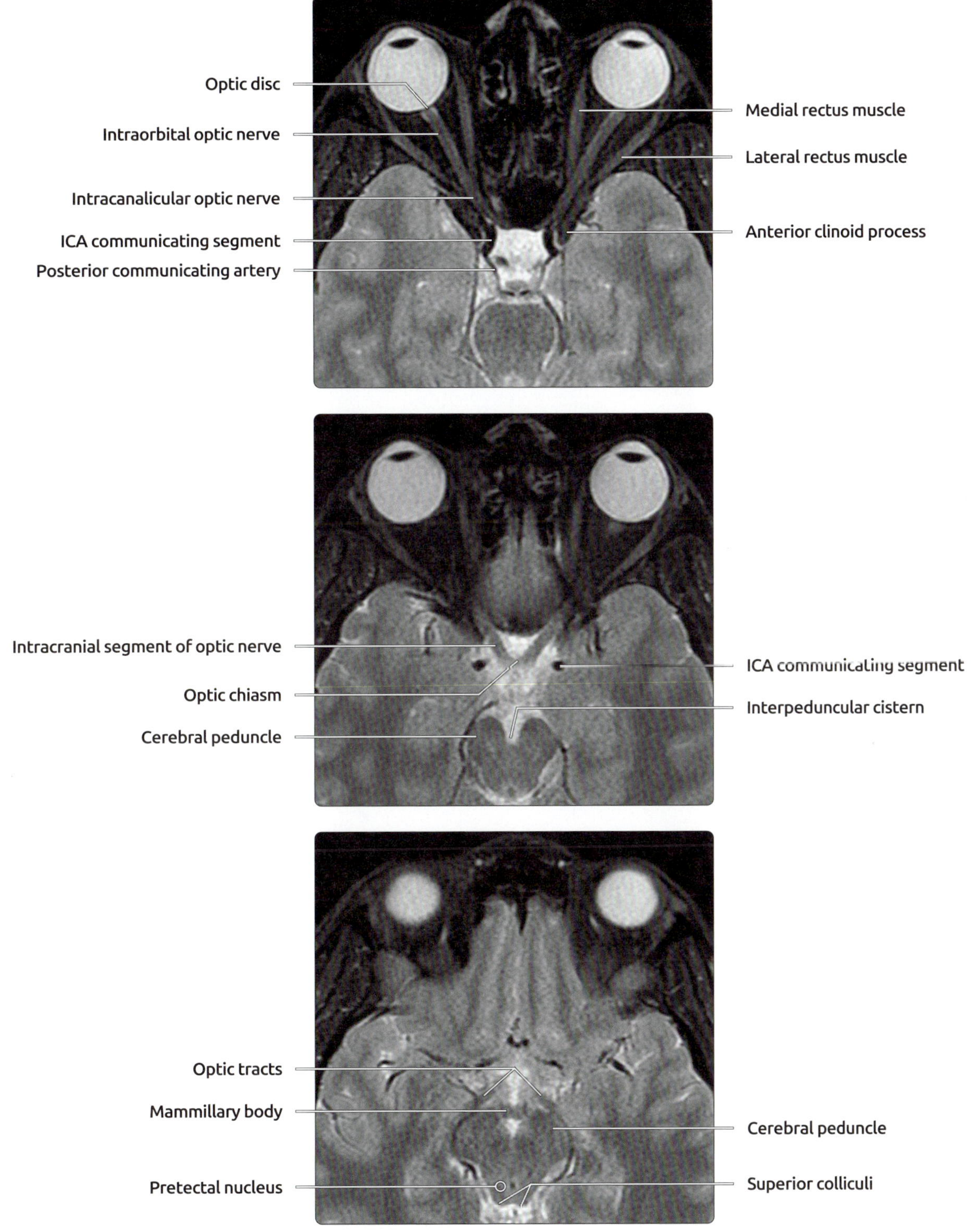

(Top) *Axial T2 FS MR through the orbits shows normal-appearing optic discs, intraorbital & intracanalicular segments of optic nerves. The intraocular segments are poorly delineated on this fat-saturated image. Note the thin sleeve of CSF-filled subarachnoid space surrounding the optic nerves. The outer dural covering of the optic nerve sheath merges with sclera anteriorly and posteriorly as periorbita at the annulus of Zinn.* **(Middle)** *Axial T2 FS MR shows the intracranial segments of both optic nerves joining to form the optic chiasm in the suprasellar cistern. The optic chiasm is usually located over the diaphragma sella (normofixed) or, rarely, over the tuberculum sella (prefixed) or dorsum sella (post fixed).* **(Bottom)** *Axial T2 FS MR shows bilateral optic tracts coursing posteriorly and laterally curving around the cerebral peduncles. The lateral band of fibers terminates in the lateral geniculate body, and the medial band terminates in the pretectal nuclei via the medial geniculate body. Pretectal nuclei are located deep to superior colliculi in the dorsal midbrain.*

CORONAL T2 FS MR

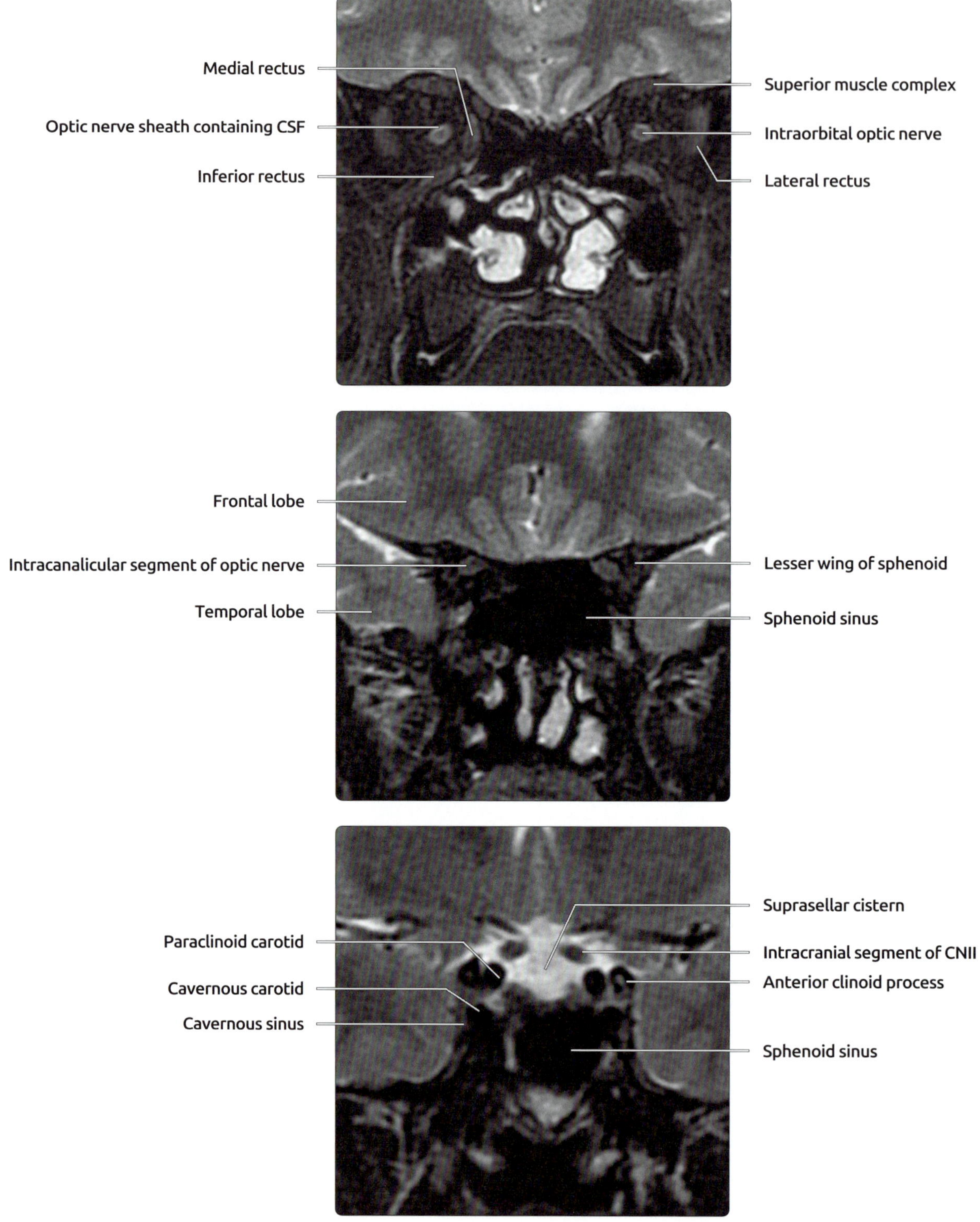

(Top) *Coronal T2 FS MR shows normal intraorbital segments of the bilateral optic nerves. A thin sleeve of CSF surrounds the optic nerves. Note that the optic nerve signal matches that of white matter.* **(Middle)** *Coronal T2 FS MR shows intracanalicular segments of the bilateral optic nerves. They usually measure between 4-9 mm. The ophthalmic artery is located inferior to CNII in the optic nerve canal (not depicted). Dura covering the optic nerve fuses with periorbita in the optic nerve canal.* **(Bottom)** *Coronal T2 FS MR shows intracranial segments of the bilateral optic nerves coursing posteriorly and medially. They are covered by pia and arachnoid membranes. The ophthalmic artery usually runs inferolateral to the nerves.*

CORONAL T2 FS MR

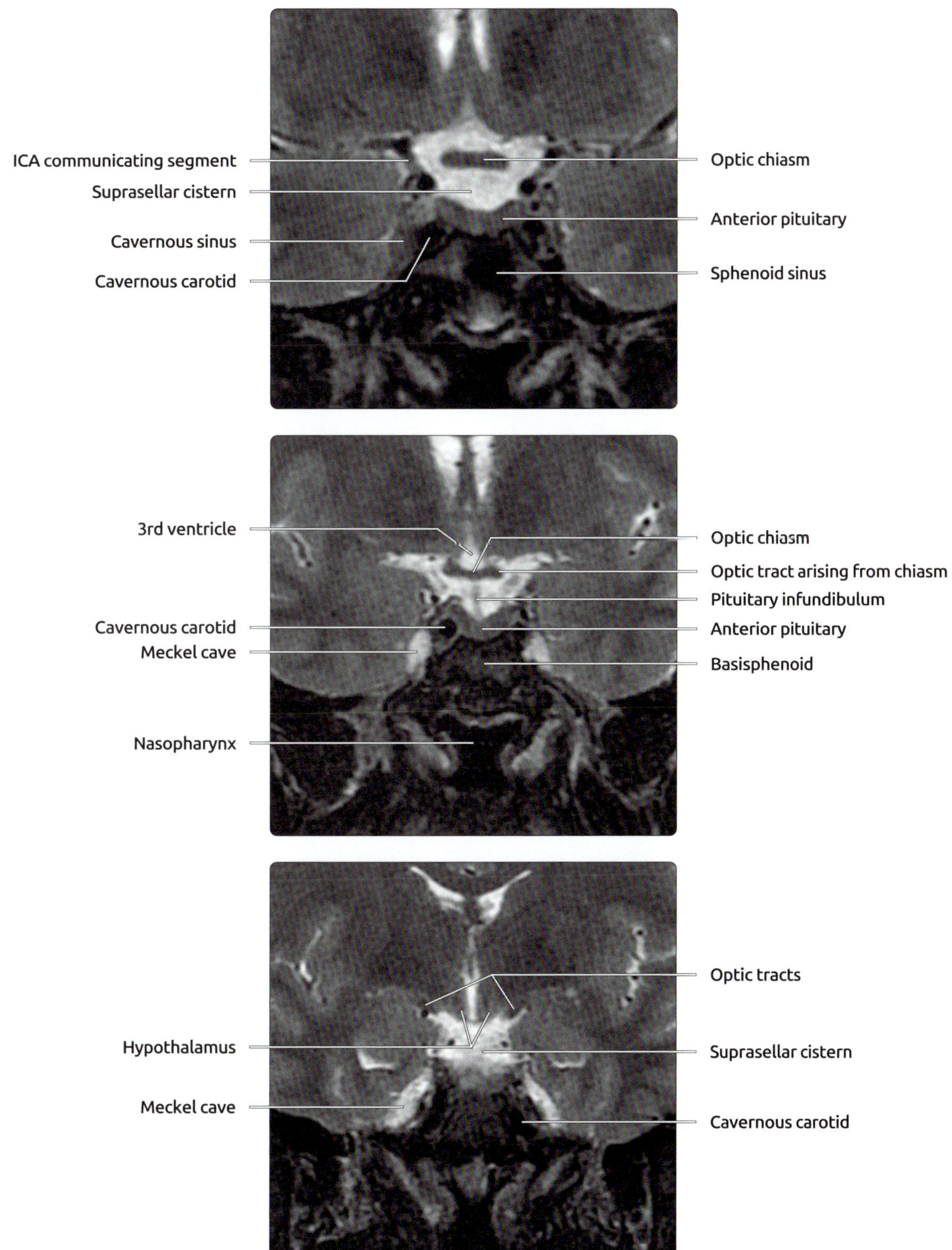

(Top) *Coronal T2 FS MR shows the horizontally oriented optic chiasm in the suprasellar cistern. It is usually located above the diaphragma sellae (normofixed). Fibers from the medial 1/2 of both retina cross over to the opposite side in the chiasm. Medial fibers in the optic tracts cross over to the opposite side at the chiasm to connect both lateral geniculate bodies (commissure of Gudden).* **(Middle)** *Coronal T2 FS MR through the posterior part of the optic chiasm shows the chiasm dividing into optic tracts. Note the optic chiasm forming part of the floor of the 3rd ventricle. The optic chiasm is closely associated with the pituitary infundibulum.* **(Bottom)** *Coronal T2 FS MR shows the bilateral optic tracts coursing posteriorly and laterally around the cerebral peduncles (not shown). The optic tracts divide into medial and lateral bands. The medial band ends in the pretectal nuclei via the medial geniculate bodies, and the lateral band ends in the lateral geniculate bodies. Note the pretectal nuclei are located deep to the superior colliculi in the dorsal midbrain (not shown).*

SAGITTAL & CORONAL T1 MR

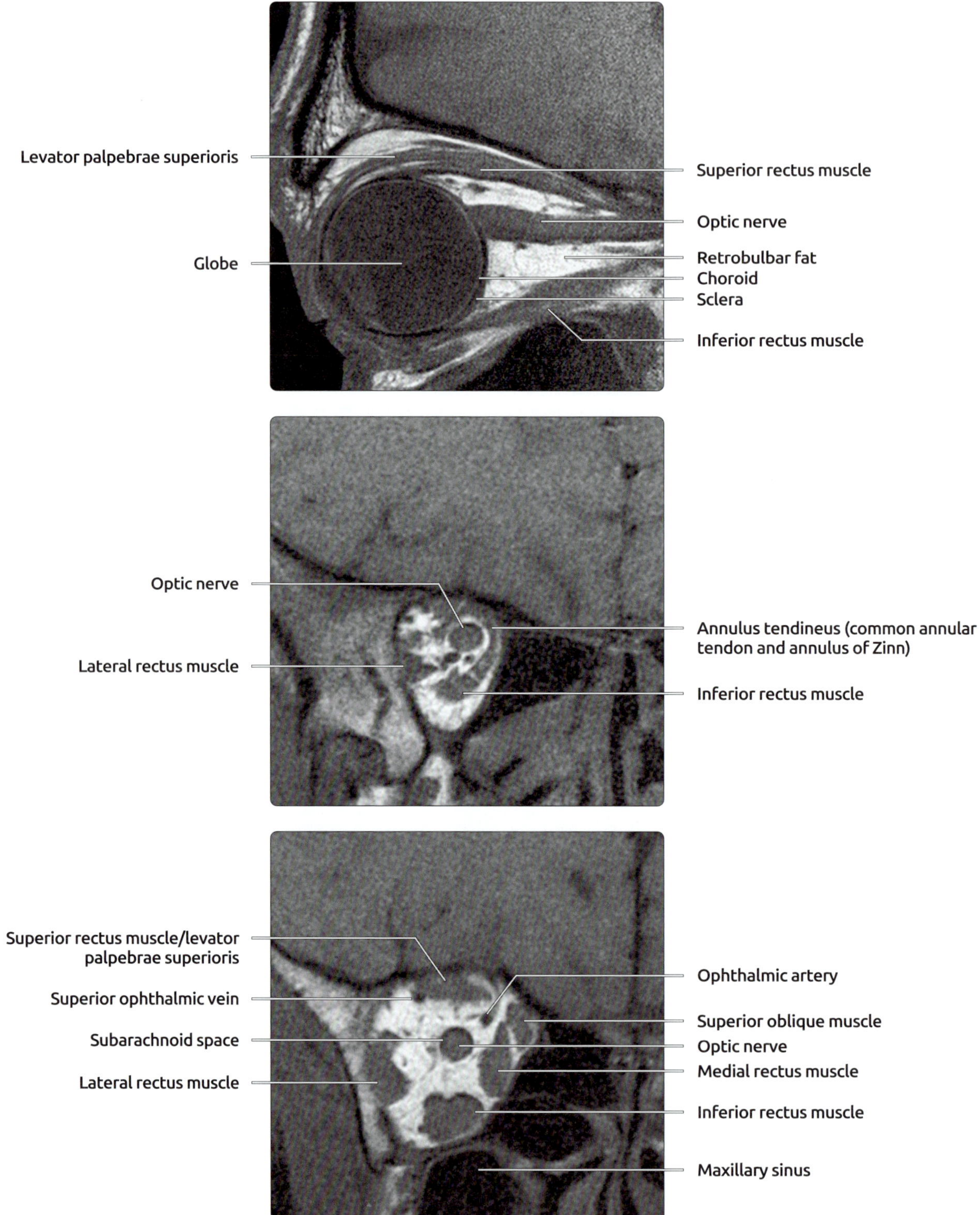

(Top) *Sagittal T1 MR through the optic nerve demonstrates the intraorbital segment of the optic nerve. The sclera of the globe is hypointense, while the pigmented choroid of the uvea is hyperintense due to T1-shortening effects of melanin.* **(Middle)** *First of 2 coronal T1 MR images through the orbit from posterior to anterior is shown. This section through the orbital apex shows the optic nerve passing through the common annular tendon, which serves as the site of origin of the rectus muscles.* **(Bottom)** *In this image, both the superolateral ophthalmic vein and the superomedial ophthalmic artery are visible. Note that the subarachnoid space is visible as a thin, black line surrounding the optic nerve, a finding often not seen on routine T1 imaging of the orbit.*

OPTIC NERVE PATHOLOGY

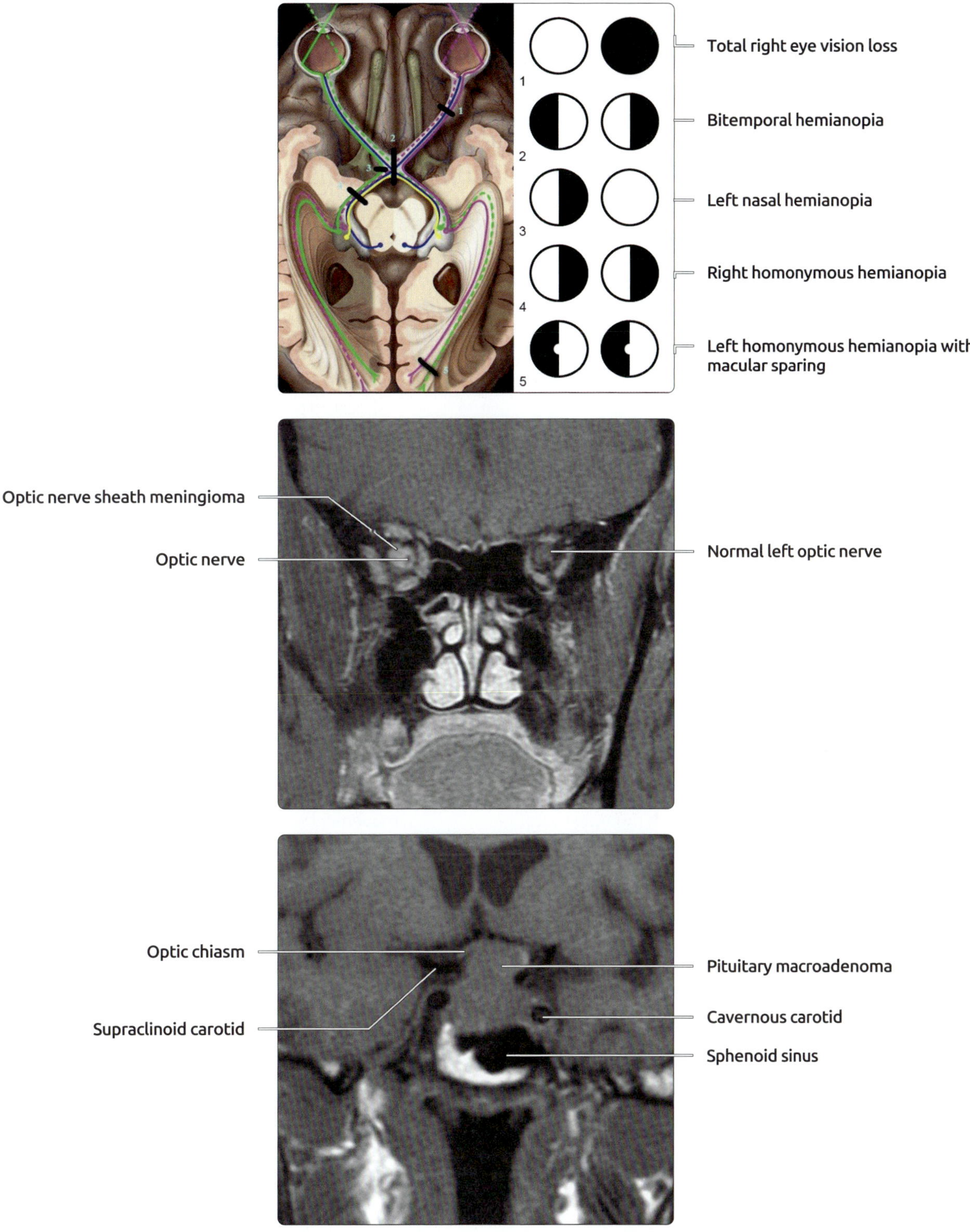

(Top) *Graphic of the optic pathway shows lesions at various levels and resultant visual field defects. The lesions are depicted at the level of the (1) optic nerve, (2) central optic chiasm, (3) peripheral optic chiasm, (4) optic tract, and (5) optic radiations.* **(Middle)** *Coronal T1 C+ FS MR of the orbit in a patient with right eye vision loss show eccentric nodular thickening of the right optic nerve sheath with the optic nerve displaced and compressed inferomedially, suggesting optic nerve sheath meningioma.* **(Bottom)** *Coronal T1 MR through the sella in a patient with bitemporal hemianopia demonstrates a large pituitary macroadenoma with mass effect on the optic chiasm, which appears to be displaced superiorly and stretched over the tumor.*

TERMINOLOGY

Abbreviations

- Oculomotor nerve (CNIII, CN3)
- Oculomotor nuclear complex (ONC)
- Extraocular muscle (EOM)
- Medial longitudinal fasciculus (MLF)
- Edinger-Westphal nucleus (EWn)
- Superior orbital fissure (SOF)

Synonyms

- 3rd cranial nerve

Definitions

- CNIII: Motor nerve to EOMs except lateral rectus (CNVI) and superior oblique muscles (CNIV); parasympathetic motor to pupillary sphincter and ciliary muscle

IMAGING ANATOMY

Overview

- Purely motor cranial nerve with general somatic efferent fibers as well as general visceral efferent (parasympathetic)
- Supplies all EOMs except superior oblique and lateral rectus muscles via general somatic efferent innervation
- Innervates pupillary sphincter and ciliary muscles via parasympathetic innervation
- Originates from ONC in posterior midbrain
- Can be divided into 7 segments: Intramesencephalic, interpeduncular cisternal, petroclinoid, trigonal, cavernous, fissural, and orbital

Oculomotor Nerve Complex

- There are paired paramedian ONCs located in posterior aspect of midbrain at level of superior colliculus
- Partially embedded in periaqueductal gray matter anterior (ventral) to cerebral aqueduct
- ONC has complex cytoarchitecture with multiple motor nuclei and parasympathetic nucleus
- Contains motor neurons of medial, inferior, and superior recti, inferior oblique, and levator palpebrae muscles
- Motor neurons are arranged into subgroups generally referred to as nuclei
- Motor nuclei are arranged in 2 paramedian clusters or stacks referred to as columns or somatic columns
- Each paramedian somatic column consists of 4 relatively distinct nuclei, providing axons to EOMs
  - **Ventral nucleus**: Ipsilateral medial rectus
  - **Central nucleus**: Contralateral superior rectus and ipsilateral inferior oblique
  - **Dorsolateral nucleus**: Ipsilateral medial rectus
  - **Dorsomedial nuclei**: Ipsilateral inferior rectus
- Just inferior to paired columns is single midline motor nucleus, **central caudal nucleus**
  - Central caudal nucleus contains motor neurons for levator palpebrae muscle, possibly provides crossed and uncrossed axons
- **EWn**
  - More complex than classically considered
    - Anatomy is confounded by differences in primates and humans
    - Afferent inputs primarily from bilateral pretectal nuclei mediating pupillary light reflex and from visual cortex mediating accommodation
    - Efferent fibers travel in CNIII and in MLF
    - Nomenclature confusing given inconsistent application of term EWn to 2 different groups of neurons that contain different cell types and provide different function
      - 1st group: Preganglionic parasympathetic component (EWpg)
      - 2nd group: Nonpreganglionic centrally projecting component (EWcp)
  - **EWnp** (parasympathetic component)
    - Provides parasympathetic motor to pupillary sphincter and ciliary muscles of eye
    - In humans, preganglionic parasympathetic neurons are located posteromedial to somatic columns near midline but do not form compact or distinct nucleus
  - **EWncp** (centrally projecting components)
    - Located posteromedial to somatic columns, in between columns and parasympathetic neurons of EWpg
    - Forms compact and distinct nucleus
    - Consists of peptidergic neurons that project to brainstem, spinal cord, and prosencephalic regions
    - Not definitely related to ocular function; may function in feeding behavior, stress responses, addiction, and pain
- **MLF**
  - Main intersegmental tract of brainstem
  - Small paramedian tract coursing from upper cervical cord to interstitial nucleus of Cajal (lateral wall of 3rd ventricle)
  - Interconnects oculomotor, trochlear, abducens, EWn, vestibular, reticular, and spinal accessory nuclei
  - Coordinates conjugate eye movements with associated movements of head and neck
  - Lesions of MLF result in internuclear ophthalmoplegia (INO)
- **Nucleus of Perlia**
  - Small linear nucleus medial to main motor nuclei near midline of midbrain
  - Function less clear; may function in ocular convergence
  - May provide some motor fibers to superior rectus
- Arterial supply to ONC and intramesencephalic nerves via group of small penetrating arteries that arise from terminal regions of basilar artery near origins of superior cerebellar and posterior cerebral arteries

Intramesencephalic Segment

- Intraaxial segment resides within midbrain and extends from ONC to interpeduncular cistern
- CNIII fascicles course anteriorly at least partially through MLF, red nucleus, substantia nigra, and medial cerebral peduncle
- Oculomotor nerve fascicles converge in posterior-to-anterior direction
- Exit midbrain into interpeduncular cistern

Interpeduncular Cisternal Segment

- Each CNIII leaves midbrain medially to cerebral peduncle in lateral part of interpeduncular fossa

- Each nerve may arise as tiny rootlets that immediately unite and extend as single root
- Cisternal segment extends from exit point of nerve along medial side of cerebral peduncle through interpeduncular and prepontine cisterns to posterior petroclinoid fold, posterior margin of oculomotor triangle
- Passes between posterior cerebral artery (PCA) above and superior cerebellar artery (SCA) below
- Courses inferior to posterior communicating artery and medial to free edge of tentorium cerebelli
- Measures ~ 2.1 mm in diameter within cistern
- Topographically, pupillary fibers are superficially located in cisternal portion of CNIII

Petroclinoid Segment

- Located between cisternal and trigonal segments
- Defined posteriorly by posterior petroclinoid fold and anteriorly by oculomotor porus (opening) of roof of cavernous sinus
- Oculomotor triangle represents floor of petroclinoid segment

Trigonal Segment

- Petroclinoid segment ends at oculomotor porus where nerve pierces roof of cavernous sinus, near center of oculomotor triangle
- Oculomotor cistern, CSF-filled arachnoid and dural cuff, begins at oculomotor porus and extends ~ 6 mm
- Trigonal segment of oculomotor nerve travels within oculomotor cistern as it enters superolateral cavernous sinus roof
- Trigonal segments terminates when nerve is incorporated into fibrous lateral wall of cavernous sinus
- Cistern and trigonal segment is recognized surgically as avascular space used to mobilize nerve during cavernous sinus surgery

Cavernous Segment

- Incorporated into lateral dural wall of cavernous sinus just under tip of anterior clinoid process
- This wall consists of 2 layers
  - Superficial dense and formed from dura
  - Deep endosteal layer that invests nerves running in lateral wall
- Cavernous segment on CNIII extends just past anterior clinoid process where SOF begins
- Carotid-oculomotor membrane: Layer of dura that lines lower margin of anterior clinoid process and extends medially to form proximal dural ring; it separates lower margin of anterior clinoid process from cavernous segment CNIII and extends medially around carotid artery
- CNIII remains most cephalad of all cranial nerves within cavernous sinus
- CNIII superolateral to cavernous internal carotid artery
- ~ 14 mm in length

Fissural Segment

- CNIII courses along lateral margin of optic strut as it passes through medial part of SOF
- Fissural segment of oculomotor nerve splits into its superior and inferior divisions
- ~ 6 mm long
- Fissural segment extends from anterior clinoid process to oculomotor foramen of SOF

Orbital Segment

- Superior and inferior branches of CNIII enter orbit through SOF and pass through annulus tendineus (annulus of Zinn)
- Annulus of Zinn partially segments SOF into lateral component and medial component; medial component is referred to as oculomotor foramen
- Superior branch supplies levator palpebrae superioris and superior rectus muscles
- Inferior branch supplies inferior rectus, medial rectus, and inferior oblique muscles
- Preganglionic parasympathetic fibers follow inferior branch to ciliary ganglion of orbit
  - Postganglionic parasympathetic fibers continue as short ciliary nerves to enter globe with optic nerve
  - In globe, short ciliary nerves to ciliary body and iris
  - Control papillary sphincter function and accommodation via ciliary muscle

ANATOMY IMAGING ISSUES

Imaging Recommendations

- Bone CT best for skull base, bony foramina
- MR for intraaxial, cisternal, cavernous segments
  - Thin-section, high-resolution T2 MR sequences in axial and coronal planes
    - Depicts cisternal CNIII surrounded by CSF with high contrast and high spatial resolution

Imaging Sweet Spots

- CNIII nuclear complex and intraaxial segment not directly visualized
  - Find periaqueductal gray matter to localize
- Identification of distal basilar artery and branches can be reliable landmark for finding cisternal CNIII; it passes between posterior cerebral artery above and SCA below

Imaging Pitfalls

- Negative MR and MRA does **not** completely exclude posterior communicating artery aneurysm
  - CTA or conventional angiography recommended to exclude this diagnosis

CLINICAL IMPLICATIONS

Clinical Importance

- Uncal herniation pushes CNIII on petroclinoid ligament
- During trauma, downward shift of brainstem upon impact can stretch CNIII over petroclinoid ligament
- CNIII susceptible to compression by PCA aneurysms
- CNIII neuropathy divided into **simple** if isolated and **complex** if with other CN involvement (CNIV and CNVI)
  - **Simple** CNIII with pupillary involvement
    - Must exclude **PCA aneurysm** as cause
    - Explanation: Parasympathetic fibers are peripherally distributed
  - Simple CNIII with pupillary sparing
    - Presumed microvascular infarction involves vessels supplying core of nerve with relative sparing of peripheral pupillary fibers

GRAPHICS

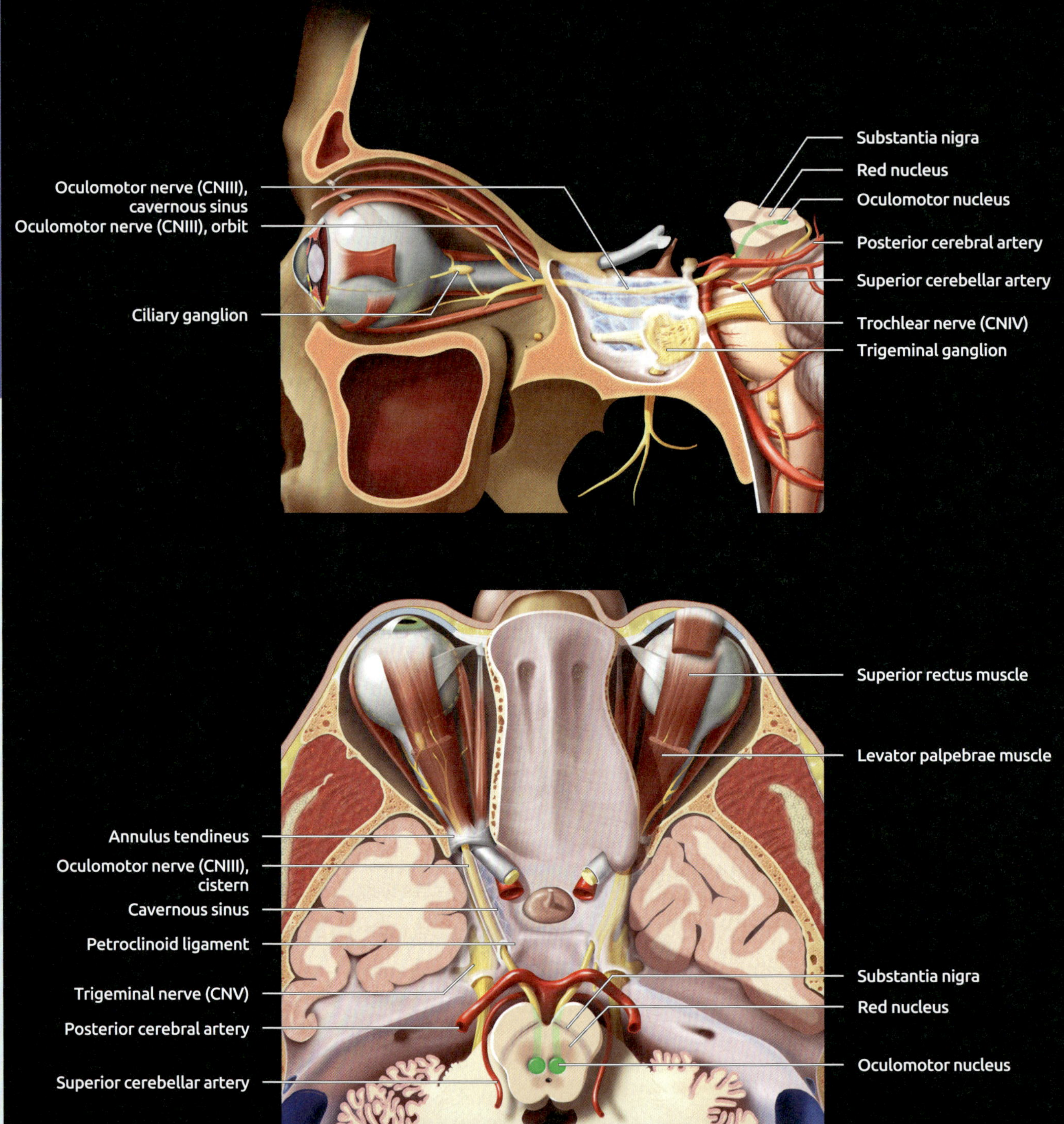

(Top) *Sagittal graphic shows the oculomotor nerve exiting from the anterior brainstem. After passing medially to the trochlear nerve (CNIV) between the superior cerebellar artery and posterior cerebral artery, it enters the cavernous sinus. CNIII is the most superior nerve coursing through the cavernous sinus. Once in orbit, it divides into the superior and inferior divisions. Preganglionic parasympathetic fibers travel with the inferior division to join the ciliary ganglion.* **(Bottom)** *Axial graphic clearly depicts CNIII originating from the oculomotor nuclei complex to travel through the medial aspect of the red nucleus and substantia nigra before exiting into the interpeduncular cistern. After traversing the cavernous sinus, surrounded by the CSF-filled oculomotor cistern, it enters the orbit through the superior orbital fissure, dividing into superior and inferior branches and passing through the annulus tendineus (annulus of Zinn).*

AXIAL T2 MR

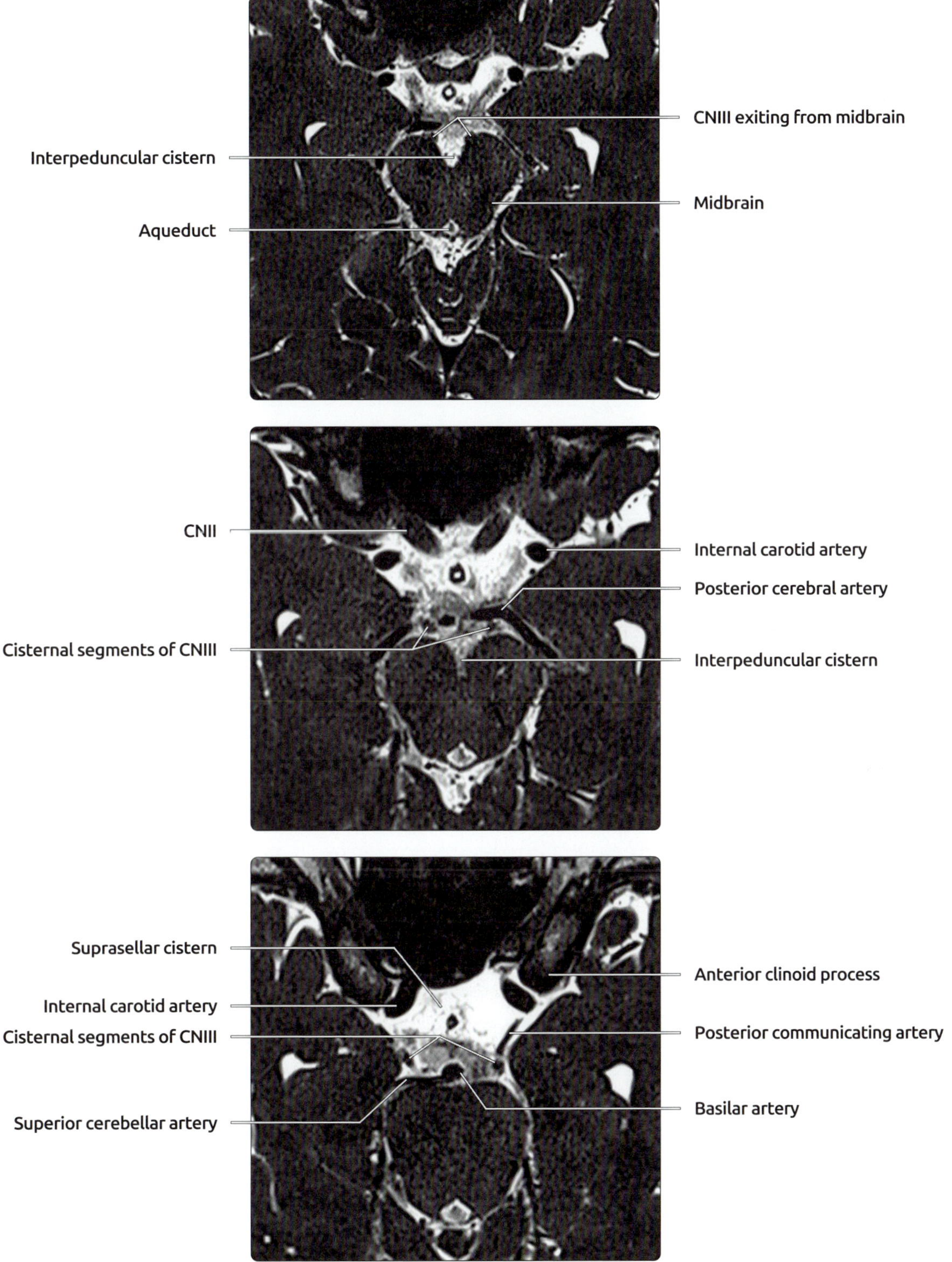

(Top) *First of 3 axial 3D T2 SPACE MR images shows bilateral CNIII emerging out of the anterior midbrain into the interpeduncular cistern. Each nerve may arise as tiny rootlets that immediately unite and extend as single root.* **(Middle)** *The cisternal segment extends from the exit point of CNIII along the medial side of the cerebral peduncle through the interpeduncular and prepontine cisterns to the posterior petroclinoid fold, posterior margin of oculomotor triangle.* **(Bottom)** *The cisternal segment of CNIII then passes between the posterior cerebral artery (PCA) above and the superior cerebellar artery (SCA) below and courses inferior to the posterior communicating artery and medial to the free edge of the tentorium cerebelli.*

AXIAL T2 & T1 MR

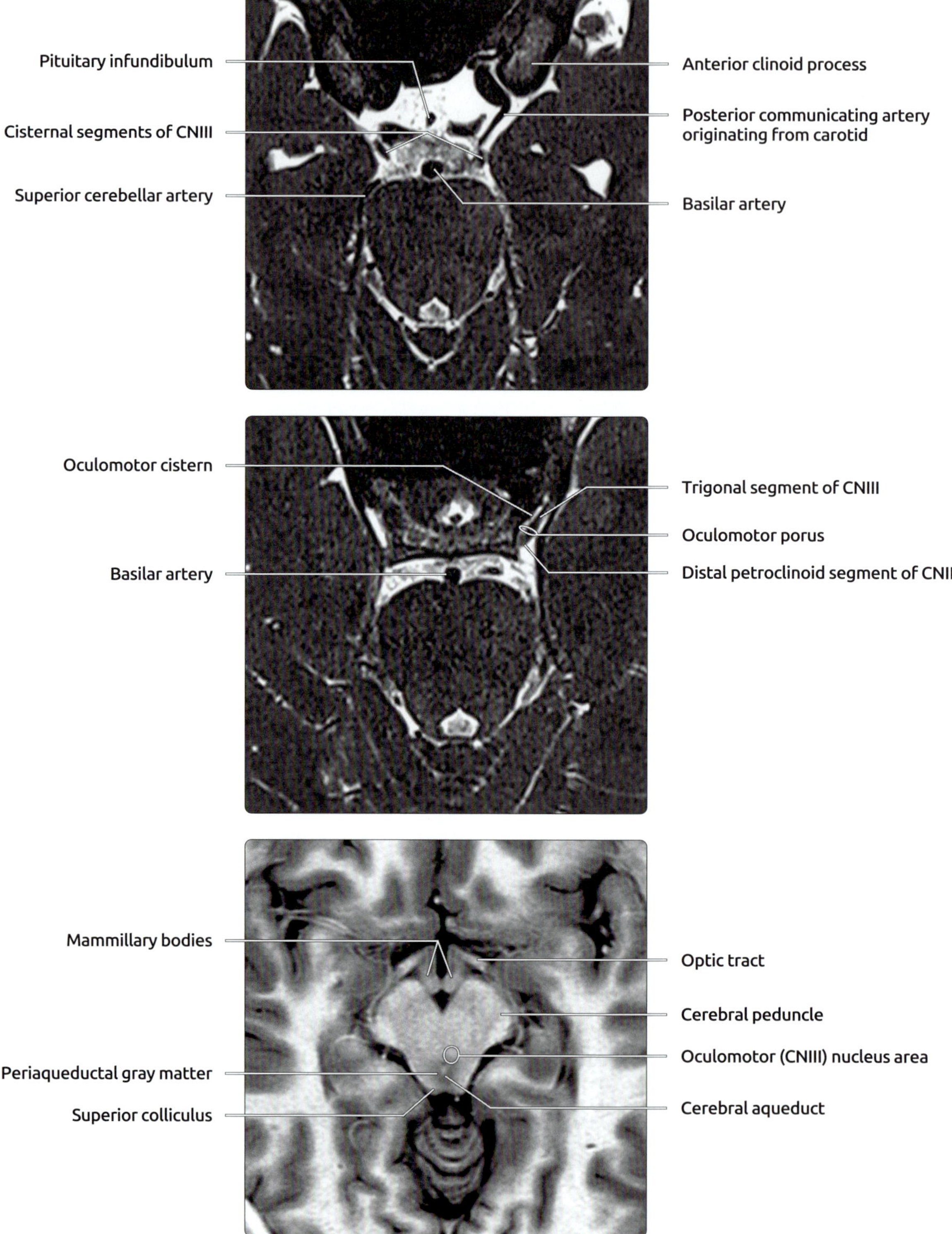

(Top) *First of 2 axial 3D T2 SPACE MR images shows the distal cisternal segments of CNIII coursing parallel and inferior to the posterior communicating artery. Topographically pupillary fibers are located superficially along the nerve and are prone to dysfunction by extrinsic compression, particularly by posterior communicating aneurysm.* **(Middle)** *The trigonal segment of CNIII begins when the distal petroclinoid segment enters the oculomotor cistern through the oculomotor porus and terminates when the nerve is incorporated into the fibrous lateral wall of the cavernous sinus.* **(Bottom)** *Axial 3D IR T1 MR through the brainstem at the level of superior colliculus is shown. The paired oculomotor nuclear complex is not directly visualized; however, since it is partially embedded in the periaqueductal gray matter anterior to the cerebral aqueduct at the level of the superior colliculus, its position can be inferred by these landmarks. The approximate location of the oculomotor nucleus is marked on the left.*

CORONAL T2 MR

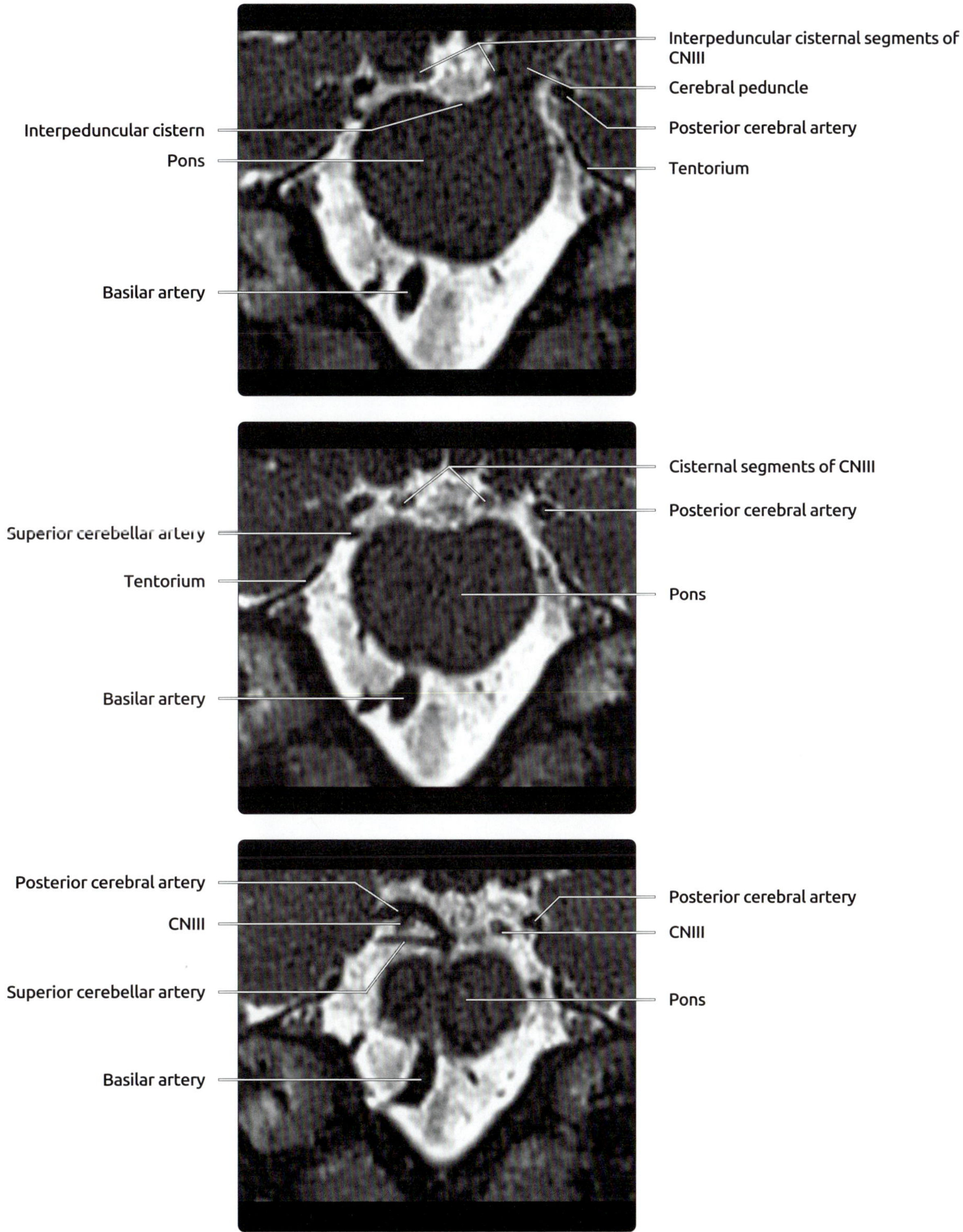

(Top) *First of 3 coronal reformat 3D T2 SPACE MR images shows CNIII emerging from the midbrain along the lateral aspect of the interpeduncular cistern. This marks the end of the intramesencephalic and the beginning of the interpeduncular segment of CNIII.* **(Middle)** *The cisternal segments of CNIII travel anteriorly and laterally to the posterior petroclinoid fold, posterior margin of oculomotor triangle.* **(Bottom)** *After emerging from the midbrain, the cisternal segments of CNIII travel anteriorly between the posterior cerebral and superior cerebellar arteries medial to CNIV.*

CORONAL T2 MR

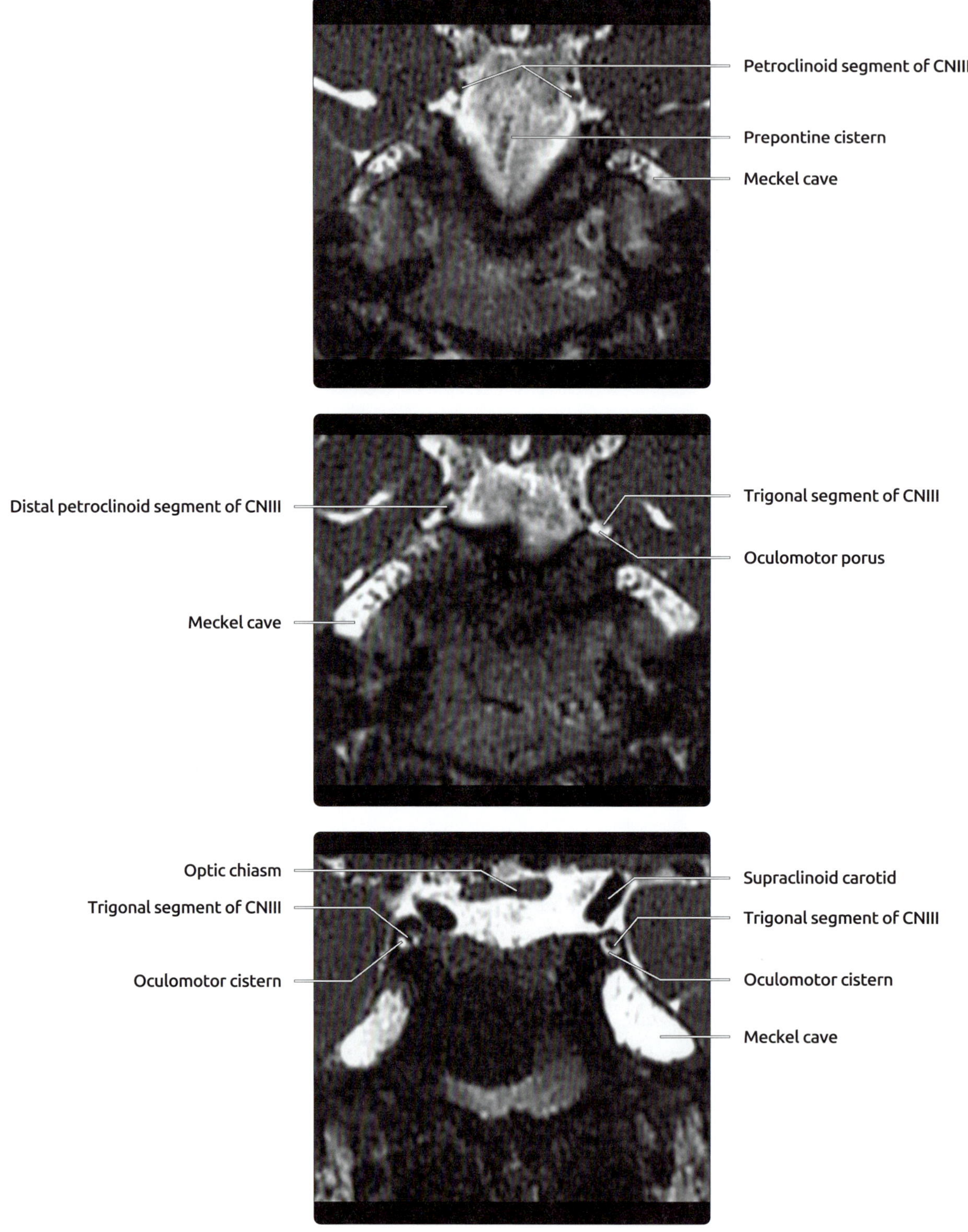

(Top) *First of 3 coronal reformat 3D T2 SPACE MR images shows the petroclinoid segments of bilateral CNIII. The petroclinoid segments are located between the cisternal and trigonal segments. The oculomotor triangle forms the floor of the petroclinoid segment.* **(Middle)** *The petroclinoid segment of CNIII is seen entering the oculomotor cistern through the oculomotor porus. The oculomotor cistern is a CSF-filled arachnoid and dural cuff, which begins at the oculomotor porus and extends ~ 6 mm.* **(Bottom)** *Bilateral CNIII trigonal segments are seen in the oculomotor cisterns. The trigonal segments terminate when the nerve is incorporated into the fibrous lateral wall of the cavernous sinus. The cavernous segment passes through the lateral wall of the cavernous sinus and through the superior orbital fissure along the lateral margin of the optic strut forming the fissural segment. The fissural segment splits into superior and inferior branches, which pass into orbit through the annulus of Zinn.*

CLINICAL CORRELATION

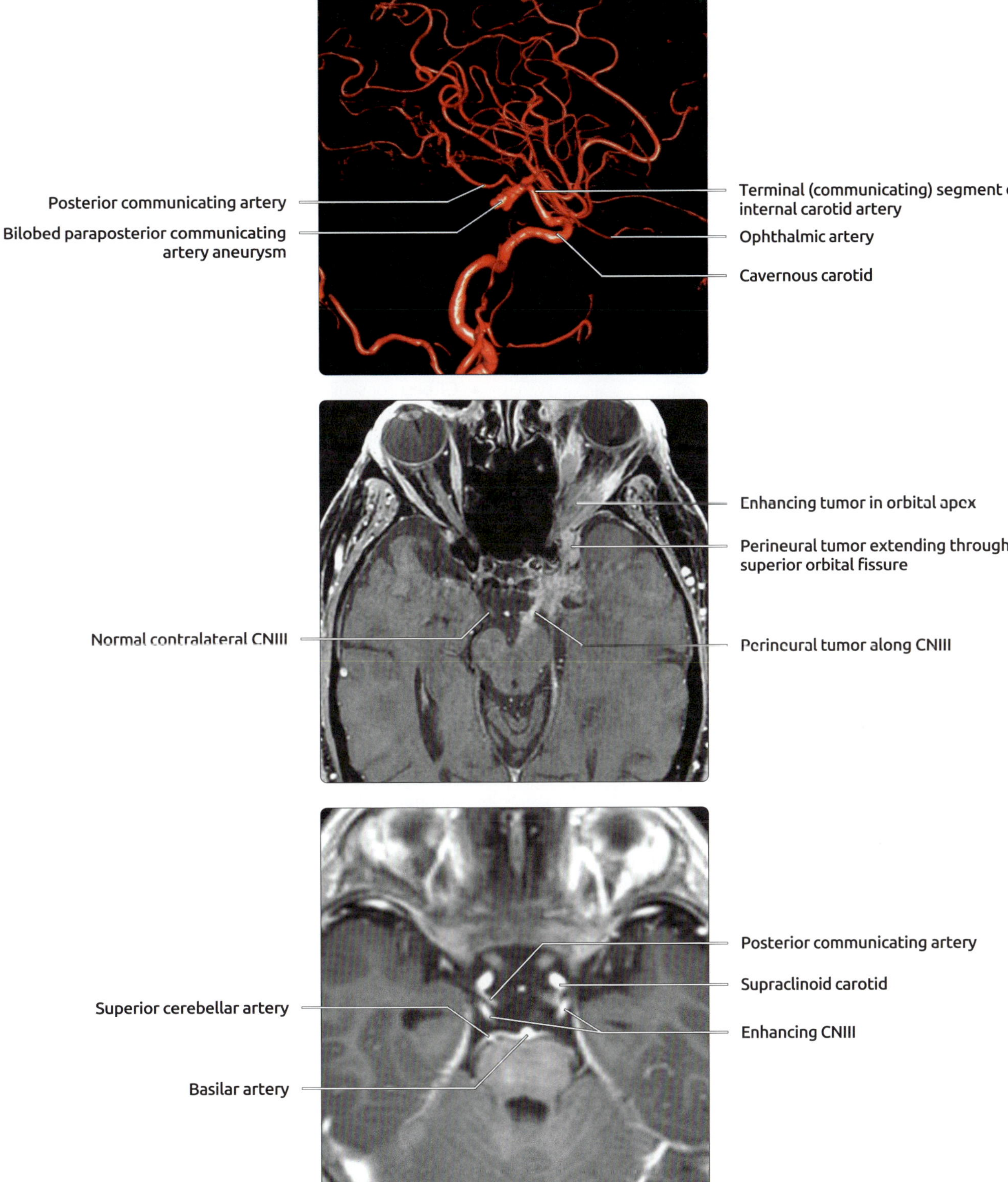

(Top) *3D volume-rendered reconstruction of catheter angiogram with right carotid injection shows a large bilobed paraposterior communicating artery (PCom) internal carotid artery aneurysm. This patient presented with CNIII palsy with involvement of superficial pupillary fibers.* **(Middle)** *Axial T1 C+ FS MR though the level of the interpeduncular cistern demonstrates abnormal thickening and enhancement of the cisternal CNIII as tumor extends in retrograde fashion along the nerve from the cavernous sinus. This middle-aged man with a history of squamous cell carcinoma of the left forehead subsequently developed progressive disease of the orbit, and perineural tumor spread to the superior orbital fissure and cavernous sinus.* **(Bottom)** *Axial 3D MPRAGE T1 C+ MR demonstrates smooth enhancement of bilateral CNIII cisternal segments in a patient with known Lyme disease.*

TERMINOLOGY

Abbreviations

- Trochlear nerve: CNIV

IMAGING ANATOMY

Overview

- Pure motor nerve (general somatic efferent) that innervates extraocular **superior oblique muscle**
- Segments: Intramesencephalic, cisternal, tentorial, cavernous, & extracranial
- Longest intracranial cranial nerve (CN) course (≈ 60 mm)
- Thinnest CN: 0.4- to 0.5-mm nerve diameter in cisternal segment

Trochlear Nuclei

- Paired nuclei located in paramedian midbrain, **ventral to cerebral aqueduct of Sylvius**, & immediately **dorsal to medial longitudinal fasciculus (MLF)**
- Caudal to oculomotor nuclei at level of inferior colliculus

Intramesencephalic Segment

- Trochlear nerve fascicles course posteriorly & inferiorly around cerebral aqueduct
    - Fibers then cross (**decussate**) within **superior medullary velum** (at roof of upper 4th ventricle)
    - **Key concept**: Each superior oblique muscle innervated by ipsilateral CNIV that originates in **contralateral** trochlear nucleus
- CNIV exits dorsal midbrain just below **inferior colliculus**
- CNIV **only CN** to **exit dorsal brainstem**

Cisternal Segment

- CNIV courses anterolaterally in through quadrigeminal & perimesencephalic cisterns
- Surrounded by CSF in subarachnoid space
- In perimesencephalic cistern, **passes between lateral** aspect of posterior cerebral artery (**PCA**) above & superior cerebellar artery (**SCA**) below, close to tentorium
    - Inferior, more lateral to CNIII, which passes between medial aspect of PCA & SCA in interpeduncular cistern

Tentorial Segment

- CNIV passes anteriorly into **trochlear groove (TG)** along lower surface of free edge of tentorium
    - TG: 4- to 6-mm long depression along tentorial medial surface near free edge of tentorium
    - Distance of TG from tentorial free edge on 7T MR study: 1.1-2.0 mm (mean: 1.5 mm)
    - Depth of TG on 7T MR study: 0.4-0.9mm (mean: 0.6 mm)
- From TG, CNIV pierces dura of **posterior petroclinoid fold** near posterior margin of **oculomotor triangle**, along rostrolateral free edge of tentorium
- Oculomotor triangle formed by 3 dural folds
    - Anterior & posterior petroclinoid folds (extending from tentorial edge at petrous apex to anterior & posterior clinoid processes, respectively)
    - Interclinoid fold (from anterior clinoid process to posterior clinoid process)
- **Trochlear cistern**: CSF sleeve around trochlear nerve (CNIV) after piercing posterior petroclinoid fold, lying posteroinferior to oculomotor (CNIII) cistern
- CNIV wedged between posterior petroclinoid fold medially & anterior petroclinoid fold laterally in trochlear cistern

Cavernous Segment

- CNIV enters roof of cavernous sinus (CS) in posterolateral apex of **oculomotor triangle**, just posterior to CNIII entry
- CNIV courses in **lateral wall** of CS inferior to CNIII, superior to CNV1

Extracranial Segment

- CNIV enters orbit through **superior orbital fissure** together with CNIII & CNVI
- Crosses over CNIII & courses medially
- Passes **above** annulus of Zinn (CNIII & CNVI go through annulus)
- Supplies motor innervation to superior oblique muscle

ANATOMY IMAGING ISSUES

Imaging Recommendations

- CT best for skull base, bony foramina
- High-resolution MR best for brainstem, cisternal, cavernous, & intraorbital imaging
- Intraorbital segment not visualized by any imaging modality or sequence
- Nerve visualization on 7T MR study: Origin at brainstem 65%, cisternal segment 93%, tentorial segment 100%, cavernous segment 74%

Imaging Sweet Spots

- CNIV nucleus & intraaxial segment not directly visualized
    - Nuclei position inferred by identifying periaqueductal gray matter & cerebral aqueduct at level of inferior colliculi on high-resolution MR

Imaging Pitfalls

- Difficult to visualize normal CNIV despite best MR imaging
- During image interrogation by radiologist, view known landmarks along its course
    - Midbrain → tentorial margin → CS → superior orbital fissure → extraconal orbit

CLINICAL IMPLICATIONS

Clinical Importance

- CNIV neuropathy divided into **simple & complex**
    - **Simple** CNIV neuropathy (isolated)
        - Most common form; usually secondary to trauma
        - Cisternal segment injury by free edge of tentorium cerebelli or from PCA or SCA aneurysm
        - Contusion of superior medullary velum
    - **Complex** CNIV neuropathy (associated with other CN injury, CNIII ± CNVI)
        - Brainstem stoke or tumor
        - CS thrombosis, tumor
        - Orbital tumor

Clinical Findings

- Paralysis of superior oblique muscle results in **extorsion** (outward rotation) of affected eye due to unopposed action of inferior oblique muscle
- Diplopia, weakness of downward gaze, neck pain from **compensatory head tilt to opposite side**

GRAPHICS

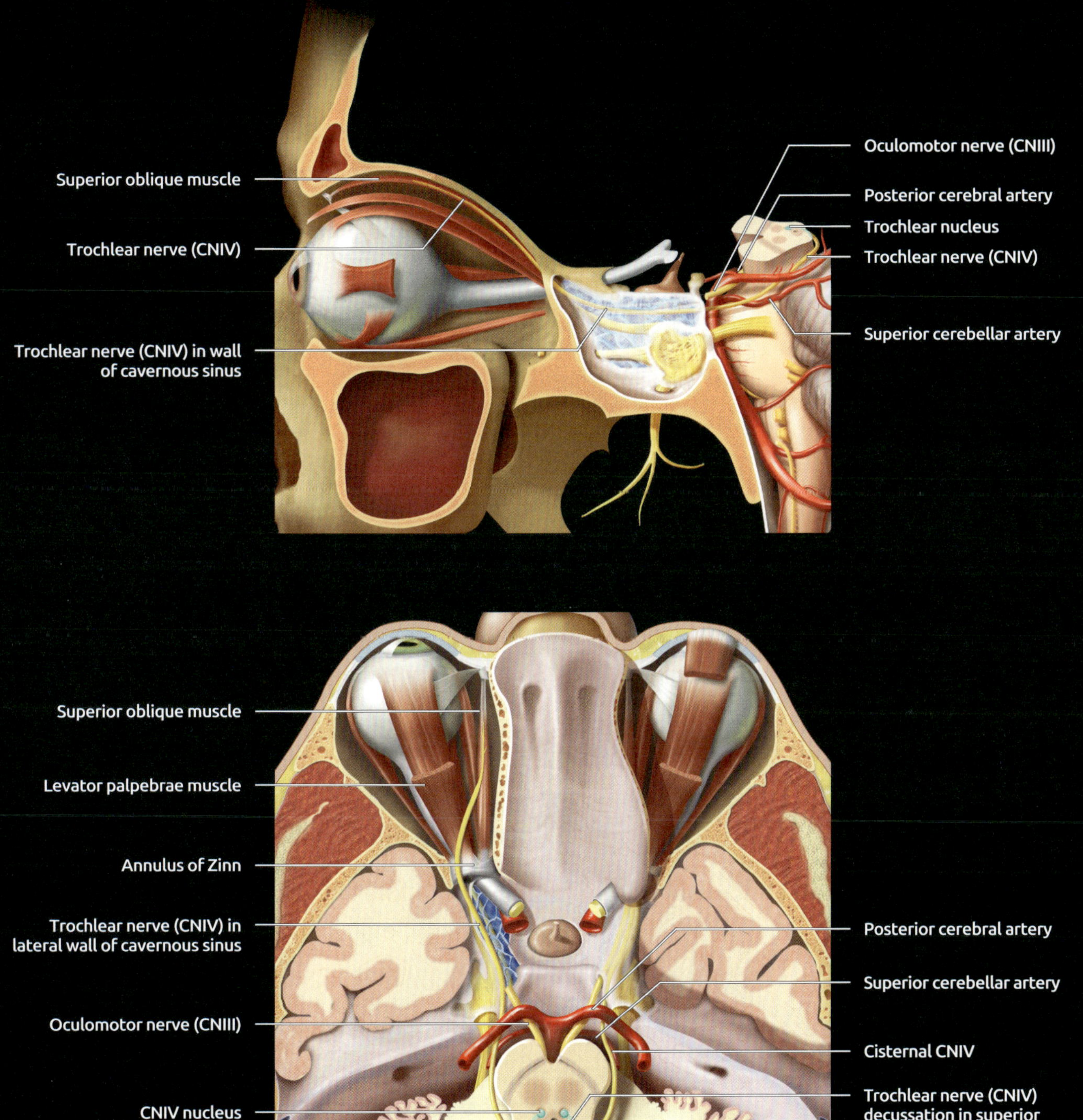

(Top) *Sagittal graphic shows that the trochlear nucleus gives rise to fibers that form the contralateral trochlear nerve. After exiting the dorsal brainstem, CNIV courses lateral to the oculomotor nerve between the posterior cerebral artery and superior cerebellar artery. After its long cisternal course, CNIV enters the cavernous sinus and runs inferolateral to CNIII and superior to the ophthalmic division of the trigeminal nerve (CNV1).* **(Bottom)** *Axial graphic shows the trochlear nerves originating from the trochlear nuclei and decussating in the superior medullary velum. CNIV runs much more lateral to the oculomotor nerve between the posterior cerebral artery and superior cerebellar artery close to tentorium, and continues inferolateral with CNIII through the cavernous sinus. It crosses over CNIII to enter orbit above the annulus of Zinn, then courses medially over the levator palpebrae muscle to innervate the superior oblique muscle.*

AXIAL AND SAGITTAL 3D T2 MR

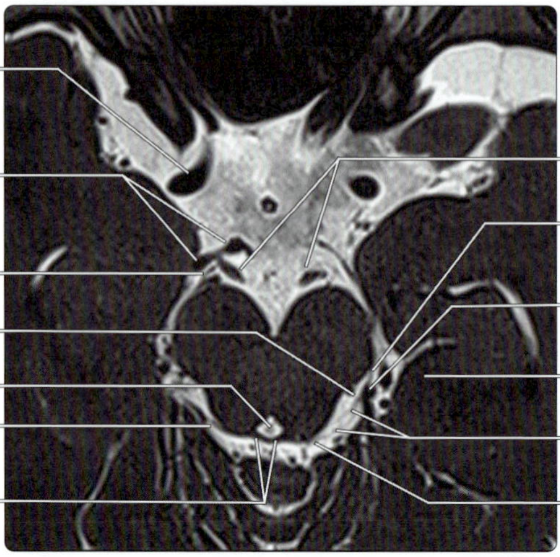

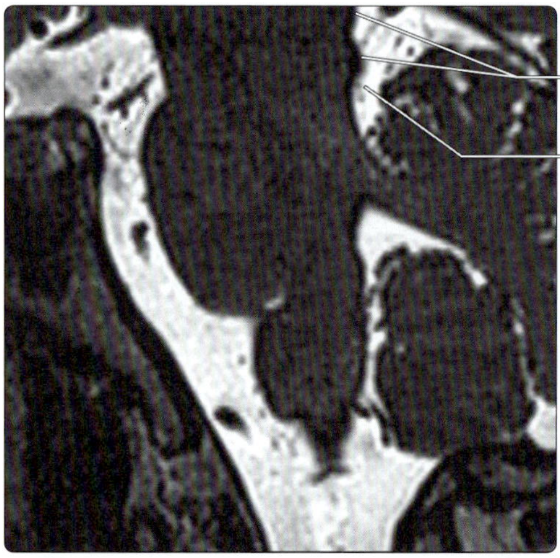

Terminal internal carotid artery
Posterior cerebral artery
Superior cerebellar artery
Left trochlear nerve (CNIV) in trochlear groove
Upper 4th ventricle
Right trochlear nerve (CNIV) origin
Superior medullary velum
Right & left oculomotor nerves (CNIII)
Left trochlear nerve (CNIV) coursing anteriorly toward trochlear cistern
Free edge of tentorium cerebelli
Parahippocampal gyrus
Left trochlear nerve (CNIV) cisternal segment
Left trochlear nerve (CNIV) origin

Superior and inferior colliculi of midbrain
Left trochlear nerve (CNIV) origin

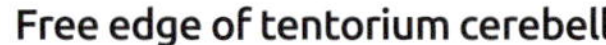

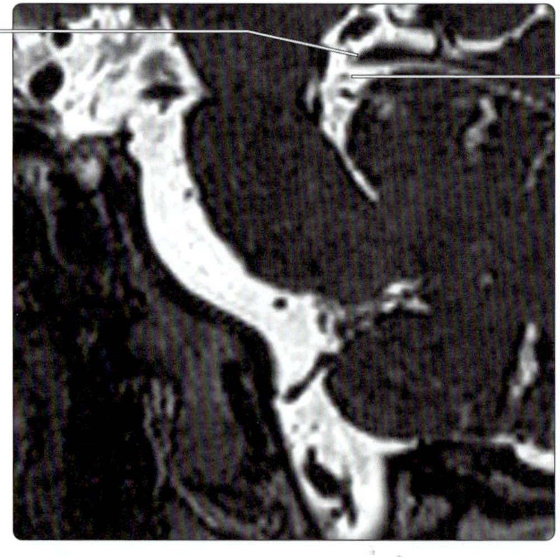

(Top) *Axial 3D T2 SPACE MR shows bilateral trochlear nerves (CNIV) exiting dorsal brainstem just below midbrain inferior colliculi. Trochlear nerve (CNIV) of each side arise in contralateral midbrain trochlear (CNIV) nucleus. Brainstem fibers of both nerves decussates within superior medullary velum and exit dorsal midbrain. Left trochlear nerve is seen passing around brainstem within quadrigeminal cistern and then perimesencephalic cistern, where it courses anteriorly below free edge of tentorium cerebelli in trochlear groove and further anteriorly to pierce posterior petroclinoid fold toward trochlear cistern. Trochlear nerve (CNIV) is thinnest and longest cranial nerve; it is unusual to see a reasonable distance of its course in a single axial section, as seen here. It can be easily confused with tiny arteries and veins. Note the bigger oculomotor nerve (CNIII) anteriorly in interpeduncular cistern.* **(Middle)** *Sagittal 3D T2 SPACE MR shows trochlear nerve origin just below inferior colliculus of midbrain. Trochlear nerve is the only cranial nerve to exit dorsal brainstem.* **(Bottom)** *Further left parasagittal reformat of 3D T2 SPACE MR shows CNIV near trochlear groove inferomedial to tentorial free edge.*

CORONAL T2 MR

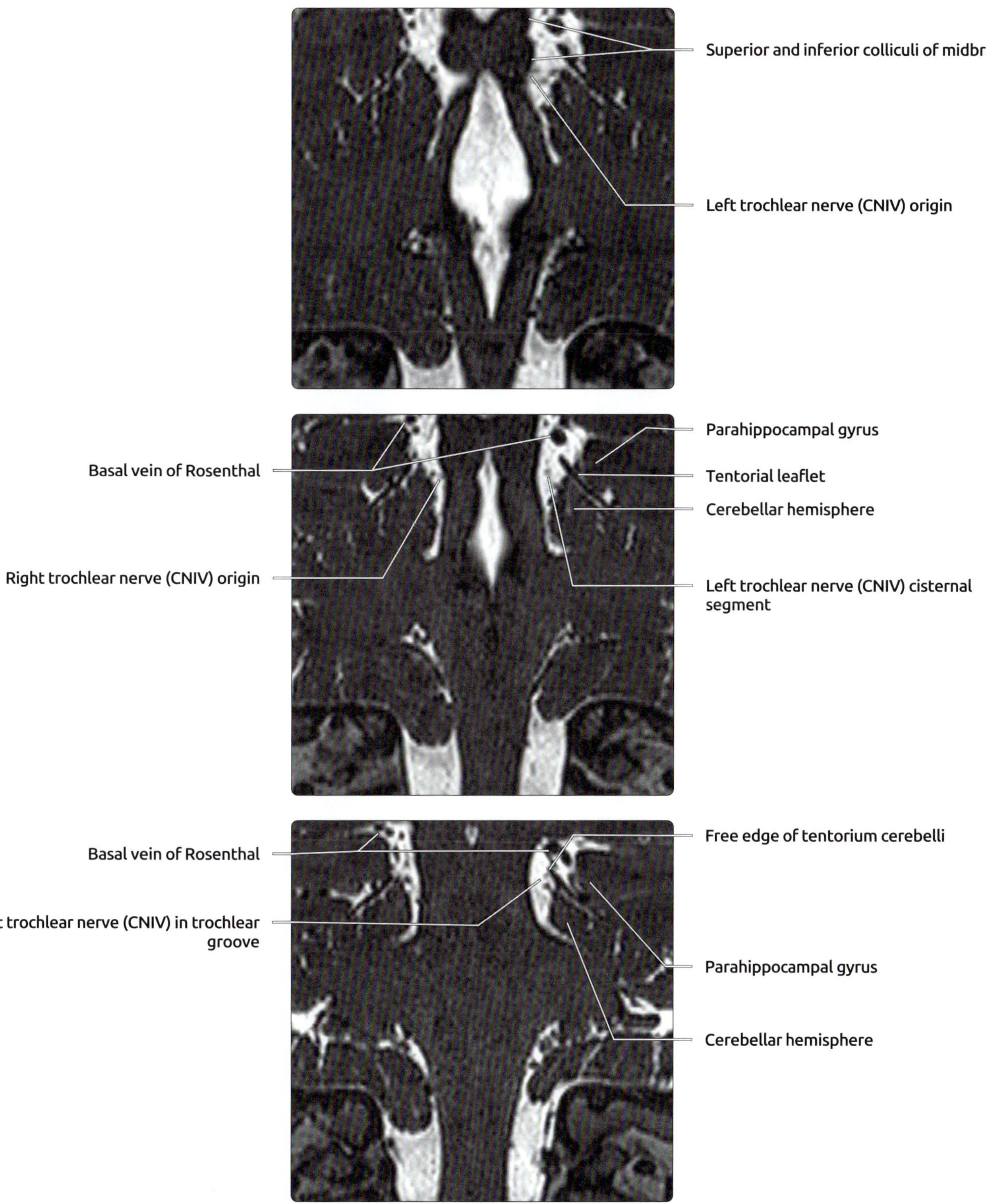

(Top) *First of 3 coronal reformatted images of a 3D T2 SPACE MR from posterior to anterior shows the left trochlear nerve (CNIV) exiting the dorsal brainstem just below the inferior colliculus into the quadrigeminal cistern.* **(Middle)** *This image shows the left trochlear nerve in the perimesencephalic cistern and the right trochlear nerve exiting the brainstem.* **(Bottom)** *Most anterior of the 3 coronal reformatted images shows the left trochlear nerve in the trochlear groove inferomedial to the tentorial free edge. Note the parahippocampal gyrus is superolateral and cerebellum inferolateral to the tentorial leaflet. The entire course of the trochlear nerves is not always visualized on clinical MR; 7T MR offers better extent of visualization, but not in its entirety. Do not confuse tiny vessels for the trochlear nerve. The trochlear nerve passes between the posterior cerebral artery (PCA) and superior cerebellar artery (SCA) laterally in the perimesencephalic cistern. CNIII passes in between the PCA and SCA near the arterial origins more medially in the anterior perimesencephalic/interpeduncular cisterns. Basal vein of Rosenthal also courses through the upper perimesencephalic cistern.*

TERMINOLOGY

Abbreviations

- Trigeminal nerve (CNV)

IMAGING ANATOMY

Overview

- Mixed nerve (both sensory, motor components)

Intraaxial Segment

- 4 nuclei (3 sensory, 1 motor) in brainstem, upper cord
  - **Mesencephalic nucleus CNV**
    - Project cephalad from pons to inferior colliculus level
    - Found anterior to upper 4th ventricle/aqueduct near lateral margin of central gray matter
    - Afferent fibers for **facial proprioception** (teeth, hard palate, and TMJ)
    - Sickle-shaped tract descending to motor nucleus
    - Controls **mastication** and **bite force**
  - **Main sensory nucleus CNV**
    - Nucleus lies lateral to entering trigeminal root
    - Provides **facial tactile sensation**
  - **Motor nucleus CNV**
    - Anteromedial to principal sensory nucleus
    - Supplies **muscles of mastication** (pterygoids, masseter, temporalis), tensor tympani, tensor veli palatini (TVP), mylohyoid, anterior belly of digastric
  - **Spinal nucleus CNV**
    - Extends from principal sensory root in pons into upper cervical cord (between C2 to C4 level)
    - Conveys **facial pain, temperature**

Cisternal (Preganglionic) Segment

- Roots: Smaller motor (1, 2, or 3), larger sensory
- Emerges from lateral pons at **root entry zone** (REZ)
- Courses anterosuperiorly through prepontine cistern
- Enters middle cranial fossa by passing beneath tentorium at apex of petrous temporal bone
- Passes through opening in dura matter called **porus trigeminus** to enter Meckel cave

Intradural Segment

- **Meckel cave** formed by meningeal layer of dura lined by arachnoid; pia covers CNV in trigeminal cave
- Preganglionic CNV ends at **trigeminal ganglion** (TG)
  - TG: Crescentic, located in anteroinferior Meckel cave

Divisions (Postganglionic) of CNV

- **Ophthalmic nerve (CNV1)**: Courses in cavernous sinus
  - Courses in lateral cavernous sinus wall below CNIV
  - Exits skull through superior orbital fissure, enters orbit
  - Divides into lacrimal, frontal, and nasociliary nerves
    - Sensory innervation of **scalp, forehead, nose, globe**
- **Maxillary nerve (CNV2)**: Courses in cavernous sinus
  - Courses in lateral cavernous sinus wall below CNV1
  - Largest nerve in pterygopalatine fossa (PPF), enters posterosuperolateral PPF from cavernous sinus lateral wall in middle cranial fossa through **foramen rotundum**
  - Provides sensory innervation to cheek, maxillary sinus, nasal cavity, maxillary alveolar ridge, palate and posterior wall of nasopharynx
  - CNV2 passes anteriorly and laterally through **upper aspect of PPF** giving rise to zygomatic nerve and posterior superior alveolar nerves
  - Continues anteriorly along roof of PPF into **inferior orbital fissure (IOF)**, gives rise to anterior and middle superior alveolar nerve branches
  - Then enters infraorbital canal in floor of orbit to become **infraorbital nerve** (terminal branch of CNV2)
  - CNV2 inferior branches passing through pterygopalatine ganglion in PPF: Greater and lesser palatine nerves
- **Mandibular nerve (CNV3)**: Does not enter cavernous sinus
  - Exits directly from Meckel cave, passing inferiorly through foramen ovale into **masticator space** (MS)
  - Carries both motor and sensory fibers; motor root bypasses TG, joins CNV3 as it exits via **foramen ovale**
  - Located near skull base medial to lateral pterygoid (LP) and lateral to TVP muscle, within **trigeminal fat pad**
  - Nonrelaying sympathetic root to otic ganglion (OG) from plexus on middle meningeal artery (MMA)
  - OG postganglionic secretomotor fibers to parotid join auriculotemporal nerve (CNV3 branch)
  - **Main trunk of CNV3** gives off meningeal branch and nerve to medial pterygoid (MP); latter provides nonrelaying motor root to OG, which supplies TVP and tensor tympani muscles
  - Main trunk soon divides into small **anterior division** and large **posterior division**
  - Anterior division: Masseteric nerve, 2 deep temporal nerves and nerve to LP motor branches, and buccal nerve sensory branch
  - **Auriculotemporal nerve** arises from 2 roots of proximal posterior division → runs backward, encircling MMA and forms single trunk → again backward, ascending behind neck of mandible above internal maxillary artery → ascends on temple behind superficial temporal vessels
    - Sensory to external ear, TMJ, parotid, temple and secretomotor to parotid via OG
  - Posterior division then divides into terminal branches: Inferior alveolar (posterior) and lingual (anterior) nerves
  - **Inferior alveolar nerve** (sensory to mandible and chin) runs downward lateral to MP → enters mandibular foramen (gives off **mylohyoid nerve** just before entering mandible) → runs in mandibular canal → finally emerges at mental foramen as mental nerve
    - Mylohyoid nerve (motor to anterior belly of digastric and mylohyoid muscles) contains all motor fibers of posterior division of CNV3
  - **Lingual nerve** (CNV3 sensory to anterior 2/3 tongue, floor of mouth) begins 1 cm below skull → runs 1st between TVP and LP → then between LP and MP → then runs anteroinferiorly between MP and mandibular ramus → then runs in direct contact with mandible medial to 3rd molar tooth → finally in lateral sublingual space compartment
  - **Chorda tympani nerve** (CT, CNVII branch) distributed through lingual nerve joins lingual nerve in MS 2 cm below skull base after exiting petrotympanic fissure
  - CT: Anterior 2/3 tongue taste; and secretomotor to submandibular/sublingual salivary glands via its preganglionic parasympathetic supply from pontine superior salivatory nucleus to submandibular ganglion

GRAPHICS

Frontal nerve branch (CNV1)
Infraorbital nerve branch (CNV2)
Ophthalmic division (CNV1)
Meckel cave with trigeminal ganglion
Mesencephalic nucleus (CNV)
Motor nucleus (CNV)
Main sensory nucleus (CNV)
Spinal nucleus (CNV)
Maxillary division (CNV2)
Mandibular division (CNV3)

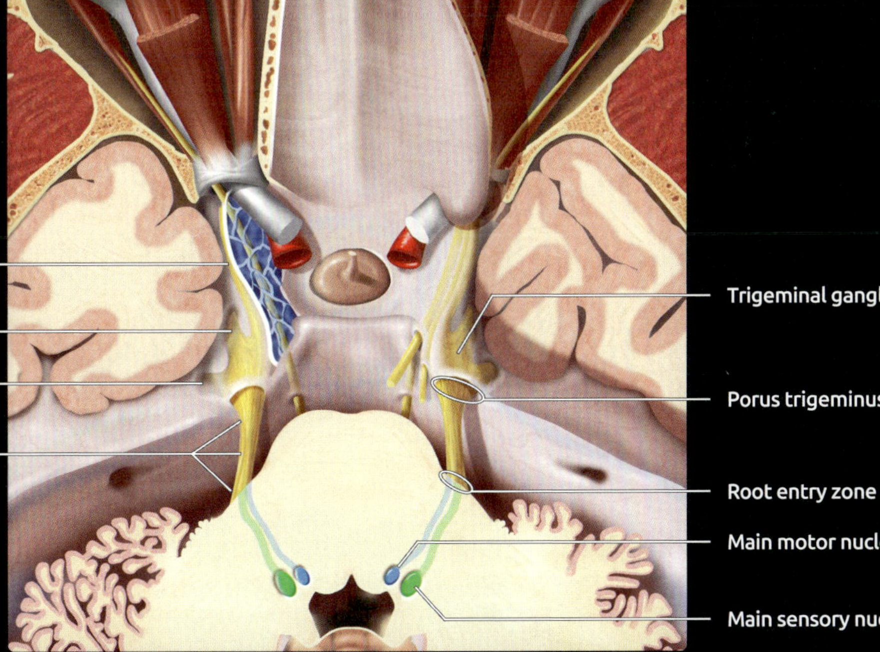

(Top) *Sagittal graphic shows the 4 nuclei of the trigeminal nerve (CNV). From superior to inferior, note the mesencephalic nucleus in the midbrain, the motor nucleus and main sensory nucleus in the pons, and the spinal nucleus extending from the lower pons into the upper cervical spinal cord. The motor root of CNV sends fibers along the mandibular division only.* **(Bottom)** *Axial graphic depicts CNV course from pontine nuclei (main sensory and motor nuclei) to the 3 main branches (CNV1, CNV2, CNV3). Notice the large preganglionic segment entering the lateral pons at the root entry/exit zone (REZ). It then enters the Meckel cave through the porus trigeminus to become the trigeminal ganglion. Vascular loop compression of the transition zone (TZ) between central and peripheral myelin is the most common cause of trigeminal neuralgia, most commonly by the superior cerebellar artery. The term REZ is often synonymously used for TZ, but REZ is actually the part of nerve that includes the TZ, central myelin root portion, and adjacent surface of the brainstem. TZ is the vulnerable anatomic area for neurovascular compression symptoms and is not always in the same position as REZ.*

GRAPHICS

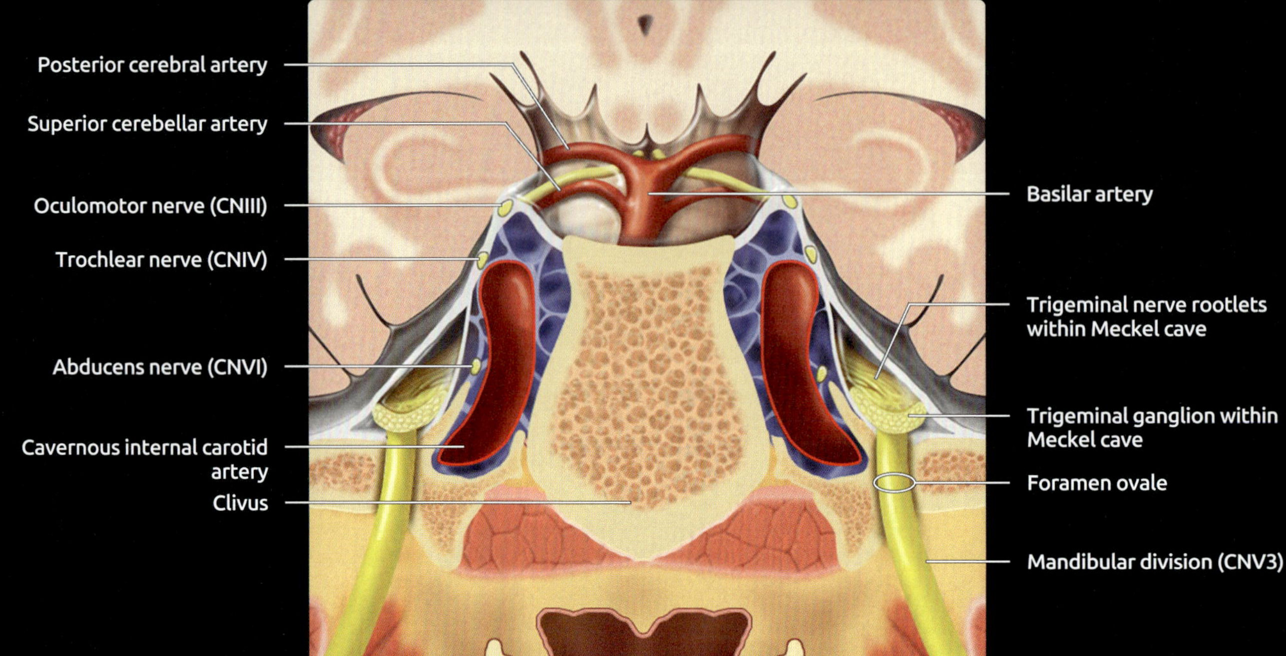

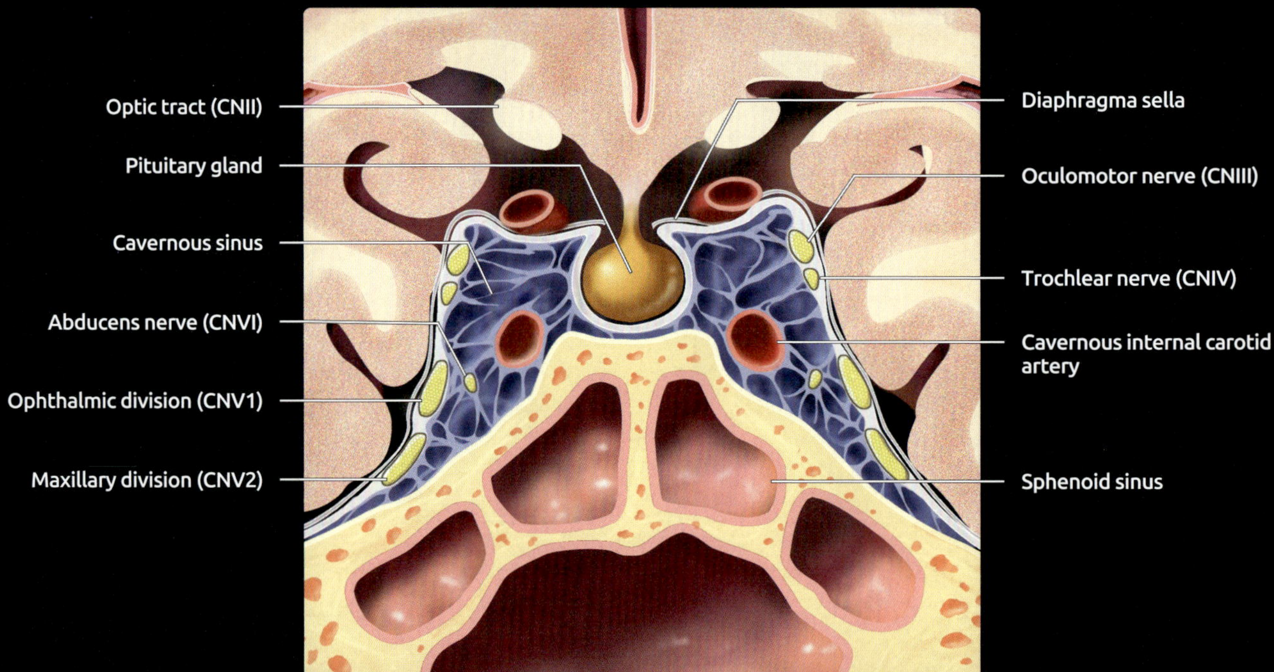

(Top) *Coronal graphic shows the mandibular division of the trigeminal nerve (CNV3), which exits directly from the Meckel cave, passing inferiorly through the foramen ovale into the masticator space and never entering the cavernous sinus. Meckel cave is actually a small anterior extension (pseudopod) of the lateral prepontine cistern, containing both the trigeminal nerve rootlets and trigeminal ganglion. Remember: CNV3 possesses the motor fibers of the trigeminal nerve. Main trunk of CNV3 gives off a motor nerve to medial pterygoid, which also supplies tensor veli palatini and tensor tympani via the otic ganglion. Anterior division of main trunk gives rise to masseteric nerve, 2 deep temporal nerves, and nerve to lateral pterygoid motor branches. Mylohyoid nerve (motor to anterior belly of digastric and mylohyoid muscles) arises from inferior alveolar nerve and contains all motor fibers of posterior division of CNV3.* **(Bottom)** *Coronal graphic through cavernous sinus shows CNV2 in the lateral wall of the cavernous sinus, just inferior to CNV1. CNV1, CNIII, and CNIV are all embedded in the lateral wall of cavernous sinus. The only centrally located intracavernous cranial nerve is abducens nerve (CNVI).*

GRAPHICS

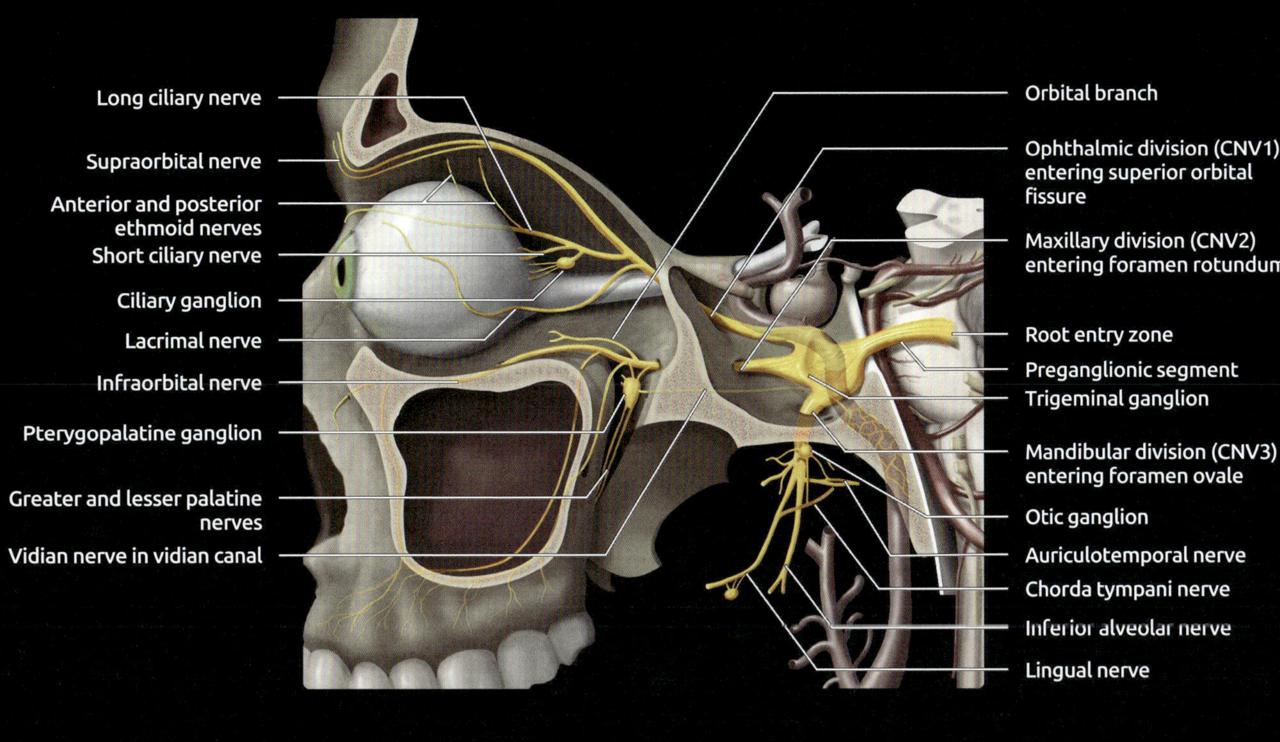

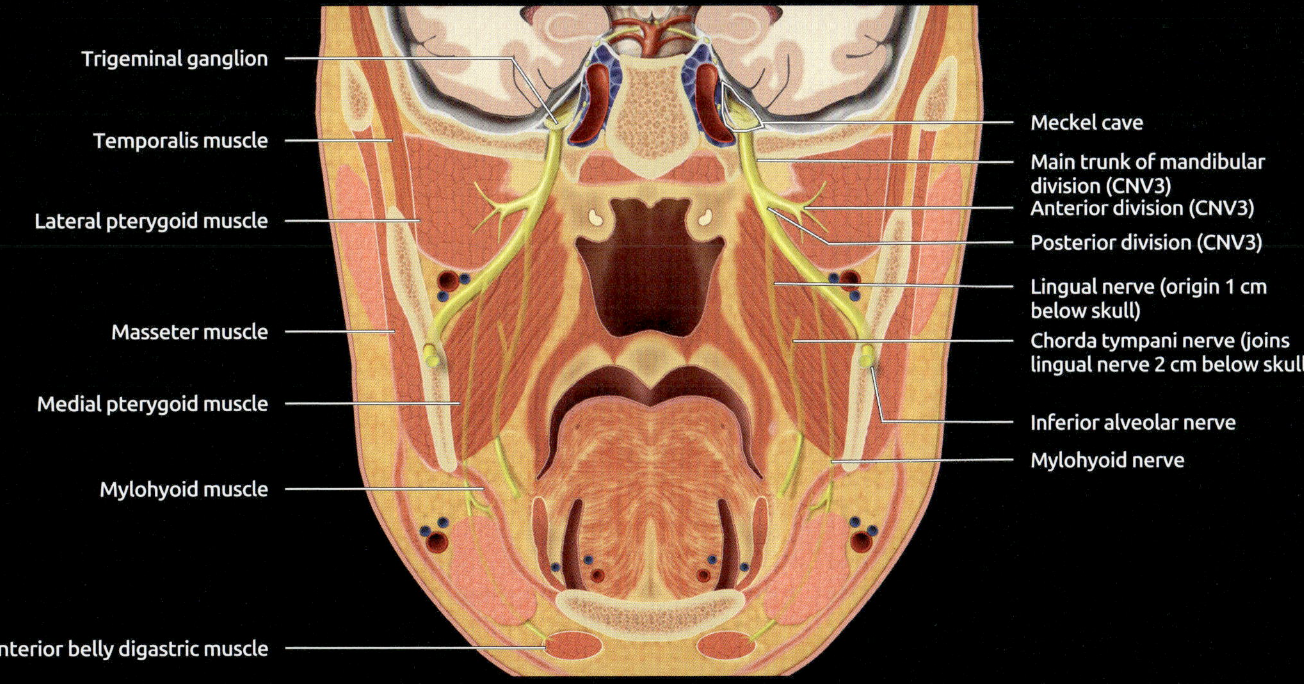

(Top) *Graphic of CNV shows major branches. Ophthalmic division (CNV1) enters orbit via superior orbital fissure, dividing into frontal, nasociliary, and lacrimal branches. Maxillary division (CNV2) enters pterygopalatine fossa via foramen rotundum, gives off multiple branches, continues into inferior orbital fissure and infraorbital canal, and terminates as infraorbital nerve. Mandibular division exits via foramen ovale. Otic ganglion (OG) lies just below skull base between CNV3 and tensor veli palatini muscle. Lesser petrosal nerve gives preganglionic parasympathetics to OG from medullary inferior salivatory nucleus, and sympathetic root is from plexus on middle meningeal artery. Postganglionic secretomotor fibers for parotid gland join auriculotemporal nerve (CNV3 branch).* **(Bottom)** *Graphic shows CNV3 exiting skull through foramen ovale without entering cavernous sinus. Main trunk gives off meningeal branch and nerve to medial pterygoid, soon dividing into small anterior division (giving rise to other masticator muscle branches and buccal sensory branch) and large posterior division, giving rise to auriculotemporal, inferior alveolar (gives off mylohyoid nerve), and lingual nerves.*

AXIAL BONE CT

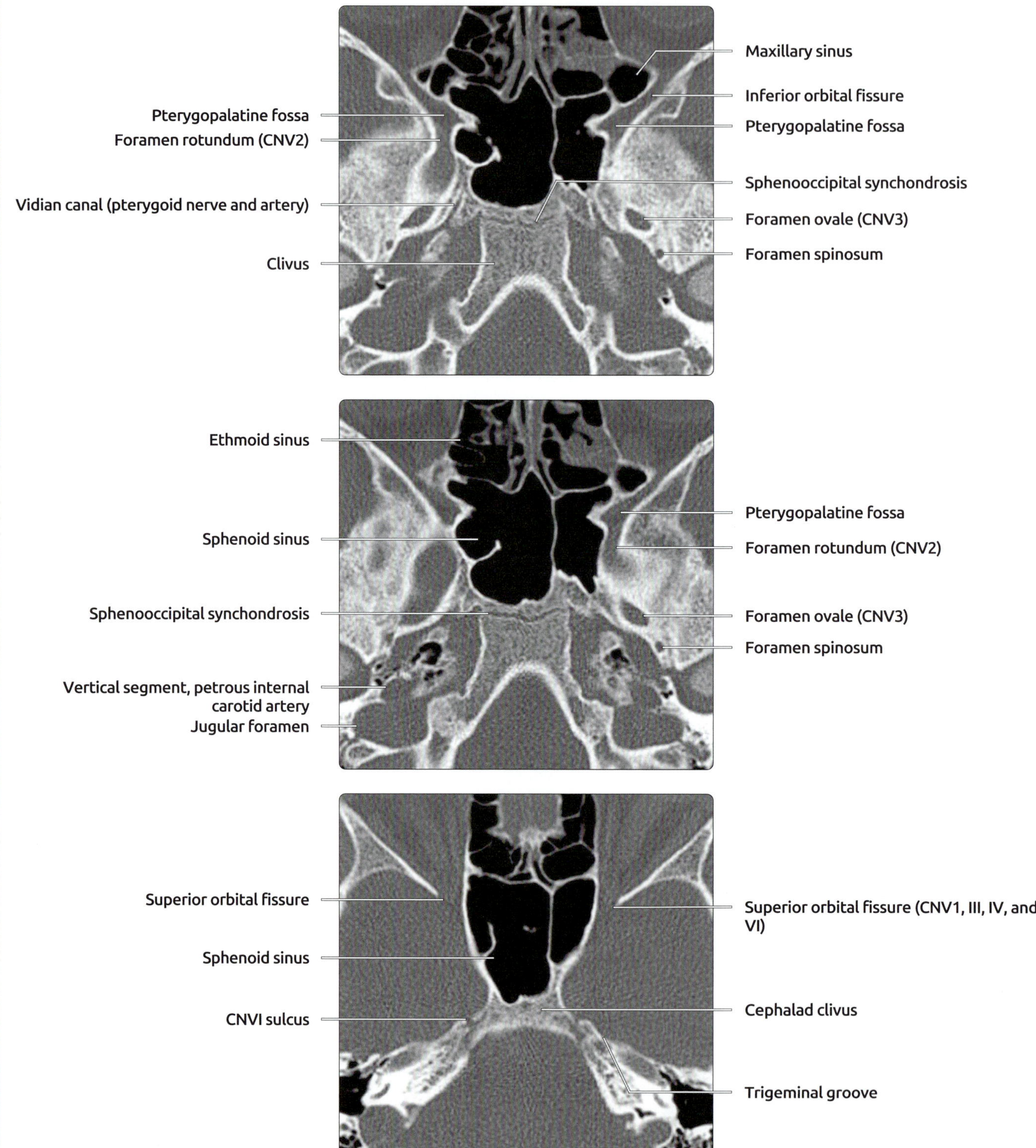

(Top) *First of 3 axial bone CT images from inferior to superior through central skull base is shown. CNV2 exits the skull base through the foramen rotundum to enter the superior margin of the pterygopalatine fossa. CNV3 exits via the foramen ovale to enter the masticator space, where it supplies motor innervation to muscles of mastication and sensory sensory innervation through inferior alveolar, lingual, and auriculotemporal nerves. Note adjacent foramen spinosum, which contains middle meningeal artery, vein, and meningeal branch of CNV3. Lesser petrosal nerve exits the middle cranial fossa via the foramen ovale, or, occasionally, via a tiny "canaliculus innominatus" in between and medial to foramen ovale and spinosum.* **(Middle)** *Foramen ovale (CNV3) and foramen rotundum (CNV2) are now best seen on the patient's left. The left foramen rotundum is seen opening into the superior pterygopalatine fossa.* **(Bottom)** *Superior orbital fissure transmits the ophthalmic division of CNV from cranium to orbit. Other structures passing through the superior orbital fissure include the oculomotor nerve (CNIII), trochlear nerve (CNIV), abducens nerve (CNVI), and the superior ophthalmic vein.*

AXIAL T2 MR

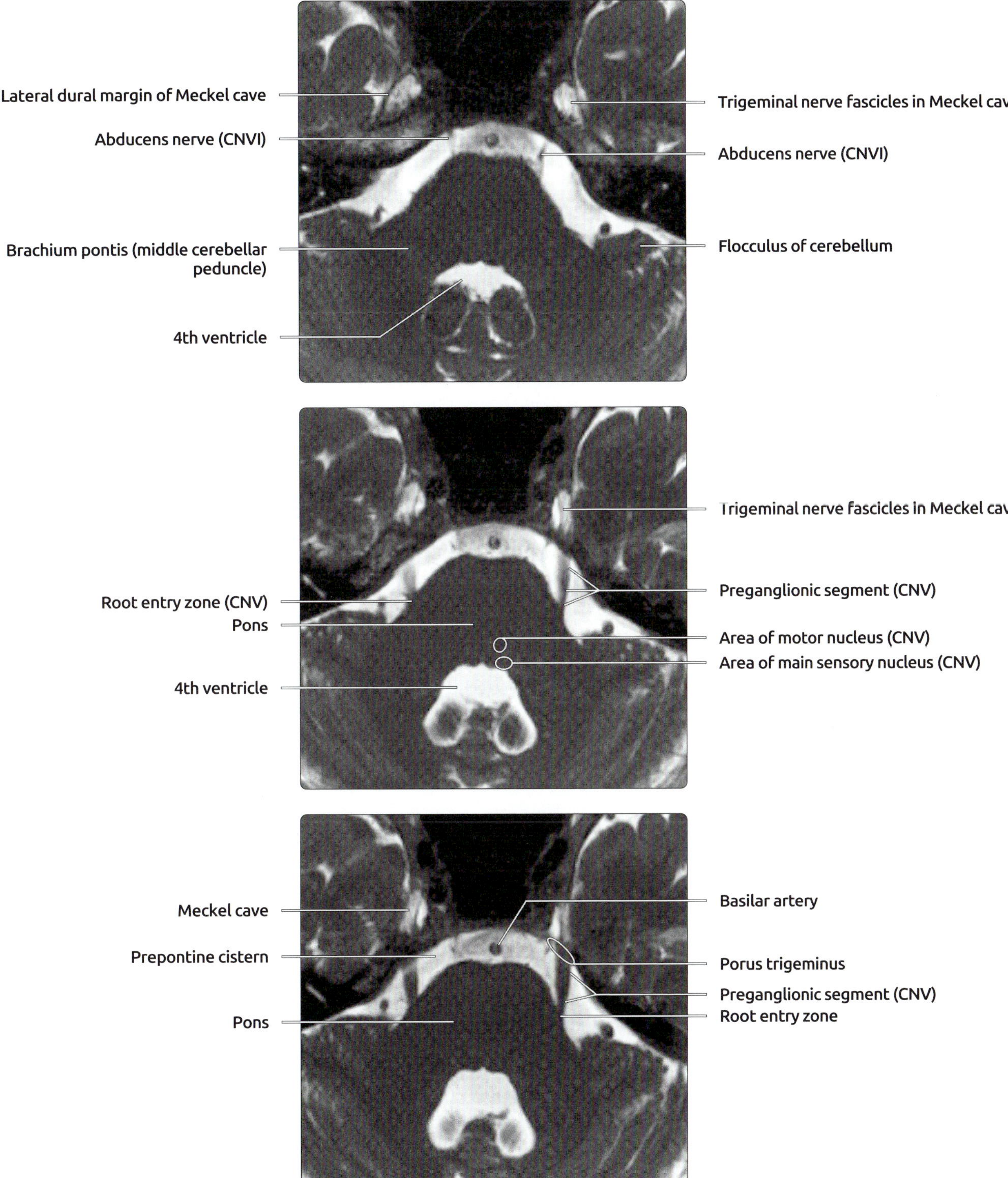

(Top) *First of 3 axial T2 MR images through CNV and the Meckel cave presented from inferior to superior shows a layer of hypointense dura mater forming the lateral wall and the roof of the Meckel cave. The right abducens nerve is seen penetrating dura to enter the Dorello canal. CNV fascicles can be seen with CSF of the Meckel cave.* **(Middle)** *Preganglionic fascicles of CNV are seen within the Meckel cave, which contains CSF, trigeminal fascicles, and trigeminal ganglion. Note main sensory and motor nuclei locations.* **(Bottom)** *In this image, the preganglionic segment of CNV is seen spanning the distance between the REZ on the lateral pons and the porus trigeminus of the Meckel cave. REZ is actually the part of nerve that includes the TZ between central and peripheral myelin, central myelin root portion, and adjacent surface of the brainstem. TZ is the vulnerable anatomic area for neurovascular compression symptoms. The cisternal portion measures ~ 8-15 mm in length, and the zone with central myelin (which is the distance from the brainstem to TZ) is shorter on the medial side (1.13 mm) than on the lateral side (2.47 mm) of the nerve.*

AXIAL T1 C+ MR

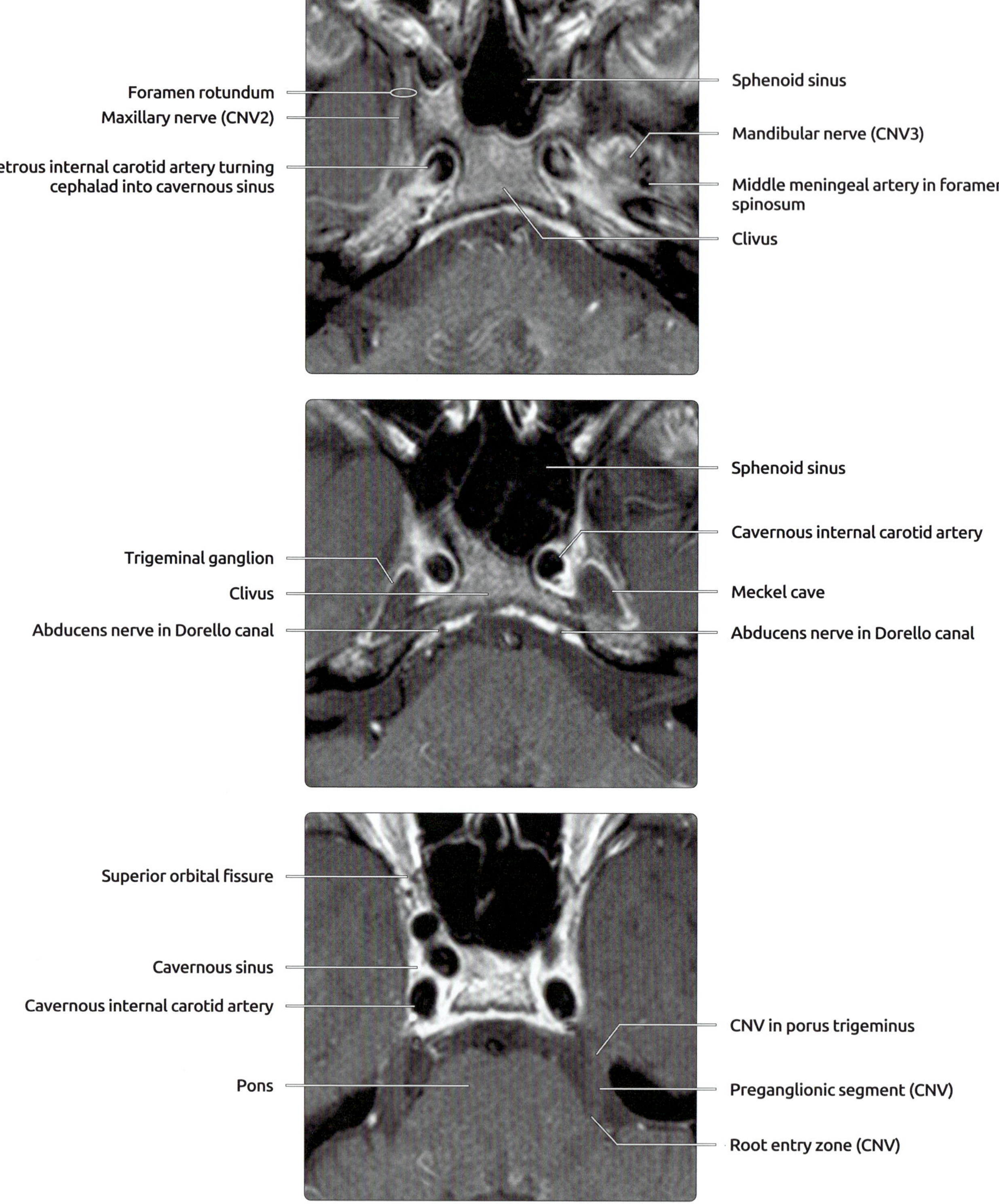

(Top) *First of 3 axial T1 C+ FS MR images presented from inferior to superior through the central skull base shows the right maxillary nerve (CNV2) passing anteriorly into the foramen rotundum and the left mandibular nerve (CNV3) passing inferiorly through the foramen ovale. Both nerves are surrounded by enhancing veins communicating with the extracranial venous system. The foramen rotundum connects the lateral wall of the cavernous sinus in the medial aspect of the middle cranial fossa with the posterosuperolateral aspect of the pterygopalatine fossa. The foramen ovale connects the middle cranial fossa floor with the masticator space.* **(Middle)** *More superior image demonstrates the ovoid shape of the CSF-filled Meckel cave. The trigeminal ganglion is the linear anteroinferior structure in the Meckel cave. It lacks a blood-nerve barrier and therefore normally enhances with contrast.* **(Bottom)** *Preganglionic segment of CNV arises from the lateral pons at the REZ. The TZ measures ~ 2 mm in length, and the distalmost part of the TZ is 3.4-5.0 mm away from the brainstem. The right internal carotid artery is tortuous within the cavernous sinus.*

CORONAL T2 MR

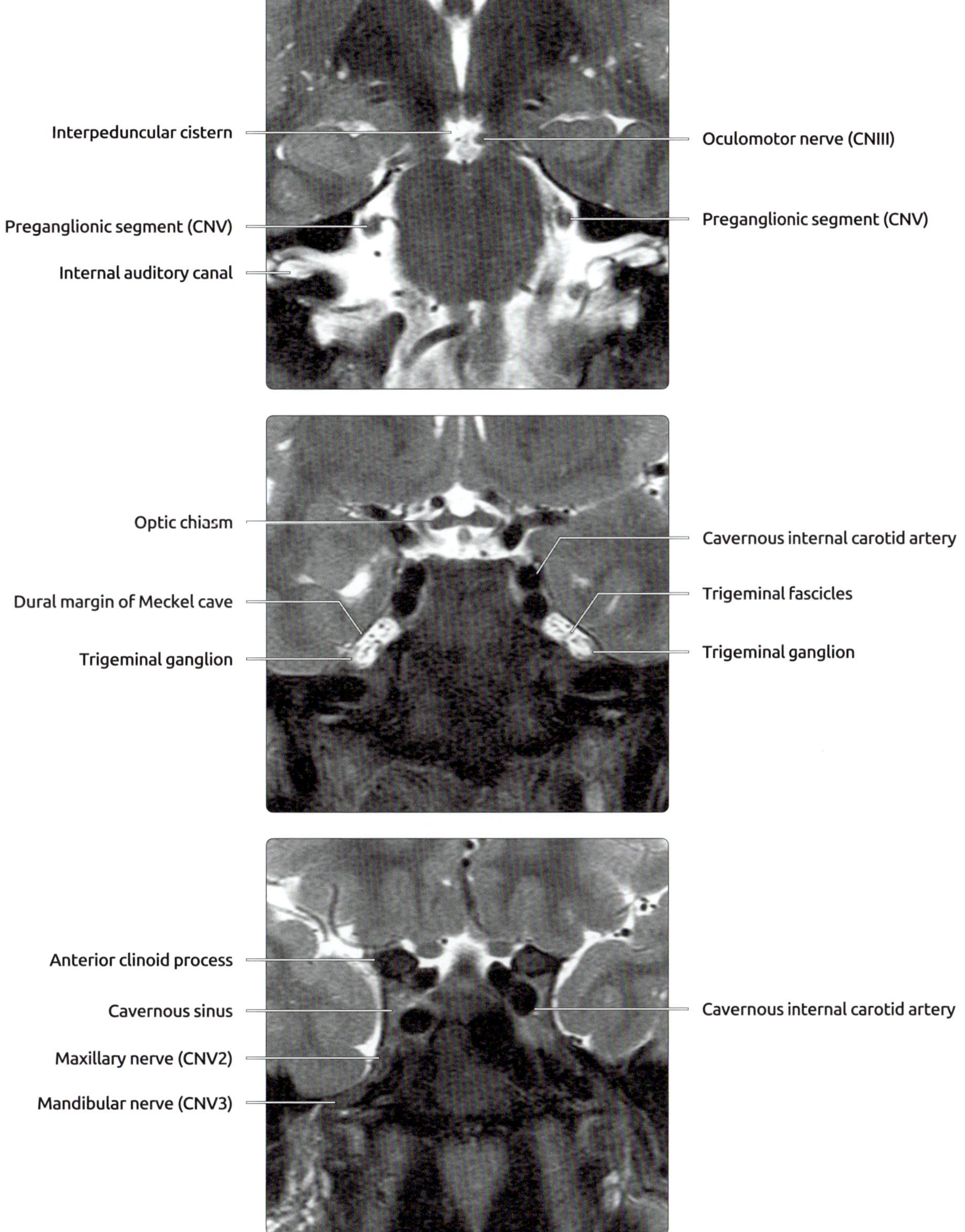

(Top) *First of 3 coronal T2 MR images presented from posterior to anterior shows the ovoid preganglionic segment of CNV surrounded by high-signal CSF. The preganglionic segment has just exited the lateral pons REZ area. One (in > 1/2 of patients), 2 (in just above 1/3 of patients) or even 3 (in ~ 1/10 of patients) small motor roots of CNV that exit the pons anterosuperomedial to the REZ of the large sensory root may be seen.* **(Middle)** *This more anterior image through the Meckel cave delineates the trigeminal fascicles of the preganglionic trigeminal nerve. The trigeminal ganglion is visible as a semilunar structure in the floor of the Meckel cave bilaterally.* **(Bottom)** *This image through the anterior cavernous sinus shows the maxillary nerve (CNV2) passing anteriorly within the lateral wall of the cavernous sinus and the mandibular nerve (CNV3) passing inferiorly to its exit point in the skull base (foramen ovale). The maxillary nerve (CNV2) passes anteriorly through the foramen rotundum into the pterygopalatine fossa, gives off many branches, and passes through the inferior orbital fissure into the infraorbital canal, terminating as an infraorbital nerve.*

CORONAL T1 C+ MR

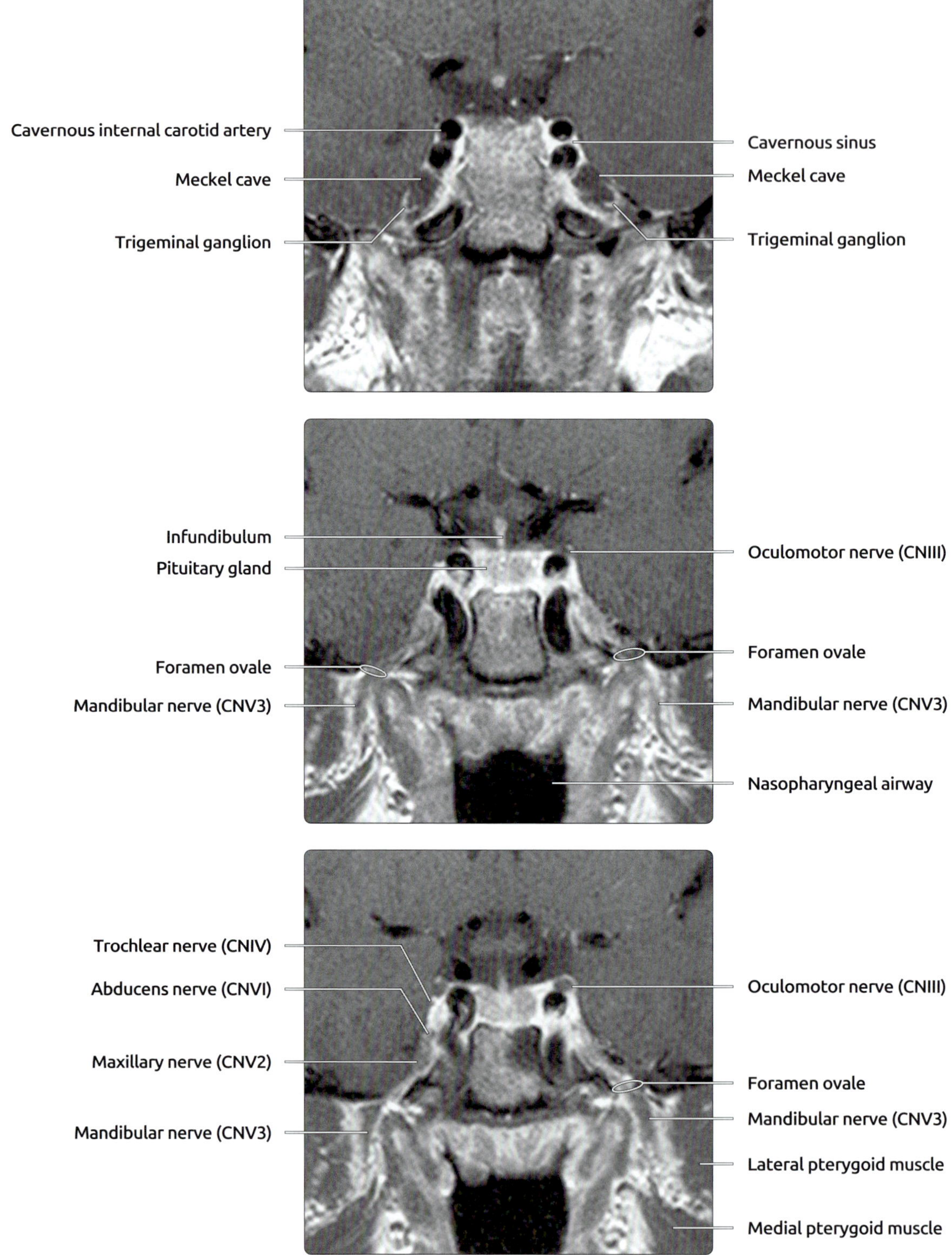

(Top) *First of 6 coronal T1 C+ MR images through the cavernous sinus presented from posterior to anterior is shown. The trigeminal ganglion is seen as a crescentic area of enhancement in the floor of the Meckel cave. Trigeminal ganglion enhances because it lacks a blood-nerve barrier.* **(Middle)** *In this image through the foramen ovale, the mandibular nerve (CNV3) is visible exiting inferiorly into the masticator space.* **(Bottom)** *In this image, the patient's left foramen ovale and mandibular nerve are seen. The motor branches from CNV3 are to the medial pterygoid, which also supplies the tensor veli palatini and tensor tympani (from the main trunk), the masseteric nerve, 2 deep temporal nerves to the temporalis and the nerve to the lateral pterygoid (from the anterior division), and the mylohyoid nerve, which supplies the mylohyoid and anterior belly of the digastric muscles (branch of inferior alveolar nerve; mylohyoid nerve contains all the motor fibers of posterior division). The main sensory branches are the meningeal branch (from main trunk), buccal nerve (from anterior division), auriculotemporal nerve, and the terminal lingual and inferior alveolar nerves (branches of posterior division).*

CORONAL T1 C+ MR

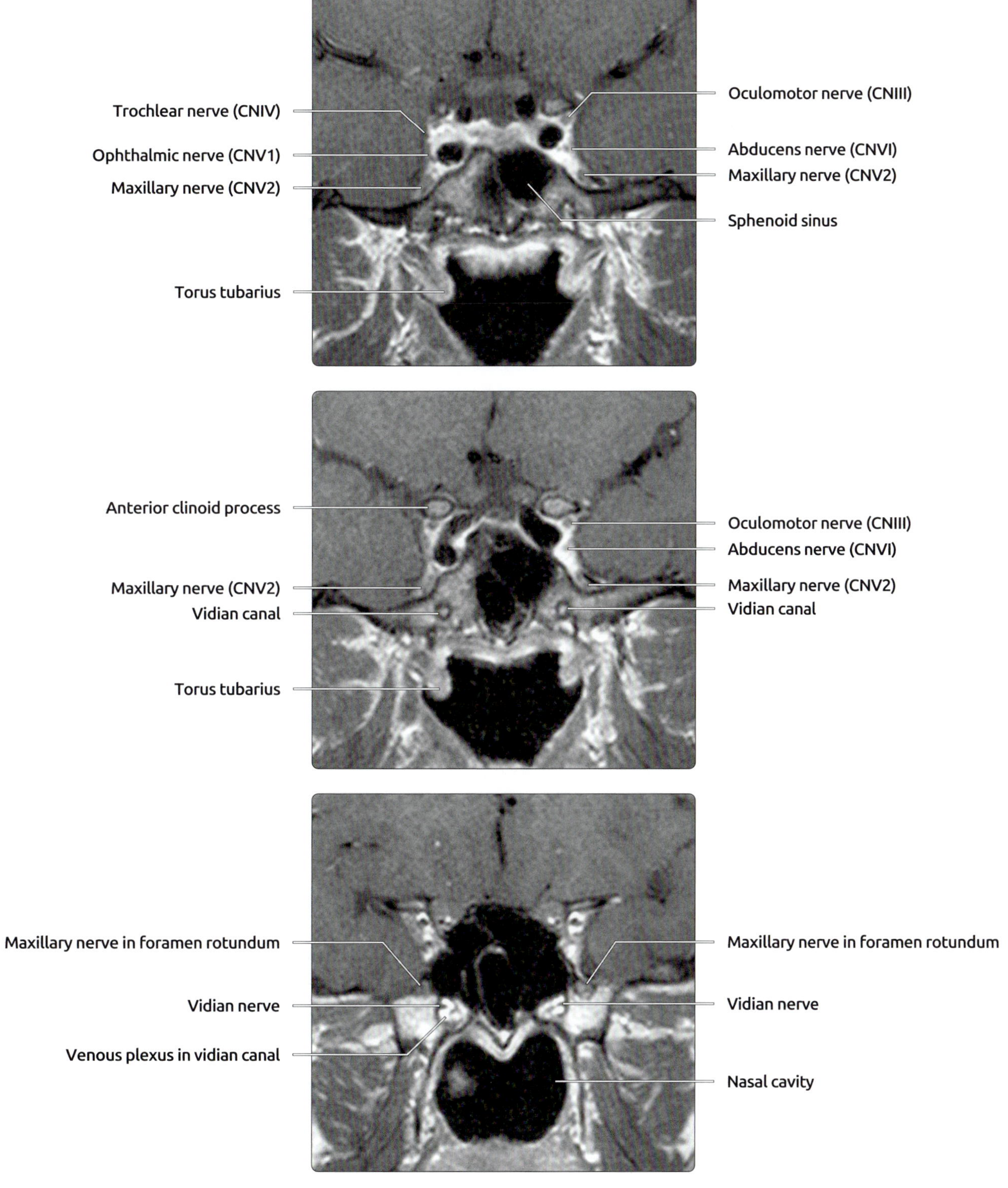

(Top) *In this MR through the anterior margin of the pituitary gland, the maxillary nerve (CNV2) is well seen bilaterally in the inferolateral wall of the cavernous sinus.* **(Middle)** *In this more anterior MR, the maxillary nerves are seen in the inferolateral wall of the cavernous sinus just prior to its entry into the foramen rotundum. Inferomedially, note the vidian canals.* **(Bottom)** *The maxillary nerve can be seen in the foramen rotundum. Notice also the vidian canal widening on its extracranial side with the vidian nerve visible surrounded by a venous plexus. Vidian nerve is formed in vidian canal by confluence of parasympathetic fibers from greater superficial petrosal nerve (GSPN), which is a branch of facial nerve in the temporal bone anterior genu region, and sympathetic fibers from deep petrosal nerve from the plexus around internal carotid artery. Foramen rotundum is situated at the base of greater wing of sphenoid, superolateral to vidian canal, which lies in the body of sphenoid bone. Practically, identify these foramina on coronal images by their relation (superolateral and inferomedial, respectively) to sphenoid sinus lateral (pterygoid) recess or an imaginary lateral recess.*

SAGITTAL T2 AND AXIAL T1 MR

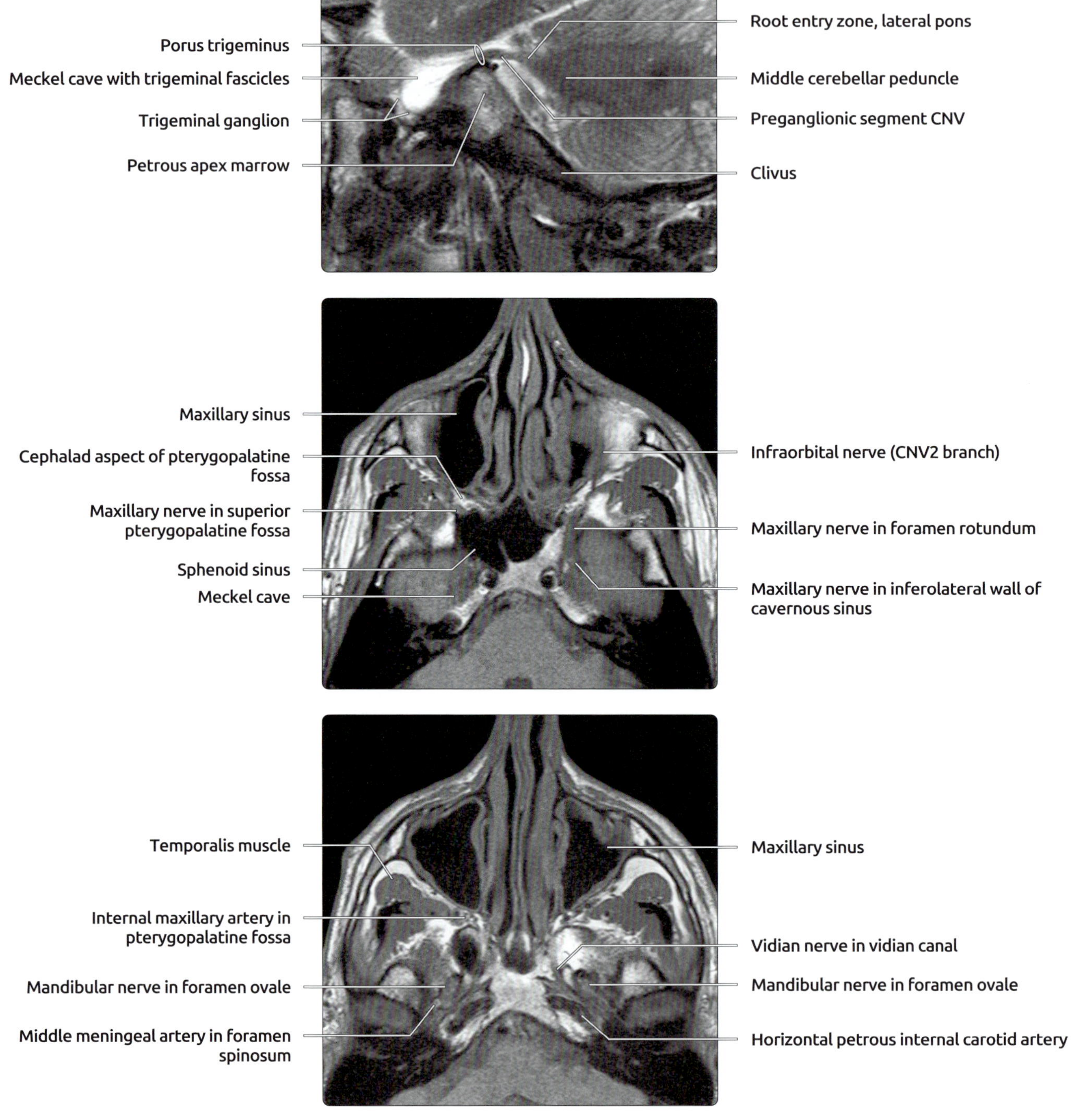

(Top) *Sagittal T2 MR along the line of the proximal trigeminal nerve shows the preganglionic segment between the REZ in the lateral pons and the trigeminal ganglion in the anteroinferior Meckel cave. The CSF within the Meckel cave communicates with the prepontine cistern through the porus trigeminus.* **(Middle)** *First of 5 axial T1 unenhanced MR images extending from the skull base to the mandibular body from superior to inferior is shown. Notice the left maxillary nerve in the foramen rotundum and how it traverses the roof of the pterygopalatine fossa. It then inclines laterally on the back of maxilla and enters the orbit through the inferior orbital fissure, after which it continues as the infraorbital nerve in the floor of the orbit that, in turn, exits the orbit through the infraorbital foramen (not shown).* **(Bottom)** *Image through the foramen ovale of the skull base is shown. Notice the mandibular nerves exiting the skull base. The vidian canal and nerve are also visible connecting the foramen lacerum to the pterygopalatine fossa. The many black dots within the pterygopalatine fossa are from the normal terminal internal maxillary artery lying anterior to the neural plane.*

AXIAL T1 MR

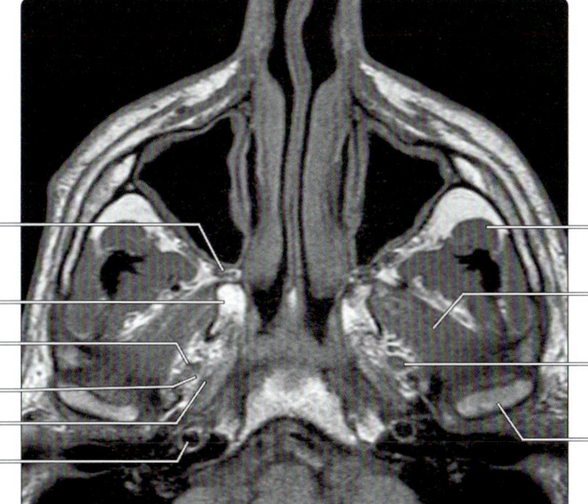

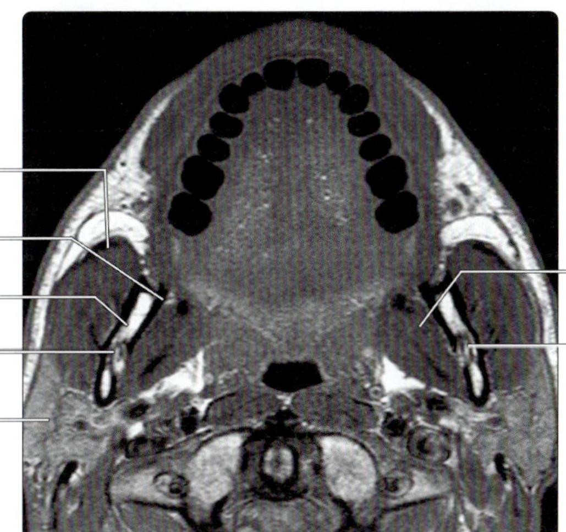

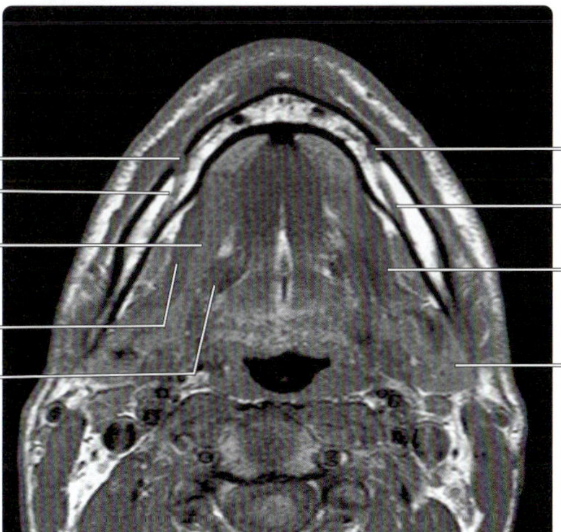

(Top) *Image just under the skull base shows mandibular nerves entering the medial upper masticator space. OG lies just below the skull base between CNV3 and tensor veli palatini muscle. Main trunk of CNV3 gives off a meningeal branch and nerve to medial pterygoid with motor root to OG and soon divides into a small anterior division (giving off masseteric, 2 deep temporal nerves to lateral pterygoid motor branches, and a buccal nerve sensory branch) and a large posterior division. Auriculotemporal nerve arises from 2 roots of the proximal posterior division, runs backward encircling the middle meningeal artery, and forms single trunk. The posterior division then divides into terminal branches, inferior alveolar (posterior) and lingual (anterior) nerves.* **(Middle)** *MR at the mandibular foramina level shows inferior alveolar nerve runs downward lateral to medial pterygoid and enters mandibular foramen, giving off mylohyoid nerve just before entering mandible.* **(Bottom)** *MR at mandible body level shows inferior alveolar nerve as it exits the mandible via the mental foramen. Lingual nerve contacts the mandible medial to 3rd molar tooth and finally enters the lateral sublingual space compartment.*

TERMINOLOGY

Abbreviations

- Abducens nerve (CNVI)

Definitions

- Motor nerve to lateral rectus muscle only

IMAGING ANATOMY

Overview

- Pure motor nerve with pontine nucleus and 5 anatomic segments

Abducens Nucleus

- Paired CNVI nuclei located in pontine tegmentum (dorsal pons) near midline, just ventral to 4th ventricle
- **Facial colliculus**: Axons of facial nerve (CNVII) loop around abducens nucleus, creating bulge in floor of 4th ventricle
  - Isolated lesion to facial colliculus can cause ipsilateral CNVI and CNVII palsy

Intraaxial Segment

- Ipsilateral axons from CNVI nucleus course anteroinferiorly through pontine tegmentum

Cisternal Segment

- Emerges from anterior brainstem near midline through groove between pons and pyramid of medulla oblongata (pontomedullary sulcus)
- Usually exits as single trunk but occasionally duplicated
- Ascends anterosuperiorly in prepontine cistern toward site where it penetrates dura along upper clivus laterally
- Posterior to anterior inferior cerebellar artery in 85%; anterior in 15%

Interdural Segment

- Extends from point where CNVI pierces inner layer dura posteriorly to its entrance into cavernous sinus (CS) anteriorly
- Thin sleeve of arachnoid (and occasionally dura) travels with nerve through this segment
- After penetrating dura, CNVI passes superiorly through basilar venous plexus
  - Basilar venous plexus: Interdural; dorsal to upper clivus and located between inner and outer (endosteal) layers of dura
- Nerve remains interdural and passes superiorly over junction of petrous apex and clivus into adjacent venous region, which is referred to as **sphenopetroclival venous confluence** [or simply petroclival confluence or **petroclival venous confluence** (PCVC)]
  - PCVC located at junction of posterior part of CS, lateral part of basilar plexus, and anterior part of superior and inferior petrosal sinuses
- In this location, PCVC and interdural segment of CNVI considered to be within **classic Dorello canal**
- Classic **Dorello canal**: Zone/space bounded by petrous apex (inferolaterally), clivus (inferomedially), and **petrosphenoidal ligament of Gruber** (superiorly)
  - Proposed modifications expanding limits to include portions of venous confluence above Gruber ligament and making posterior petroclinoid fold as superior boundary

Cavernous Segment

- After exiting Dorello canal, CNVI enters CS and passes laterally around proximal aspect of cavernous internal carotid artery (ICA)
- CNVI: **Only cranial nerve to lie within CS**, passing lateral to cavernous ICA
- Cranial nerves III, IV, V1, and V2: All embedded within lateral wall of CS

Extracranial (Intraorbital) Segment

- CNVI enters orbit through **superior orbital fissure (SOF)** together with CNIII and CNIV
- Passes through annulus of Zinn
- Supplies **motor innervation** to **lateral rectus muscle**

ANATOMY IMAGING ISSUES

Imaging Recommendations

- MR for intraaxial, cisternal, interdural, and cavernous segments
  - Thin-section high-resolution T2 and contrast-enhanced T1 in axial and coronal planes
    - Depicts small structures, including cranial nerves, surrounded by CSF with high contrast and high spatial resolution
- Bone CT best for skull base and its bony foramina

Imaging Sweet Spots

- Axial and coronal MR sequences should include brainstem, 4th ventricle, CS, and orbit
- CNVI nucleus and intraaxial segment not directly visualized
  - CNVI location inferred by identifying facial colliculus in 4th ventricle floor on high-resolution thin-section T2 MR
- Cisternal segment routinely visualized on high-resolution T2 MR
- CNVI entrance into Dorello canal may be visualized due to evagination of CSF into proximal canal
  - **CSF sleeve in Dorello canal > 2x width of CNVI**, highly associated with idiopathic intracranial hypertension (**IIH/pseudotumor cerebri**)
- Enhancement of basilar plexus may demonstrate CNVI as tiny, linear, nonenhancing structures

Imaging Pitfalls

- Use of fat saturation on postcontrast T1 MR sequences can amplify blooming (susceptibility) artifact around well-aerated sphenoid sinus
  - CS and orbital apex subtle lesions may be obscured by this artifact
  - Remove fat saturation and repeat T1 postcontrast MR if this artifact obscures key areas of interest

CLINICAL IMPLICATIONS

Clinical Importance

- In abducens neuropathy, affected eye will not **abduct**
- CNVI neuropathy divided into **simple** if isolated and **complex** if associated with other cranial nerve involvement
  - Simple **CNVI neuropathy most common ocular motor nerve palsy**
  - Usually presents as complex cranial neuropathy
    - Pontine lesions affect CNVI with CNVII
    - CS, SOF lesions affect CNVI with CNIII, CNIV, and CNV1

GRAPHICS

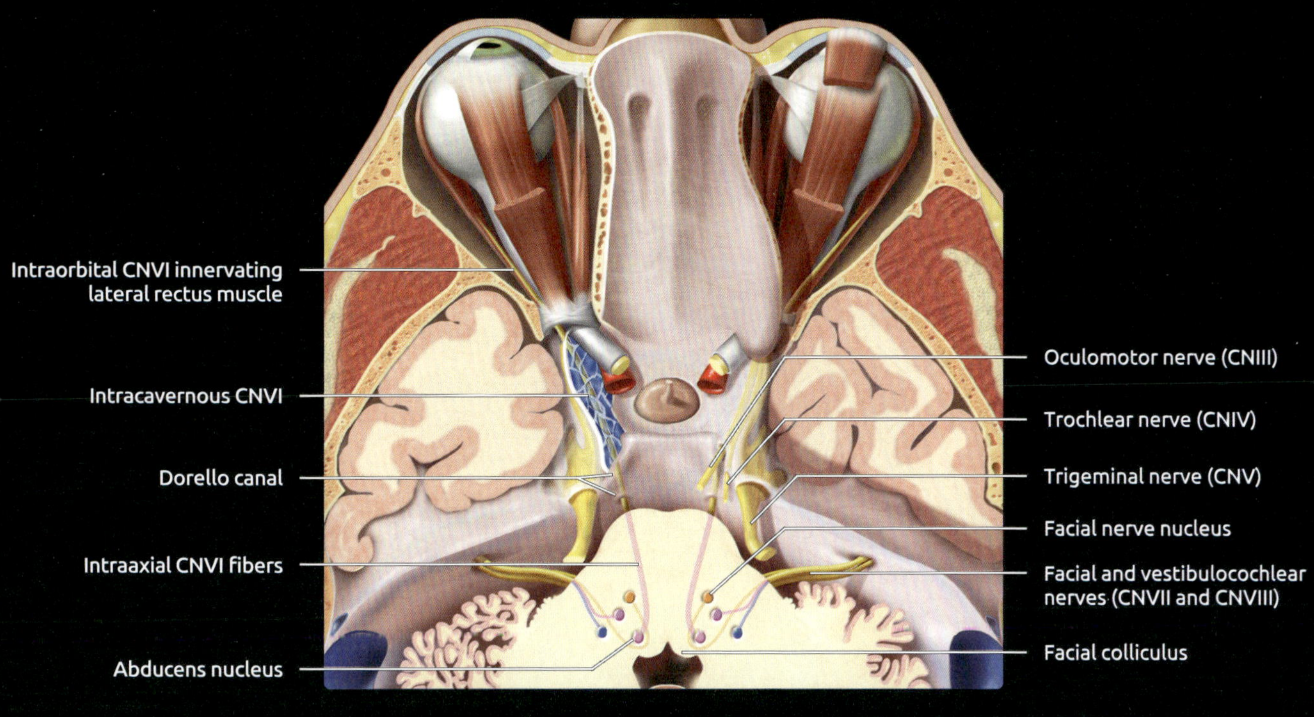

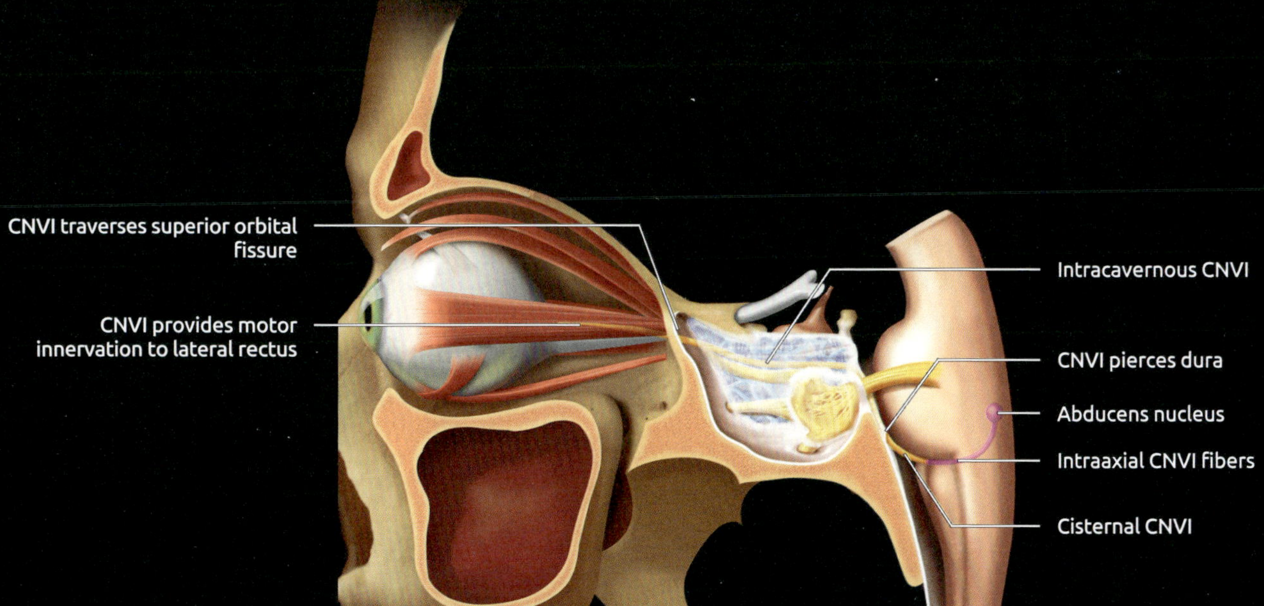

(Top) *Axial graphic shows the entire length of the abducens nerve from its pontine tegmentum nuclear origin to its motor endplate in the lateral rectus muscle. Follow its progress from the nucleus to its exit at the anteromedial bulbopontine sulcus. From there, note the dural penetration into the Dorello canal leading to its intracavernous portion. Finally, it passes through the superior orbital fissure and the ring of Zinn into the orbit.* **(Bottom)** *Sagittal graphic shows the abducens nerve depicted from its origin in the pontine tegmentum to its motor endplate in the lateral rectus muscle. Notice the intraaxial CNVI fibers descend before exiting the bulbopontine sulcus anteriorly. Prepontine cistern CNVI then ascends to pierce the dura into the Dorello canal. Intracavernous CNVI proceeds anteriorly to pass through the superior orbital fissure and the annulus of Zinn before innervating the lateral rectus muscle in orbit.*

AXIAL T2 AND T1 C+ MR

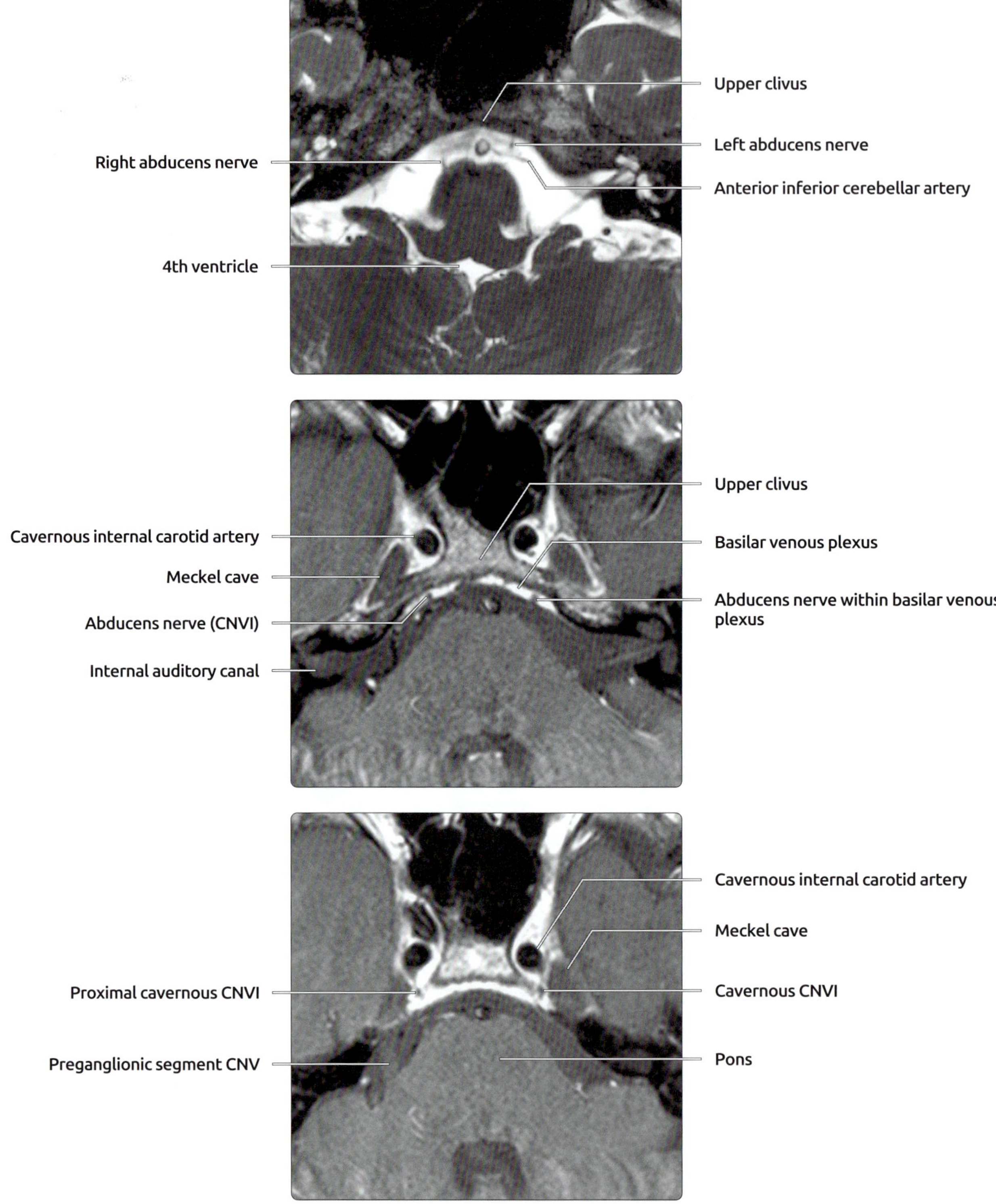

(Top) *Axial T2 MR near the level of the internal auditory canal shows the appearance of the abducens nerve in the prepontine cistern. On the patient's right, CNVI is just exiting the bulbopontine sulcus, while on the left, it is poised to penetrate the dura. Both nerves are rising in the prepontine cistern.* **(Middle)** *Axial T1 C+ MR demonstrates the interdural segment of the abducens nerve within the Dorello canal surrounded by brightly enhancing basilar venous plexus.* **(Bottom)** *Axial T1 C+ MR just above the internal auditory canal shows the abducens nerves passing through the superior basilar venous plexus to enter the posterior margin of the cavernous sinus. At this point, CNVI is arching over the petrous apex below the petrosphenoidal ligament of Gruber into the upper posterior region of the cavernous sinus.*

SAGITTAL T2 MR

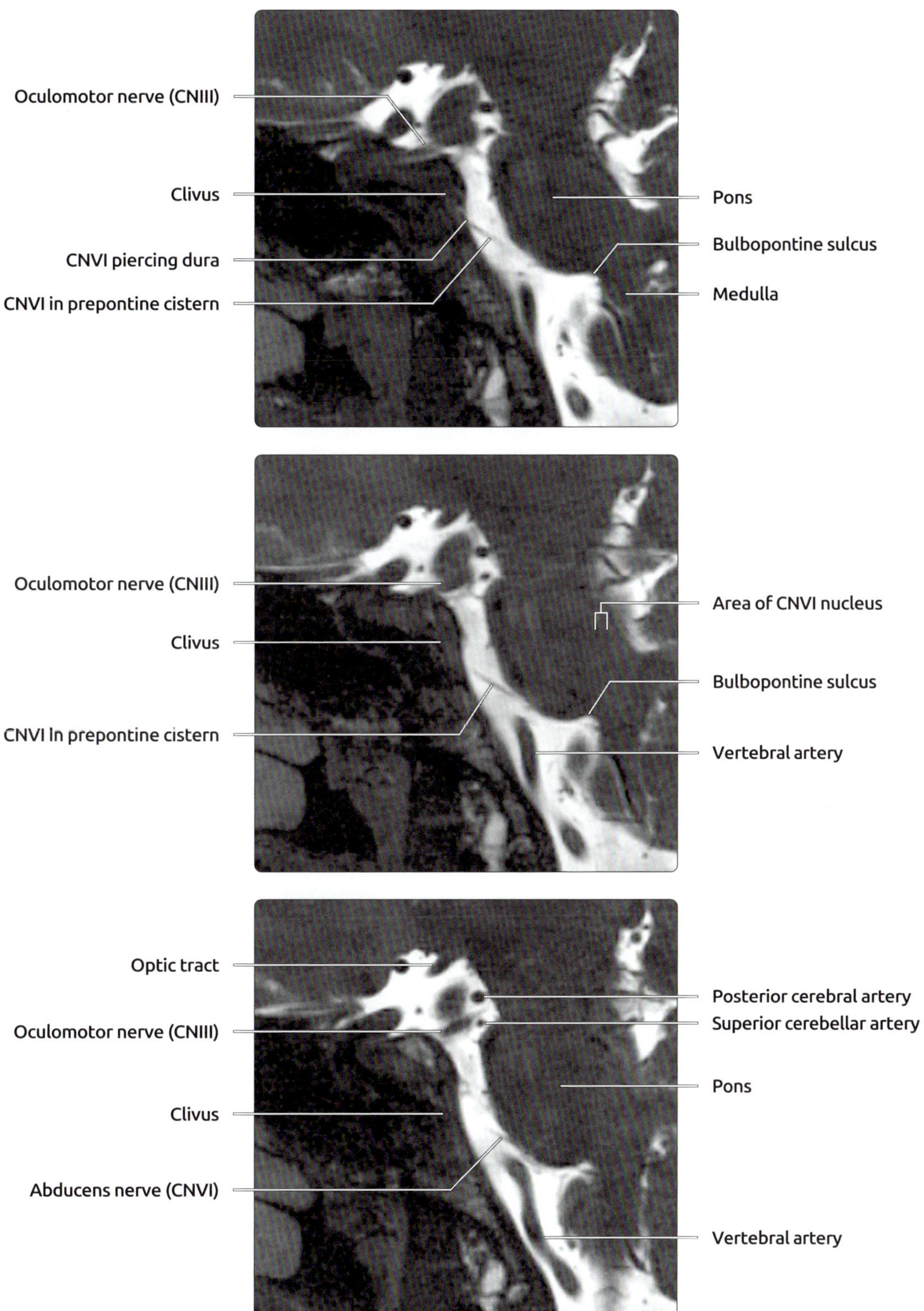

(Top) *First of 3 sagittal T2 MR images presented from lateral to medial reveals the abducens nerve traversing the prepontine cistern toward the clivus. In this image, the abducens nerve is visible penetrating the dura to enter the Dorello canal, which lies between the cranial dura and periosteum surrounded by the basilar venous plexus.* **(Middle)** *Image of the brainstem area shows the abducens nerve coursing anterosuperiorly from its exit point from the brainstem (bulbopontine sulcus) toward its point of dural penetration into the Dorello canal. Notice the approximate location of the CNVI nucleus and the steep course that the intraaxial fibers take to reach the bulbopontine sulcus.* **(Bottom)** *Image of the brainstem and prepontine cisterns shows the proximal cisternal CNVI closely associated with the belly of the pons. CNIII (oculomotor nerve) is seen passing between the posterior cerebral artery (PCA) and superior cerebellar artery (SCA). More laterally in the perimesencephalic cistern, CNIV (trochlear nerve) also passes between the PCA and SCA (not shown).*

TERMINOLOGY

Abbreviations

- Facial nerve (CNVII)

Definitions

- CNVII: Cranial nerve carrying motor nerves to muscles of facial expression; parasympathetics to lacrimal, submandibular, & sublingual glands; and taste from anterior 2/3 of tongue

IMAGING ANATOMY

Overview

- Mixed nerve: Motor, parasympathetic, and special sensory (taste)
- 2 roots: Motor and sensory (nervus intermedius) roots
  - Nervus intermedius exits lateral brainstem between motor root of CNVII and CNVIII, hence its name
- 3 nuclei and 4 segments: Intraaxial, cisternal, intratemporal, and extracranial (parotid)
- Blood supply from petrosal branch of **middle meningeal artery** & stylomastoid branch of **posterior auricular artery**

Nuclei and Intraaxial Segment

- 3 nuclei (1 motor, 2 sensory)
- **Motor nucleus of facial nerve**
  - Located in ventrolateral pontine tegmentum
  - Efferent fibers loop dorsally around CNVI nucleus in floor of 4th ventricle, forming facial colliculus
  - Fibers then course anterolaterally to exit lateral brainstem at pontomedullary junction
- **Superior salivatory nucleus**
  - Located lateral to CNVII motor nucleus in pons
  - Efferent **parasympathetic fibers** exit brainstem posterior to CNVII as nervus intermedius
    - To submandibular, sublingual, and lacrimal glands
- **Solitarius tract nucleus**
  - Taste sensation fibers from anterior 2/3 of tongue
  - **Cell bodies** of these fibers in **geniculate ganglion**
  - Fibers travel within nervus intermedius

Cisternal Segment

- 2 roots in cisternal CNVII
  - Larger motor root anteriorly
  - Smaller sensory nervus intermedius posteriorly
- Emerge from lateral brainstem at **root exit zone** in pontomedullary junction to enter cerebellopontine angle (CPA) cistern
  - CNVIII exits brainstem posterior to CNVII
- 2 roots join together and pass anterolaterally through CPA cistern with CNVIII to internal auditory canal (IAC)

Intratemporal Segment

- Further divided in temporal bone into 4 segments: IAC, labyrinthine, tympanic, & mastoid
- **IAC segment**: Porus acusticus to IAC fundus; anterosuperior position above crista falciformis
- **Labyrinthine segment**: Connects fundal CNVII to geniculate ganglion (anterior genu)
- **Tympanic segment**: Connects anterior to posterior genu, passing under lateral semicircular canal
- **Mastoid segment**: Inferiorly directed from posterior genu to stylomastoid foramen

Extracranial Segment

- Main CNVII exits skull base through **stylomastoid foramen** to enter parotid space
- Parotid CNVII passes lateral to retromandibular vein
- Ramifies within parotid, passes anteriorly to innervate muscles of facial expression

CNVII Branches

- **Greater (superficial) petrosal nerve**
  - Arises at geniculate ganglion, passes anteromedially, exits temporal bone via facial hiatus
  - Carries **parasympathetic** fibers to **lacrimal gland**
  - Joined by deep petrosal nerve (sympathetic fibers) in foramen lacerum to form **vidian nerve**
- **Nerve to stapedius**
  - Arises from high mastoid segment of CNVII behind pyramidal eminence
  - Provides **motor** innervation to **stapedius muscle**
- **Chorda tympani**
  - Arises from lower mastoid segment
  - Courses across middle ear to exit anterior temporal bone
  - Carries **taste** fibers from **anterior 2/3 of tongue**
  - Carries **parasympathetic** fibers to **submandibular & sublingual glands** via submandibular ganglion
- **Terminal motor branches** to muscles of facial expression
  - Superior to inferior: Temporal, zygomatic, buccal, mandibular, cervical

ANATOMY IMAGING ISSUES

Imaging Recommendations

- High-resolution bone CT best for intratemporal CNVII
- MR for intraaxial, cisternal, IAC, and extracranial segments
  - 3D heavily T2 sequence, thin-section axial and coronal T2, precontrast and postcontrast fat-saturated T1
- Include brainstem, CPA cistern, IAC, temporal bone, and **parotid** when MR completed for CNVII palsy
- Do not image typical Bell palsy

Imaging Pitfalls

- Enhancement of geniculate ganglion, tympanic & mastoid segments of CNVII normal on postcontrast T1 MR; can be asymmetric intensity of enhancement on right & left
  - Secondary to circumneural arteriovenous plexus
- Cisternal, IAC, labyrinthine, and parotid segments do not normally enhance on MR
  - Faint enhancement may be seen depending on MR scanner, sequence, & type of contrast used
  - Be familiar with normal images in different institutions
- Always check parotid in peripheral CNVII paralysis

Clinical Issues

- Facial nerve paralysis can be central or peripheral
  - **Central**: Supranuclear injury; paralysis of contralateral muscles of facial expression with **forehead sparing**
  - **Peripheral**: Injury to CNVII from brainstem nucleus peripherally, resulting in paralysis of all ipsilateral muscles of facial expression

GRAPHICS

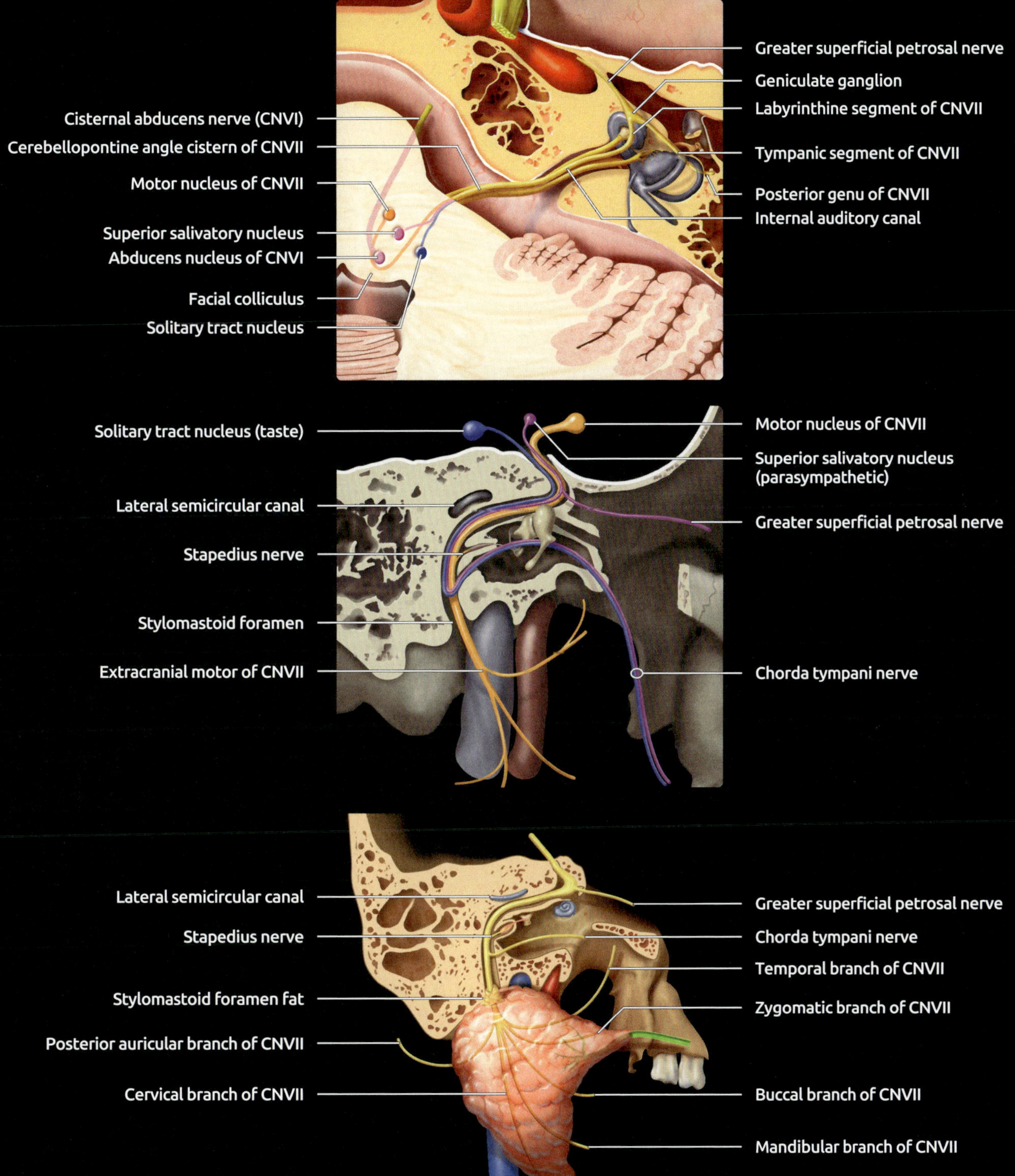

(Top) *Axial graphic shows CNVII nuclei. The motor nucleus sends out its fibers to circle the CNVI nucleus before reaching the root exit zone at the pontomedullary junction. The superior salivatory nucleus sends parasympathetic secretomotor fibers to the lacrimal, submandibular, and sublingual glands. The solitary tract nucleus receives taste information from the anterior 2/3 of the tongue.* **(Middle)** *Sagittal graphic depicts CNVII within the temporal bone. Motor fibers pass through the temporal bone, dropping stapedius nerve to stapedius muscle, then exits via the stylomastoid foramen to the extracranial CNVII (entirely motor). Parasympathetic fibers from the superior salivatory nucleus reach the lacrimal gland via the greater superficial petrosal nerve and the submandibular-sublingual glands via the chorda tympanic nerve. The anterior 2/3 of tongue taste fibers come via the chorda tympani nerve.* **(Bottom)** *Sagittal graphic depicts the extracranial motor branches of CNVII.*

AXIAL BONE CT

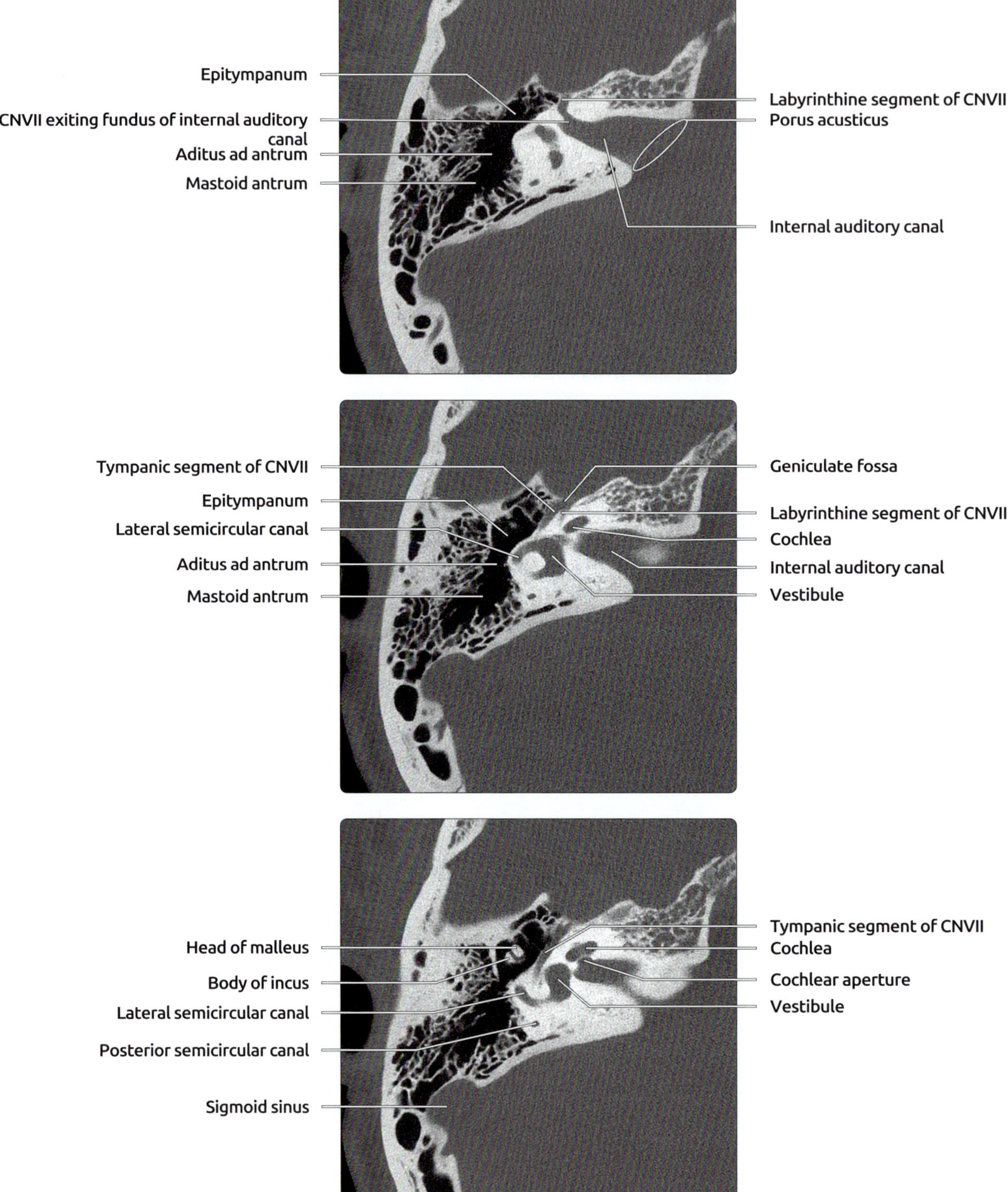

(Top) *First of 5 high-resolution NECT bone window images of the right temporal bone from superior to inferior demonstrates the CNVII canal for the labyrinthine segment coursing anterolaterally from the fundus of the internal auditory canal (IAC) to the geniculate fossa. The labyrinthine segment is the shortest and narrowest segment.* **(Middle)** *This image demonstrates the geniculate fossa, which lodges the geniculate ganglion. The greater (superficial) petrosal nerve (not shown) arises here and travels anteromedially toward the foramen lacerum.* **(Bottom)** *This image demonstrates the tympanic segment of CNVII arising from the geniculate ganglion and traversing posteriorly and laterally to take a 2nd turn downward, forming the posterior genu (not shown).*

AXIAL BONE CT

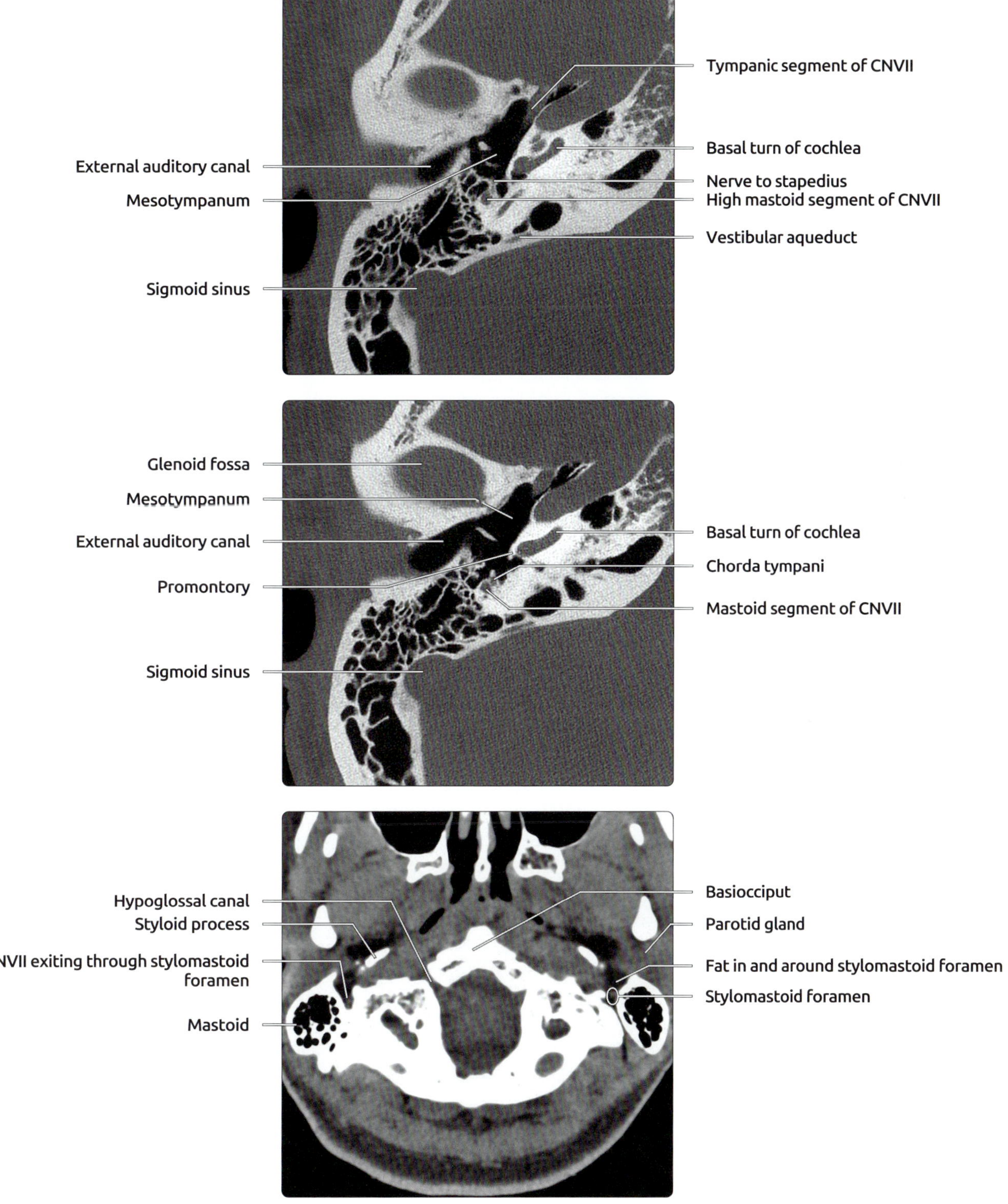

(Top) *This image demonstrates the high mastoid segment of CNVII canal posteriorly, which then descends toward the stylomastoid foramen. Nerve to stapedius arises at this level.* **(Middle)** *This image demonstrates the midmastoid segment of CNVII with adjacent chorda tympani.* **(Bottom)** *Axial soft tissue window NECT through the skull base demonstrates bilateral fat-containing stylomastoid foramen. CNVII exits from bone canal into the parotid space through this foramen.*

CORONAL BONE CT

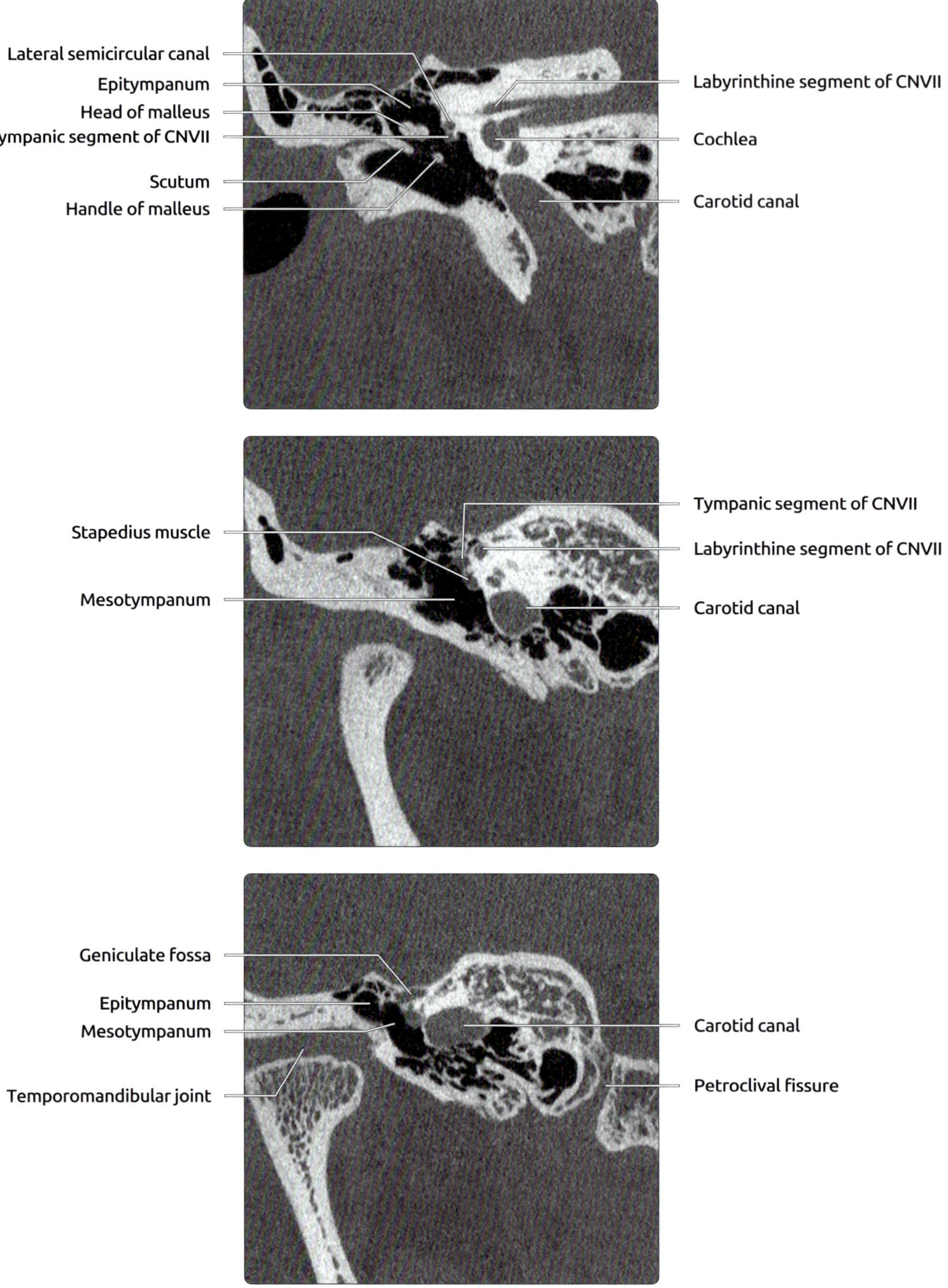

(Top) *First of 6 coronal reformatted high-resolution NECT bone window images show the labyrinthine segment of CNVII canal arising from the superior aspect of the fundus of the IAC.* **(Middle)** *This image shows the snake eye appearance of labyrinthine and tympanic segments coursing adjacent to each other. The labyrinthine segment courses posteriorly toward the geniculate fossa, and the tympanic segment courses anteriorly away from the geniculate fossa.* **(Bottom)** *This image shows the geniculate fossa, which lodges the geniculate ganglion.*

CORONAL BONE CT

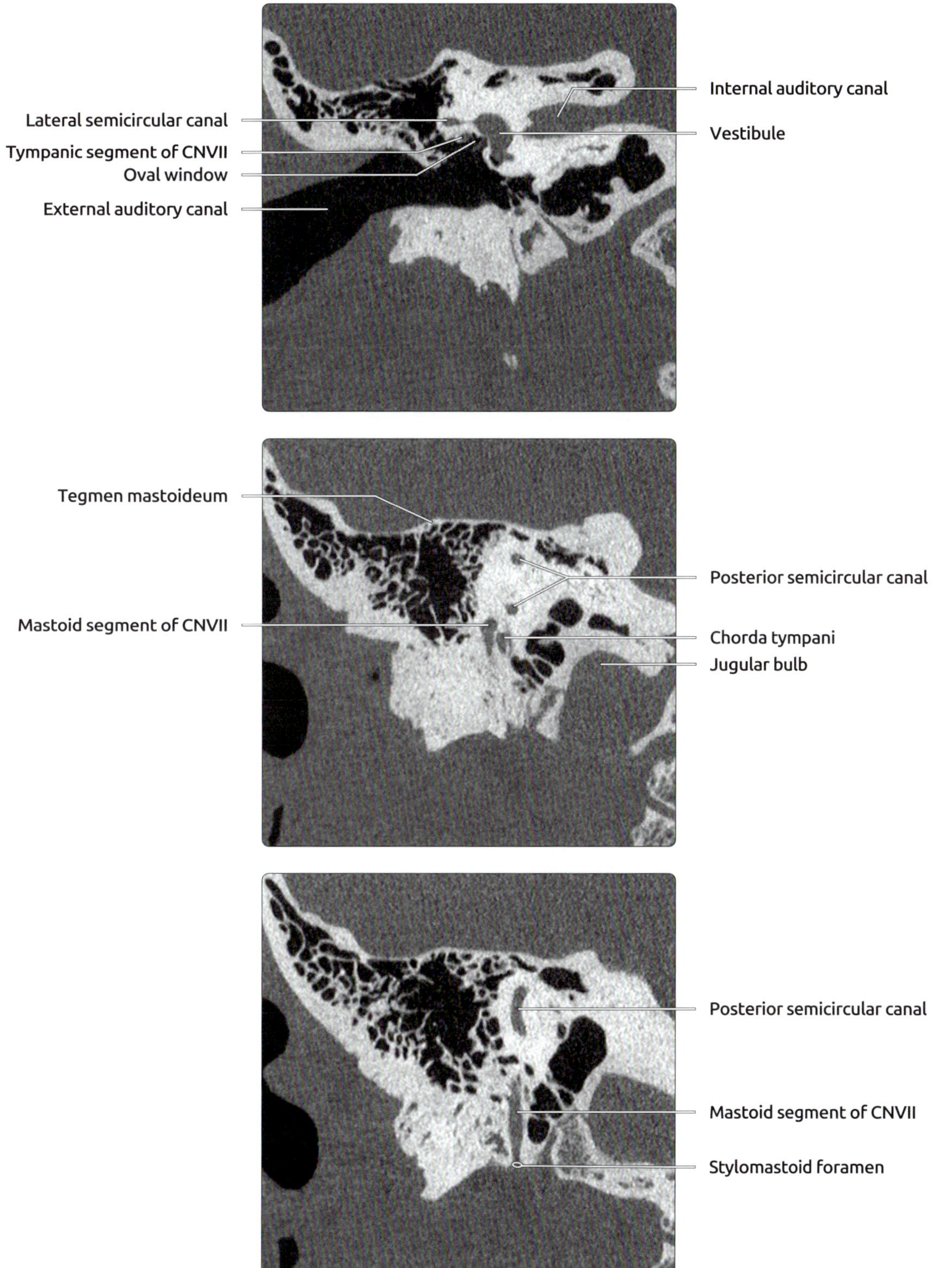

(Top) *This image shows the lateral semicircular canal, the tympanic segment of CNVII canal, and oval window from superior to inferior along the medial wall of the middle ear cavity.* **(Middle)** *This image shows the descending mastoid segment of the CNVII canal. The chorda tympani leaves the CNVII canal 6 mm above the stylomastoid foramen and enters the middle ear cavity through the posterior canaliculus (not shown).* **(Bottom)** *This image shows the distal part of the CNVII mastoid segment exiting through the stylomastoid foramen into the parotid space.*

AXIAL T2 MR

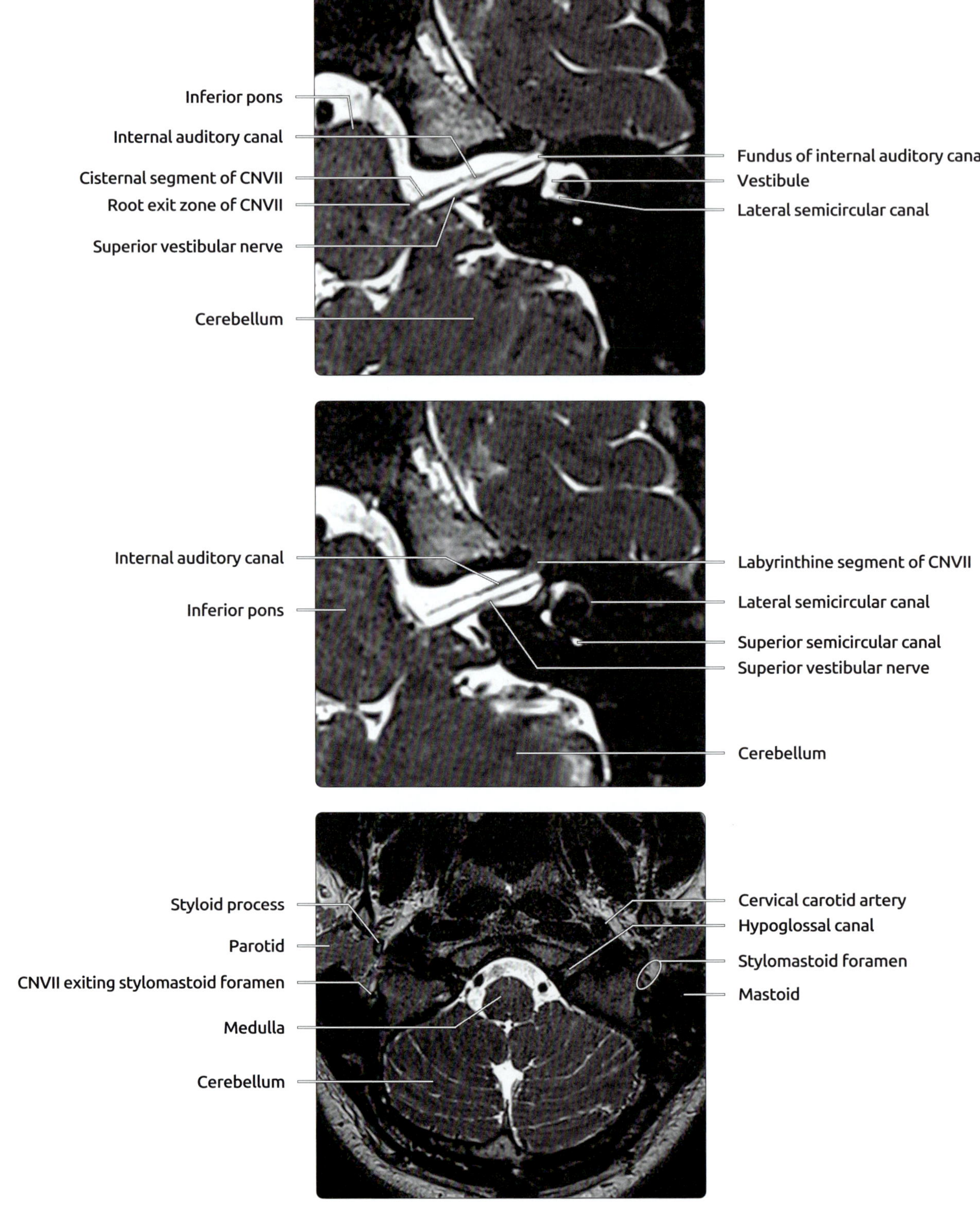

(Top) *First of 2 axial 3D T2 SPACE MR images through the left IAC shows CNVII arising from the lateral pontomedullary junction at the root exit zone. It then traverses the cerebellopontine angle cistern and enters the IAC through the porus acusticus. Note that posterior to it is the superior vestibular nerve.* **(Middle)** *This image shows the IAC and labyrinthine segments of CNVII in the anterosuperior quadrant.* **(Bottom)** *Axial 3D T2 SPACE MR through the skull base at the level of stylomastoid foramina shows bilateral facial nerve mastoid segment exiting the bony canal and entering the parotid space. Note the fat surrounding the facial nerves bilaterally at this level.*

OBLIQUE SAGITTAL T2 MR

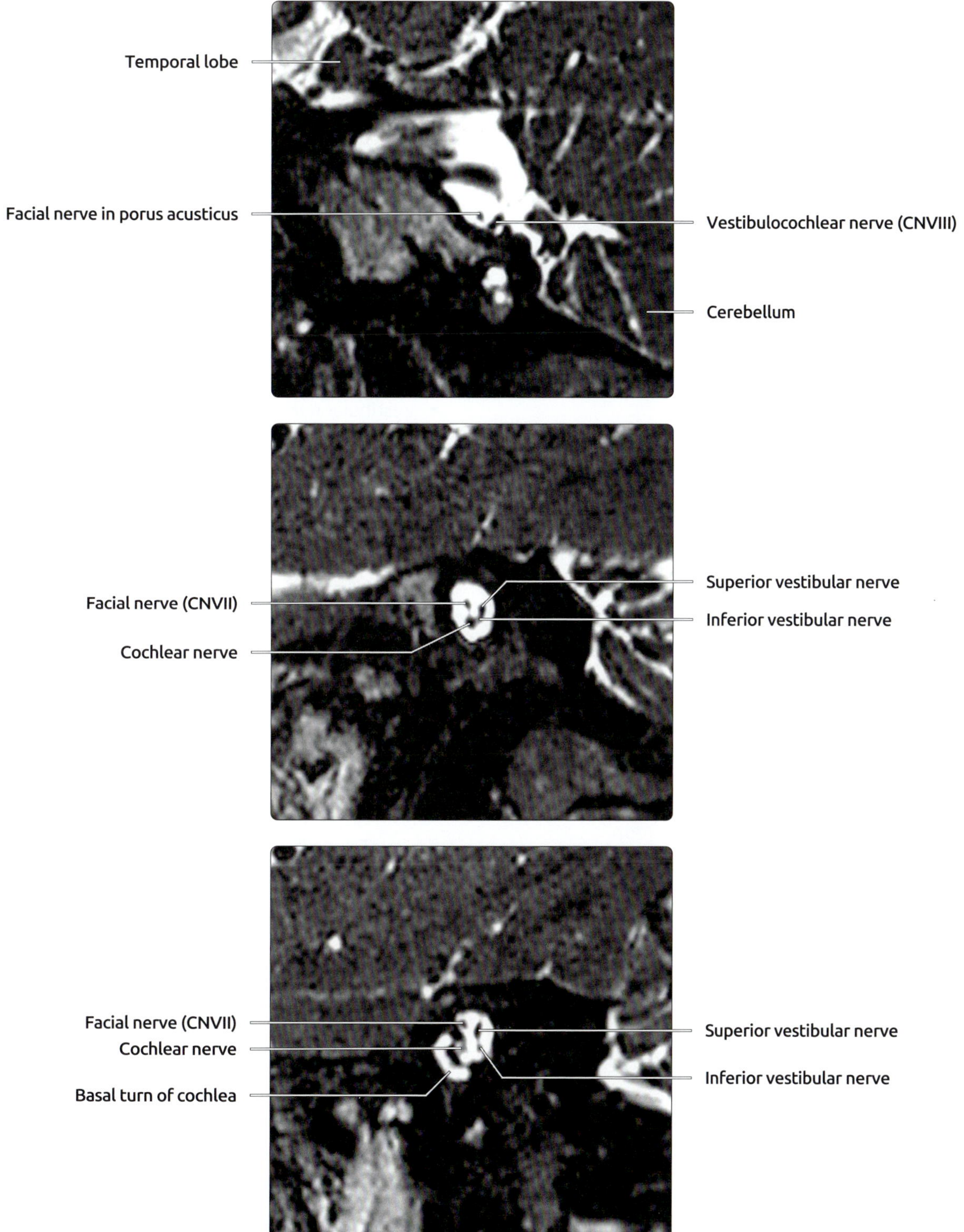

(Top) *First of 3 sagittal oblique MR images of the IAC from medial to lateral is shown. This image through the porus acusticus shows the anteriorly traversing facial nerve trunk, and immediately posterior to it is the vestibulocochlear nerve, both entering the IAC.* **(Middle)** *This image through the middle of the IAC shows the appearance of a ball in the catcher's mitt where the ball is CNVII and the catcher's mitt is formed by the vestibulocochlear nerve complex.* **(Bottom)** *This image through the fundus of the IAC shows CNVII in the anterosuperior quadrant above the crista falciformis. Note the anteroinferiorly located cochlear nerve, posterosuperiorly located superior vestibular nerve, and posteroinferiorly located inferior vestibular nerve.*

TERMINOLOGY

Abbreviations

- Vestibulocochlear nerve (CNVIII)

Synonyms

- 8th cranial nerve, CN8

Definitions

- CNVIII: Afferent sensory nerve of hearing & balance

IMAGING ANATOMY

Overview

- Sensory (special sensory afferent) nerve consisting of 2 parts
  - Vestibular part: Balance
  - Cochlear part: Hearing
- CNVIII best described from peripheral to central

Cochlear Nerve

- Connects organ of Corti to cochlear nuclei & related nuclei of brainstem
- Arises from bipolar neurons located in **spiral ganglion** within modiolus of cochlea
  - Peripheral fibers pass to organ of Corti in cochlear duct (scala media) within cochlea
  - Central fibers coalesce & pass as auditory component of CNVIII (cochlear nerve) to brainstem
- Central fibers pass from modiolus through cochlear aperture into internal auditory canal (IAC)
  - **Cochlear aperture** defined as bony opening into anteroinferior quadrant of fundus of IAC
  - Maximum diameter of cochlear aperture: ~ 2 mm
- **Cochlear nerve** passes from IAC fundus to porus acusticus within **anteroinferior quadrant of IAC**
- Near porus acusticus, cochlear nerve joins together with superior & inferior vestibular nerves to form vestibulocochlear nerve (CNVIII)
- CNVIII crosses cerebellopontine angle (CPA) cistern posterior to facial nerve
- CNVIII enters lateral brainstem at pontomedullary junction posterior to facial nerve
- Cochlear nerve fibers bifurcate, ending in dorsal & ventral cochlear nuclei
- **Dorsal & ventral cochlear nuclei**
  - Cochlear nuclei found on lateral surface of inferior cerebellar peduncle (**restiform body**)

Vestibular Nerve

- Arises from bipolar neurons located in vestibular (**Scarpa**) ganglion located within vestibular nerve in fundal portion of IAC
  - Vestibular ganglion not visible on imaging
  - Peripheral fibers pass to sensory epithelium of utricle, saccule, & semicircular canals
    - Traverse multiple foramina in **macula cribrosa** in lateral wall of IAC fundus
    - Larger superior division supplies ampullary crests in lateral & superior semicircular ducts via **lateral & anterior ampullary nerves**
    - Smaller inferior division supplies remainder of saccule & posterior semicircular canal ampullary crest via **saccular & singular nerves**
  - Central fibers coalesce to form superior & inferior vestibular nerves that pass medially to brainstem
- Fundus of IAC
  - Superior & inferior vestibular nerves are separated by **falciform crest** (transverse crest)
  - Superior vestibular nerve separated from facial nerve anteriorly by vertical bony structure called **Bill bar**
- Superior & inferior vestibular nerves pass medially from IAC fundus to porus acusticus within posterosuperior & posteroinferior quadrants of IAC
- Near porus acusticus, superior & inferior vestibular nerves join together with cochlear nerve to form vestibulocochlear nerve (CNVIII)
- Vestibular nerve fibers divide into ascending & descending branches, which mainly terminate in vestibular nuclear complex
- **Vestibular nuclear complex**
  - 4 nuclei (lateral, superior, medial, & inferior)
  - Located beneath lateral recess along floor of 4th ventricle (rhomboid fossa) in lower pons
  - Complex connections exist between vestibular nuclei, cerebellum, spinal cord (vestibulospinal tract), & nuclei controlling eye movement through medial longitudinal fasciculus (MLF)

ANATOMY IMAGING ISSUES

Imaging Recommendations

- Sensorineural hearing loss (SNHL)
  - **Intracochlear lesion suspected**
    - CT & MR imaging complimentary to each other
    - Congenital lesions of membranous labyrinth seen as abnormalities of fluid spaces on MR or in bony labyrinth shape on T-bone CT
    - T-bone CT better for otosclerosis, Paget disease, labyrinthine ossificans, or if trauma suspected
    - Only MR will demonstrate labyrinthitis or intralabyrinthine tumor
  - **CNVIII lesion suspected (CPA-IAC)**
    - MR imaging method of choice
    - Thin-section high-resolution T2 sequence in axial & coronal planes may be used to screen patients with unilateral SNHL
    - T1 C+ MR remains gold standard

Imaging Sweet Spots

- Unilateral SNHL
  - Focus on brainstem (inferior cerebellar peduncle)-CPA-IAC-cochlea
  - Central acoustic pathway (intraaxial pathways above cochlear nuclei) rarely site of offending lesion
- Cisternal & IAC segments of CNVIII routinely visualized on high-resolution T2 MR

Imaging Pitfalls

- Beware small lesions of IAC (≤ 2 mm)
  - Follow-up imaging recommended, as may be transient finding where surgery not needed

GRAPHICS

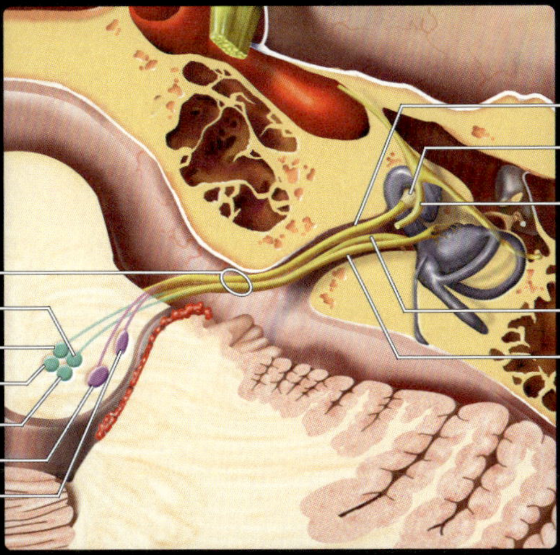

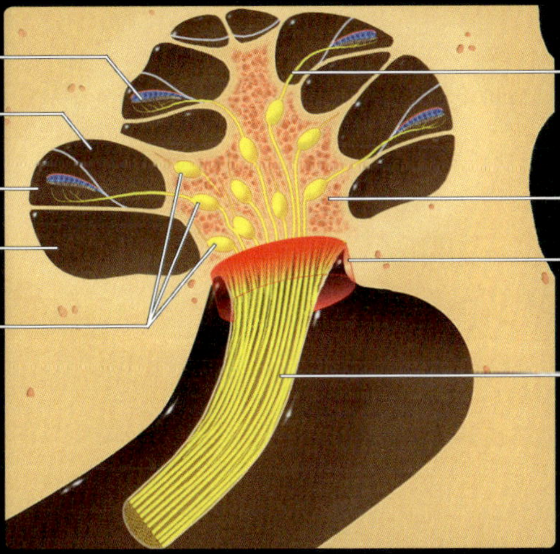

Cochlear nerve
Cochlear modiolus
Facial nerve, labyrinthine segment
Vestibulocochlear nerve (CNVIII)
Inferior vestibular nucleus
Superior vestibular nucleus
Medial vestibular nucleus
Lateral vestibular nucleus
Dorsal cochlear nucleus
Ventral cochlear nucleus
Inferior vestibular nerve
Superior vestibular nerve

Organ of Corti
Scala vestibuli
Scala media
Scala tympani
Spiral ganglia
Distal axon from spiral ganglia
Modiolus
Cochlear aperture (cochlear foramen)
Cochlear nerve

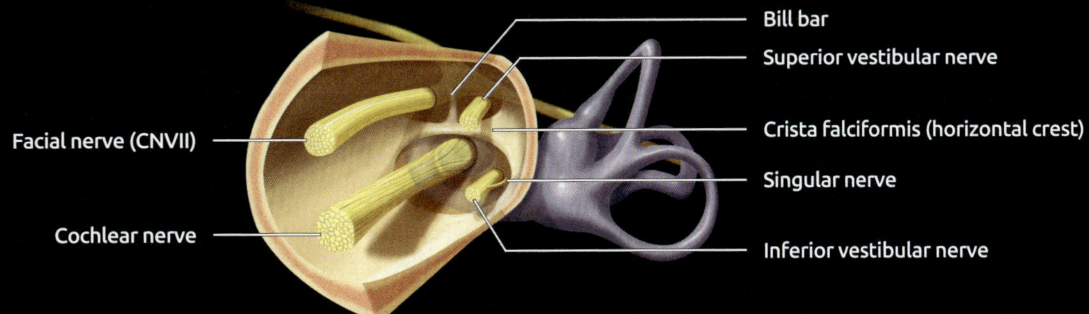

(Top) *Axial graphic of the cerebellopontine angle (CPA), internal auditory canal (IAC), & inner ear is shown. Cochlear component of CNVIII begins in bipolar cell bodies in spiral ganglion of cochlear modiolus. Central fibers run in the cochlear nerve to dorsal & ventral cochlear nuclei in the inferior cerebellar peduncle. The inferior & superior vestibular nerves begin in cell bodies in the vestibular ganglion &, from there, course centrally to 4 vestibular nuclei.* **(Middle)** *Axial graphic of the magnified cochlea, modiolus, & cochlear nerve is shown. Notice the bipolar spiral ganglion cells within modiolus contribute distal fibers to the organ of Corti as well as proximal axons that constitute the cochlear nerve.* **(Bottom)** *Graphic depicting the fundus of the IAC is shown. Notice the crista falciformis separates the cochlear nerve & inferior vestibular nerve below from CNVII & superior vestibular nerve above. Also note the Bill bar separating CNVII from the superior vestibular nerve.*

AXIAL BONE CT

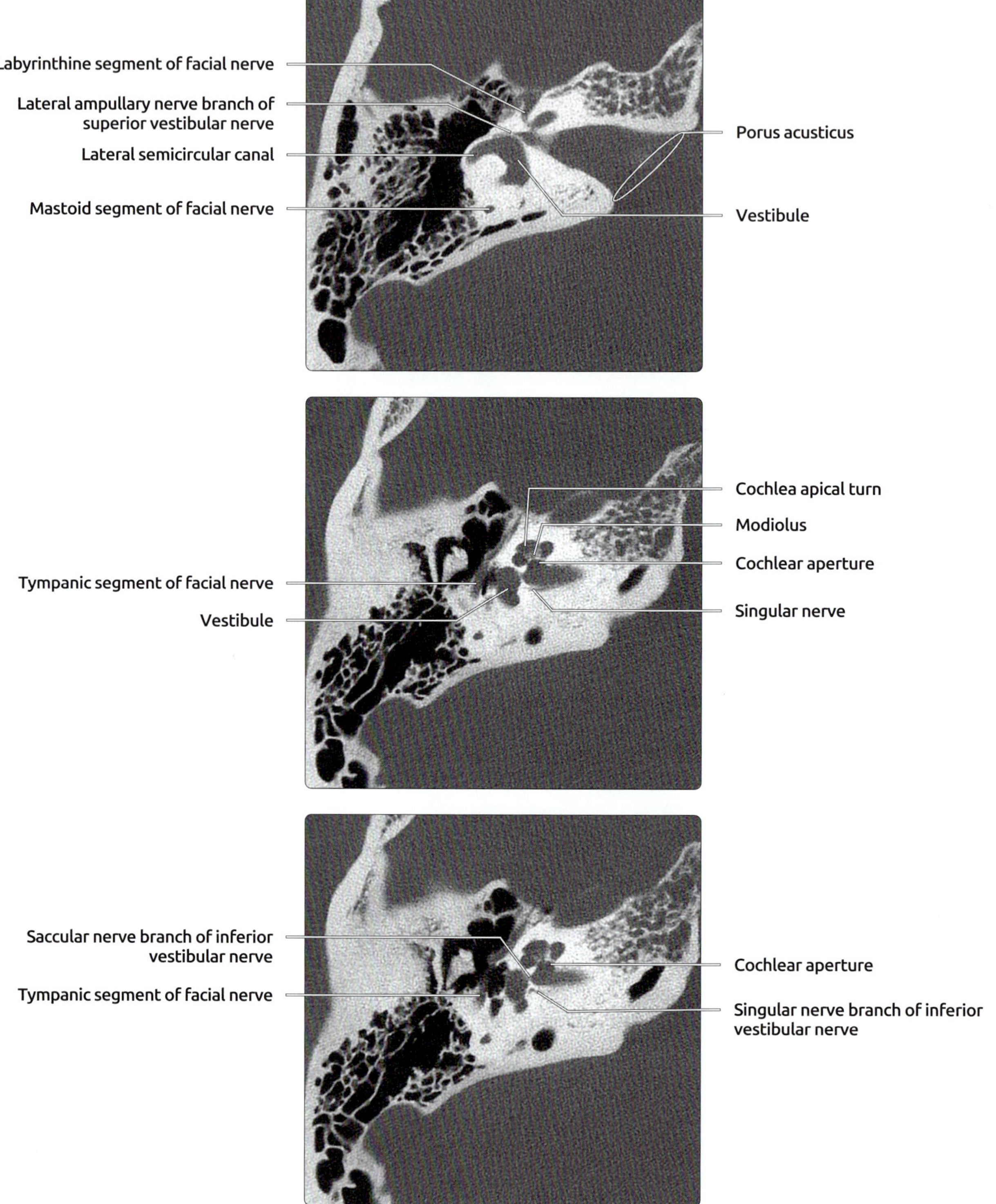

(Top) *First of 3 axial high-resolution NECT bone window images of the right temporal bone shows the lateral ampullary nerve, which is a branch of the superior vestibular nerve & supplies the ampullary crest in the lateral semicircular canal. The other branch is the anterior ampullary nerve (not shown), which supplies the anterior (superior) semicircular canal ampullary crest.* **(Middle)** *This image shows a singulare nerve, which is a branch of the inferior vestibular nerve & supplies the posterior ampullary crest. Also note modiolus in the cochlea, which contains spiral ganglia. The peripheral fibers of the spiral ganglia connect to the organ of Corti, & the central fibers pass through the cochlear aperture & coalesce to form the cochlear nerve, which connects to the brainstem dorsal & ventral cochlear nuclei.* **(Bottom)** *This image shows another branch of the inferior vestibular nerve, the saccular nerve, which supplies the saccule. Also note the singular canal with a singular nerve & the cochlear aperture.*

AXIAL T2 MR

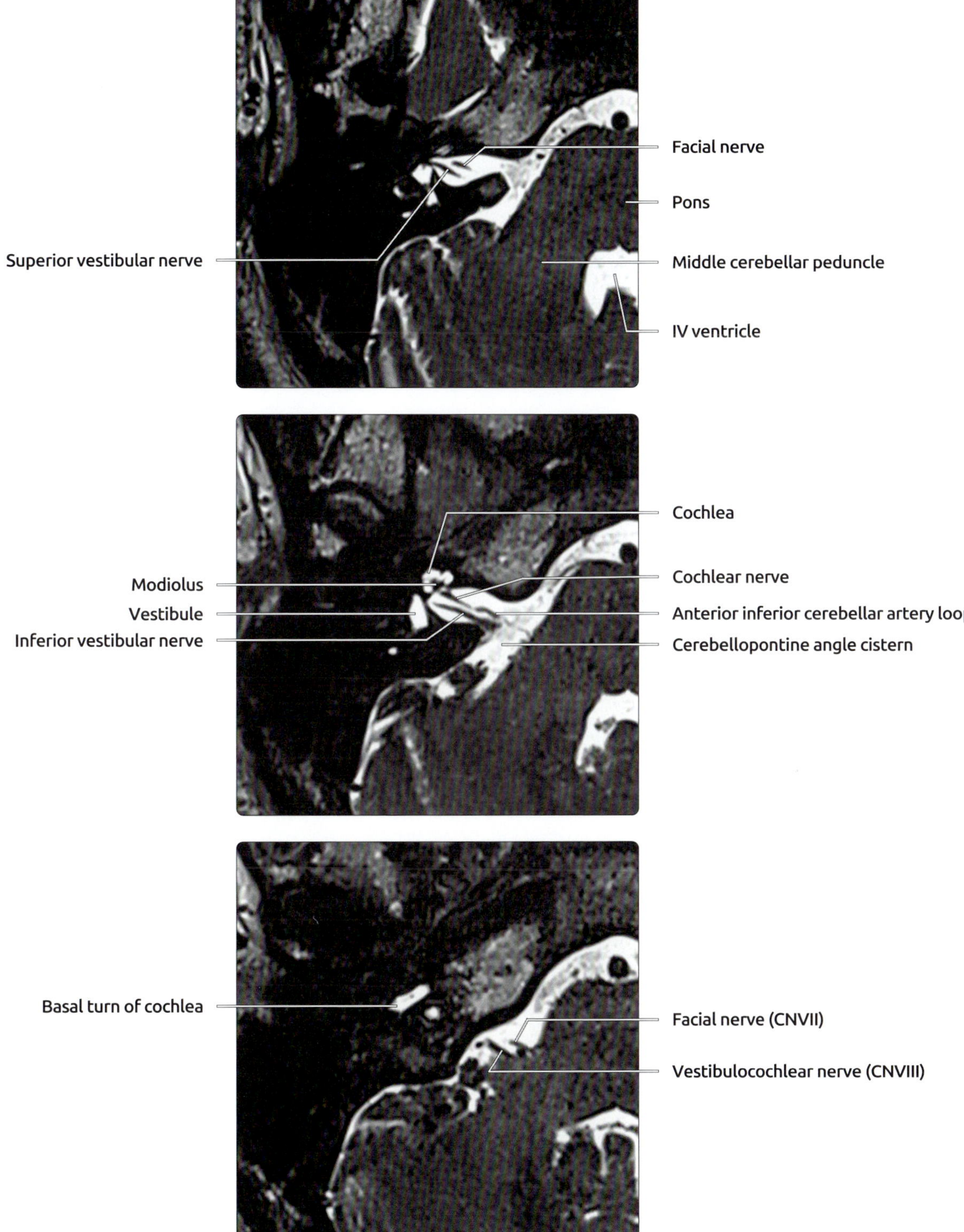

(Top) *First of 3 T2 SPACE 3D axial images through the superior aspect of the right IAC shows the facial nerve located anteriorly & the superior vestibular nerve located posteriorly.* **(Middle)** *This image through the inferior aspect of the IAC shows the anteriorly located cochlear nerve exiting through the cochlear aperture. The modiolus appears dark on the T2-weighted image, which contains the spiral ganglion. Posteriorly, the inferior vestibular nerve & a loop of the anteroinferior cerebellar artery in the medial aspect of the canal are also depicted.* **(Bottom)** *This image shows the CPA cisternal segment of facial nerve anteriorly & CPA cisternal segment of vestibulocochlear nerve posteriorly; they enter the brainstem at the lateral pontomedullary junction.*

CORONAL T2 MR

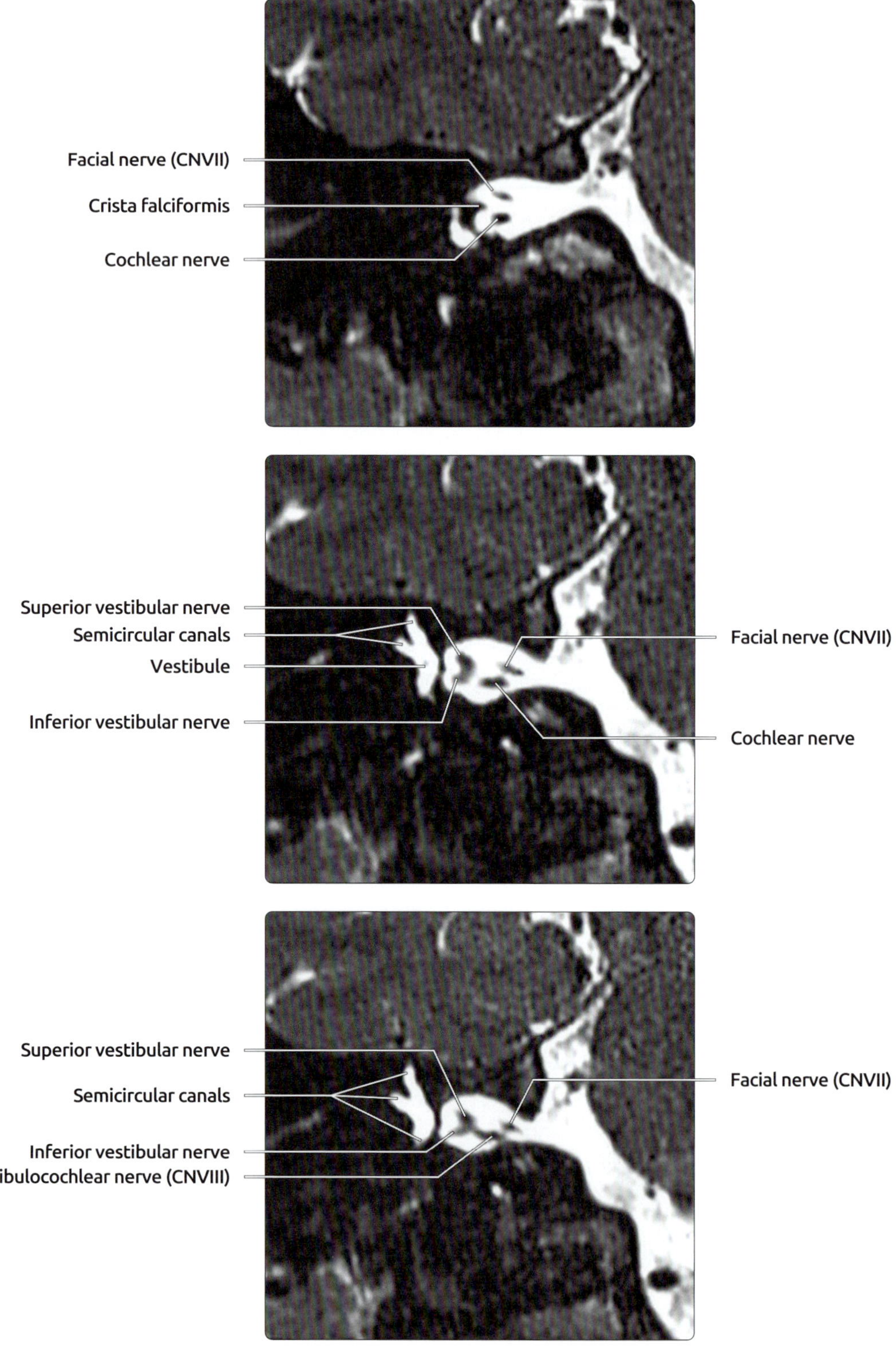

(Top) *First of 3 coronal T2 SPACE MR reformatted images of the right temporal bone through the anterior aspect of the IAC shows the superior facial nerve and the inferior cochlear nerve in the fundus region. Note a small bone projection, the crista falciformis, which separates the IAC into the superior and inferior halves at the fundus. These are further divided into 4 quadrants by a vertically oriented Bill bar.* **(Middle)** *This image through the middle of the IAC shows all 4 nerves, including the superior & inferior vestibular nerves & facial & cochlear nerves.* **(Bottom)** *This image through the posterior aspect of the canal shows convergence of the cochlear, superior, & inferior vestibular nerves, which form a common trunk of the vestibulocochlear nerve at the porus acusticus. The facial nerve is seen anterior & superior to the vestibulocochlear nerve at the porus acusticus.*

OBLIQUE SAGITTAL T2 MR

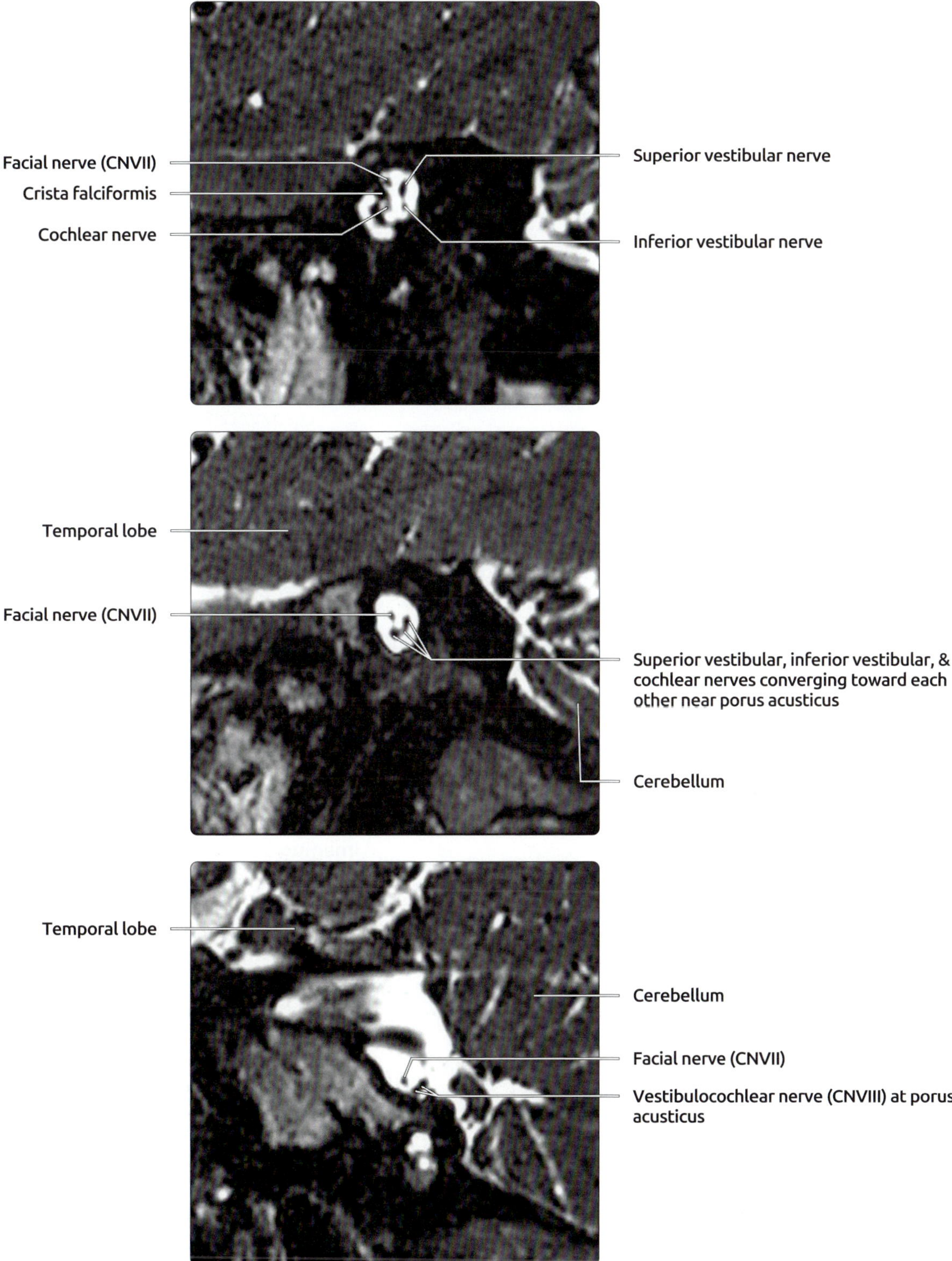

(Top) *First of 3 sagittal oblique T2 SPACE 3D reformatted images of the temporal bone through the fundus of the IAC shows all 4 nerves, including anterosuperiorly located facial nerve, anteroinferiorly located cochlear nerve, posterosuperiorly located superior vestibular nerve, & posteroinferiorly located inferior vestibular nerve. Note that the crista falciformis divides the canal into superior and inferior halves. The anterior and posterior division is by the Bill bar (not seen on imaging).* **(Middle)** *This image through the mid-IAC shows the convergence of the cochlear, superior, & inferior vestibular nerves forming the appearance of a catcher's mitt with the facial nerve as the ball in it.* **(Bottom)** *This image at the porus acusticus shows the vestibulocochlear nerve posterior and inferior to the facial nerve.*

CNIX (Glossopharyngeal Nerve)

TERMINOLOGY

Abbreviations

- Glossopharyngeal nerve (CNIX)

Synonyms

- 9th cranial nerve, CN9

Definitions

- Mixed nerve with complex functions
  - Taste & sensation to posterior 1/3 of tongue
  - Sensory nerve to middle ear & pharynx
  - Parasympathetic to parotid gland
  - Motor to stylopharyngeus muscle
  - Viscerosensory to carotid body & sinus

IMAGING ANATOMY

Overview

- 4 segments: Intraaxial, cisternal, skull base, & extracranial

Intraaxial Segment

- Glossopharyngeal nuclei in upper & middle medulla
  - **Motor fibers** to stylopharyngeus muscle from **nucleus ambiguus**
  - **Sensory fibers** from tympanic membrane, soft palate, tongue base, & pharynx terminate in **spinal nucleus CNV**
  - **Taste fibers** from posterior 1/3 of tongue terminate in **solitary tract nucleus**
  - **Parasympathetic fibers** to parotid gland originate in **inferior salivatory nucleus**

Cisternal Segment

- Exits lateral medulla in **postolivary sulcus** as 3-5 rootlets uniting to form cisternal segment just above vagus nerve
- Mean length from medulla to jugular foramen: ~ 14-18 mm
- Transition zone (TZ) located ~ 1.1-1.8 mm from medulla or root entry/exit zone (REZ)
  - TZ: Area between central & peripheral myelin with increased vulnerability to mechanical irritation & relevant in neurovascular compression
  - REZ: Portion of nerve, including TZ, central myelin root portion, & adjacent brainstem surface
  - Glossopharyngeal neuralgia caused by neurovascular compression: 95% in proximal REZ, overlapping proximal location of TZ
- Travels anterolaterally through basal cistern with vagus nerve & bulbar portion of accessory nerve
- Passes through glossopharyngeal meatus into **pars nervosa** portion of **jugular foramen**

Skull Base Segment

- Passes through anterior **pars nervosa**
  - Accompanied by inferior petrosal sinus
  - CNX & CNXI posteriorly within pars vascularis portion of jugular foramen
  - Superior & inferior sensory ganglia of CNIX found within jugular foramen

Extracranial Segment

- Exits into anterior **nasopharyngeal carotid space**
- Passes lateral to internal carotid artery, innervates stylopharyngeus, & contributes to carotid sinus nerve
- Gives branches to pharyngeal plexus & terminates as tonsillar & lingual branches

Extracranial Branches

- **Tympanic branch (Jacobson nerve)**
  - Sensation from middle ear & parasympathetic to parotid gland via lesser petrosal nerve & otic ganglion
  - Arises from inferior sensory ganglion in jugular foramen
  - Via **inferior tympanic canaliculus** to hypotympanum
    - Aberrant internal carotid artery enters via this canal
  - Forms tympanic plexus on cochlear promontory
    - Associated glomus bodies form glomus tympanicum paraganglioma
- **Stylopharyngeus branch**
  - Motor to stylopharyngeus muscle; arises from CNIX between stylopharyngeus & styloglossus muscles
- **Carotid sinus nerve**
  - Supplies viscerosensory fibers to carotid sinus & body
  - Conducts impulses from mechanoreceptors of sinus & chemoreceptors of carotid body to medulla
- **Pharyngeal branches**
  - Sensory input from posterior oropharynx & soft palate (pharyngeal plexus)
- **Lingual branch**
  - Sensory input & taste from posterior 1/3 of tongue

ANATOMY IMAGING ISSUES

Imaging Recommendations

- MR imaging method of choice
  - Superior sensitivity for skull base, meningeal, cisternal, & brainstem pathology
  - T2 (including 3D high-resolution, heavily T2-weighted), T1 without fat saturation, & contrast-enhanced T1 sequences with fat saturation in axial & coronal planes
- Supplemental bone CT for complex skull base pathology

Imaging Sweet Spots

- Image from pontomedullary junction to hyoid bone
- CNIX nuclei & intraaxial segment not directly visualized
  - Position inferred by identifying upper medulla, posterior to postolivary sulcus
  - Cisternal segment not always visualized on routine MR
    - High-resolution thin-section T2 sequences often identify cisternal segments of CNIX-XI nerve complex
    - Bone algorithm CT for bony anatomy of pars nervosa
- Extracranial segment not visualized

Imaging Pitfalls

- Remember to image entire extracranial course of CNIX beyond skull base

CLINICAL IMPLICATIONS

Clinical Importance

- Complex CNIX-XI neuropathies (Vernet syndrome) caused by disease in medulla, basal cistern, jugular foramen, or nasopharyngeal carotid space
  - Isolated CNIX neuropathy exceedingly rare
- Glossopharyngeal neuralgia mostly from compression by PICA > vertebral > AICA; minority from trauma, neoplasm, infection, multiple sclerosis, or elongated styloid process (Eagle syndrome)

GRAPHICS

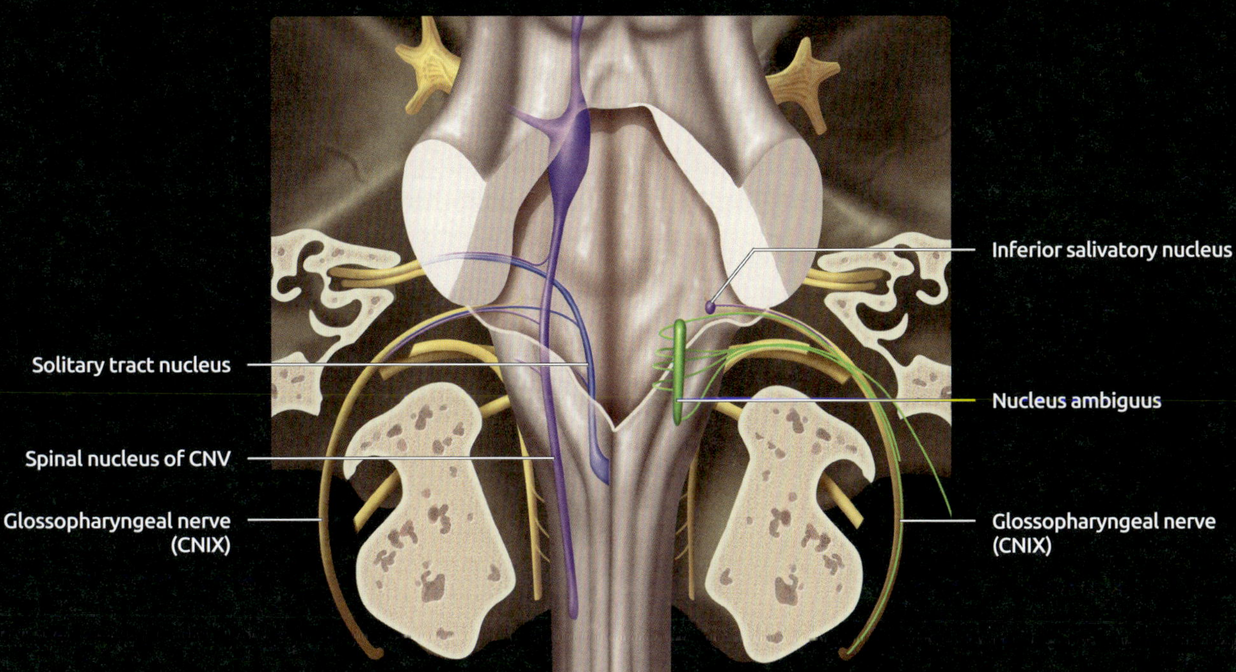

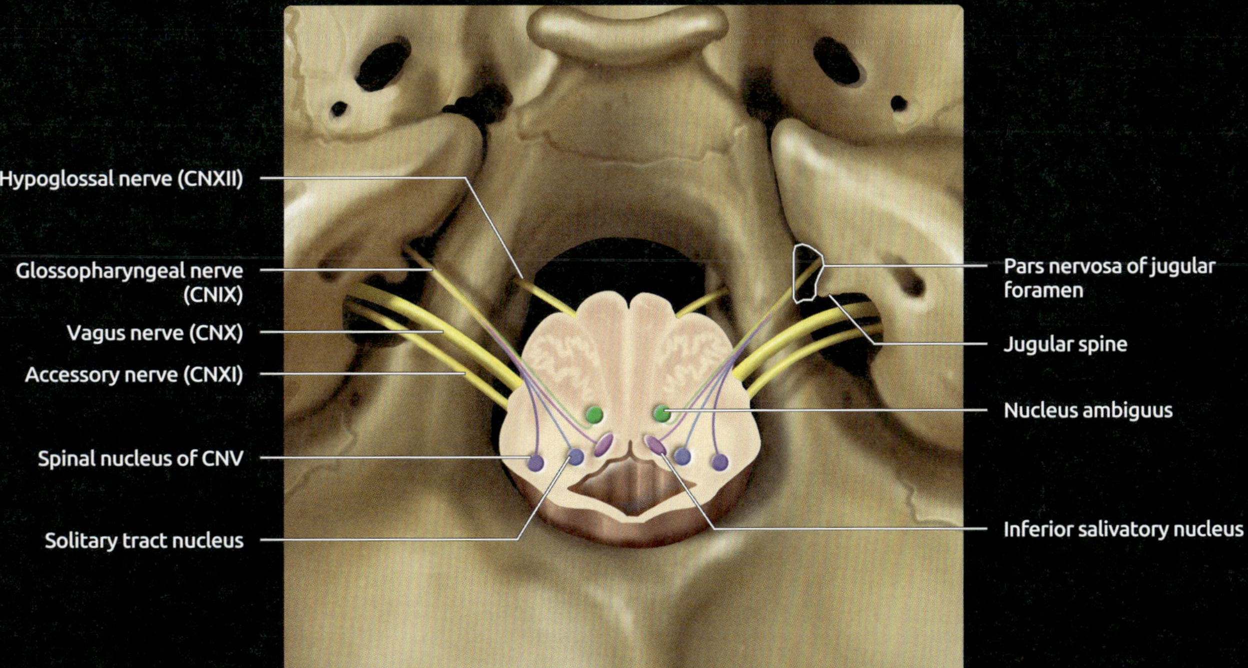

(Top) *Posterior view of the brainstem emphasizes the 4 nuclei participating in the functions of the glossopharyngeal nerve. Notice the 2 efferent nuclei, the nucleus ambiguus and inferior salivatory nucleus labeled on the right. The nucleus ambiguus supplies motor fibers to the stylopharyngeus muscle, while the inferior salivatory nucleus supplies parasympathetic fibers to the parotid gland. On the left, the afferent nuclei are the solitary tract nucleus and the spinal nucleus of CNV. The solitary tract nucleus receives taste fibers from the tongue base, while the spinal nucleus of CNV receives sensation from the middle ear, soft palate, tongue base, and pharynx.* **(Bottom)** *Axial graphic through the medullary brainstem from above shows the 4 nuclei of the glossopharyngeal nerve.*

GRAPHIC, EXTRACRANIAL

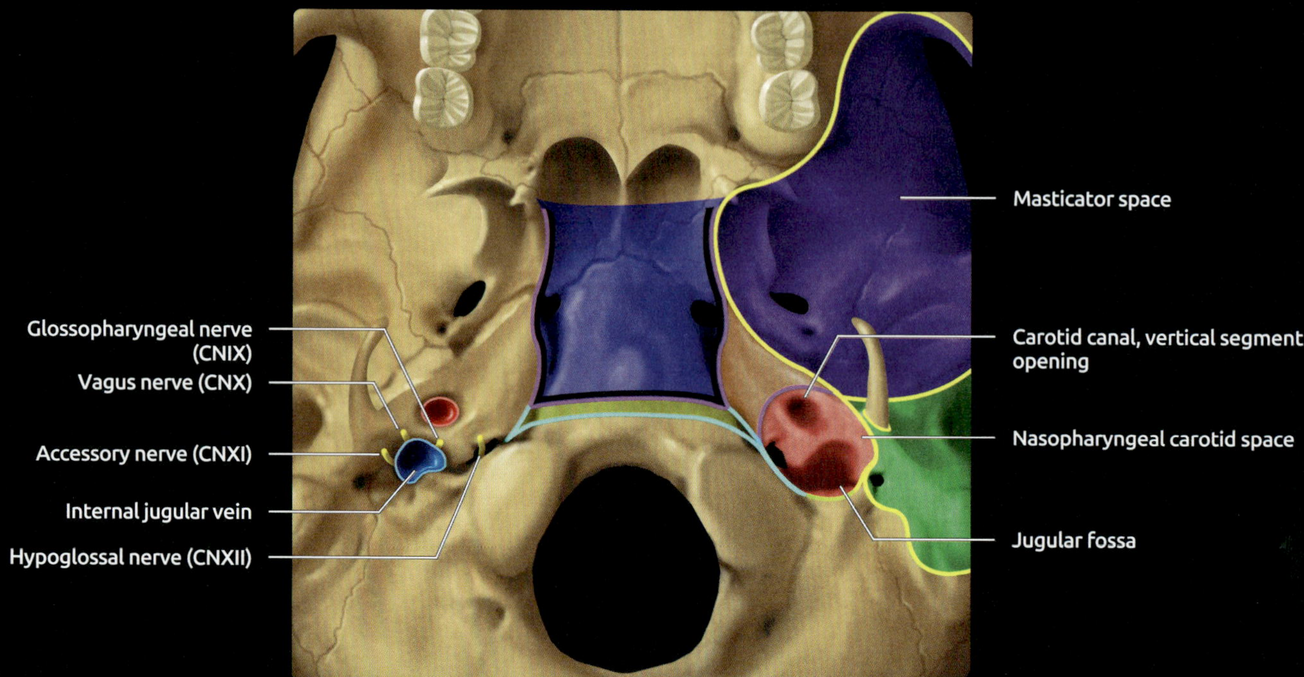

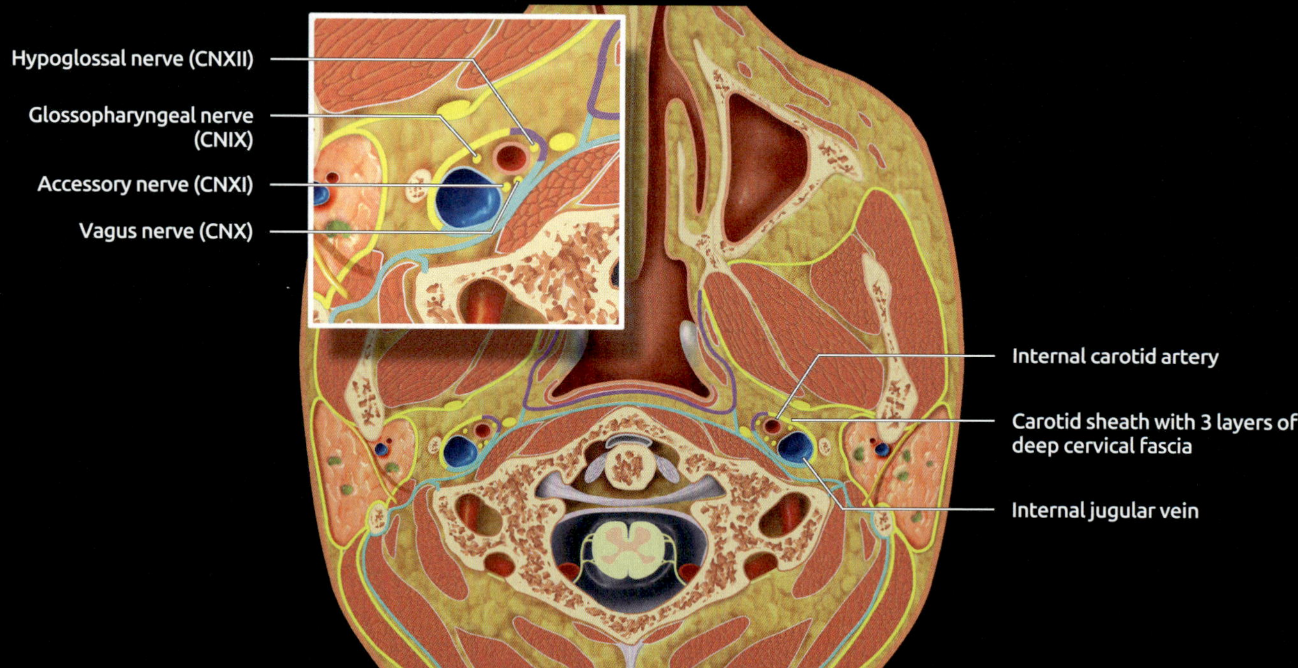

(Top) *Graphic of the skull base viewed from below depicts the 4 cranial nerves emerging into the nasopharyngeal carotid space. The glossopharyngeal nerve is just anteromedial to the internal jugular vein as it exits the pars nervosa of the jugular foramen.* **(Bottom)** *Axial graphic of nasopharyngeal carotid spaces shows the extracranial glossopharyngeal nerve situated anteriorly in the gap between the internal carotid artery and the internal jugular vein. Notice that at this level, CNX, CNXI, and CNXII are all still within the carotid space. The glossopharyngeal nerve exits the carotid space at the level of the high oropharynx.*

GRAPHIC, EXTRACRANIAL

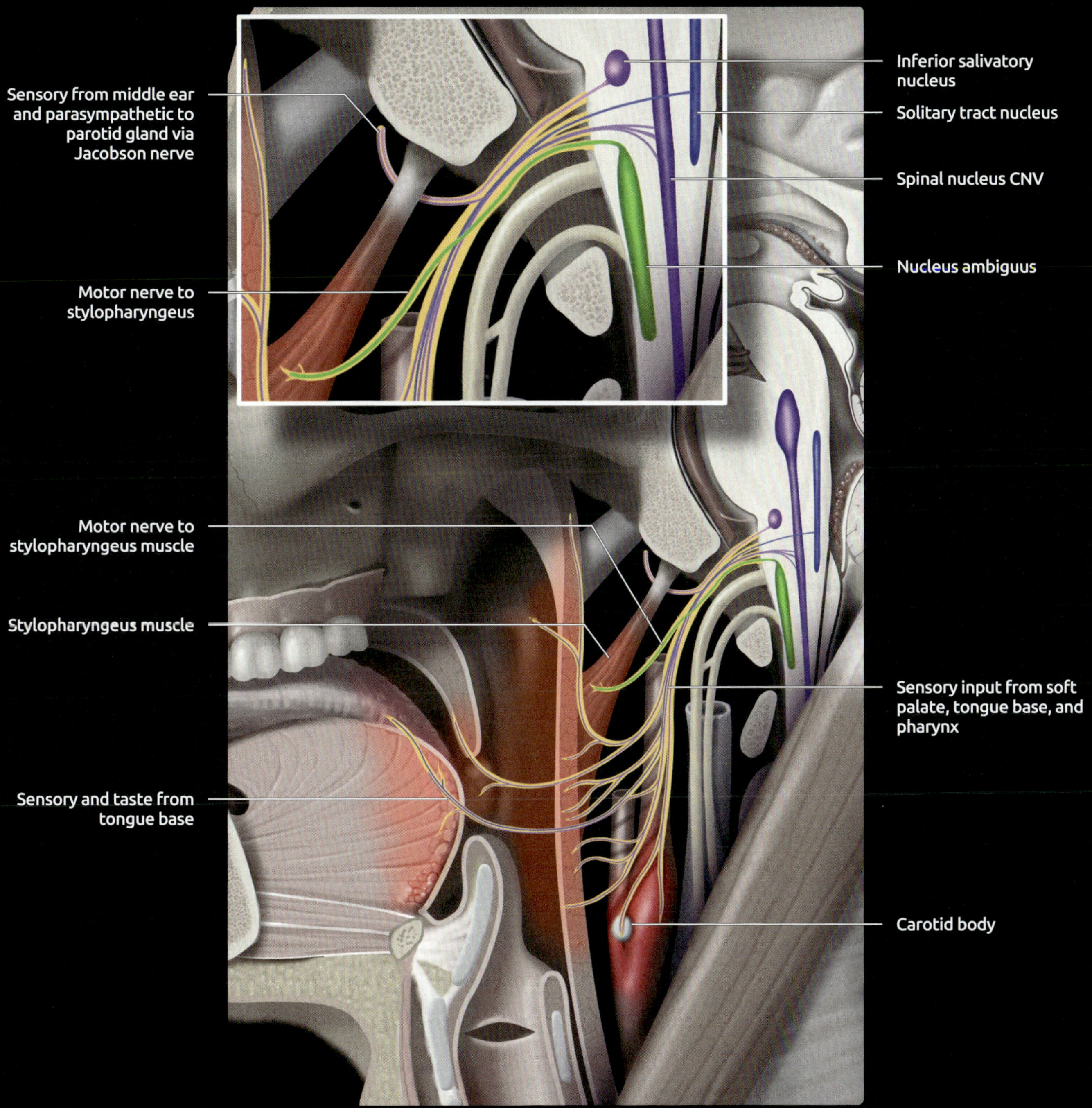

Sagittal graphic emphasizing the extracranial component of the glossopharyngeal nerve (CNIX) is shown. Only 1 muscle is innervated by the fibers in CNIX from the nucleus ambiguus, the stylopharyngeus. Sensory information from the middle ear, tongue base, soft palate, and oropharyngeal surface are transmitted via CNIX to the spinal nucleus of the trigeminal nerve. Taste sensation from the tongue base travels via CNIX to the solitary tract nucleus. Parasympathetic secretomotor fibers from the inferior salivatory nucleus bound for the parotid gland also travel in CNIX.

AXIAL BONE CT

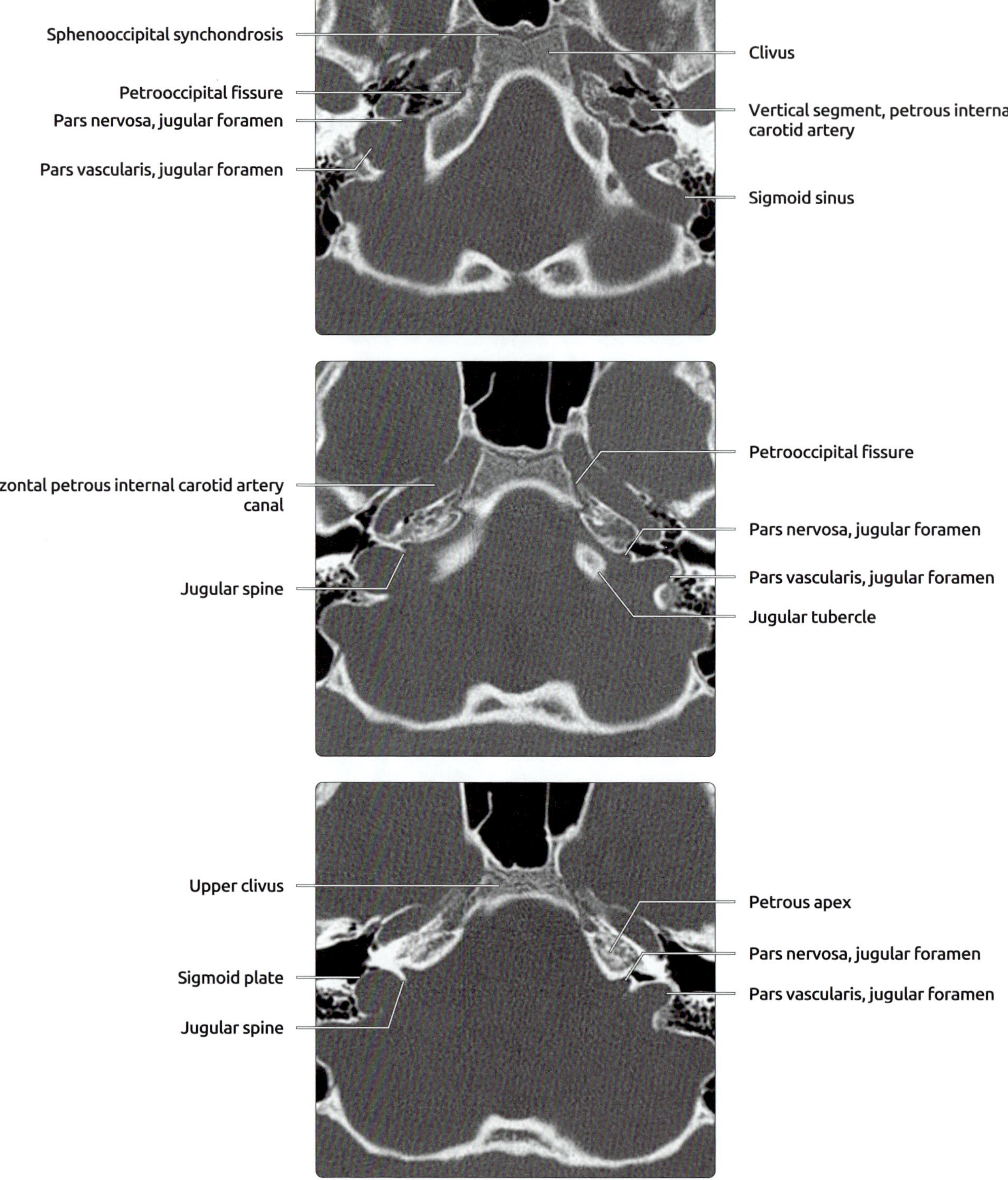

(Top) *First of 3 axial bone CT images presented from inferior to superior through the posterior skull base emphasizes the bony anatomy of the jugular foramen. The jugular foramen is located on the floor of the posterior cranial fossa between the petrous temporal bone anterolaterally and occipital bone posteromedially; therefore, it is a venous channel between these bones.* **(Middle)** *The jugular foramen is seen here as 2 discrete pieces, the smaller anteromedial pars nervosa and larger posterolateral pars vascularis, separated by the jugular spine of the petrous bone.* **(Bottom)** *The 2 parts of the jugular foramen are visibile. The pars nervosa transmits the glossopharyngeal nerve (CNIX), Jacobson nerve, and inferior petrosal sinus. The pars vascularis transmits the vagus (CNX) and accessory (CNXI) cranial nerves, Arnold nerve, and sigmoid sinus, which becomes the internal jugular vein.*

AXIAL T2 MR

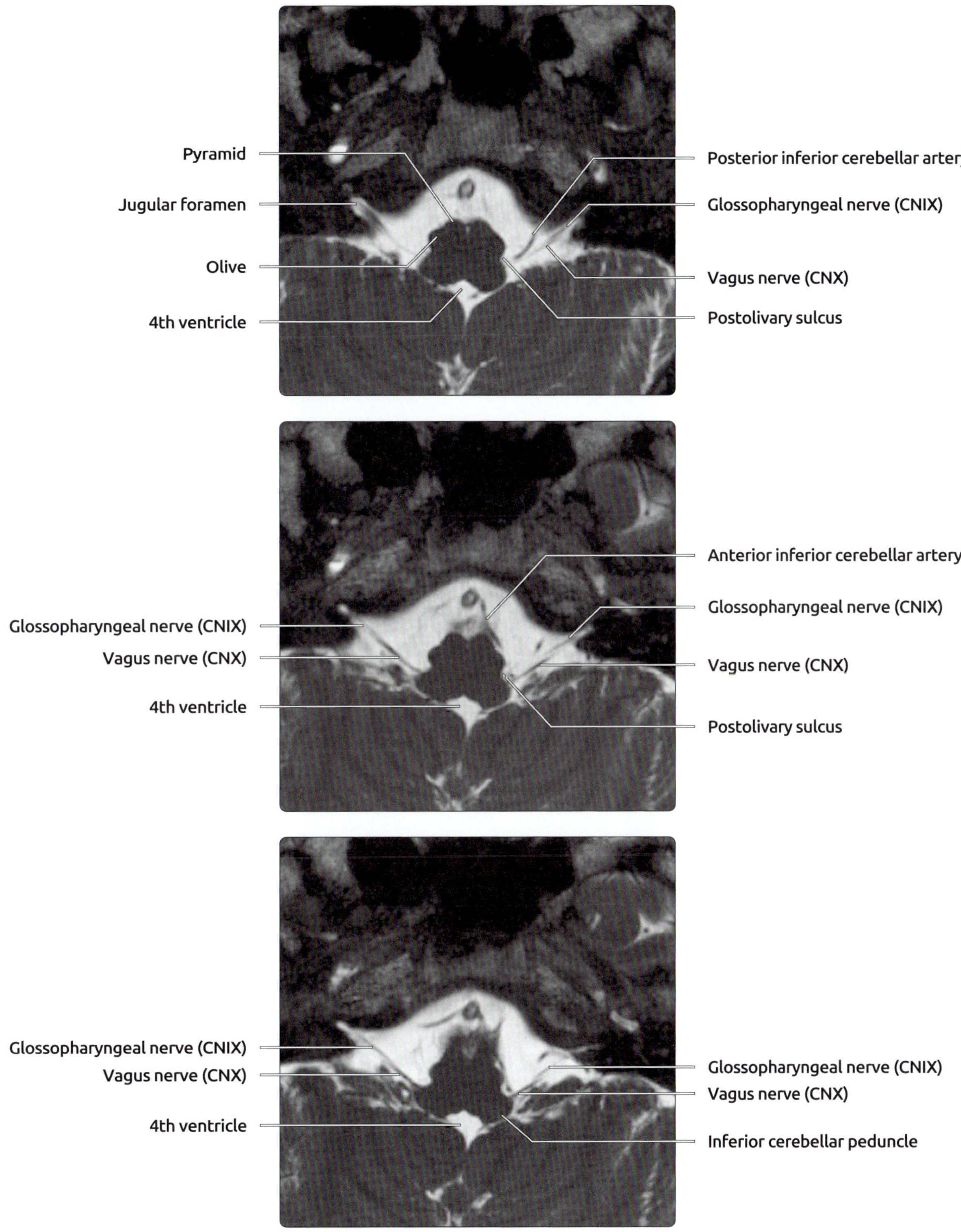

(Top) *First of 3 axial high-resolution T2 MR images through the brainstem medulla presented from inferior to superior is shown. The glossopharyngeal nerve is seen passing laterally into the pars nervosa of the jugular foramen.* **(Middle)** *The glossopharyngeal nerve (CNIX), vagus nerve (CNX), and bulbar accessory nerve (CNXI) all exit the medulla laterally in the postolivary sulcus. CNIX is the most cephalad of these. With routine MR imaging it is not possible to see these 3 cranial nerves individually.* **(Bottom)** *In the upper medulla, the vagus nerve is well seen leaving the brainstem via the postolivary sulcus. The glossopharyngeal nerve is seen more laterally, as it has already exited the brainstem above the vagus nerve.*

AXIAL T2 MR

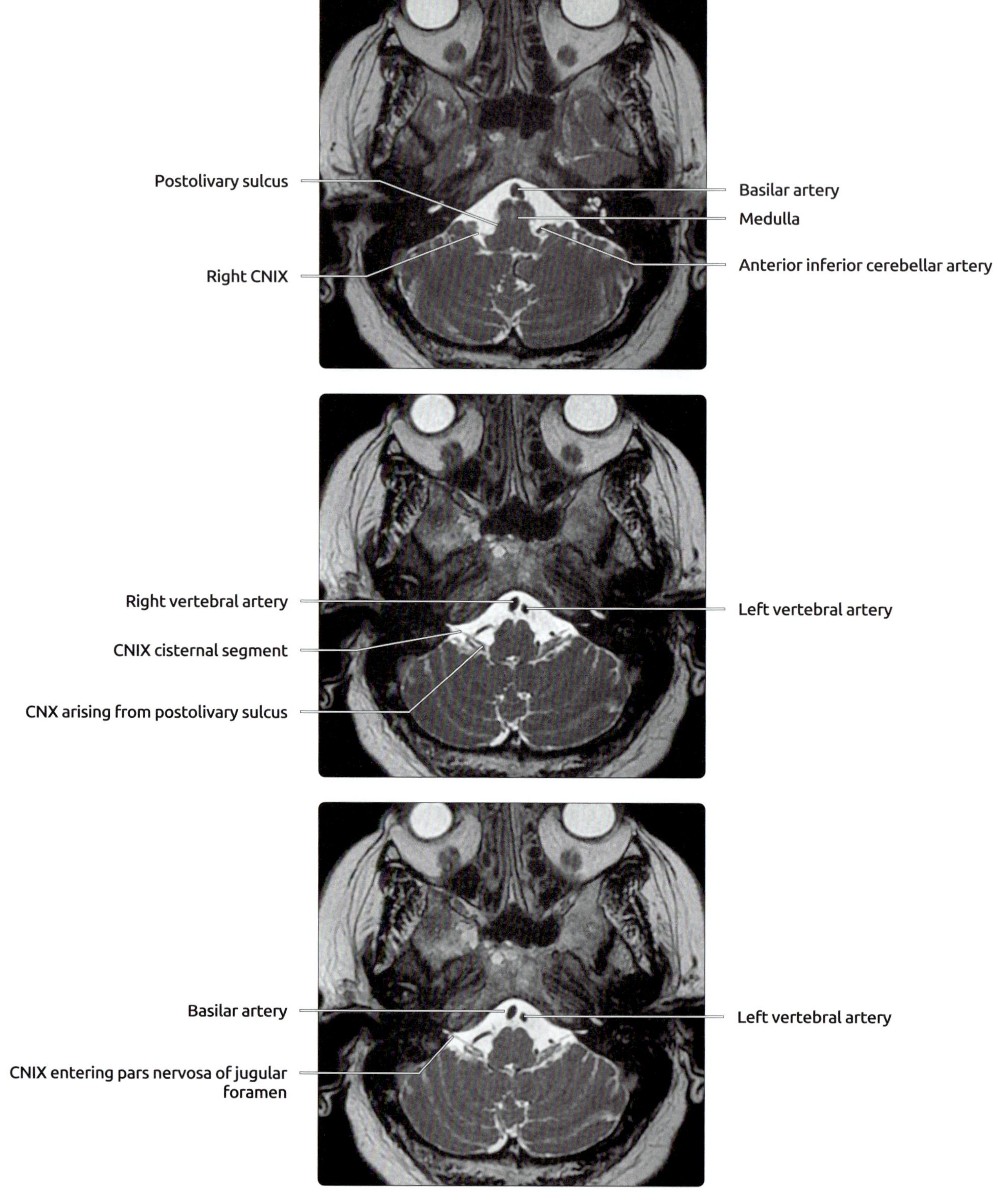

(Top) *First of 4 axial heavily T2-weighted MR images from superior to inferior is shown, demonstrating the right glossopharyngeal nerve (CNIX) exiting the medulla laterally in the postolivary sulcus. A high-resolution 3D heavily T2-weighted sequence, such as CISS, FIESTA, or DRIVE, is key to evaluating these nerves.* **(Middle)** *The vagus nerve (CNX) and bulbar accessory nerve (CNXI) also exit the medulla in the postolivary sulcus. CNIX arises cephalad to these. This image demonstrates the right vagus nerve arising from the brainstem via the postolivary sulcus. The cisternal segment of the right CNIX is seen more laterally, as it already exited the brainstem above the vagus nerve.* **(Bottom)** *Axial T2-weighted MR in the same patient shows the right CNIX entering the pars nervosa of the jugular foramen.*

AXIAL AND CORONAL T2 MR

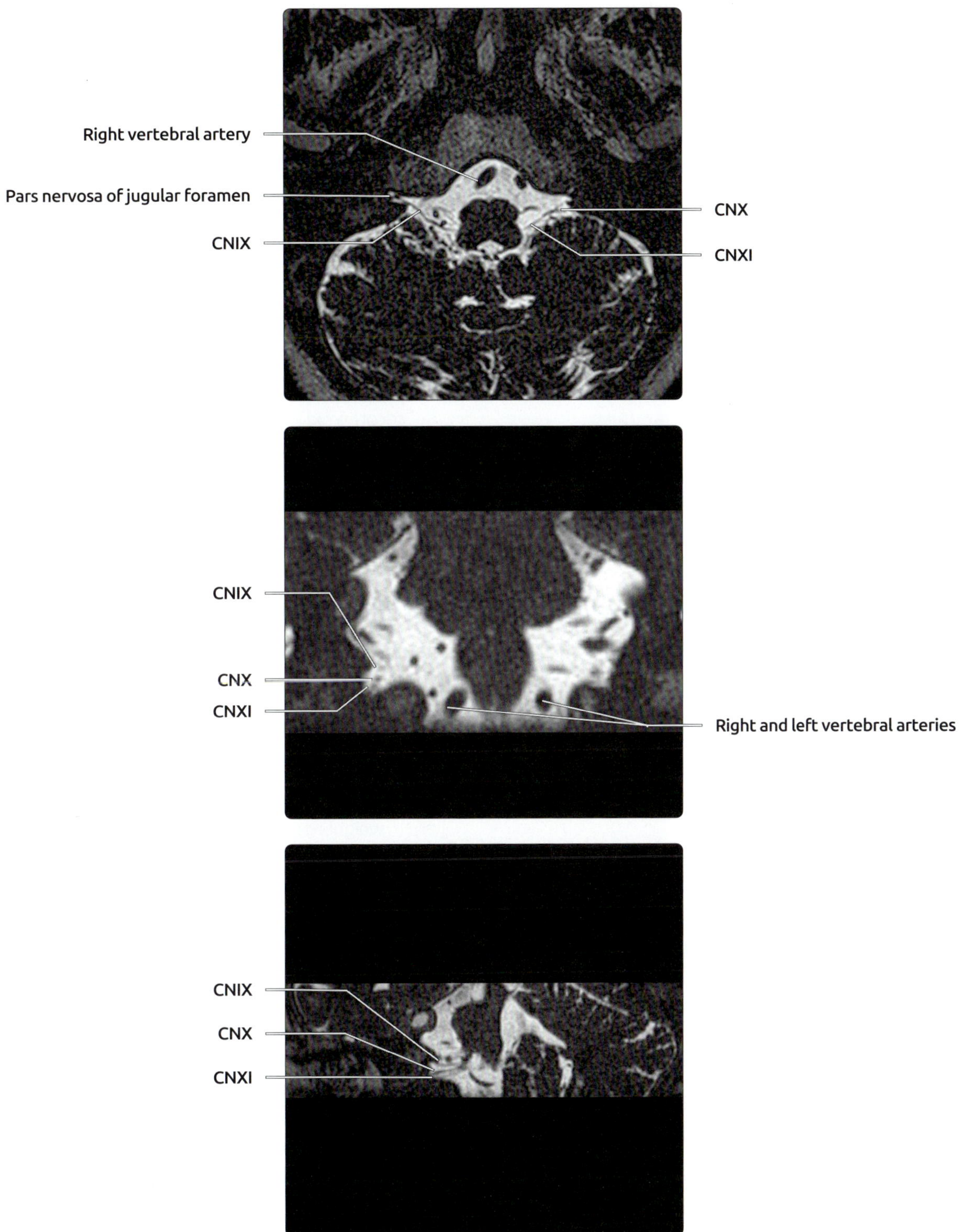

(Top) *MR in another patient demonstrates the course of the right glossopharyngeal nerve (CNIX) in the cistern entering the pars nervosa of the jugular foramen. The vagus nerve (CNX) and accessory nerve (CNXI) are both seen on the left side.* **(Middle)** *Coronal reformat from a 3D heavily T2-weighted MR demonstrates the cisternal segments of the right CNIX, CNX, and CNXI as they enter the jugular foramen on the right. The segments may not always be as clearly visualized, as they are not on the left side in this image.* **(Bottom)** *Oblique coronal reformat from a 3D heavily T2-weighted MR shows the cisternal segments of CNIX, CNX, and CNXI as they enter the jugular foramen on the right. CNIX enters the jugular foramen through the glossopharyngeal meatus, whereas CNX and CNXI enter through the vagal meatus, and the fibers of CNX and CNXI intermix with each other within the jugular foramen and are classified together as the CNX/XI complex.*

TERMINOLOGY

Abbreviations

- Vagus nerve (CNX)

Definitions

- CNX: Longest & one of most complex cranial nerves (CNs) with complex functions, including parasympathetic (PS) innervation of neck, thoracic & abdominal viscera
- Involved in autonomic regulation of cardiovascular, respiratory, & gastrointestinal systems
- Additional innervation
  - Motor to majority of soft palate, pharynx, larynx, & palatoglossus tongue muscle
  - Visceral sensation from larynx, esophagus, trachea, thoracic & abdominal viscera
  - Sensory nerve to external tympanic membrane (TM), external auditory canal (EAC), & external ear
  - Taste from epiglottis

IMAGING ANATOMY

Overview

- Longest of CNs, extending from medulla to colon
- Segments: Intraaxial, cisternal, skull base, & extracranial

Intraaxial Segment

- Vagal nuclei in upper & middle medulla
  - **Motor fibers** originate in **nucleus ambiguus**
  - **Taste** from epiglottis goes to **solitary tract nucleus**
  - **Sensory fibers** from viscera go to **dorsal motor vagal nucleus** (afferent component)
  - **PS or visceral motor fibers** project from **dorsal motor vagal nucleus** (efferent component)
  - Sensations from meninges, laryngeal mucosa, & ear to spinal nucleus CNV

Cisternal Segment

- Nerve fibers exit lateral medulla in **postolivary sulcus** inferior to CNIX & superior to bulbar portion of CNXI

Skull Base Segment

- Enters **pars vascularis** portion of jugular foramen (JF)
  - With CNXI (shared fibrous sheath) & jugular bulb
  - **Superior vagal (jugular) ganglion** found within JF

Extracranial Segment

- Exits JF into nasopharyngeal **carotid space**
- **Inferior vagal (nodose) ganglion** lies just below skull base
- Travels posterolateral to carotid artery into thorax
  - Goes anterior to aortic arch on left & subclavian artery (SCA) on right
- Forms plexus around esophagus & major blood vessels to heart & lungs
- Esophageal plexus nerves provide PS supply to stomach
- Innervation to intestines & visceral organs follows arterial blood supply

Extracranial Branches in Head & Neck

- **Auricular branch (Arnold nerve)**
  - Sensation from external surface of TM, EAC, & external ear
  - From superior vagal ganglion within JF (also has CNIX branches), passes through **mastoid canaliculus** from posterolateral JF to mastoid segment CNVII canal, enters EAC via tympanomastoid fissure
- **Pharyngeal branches**
  - **Pharyngeal plexus** exits just below skull base
  - Sensory to epiglottis, trachea, & esophagus
  - Motor to soft palate [except tensor veli palatini muscle (CNV3)] & pharyngeal constrictor muscles
- **Superior laryngeal nerve**
  - Motor to **cricothyroid** muscle (external branch)
  - Sensory internal branch to hypopharynx & supraglottis
- **Recurrent laryngeal nerve (RLN)**
  - On right, recurs at cervicothoracic junction, passes posteriorly around SCA
  - On left, recurs in mediastinum, passes posteriorly under aorta at aortopulmonary window (APW)
  - Travels in **tracheoesophageal groove** (TEG) posteromedial to thyroid lobe & enters larynx at cricothyroid joint level
  - Motor to all laryngeal muscles except cricothyroids
  - Sensory to mucosa of infraglottis
- **Carotid sinus branch (Hering nerve)**
  - Formed by small CNIX branch & branch from CNX
  - Supplies carotid sinus wall baroreceptors & carotid body chemoreceptors

ANATOMY IMAGING ISSUES

Imaging Recommendations

- **Proximal vagal neuropathy**
  - Image from medulla to hyoid bone
  - MR imaging method of choice: Superior sensitivity for skull base, meningeal, cisternal, & brainstem pathology
    - Must have axial, coronal T2, T1 (without fat saturation & contrast-enhanced with fat saturation), heavily T2-weighted steady state (e.g., FIESTA/CISS) sequence
    - May be indistinguishable sometimes from CNXI & IX
    - Bone CT complementary in skull base pathology
- **Distal vagal neuropathy**
  - Image skull base to mediastinum; **to carina for left side**
  - Key areas to evaluate: Carotid space, TEG, APW
  - CECT imaging method of choice

CLINICAL IMPLICATIONS

Clinical Importance

- **Vagal nerve dysfunction: Proximal symptom complex**
  - Injury site: Between medulla & hyoid bone
  - Multiple CNs involved (CNIX-XII, Vernet syndrome) with oropharyngeal & laryngeal dysfunction, including deviation of uvula to opposite side & ipsilateral loss of pharyngeal reflex & vocal cord (VC) paralysis
- **Vagal nerve dysfunction: Distal symptom complex**
  - Injury site: Below hyoid bone
  - Isolated larynx dysfunction with VC paralysis (RLN involvement > > infrahyoid CNX)
  - Imaging features of VC paralysis: Medialization of ipsilateral true VC, anteromedial arytenoid cartilage rotation, enlarged laryngeal ventricle = sail sign, medialized, thickened aryepiglottic fold, enlarged pyriform sinus

GRAPHICS, PROXIMAL CNX

Dorsal vagal nucleus (afferent visceral sensory)

Glossopharyngeal nerve (CNIX)

Accessory nerve (CNXI)

Solitary tract nucleus (taste from epiglottis and visceral afferent)

Spinal nucleus CNV

Hypoglossal nerve (CNXII)

Vagus nerve (CNX)

Dorsal vagal nucleus (efferent visceral motor or parasympathetic)

Nucleus ambiguus (efferent motor)

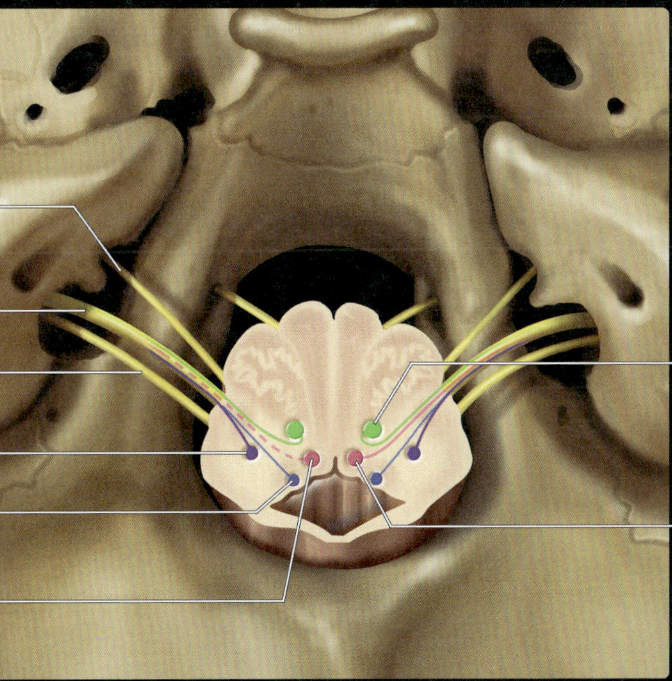

Glossopharyngeal nerve (CNIX)

Vagus nerve (CNX)

Accessory nerve (CNXI)

Spinal nucleus CNV

Solitary tract nucleus (taste from epiglottis and visceral afferent)

Dorsal vagal nucleus (afferent visceral sensory)

Nucleus ambiguus (efferent motor)

Dorsal vagal nucleus (efferent visceral motor or parasympathetic)

(Top) *Graphic of the brainstem viewed from behind shows critical nuclear columns of CNX. Note the nucleus ambiguus supplies motor fibers to CNX. The dorsal vagal nucleus is a mixed nucleus, sending efferent parasympathetic fibers to the viscera while receiving afferent sensory fibers from these same viscera. The solitary tract nucleus receives taste information from the epiglottis and vallecula via CNX.* **(Bottom)** *Axial graphic through the medulla shows principal nuclei associated with vagus nerve function. Skeletal motor fibers to the pharynx and larynx come from the nucleus ambiguus. This nucleus also contributes to CNIX and CNXI. Parasympathetic fibers to the viscera are associated with the dorsal motor nucleus of the vagus nerve (solid pink line). Sensory information transmitted from the viscera is also transmitted to the dorsal nucleus of the vagus nerve (dashed pink line). Via the vagus nerve, the solitary tract nucleus receives taste information from the epiglottis and afferent information from the aortic bodies and sinoatrial node, in addition to various visceral afferents via other cranial nerves.*

GRAPHIC, EXTRACRANIAL VAGUS NERVE

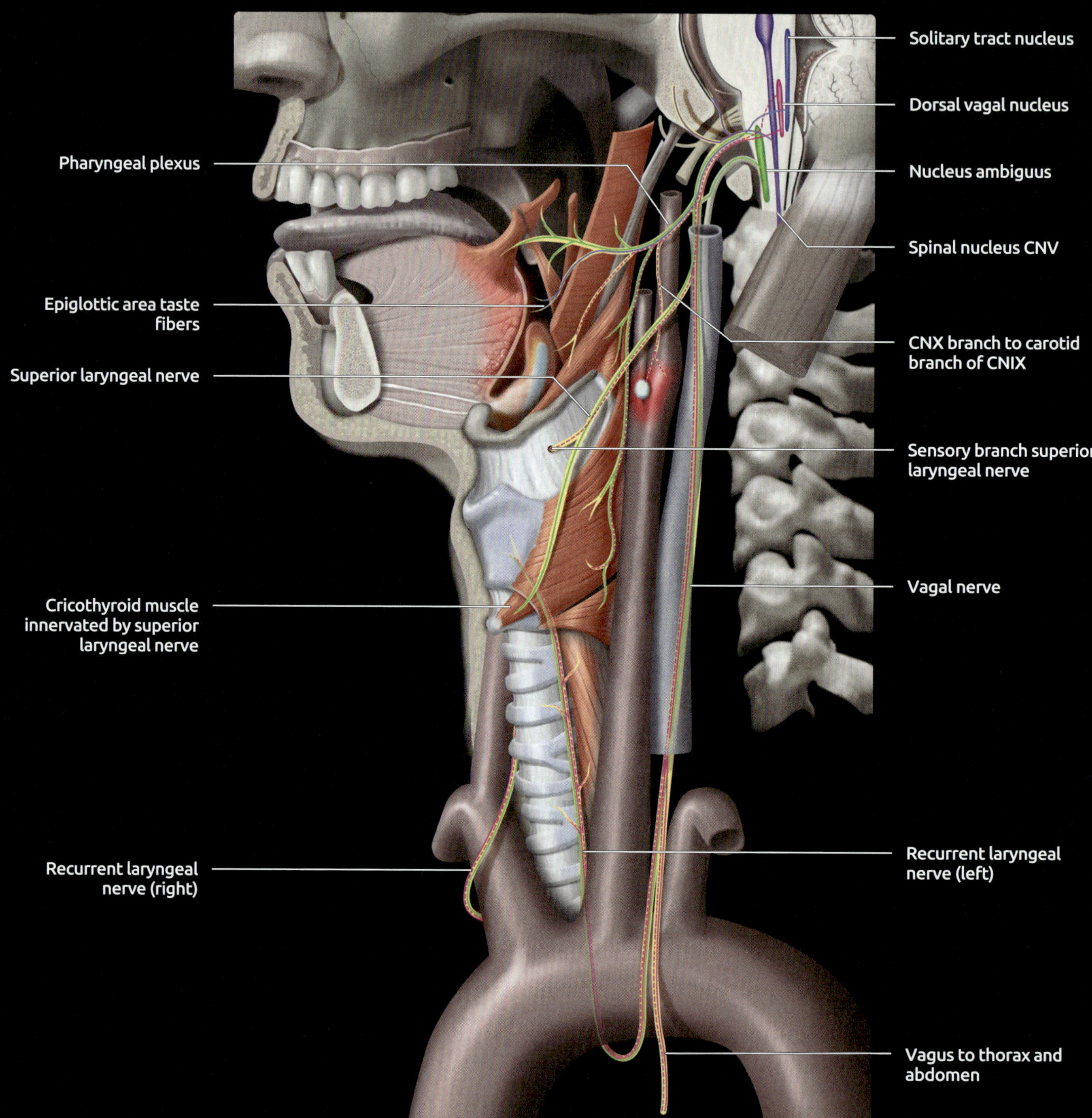

Lateral graphic shows the neck and upper mediastinal portions of CNX, including the 4 brainstem nuclei. The nucleus ambiguus supplies efferent motor innervation (green lines) via the pharyngeal plexus to the soft palate and pharynx (superior, middle, and inferior constrictor muscles) and via the recurrent laryngeal nerves to all laryngeal muscles except the cricothyroids. The dual-functioning dorsal vagal nucleus both sends out efferent fibers for involuntary motor activity in the viscera (solid pink line) and receives sensations from these same viscera (dashed pink line). The solitary tract nucleus receives taste information from the region of the epiglottis and vallecula. The spinal nucleus of CNV receives external ear and skull base-meninges sensory information. Only the visceral motor and sensory fibers from dorsal vagal nucleus continue on CNX to the rest of the body.

GRAPHICS, EXTRACRANIAL CNX

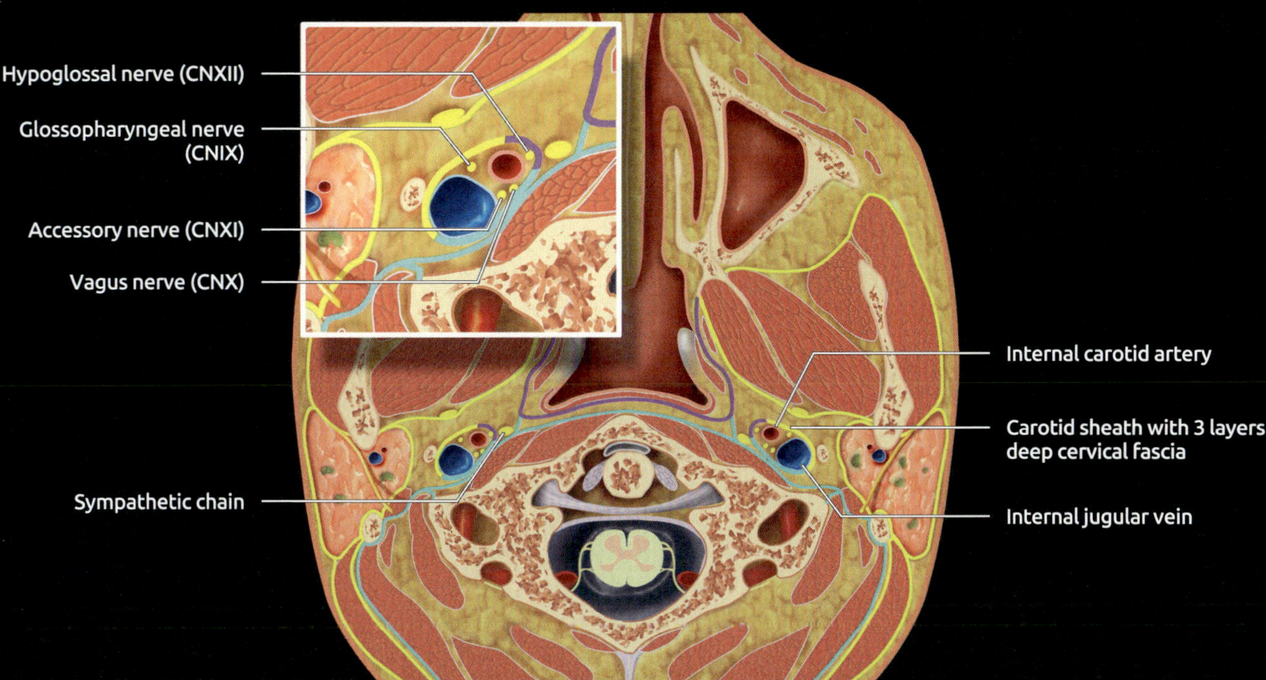

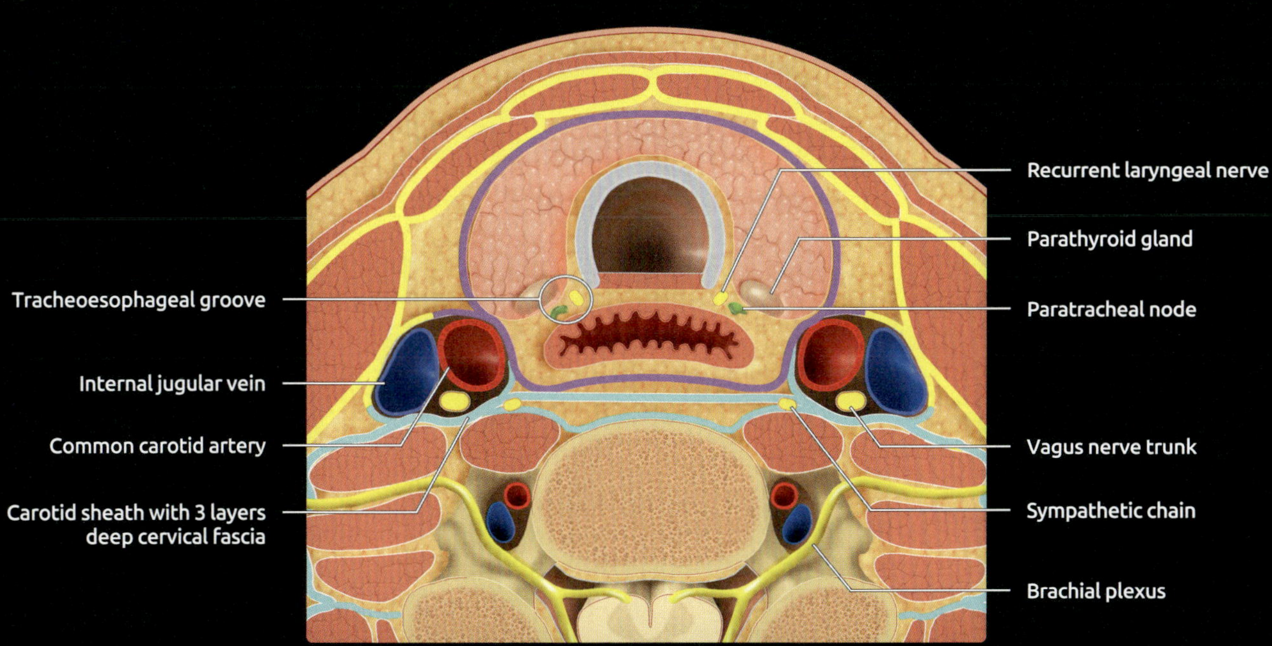

(Top) *Axial graphic of the nasopharyngeal carotid spaces shows the extracranial vagus nerve situated posteriorly in the gap between the internal carotid artery and the internal jugular vein. Notice that at this level, CNIX, CNXI, and CNXII are all still within the carotid space.* **(Bottom)** *Axial graphic through the infrahyoid carotid spaces at the level of the thyroid gland demonstrates the vagus trunk is the only remaining cranial nerve within the carotid space. It remains in the posterior gap between the common carotid artery and the internal jugular vein. Note the recurrent laryngeal nerve in the tracheoesophageal groove with the visceral space. Remember the left recurrent laryngeal nerve turns cephalad in the aortopulmonic window in the mediastinum, whereas the right recurrent nerve turns at the cervicothoracic junction around the subclavian artery.*

AXIAL BONE CT

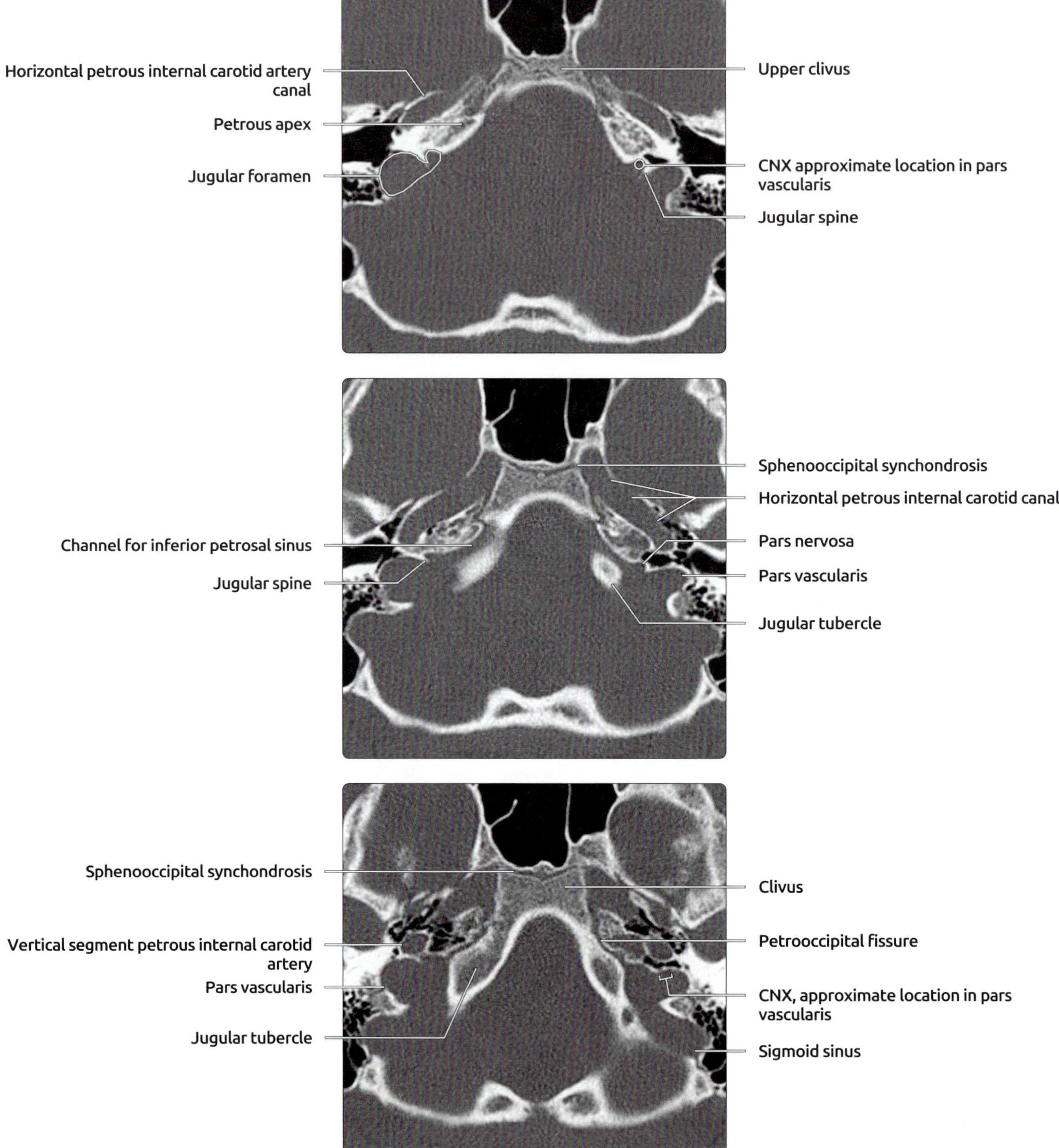

(Top) *First of 3 axial bone CT images of the skull base presented from superior to inferior is shown. The jugular foramen is divided by the jugular spine into the anteromedial smaller pars nervosa, and posterolateral pars vascularis. The pars vascularis transmits the vagus and accessory cranial nerves, Arnold nerve, and jugular bulb, which becomes the internal jugular vein.* **(Middle)** *In this image, the pars nervosa is seen to connect anteromedially to the inferior petrosal sinus. CNIX, the Jacobsen nerve, and the inferior petrosal sinus are all found within the pars nervosa.* **(Bottom)** *Image through the lower jugular foramen shows the sigmoid sinuses emptying into the pars vascularis of the jugular foramen. Notice the jugular foramen is located on the floor of the posterior cranial fossa in the seam between the petrous temporal bone anterolaterally and occipital bone posteromedially.*

AXIAL T2 MR

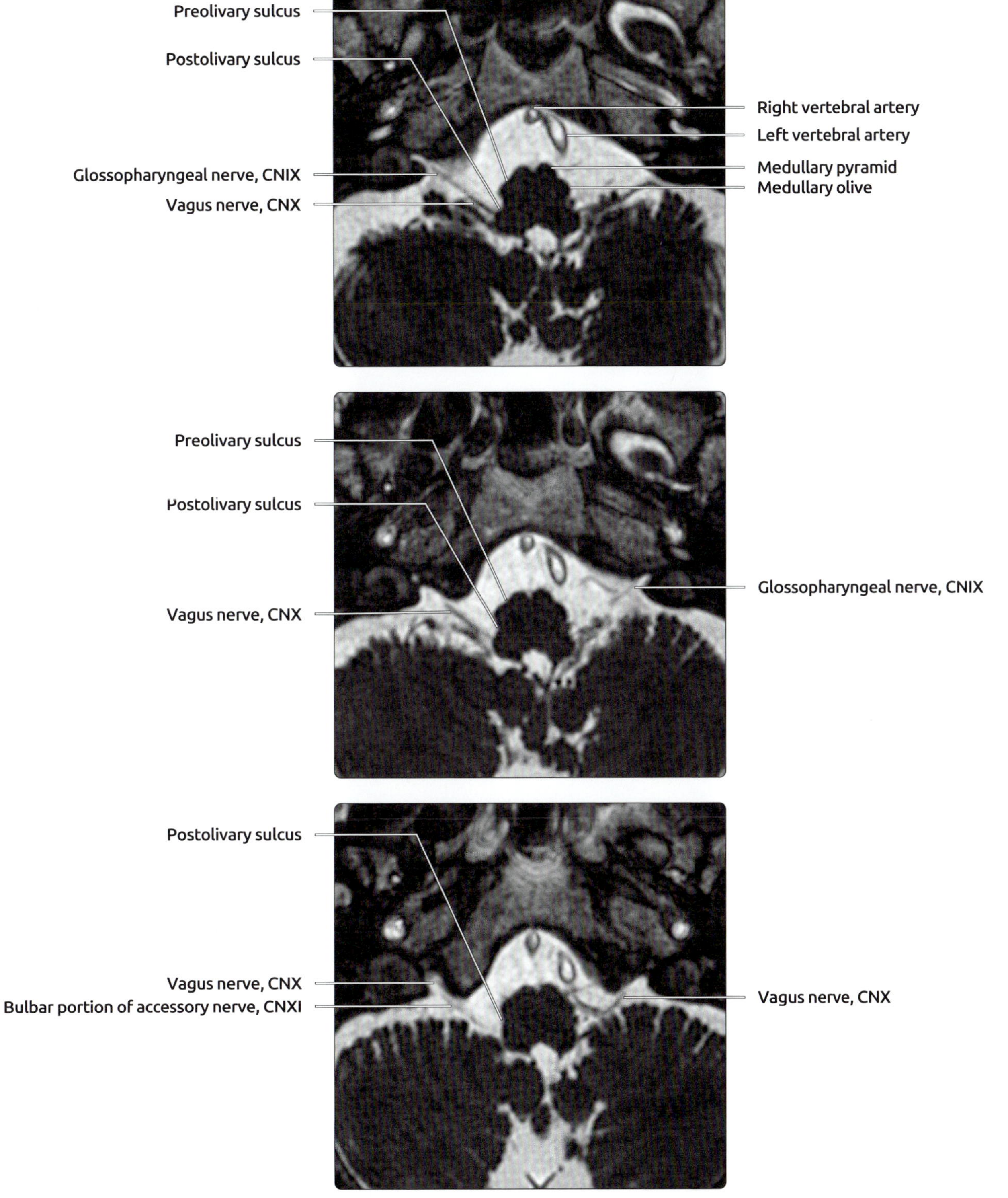

(Top) *First of 3 axial T2 MR images of the low brainstem presented from superior to inferior is shown. The vagus nerve is seen exiting the lateral medulla in the postolivary sulcus inferior to the glossopharyngeal nerve.* **(Middle)** *In this image, the vagus nerve is seen exiting the postolivary sulcus into the lateral basal cistern bilaterally. A portion of the cisternal glossopharyngeal nerve, CNIX, is seen on the left.* **(Bottom)** *At the level of the lower aspect of the jugular foramen, the cisternal portion of the bulbar portion of the accessory nerve, CNXI, is seen close to the postolivary sulcus. The vagus nerve is seen entering the jugular foramen laterally. Without thin-section focused T2 MR imaging, it is often difficult to separate the glossopharyngeal nerve, vagus nerve, and bulbar root of the accessory nerve in the basal cisterns.*

PATHOLOGY EXAMPLES

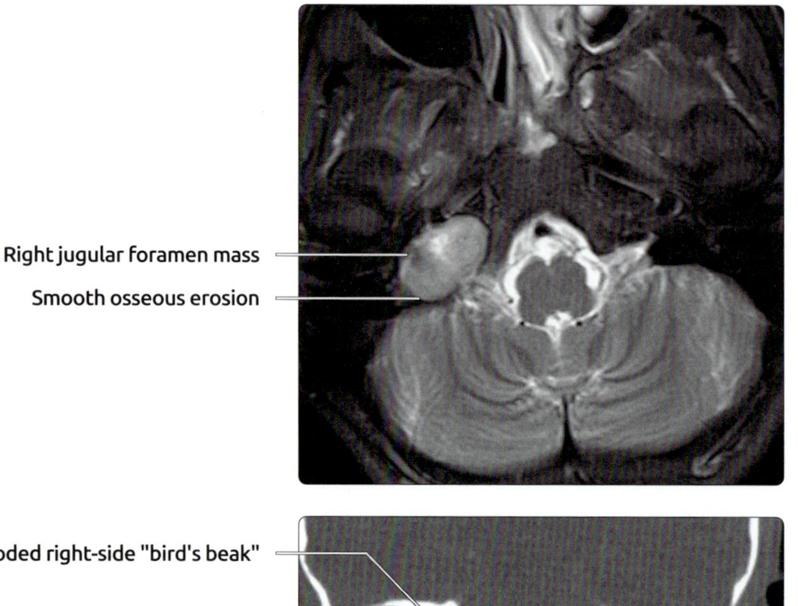

Eroded right-side "bird's beak"

Smooth osseous erosion

Jugular foramen mass

Hypoglossal canal

Intact left-side "bird's beak"

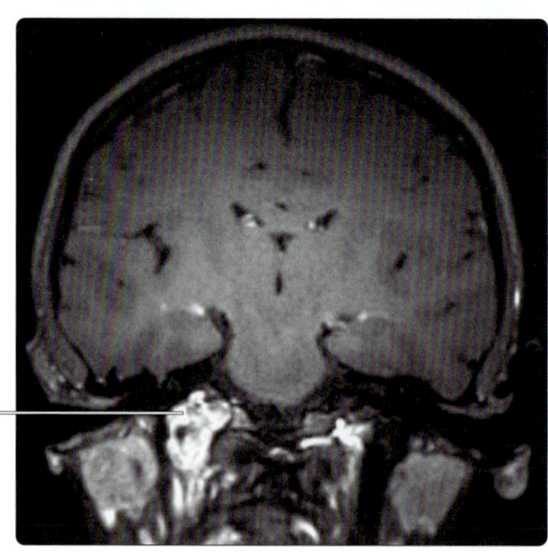

(Top) *Axial T2 FS MR demonstrates a hyperintense right jugular foramen mass with adjacent osseous remodeling. Note the lack of flow voids, which will be a feature of a paraganglioma, another differential consideration for a jugular foramen mass.* **(Middle)** *Coronal CT shows a large right jugular foramen mass with smooth erosion or remodeling of the jugular foramen bony margins. The right lateral jugular tubercle (also called the "bird's beak") is eroded, whereas the left side is intact. The primary differential for a mass with these features is a schwannoma.* **(Bottom)** *Coronal T1 C+ FS MR demonstrates a lobulated, heterogeneously enhancing mass arising from the right jugular foramen. Note the typical superomedial vector of spread toward the brainstem; contrast this with a paraganglioma that tends to grow superolaterally toward the middle ear.*

VAGAL NERVE NUCLEI

Nucleus	Function		Structure Innervated	Named Branch	Other Cranial Nerve Functions From This Nucleus
Nucleus ambiguus	Efferent	Motor	Soft palate muscles Pharyngeal constrictors Laryngeal muscles Palatoglossus	• Pharyngeal plexus: Motor to pharyngeal constrictors and all soft palate muscles except tensor veli palatini (CNV3), namely palatopharyngeus, salpingopharyngeus, levator veli palatini, palatoglossus, and muscles of the uvula • Superior laryngeal nerve external branch: Cricothyroid muscle and inferior constrictor • Recurrent laryngeal nerve: Motor to all laryngeal muscles except cricothyroid	• Efferent of CNIX and CNXI • Stylopharyngeus muscle: CNIX
Dorsal vagal nucleus	Efferent	Visceral motor or parasym-pathetic	Heart, lungs, gastrointestinal smooth muscles, and glands		
	Afferent	Visceral sensory	Larynx, esophagus, trachea, thoracic and abdominal viscera	• Pharyngeal plexus for epiglottis, trachea, and esophagus • Superior laryngeal nerve (internal branch): Sensory to hypopharynx, glottis, and supraglottis • Recurrent laryngeal nerve: Sensory to infraglottis	
Solitary tract nucleus	Afferent	Taste from epiglottis	Epiglottis		• Taste from tongue: Anterior 2/3rd via chorda tympani, branch of facial nerve • Posterior 1/3rd via CNIX
		Visceral afferent	Aortic bodies Sinoatrial node		• Carotid body and carotid sinus via CNIX • Gag reflex, carotid sinus reflex, vomiting reflex, and cough reflex
Spinal nucleus CNV	Afferent	Sensory	Dura of posterior fossa, laryngeal mucosa, and ear	• Arnold nerve: Sensory from external surface of tympanic membrane, external auditory canal, external ear (deep touch, pain, temperature)	Also receives sensory from CNV, CNVII, CNIX, CNX: Overall, touch, pain, and temperature from ipsilateral face

Table depicting the vagus nerve nuclei with the structures innervated and some of the interactions of these nuclei with other cranial nerves is shown.

CNXI (Accessory Nerve)

TERMINOLOGY

Abbreviations

- Accessory nerve (CNXI)

Synonyms

- 11th cranial nerve (CN), CN11

Definitions

- CNXI: Pure motor CN, supplying sternocleidomastoid (SCM), trapezius muscles (through spinal component) and palatal, pharyngeal, and laryngeal muscles (through cranial component)

IMAGING ANATOMY

Overview

- Motor CN only
- 4 CNXI segments are defined
  - Intraaxial, cisternal, skull base, and extracranial

Intraaxial Segment

- 2 distinct nuclear origins
  - **Bulbar** (cranial) motor fibers originate in lower **nucleus ambiguus**
    - Fibers course anterolaterally to exit lateral medulla in postolivary sulcus inferior to CNIX and CNX
  - **Spinal** motor fibers originate from **spinal nucleus** of accessory nerve
    - Narrow column of cells along lateral aspect of anterior horn from C1 to C5
    - Nerve fibers emerge from lateral aspect of cervical spinal cord between anterior and posterior roots
    - Fibers combine, forming bundle that ascends, entering posterior cranial fossa via **foramen magnum**

Cisternal Segment

- Bulbar portion travels anterolaterally through basal cistern along similar course as CNIX and CNX
- Spinal portion enters lower lateral basal cistern, exits through jugular foramen
- Bulbar root joins spinal component of accessory nerve either in lower cistern or within jugular foramen

Skull Base Segment

- Passes through posterior **pars vascularis portion of jugular foramen**
  - CNX and jugular bulb are also in pars vascularis
- Bulbar and spinal portions remain together in jugular foramen

Extracranial Segment

- Fibers from bulbar portion (nucleus ambiguus) separate from main nerve and merge with vagus nerve
  - Travel via CNX to supply muscles of
    - Palate: Levator veli palatini, palatoglossus, palatopharyngeus, and musculus uvulae
    - Pharynx: Superior constrictor and soft palate via pharyngeal plexus
    - Larynx: Except cricothyroid muscle via recurrent laryngeal nerve
- Fibers from spinal portion remain in extracranial CNXI
  - Diverges posterolaterally from carotid space
  - Enters deep surface of upper portion of SCM, anastomoses with C2 &/or C3 fibers, exits posterior border around midportion of SCM
  - Continues across floor of posterior cervical space to anterior border of trapezius
  - Often forms plexus along with branches from C2 to C4 before entering and terminating in trapezius
  - **Innervates SCM and trapezius muscles**
  - Rarely terminates in SCM, trapezius being supplied by cervical nerves

ANATOMY IMAGING ISSUES

Imaging Recommendations

- MR imaging method of choice
  - Superior sensitivity to skull base, meningeal, cisternal, and brainstem pathology
  - Sequences should include combination of T2, T1 without fat saturation, and contrast-enhanced T1 with fat saturation in axial and coronal planes
- Bone CT used to supplement MR when complex skull base pathology is present

Imaging Sweet Spots

- CNXI nuclei and intraaxial segment not directly visualized
- Cisternal segment is often not visualized on routine MR imaging
  - High-resolution thin-section T2 MR sequence usually demonstrates CNIX-XI nerve complex passing through basal cisterns from postolivary sulcus to pars vascularis of jugular foramen
- Bone CT clearly demonstrates bony anatomy of pars vascularis of jugular foramen
- Extracranial CNXI segment not identifiable in conventional imaging
  - Location inferred from its constant position deep to SCM muscle in floor of posterior cervical space
  - MR neurography techniques, such as 3D CRANI and PSIF, can demonstrate extracranial course

Imaging Pitfalls

- Hypertrophic levator scapulae muscle following serious CNXI injury may mimic tumor
- **Do not mistake this enlarged muscle for mass**

CLINICAL IMPLICATIONS

Clinical Importance

- CNXI innervates SCM and trapezius muscles

Function Dysfunction

- CNXI dysfunction: Isolated CNXI injury
  - Most common cause is radical neck dissection because jugular nodal chain intimately associated with CNXI
  - Initial symptoms of spinal accessory neuropathy
    - Downward and lateral rotation of scapula
    - Shoulder droop resulting from loss of trapezius tone
  - Long-term findings in spinal accessory neuropathy
    - Within 6 months results in **atrophy** of ipsilateral SCM and trapezius muscles
    - **Compensatory hypertrophy** of ipsilateral **levator scapulae muscle** occurs over months

GRAPHICS

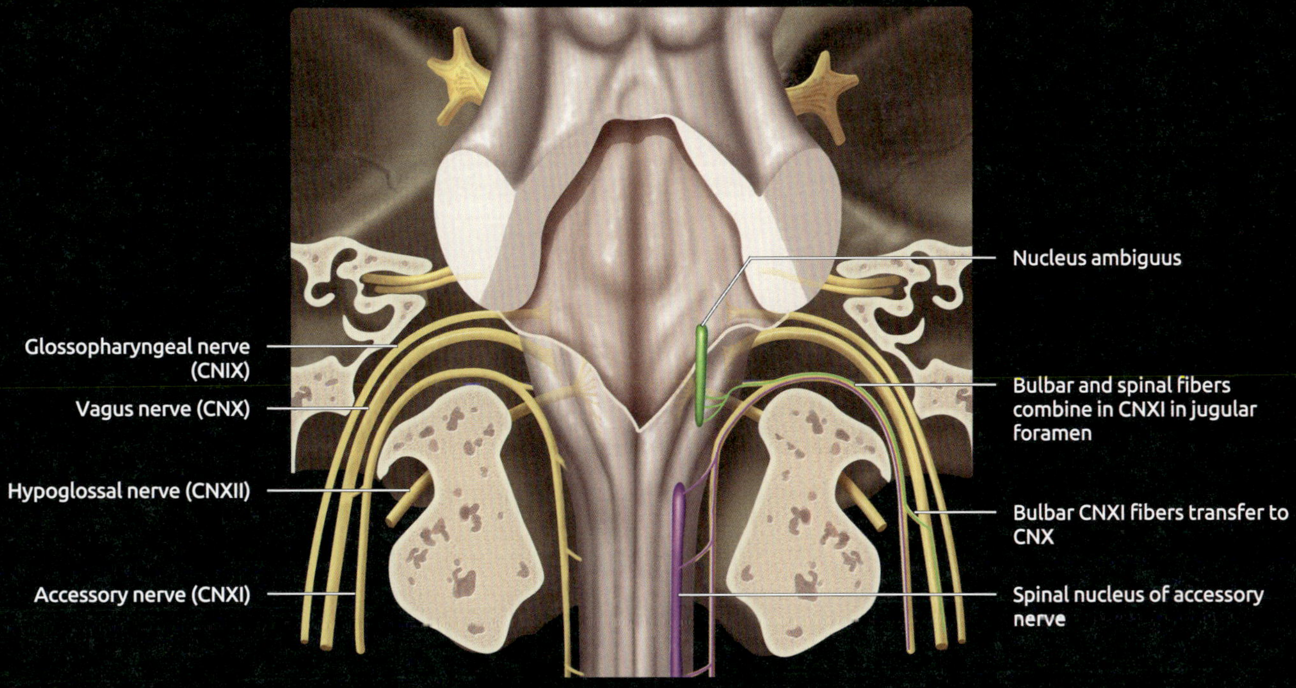

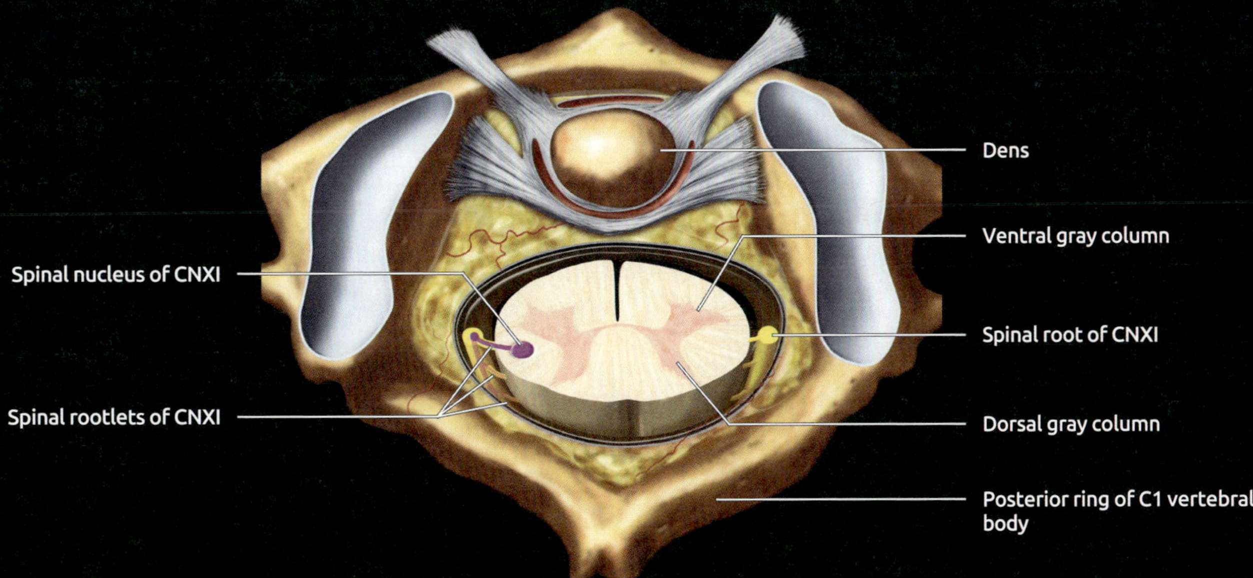

(Top) *Graphic of the posterior brainstem reveals both the spinal and the bulbar roots of the accessory nerve (CNXI). Note the lower nucleus ambiguus gives rise to multiple rootlets of the bulbar root of CNXI. Both the spinal and the bulbar roots combine in the lateral basal cistern and jugular foramen. The spinal root continues as extracranial CNXI to innervate the sternocleidomastoid and trapezius muscles. The bulbar root fibers cross to the vagus nerve extracranially or within the jugular foramen to supply motor innervation to the pharynx (superior constrictor and soft palate) and the larynx (except the cricothyroid muscle).* **(Bottom)** *Axial graphic shows the upper cervical spinal cord cut to reveal the spinal nucleus of the accessory nerve giving rise to multiple rootlets that unite to form the spinal root of the accessory nerve. The rootlets exit the posterolateral sulcus just anterior to the posterior cervical roots.*

GRAPHIC, INTRACRANIAL AND EXTRACRANIAL

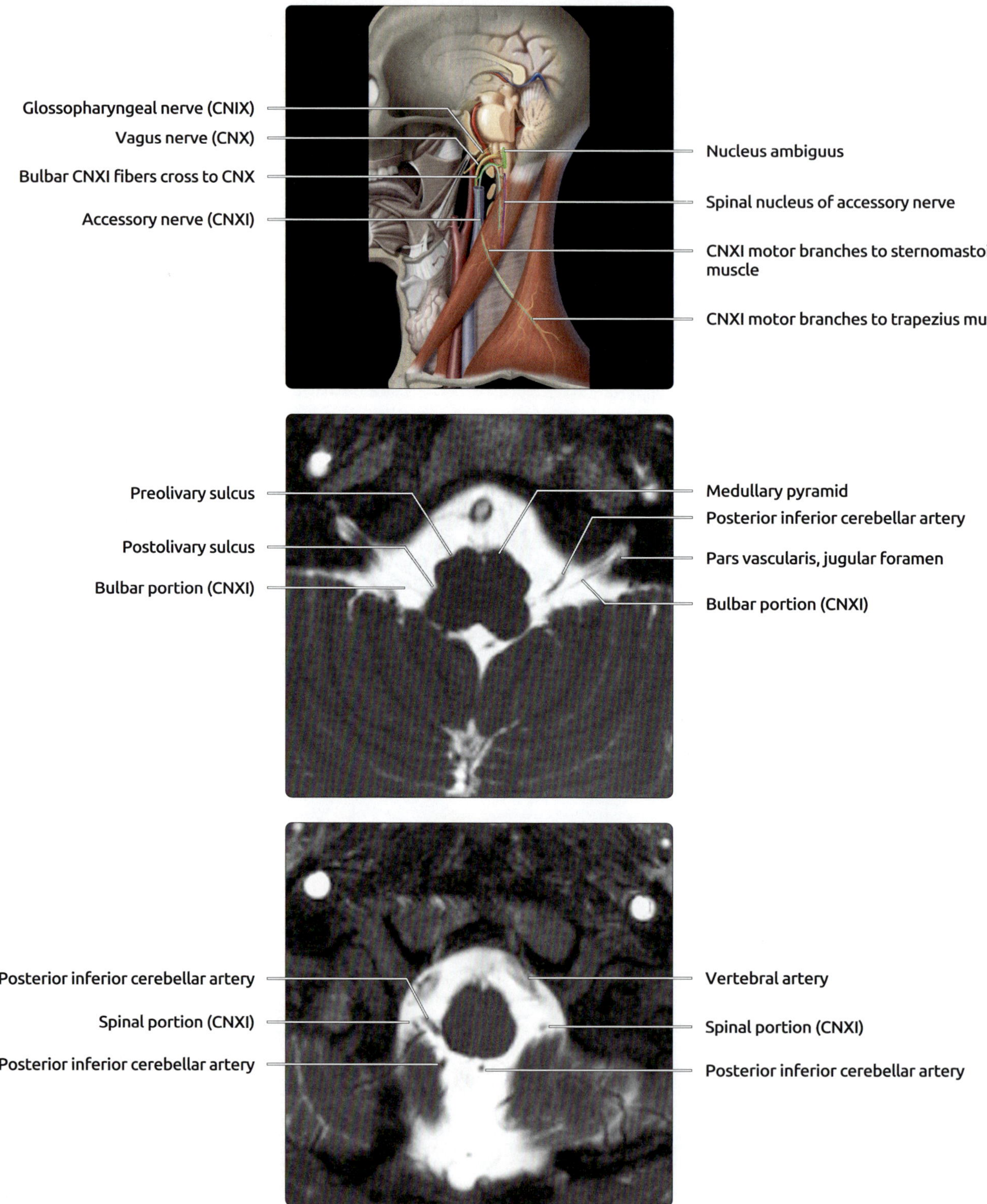

(Top) *Overview graphic of the intracranial and extracranial accessory nerve (CNXI) shows the lower nucleus ambiguus at the origin of the bulbar root of CNXI, while the spinal nucleus gives rise to the spinal root. Both roots combine in the jugular foramen. Extracranially, the bulbar fibers cross to the vagus nerve to eventually provide motor innervation via the pharyngeal plexus to the soft palate and superior constrictor muscles and via the recurrent laryngeal nerve to the majority of the endolaryngeal muscles. The spinal fibers that remain in the accessory nerve provide motor innervation to the sternocleidomastoid and trapezius muscles. Notice extracranial CNXI runs along the floor of the posterior cervical space.* **(Middle)** *Axial T2 MR at the level of the medulla shows the bulbar portion of CNXI emerging from the postolivary sulcus just inferior to CNX. The bulbar portion travels anterolaterally through the basal cistern together with CNX and CNIX.* **(Bottom)** *Axial T2 MR through the lower medulla shows the spinal root of CNXI ascending through the foramen magnum to join the bulbar root before entering the pars nervosa of the jugular foramen.*

AXIAL BONE CT AND T2 MR

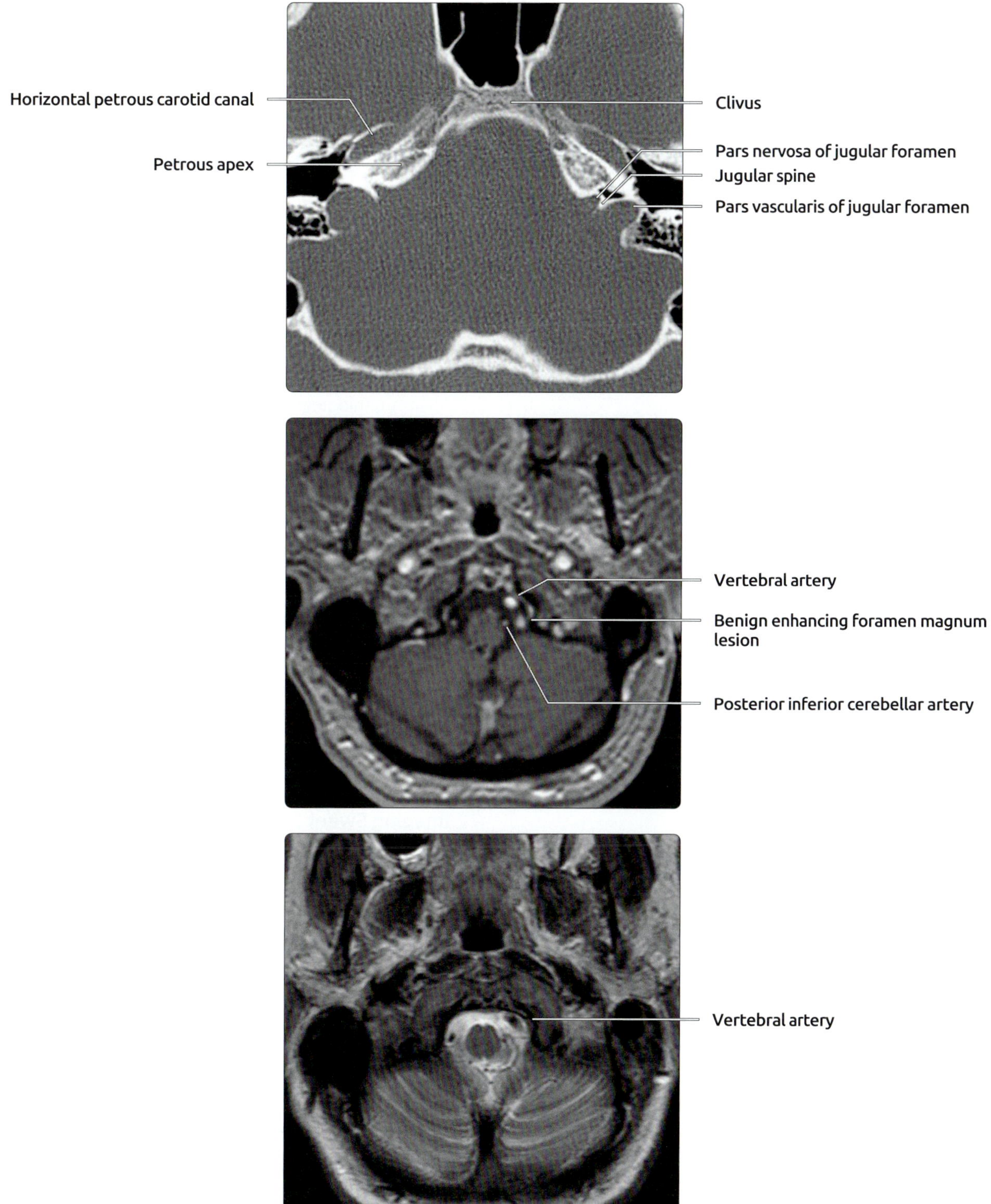

(Top) *Axial bone CT through the jugular foramen shows the anteromedial pars nervosa, the jugular spine, and the posterolateral pars vascularis. The pars nervosa transmits CNIX, the Jacobsen nerve, and the inferior petrosal sinus. The pars vascularis transmits CNX, CNXI, the Arnold nerve, and the sigmoid sinus, which becomes the internal jugular vein.* **(Middle)** *Axial view of a contrast-enhanced MPRAGE sequence shows an enhancing nodule posterior to the left vertebral artery. Enhancing T2-hyperintense small lesions located posterior to the intradural vertebral artery at the foramen magnum have been previously described as benign enhancing foramen magnum lesions (BEFMLs) and recently reported as fibrotic arachnoid nodules adherent to the dorsal aspect of the spinal accessory nerve. On the right side, the nondominant vertebral artery terminates as the posterior inferior cerebellar artery.* **(Bottom)** *Axial T2 MR at the same level fails to demonstrate BEFML seen in the contrast-enhanced sequence. BEFMLs are T2 hyperintense and are not identified on routine spin-echo T2-weighted images, as it blends with T2-hyperintense CSF.*

TERMINOLOGY

Abbreviations

- Hypoglossal nerve (CNXII)

Definitions

- Motor nerve supplying intrinsic and extrinsic tongue muscles

IMAGING ANATOMY

Overview

- Motor cranial nerve to intrinsic and extrinsic tongue muscles
  - **Palatoglossus**: Only extrinsic muscle **not** innervated by CNXII (but by CNX)
- Hypoglossal nerve anatomic segments
  - Intraaxial segment
  - Cisternal segment
  - Skull base segment
  - Extracranial

Intraaxial Segment

- **Hypoglossal nucleus**
  - In dorsal medulla, medial to dorsal vagal nucleus
  - Long, thin nucleus approximately same length as ventrolateral olive (15- to 18-mm craniocaudal dimension)
  - Extends from level of hypoglossal eminence (trigone) in floor of 4th ventricle just inferior to medullary striae of 4th ventricle to proximal medulla
- Hypoglossal intraaxial axonal course
  - Efferent fibers from hypoglossal nucleus extend ventrally through medulla, lateral to medial lemniscus
  - Efferent fibers exit between olivary nucleus and pyramid (root exit zone) at **ventrolateral sulcus** (a.k.a. **preolivary sulcus)**

Cisternal Segment

- Efferent fibers coalesce to form multiple (6-14) **rootlets**
  - In premedullary cistern, course between posterior inferior cerebellar artery and vertebral artery
- Rootlets fuse into hypoglossal nerve (2-4 trunks) as it exits skull base through hypoglossal canal
- Hypoglossal filaments may merge with vagal fibers
- Total length of cisternal segment ranges from 8-15 mm; mean width of cisternal segment ranges from 0.3-0.6 mm

Skull Base Segment

- Hypoglossal nerve exits occipital bone via **hypoglossal canal**, surrounded by venous plexus
  - Canal in occipital bone caudal to jugular foramen
    - "Empties" into medial nasopharyngeal carotid space
    - Osseous septa may bisect hypoglossal canal
  - Mean length of hypoglossal canal ranges from 9.5-16.0 mm; mean width ranges from 1.3-3.0 mm

Extracranial Segment

- **Carotid space component of CNXII**
  - Hypoglossal canal "empties" into medial nasopharyngeal carotid space
  - Hypoglossal nerve immediately gives off **dural branches** after exiting hypoglossal canal
  - Descends in posterior carotid space, closely apposed with CNX
  - Exits carotid space anteriorly between jugular vein and internal carotid artery, crosses lateral surface of external carotid artery at inferior margin of posterior belly of digastric muscle
- **Transspatial component of CNXII**
  - From carotid space, nerve runs anteroinferiorly toward hyoid bone, lateral to carotid bifurcation
  - At level of occipital artery base, nerve turns anterior, continuing as muscular branch below posterior belly of digastric muscle, medial to submandibular gland
  - Gives off superior root of ansa cervicalis from horizontal segment of nerve to anastomose with lower root
- Distal branches of imaging importance
  - **Muscular branch** travels on lateral margin of hyoglossus muscle in posterior sublingual space close to lingual artery, medial to mylohyoid muscle
    - Innervates extrinsic (styloglossus, hyoglossus, and genioglossus) and intrinsic tongue muscles
    - **Geniohyoid** innervated by **C1** spinal nerve
  - **Ansa cervicalis**: Formed from superior and inferior (C1-C3 spinal nerves) roots
    - Innervates infrahyoid strap muscles (sternothyroid, sternohyoid, omohyoid)
- Difficult to directly identify nerve extracranially; position inferred by adjacent anatomical structures

ANATOMY IMAGING ISSUES

Imaging Recommendations

- MR preferred study: Best for brainstem, cisterns, skull base, and suprahyoid neck
  - Should include heavily T2-weighted sequence
- CECT of suprahyoid neck (cover from orbital roof to below hyoid) with bone algorithm of skull base

Imaging Sweet Spots

- Include nerve from brainstem to hyoid bone
- Asymmetric appearance of tongue gives clue to denervation
  - Acute/subacute: Denervated hemitongue may show low T1 and high T2 intensity with enhancement
  - Chronic: Tongue atrophy (fatty infiltration and volume loss); infrahyoid strap muscle atrophy

Imaging Pitfalls

- Denervated hemitongue may appear enlarged due to edema (acute) or flaccidity (chronic); may mimic infiltrative tongue mass
- Not imaging hyoid bone will result in missed diagnoses

CLINICAL IMPLICATIONS

Clinical Importance

- Unilateral lesion causes tongue protrusion to "side of lesion"
- Nearly 50% of CNXII neuropathies from neoplastic processes, mostly malignant
- Rare, persistent, primitive hypoglossal artery arises from cervical internal carotid artery C1-C2 level and passes through hypoglossal canal into posterior fossa; anastomoses with vertebrobasilar system

GRAPHICS, INTRACRANIAL

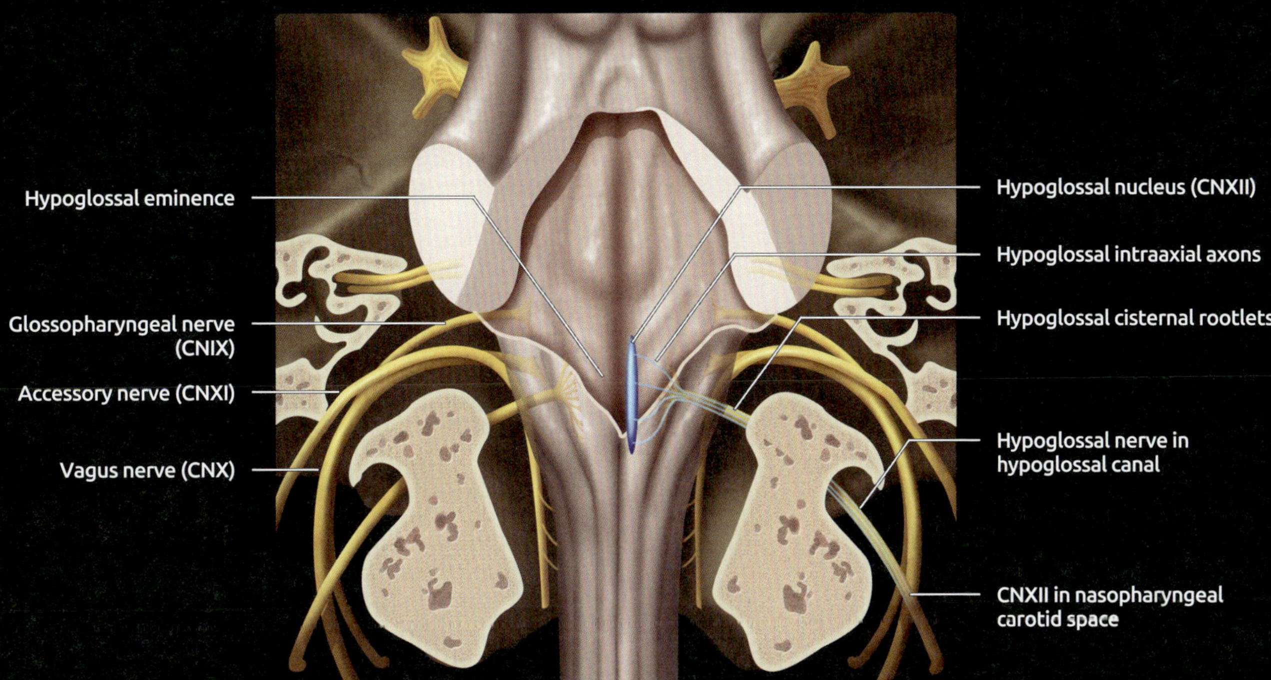

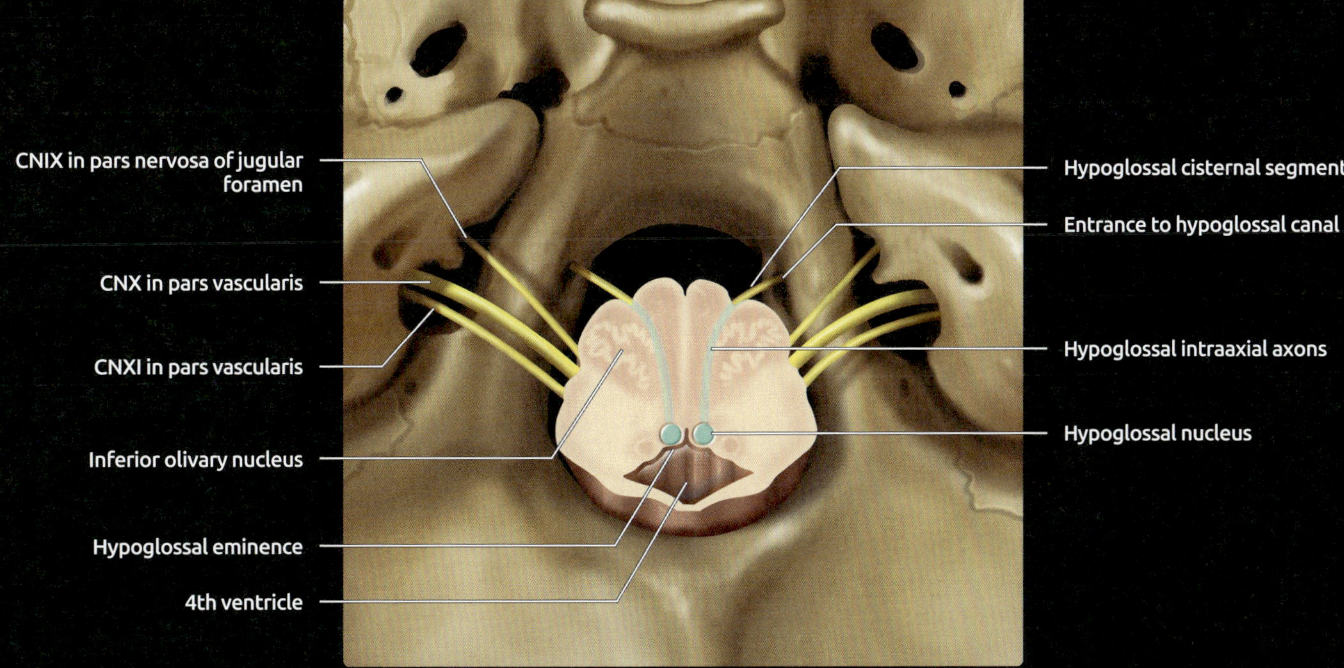

(Top) *Graphic of the lower brainstem seen from behind illustrates key features of the proximal hypoglossal nerve. Notice the hypoglossal nucleus in the dorsal paramedian medulla feeding intraaxial axons that exit the preolivary sulcus into the anterolateral basal cistern. Cisternal rootlets fuse into the hypoglossal nerve that traverses the skull base through the hypoglossal canal. Exiting the hypoglossal canal, CNXII immediately enters the nasopharyngeal carotid space.* **(Bottom)** *Axial graphic through the lower medulla shows the hypoglossal nucleus feeding intraaxial axons that dive ventrally to curve around the inferior olivary nucleus to exit the medulla ventrolaterally via the preolivary sulcus. Note that the hypoglossal nucleus gives the floor of the 4th ventricle an arch (hypoglossal eminence/trigone). The cisternal rootlets combine in the hypoglossal canal to become the hypoglossal nerve (CNXII). Note the hypoglossal canal is anterior and inferior to the jugular foramen.*

GRAPHIC, EXTRACRANIAL

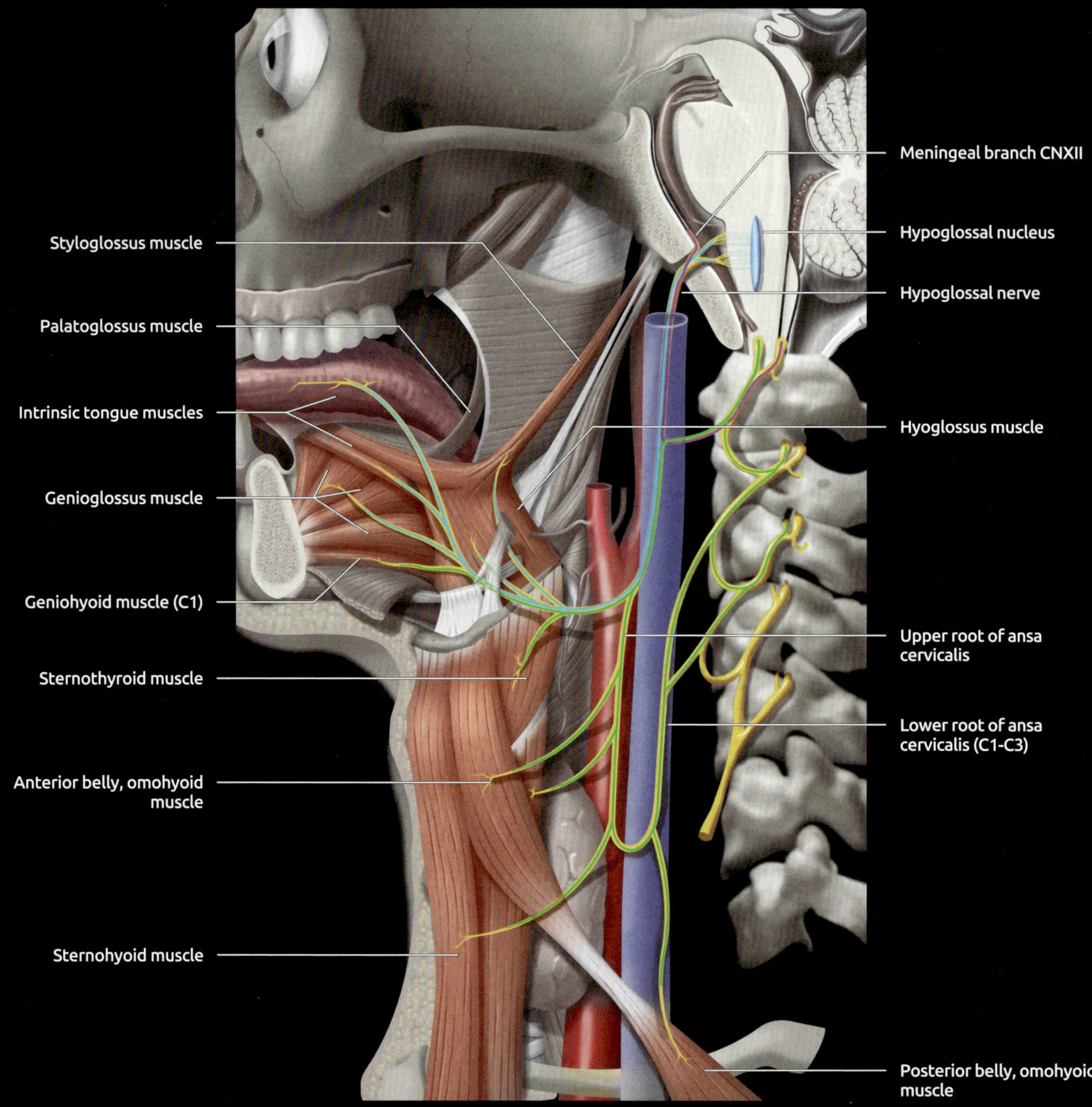

Lateral graphic depicts the entire course of the hypoglossal nerve. The nerve originates in the hypoglossal nucleus in the floor of the 4th ventricle. As CNXII exits the skull base, it immediately enters the nasopharyngeal carotid space just medial to the internal carotid artery. It travels inferiorly in the carotid space to exit anteriorly between the carotid artery and the internal jugular vein. CNXII supplies motor innervation to intrinsic and extrinsic (styloglossus, hyoglossus, genioglossus) tongue muscles. C1 spinal nerve supplies motor to the geniohyoid muscle. Ansa cervicalis (C1-C3 spinal nerves) supplies motor innervation to the infrahyoid strap muscles, including sternothyroid, sternohyoid, and omohyoid muscles. Also note the meningeal sensory branch from C1 following CNXII retrograde to supply clival meninges.

AXIAL T2 MR

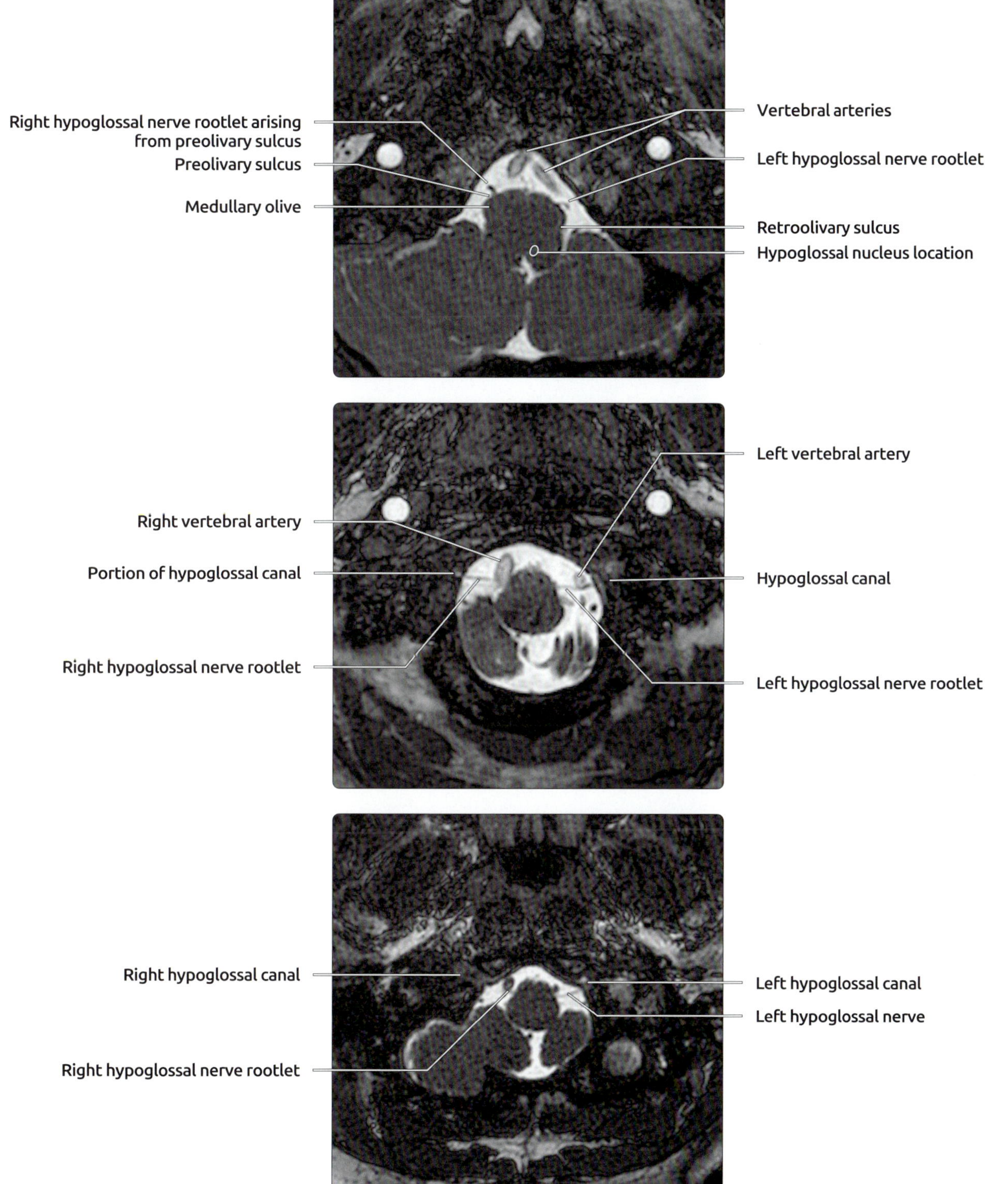

(Top) *Superior of 2 axial T2 MR images in the same patient through the lower medulla demonstrates the origin of hypoglossal nerves from the preolivary sulcus. The nerves arise as rootlets that coalesce into 2-4 trunks, which exit through the hypoglossal canal. The trunks abut or pass near the vertebral arteries in the basal cisterns.* **(Middle)** *Second axial MR at the lower medulla shows the cisternal segments of bilateral hypoglossal nerves after they emerge from the medulla in the preolivary sulcus as rootlets. Rootlets on either side fuse into the corresponding side hypoglossal nerve and exit the skull base through the hypoglossal canal. Close proximity of these rootlets with the vertebral arteries is seen in this view.* **(Bottom)** *Axial heavily T2-weighted MR in another patient through the lower medulla demonstrates a cisternal rootlet on the left from the origin to the hypoglossal canal. Note the hypoglossal canal on the right seen with an intermediate signal intensity.*

CORONAL BONE CT

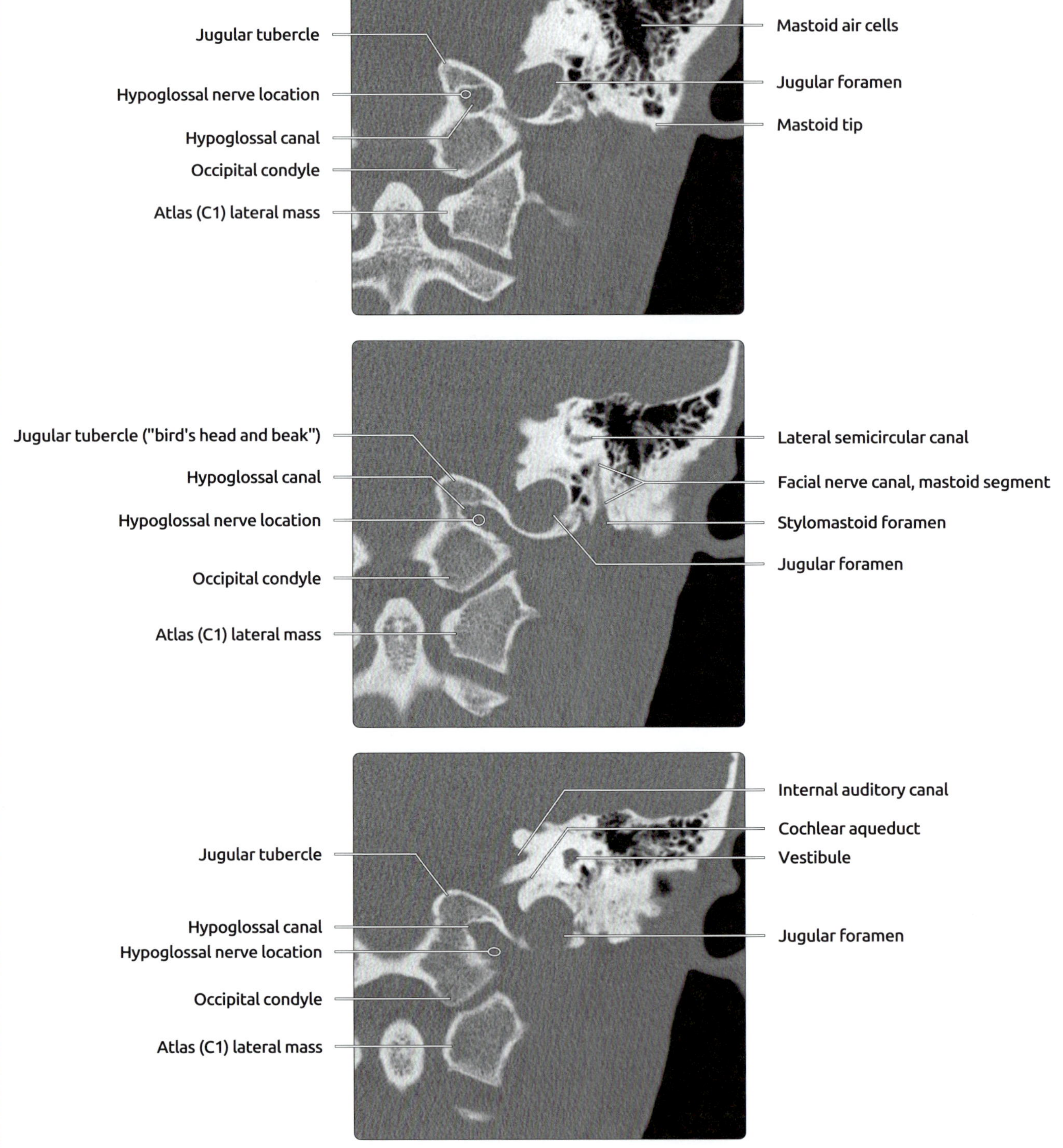

(Top) *First of 3 coronal bone CT images presented from posterior to anterior shows the hypoglossal canal as a complete bony circle, indicating that the image is at the level of the entry into the canal. The location of CNXII is in the upper medial quadrant within the hypoglossal canal.* **(Middle)** *In this image of the midhypoglossal canal, the surrounding bone appears as a "bird's head and beak" with the head and beak made up of the jugular tubercle. The jugular foramen is directly lateral to the hypoglossal canal.* **(Bottom)** *At the level of the distal hypoglossal canal, the hypoglossal nerve leaves the skull base to emerge inferiorly into the nasopharyngeal carotid space. Notice the lateral jugular foramen also empties its contents into the carotid space, including the jugular vein and cranial nerves IX, X, and XI.*

CORONAL T1 C+ MR

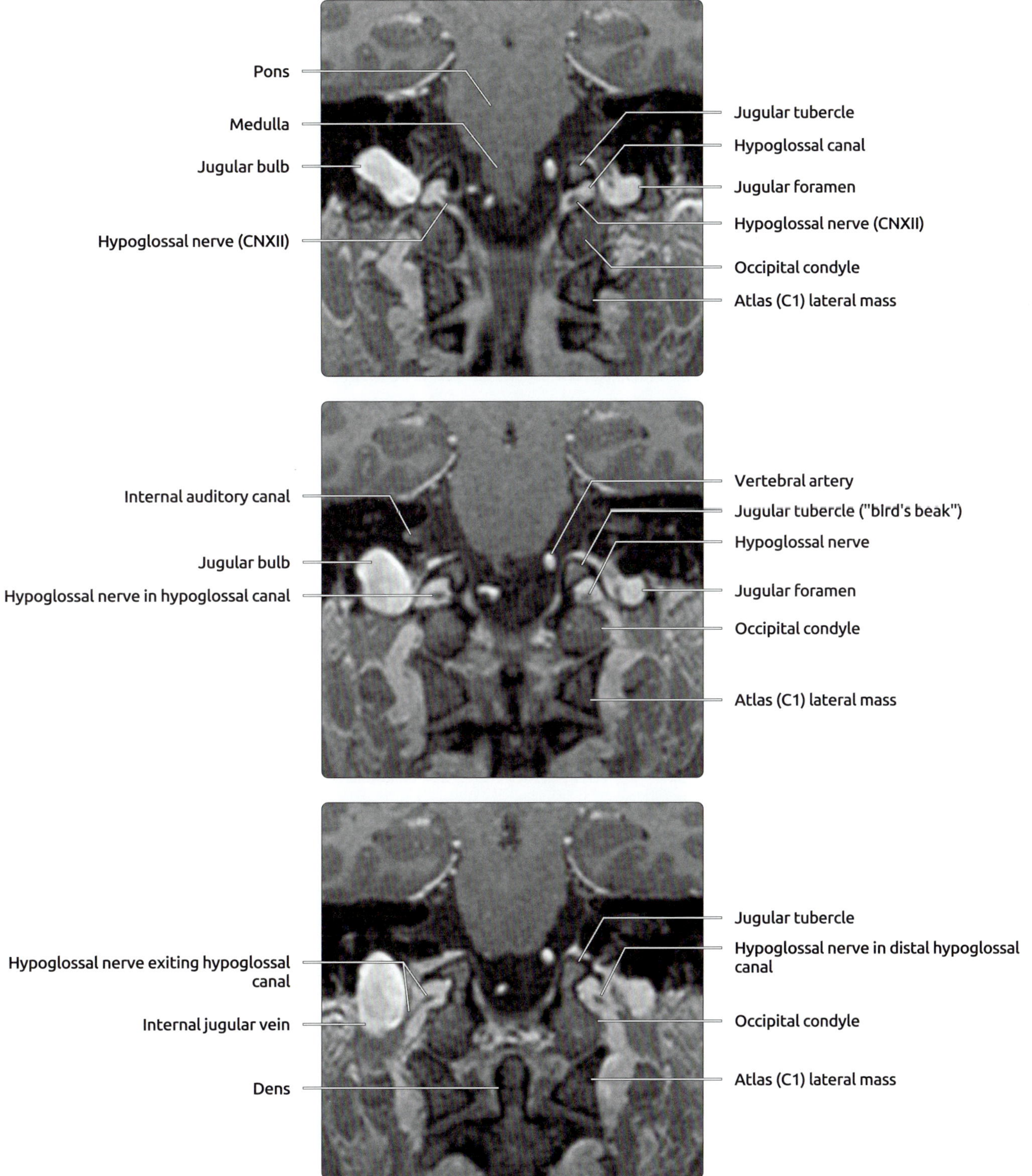

(Top) *First of 3 sequential coronal T1 C+ MR images presented from posterior to anterior is shown. In this MR, the hypoglossal nerve is seen entering the proximal hypoglossal canal. The hypointense hypoglossal nerve is surrounded by the strongly enhancing venous plexus and is therefore easily seen on thin-section enhanced MR. The hypoglossal canal also carries a branch of the ascending pharyngeal artery.* **(Middle)** *In this coronal MR of the midhypoglossal canal, the low-signal hypoglossal nerve is visible surrounded by the enhancing venous plexus just beneath the "bird's beak" of the jugular tubercle.* **(Bottom)** *In this coronal MR through the distal hypoglossal canal, the hypoglossal nerves can be seen exiting inferolaterally into the nasopharyngeal carotid space. Notice also the internal jugular vein exiting inferiorly on the patient's right into this same nasopharyngeal carotid space.*

AXIAL BONE CT AND CTA

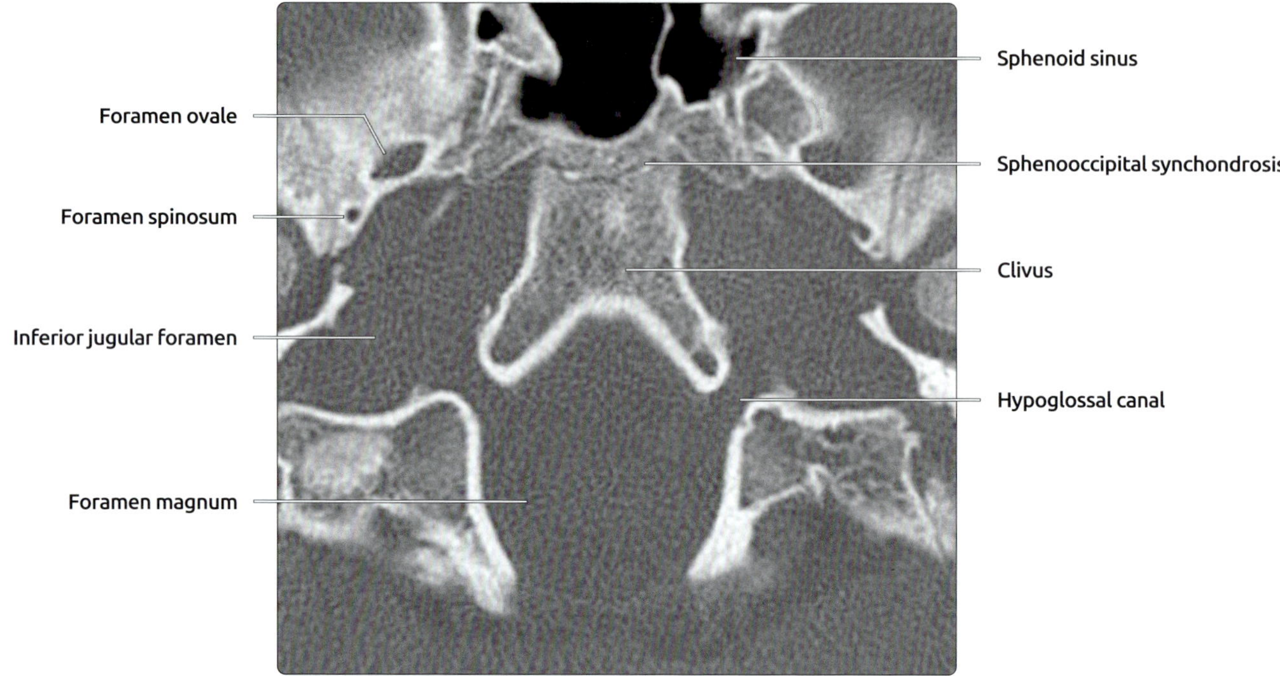

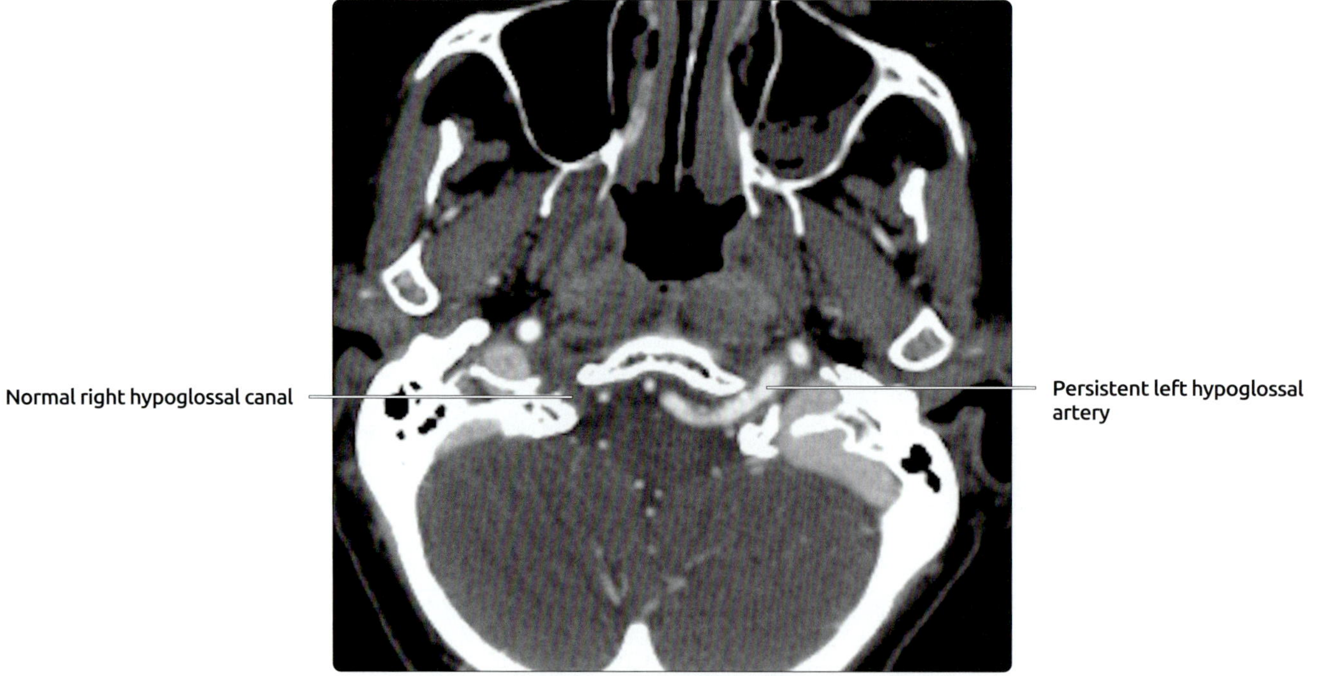

(Top) *Axial bone CT at the level of the hypoglossal canal is shown. Notice the margins of the hypoglossal canals are well corticated.* **(Bottom)** *Axial CTA through the skull base demonstrates a persistent carotid basilar connection, a persistent hypoglossal artery traversing the left hypoglossal canal. The normal right hypoglossal canal can also be seen.*

PATHOLOGY

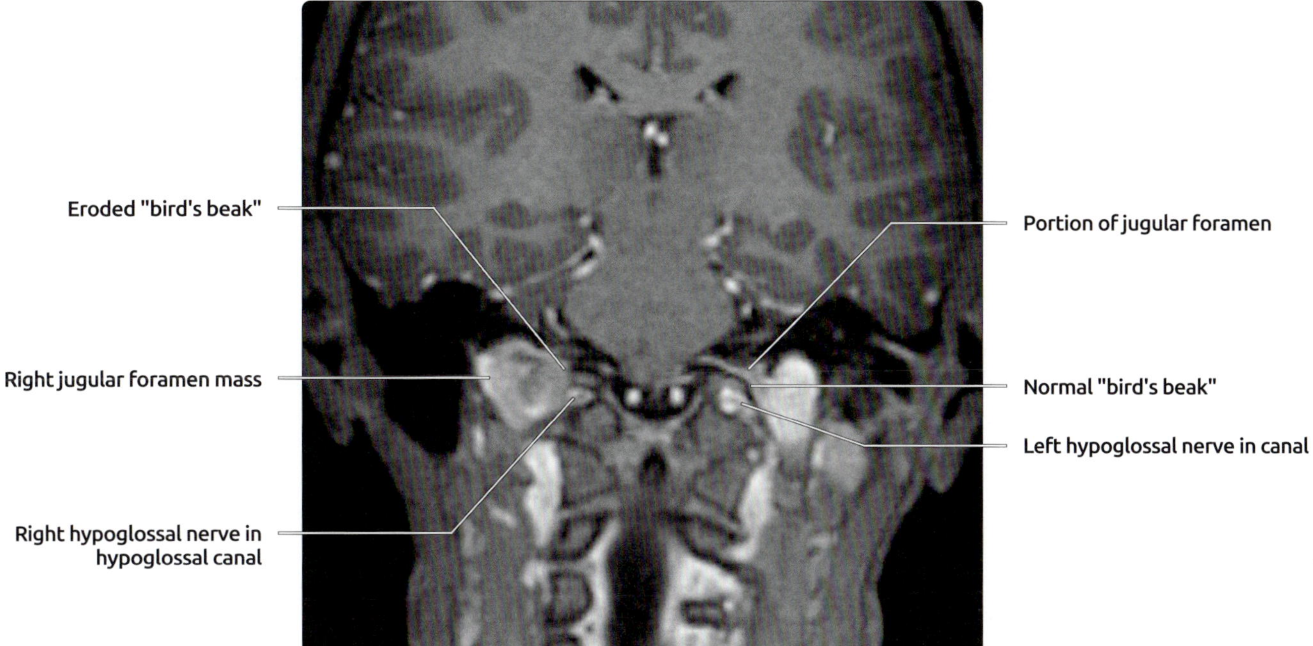

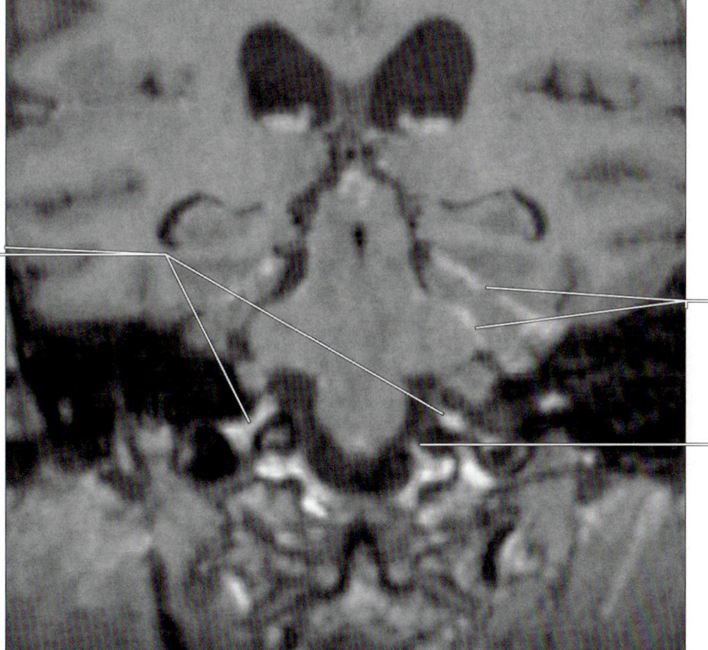

(Top) *Coronal T1 FS MR demonstrates a heterogeneously enhancing skull base mass along the right jugular foramen. Note the smooth erosion of the right lateral jugular tubercle ("bird's beak") and the intact hypoglossal canal with the nerve below the "bird's beak."* **(Bottom)** *Coronal T1 FS MR demonstrates abnormal leptomeningeal enhancement, including leptomeningeal spread along the left hypoglossal nerve cisternal segment entering into the hypoglossal canal. Again note abnormal leptomeningeal enhancement seen along bilateral jugular foramina above the "bird's beaks."*

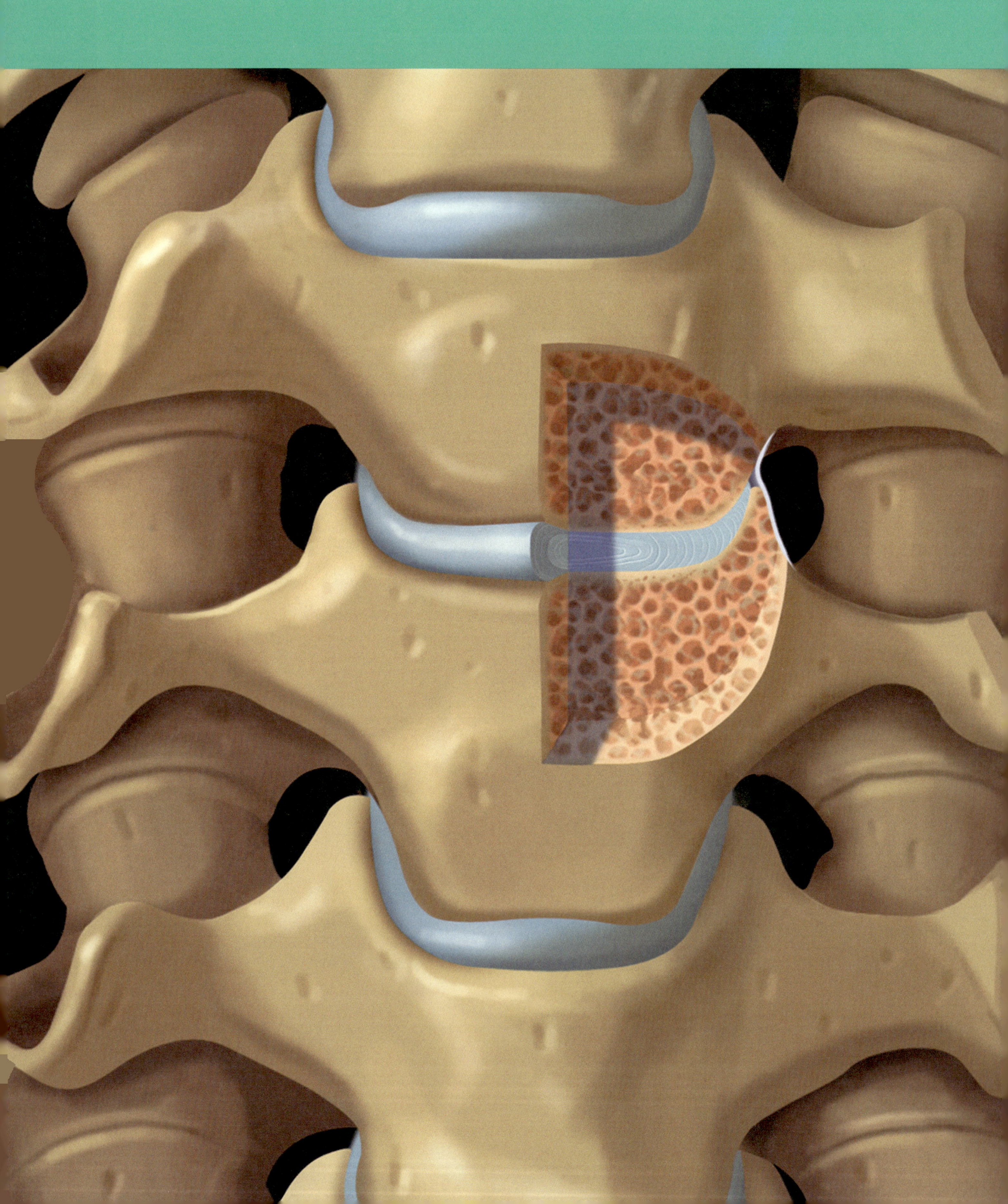

SECTION 9
Spine

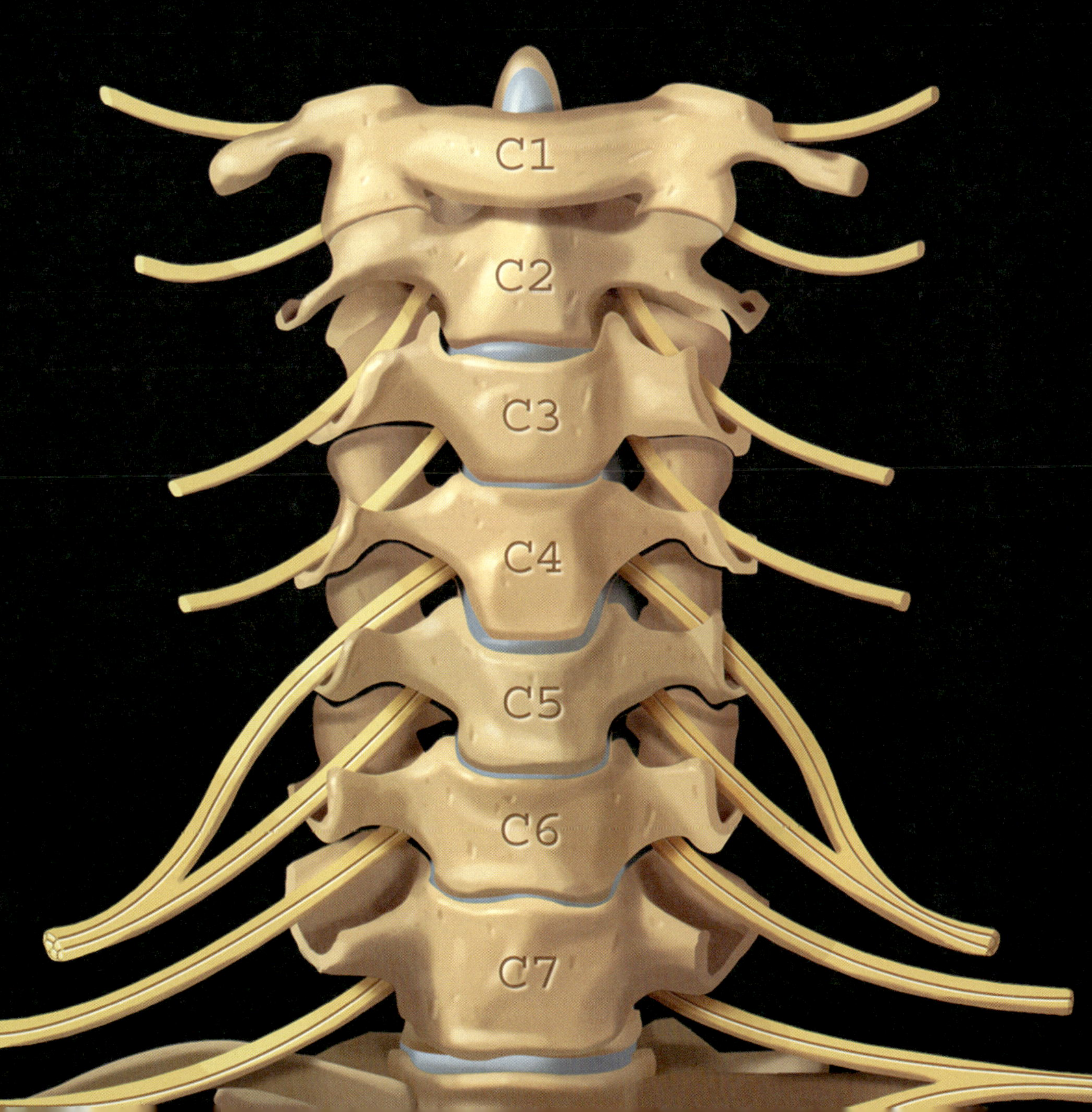

TERMINOLOGY

Definitions

- Craniocervical junction (CCJ): C1, C2, and articulation with skull base

GROSS ANATOMY

Components

- **Bones**
  - **Occipital bone**
    - Occipital condyles: Paired, oval-shaped prominences of inferior lateral exoccipital portion of occipital bone
    - Articular facet projects laterally
    - **Basion**: Anterior margin of foramen magnum: Inferior tip of clivus (formed by basiocciput)
    - **Opisthion**: Posterior margin of foramen magnum: Most inferior aspect of squamous occipital bone
  - **C1 (atlas)**
    - Composed of anterior and posterior arches; no body
    - Paired lateral masses with their superior and inferior articular facets
    - Large transverse processes with transverse foramen
  - **C2 (axis)**
    - Body and superiorly projecting odontoid process
    - Superior facet positioned relatively anteriorly; inferior facet posterior with elongated pars interarticularis
- **Joints**
  - **Atlantooccipital joints**
    - Inferior articular facet of occipital condyle: Oval, convex surface; projects laterally
    - Superior articular facet of C1: Oval, concave anteroposteriorly; projects medially
  - **Median atlantoaxial joints**
    - Pivot-type joint between dens + ring formed by anterior arch + transverse ligament of C1
    - Synovial cavities between transverse ligament/odontoid and atlas/odontoid articulations
  - **Lateral atlantoaxial joints**
    - Inferior articular facet of C1: Concave mediolaterally; projects medially in coronal plane
    - Superior articular facet of C2: Convex surface; projects laterally
- **Ligaments**
  - **Anterior atlantooccipital membrane (AAOM)**: a.k.a. anterior atlantooccipital ligament
    - Connects upper margin of C1 anterior arch to basion
    - Located posterior to longus capitis muscle
    - Forms anterior margin of **supradental space**
  - **Superficial anterior atlantooccipital ligament (SAAOL)**: Midline cord-like ligament extending from anterior tubercle of C1 to basion
    - Located posterior to longus capitis muscle and just anterior to AAOM
  - **Anterior longitudinal ligament (ALL)**
    - Extends from basiocciput of skull to anterior tubercle of C1 and then along front of body of C2 toward front of upper sacrum
    - Between C1 and basion, ALL continuous laterally with AAOM
  - **Odontoid ligaments**
    - **Apical ligament**: Small fibrous band extending from dens tip to basion; elastic fibers around **notochordal remnant** core (rudimentary nucleus pulposus)
    - **Alar ligaments**: Thick, horizontally directed ligaments extending from lateral surface of dens tip to anteromedial occipital condyles
  - **Cruciate ligament**
    - **Transverse atlantal ligament (TAL)**: Horizontal component between lateral masses of C1; passes posterior to dens to support it like pillow from behind
      - ◻ Strongest and thickest CCJ ligament
      - ◻ TAL disruption: Dens may move posteriorly and compress spinal cord
    - **Craniocaudal component**: Fibrous band from TAL superiorly to foramen magnum **(crus superioris)** and inferiorly to posterior body of C2 **(crus inferioris)**
  - **Tectorial membrane (membrana tectoria)**
    - Superior continuation of **posterior longitudinal ligament** above body of C2 level; attaches to anterior rim of foramen magnum
    - Located posterior to dens and cruciate ligament; intimately contacts dura
    - Forms posterior margin of **supradental space**
  - **Posterior atlantooccipital membrane**
    - Superior continuation of **ligamentum flavum**
    - Posterior arch of C1 to posterior margin of foramen magnum; surrounded by normal fat
    - Deficit laterally where vertebral artery enters on superior surface of C1
  - **Ligamentum nuchae**
    - Superior continuation of **supraspinous ligament**
    - From C7 spinous process to external occipital protuberance (EOP), restricts hyperflexion
    - **Dorsal raphe**: Thick **funicular** segment posteriorly (low signal on all MR sequences)
      - ◻ Extends from C7 spinous process to EOP
    - **Medial septum**: Thin **lamellar membranous** portion (shows surrounding fat signal on MR)
      - ◻ Extends from anterior surface of dorsal raphe into deep neck, reaching ligamentum flavum
      - ◻ Blends into posterior atlantooccipital membrane and posterior atlantoaxial membrane and **attaches to posterior spinal dura** via **myodural bridges**
      - ◻ On sagittal STIR MR, do not mistake normal bright venous plexus at anterior aspect of interspinous ligament for injury
  - **Myodural bridges**
    - Especially in children, traction on myodural bridges may pull dura away from arachnoid, leading to spinal subdural hemorrhage
    - Traction on intradural dentate ligaments & nerve roots may transmit forces to spinal cord & brainstem
- **Supradental (supraodontoid) space**
  - Extradural space filled with fat, central varicose veins connected to peripheral cavernous sinus-like veins, and apical arterial arcade at anterior CCJ superior to dens
  - Also contains apical ligament, crus superioris of cruciate ligament, and subtectorial membrane
  - Anterior and posterior borders: AAOM and tectorial membrane
  - Superior border: Clivus/basion; inferior border: Dens

- Inferolateral border: Alar ligaments; lateral border: Occipital condyles
- Supradental space normal fat density obscured due to edema/hemorrhage in CCJ ligamentous injury
  - Correlates well with tectorial membrane injury (supradental space sign)
- **Subtle signs of CCJ ligamentous injury**
  - **Supradental space sign**
  - Loss of normal **fat** density **along posterior atlantooccipital membrane** due to edema/hemorrhage
  - Intracranial **retroclival hematoma** with **elevation of tectorial membrane**

IMAGING ANATOMY

Overview

- **Basion-dens interval (BDI)**: Sagittal CT: < 9.1 mm, 8.5 mm in 95%; range 1.4-9.1 mm (< 12 mm on plain radiograph)
  - Between basion tip and tip of dens; reliable measurement for CCJ distraction injury
  - In children: < 9.5 mm with ossified dens tip & < 11.6 mm without ossified dens tip
- **Atlantooccipital interval (AOI)**: Parasagittal CT: < 1.4 mm; range 0.5-1.8 mm (no data on plain radiograph for adults)
  - Measured perpendicular to articular surfaces of occipital condyle and lateral mass of C1
  - Drawn at center of this atlantooccipital joint by correlating sagittal and coronal images
  - In children: < 2.5 mm; range 0.4-3.3 mm (< 5 mm on plain radiograph)
- **Anterior atlantodental interval (ADI)**: Sagittal CT: < 2 mm; range 0.5-2.4 mm (< 3.0 mm in men and < 2.5 mm in women on plain radiograph)
  - At midline of anterior atlantoaxial joint between anterior arch of C1 and dens
  - In children: < 2.6 mm; range 0.4-3.2 mm (< 4-5 mm on plain radiograph)
- **Powers ratio**: Sagittal CT: < 0.9; range 0.6-1.2 (< 1 on plain radiograph)
  - Ratio of distance from basion tip to C1 spinolaminar line: Opisthion tip to C1 anterior arch posterior aspect midpoint
- **Basion-axis (posterior axial line) interval (BAI)**: Sagittal CT: Posterior axial line < 12 mm posterior to basion, or < 4 mm anterior to basion; range minus 8.7-26 mm (< 12 mm on plain radiograph)
  - Between basion tip and posterior axial line
  - Not reliable; varies significantly depending on drawing posterior axial line including vs. not including osteophytic projection from posterior aspect of dens
- **C1-C2 interspinous space**
  - ≤ 12 mm on lateral radiograph
  - **Interspinous ratio**: C1-C2 interspinous space measurement:C2-C3 interspinous space measurement
    - Normal interspinous ratio < 2.5
- **Wackenheim (clivus-canal) line**
  - Along posterior clivus (dorsum sellae to basion)
  - Posterior odontoid tip should lie anteroinferior to this
- **Welcher basal angle**
  - Angle between lines drawn along planes of sphenoid bone (nasion-tip of dorsum sellae line) and posterior clivus [dorsum sellae-basion line (Wackenheim line)]
  - Normal < 140° (average 132°), ↑ in platybasia
- **Chamberlain line**
  - Between hard palate and opisthion
  - Odontoid tip ≥ 5 mm above line abnormal
- **McGregor line**
  - Between hard palate to base of occipital bone
  - Odontoid tip ≥ 7 mm above line abnormal
- **Clivus canal angle**
  - Junction of Wackenheim line and posterior axial line (line along posterior C2 body and dens); 150° (flexion) to 180° (extension)
  - Abnormal < 150° (chance for ventral cord compression)
- **McRae line**
  - Drawn between basion and opisthion
  - Normal 35-mm diameter; dens tip below this line
- **Boogaard angle**
  - Angle between McRae line and Wackenheim line
  - Normal angle 126° ± 6°; > 136° in platybasia
- **Klaus height index**
  - Distance between tip of dens and **Twining line** (line between tuberculum sellae and internal occipital protuberance)
  - Normal height 40 mm; < 36 mm in basilar impression
- **Harris ring**
  - Ring-like opacity on C2 on lateral view radiograph
  - Formed by superimposition of lateral masses of C2 on body of C2, at base of dens region
  - Harris ring disruption seen in dens fractures especially type III, less commonly in type II
  - ↑ AP diameter of Harris ring with significant comminution of body of C2
    - May be associated with **fat C2 sign** on lateral view: ↑ AP diameter of body of C2 compared to body of C3
  - Harris ring normally incomplete at its inferior aspect and sometimes superiorly as well
  - **Break in anterior** or **posterior margin** of Harris ring: Possible **fracture** of odontoid base or body of C2
- **Pediatric pseudosubluxation**
  - Physiologic anterior displacement seen in 40% at C2-C3 level and 14% at C3-C4 level up to age 8
  - **Swischuk line**: Line joining anterior margin of posterior arch of C1 and C3
    - Pseudosubuxation: Anterior margin of C2 posterior arch within 1-2 mm of Swischuk line
    - True subluxation (Hangman fracture): Anterior margin of C2 posterior arch > 2 mm posterior to Swischuk line
- **Pediatric physiologic anterior wedging**
  - Most prominent at C3, may have up to 3-mm wedging
- **Frontal assessment of CCJ**
  - Lateral masses of C1 and C2 should align
  - Overlapping lateral masses can be normal variant in children
  - **Rule of Spence**
    - AP open-mouth radiograph: In C1 Jefferson burst fracture, combined sum of C1 lateral mass displacement in relation to C2 on either side measuring 6.9 mm **predicts TAL disruption**
  - **Atlantooccipital joint angle**
    - Angle formed at junction of lines traversing joints
    - 125-130° normal, < 124° condyle hypoplasia

GRAPHICS

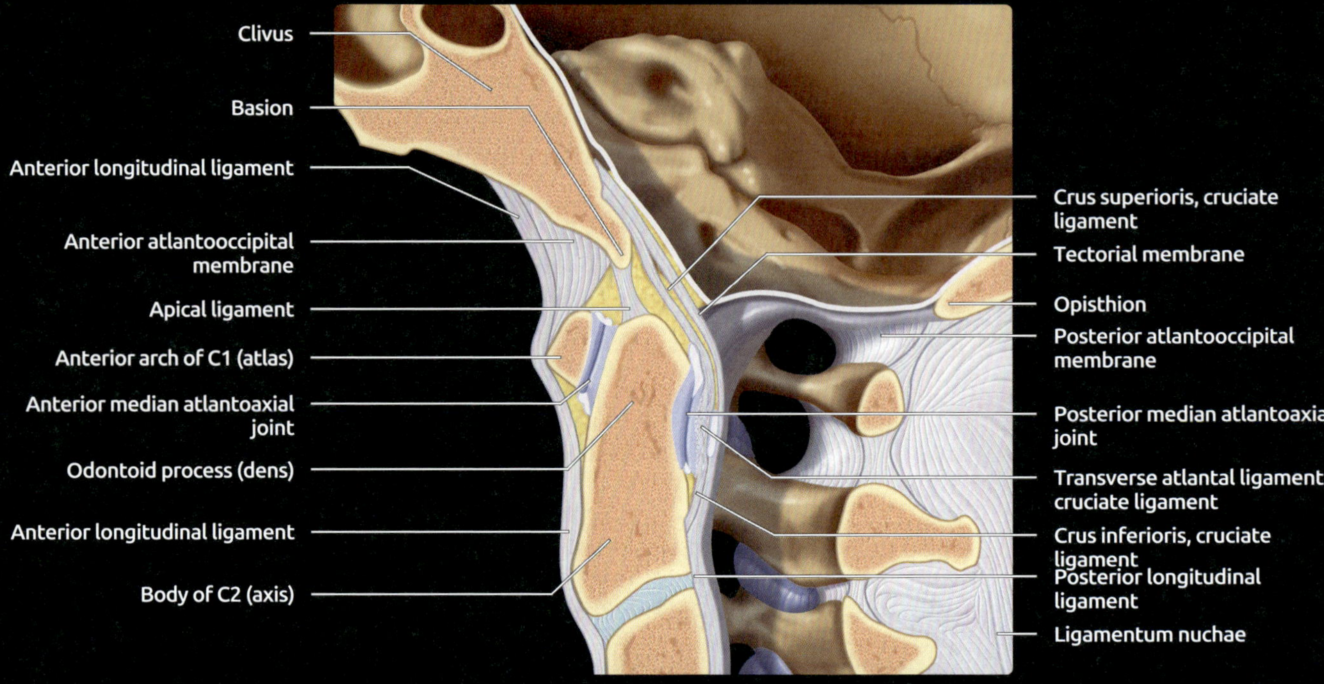

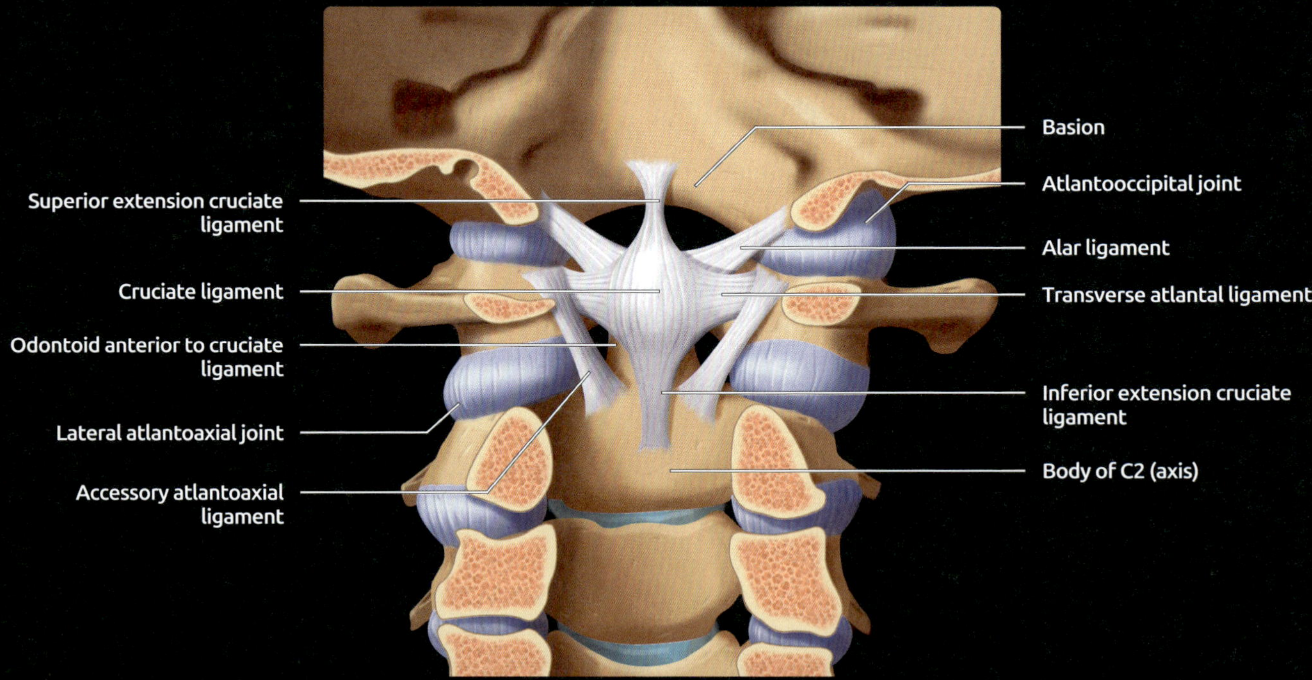

(Top) *Sagittal midline graphic of the craniocervical junction (CCJ) is shown. The complex articulations and ligamentous attachments are highlighted. The midline atlantoaxial articulations consist of anterior and posterior median atlantoaxial joints. The anterior joint is between the posterior aspect of the anterior C1 arch and the ventral aspect of odontoid process. The posterior joint is between the dorsal aspect of the odontoid process and the cruciate ligament. The midline view shows a series of ligamentous connection to the skull base, including the anterior atlantooccipital membrane, apical ligament, superior component of cruciate ligament, tectorial membrane, and posterior atlantooccipital membrane.* **(Bottom)** *Posterior graphic shows the CCJ with posterior elements cut away to define the components of the cruciate ligament and alar ligaments.*

C1 GRAPHICS

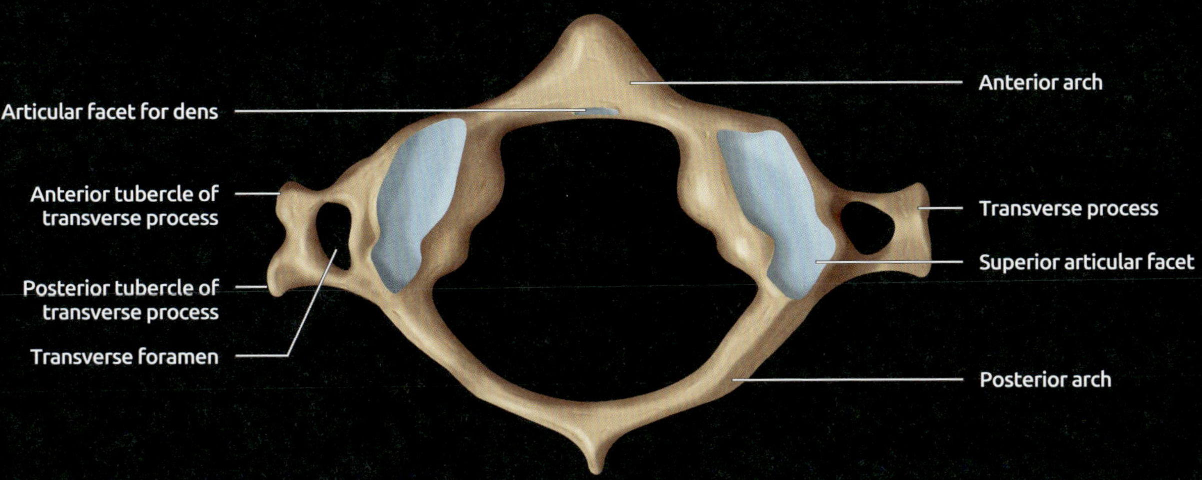

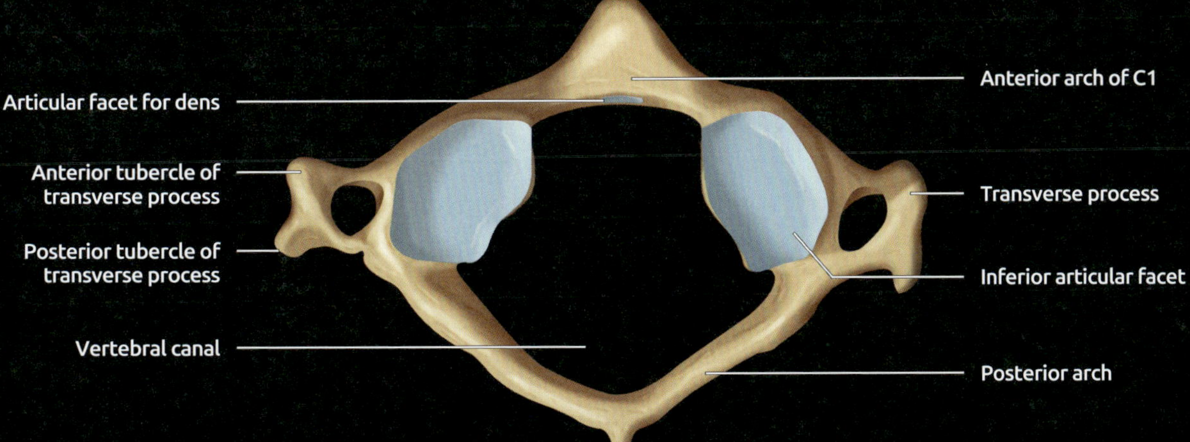

(Top) *Axial graphic shows atlas viewed from above. The characteristic ring shape is shown, composed of anterior and posterior arches and paired large lateral masses. The superior articular facet is concave anteroposteriorly and projects medially for articulation with the convex surface of the occipital condyle at the atlantooccipital joint. The anterior arch articulates with the odontoid process at the anterior median atlantoaxial joint.* **(Bottom)** *Axial graphic shows the atlas viewed from below. The large inferior facet surface is concave mediolaterally and projects medially for articulation with the convex surface of the superior articular facet of C2. The canal of the atlas is ~ 3 cm in AP diameter. Spinal cord, odontoid process, and free space for cord are each ~ 1 cm in diameter. The size of the anterior midline tubercle of the anterior arch and the spinous process of the posterior arch are quite variable.*

C2 GRAPHICS

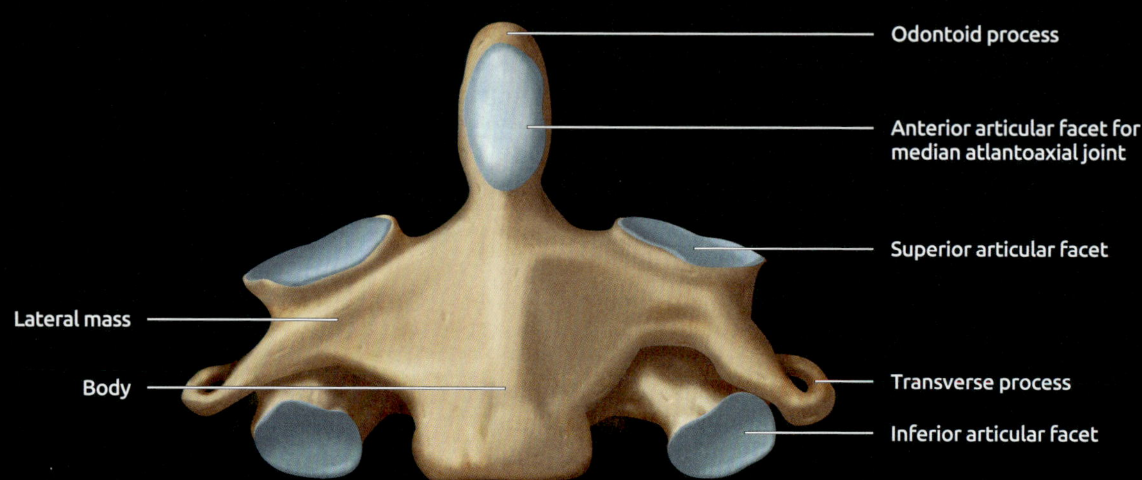

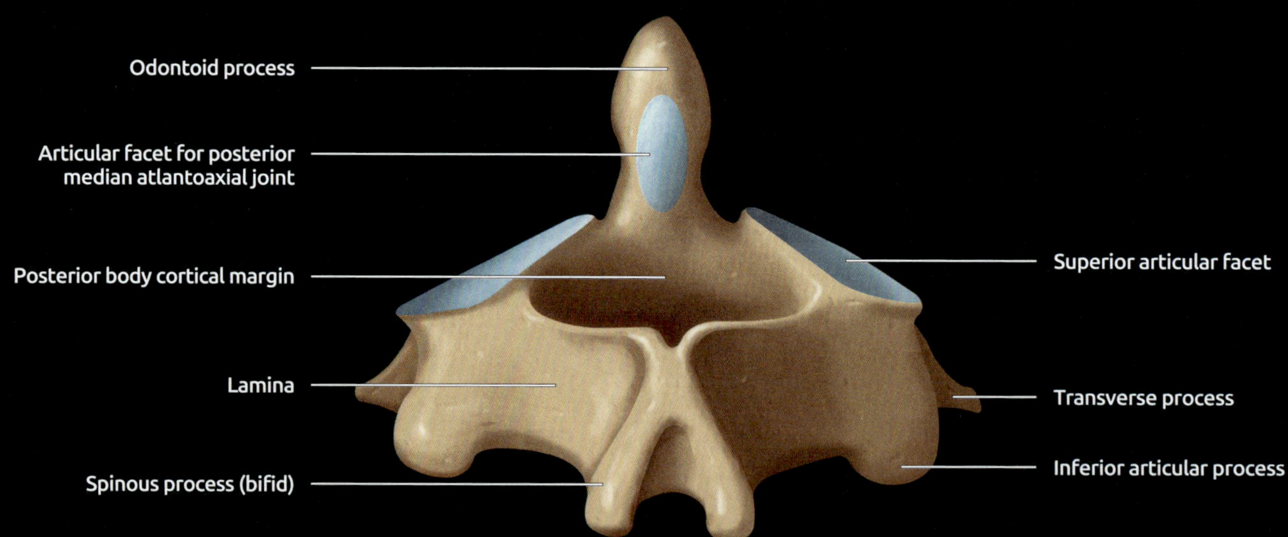

(Top) *Axis viewed from the anterior perspective is shown. The odontoid process is the "purloined" embryologic centrum of C1, which is incorporated into C2, giving C2 its unique morphology. The C2 body laterally is defined by large lateral masses for articulation with the inferior facet of C1. The elongated pars interarticularis of C2 ends with the inferior articular process for articulation with the superior articular facet of C3.* **(Bottom)** *Axis viewed from the posterior perspective is shown. The odontoid process has anterior and posterior joints for articulation with C1. The anterior median joint articulates with the C1 arch, while the posterior median joint (shown here) involves the transverse ligament.*

CRANIOMETRY GRAPHICS

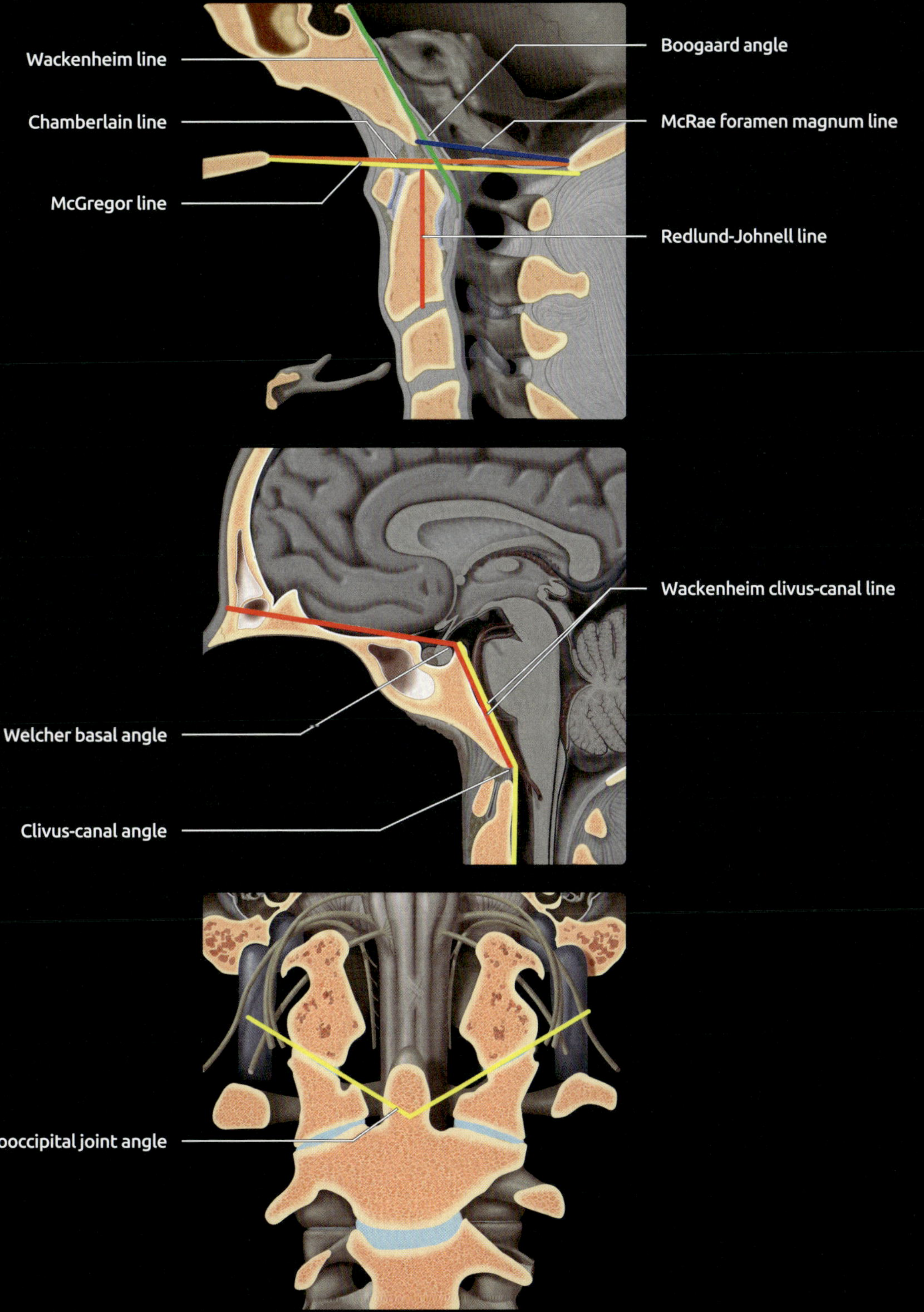

(Top) *Sagittal graphic shows important skull base craniometry. Wackenheim line (green) is drawn along posterior surface of clivus. McRae foramen magnum line (blue) is drawn between basion and opisthion. Boogaard angle is measured between McRae line and Wackenheim line. Chamberlain line (orange) is drawn between hard palate and opisthion. McGregor line (yellow) is drawn from hard palate to caudal point (base) of occipital bone. Redlund-Johnell line (red) is drawn from base of C2 to McGregor line.* **(Middle)** *Sagittal midline graphic shows Welcher basal angle between the lines drawn along plane of sphenoid bone and along clivus [nasion to tip of dorsum sellae (DS) and tip of DS to basion (Wackenheim clival line)] as per modified MR method of basal angle measurement. Instead of DS, other methods of basal angle measurement use center of sella or tuberculum sellae as center point of angle. Clivus canal angle measurement at junction of Wackenheim line and posterior axial line (line along posterior C2 body and dens) is also shown.* **(Bottom)** *Coronal graphic of the CCJ shows measurement of atlantooccipital joint angle; < 124° may reflect condyle hypoplasia.*

SAGITTAL BONE CT & CORONAL PD MR

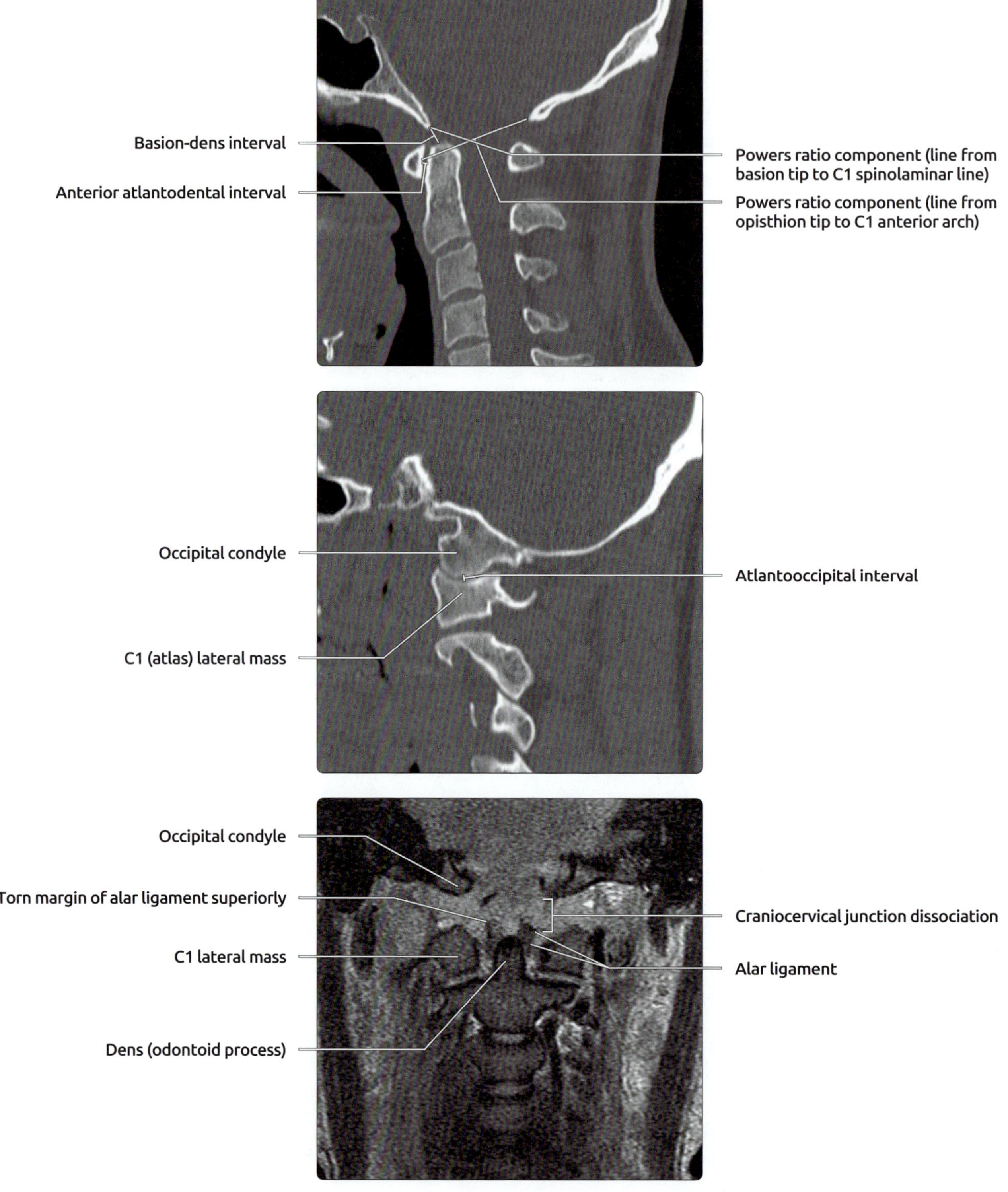

(Top) *Sagittal bone CT shows CCJ measurements. Basion-dens interval (BDI) is measured between basion tip and tip of dens. Powers ratio is the ratio between distance from basion tip to C1 spinolaminar line and from opisthion tip to C1 anterior arch posterior aspect midpoint. Anterior atlantodental interval (ADI) is also shown. Basion-axis (posterior axial line) interval (BAI) is between basion tip and line projected superiorly along posterior C2 margin. BAI is not not reliable; varies depending on drawing posterior axial line including vs. not including posterior osteophytic projection from upper dens.* **(Middle)** *Sagittal CT shows atlantooccipital interval (AOI) measurement done perpendicular to the articular surfaces of occipital condyle and lateral mass of C1. AOI is measured at the center of the atlantooccipital joint by correlating sagittal and coronal images.* **(Bottom)** *Coronal thin-section high-resolution PD MR in a patient with severe CCJ distraction injury shows the dissociation of the skull base from the cervical spine with wide gap. Note that the bilateral alar ligaments are torn superiorly and are not attached to the occipital condyles but still attached to the odontoid process.*

BONE CT & T1 MR CRANIOMETRY

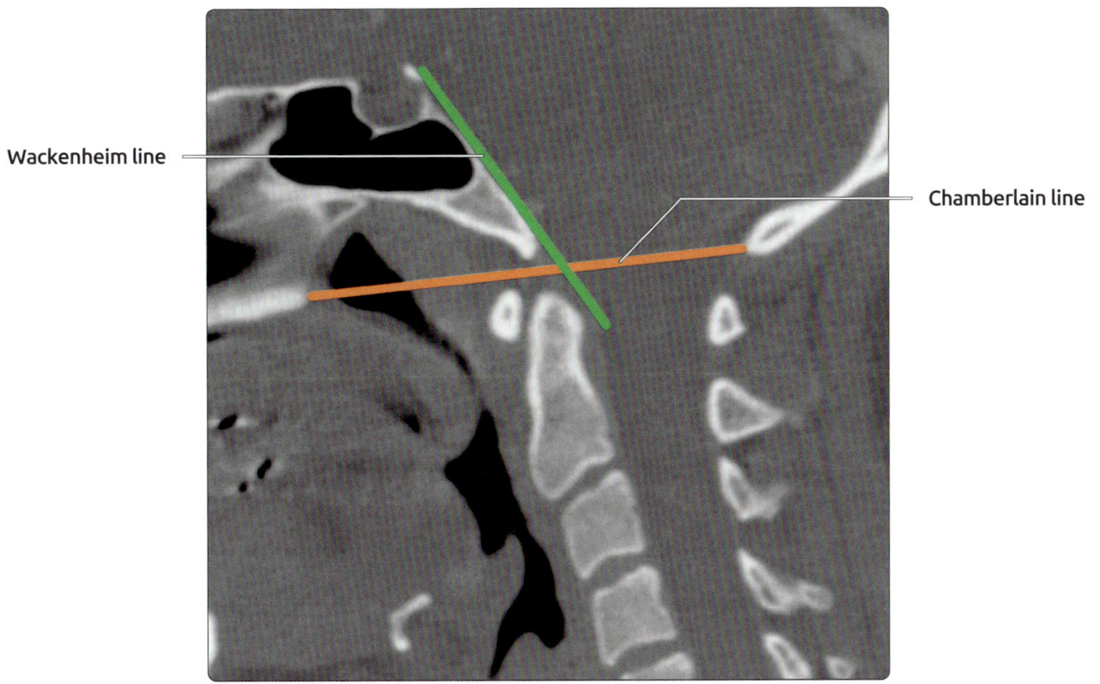

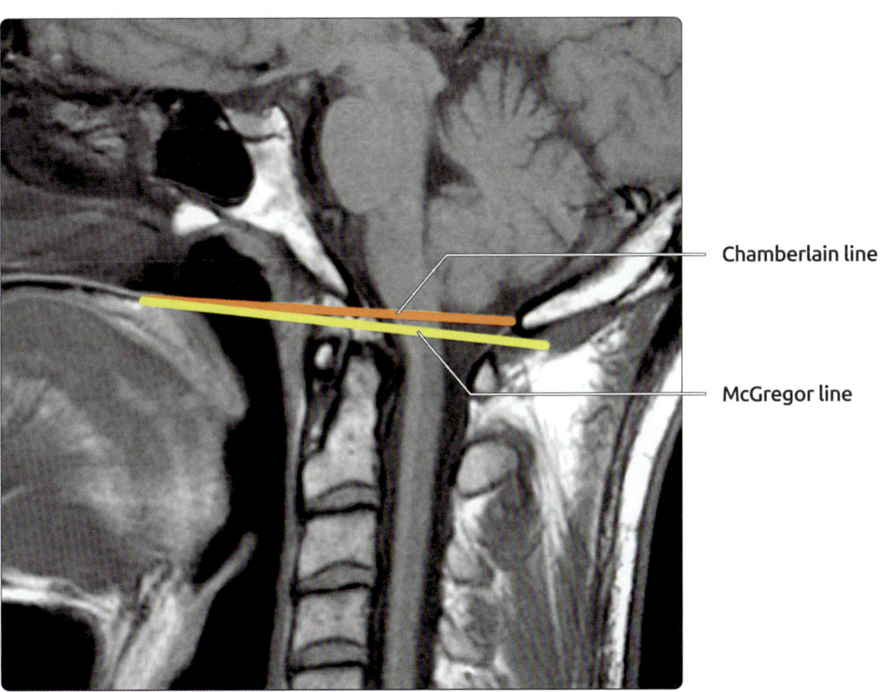

(Top) *Sagittal CT reformat in the midline is shown. The Chamberlain line is shown in orange extending from the hard palate to the opisthion. Projection of up to 1/3 of the dens (5 mm) above this line is normal. The Wackenheim line is shown in green along the clivus. The dens should lie immediately inferior to this line, and any intersection is considered abnormal.* **(Bottom)** *Sagittal T1 MR shows the Chamberlain line in orange. The odontoid tip ≥ 5 mm above the line defines the basilar impression. The McGregor line is shown in yellow. This line has the same significance as the Chamberlain line, with the odontoid tip ≥ 7 mm above the line, defining the basilar impression.*

LATERAL RADIOGRAPHY CRANIOMETRY

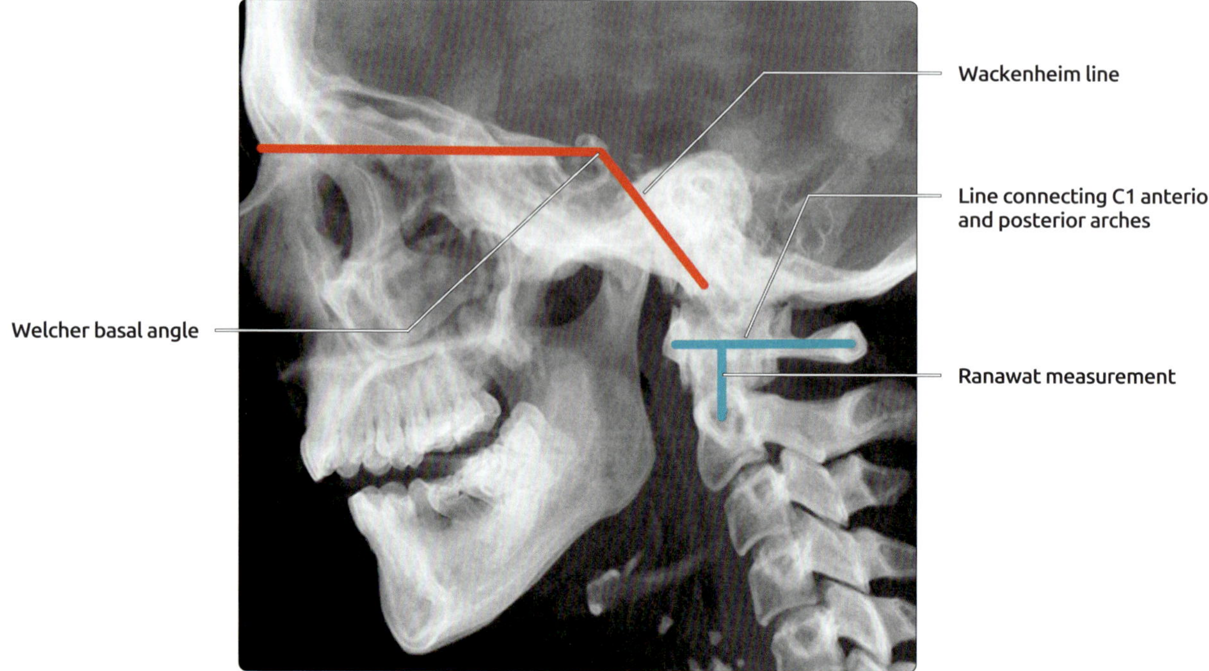

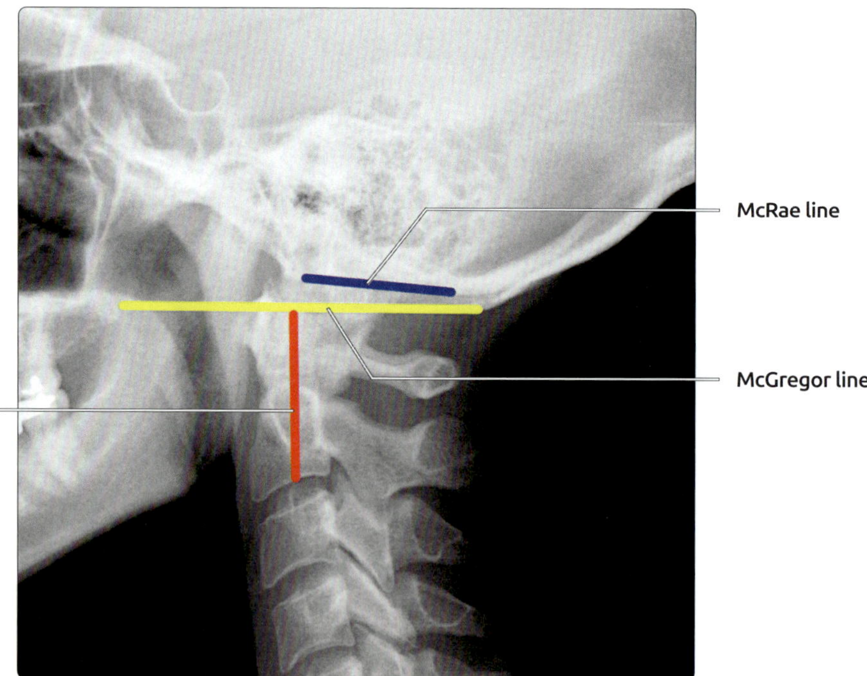

(Top) *In this lateral plain film radiograph, the Welcher basal angle is shown in red. Platybasia exists if the angle is > 140° (normal is < 140°). Ranawat measurement is shown in blue and is used to assess collapse at the C1-C2 articulation. Ranawat measurement is taken from the center of sclerotic Harris ring of C2 to the line drawn along the axis of the C1 vertebra (connecting the C1 anterior and posterior arches). Normal is ~ 17 mm in men and ~ 15 mm in women; < 13 mm in basilar invagination.* **(Bottom)** *In this lateral plain film radiograph, the McRae line is shown in blue. Normal is ~ 35-mm diameter. The normal odontoid process does not extend above this line. The Redlund-Johnell measurement is shown in red. This measurement is from the base of the C2 body to the McGregor line (shown in yellow). Normal is ~ 34 mm in men and ~ 28 mm in women.*

LATERAL RADIOGRAPHY

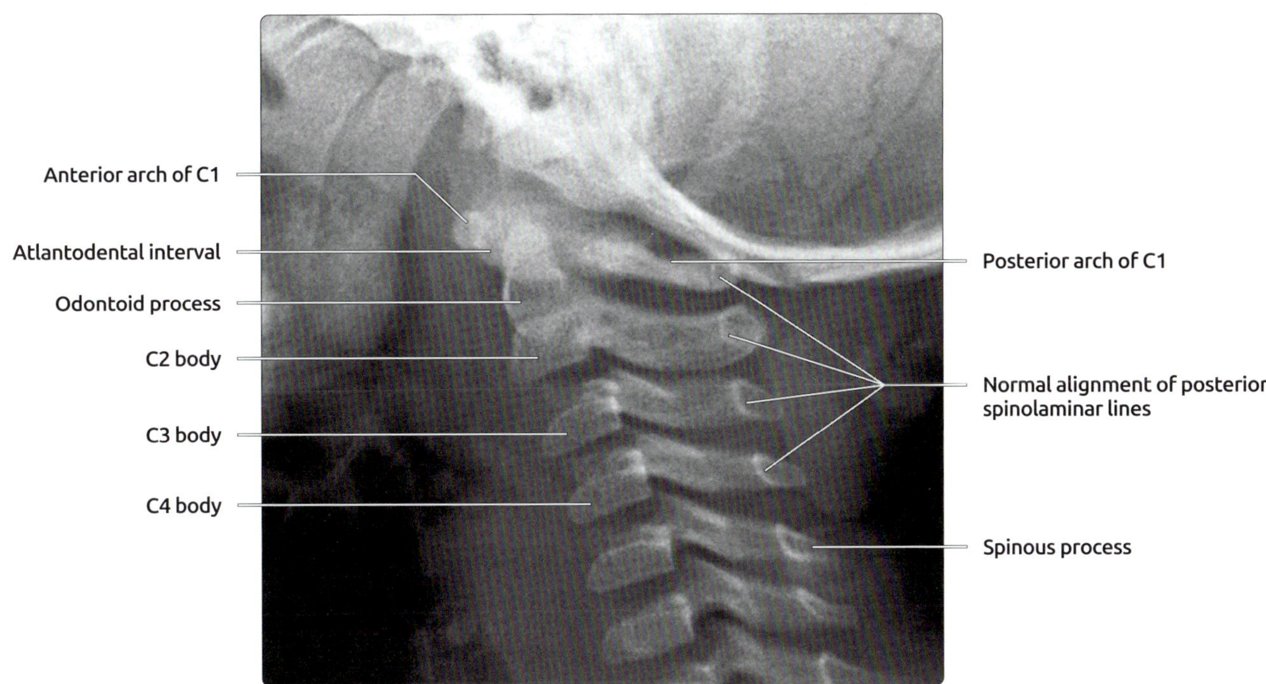

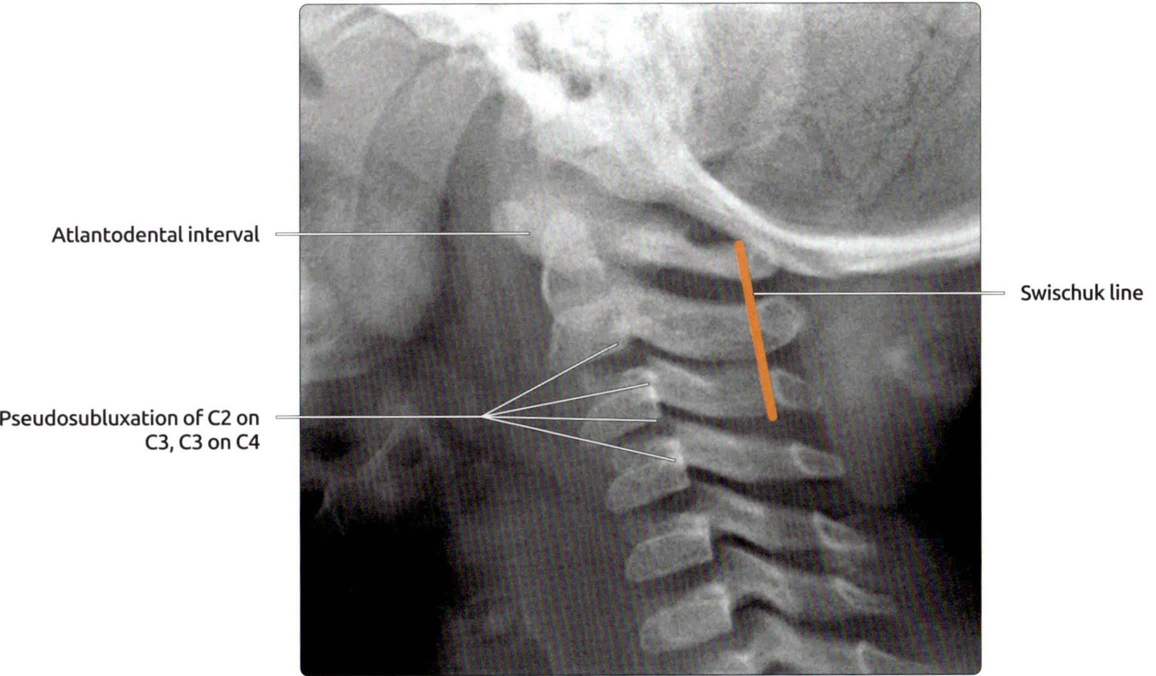

(Top) *Lateral plain film radiograph of the cervical spine in a child shows physiologic anterior displacement of C2 with respect to C3, and C3 with respect to C4, the so-called pseudosubluxation. Physiologic subluxation is differentiated from pathologic anterior displacement by the absence of prevertebral soft tissue swelling, reduction on extension, and assessment of the Swischuk line.* **(Bottom)** *Swischuk line is drawn joining the anterior margin of posterior arches of C1 and C3. In pseudosubuxation, the anterior margin of C2 posterior arch will be within 1-2 mm of Swischuk line on flexion and extension. In true subluxation (as in hangman fracture), the anterior margin of C2 posterior arch will be > 2 mm posterior to Swischuk line. The ADI is < 3.5 mm in children and < 3 mm in adults.*

RADIOGRAPHY

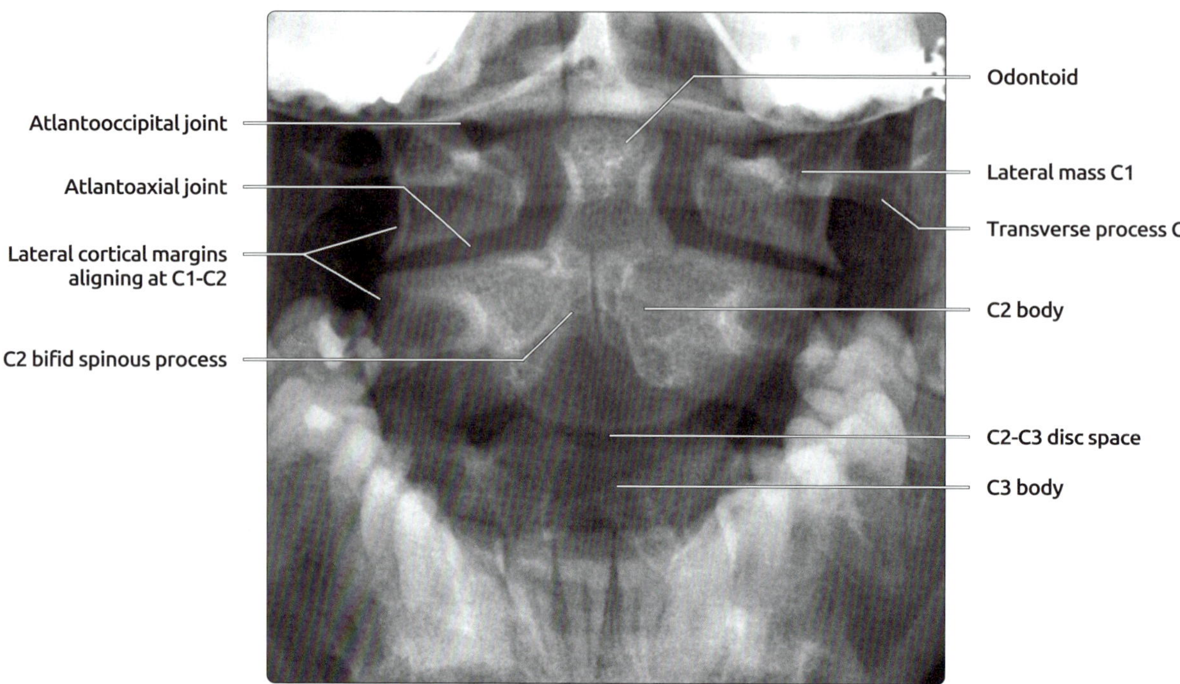

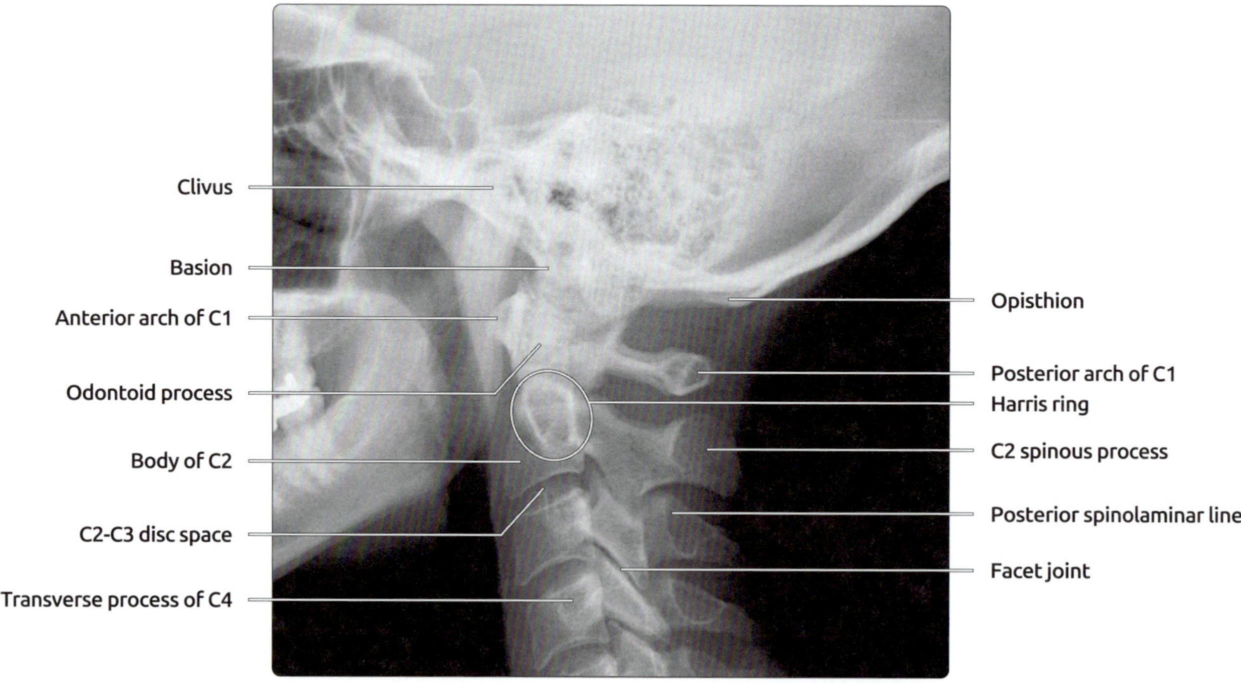

(Top) *AP open-mouth view shows the odontoid process. With proper positioning, the odontoid process is visualized in the midline with symmetrically placed lateral C1 masses on either side. The medial space between the odontoid and C1 lateral masses should be symmetric as well. The lateral cortical margins of the C1 and C2 lateral masses should align. The atlantoaxial joints are visible bilaterally with smooth cortical margins. The bifid C2 process should not be confused for fracture.* **(Bottom)** *Lateral radiograph shows the CCJ. There is smooth anatomic alignment of the posterior vertebral body margins and the posterior spinolaminar line of the posterior elements. The anterior arch of C1 should assume a well-defined oval appearance with sharp margination between the anterior C1 arch and the odontoid process. Harris ring is a sclerotic ring-like opacity on C2 on lateral radiograph, formed by superimposition of lateral masses of C2 on body of C2. Harris ring can be normally incomplete at its inferior aspect and sometimes superiorly as well. Break in anterior or posterior margin of Harris ring suggests possible fracture of odontoid base or body of C2.*

CORONAL BONE CT

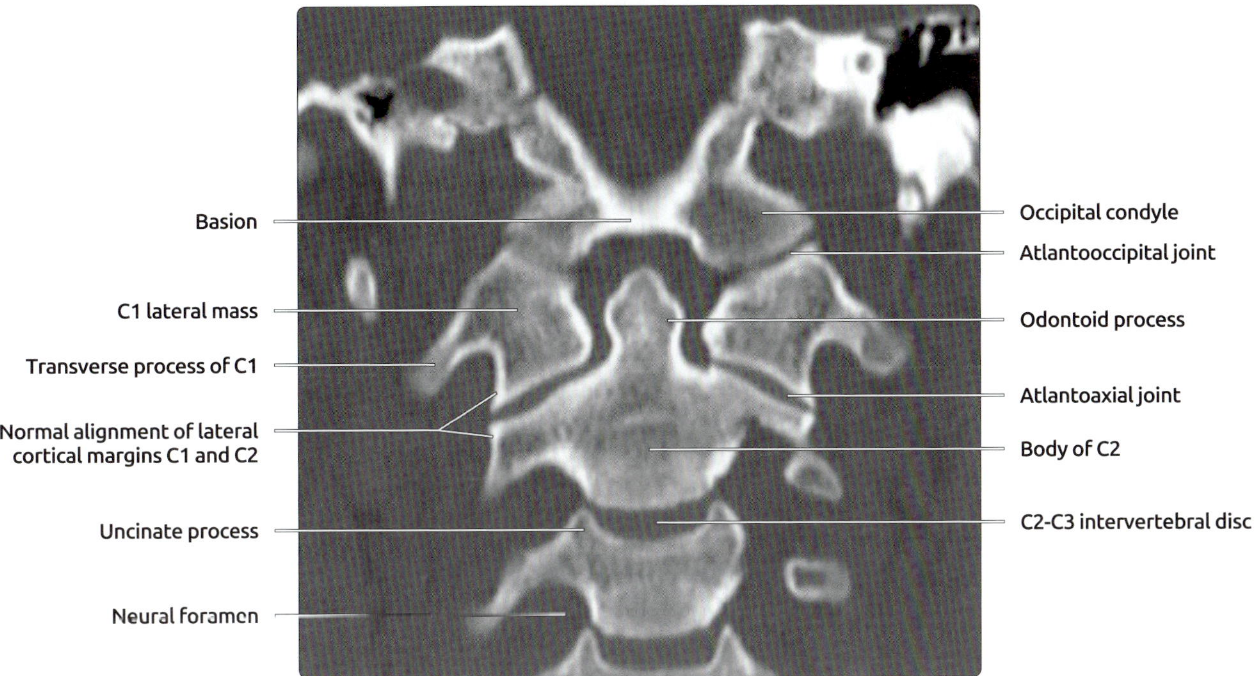

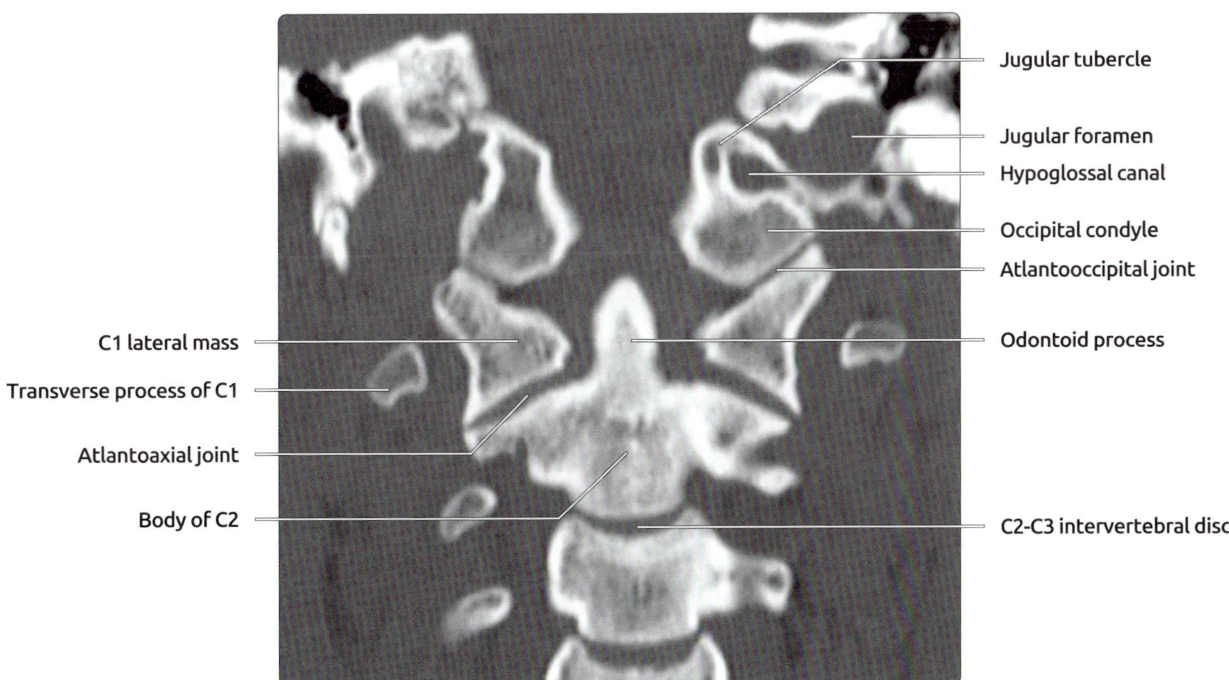

(Top) *First of 2 coronal bone CT reconstructions of the CCJ presented from anterior to posterior is shown. The odontoid process is visualized in the midline as a sharply corticated, bony peg with symmetrically placed lateral C1 masses on either side. The lateral cortical margins of the C1 lateral masses and the C2 lateral masses should align. The atlantooccipital and atlantoaxial joints are visible bilaterally with even joint margins and sharp cortical margins.* **(Bottom)** *More posterior view of the CCJ is shown. Both atlantooccipital joints are now well defined with smooth cortical margins sloping superolateral to inferomedial. The atlantoaxial joints are smoothly sloping inferolateral to superomedial. Note the double-eagle appearance (jugular tubercle on occipital condyle on both sides) sitting on mountain top (C2 vertebra with odontoid process), which is very useful to identify the jugular foramen and hypoglossal canal on coronal CT/MR. Occipital condyle forms the upper torso of the eagle, and jugular tubercle forms its beak, head, and neck. Jugular foramen is seen superolateral to the beak and head of the eagle. Hypoglossal canal is seen underneath the beak and neck.*

AXIAL BONE CT

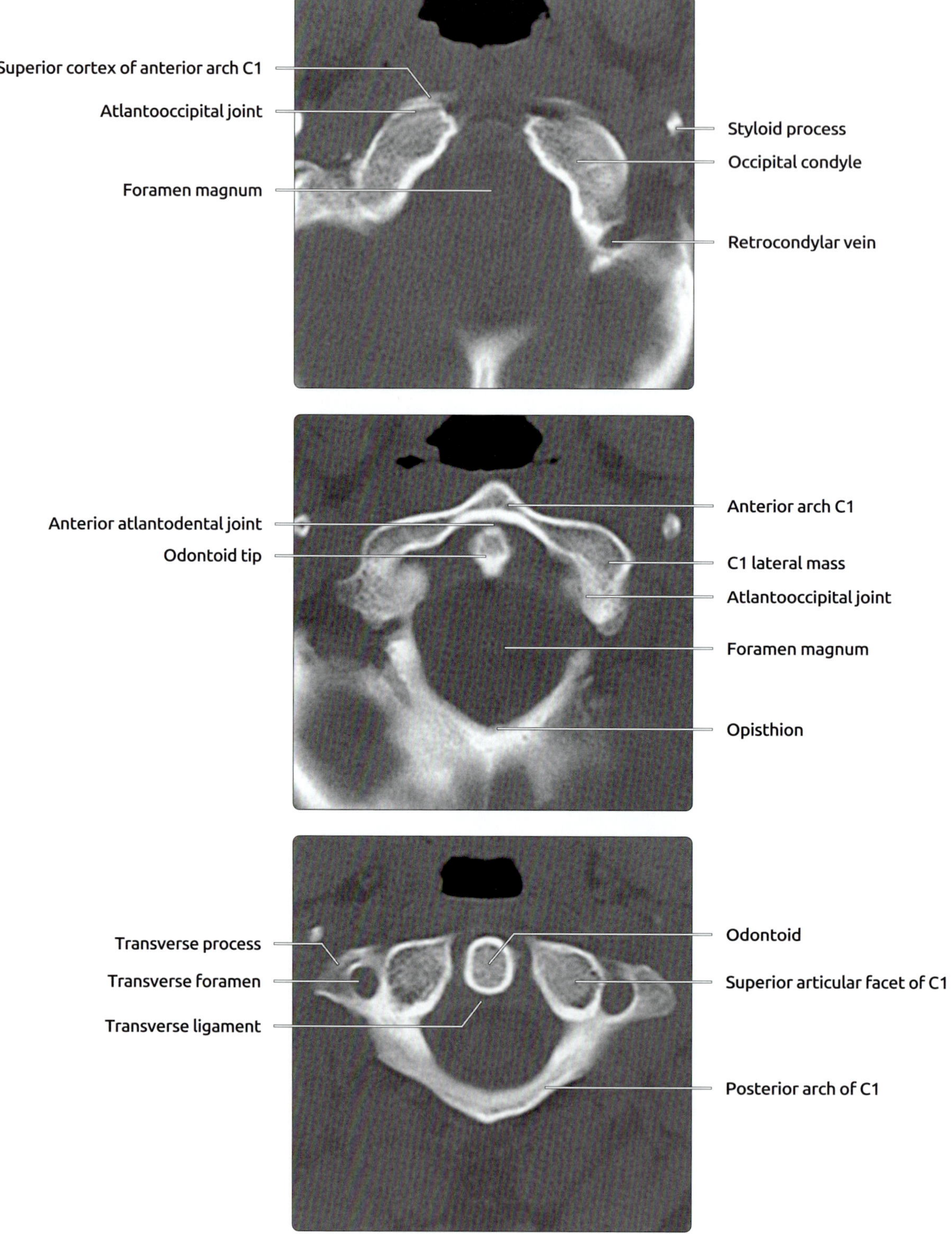

(Top) *First of 6 axial bone CT images through the CCJ presented from superior to inferior is shown. The anterolateral margin of the foramen magnum is formed by the prominent occipital condyles, which articulate with the superior articular facets of the C1 lateral masses.* **(Middle)** *More inferior image of the CCJ is shown. The anterior arch of C1 is now well defined with the odontoid process of C2 coming into plane. The atlantooccipital joint is seen in oblique section and therefore has poorly defined margins. The odontoid is tightly applied to the posterior margin of the C1 arch, held in place by the strong transverse component of the cruciate ligament.* **(Bottom)** *Image at the level of the atlas is shown. The unique morphology of the C1 is defined with its large transverse process with transverse foramen and ring shape.*

AXIAL BONE CT

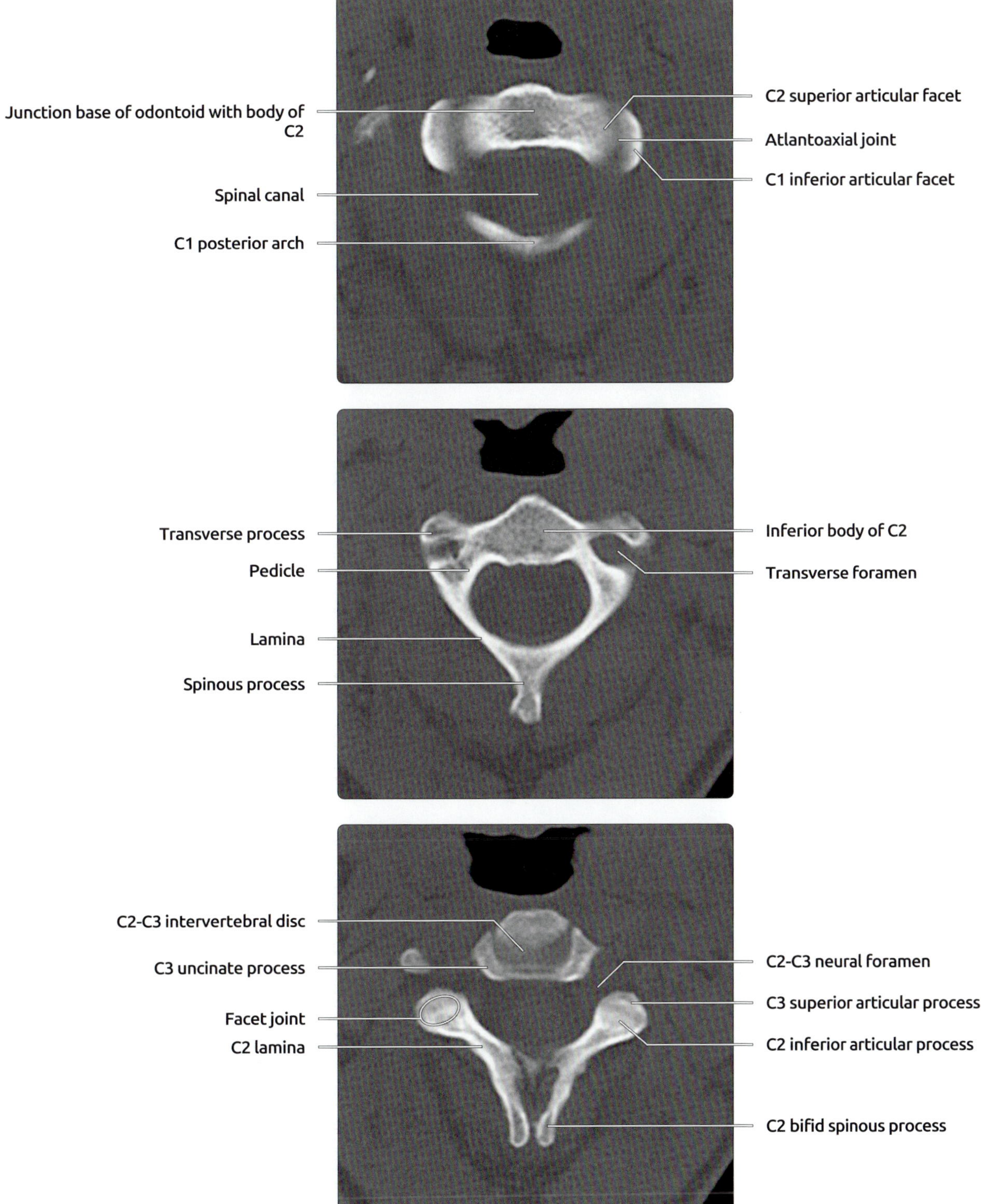

(Top) *Image through lateral atlantoaxial joints is shown. This section defines the junction of the odontoid process with the body of C2. The obliquely oriented atlantoaxial joints are partially seen with the C1 component lateral to the joint space and the C2 component medially.* **(Middle)** *Image through inferior C2 body level shows large C2 vertebral body and vertebral arch formed by gracile pedicles and laminae.* **(Bottom)** *Image through C2-C3 intervertebral disc level is shown. The C2-C3 neural foramen is well defined with the posterior margin formed by the superior articular process of C3. The spinous process of C2 is large and typically bifid. The C2-C3 disc assumes the characteristic cervical cup-shaped morphology bounded by uncinate processes.*

3D-VRT NECT

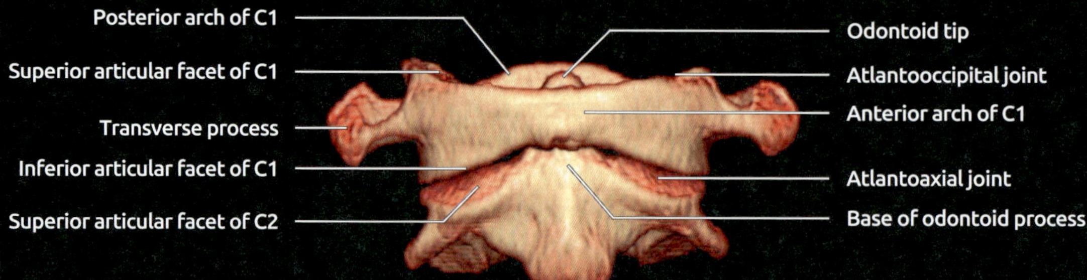

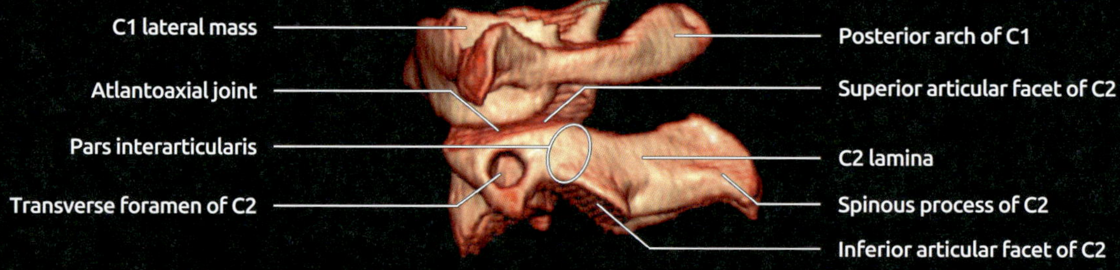

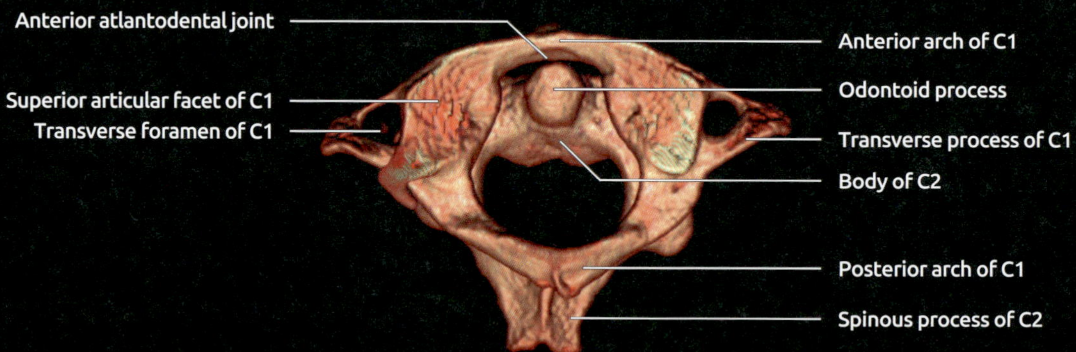

(Top) *Anterior 3D-VRT NECT examination is shown. The unique ability of the C1-C2 articulation to provide rotation is apparent in this projection with the bony peg of the odontoid process forming the pivot point for the C1 ring.* **(Middle)** *Lateral 3D-VRT NECT examination is shown. The complex lateral components of C1 and C2 bodies are highlighted in this projection. The superior facet of C2 is anteriorly positioned to articulate with the inferior articular facet of C1, while the inferior articular facet of C2 is more posterior, forming the top of the cervical articular "pillar." The articular facets are separated by the elongated pars interarticularis.* **(Bottom)** *Superior 3D-VRT NECT examination depicts the relationship of the C1 ring with underlying C2 odontoid and lateral masses.*

SAGITTAL T1 MR

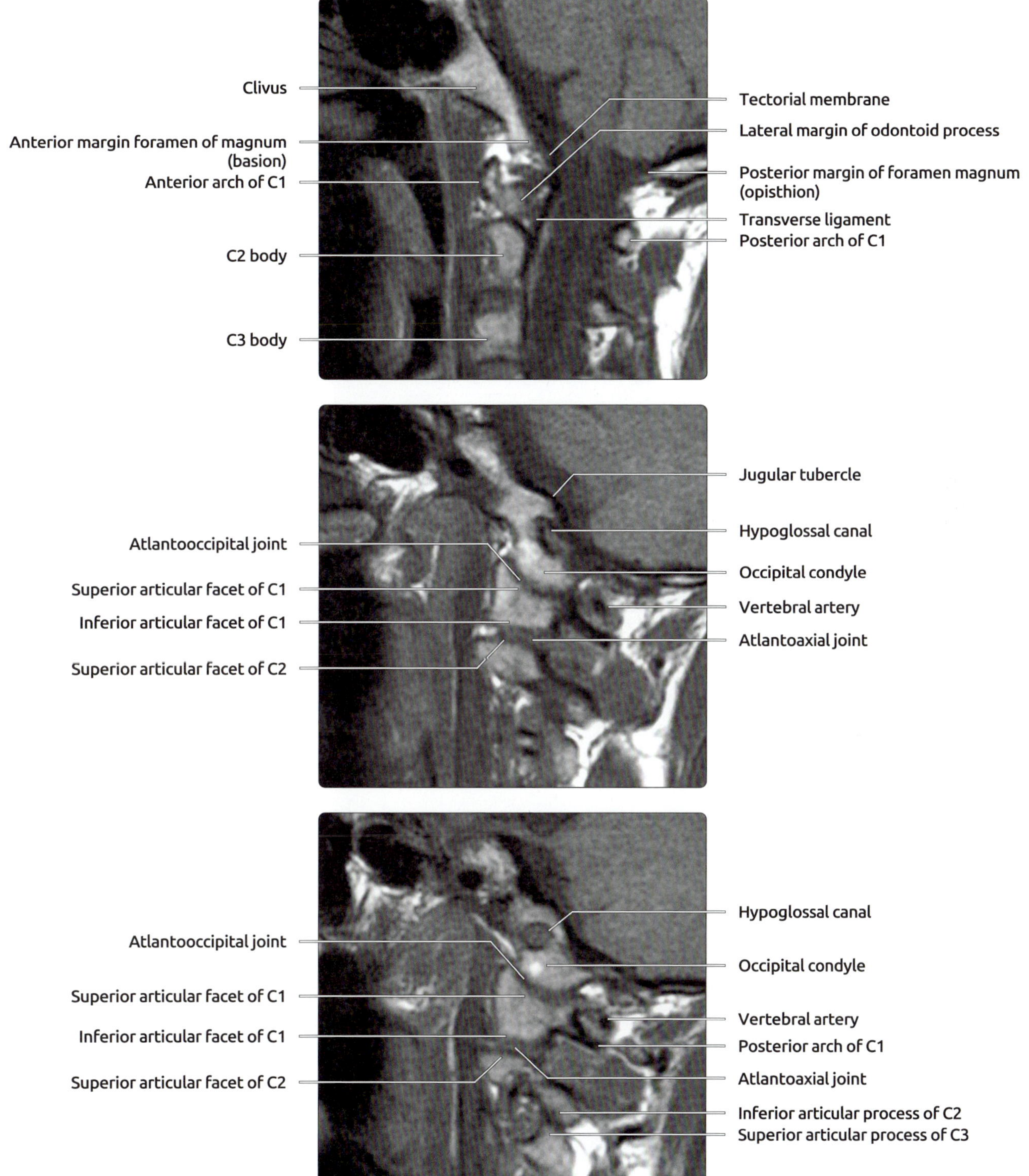

(Top) *First of 3 parasagittal T1 MR images from medial to lateral through the atlantooccipital joint is shown. This image extends through the lateral cortical margin of the odontoid, which is incompletely visualized. The anterior arch of C1 is obliquely visualized as it curves posterolaterally. The lateral extension of the cruciate ligament, the transverse ligament, is prominent.* **(Middle)** *The relationship of the occipital condyle, C1 lateral mass, and atlantoaxial joint is highlighted in this image. The articular surface of the occipital condyle is convex and the superior facet of C1 is concave, allowing for flexion/extension.* **(Bottom)** *More lateral image of the CCJ is shown. The atlantooccipital joint and atlantoaxial joints are visible with sharp, smooth cortical margins.*

SAGITTAL CT & MR

Supradental space
Anterior atlantooccipital membrane
Apical ligament
Anterior arch of C1
Anterior atlantodental joint
Base of odontoid process
C2-C3 intervertebral disc
Basion
Tectorial membrane
Odontoid tip
Transverse atlantal ligament, cruciate ligament
Opisthion
Posterior atlantooccipital membrane
Posterior arch of C1
C2 spinous process
Posterior longitudinal ligament

Supradental space fat
Anterior atlantooccipital membrane
Anterior arch of C1
Anterior atlantodental joint
Anterior longitudinal ligament
Base of odontoid process
C2-C3 intervertebral disc
Basion
Apical ligament
Tectorial membrane
Opisthion
Posterior atlantooccipital membrane
Transverse atlantal ligament, cruciate ligament
Posterior arch of C1
Spinous process of C2

Anterior atlantooccipital membrane
Apical ligament
Anterior arch of C1
Anterior longitudinal ligament
Base of odontoid process
C2-3 intervertebral disc
Basion
Crus superioris, cruciate ligament
Tectorial membrane
Odontoid tip
Posterior atlantooccipital membrane
Transverse atlantal ligament, cruciate ligament
Posterior arch of C1
Posterior longitudinal ligament

(Top) *Sagittal midline CT reformat shows ligamentous structures visible at CCJ. Apical ligament is visible as a linear band between the odontoid tip and clivus. The tectorial membrane is the superior extension of the posterior longitudinal ligament. The anterior atlantooccipital membrane is continuous with the anterior longitudinal ligament. Supradental (supraodontoid) space is filled with fat, veins, and apical arterial arcade superior to the dens. It also contains the apical ligament, crus superioris of cruciate ligament and subtectorial membrane. Anterior and posterior borders are anterior atlantooccipital membrane and tectorial membrane, respectively. Obliteration of normal supradental space fat, and fat along posterior atlantooccipital membrane (between posterior arch of C1 and opisthion) suggest edema/hemorrhage.* **(Middle)** *Sagittal T1 MR midline image of the CCJ shows ligamentous structures. Transverse atlantal ligament (thick part of cruciate ligament) is a low-signal band dorsal to the odontoid.* **(Bottom)** *Sagittal T2 MR of the CCJ is shown. Tectorial membrane, crus superioris of cruciate ligament, apical ligament, and anterior atlantooccipital membranes are evident.*

AXIAL T2 MR

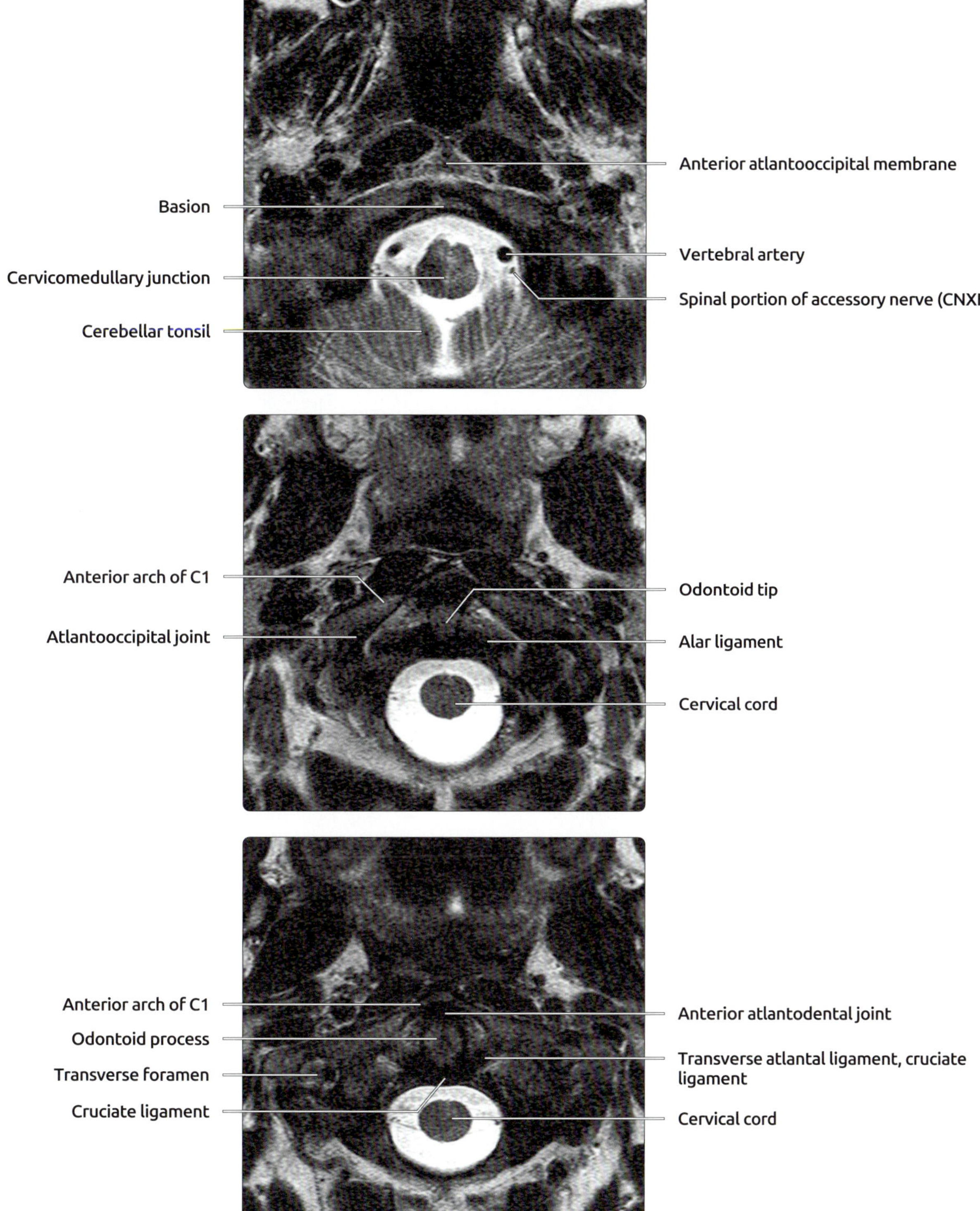

(Top) *First of 3 axial T2 MR images through the CCJ from superior to inferior shows the anterior margin of the foramen magnum, the cervicomedullary junction, and adjacent vertebral artery flow voids.* **(Middle)** *Image at level of C1 anterior arch is shown. The odontoid tip is seen as rounded, intermediate signal in the midline, ventral to the cervical cord. The anterior arch of C1 is visible with its well-defined cortical margins. The alar ligaments are identified as low signal intensity bands extending laterally from the lateral margins of the odontoid process toward the occipital condyles.* **(Bottom)** *More inferior MR through the atlantodental joint shows the anterior atlantodental joint along the ventral margin of the odontoid process. The cruciate ligament (transverse atlantal ligament component) is seen as low-signal bands curving over the dorsal margin of odontoid. Transverse atlantal ligament extends between the lateral masses of C1 and on the way passes passes posterior to dens to support it like a pillow from behind. It is the strongest and thickest CCJ ligament. Dens may move posteriorly and compress spinal cord with disruption of the transverse atlantal ligament.*

TERMINOLOGY

Definitions

- Cervical spine consists of 7 uppermost spinal bones, including atlas (C1) and axis (C2); subaxial cervical spine = C3-C7

GROSS ANATOMY

Overview

- Consists of 7 vertebrae (C1-C7)
  - **Craniocervical junction (CCJ)**: C1, C2, and articulation with skull base constitutes CCJ
  - **Subaxial spine**: C3-C7
    - C3-C6 typical cervical vertebrae
    - C7 has features that differ slightly from C3-C6

Components of Subaxial Cervical Spine

- **Bones C3-C7**
  - **Body**
    - Small, broader transversely than in AP dimension
    - Posterolateral edges of superior surface are turned upward = uncinate processes
  - **Vertebral arch**
    - Pedicle: Delicate, projects posterolaterally
    - Lamina: Thin and narrow
    - Vertebral foramen: Large, triangular-shaped
  - **Transverse process**
    - Projects laterally; contains vertebral artery foramen
    - Anterior and posterior tubercles are separated by superolateral groove (lateral neural recess) for exiting spinal nerve
  - **Articular processes**
    - Superior and inferior articular processes with articular facets oriented ~ 45° superiorly from transverse plane
    - Form paired osseous shafts posterolateral to vertebral bodies = articular pillars
  - Spinous process: Short and bifid
  - **C7 unique features**
    - Spinous process: Long, prominent
    - Transverse process: Short and project inferolaterally compared with T1 spinous processes, which are long and project superolaterally
- **Intervertebral foramen**
  - Oriented anterolaterally below pedicles at ~ 45° to sagittal plane
  - Oblique reformats of CT best demonstrate foramina en face
    - Multiple neural foramina are seen in same slice allowing relative comparison with regard to degree of narrowing
- **Joints**
  - Intervertebral disc
    - Narrowest in cervical region
    - Thinner posteriorly than anteriorly
    - Does not extend to lateral margins of vertebral bodies in cervical spine → joints of Luschka
  - **Uncovertebral joint** (joints of Luschka)
    - Oblique, cleft-like cavities between superior surfaces of uncinate processes and lateral lips of inferior articular surface of next superior vertebrae
    - Lined by cartilaginous endplate of vertebral body
    - No true synovial lining present; contains serum, simulating synovial fluid
    - Uncinate process develops during childhood with uncovertebral joint forming by fibrillation and fissuring in fibers of annulus fibrosus
  - **Facet (zygapophyseal) joints**
    - Facet joints oriented ~ 45° superiorly from transverse plane in upper cervical spine; assume more vertical orientation toward C7
    - Formed by articulation between superior and inferior articular processes = articular pillars
    - Forms 2 sides of flexible tripod of bone (vertebral bodies, right and left articular pillars) for support of cranium
- **Ligaments**
  - Anterior and posterior longitudinal, ligamentum flavum, interspinous and supraspinous ligaments
  - Additional ligaments of CCJ include apical, alar, and cruciate ligaments
- **Biomechanics**
  - Subaxial cervical spine shows free motion range relative to remainder of presacral spine
    - Cervical extension checked by anterior longitudinal ligament and musculature
    - Cervical flexion checked by articular pillars and intertransverse ligaments

IMAGING ANATOMY

Lateral Assessment of Subaxial Spine

- Principles apply equally to radiography, CT or MR
- **Prevertebral soft tissues**: Distance between air column and anterior aspect of vertebral body
  - Adults: < 7 mm at C2 and < 22 mm at C6
  - Children: < 14 mm at C6
- Bony alignment
  - **Anterior vertebral line**: Smooth curve paralleling anterior vertebral cortex
    - Less important than posterior cortical line
  - **Posterior vertebral line**: Smooth curve paralleling posterior vertebral cortex
    - Translation > 3.5 mm is abnormal
    - Flexion and extension allow physiological offset < 3 mm of posterior cortical margin of successive vertebral bodies
  - **Spinolaminar line**: Smooth curve from opisthion to C7 formed by junction of laminae with spinous processes
  - **Spinous process angulation**: Cervical spinous processes should converge toward common point posteriorly
    - Widening is present when distance is > 1.5x interspinous distance of adjacent spinal segments

Frontal Assessment of Subaxial Spine

- Lateral masses: Bilateral smooth undulating margins
- Spinous processes: Midline
  - Lateral rotation of 1 spinous process with respect to others is abnormal
- Interspinous distance: Symmetric throughout
  - Interspinous distance 1.5x distance of level above or below is abnormal

GRAPHICS

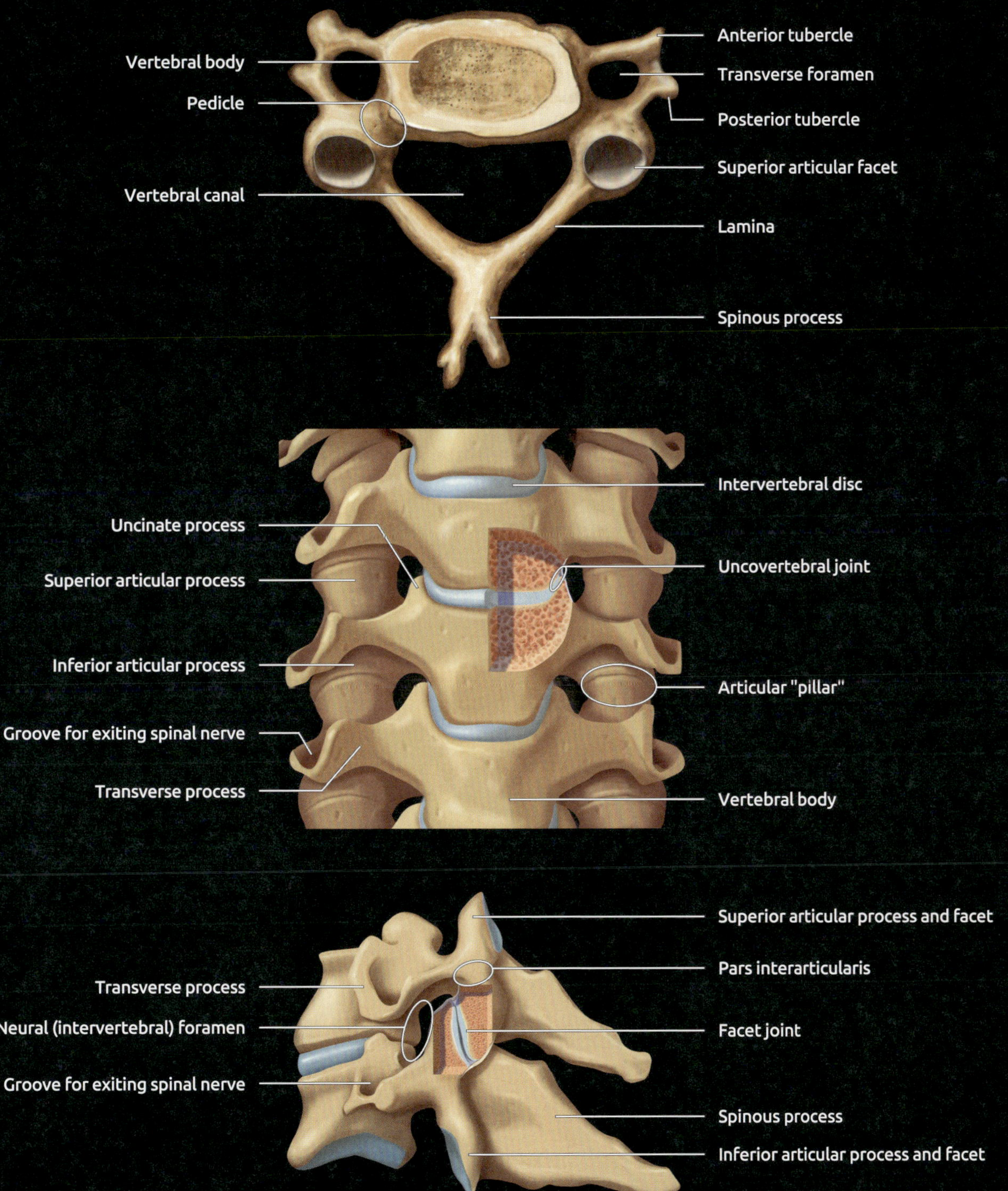

(Top) *Graphic of a typical cervical vertebra viewed from above demonstrates important morphology. Vertebral body is broader transversely than in AP dimension, central vertebral canal is large and triangular in shape, pedicles are directed posterolaterally, and laminae are delicate and give rise to a spinous process with a bifid tip. Lateral masses contain the vertebral foramen for passage of vertebral artery and veins.* **(Middle)** *Frontal graphic of subaxial cervical spine with cutout shows intervertebral disc and uncovertebral joints. Paired lateral articular "pillars" are formed by articulation between superior and inferior articular processes.* **(Bottom)** *Lateral graphic of 2 consecutive typical cervical vertebrae with cutout shows facet (zygapophyseal) joint detail. Note also the prominent groove on the superior surface of the transverse process for exiting spinal nerves.*

GRAPHICS

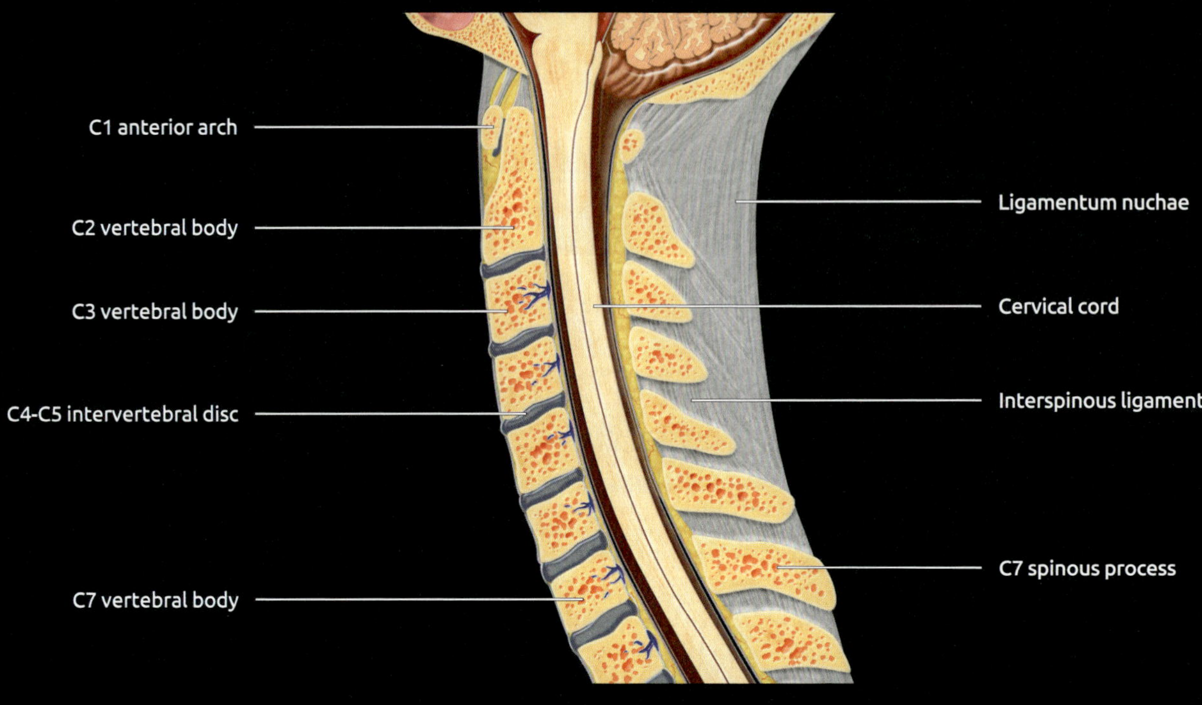

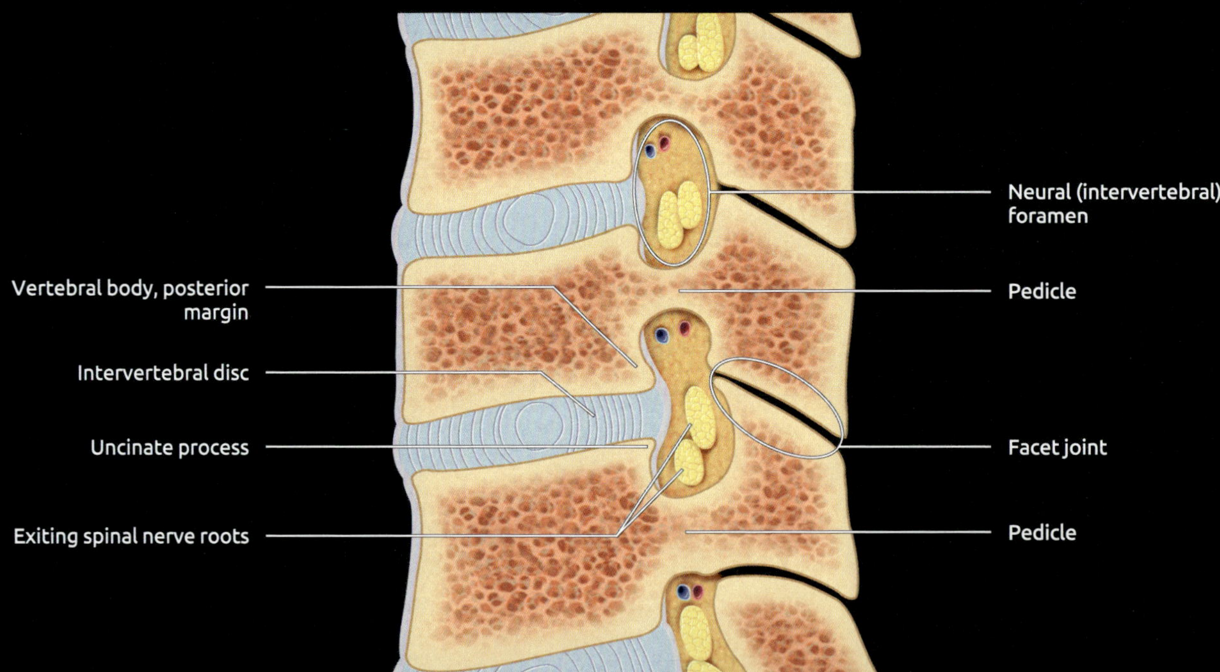

(Top) *Sagittal midline graphic of the cervical spine and cord shows a gentle lordotic curve and smooth alignment of the adjacent vertebrae. C1, C2, and their articulation with the skull base constitutes the craniocervical junction. C3-C7 constitutes the subaxial cervical spine. C3-C6 are regarded as typical cervical vertebrae, whereas C7 has features that differ slightly from C3-C6, including a long, prominent spinous process.* **(Bottom)** *Sagittal graphic through the cervical neural foramen shows position of exiting spinal nerves within the lower part of the neural foramen. Neural foramina are oriented anterolaterally (compare with thoracic and lumbar regions). Anterior boundary of the neural foramen include the uncinate process, intervertebral disc, and vertebral body from inferior to superior. Pedicles form superior and inferior boundaries. Posterior boundary is the facet joint complex.*

GRAPHIC & 3D-VRT NECT

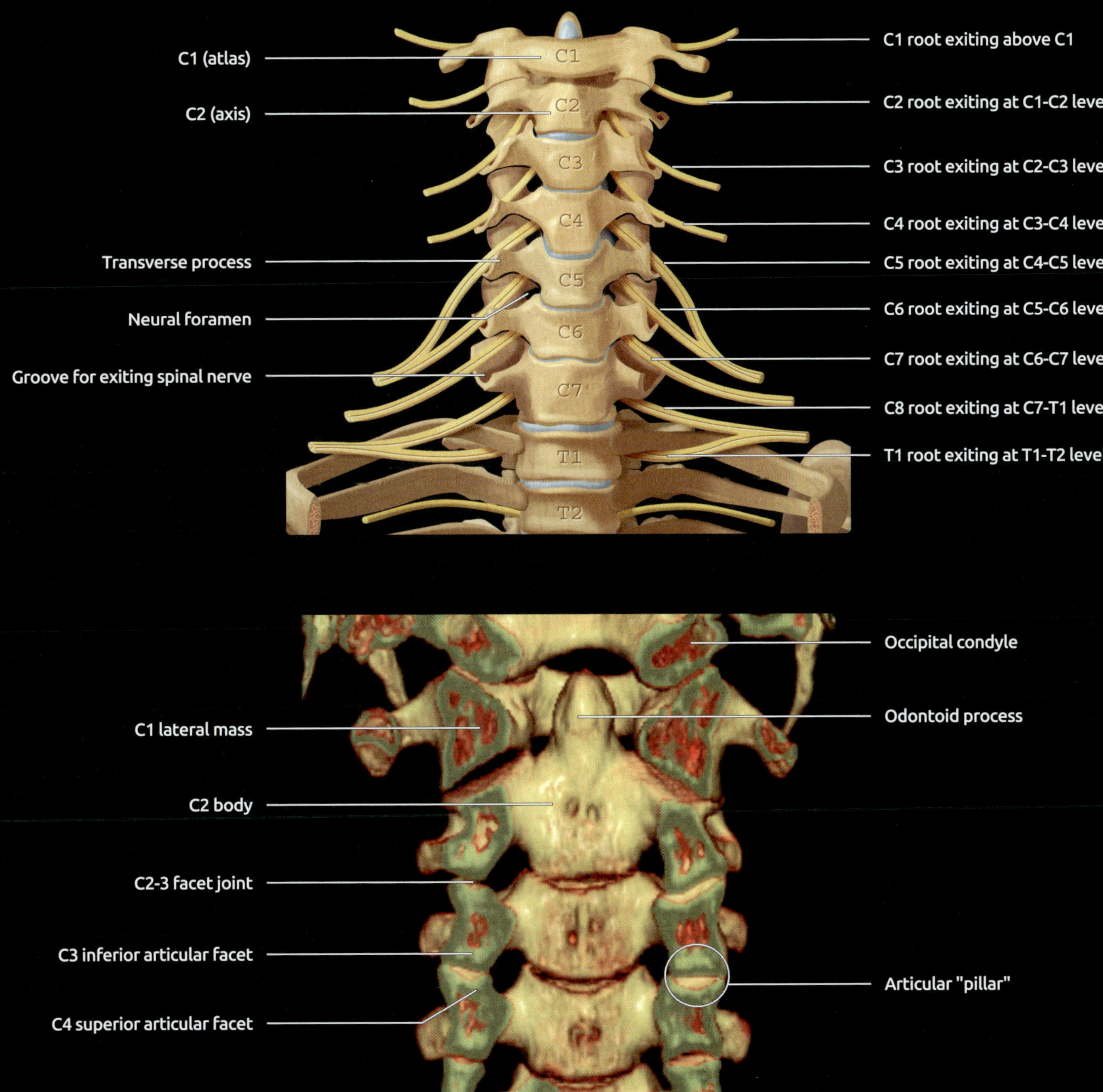

(Top) *Coronal graphic of the cervical spine shows vertebrae and corresponding cervical nerves. The vertebra are numbered and are shown with their exiting nerves. There are 8 cervical nerves with C1 nerve exiting above the C1 body and C2 nerve exiting at the C1-C2 level. The C8 nerve exits at C7-T1. Below this level, the thoracic roots exit below their respective numbered vertebra. The roots exit inferiorly within the neural foramen, along the bony groove in the transverse process.* **(Bottom)** *Coronal 3D-VRT shows the cervical spine viewed posteriorly with the dorsal elements partially removed to reveal the dorsal vertebral body surface. The concept of the cervical articular pillars is well shown in this view with the facets forming paired columns of bone with superior and inferior articulating facets.*

GRAPHIC & LATERAL RADIOGRAPH

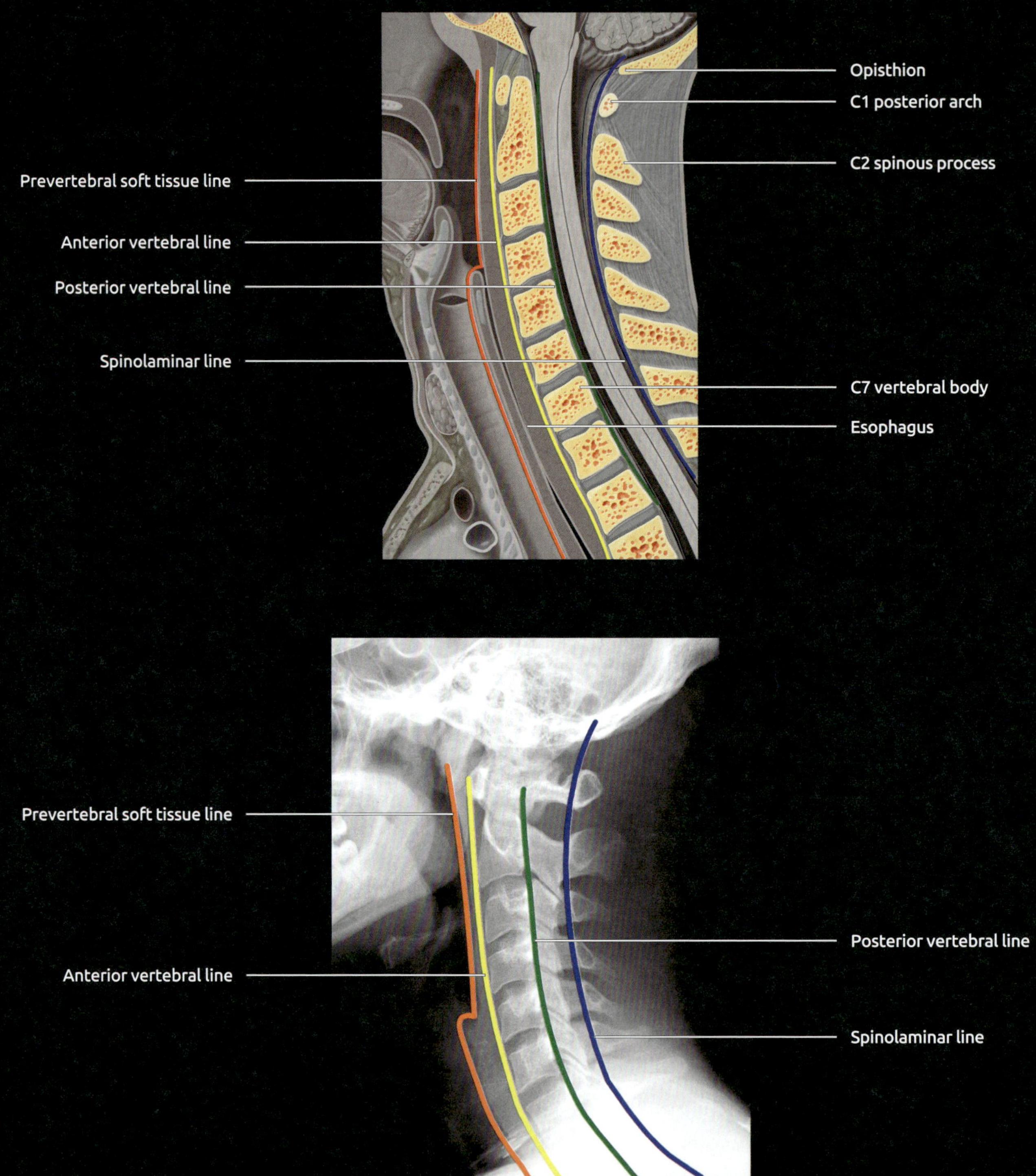

(Top) *Sagittal midline graphic of the cervical spine is shown. The normal cervical spine shows a smooth lordotic curve with smooth alignment of a series of lines going from ventral to dorsal, including prevertebral soft tissues (orange), anterior vertebral body cortical margins (yellow), posterior vertebral body margins (green), and posterior spinolaminar line (blue). In adults, the prevertebral soft tissues measure < 7 mm at C2 and < 22 mm at C6. In children, they measure < 14 mm at C6.* **(Bottom)** *Lateral radiograph of the cervical spine shows normal alignment. A series of gently curving lines make up the normal cervical curvature, extending from prevertebral soft tissues to the posterior spinolaminar line. In addition, the cervical spinous processes should all converge toward a common point posteriorly.*

RADIOGRAPHY

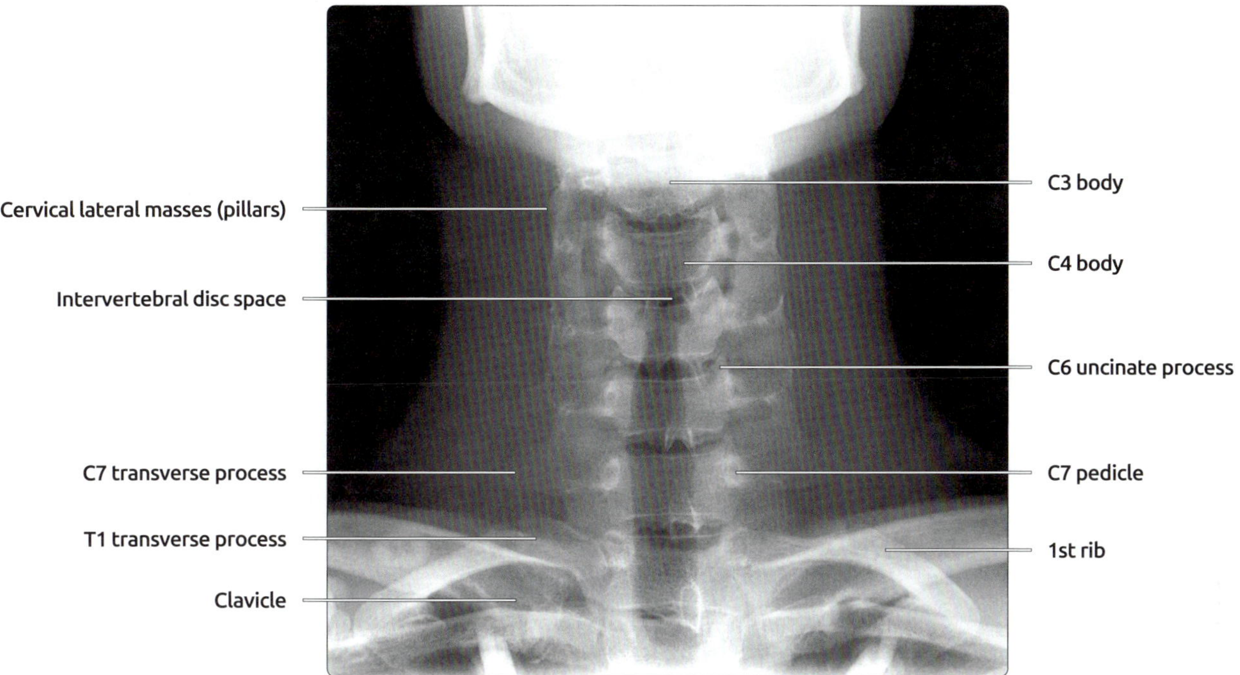

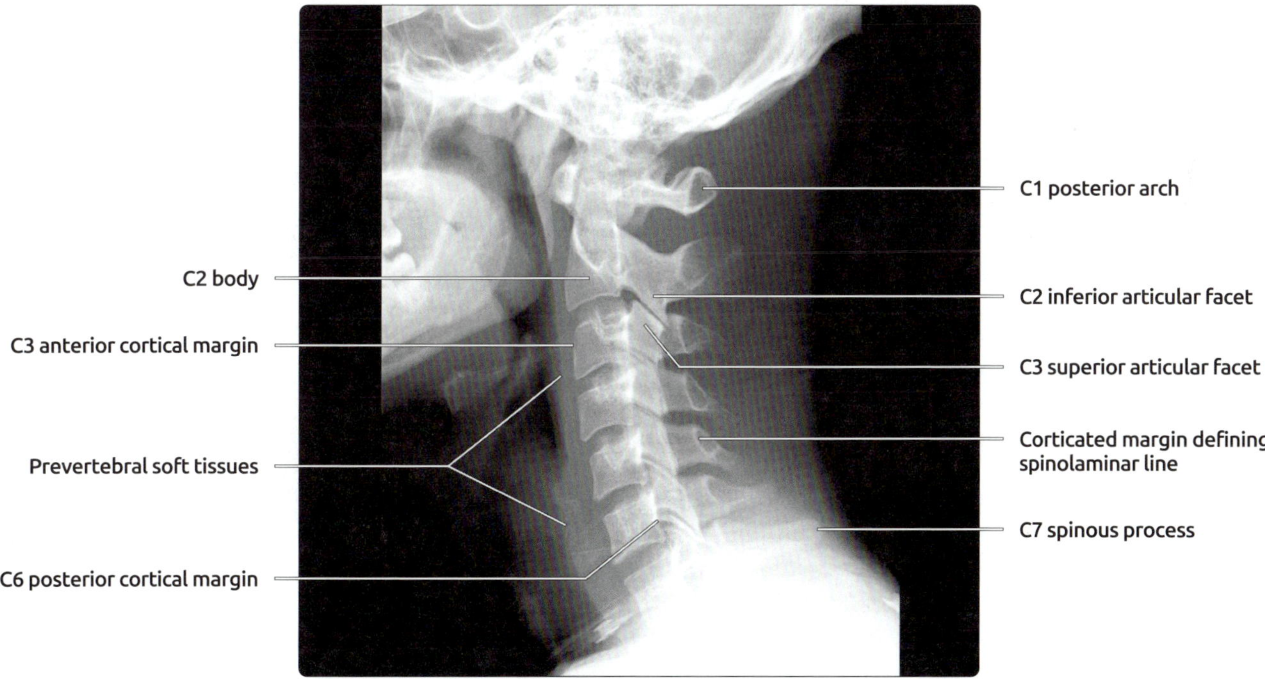

(Top) *AP plain film of the cervical spine is shown. The articular facets are viewed obliquely in this projection and therefore not defined, giving the appearance of smoothly undulating lateral columns of bone. The superior and inferior vertebral endplate margins are sharp with regular spacing of the intervertebral discs. The spinous processes are midline. C7 transverse process is directed inferolaterally compared with T1, which is directed superolaterally.* **(Bottom)** *Lateral radiograph of the cervical spine is shown. The prevertebral soft tissues should form a defined, abrupt "shelf" at ~ C4/C5 where the hypopharynx/esophagus begins, hence thickening the prevertebral soft tissues. The bony cervical spine is aligned from anteriorly to posteriorly with the anterior vertebral body margins, the posterior vertebral body margins, and ventral margins of the spinous processes (spinolaminar line).*

RADIOGRAPHY & 3D-VRT NECT

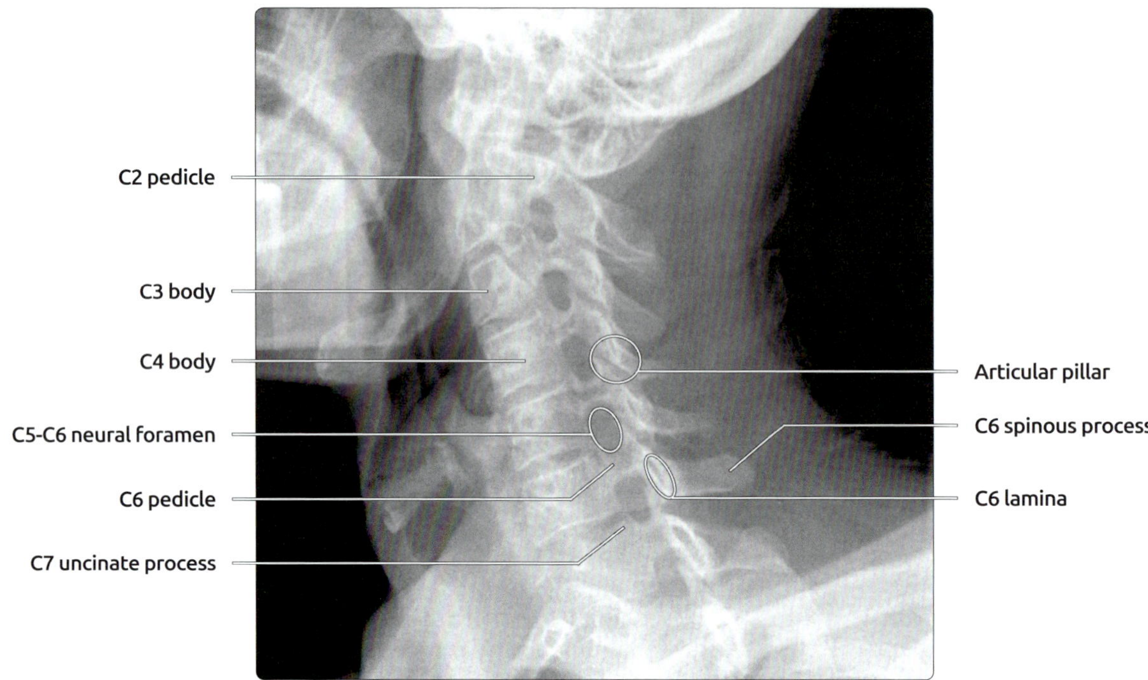

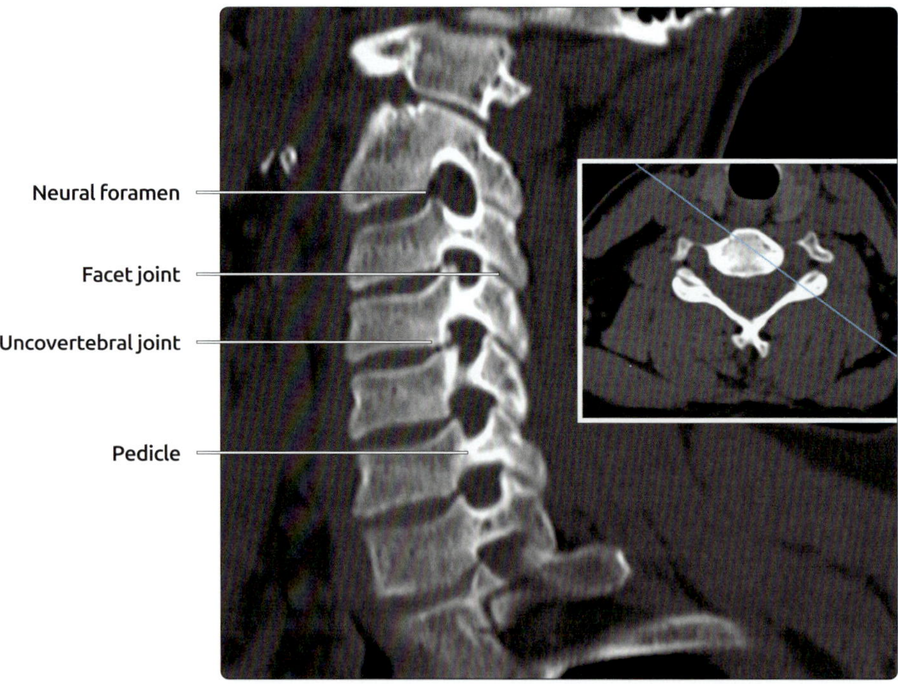

(Top) *Oblique radiograph of the cervical spine best demonstrates the neural foramina, as these are oriented obliquely at ~ 45° from the sagittal plane. With the patient rotated to the left, the radiograph demonstrates the right-sided foramina. The anterior boundary of the neural foramina includes the uncinate process, intervertebral disc, and vertebral body. The posterior boundary is the facet joint complex. The articular pillar facet joints are viewed obliquely and hence are not well defined. The lamina are seen end on and hence sharply corticated.* **(Bottom)** *Coronal oblique reformat CT of the cervical spine best demonstrates neural foramina, which are oriented obliquely at ~ 45° from the coronal and sagittal planes. The coronal oblique plane goes perpendicular to the plane of neural foramina on axial image (inset).*

3D-VRT NECT

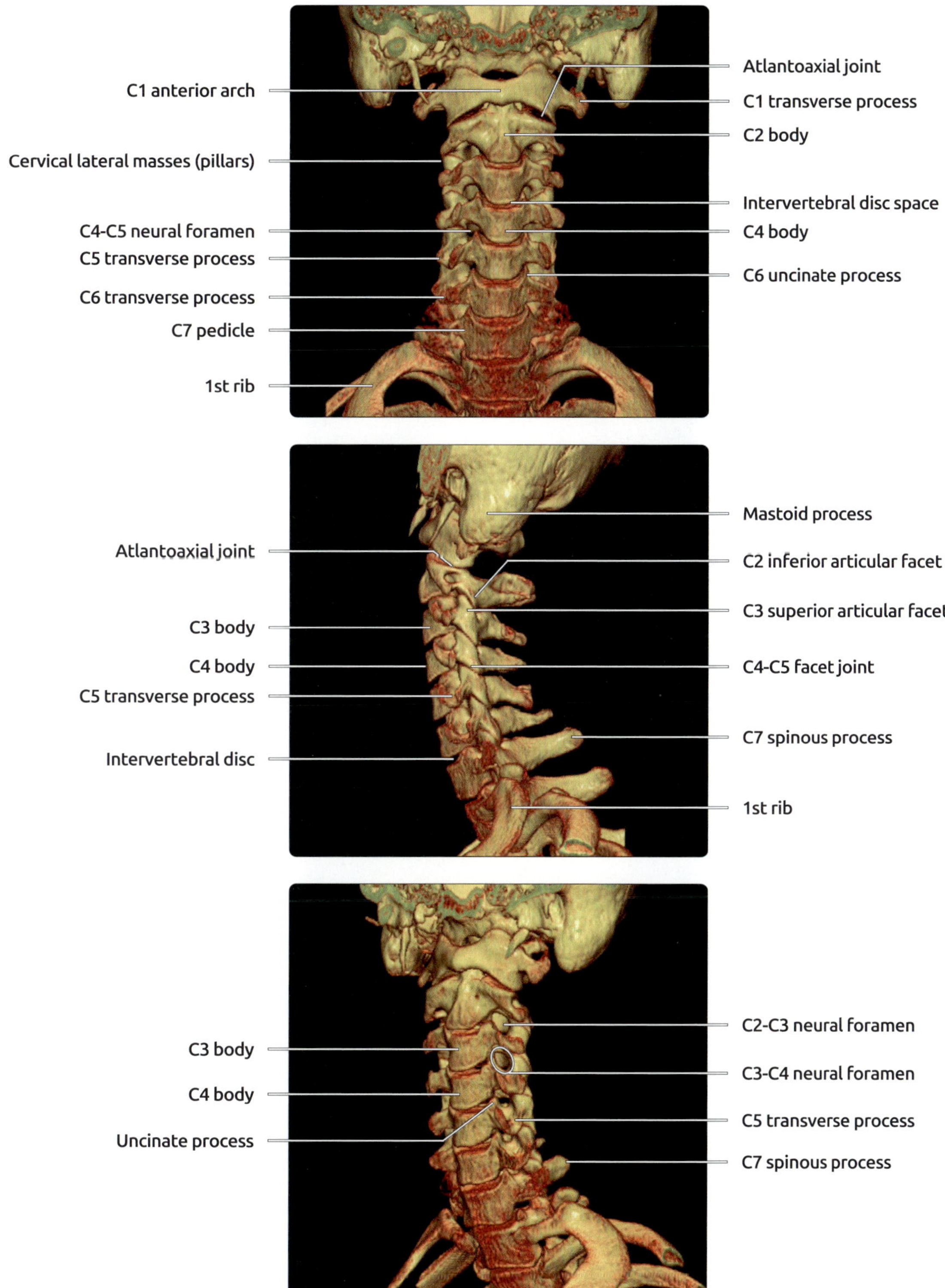

(Top) *Anterior 3D-VRT NECT of the cervical spine is shown. The wide neural foramina with the groove or sulcus on the superior surface of the transverse processes for the exiting nerves are well seen. The transverse processes with the tubercles for muscle attachments are well identified from C3-C7 levels. The uncinate processes are acquired, superior bony projections along the posterolateral margins of the vertebral bodies and form the uncovertebral joints with the adjacent superior vertebral body.* **(Middle)** *Lateral 3D-VRT NECT of the cervical spine is shown. The facet joints are seen in profile angled ~ 45° superiorly from the transverse plane. They align in a smooth interlocking fashion with the superior articular facets directed posteriorly and the inferior articular facets directed anteriorly.* **(Bottom)** *Oblique 3D-VRT NECT of the cervical spine shows the neural foramina end on. The groove on the superior surface of the transverse processes for the exiting spinal nerves is well shown.*

AXIAL BONE CT

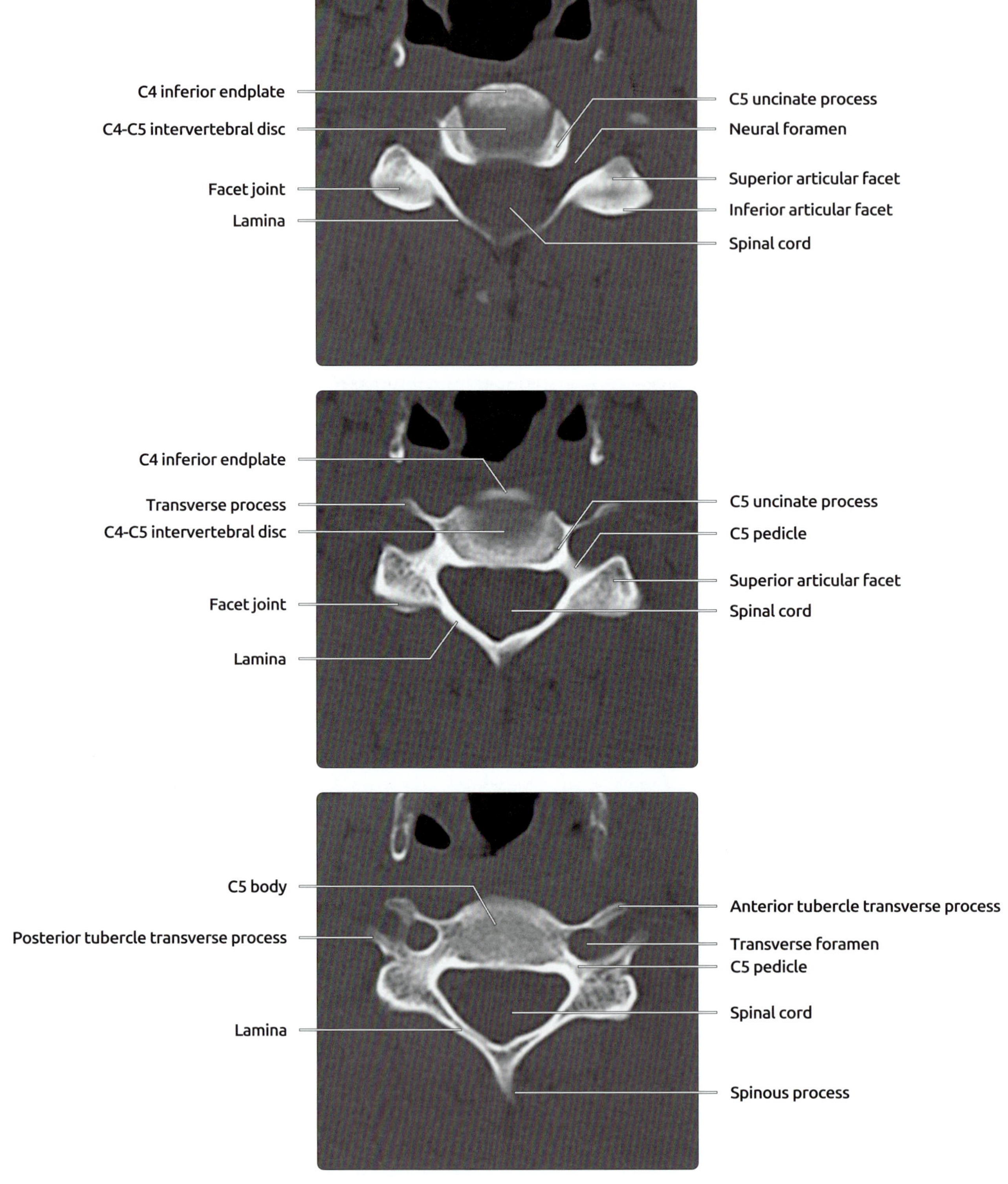

(Top) *First of 6 axial bone CT images presented from superior to inferior through the cervical spine starting at the C4-C5 level is shown. The cup-shaped intervertebral disc of the cervical region is seen centrally, bounded along the posterolateral margin by the uncinate processes. The uncinate process defines the joint of Luschka between adjacent vertebral segments. The neural foramina exit at ~ 45° in an anterolateral direction, bounded posteriorly by the superior articular process.* **(Middle)** *Axial bone CT through the inferior margin of the intervertebral disc is shown. The gracile pedicles arise obliquely from the posterolateral margins of the vertebral bodies. The bony canal is large relative to the posterior elements and assumes a triangular configuration.* **(Bottom)** *Axial bone CT through the C5 body level is shown. The transverse process contains the transverse foramen for the vertebral artery.*

AXIAL BONE CT

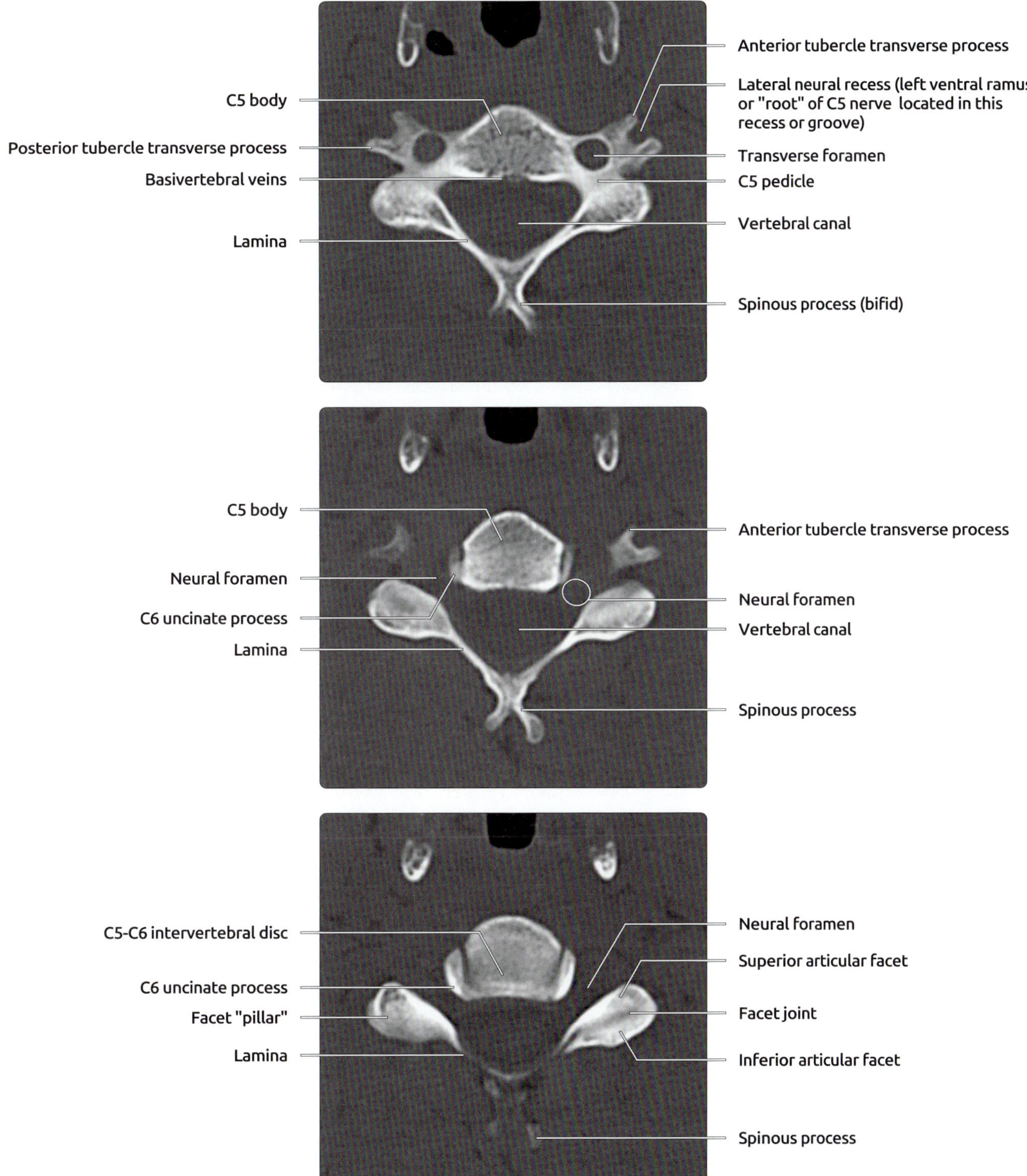

(Top) *Axial bone CT through the mid-C5 body at the pedicle level is shown. The transverse foramina are prominent at this level with the round, sharply marginated transverse foramen encompassing the vertical course of the vertebral artery. The anterior and posterior tubercles give rise to muscle attachments in the neck. The vertebral body is interrupted along the posterior cortical margin for the passage of the basivertebral venous complex.* **(Middle)** *Axial bone CT at the inferior C5 body level is shown. The uncinate process arising off of the next inferior vertebral body is coming into view. The inferior margins of the transverse processes are incompletely visualized. The spinous process is well seen, joining with the thin lamina.* **(Bottom)** *Axial bone CT at the C5-C6 level shows the next neural foraminal level bounded by the uncovertebral joint anteriorly and facet posteriorly.*

CORONAL CT MYELOGRAM

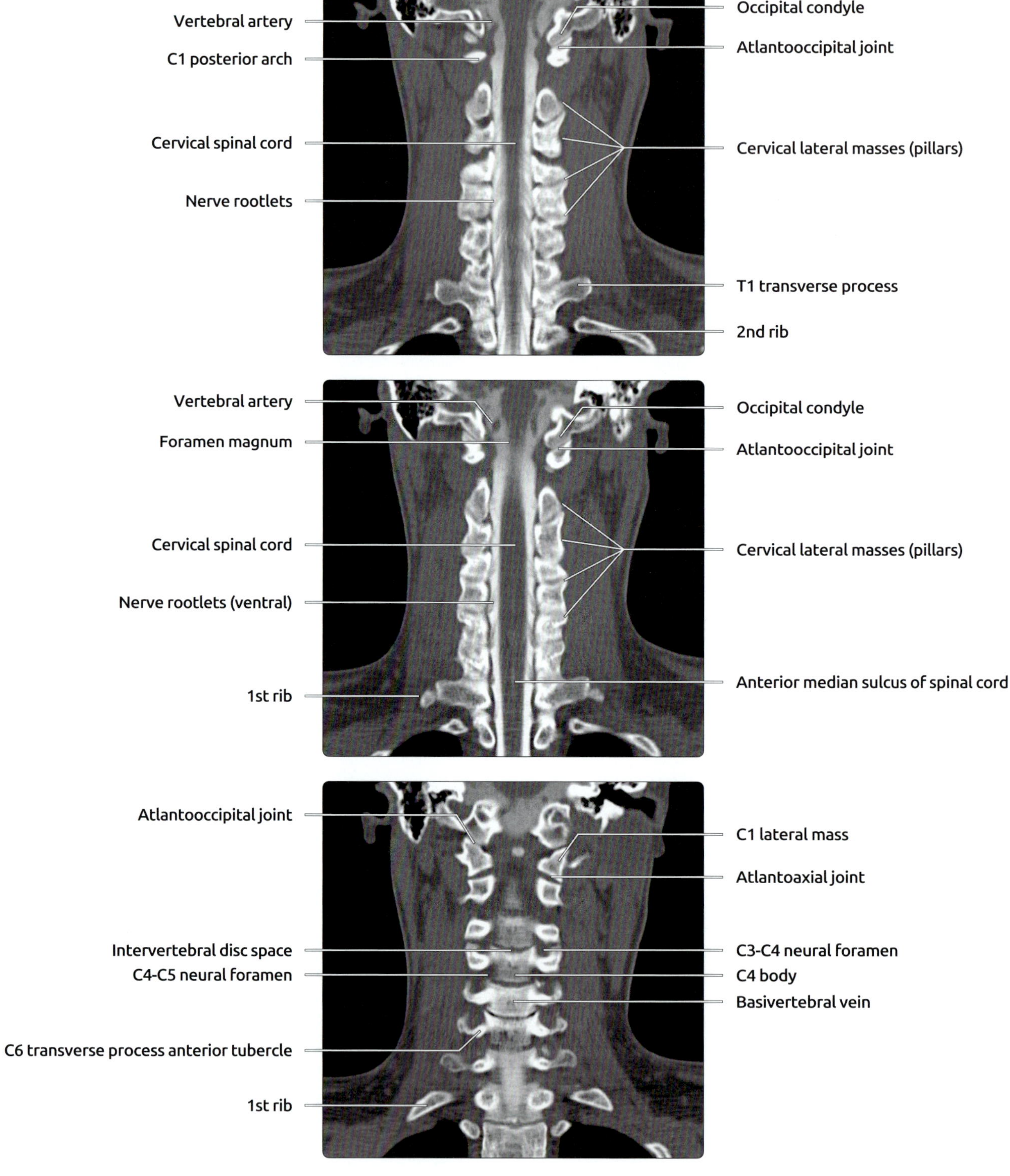

(Top) *First of 3 coronal reformatted CT myelogram images displayed from posterior to anterior is shown. This most posterior view shows the spinal cord with exiting nerve rootlets at each segmental level traversing in a craniocaudal direction within the thecal sac. T1 transverse process is prominent and directed superolaterally.* **(Middle)** *More anterior view shows the ventral margin of the cervical spinal cord with the anterior median sulcus, which would contain the anterior spinal artery. The ventral nerve rootlets are also visible. The articular pillars of the facet joints are well shown, giving a view similar to an AP radiograph of the undulating lateral margin of the cervical pillars.* **(Bottom)** *More anterior view shows transverse processes with adjacent neural foramina. The posterior margins of the vertebral bodies show the midline basivertebral veins.*

SAGITTAL CT MYELOGRAM

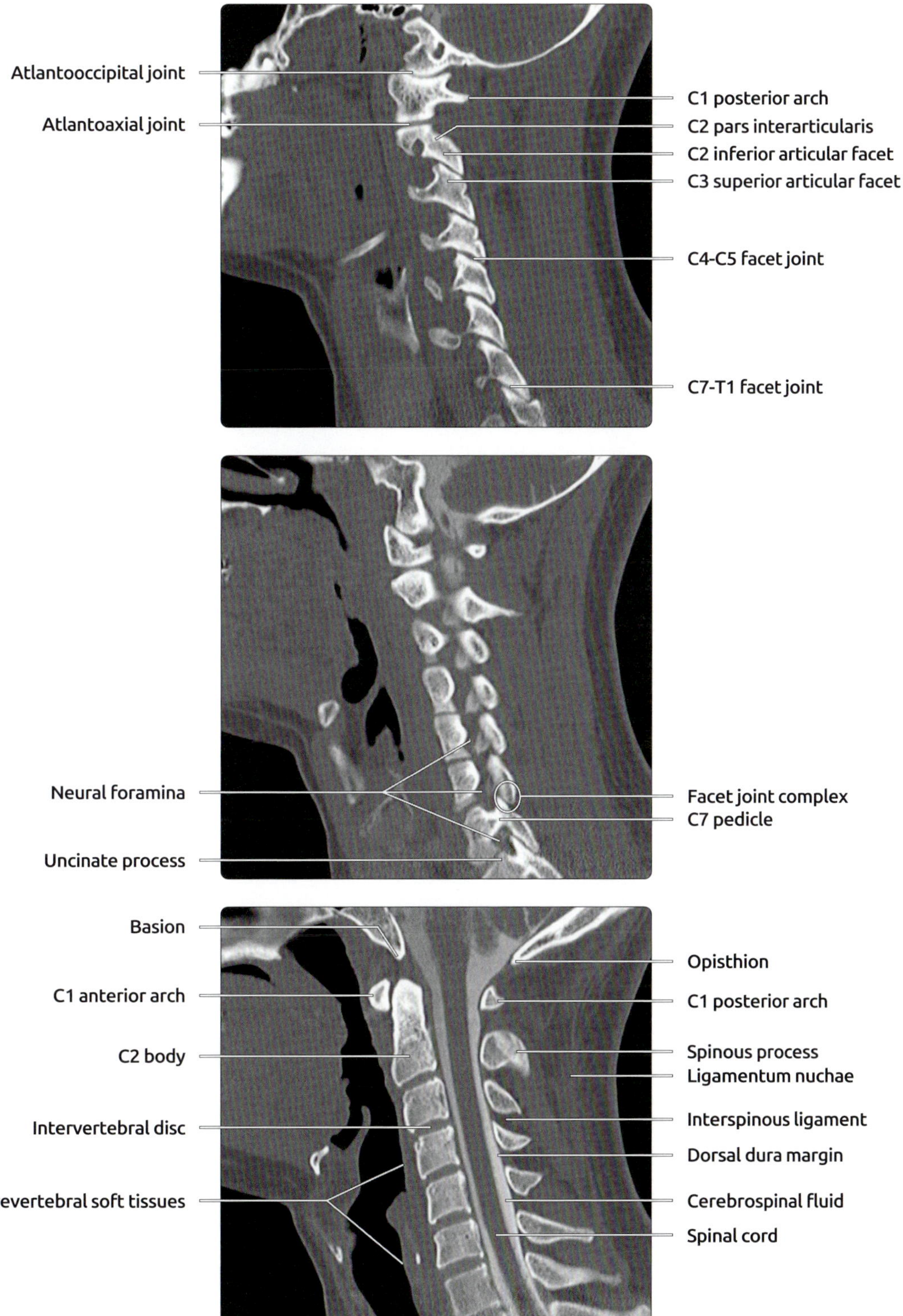

(Top) *First of 3 sagittal reformatted CT myelogram images is shown. Paramedian sagittal section through the articular pillar shows the facet joints in profile. Superior articular facets are directed posteriorly, while inferior facets are directed anteriorly. The curvilinear shape of the atlantooccipital joint is visible, allowing for flexion/extension.* **(Middle)** *More medial section through obliquely oriented neural foramina, which are bounded above and below by pedicles, anteriorly by uncovertebral joint, disc and vertebral body, and posteriorly by facet joint complex, is shown.* **(Bottom)** *Midline section shows the spinal cord outlined by the high attenuation of the contrast within the CSF. Vertebral alignment is normal, and prevertebral soft tissues demonstrate an abrupt "shelf" at ~ the C4-C5 level, where the esophagus begins.*

SAGITTAL T1 MR

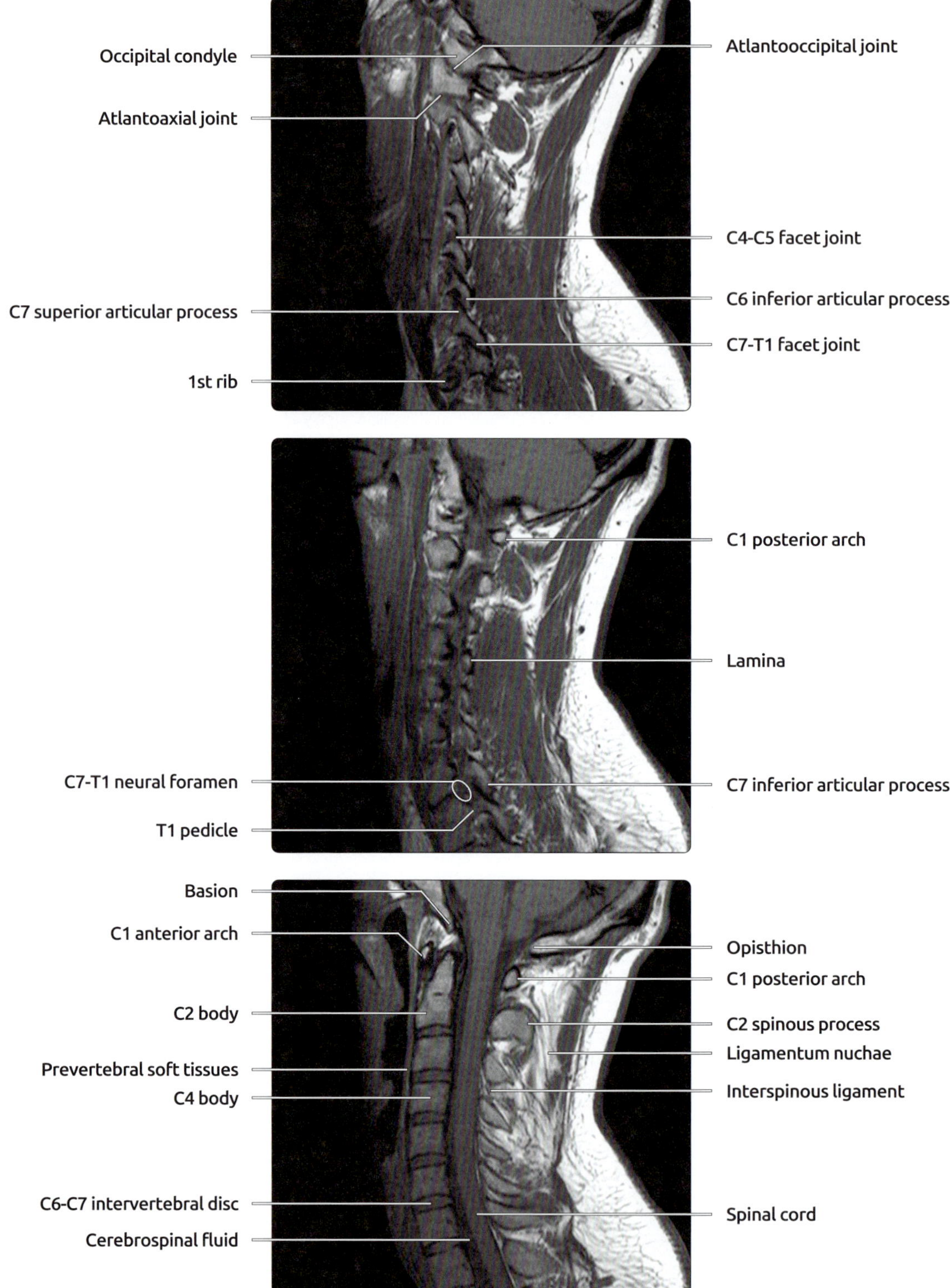

(Top) *First of 3 sagittal T1 MR images viewed from lateral to medial is shown. View through the articular pillar shows the facet joints in profile. Margins of the facet joints are well corticated and seen as thin hypointense lines.* **(Middle)** *More medial section through obliquely oriented neural foramina is shown.* **(Bottom)** *Midline image shows the well-defined, low-signal cortical margins of the vertebral bodies, which merge along their anterior and posterior margins with the hypointense anterior and posterior longitudinal ligaments, respectively. Vertebral marrow signal is hyperintense relative to intervening discs on T1 MR. CSF is hypointense.*

SAGITTAL T2 MR

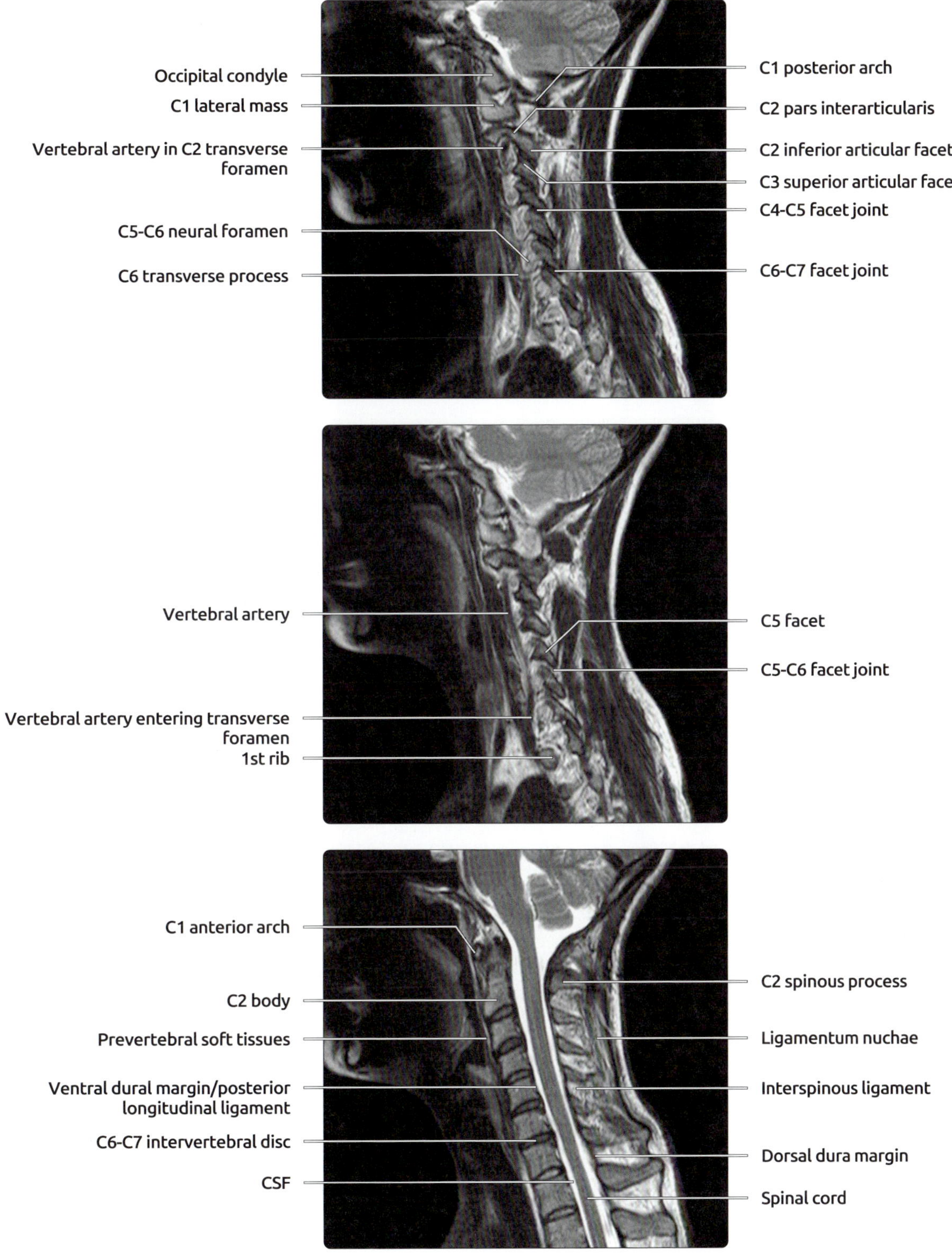

(Top) *First of 3 sagittal T2 MR images viewed from lateral to medial is shown. View through the articular pillars shows normal alignment of the facet joints. The rhomboidal configuration of the cervical facets is noted with their complementary superior and inferior articular facets. The exiting spinal nerves run in the groove along the superior aspect of transverse processes.* **(Middle)** *More medial section shows the overlapping facets at each level and the flow void of the vertebral artery within the transverse foramen.* **(Bottom)** *Midline image shows the relationship of the cervical cord, vertebral bodies, and spinous processes with smooth straight margins and alignment. The posterior dural margin merges with the low signal of the ligamentum flavum and spinous process cortex. The anterior dural margin merges with the posterior body cortex and posterior longitudinal ligament.*

AXIAL GRE MR

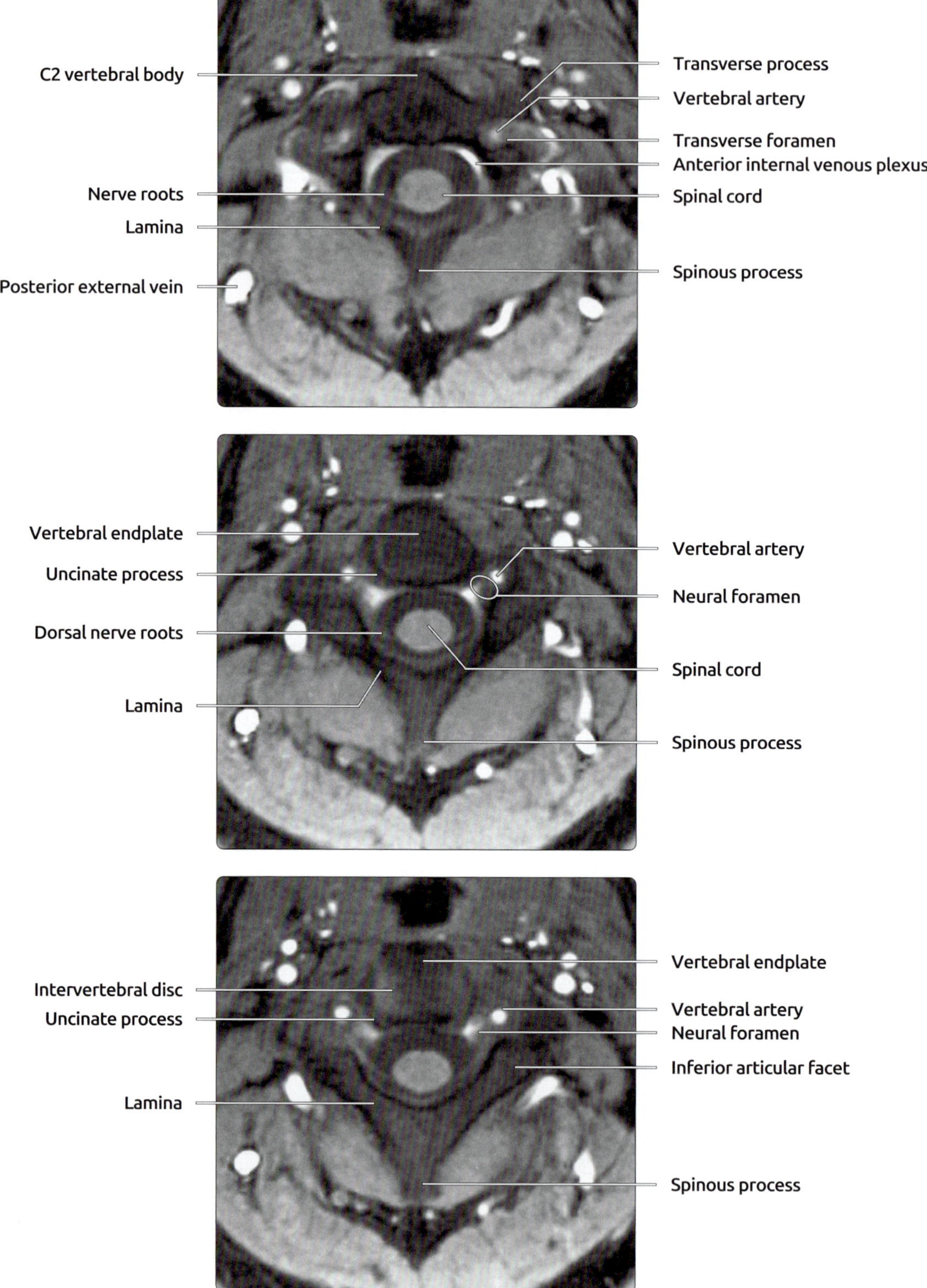

(Top) *First of 6 axial gradient-echo MR images with large flip angle (giving dark CSF signal) from superior to inferior beginning at the inferior C2 body level is shown. The prominent transverse foramen with the vertebral artery is apparent. Flow-related enhancement is also visible in the cervical dorsal veins as well as the epidural veins (anterior internal venous plexus).* **(Middle)** *Image at the inferior endplate of C2 is shown. The neural foramina are directed at 45° anterolaterally and show flow-related enhancement in epidural/foraminal venous plexus and the ascending vertebral arteries. The spinal cord and dural margins are well defined and smooth. The dorsal nerve rootlets are barely visible within the dorsal thecal sac.* **(Bottom)** *Image at the C2-C3 disc level is shown. The inferior articular facet of C2 and the prominent C2 spinous process are visible.*

AXIAL GRE MR

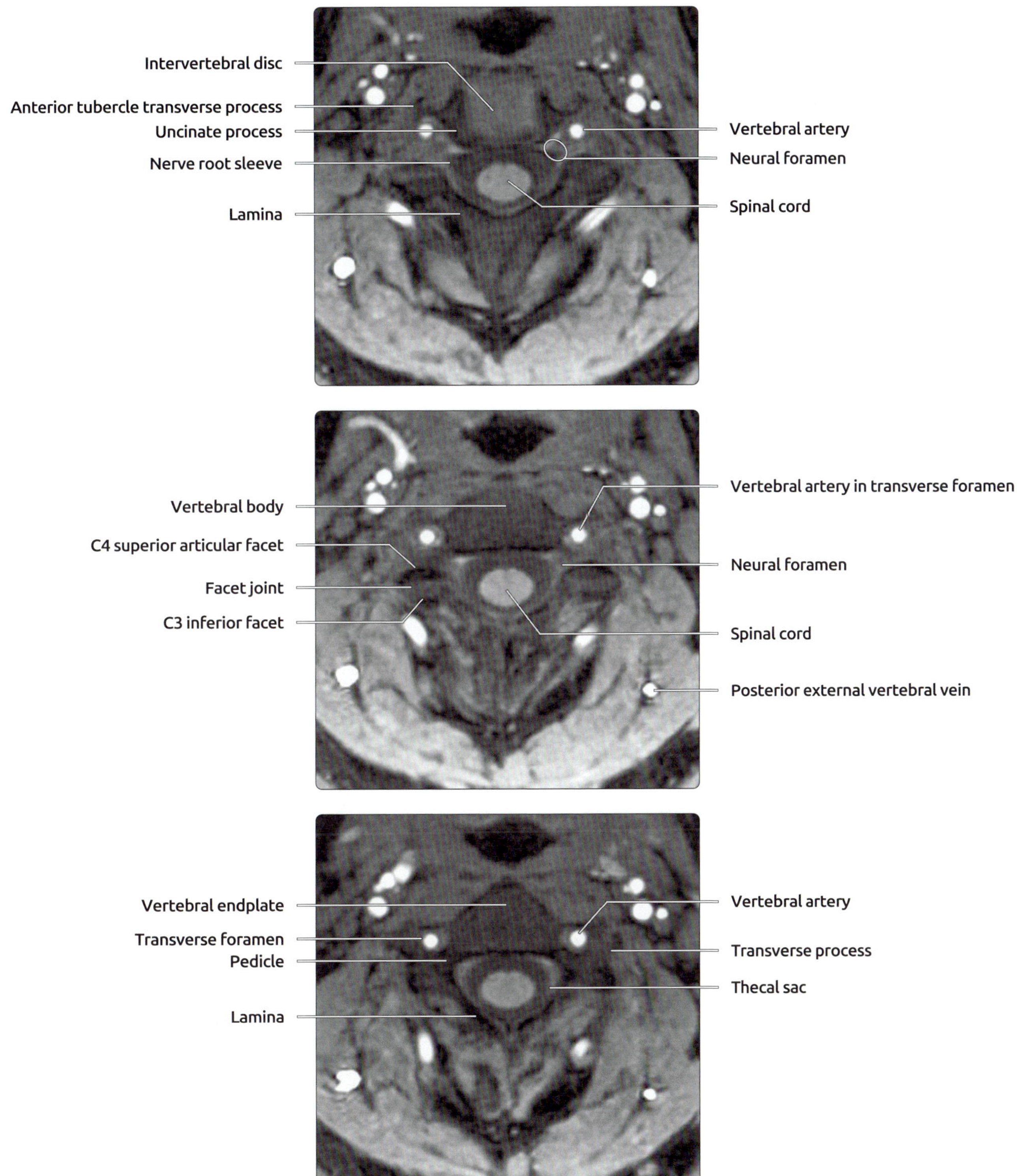

(Top) *Image through C2-C3 intervertebral disc is shown. The intermediate-signal, square-shaped intervertebral disc is evident with the bounding lower signal uncinate processes. The low-signal, CSF-containing, triangular-shaped root sleeves are seen extending anterolaterally into the neural foramina.* **(Middle)** *Image through the superior C3 vertebral body shows the C3-C4 facet joint with the anterior low-signal superior facet of C4, the intermediate-signal linear joint space, and the dorsal-positioned low-signal inferior facet of C3.* **(Bottom)** *Image through the C3 pedicles, which project posterolaterally from the vertebral body, is shown. The delicate laminae complete the triangular-shaped vertebral foramen containing the thecal sac and contents. The transverse foramina containing the vertebral arteries are prominent within the transverse processes.*

AXIAL T2 MR

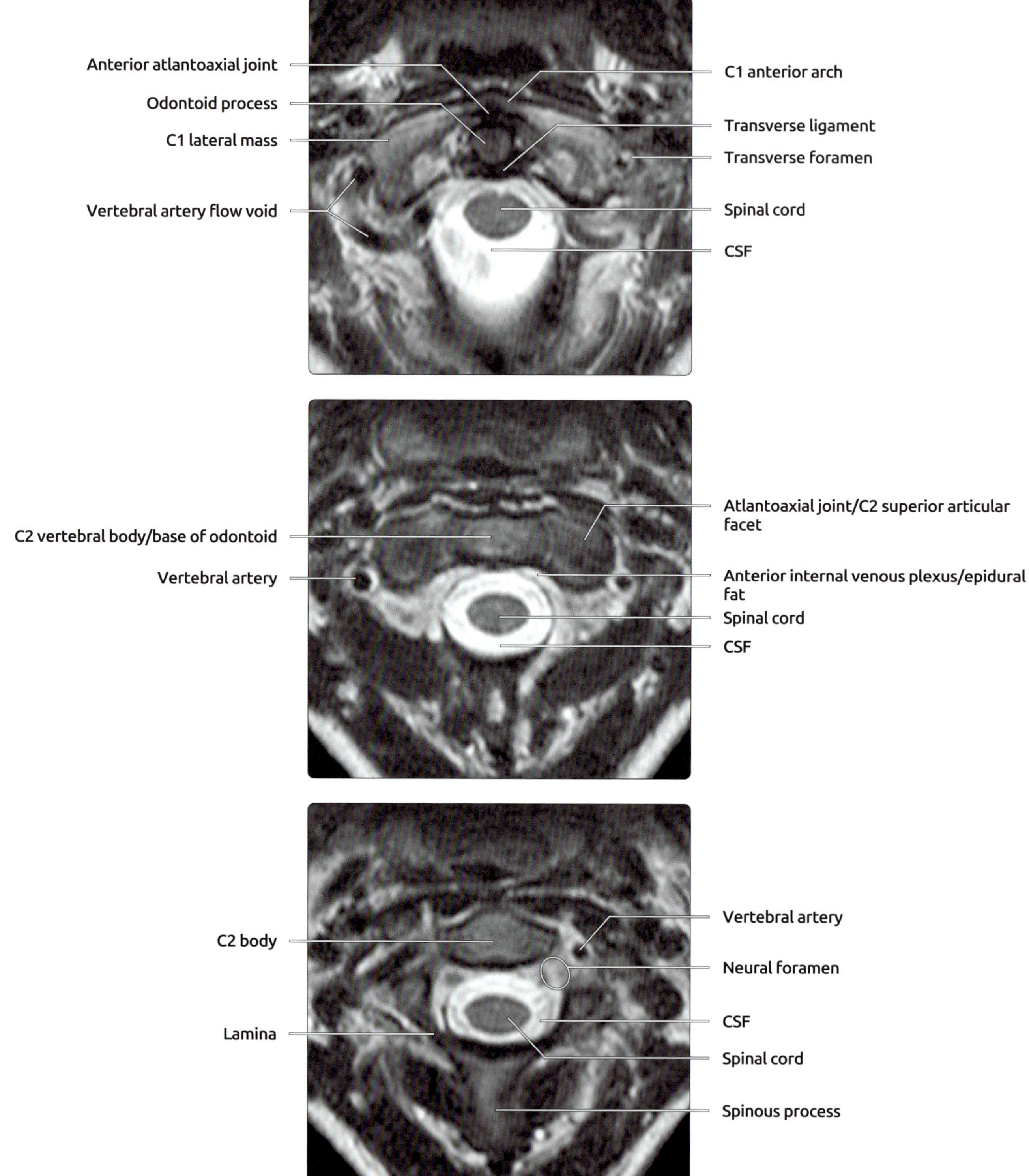

(Top) *First of 6 axial T2 MR images from superior to inferior beginning at the level of the anterior arch of C1 is shown. The anterior atlantodental joint is well identified, bounded by the low-signal cortical margins of the anterior odontoid and anterior arch of C1. Posterior to the odontoid is the low-signal transverse ligament complex.* **(Middle)** *Image at odontoid/C2 body level is shown. The base of the odontoid is at the level of the lateral atlantoaxial articulation. This joint is sloped, being more superior at the medial margin. The vertebral arteries are identified by their flow voids, located just lateral to the lateral masses, passing superiorly toward the C1 transverse foramen.* **(Bottom)** *Image at the C2 body level is shown. The relationship of the vertically oriented vertebral artery to the neural foramen is highlighted in this section.*

AXIAL T2 MR

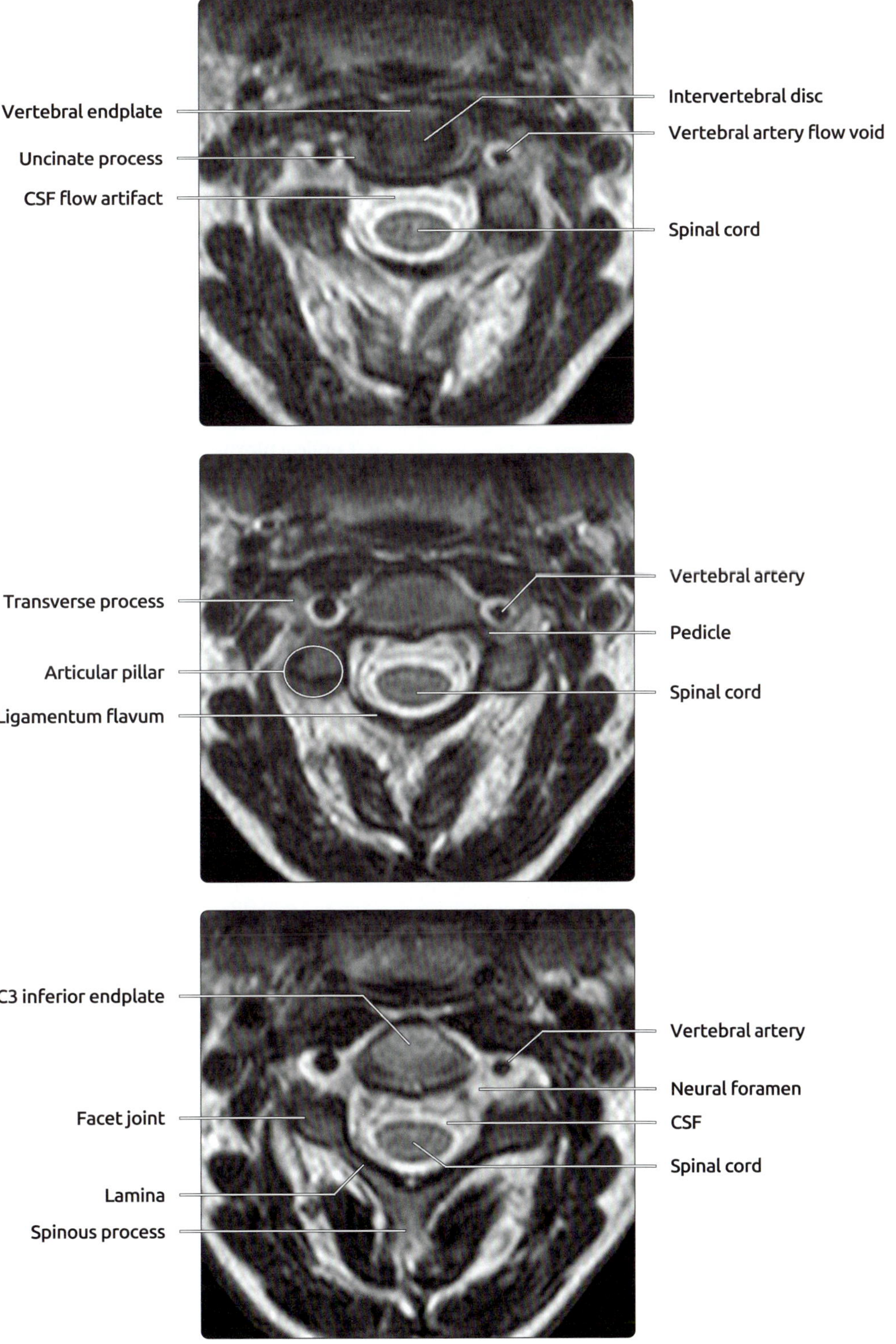

(Top) *Image at the C2-C3 disc level is shown. The intervertebral disc is fully visualized as low signal with the bounding posterior lateral uncovertebral joints.* **(Middle)** *Image through the pedicles of C3 is shown. Pedicles are delicate and are directed posterolaterally from the vertebral body. The articular pillars are formed by the superior and inferior articular processes and intervening facet joints. Prominent vertebral artery flow voids are seen within the transverse foramina of the transverse processes.* **(Bottom)** *Image through the neural foramina of C3, which are oriented ~ 45° anterolaterally, is shown. The posterior margin of the neural foramen is the facet joint; the ventral margin is the disc and uncinate process.*

TERMINOLOGY

Abbreviations

- Brachial plexus (BP)

Definitions

- Collection of interconnecting nerves of lower cervical spine (C5-C8) and 1st thoracic nerve (T1) that provides cutaneous and motor innervation of upper extremity

GROSS ANATOMY

Overview

- **Cervical cord**
  - Internally, cervical spinal cord arranged so that white matter tracts are positioned in periphery of cord
  - Gray matter formed by neuronal cell bodies arranged in vertical columns located centrally within cord
  - Gray matter columns form H-shaped arrangement in axial plane (in cross section)
    - Lateral sagittally oriented components referred to as horns
    - Transverse coronal components referred to as gray commissures
  - Ventral (anterior) horns: Thicker, shorter, and contain multipolar motor neurons
  - Dorsal (posterior) horns: Thinner, longer, and contain cell bodies that receive sensory axons from dorsal root ganglions (DRGs)
- **Cervical nerve rootlets, nerve roots, and proximal nerves**
  - At each cervical level, ventral horns give rise to motor axons that exit ipsilateral ventrolateral sulci of cervical cord as several tiny (< 1-mm) **nerve rootlets**
  - Ventral nerve rootlets at each level coalesce within few millimeters of cord to form ipsilateral **ventral root** (~ 1 mm)
  - Similarly, dorsal horns receive multiple tiny nerve rootlets at posterolateral sulcus of cord
  - Dorsal nerve rootlets also coalesce within few millimeters of cord to form **dorsal root**
  - Dorsal root extends laterally from cord, passes and merges with **DRG** within **lower aspect of neural foramen (NF)**
  - Within lateral aspect of cervical NF, DRG fuses with ventral root to become **spinal nerve proper**
  - Immediately after proper spinal nerve formation, small, posteriorly oriented **dorsal ramus** emerges
    - Dorsal ramus supplies motor and sensory innervation to posterior paraspinous muscles and cervical soft tissues
  - Larger remaining segment of spinal nerve represents **ventral ramus**
    - Ventral ramus typically main part of spinal nerve in cervical region; often referred to as simply **spinal nerve** itself
    - Large ventral rami of nerves C5-T1 also referred to as **roots of BP**
  - On sagittal MR and CT, spinal DRG and contiguous cervical spinal nerve/BP root seen along lower aspect of NF
    - Bird's dropping-appearing filling defect of DRG in bright NF fat on sagittal T1WI MR
  - In contrast, thoracic and lumbar DRG and contiguous spinal nerves seen along upper aspect of NF
    - Bird's eye-appearing filling defect of DRG in bright NF fat on sagittal T1WI MR
  - **1st cervical nerve (C1)** exits spinal canal between occiput and C1
    - C1 nerve exits above C1 vertebra (atlas)
    - C2 nerve exits between C1 and C2 vertebrae, and so forth
    - C8 nerve exits between C7 and T1 vertebrae
  - Arrangement of **cervical nerve roots** passing laterally to DRG in lower aspect of NF just **above pedicle**, and **thoracic (and lumbar) nerve roots** just **below pedicle** to DRG in upper aspect of NF
    - Allows for 8 cervical nerves with only 7 cervical vertebrae
  - C8 nerve exits above T1 pedicle to lower C7-T1 NF
  - T1 nerve exits below T1 pedicle to upper T1-T2 NF
  - T2 nerve exits below T2 pedicle to upper T2-T3 NF
- **Cervical plexus**
  - Formed from ventral rami of C1-C4 ± minor branch of C5
  - Has ascending superficial, descending superficial, deep branches
  - Supplies nuchal muscles, diaphragm, cutaneous head/neck tissues
- **BP**
  - Formed from **ventral rami of C5-T1** ± minor branches from C4 and T2
  - BP divided into anatomic segments moving from medial to lateral: Rami/roots, trunks, divisions, cords, terminal branches
    - Relationships of these segments with adjacent anatomic structures variable
  - **Ventral rami/roots of BP**
    - Originate from spinal cord levels C5-T1
    - Roots of BP represent ventral rami of nerves C5-T1
    - Term BP "root" in this context is not to be confused with ventral and dorsal nerve roots in spinal canal discussed previously
      - Latter roots represent small nerves within spinal canal and within proximal NF before joining DRG
    - Some nerves arise directly from roots
      - **Dorsal scapular nerve** (C5)
      - **Long thoracic nerve** (C5, C6, C7)
      - **Phrenic nerve** (C3, C4, C5; mainly C4)
    - On coronal MR, **T1 root** easily seen as horizontal linear structure surrounded by **fat** close to **lung apex**
      - **Good starting point** to identify BP roots; then count C8, C7, C6, C5 upwards
      - Stellate ganglion can also be seen at this level
  - **Trunks**
    - Within interscalene triangle, upper roots of BP (C5-C6) fuse to form **superior (upper) trunk**
    - Only **upper trunk** gives off branches
      - **Suprascapular nerve** (C5, C6)
      - **Nerve to subclavius muscle** (C5, C6)
    - C7 root continues laterally as **middle trunk**
    - Lower roots (C8-T1) fuse to form **inferior (lower) trunk**
  - **Divisions**

- As BP passes laterally beyond interscalene triangle over lateral margin of 1st rib in **retroclavicular** location, and begins to descend toward axilla
  - Each trunk divides into 2 main nerve branches: **Anterior and posterior divisions**
- Subsequently, each BP contains total of 6 divisions: 3 anterior and 3 posterior
- Anterior divisions innervate anterior (flexor) muscles
- Posterior divisions innervate posterior (extensor) muscles
- **No named branches** arising directly from divisions
- Divisions located at level of clavicle and above junction of subclavian and axillary arteries

- **Cords**
  - As BP passes into axilla, divisions fuse again to form **cords**
  - Cords intimately associated with **axillary artery**; named by their relationship to artery itself
  - **Lateral cord** (anterior divisions of superior, middle trunks) innervates anterior (flexor) muscles
  - **Medial cord** (anterior division of inferior trunk) innervates anterior (flexor) muscles
  - **Posterior cord** (posterior divisions of all 3 trunks) innervates posterior (extensor) muscles
- **Branches (terminal)**
  - Cords form terminal **branches** of BP at approximately level of **lateral margin of pectoralis minor** muscle
  - **Lateral cord branches**
    - **Musculocutaneous nerve** (C5, C6, C7)
    - **Lateral pectoral nerve** (C5, C6, C7)
    - **Lateral root of median nerve** (C5, C6, C7)
  - **Medial cord branches**
    - **Ulnar nerve** (C7, C8,T1)
    - **Medial pectoral nerve** (C8, T1)
    - **Medial cutaneous nerve of arm** (C8, T1)
    - **Medial cutaneous nerve of forearm** (C8, T1)
    - **Medial root of median nerve** (C8, T1)
    - Note: **Median nerve** (C5-T1) formed by confluence of contributions from both medial and lateral cords
  - **Posterior cord branches**
    - **Radial nerve** (C5, C6, C7, C8, T1)
    - **Axillary nerve** (C5, C6)
    - **Thoracodorsal nerve (nerve to latissimus dorsi)** (C6, C7, C8)
    - Upper and lower **subscapular nerves** (C5, C6)

Anatomy Relationships

- **NF**
  - C5 nerve passes through NF at C4-C5
    - C6 nerve passes through NF at C5-C6
    - C7 nerve passes through C6-C7 NF
    - C8 nerve passes through NF at C7-T1
    - T1 nerve passes through NF at T1-T2
  - Within NF, DRG most conspicuous neural structure: Bulbous enlargement of dorsal root
  - Within NF, nerves of **C5, C6, and C7** positioned immediately posterior to vertebral artery
- **Lateral neural sulcus**
  - Transverse processes of C3-C6 have similar anatomic appearance with transverse foramen that transmits vertebral artery and lateral neural sulcus (superolateral groove of transverse process), where corresponding cervical nerve is positioned
    - e.g., after exiting NF at C4-C5, C5 nerve descends and passes laterally to lateral neural sulcus of transverse process of C5 vertebra
  - When vertebrae of C3-C6 are viewed in axial plane through transverse process, vertebral artery separated from proximal ventral ramus by small bony bar that separates transverse foramen from lateral neural sulcus
- **Interscalene triangle**
  - Anterior scalene muscle arises from anterior tubercles of transverse processes of C3-C6 cervical vertebrae and inserts on superior surface of 1st rib anteriorly
  - Middle scalene muscle arises from posterior tubercles of transverse processes of C2-C7 vertebrae and attaches to 1st rib laterally
  - Borders of interscalene triangle
    - Anterior border: Posterior margin of anterior scalene muscle
    - Posterior border: Anterior edge of middle scalene muscle
    - Inferior border (base): Superior margin of 1st rib, between separate attachments for 2 muscles
    - Interscalene triangle can also be considered 3D space with both lateral and medial borders as well
    - Medial border represented by plane extending from medial margins of anterior and middle scalene muscles, and lateral border as plane between lateral margins of both muscles
  - Widest portion of triangle at base, along 1st rib
    - Distance between attachments of anterior and middle scalene muscles to ribs is ~ 1 cm (range: 1.0-2.5 cm)
  - Interscalene triangle contains variable amounts of fat
    - Interscalene fat most conspicuous in lower aspect of triangle
    - More superiorly, anterior and middle scalene muscles closely approximated, and distinct fat separating muscles may be minimal or absent
    - Presence of fat, particularly perineural fat, useful for identifying proximal components of BP within interscalene triangle on MR and CT scans
  - BP **roots of C5-C7** located **within** upper aspect of interscalene triangle
    - Begin to form upper and middle trunks as they pass through triangle itself
  - BP **roots of C8-T1** are actually **medial to triangle initially**
    - Begin to form lower trunk as they enter medial margin of interscalene triangle
  - Interscalene triangle considered to contain upper, middle, and lower trunks of BP
- **Subclavian artery**
  - Gives off vertebral artery and internal thoracic artery before entering interscalene triangle
  - Passes through **base of interscalene triangle**, passing just over superior margin of 1st rib
  - Within triangle, subclavian artery intimately associated with proximal BP

- **C5-C7 roots** located **superior** to artery; **C8 and T1 roots** often more **posterior** to artery
  - Subclavian artery and BP **separated from subclavian vein** by **anterior scalene muscle** itself
  - Subclavian artery transitions to axillary artery at lateral margin of 1st rib
- **Axillary artery**
  - As subclavian artery passes 1st rib, it becomes axillary artery
  - Components of BP **above proximal axillary artery** generally consist of anterior and posterior **divisions**
  - Divisions then form cords intimately associated with axillary artery; named by their relationship to artery itself
  - **Cords** generally formed **prior to reaching sagittal plane** that passes through **coracoid process** of scapula
- **Phrenic nerve**
  - Arises primarily as branch from C4 ventral ramus with variable contributions from C5 and, occasionally, C3
  - Passes around lateral margin of anterior scalene muscle and descends in neck along **anterior surface of anterior scalene**
  - Near base of anterior scalene muscle, phrenic nerve passes **between subclavian vein and subclavian artery** before passing **anterior to internal thoracic artery** and entering mediastinum
  - Supplies motor and sensory innervation to diaphragm

IMAGING ANATOMY

Overview

- Knowledge of normal BP anatomy and relationship of BP components to surrounding structures critical for evaluating BP
- Components of BP complex difficult to identify and fully evaluate with single MR sequence or in single plane
- Surrounding perineural fat often provides excellent visualization of nerves on T1WI and allows them to be distinguished from adjacent soft tissues
- Corresponding T2WI, STIR sequences best for evaluating intrinsic signal and architecture of nerves
- Characteristics of normal nerve on MR
  - In cross section, nerve appears as well-defined oval structure
  - Discrete fascicles identified with high-resolution imaging
    - Fascicles uniform in size, shape
  - Isointense to adjacent muscle tissue on T1WI
  - Slightly hyperintense to adjacent muscle on fat-saturated T2WI, STIR
  - Normal nerves should be similar in signal intensity compared to adjacent normal nerves and contralateral normal nerves
  - While DRG enhances with IV gadolinium, major components of BP should not enhance normally

ANATOMY IMAGING ISSUES

Imaging Recommendations

- **3D STIR (fat suppression) with gadolinium contrast (better water suppression, nerve visualization, and lesion enhancement)**
  - Reformatted in multiplanar maximum-intensity projections **(MIP)** and volumetric **3D** reconstructions
- Diffusion-weighted imaging with background signal suppression **(DWIBS)**-based MR neurography
- Diffusion tensor imaging **(DTI)** tractography
- MR of cervical spine can be useful primary examination to evaluate for spinal cord pathology as well as common degenerative findings, including spinal stenosis and NF stenosis, that create BP symptoms
- CECT of neck/chest for evaluation of neck/apical pulmonary masses (Pancoast tumor) that involve BP
- CT myelography can be effective tool to evaluate for traumatic nerve root avulsion and associated traumatic pseudomeningoceles
- CT of cervical spine with bone windows preferred for cervical spine fracture
- CTA of neck can demonstrate relationship of proximal BP masses with vertebral arteries
- High-frequency transducer US provides excellent spatial resolution to visualize small components of BP
  - Seen as long, tubular, hypoechoic structures against background of echogenic fat on longitudinal scan
  - Several small ovoid/round hypoechoic nodules in lower posterior triangle between scalenus anterior and scalenus medius muscles on transverse scan
  - Lack of flow distinguishes them from vascular structures

Imaging Approaches

- Best imaging sequences: 3D STIR with contrast and reconstructions, coronal T1, oblique sagittal T1
- Best imaging reconstruction planes: Coronal and oblique sagittal planes from C3 (rostral) through T2 (caudal), nerve roots (medial) through axilla (lateral)
- Optional sequences
  - Oblique sagittal and coronal contrast-enhanced fat-saturated T1 (for cases of known or suspected neoplasm, scar, or infection)
  - Coronal technique with larger field of view (FOV) can include contralateral BP for comparison

Imaging Pitfalls

- Too-large FOV reduces spatial resolution, compromises visualization of internal BP architecture
- Technically simpler to evaluate supraclavicular plexus than infraclavicular plexus
- Motion artifact (especially respiratory motion of chest) degrades image quality
- Subclavian/axillary vessels (especially veins) can show linear high signal on fast spin-echo or inversion recovery sequences and can be difficult to separate from BP
  - Saturation bands can help decrease vascular signal
  - **3D STIR SPACE/3D STIR VISTA with contrast**: Normal BP signal not affected, while high signals from vessels completely suppressed
- Enhancing vascular structures and normal perineural venous plexus mimic pathologically enhancing BP

CLINICAL IMPLICATIONS

Clinical Importance

- Variety of pathologies affect BP, including idiopathic inflammation, traumatic injuries, neoplasm, and compression syndromes
- Combination of neurologic evaluation and MR key to identify and localize lesion as well as plan treatment

GRAPHICS: OVERVIEW

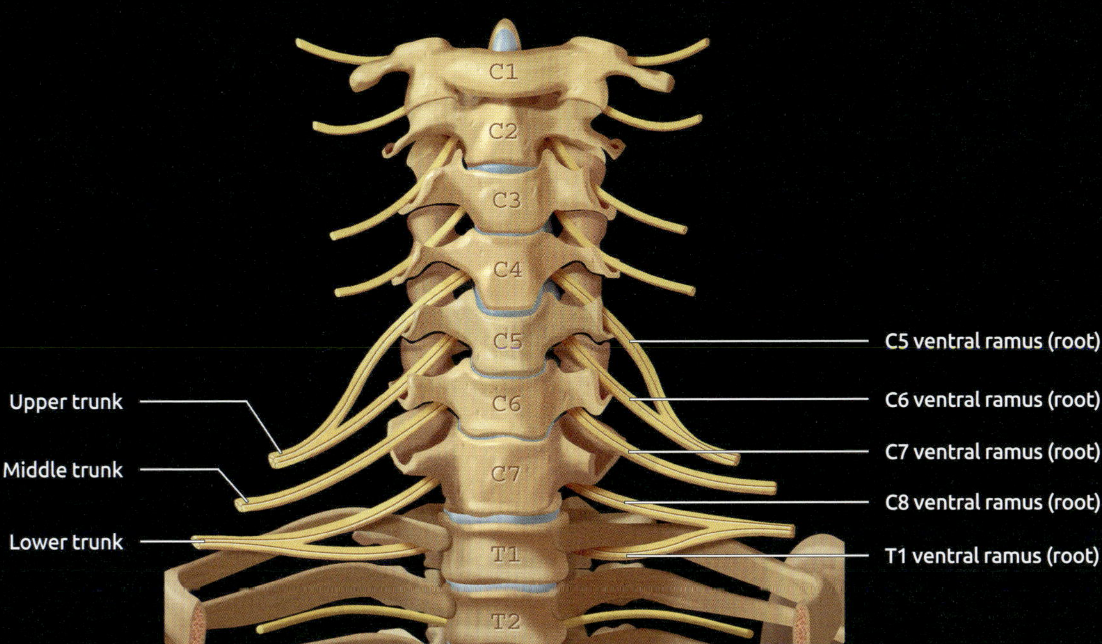

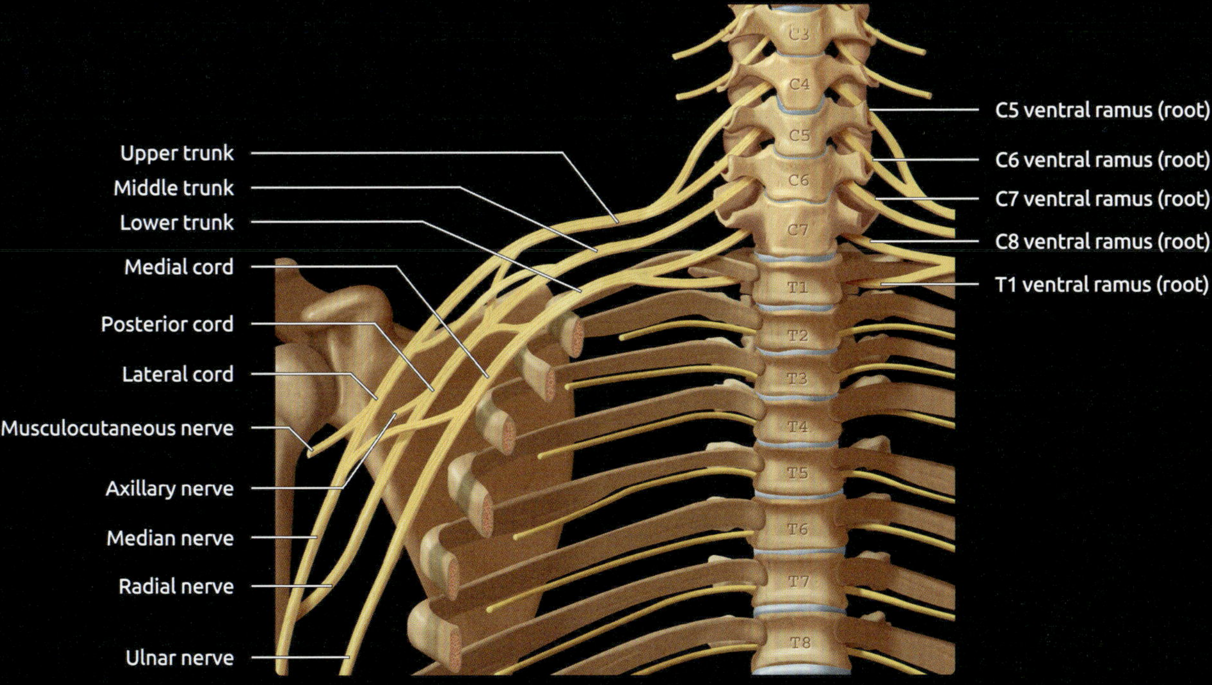

(Top) *Coronal graphic demonstrates an overview of the cervical spine and supraclavicular brachial plexus. This shows the basic arrangement of the cervical ventral primary rami combining to form the brachial plexus. The C1-C7 cervical nerves exit above the same numbered pedicle, C8 nerve exits above the T1 pedicle, and more caudal roots exit below their numbered pedicle.* **(Bottom)** *Coronal graphic of the brachial plexus demonstrates an overview of the more distal plexus elements extending into the axilla. The trunks recombine into posterior and anterior divisions that form the cords. The posterior cord forms the radial, axillary, thoracodorsal, and upper and lower subscapular nerves. The medial cord forms the ulnar nerve, medial pectoral nerve, medial cutaneous nerve of arm and medial cutaneous nerve of forearm, and also gives off the medial root of median nerve. The lateral cord forms the musculocutaneous nerve and lateral pectoral nerve and also gives off the lateral root of median nerve. Note that the median nerve is formed from branches of both the lateral and medial cords.*

GRAPHIC: BRACHIAL PLEXUS

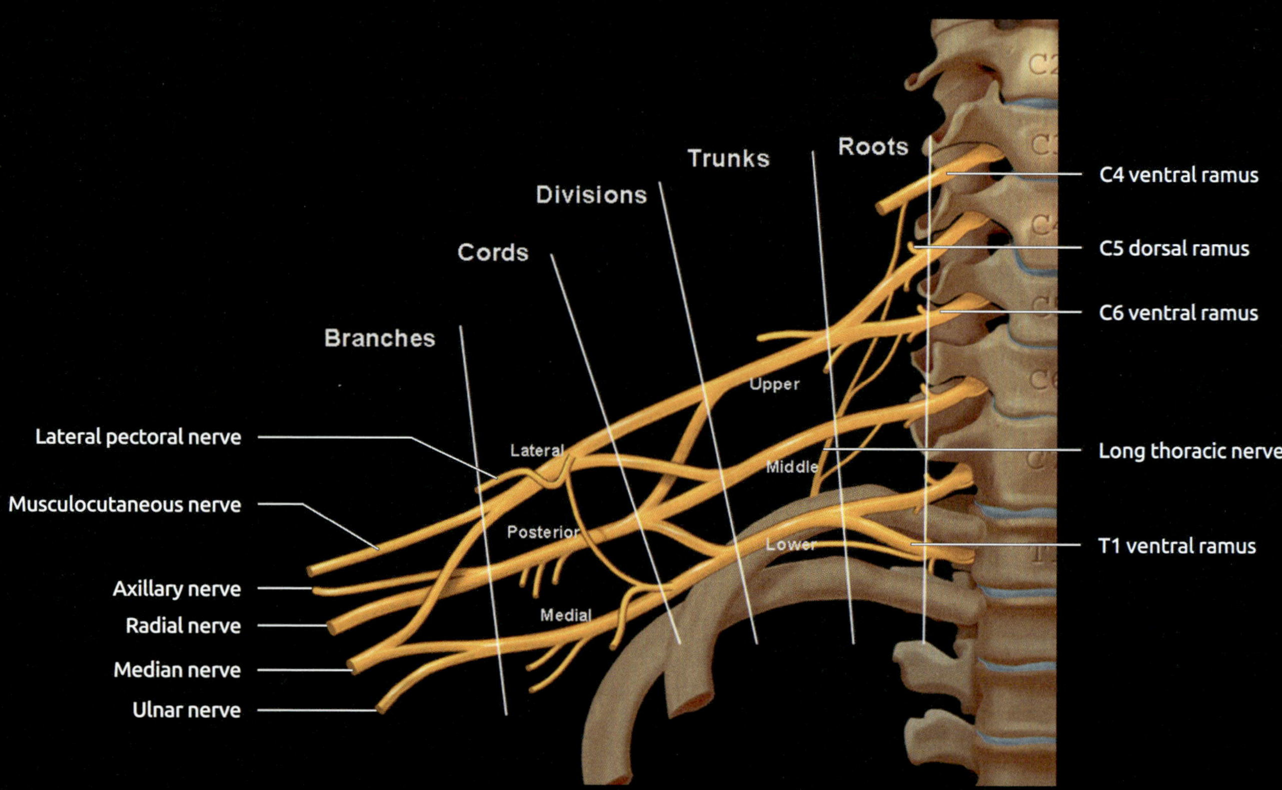

Graphic shows the components of the brachial plexus. The exiting nerves quickly divide into small dorsal rami and larger ventral rami. The ventral rami (roots) of C5-T1 pass into the scalene triangle and merge into trunks. Branches arising directly from the brachial plexus roots are the dorsal scapular nerve (C5), long thoracic nerve (C5, C6, C7) and phrenic nerve (C3, C4, C5; mainly C4). The upper trunk is formed by C5 and C6 ventral rami or roots. Only the upper trunk gives off branches, namely suprascapular nerve and nerve to subclavius muscle. The middle trunk is formed by continuation of the C7 root. The lower trunk is formed by the coalescence of C8 and T1 roots. Each trunk divides into a ventral and dorsal division. Divisions do not have any named branches. The 3 dorsal divisions merge into the posterior cord. Ventral divisions of the upper and middle trunks unite to form the lateral cord. The ventral division of the lower trunk merges and forms the medial cord. The cords ultimately give rise to the terminal branches of the upper extremity.

CORONAL RELATIONSHIPS OF BRACHIAL PLEXUS

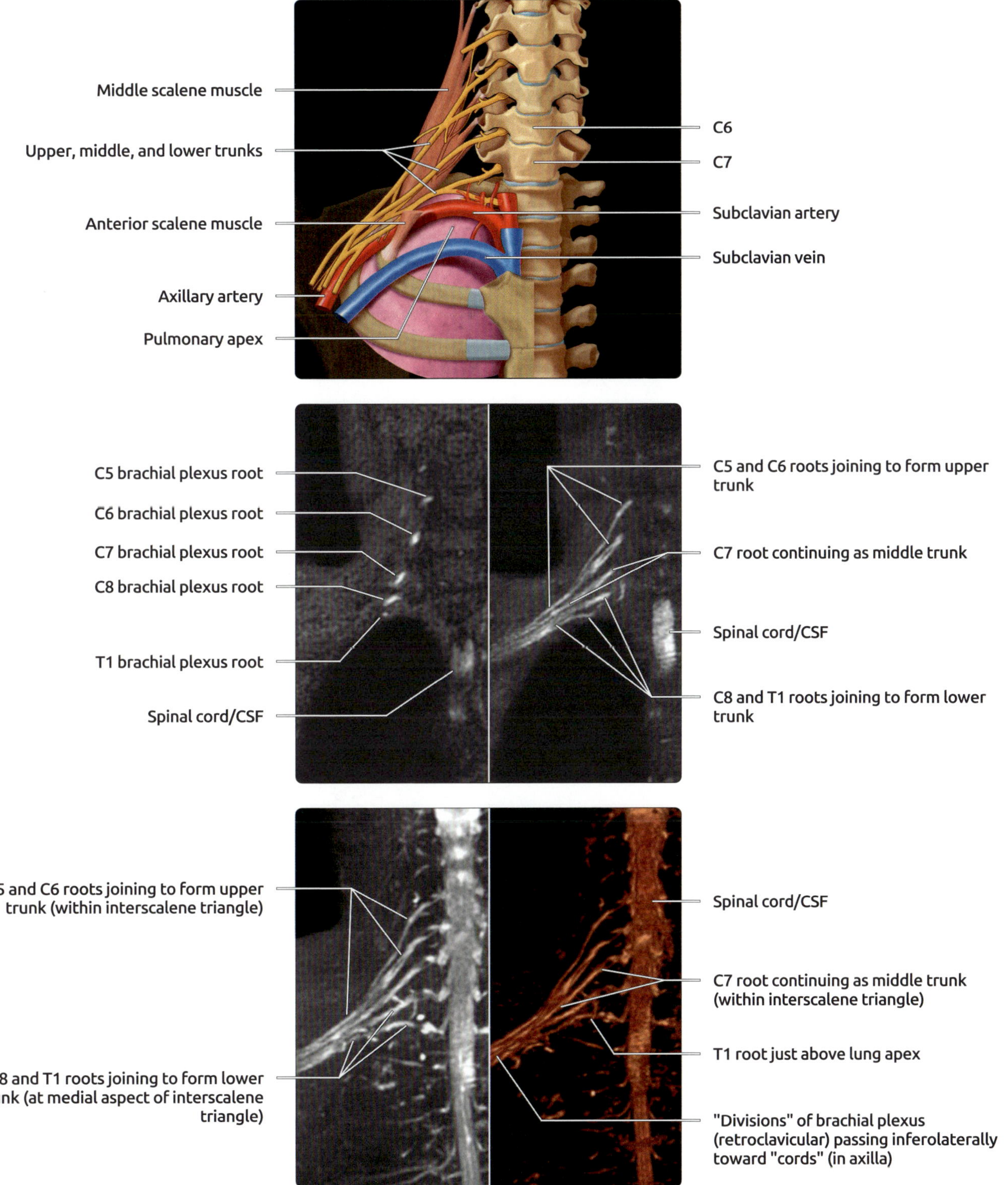

(Top) *Graphic demonstrates the relationship of the proximal brachial plexus to the vertebral bodies, middle scalene muscle, subclavian artery, and pulmonary apex. Anterior scalene has been removed to expose the scalene triangle, the region between scalene muscles. Note subclavian vein passes anterior to the inferior attachment of anterior scalene muscle, and the subclavian artery passes posterior to this attachment. The subclavian artery can serve as a marker to find brachial plexus elements on imaging. Note that if an apical lung tumor invades superiorly, it often involves the subclavian artery before it involves the brachial plexus.* **(Middle)** *Thin source image (right) of postcontrast 3D STIR MR shows the hyperintense distal aspects of the roots of the right brachial plexus. 3D STIR (fat suppression) with gadolinium contrast (better water/vessel signal suppression, nerve visualization and lesion enhancement) is a very efficient way of doing high-resolution brachial plexus MR. 15-mm maximum-intensity projection (MIP) image (left) shows roots joining to form trunks.* **(Bottom)** *3D volumetric grayscale (right) and colored (left) images from same 3D STIR MR with contrast show the brachial plexus.*

AXIAL ANATOMY: PROXIMAL CERVICAL NERVES

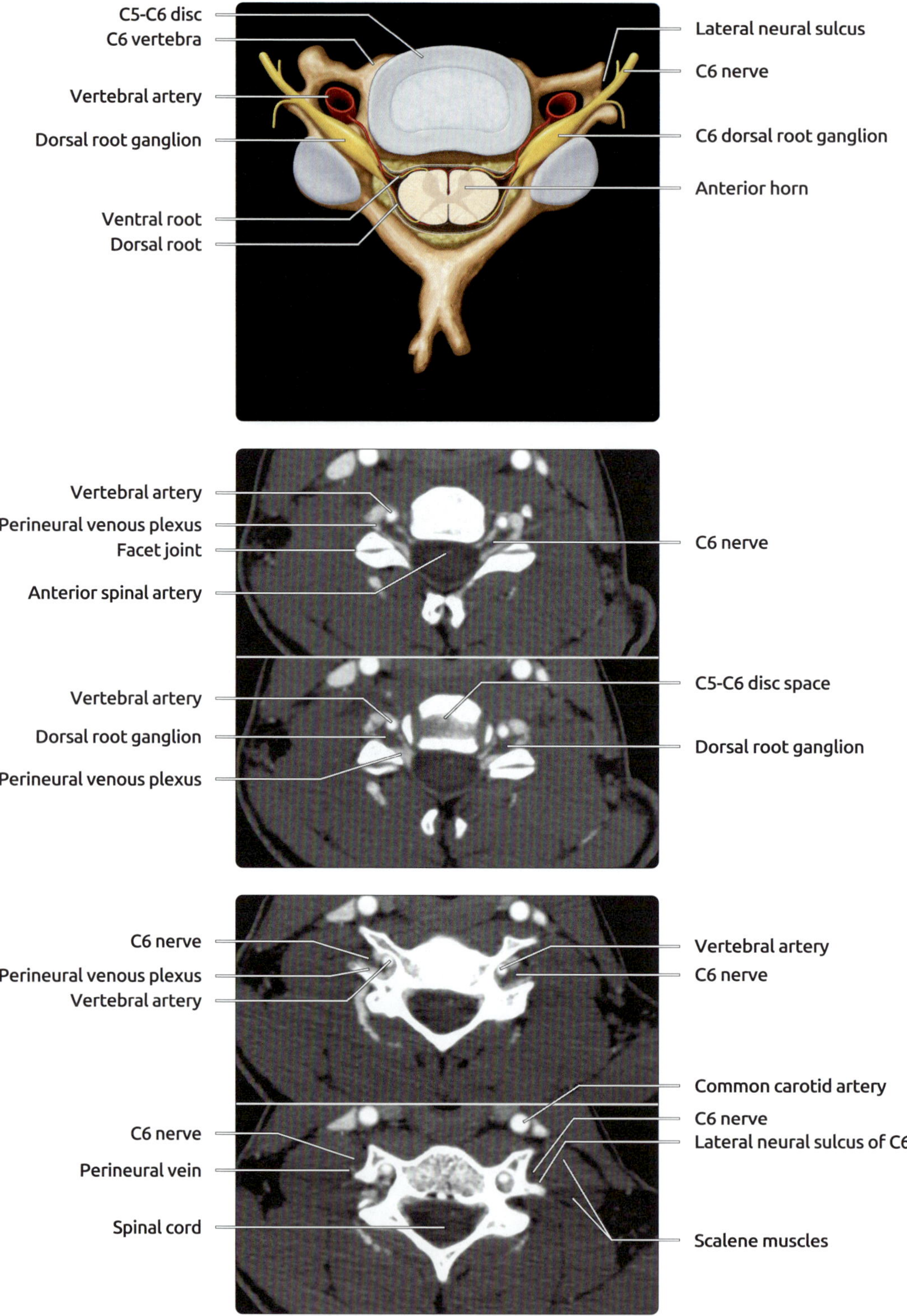

(Top) *Graphic demonstrates ventral and dorsal roots of C6 nerve merging in upper medial neural foramen (NF). Localized expansion of the dorsal nerve is the dorsal root ganglion (DRG). Note the intimate relationship of the DRG to the vertebral artery as it passes through NF. The extraforaminal nerve descends slightly toward the lateral neural sulcus that cradles the nerve before it extends into the scalene triangle. When the nerve is within lateral neural sulcus, it is separated from the vertebral artery within transverse foramen by thin bony bridge of the lateral process.* **(Middle)** *Axial CTA images descending through C5-C6 disc space show there is prominent enhancement of epidural and perineural venous plexus that surround exiting nerves.* **(Bottom)** *Axial images continue to descend from disc space at C5-C6 into C6 vertebrae. As the nerve begins to exit NF, it moves inferiorly and laterally and begins to separate from vertebral artery. The extraforaminal nerve will pass lateral to the transverse process within a shallow groove known as lateral neural sulcus, which is a reliable landmark for cervical nerves C3-C6. In many patients, it is difficult to fully distinguish separate scalene muscles on imaging.*

CORONAL STIR MR

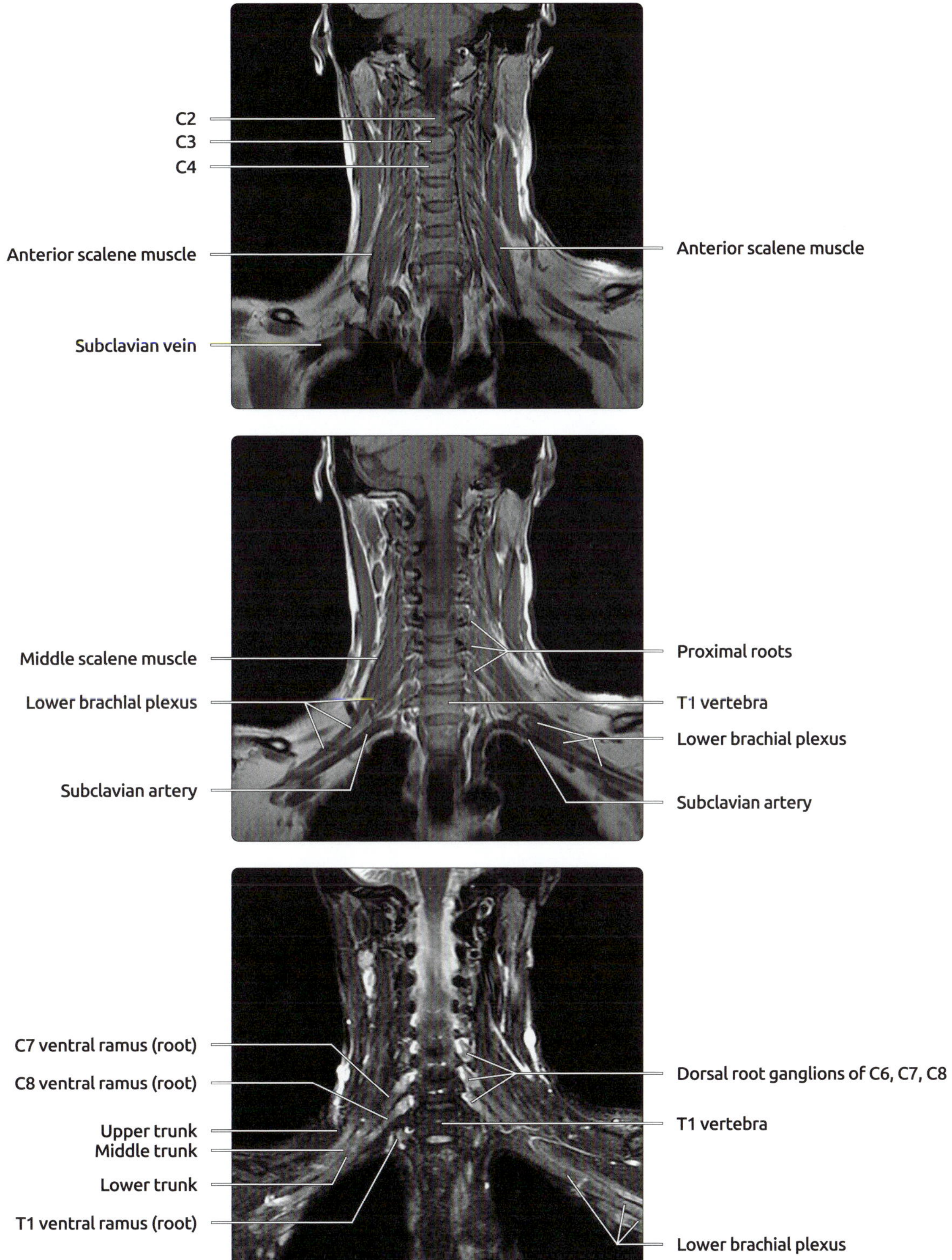

(Top) *Coronal T1 MR shows vertebral bodies (upper) and anterior scalene muscles (lower). Anterior scalene muscles arise from transverse processes of cervical vertebrae and attach to 1st rib laterally. Subclavian vein passes anteriorly to attachment of anterior scalene.* **(Middle)** *Coronal T1 MR reveals the difficulty in distinguishing normal nerve tissue from adjacent muscle. Oblique bands of hypointense tissue traverse the ventral face of middle scalene muscle, but the nerves are difficult to separate from oblique tendinous attachments of the muscle itself. There is minimal interscalene fat to provide satisfactory contrast. Subclavian artery is a useful landmark for determining best plane for proximal components of brachial plexus, particularly the trunks. The trunks will pass above the subclavian artery as it passes over the 1st rib.* **(Bottom)** *Coronal STIR MR shows relative hyperintensity of normal nerves to muscle. Fat has been suppressed to enhance contrast resolution of nerves. Note DRGs are easily identified as focal enlargements of proximal nerves within NF. Given complex curvature of components, it is difficult to obtain a full view of the brachial plexus in a single slice on 2D MR.*

AXIAL STIR MR

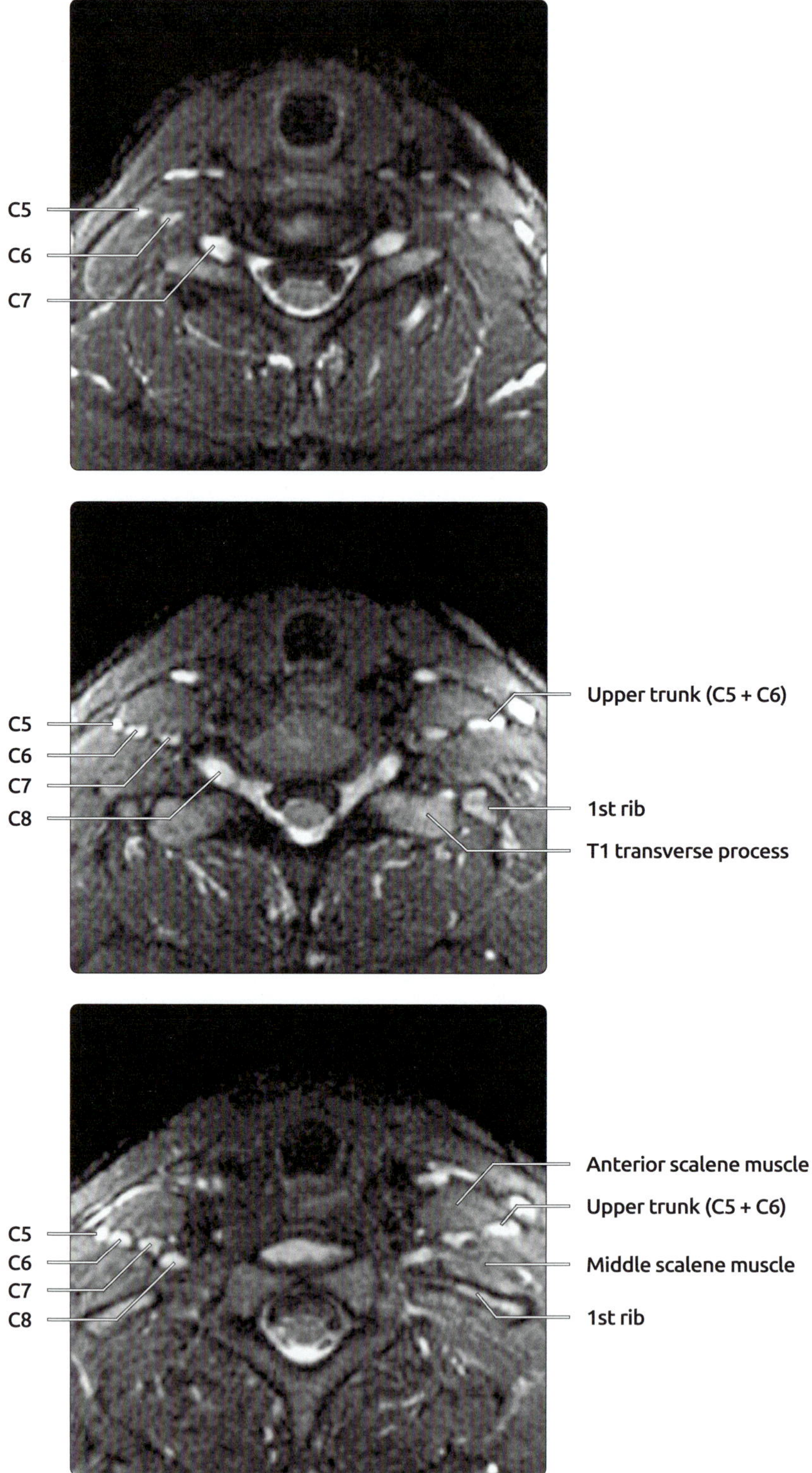

(Top) *First of 3 axial STIR MR images presented from rostral to caudal shows the upper brachial plexus elements [C5-C7 ventral primary rami (VPR)] traveling between the anterior and middle scalene muscles in preparation to form the brachial plexus.* **(Middle)** *Image at the C7/T1 level depicts the linear alignment of the C5-C8 VPR. C5 and C6 are closely approximated and form the left upper trunk.* **(Bottom)** *Imaging more caudal at C7/T1 level depicts the upper trunk on the left. Note that the brachial plexus elements exit the neck between the anterior and middle scalene muscles.*

OBLIQUE SAGITTAL STIR MR

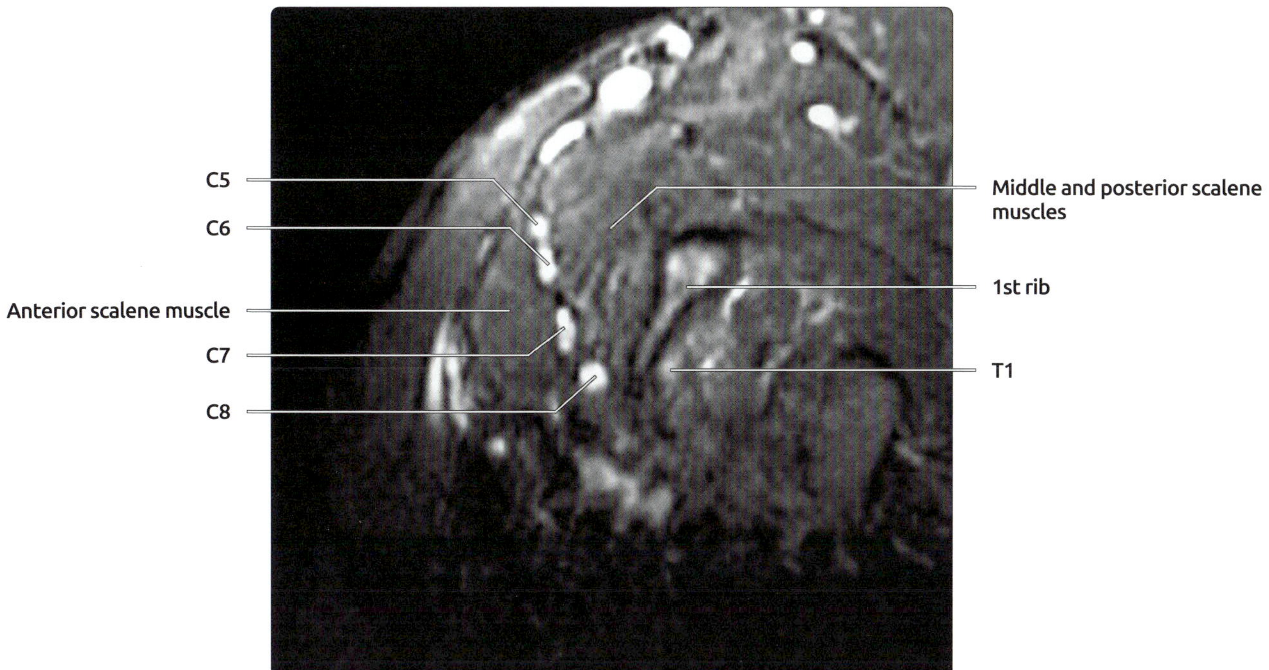

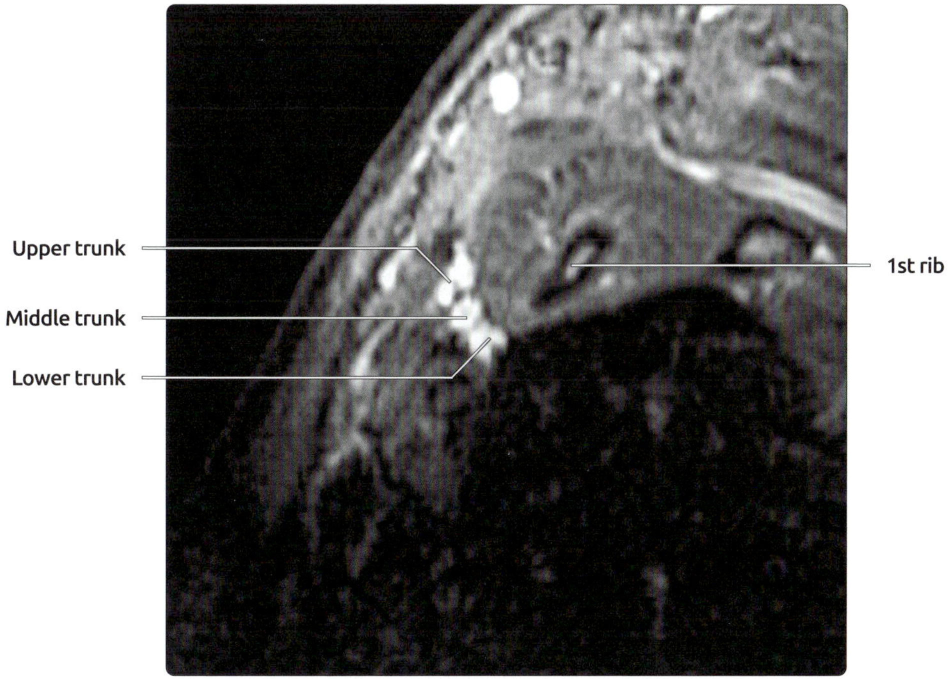

(Top) *First of 4 oblique sagittal STIR MR images presented from medial to lateral demonstrates the ventral primary rami of C5-T1 proximal to the trunks. C8 exits above the 1st rib while T1 exits below. The brachial plexus is normally sandwiched between the anterior and middle scalene muscles.* **(Bottom)** *A slightly more lateral slice demonstrates the formation of the upper, middle, and lower trunks arranged in a vertical line between the scalene muscles. The C5 and C6 VPR can be still resolved as distinct elements within the upper trunk at this level.*

OBLIQUE SAGITTAL STIR MR

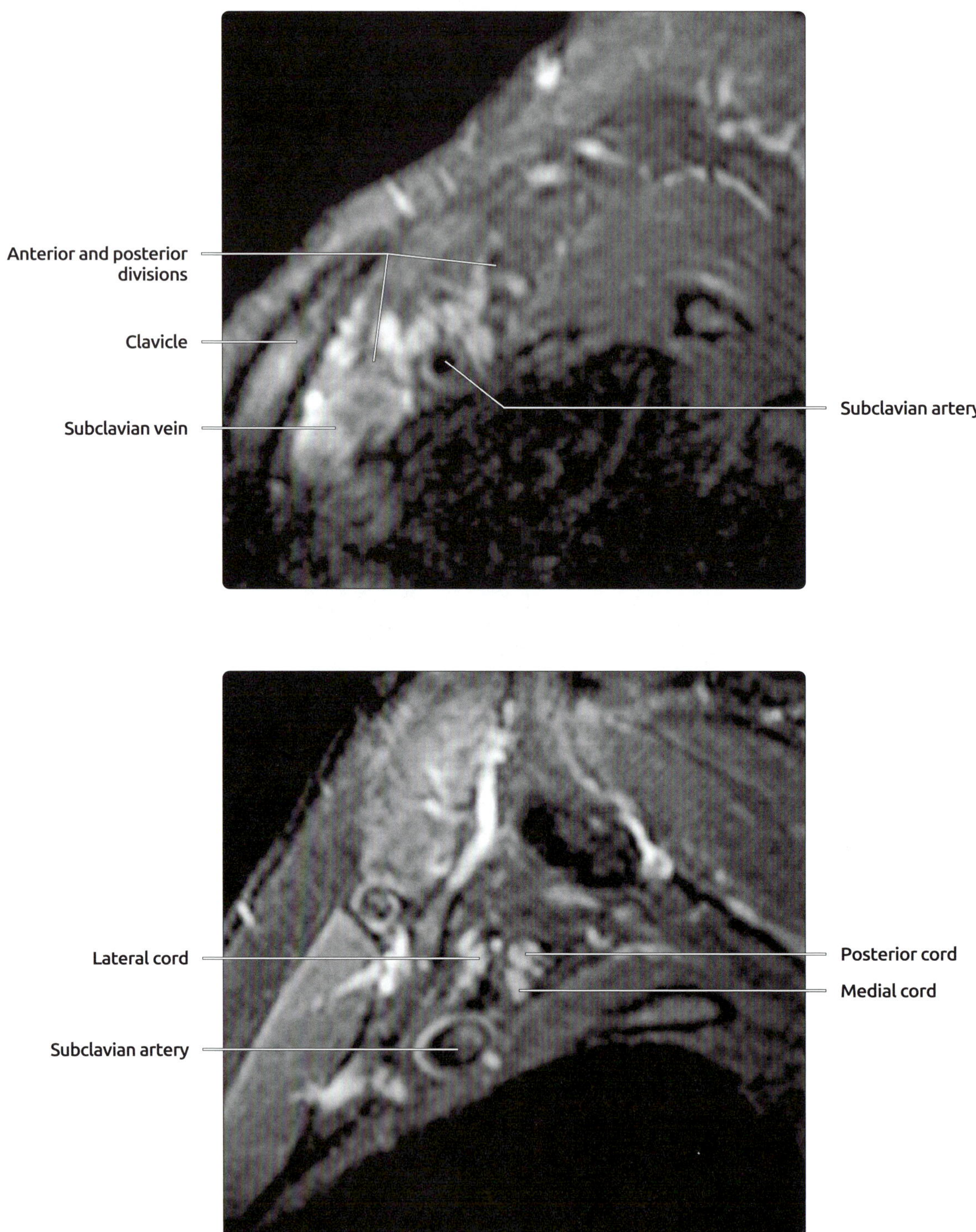

(Top) *Image at the division level shows mixing and matching of the trunks into anterior and posterior divisions. Note that the divisions are retroclavicular. The posterior divisions will form the posterior cord, and the anterior divisions will form the lateral and medial cords. It is generally not possible to follow individual branches of the divisions from trunk to cord.* **(Bottom)** *Image demonstrates the formation of the 3 cords (lateral, medial, and posterior). The most important terminal branch of the lateral cord is the musculocutaneous nerve. The posterior cord forms the axillary and radial nerve terminal branches. The medial cord terminates as the ulnar nerve.*

ANATOMIC-PATHOLOGIC CORRELATION

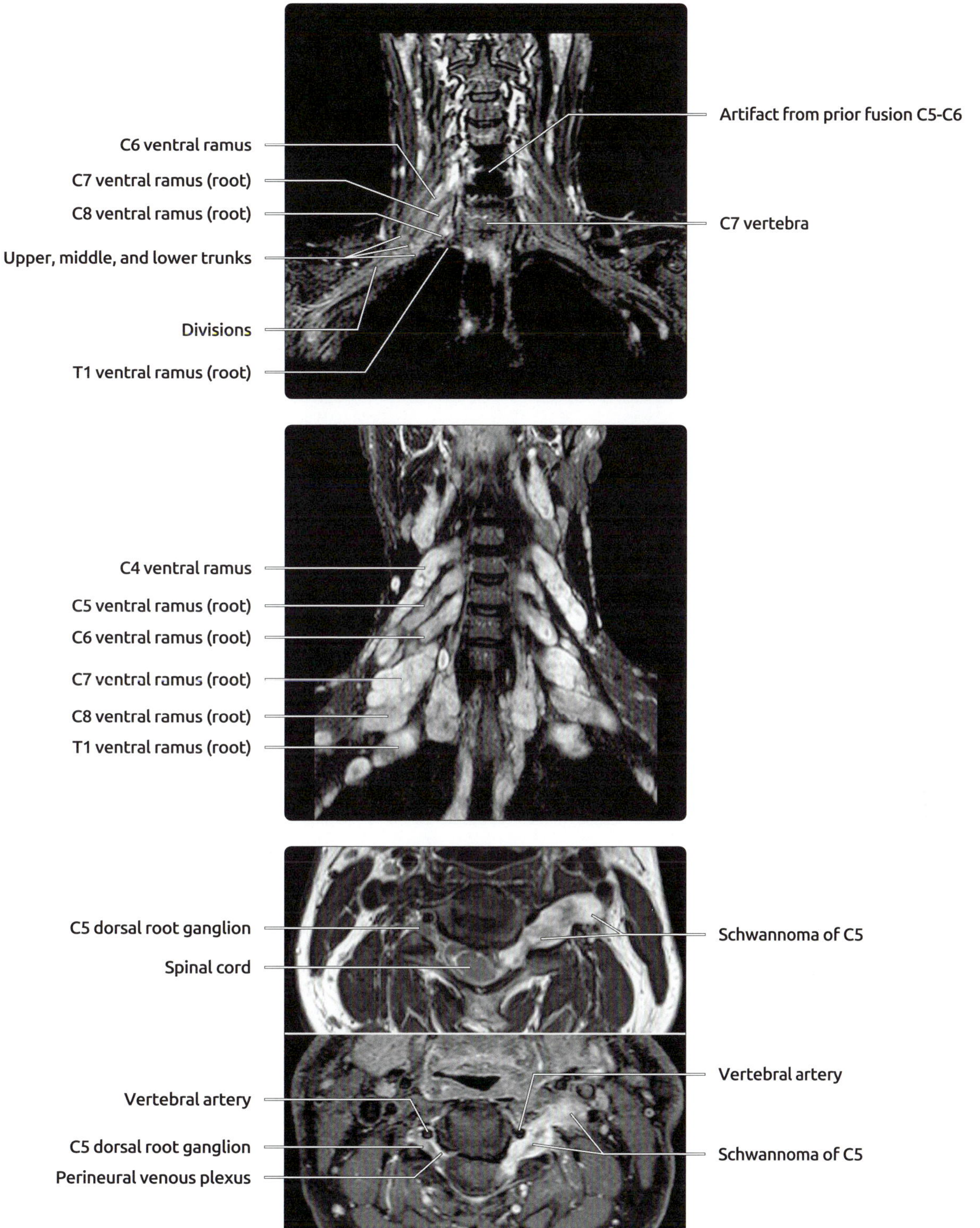

(Top) *Coronal T2 FS MR demonstrates mild relative hyperintensity in the brachial plexus diffusely in the right side of this patient with idiopathic plexitis. On coronal MR, T1 root is easily seen as a horizontal linear structure surrounded by fat close to lung apex. This is a good starting point to identify brachial plexus roots and then count C8, C7, C6, C5 upward. Stellate ganglion can also be seen at this level.* **(Middle)** *Coronal STIR MR depicts massive enlargement of all of the proximal cervical nerves and supraclavicular components of the brachial plexus in this patient with neurofibromatosis type 1. In this case, essentially all the nerves have given rise to neurofibromas.* **(Bottom)** *Axial T2 and contrast-enhanced T1 FS MR images through the C4-C5 NF demonstrate a solitary, enlarged, fusiform enhancing mass along the proximal C5 nerve on the patient's left. Notice the lesion's relationship to the left vertebral artery; the lesion pushes the vertebral artery anteriorly. Notice the DRG on the unaffected side enhances normally.*

TRANSVERSE AND LONGITUDINAL ULTRASOUND

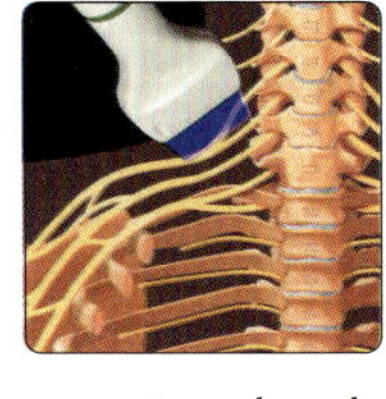

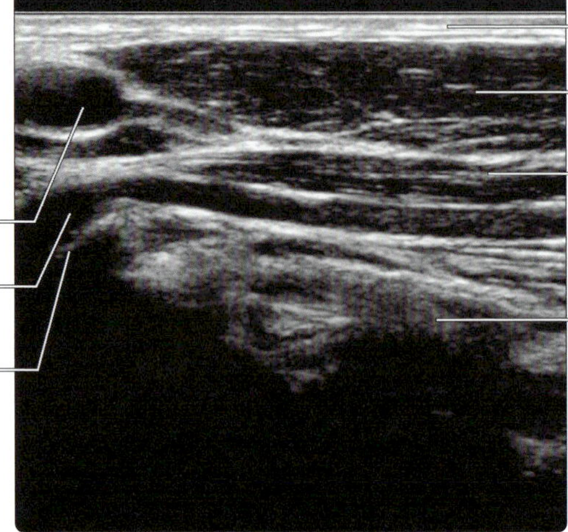

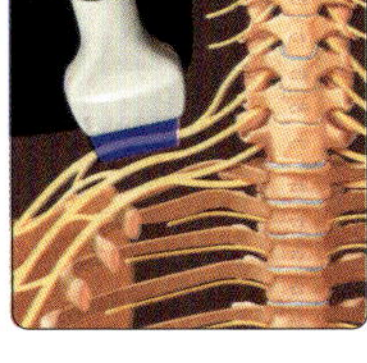

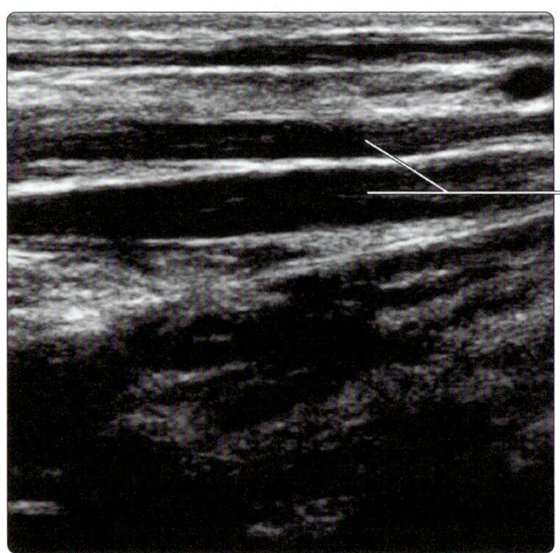

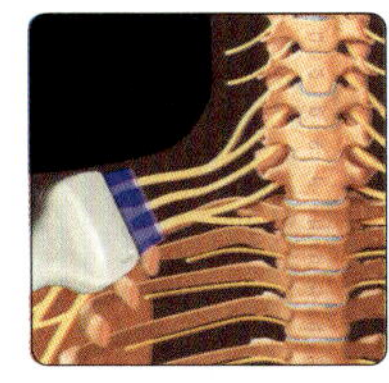

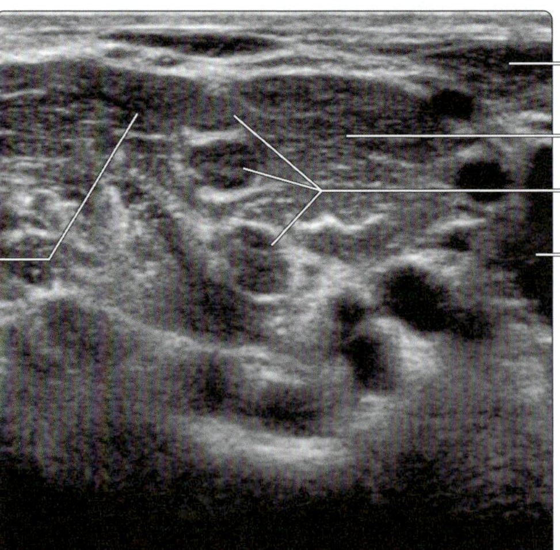

(Top) *Longitudinal grayscale ultrasound of the posterior triangle of the neck shows the root and trunk of the brachial plexus, which appears as a thin, tubular, hypoechoic structure related superficially to the scalenus anterior muscle and deeply to the cervical vertebrae.* **(Middle)** *Longitudinal grayscale ultrasound of the right posterior triangle/supraclavicular fossa confirms the elongated linear, hypoechoic, thickened elements of the brachial plexus. The patient had past history of neck irradiation for metastatic neck nodes, and the nerve thickening is likely secondary to postradiation change.* **(Bottom)** *Transverse grayscale ultrasound of the right lower posterior triangle/supraclavicular fossa shows round smooth hypoechoic "nodules" between the scalenus anterior and medius muscles, representing thickened brachial plexus elements viewed in cross section. If there is a question, rotate the transducer to elongate the nerve.*

TRANSVERSE AND LONGITUDINAL ULTRASOUND

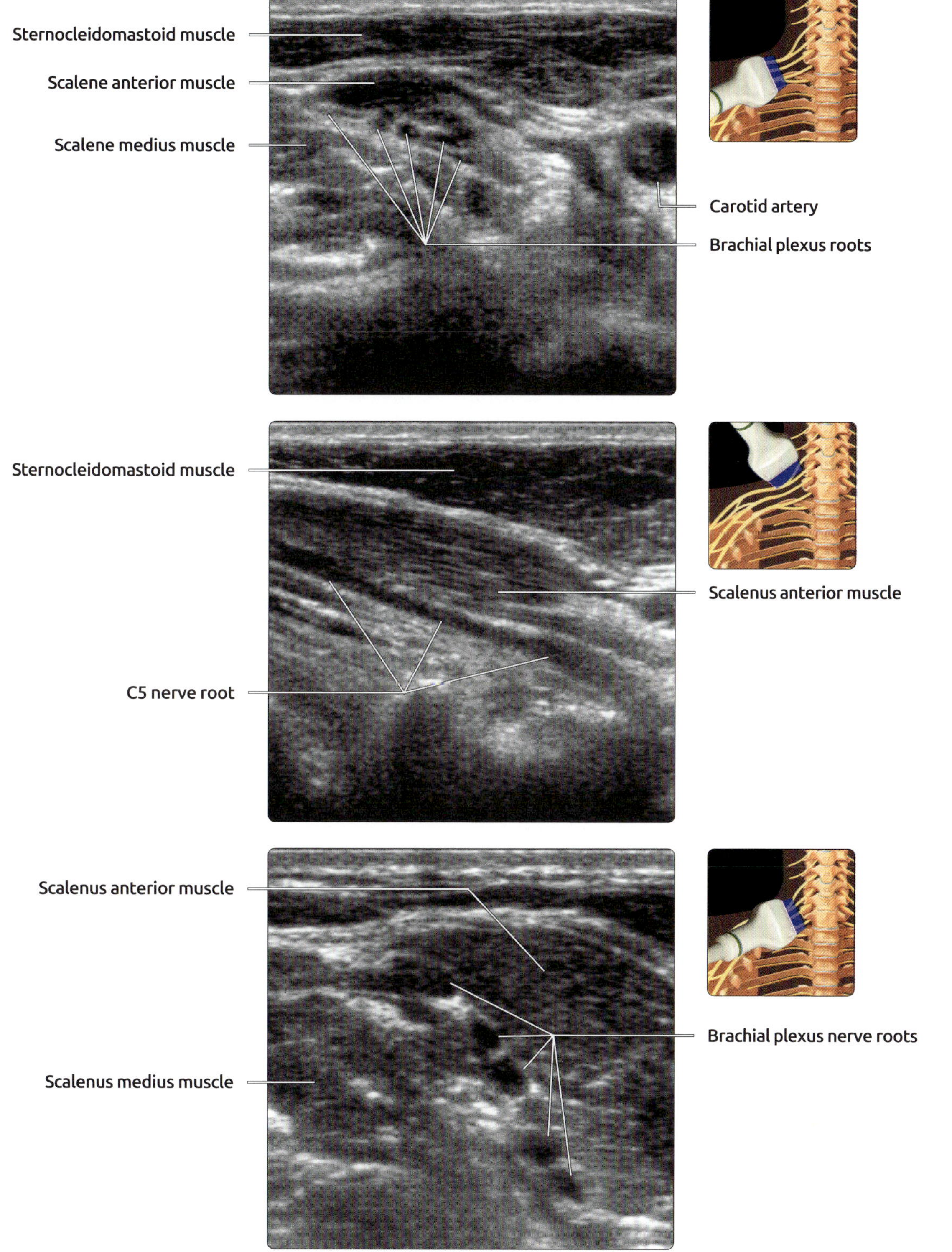

(Top) *Transverse ultrasound of the anterolateral lower neck shows the hypoechoic roots of the brachial plexus as they exit the NF and move to the scalene triangle.* **(Middle)** *Longitudinal ultrasound shows the longitudinal section of the hypoechoic C5 nerve root as it exits from the foramen and descends to the intrascalene area.* **(Bottom)** *Transverse ultrasound at the entry into the interscalene triangle shows 5 hypoechoic roots of the brachial plexus between the scalenus anterior and medius muscles. The hypoechoic roots are clearly seen against the adjacent hyperechoic intermuscular fat.*

INDEX

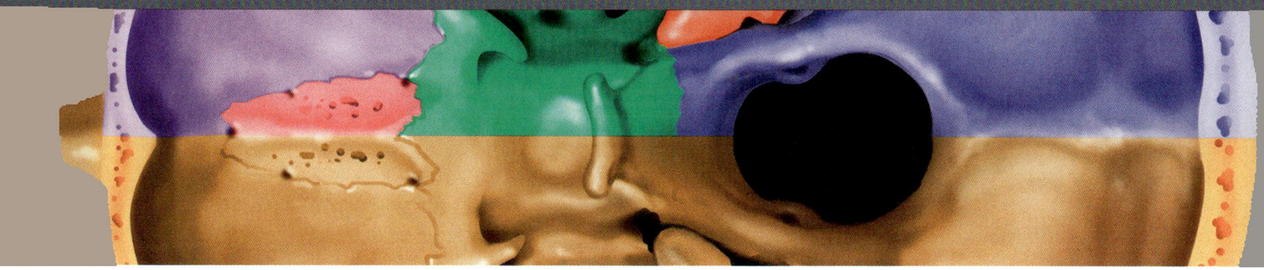

A

INDEX

B

INDEX

C

INDEX

INDEX

INDEX

D

E

F

G

H

I

INDEX

J

K

L

M

N

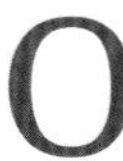

P

INDEX

Q

R

S

INDEX

INDEX

T

INDEX

U

V

W

Z